Balance Function Assessment and Management

Second Edition

Balance Function
Assessment and Management

Second Edition

Gary P. Jacobson, PhD
Neil T. Shepard, PhD

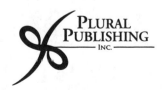

PLURAL
PUBLISHING
INC.

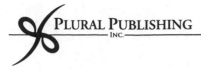

PLURAL PUBLISHING
INC.

5521 Ruffin Road
San Diego, CA 92123

e-mail: info@pluralpublishing.com
website: http://www.pluralpublishing.com

Typeset in 10 ½/13 Palatino by Flanagan's Publishing Services, Inc.
Printed in the United States of America by McNaughton and Gunn, Inc.
19 18 17 16   2 3 4 5

Library of Congress Cataloging-in-Publication Data

Balance function assessment and management / [edited by] Gary P. Jacobson, Neil T. Shepard. — Second edition.
    p. ; cm.
Includes bibliographical references and index.
ISBN 978-1-59756-547-9 (alk. paper) — ISBN 1-59756-547-4 (alk. paper)
I. Jacobson, Gary P., editor. II. Shepard, Neil T., editor.
[DNLM: 1. Vestibular Diseases—diagnosis. 2. Vestibular Diseases—therapy.
3. Vestibular Function Tests—methods. WV 255]
RF260
617.8'82—dc23
                                                    2014035796

CONTENTS

LIST OF VIDEOS

 To access the videos, please visit the companion website.

PREFACE

Why do a second edition? Subsequent editions make it possible to keep a textbook contemporary. This may mean that some topics are removed while others are added. Much has transpired in the area of clinical vestibular sciences and balance since publication of the first edition of this book. For instance, both ocular vestibular-evoked myogenic potentials (oVEMPs), and the video head impulse test (vHIT) have been added to the tools available to the clinical neurophysiologist. To these contributions we have added content describing topics as diverse as the ontogeny of the vestibular system, the effects of age on balance function, compensatory mechanisms following unilateral peripheral vestibular system impairment, and techniques for assessing vestibular system function in children. These chapters have been authored by national and internationally known experts. It is our hope that this updated text will become even more useful than it is currently.

The editors are grateful to the new and returning authors for their outstanding contributions to the 2nd edition of *Balance Function Assessment and Management*.

Last, the editors would like to thank, once again, our families for providing us with the time required to complete this work.

ABOUT THE EDITORS

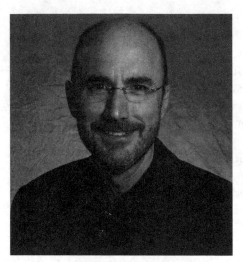

Gary P. Jacobson, PhD

Gary Jacobson is professor in the Department of Hearing and Speech Sciences, and director, Division of Audiology and codirector, Division of Vestibular Sciences, Vanderbilt Bill Wilkerson Center for Otolaryngology and Communication Sciences (Nashville, Tennessee).

He completed his undergraduate studies at California State University at Fullerton. He received his MS in Communicative Disorders (Audiology) at the University of Wisconsin-Stevens Point, and received his PhD from Kent State University. Dr. Jacobson is a past president of the American Society of Neurophysiological Monitoring. He is the past editor of the *American Journal of Audiology* (American Speech-Language-Hearing Association) and the current editor-in-chief of the *Journal of the American Academy of Audiology*. He has authored and coauthored over 150 publications that cover the areas of tinnitus, dizziness, auditory function, outcome measures development, brain mapping, and intraoperative neurophysiology. He is a fellow of the American Speech-Language-Hearing Association, and a recipient of both the Jerger Career Award for Research in Audiology from the American Academy of Audiology and the Honors of the American Speech-Language-Hearing Association.

Neil Shepard is director of the Dizziness and Balance Disorders Program at Mayo Clinic–Rochester, Minnesota, and a professor of audiology in the Mayo Clinic School of Medicine. He received his undergraduate and master's training in electrical and biomedical engineering from University of Kentucky (Lexington, Kentucky) and Massachusetts Institute of Technology (Cambridge, Massachusetts). He completed his PhD in auditory electrophysiology and clinical audiology from the University of Iowa (Iowa City, Iowa) in 1979. He has specialized in clinical electrophysiology for both the auditory and vestibular systems. Activity over the last 34 years has concentrated on the clinical assessment and rehabilitation of patients with balance disorders and clinical research endeavors related to both assessment and rehabilitation.

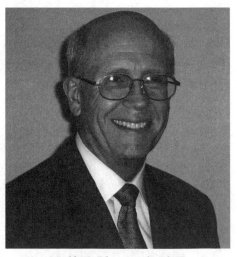

Neil T. Shepard, PhD

CONTRIBUTORS

Kamran Barin, PhD
Assistant Professor, Emeritus
Department of Otolaryngology
Ohio State University
Columbus, Ohio
Consultant
GN Otometrics
Taastrup, Denmark
Chapters 4, 12, and 13

Adolfo M. Bronstein, MD, PhD, FRCP
Professor, Consultant Neurologist
Head of Neuro-otology Unit
Division of Brain Sciences
Imperial College
London, England
United Kingdom
Chapter 22

Ann M. Burgess, PhD
Postdoctoral Research Fellow
School of Psychology
University of Sydney
Sydney
Australia
Chapter 16

Richard A. Clendaniel, PT, PhD
Doctor of Physical Therapy Division
Duke University School of Medicine
Durham, North Carolina
Chapter 26

Ian S. Curthoys
Emeritus Professor, Vestibular Function
School of Psychology
University of Sydney NSW
Sydney, New South Wales
Australia
Chapter 16

J. Andrew Dundas
Assistant Professor, Otolaryngology

Director, Division of Audiology
University of California, San Francisco Medical
    Center
San Francisco, California
Chapters 5 and 7

Scott D. Z. Eggers, MD
Consultant and Assistant Professor
Department of Neurology
Mayo Clinic
Rochester, Minnesota
Chapters 2 and 10

Lauren L. English, AuD
Audiologist
Vanderbilt Bill Wilkerson Center
Vanderbilt University Medical Center
Nashville, Tennessee
Chapter 24

Joseph M. Furman, MD, PhD
Professor
Departments of Otolaryngology, Neurology,
    Bioengineering, and Physical Therapy
University of Pittsburgh School of Medicine
Pittsburgh, Pennsylvania
Chapters 29 and 31

Joel A. Goebel, MD, FACS
Professor and Vice Chairman, Otolaryngology-
    Head and Neck Surgery
Director, Dizziness and Balance Center
Washington University School of Medicine
St. Louis, Missouri
Chapter 6

Adam M. Goulson, AuD
Clinical Audiologist
Mayo Clinic
Rochester, Minnesota
Chapters 14 and 15

Sarah L. Grantham, AuD
Associate Director
Vanderbilt Balance Disorders Clinic
Vanderbilt Bill Wilkerson Center
Nashville, Tennessee
Chapter 24 and 34

Jill M. Gruenwald, AuD, CCC-A
Clinical Audiologist
Vanderbilt Bill Wilkerson Center
Nashville, Tennessee
Chapter 24

Courtney D. Hall, PT, PhD
Research Health Scientist
James H. Quillen VA Medical Center
Associate Professor
East Tennessee State University
Johnson City, Tennessee
Chapter 32

G. Michael Halmagyi, MD, FRACP
Clinical Professor
Neurology Department
Royal Prince Alfred Hospital
Sydney
Australia
Chapter 16

Gary P. Jacobson, PhD, FASHA
Professor, Director
Division of Audiology
Vanderbilt University Medical Center
Nashville, Tennessee
Chapters 5, 7, 8, 21, 24, 33, and 34

Kristen Janky, AuD, PhD
Director, Clinical Vestibular Lab
Coordinator, Clinical Vestibular Services
Department of Audiology
Boys Town National Research Hospital
Omaha, Nebraska
Chapter 25

Sherri M. Jones, PhD
Professor and Chair
Department of Special Education and
    Communication Disorders
College of Education and Human Sciences

University of Nebraska–Lincoln
Lincoln, Nebraska
Chapters 3 and 20

Timothy A. Jones, PhD
Professor
Department of Special Education and
    Communication Disorders
College of Education and Human Sciences
University of Nebraska–Lincoln
Lincoln, Nebraska
Chapters 3 and 20

Paul R. Kileny, PhD, FAAA, F-ASHA, BCS-IOM
Professor
Academic Program Director
Audiology and Electrophysiology
University of Michigan Health System
Ann Arbor, Michigan
Chapter 23

Leonardo Manzari, MD
MSA ENT Academy Center
Cassino (FR)
Italy
Chapter 16

Hamish G. MacDougall, PhD
GPRWMF Research Fellow
Faculty of Science, School of Psychology
University of Sydney
Sydney
Australia
Chapter 16

Devin L. McCaslin, PhD
Associate Professor
Division of Audiology
Vanderbilt Bill Wilkerson Center
Nashville, Tennessee
Chapters 5, 7, 21, 24, 33, and 34

Leigh A. McGarvie
Biomedical Engineer
Institute of Clinical Neurosciences
Royal Prince Alfred Hospital
Sydney
Australia
Chapter 16

James H. McPherson, MS
Audiologist
Mayo Clinic
Rochester, Minnesota
Chapters 14 and 15

Dara Meldrum, MSC, BSC
Lecturer, Physiotherapy
Royal College of Surgeons in Ireland
Dublin, Ireland
Chapter 32

Lewis M. Nashner, ScD
Adjunct Professor
Vanderbilt University
Nashville, Tennessee
Director of Business Development
Bertec, Inc.
Columbus, Ohio
CEO
BalanceTek Corporation
Boston, Massachusetts
Chapters 17 and 18

Brian Neff, MD
Assistant Professor, Consultant
Department of Otolaryngology-Head and Neck
 Surgery
Mayo Clinic Medical School
Rochester, Minnesota
Chapter 27

Craig W. Newman, PhD
Section Head, Audiology
Head and Neck Institute, Cleveland Clinic
Professor, Department of Surgery
Cleveland Clinic Lerner College of Medicine of
 Case Western Reserve University
Cleveland, Ohio
Chapter 8

Erin G. Piker, AuD, PhD
Assistant Professor
Division of Otolaryngology-Head and Neck
 Surgery
Duke University Medical Center
Durham, North Carolina
Chapters 5, 8, and 24

Richard A. Roberts, PhD
Director
Vestibular Services
Alabama Hearing and Balance Associates, Inc.
Foley, Alabama
Chapter 11

Lauren T. Roland, MD
Resident Physician
Otolaryngology-Head and Neck Surgery
Washington University in St. Louis
St. Louis, Missouri
Chapter 6

Michael C. Schubert
Associate Professor
Department of Otolaryngology-Head and Neck
 Surgery
Department of Physical Medicine and
 Rehabilitation
Johns Hopkins University School of Medicine
Baltimore, Maryland
Chapters 1, 9, and 10

Neil T. Shepard, PhD
Chair, Division of Audiology
Department of Otolaryngology
Director, Dizziness and Balance Disorder
 Program
Professor of Audiology
Mayo Clinic School of Medicine
Rochester, Minnesota
Chapters 1, 5, 9, 10, 14, 15, 19, 25, and 34

Belinda C. Sinks, AuD
Dizziness and Balance Center
Department of Otolaryngology-Head and Neck
 Surgery
Washington University School of Medicine
St. Louis, Missouri
Chapter 6

Jeffrey P. Staab, MD, MS
Associate Professor, Psychiatry
Department of Psychiatry and Psychology
Mayo Clinic
Rochester, Minnesota
Chapter 30

David Szmulewicz, MBBS, FRACP
Head of Balance Disorders and Ataxia Service
Royal Victorian Eye and Ear Hospital
University of Melbourne
Victoria
Australia
Chapter 16

Steven A. Telian, MD
John L. Kemink Professor of Neurotology
University of Michigan
Ann Arbor, Michigan
Chapter 28

Konrad P. Weber, MD
Senior Physician, Neuro-Ophthalmology
Departments of Neurology and Ophthalmology
University Hospital Zurich
Zurich
Switzerland
Chapter 16

Susan L. Whitney, DPT, PhD, NCS, ATC, FAPA
Professor, Physical Therapy
School of Health and Rehabilitation
University of Pittsburgh
Pittsburgh, Pennsylvania
Chapters 29 and 31

R. Mark Wiet, MD
Assistant Professor
Department of Otorhinolaryngology-Head and
    Neck Surgery
Section Head
Otology, Neurotology, and Lateral Skull Base
    Surgery
Rush University Medical Center
Chicago, Illinois
Associate Surgeon
Ear Institute of Chicago
Hinsdale, Illinois
Chapters 27 and 28

Practical Anatomy and Physiology of the Vestibular System

Michael C. Schubert and Neil T. Shepard

INTRODUCTION

The vestibular system is responsible for sensing motion of the head to maintain postural control and stability of images on the fovea of the retina during that motion. When functioning normally, the vestibular receptors in the inner ear provide amazing precision in the representation of head motion in three dimensions. This information is then used by the central vestibular pathways to control reflexes and perceptions that are mediated by the vestibular system. Disorders of vestibular function result in abnormalities in these reflexes and lead to sensations that reflect abnormal information about motion from the vestibular receptors.

Normal activities of daily life (such as running) can have head velocities of up to 550 degrees per second, head accelerations of up to 6000 degrees per square second, and frequency content of head motion from <1 to 20 Hz (Das, Zivotofsky, DiScenna, & Leigh, 1995; Grossman, Leigh, Abel, Lanska, & Thurston, 1988). Only the vestibular system can detect head motion over this range of velocity, acceleration, and frequency (Waespe & Henn, 1987). Additionally, the latency of the vestibulo-ocular reflex (VOR) has been reported to be as short as 5 to 7 ms (Huterer & Cullen 2002; Minor, Lasker, Backous, & Hullar 1999). As a result the vestibular system remains critical not only for detection of head motion, but generation of the appropriate motor command to represent that head motion.

This chapter reviews the anatomy and physiology of the vestibular system and offers examples of how the neurophysiology of the vestibular system can be examined practically.

PERIPHERAL VESTIBULAR ANATOMY

Within the petrous portion of each temporal bone lies the membranous vestibular labyrinth. Each labyrinth contains five neural structures that detect head acceleration: three semicircular canals and two otolith organs (Figure 1–1). Three semicircular canals (SCC) (horizontal, anterior, and posterior) respond to angular acceleration and are approximately orthogonal with respect to each other. Alignment of the SCCs in the temporal bone is such that each canal has a contralateral coplanar mate. The horizontal canals form a coplanar or functional pair, whereas the posterior and contralateral anterior SCC form coplanar or functional pairs. The anterior aspect of the lateral SCC is inclined approximately 20 degrees upward from a plane connecting the boney external auditory canal to the floor of the boney rim of the orbit—Reid's baseline (Della Santina, Potyagaylo, Migliaccio, Minor, & Carey, 2005). The orientation of

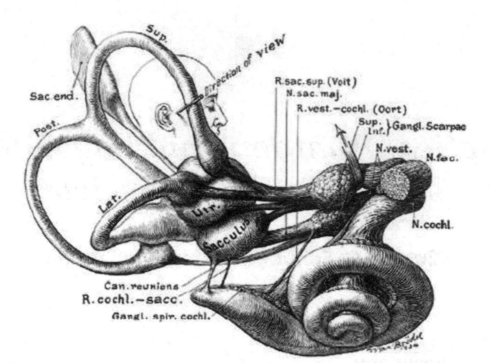

Figure 1–1. Anatomy of the vestibular labyrinth. Structures include the utricle (Utr.), sacculus, anterior (or superior) semicircular canal (Sup.), posterior semicircular canal (Post.), and the lateral (or horizontal) semicircular canal (Lat.). Note the superior vestibular nerve innervating the anterior and lateral semicircular canals as well as the utricle. The inferior vestibular nerve innervates the posterior semicircular canal and the saccule. The cell bodies of the vestibular nerves are located in Scarpa's ganglion (Gangl. Scarpae). Drawing from original art in the Max Brödel Archives (No. 933), Department of Art as Applied to Medicine, The Johns Hopkins University School of Medicine. http://www.hopkins medicine.org/medart/history/Archives.html and from M. C. Schubert and L. B. Minor, Vestibulo-Ocular Physiology Underlying Vestibular Hypofunction. *Physical Therapy*, (2004), *84*(4), 373–385, with permission of the American Physical Therapy Association. This material is copyrighted, and any further reproduction or distribution is prohibited.

the vestibular labyrinth with respect to the skull is shown in Figure 1–2.

The posterior and anterior SCCs are inclined about 92 and 90 degrees from the plane of the horizontal SCC (Della Santina et al., 2005). Specifically the range of angles between the planes of the canals is quite large. The angle between the horizontal-posterior planes ranges from 75.8 to 98.0 degrees; the range between the horizontal-anterior planes is 77.0 to 98.4 degrees; and for the posterior-anterior planes the range is 75.8 to 100.1 (Bradshaw et al., 2010). As a result of the anatomical variations the SCCs are not precisely orthogonal with earth vertical or earth horizontal, and angular rotation of the head stimulates each canal to varying degrees (Cremer et al., 1998).

There are clinical implications for the treatment of benign paroxysmal positional vertigo (BPPV) as all of the maneuvers are based on the premise that the SCC canals are orthogonal to one another and the vertical canals are at 45-degree angles to the midsagittal plane. When the maneuver say for posterior canal BPPV is not effective on the first or second try, slight reorientation of the head relative to the midsagittal plane and the earth horizontal plane should be considered (i.e., the amount of head rotation may need to be modified) . The SCCs are filled with endolymph that has a density slightly greater than that of water. Endolymph contains a high concentration of potassium, with a lower concentration of sodium (Smith, Lowry, & Wu, 1965).

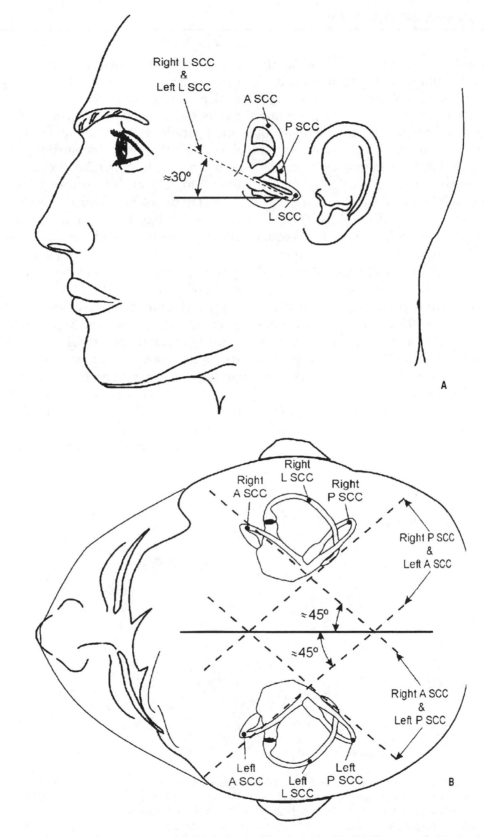

Figure 1–2. A. The line drawing shows the sagittal view of the head with the boney vestibular labyrinth ghosted into the position in the skull for the left ear. Reid's baseline, an anatomical landmark used in radiography has been drawn in on the figure for reference. **B.** The line drawing shows both right and left vestibular labyrinths ghosted on a horizontal axial plane view of the skull. The presumed angle orientations are shown. *L SCC* = lateral semicircular canal; *P SCC* = posterior semicircular canal; *A SCC* = anterior semicircular canal. Reprinted with permission.

3

The SCCs enlarge at one end to form the ampulla. Within the ampulla, a gelatinous goblet-shaped structure called the cupula serves as a barrier separating the semicircular canal from the vestibule. The cupula extends completely across the lumen of the semicircular canal filling the full cross section of the ampulla (Hillman & McLaren, 1979; Scherer, 2001), and data suggest the apex is attached by glycosaminoglycans (Holman, Tran, Arungundram, Balagurumathan, & Rabbitt, 2012; Holman et al., 2013). The cupula has a specific gravity that is equal to that of the endolymph. As a result, the cupula is not responsive to static position changes of the head in the gravitational field. Positioned beneath the cupula is the crista, which extends perpendicularly across the canal in a saddle shape. The crista contains the supporting cells and the cell bodies, commonly known as hair cells, of the stereocilia and the single kinocillium on each of the hair cells, as well as the vestibular afferents (Figure 1–3).

Kinocilia and stereocilia extend into the cupula and are the physical structures that respond to cupular deformation (Figure 1–4). If you remove a cupula and view the underneath surface you find that it is perforated with openings ranging from 3 to 5 microns in diameter. This is the same size range as that of the hair cell bundles of kinocilia and stereocilia (Harada, 1988). These openings in the base of the cupula represent a channel that runs the length of the cupula to allow for circulation of the endolymph to contact the surface of the hair cells (the cuticular plate) into which the stereocilia extend (Lim & Anniko, 1985). Deformation of the cupula occurs from attempted motion of the endolymph (the cupula occludes the canal so continual endolymph current flow is not possible), which enables a billowing (like a sail) of the central portion of the cupula with minimal movement at base on the crista or at the apex. This billowing occurs from the pressure differential that results from the attempted endolymph flow movement. Due to the maximum cupular deformation occurring in the center, a maximum shear force is created at the surface of the crista (Yamauchi et al., 2002). This results in the movement of the stereocilia bundle that causes opening (or closing) of the transduction channels of hair cells,

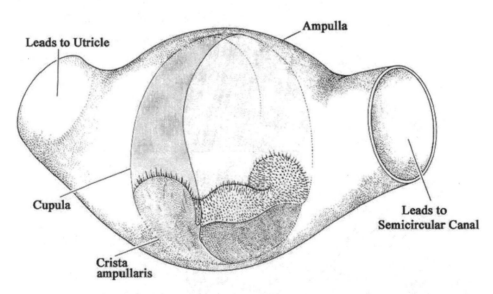

Figure 1–3. The semicircular canals enlarge at one end to form the ampulla. The cupula of the ampulla is a flexible barrier that partitions the canal. The crista ampullaris contains the sensory hair cells. The hair cells generate action potentials in response to cupular deflection. Drawing adapted with permission from Patricia Wynne (patriciawynne.com). Reprinted from M. C. Schubert and L. B. Minor, Vestibulo-Ocular Physiology Underlying Vestibular Hypofunction. *Physical Therapy*, (2004), *84*(4), 373–385, with permission of the American Physical Therapy Association. This material is copyrighted, and any further reproduction or distribution is prohibited.

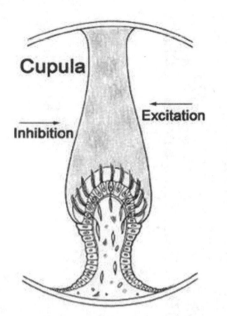

Figure 1–4. Cross section of crista ampullaris showing kinocilia and stereocilia of hair cells projecting into the cupula. Deflection of the stereocilia toward the kinocilia causes excitation; deflection in the opposite direction causes inhibition. Drawing adapted with permission from Patricia Wynne (patriciawynne.com). Reprinted from M. C. Schubert and L. B. Minor, Vestibulo-Ocular Physiology Underlying Vestibular Hypofunction. *Physical Therapy*, (2004), *84*(4), 373–385, with permission of the American Physical Therapy Association. This material is copyrighted, and any further reproduction or distribution is prohibited.

which changes the membrane potential of the hair cells. Deflection of the stereocilia toward the single kinocilia in each hair cell leads to excitation (depolarization), whereas motion of the stereocilia away from the kinocilia causes inhibition (hyperpolarization). Hair cells are oriented in the horizontal SCC so that endolymph motion toward the ampulla (utricle) causes excitation. In contrast, hair cells of the vertical SCCs (posterior and anterior) are oriented so that depolarization occurs when endolymph moves *away* from the ampulla (utricle). Having the hair cells oriented in this manner is referred to as morphologic polarization. Figure 1–5 diagrammatically illustrates this by taking the surface of the crista, flattening it, and looking down on it from above. This is shown for both the horizontal canal in part A and for the two vertical canals in part B. Each of the SCCs responds best to motion in its own plane, with coplanar pairs exhibiting a push-pull dynamic. For example, as the

head is turned to the right, the hair cells in the right horizontal SCC are excited, whereas the hair cells in the left horizontal SCC are inhibited (Goldberg & Fernandez, 1971). The brain detects the direction of head movement by comparing input from the coplanar labyrinthine mates.

The saccule and utricle make up the otolith organs of the membranous labyrinth. Sensory hair cells project into a gelatinous material that has calcium carbonate crystals (otoconia) embedded in it, which provide the otolith organs with an inertial mass (Figure 1–6). The presence of the otoconia increases the specific gravity above that of the endolymph. As a result, the maculae (the surfaces of the otolithic organs that contain the hair cells) are responsive to linear acceleration, including the force of gravity as the head is placed in different static positions. The utricle and the saccule have central regions known as the striola, dividing the otolith organs into two parts. This division is used to set up the morphologic polarization for the otolith organs. The kinocilia of the utricular hair cells are oriented toward their striola, whereas the kinocilia of the saccular hair cells are oriented away from their striola. Motion toward the kinocilia causes excitation. Utricular excitation occurs during horizontal linear acceleration or static head tilt, and saccular excitation occurs during vertical linear acceleration. The striola is not a straight line but is a curved region; therefore, as the utricle or saccule is stimulated by a linear movement in any direction there will be a portion of the utricle (saccule) that is excited and a portion that is inhibited. In effect each of the four otolith organs is its own functional pair along with the unit in the other ear (Rabbitt, Damiano, & Grant, 2004).

The cell bodies of vestibular nerve afferents are located in the superior or inferior divisions of Scarpa's ganglia, which lie within the internal auditory canal near the emergence of the vestibular nerve into the cerebellopontine angle (Brodal, 1981). From the vestibular labyrinth, the afferent information travels ipsilateral in one of two branches of the vestibular nerve. The superior vestibular nerve innervates the horizontal and anterior SCC as well as the utricle. The inferior vestibular nerve innervates the posterior SCC and the saccule (Naito, Newman, Lee, Beykirch, & Honrunbia, 1995). The posterior canal has been reported to have a double innervation; therefore, it may have branches from both superior and inferior

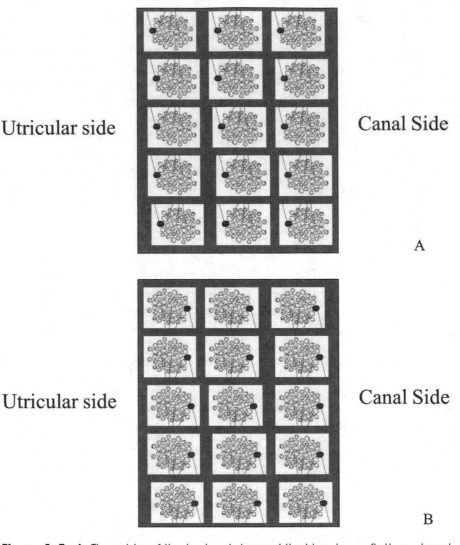

Utricular side   Canal Side

A

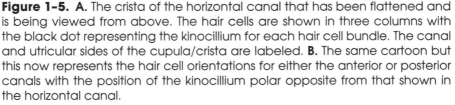

Utricular side   Canal Side

B

Figure 1–5. A. The crista of the horizontal canal that has been flattened and is being viewed from above. The hair cells are shown in three columns with the black dot representing the kinocillium for each hair cell bundle. The canal and utricular sides of the cupula/crista are labeled. **B.** The same cartoon but this now represents the hair cell orientations for either the anterior or posterior canals with the position of the kinocillium polar opposite from that shown in the horizontal canal.

vestibular nerves (Arbusow et al., 1999). It is estimated that between 15,000 and 25,000 vestibular nerve fibers exist in humans (Lopez, Honrubia, & Baloh, 1997; Park, Tang, Lopez, & Ishiyama, 2001; Richter, 1980). Nerve fiber counts vary among studies likely as a function of age, although rate of decline of the number of afferent fibers also appears to be variable.

The branches of the vestibular nerve travel together into the pontomedullary junction where they bifurcate. Primary vestibular afferents in the superior division of the vestibular nerve include axons that synapse in the superior and medial vestibular nuclei or the uvula, nodulus, flocculus, or fastigial nucleus of the cerebellum (Brodal & Brodal, 1985; Furuya, Kawano, & Shimazu, 1975; Goldberg, 2000; Korte & Mugnaini, 1979). Primary vestibular afferents from the inferior branch synapse with neurons in either the medial, lateral, or inferior vestibu-

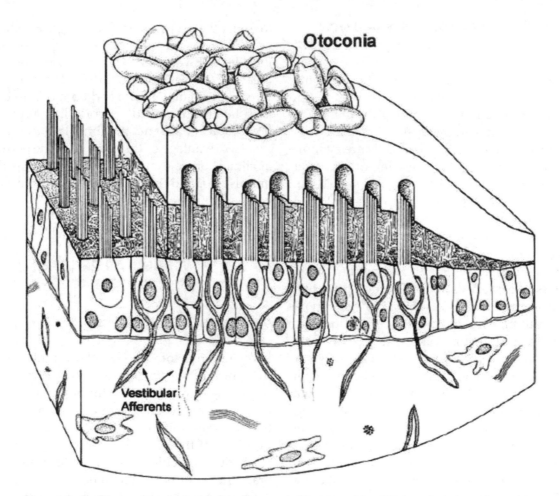

Figure 1-6. Otoconia are embedded in a gelatinous matrix of the maculae and provide an inertial mass. Linear acceleration shifts the gelatinous matrix and excites or inhibits the vestibular afferents depending on the direction in which the stereocilia are deflected. Drawing adapted with permission from Patricia Wynne (patriciawynne.com). Reprinted from M. C. Schubert and L. B. Minor, Vestibulo-Ocular Physiology Underlying Vestibular Hypofunction. *Physical Therapy*, (2004), *84*(4), 373–385, with permission of the American Physical Therapy Association. This material is copyrighted, and any further reproduction or distribution is prohibited.

lar nuclei, which, along with the superior vestibular nuclei and other subnuclei, comprise the vestibular nuclear complex (Naito et al., 1995).

Blood supply to the vestibular end organ follows the afferent innervation and is provided through the labyrinthine artery which commonly arises from the anterior inferior cerebellar artery (AICA), but may arise from either the superior cerebellar artery or basilar artery (Baloh & Honrubia, 1990). The labyrinthine artery bifurcates, with the first branch supplying the superior vestibular artery to nourish the utricle, and superior and horizontal semicircu-lar canals, as well as a small portion of the saccule. The second branch is the common cochlear artery which splits in two divisions, one of which supplies the cochlea (with further bifurcation). The other, the posterior vestibular artery, supplies the posterior semicircular canal and a majority of the saccule. Venous drainage follows a trajectory similar to the arterial supply. The superior (anterior) vestibular vein drains the superior and horizontal SCC as well as the utriculus, whereas the inferior (posterior) vestibular vein drains the sacculus, posterior canal, and most of the cochlea.

VESTIBULAR AFFERENT PHYSIOLOGY

Two types of hair cells exist within the vestibular periphery: Type I hair cells are flask shaped and have a chalice-shaped nerve ending on them. One calyx nerve ending can synapse with just one or two to four hair cells. Type II hair cells are cylindrical in shape and have multiple efferent and afferent bouton nerve synapses (Lysakowski, Minor, Fernandez, & Goldberg, 1995). Type I and Type II hair cells generally are associated with irregular and regular vestibular afferents, respectively. The naming of the afferents as irregular or regular refers to the discharge regularity determined by the spacing of the interspike intervals between action potentials. Although both primary vestibular afferent types (healthy vestibular system) have a resting firing rate that is typically 70 to 100 spikes per second (Goldberg & Fernandez, 1971; Lysakowski et al., 1995), the irregular afferents do not have a periodic firing pattern. As a result, the information carried by irregular and regular afferents varies over the spectral range of frequency and acceleration that encompasses natural head movements. In general, irregular afferents are more sensitive to rotations during large head accelerations than are regular afferents (Lysakowski et al., 1995). This heightened sensitivity of the irregular afferents may be more critical for the rapid detection of head movements as well as initiation of the VOR (Lysakowski et al., 1995; Minor et al., 1999). Data also suggest the irregular afferents provide an important role in viewing distance-related changes in the angular vestibulo-ocular reflex (aVOR) (Chen-Huang & McCrea, 1998). The regular afferents, in contrast, provide a signal that is proportional to head velocity over a broader spectral range (Lysakowski et al., 1995). In addition, the regular afferents may be the primary source of input to the VOR for steady-state responses to sinusoidal rotations because temporarily silencing the irregular afferents has no effect on the VOR during low-frequency and small head accelerations.

During head rotation, primary vestibular afferents can be excited up to 400 spikes per second for an ipsilateral rotation (Uchino, Hirai, & Suzuki, 1982), whereas the contralateral vestibular afferents are inhibited to zero spikes per second. The asymmetry in excitation versus inhibition with the ability to excite the system significantly greater than it can be inhibited is representative of Ewald's second and third laws (Ewald, 1892). This property of excitation greater than inhibition holds for the function of all three semicircular canals and both otolith organs in each labyrinth. Ewald's second law applies to the horizontal canals and the third law to the vertical canals. Advantage of this is taken in the performance of clinical office examination tests such as the head impulse test and the head-shake test both discussed below and in more detail in Chapter 7.

VESTIBULAR REFLEXES

Vestibulo-Ocular Reflex

Investigations of the VOR routinely study the dynamics of the response considering the neurophysiologic substrate of the system as a simple three-neuron arc. Although convenient to learn the basic neurophysiologic principles, intricate communications of the central vestibular system with the cerebellum, reticular formation, thalamus, and cerebral cortex (Buttner & Buettner, 1978; Grusser, Pause, & Schreiter, 1990; Thier & Erickson, 1992) are overly simplistic. In addition, the output of the VOR is linear with regard to detection of head motion at low acceleration and low velocity but becomes nonlinear with higher head accelerations and head velocities (Lasker, Hullar, & Minor, 2000; Minor et al., 1999).

For the purpose of this chapter we consider the VOR as a three-neuron arc. The primary purpose of the VOR is to elicit rapid compensatory eye movements that maintain stability of images on the fovea (that part of the macula of the retina that is the most sensitive for clear visual viewing of objects in the visual field) during head motion. Prior to discussion of the VOR in more detail, a brief review of the extraocular muscles and their intervention is needed. There are six extraocular muscles that control the position of the eye in the orbit. All of the muscles approach the globe from a region posterior and medial to the axis of primary viewing except for the superior and inferior oblique muscles. Both of the oblique muscles approach their insertion into the globe from an anterior and medial perspective relative to the axis of primary gaze. Because of the orientations of the muscles with respect to axis of primary gaze, only the medial and lateral recti muscles when contracted produce a pure medial-lateral movement of the eye (yaw) as long as the axis of primary gaze is directed upward, parallel to the plane of the horizontal canals. All of the other muscles when contracted produce complex movements of the eye in the yaw, pitch, and roll planes, even when the axis of gaze is parallel to the vertical canals. As it turns out the orientations of the eye muscles are in planes that are roughly parallel to the respective semicircular canals that are the primary activators of the muscles on the ipsilateral side. Therefore, the horizontal canals are in a plane parallel to the plane of insertion of the medial and lateral recti muscles. The anterior canal aligned with the superior and inferior recti and the posterior canal with the superior and inferior oblique muscles (Cohen & Raphan, 2004). These anatomical relationships and the resultant movements of the eye when the various canals are stimulated for the basis behind Ewald's first law (see Table 1–1 for a summary of Ewald's laws). This law states that the eyes (and head) move in the plane of the canal being stimulated. The impact of this clinically is seen by the change in nystagmus that can be seen by chang-

ing the position of the eye in the orbit. This principle is used in the investigation of BPPV by having the individual look toward and away from the underneath ear during the Dix-Hallpike test to help bring out the torsional or the vertical component of the complex nystagmus that is generated with posterior canal BPPV (see Chapter 26).

In the case of the horizontal SCC, primary vestibular afferents from the horizontal SCC synapse in the ipsilateral medial and ventrolateral vestibular nuclei. Some of the secondary vestibular neurons receiving innervation from the ipsilateral labyrinth have axons that decussate and synapse in the contralateral abducens nucleus, whereas others ascend ipsilaterally to the oculomotor nucleus. Motoneurons from the abducens nucleus and the medial rectus subdivision of the oculomotor nucleus then synapse at the neuromuscular junction of the lateral rectus and medial rectus muscles, respectively. Similar patterns of connectivity exist for the anterior and posterior SCC, each of which synapses with the vestibular nuclei, cranial nerves (III, IV, or VI), the medial longitudinal fasciculus, and collateral neural inputs from the reticular formation in the brainstem. A detailed description of these synapses and central VOR pathways is provided in Chapter 2.

Table 1–1. Summary of Ewald's Laws

Ewald's Law 1	Stimulation of a semicircular canal causes eye rotation (with respect to the head) in the plane of the canal being stimulated.
Ewald's Law 2	In the horizontal canals, movement of the endolymph toward the utricle (utriculopetal) causes greater neural activity (cupular excitation) than does movement of the endolymph away from the utricle (utriculofugal). Thus, neural activity from excitation is greater than neural activity due to inhibition.
Ewald's Law 3	In the vertical canals, movement of the endolymph away the utricle (utriculofugal) causes greater neural activity than utriculopetal movement of the endolymph (i.e., the opposite of the horizontal canals). Differences in arrangement of the hair cells on the crista (morphological polarization, see text and Figure 1–5) are the reason for differences in neural excitation between the vertical and horizontal semicircular canals.
Extension of Ewald's Laws 2 and 3	For the otolith organs, the principle of excitation causing greater neural activity than inhibition also applies as a result of the arrangement of the hair cells on the macula of the utricle and saccule.

VESTIBULO-OCULAR REFLEX AND VESTIBULO-OCULAR REFLEX GAIN AND PHASE

For the vestibulo-ocular reflex (VOR) to maintain stability of an image on the fovea of the retina during rapid head movements, it must generate rapid compensatory eye movements (in the direction opposite the head rotation). Normally, as the head moves in one direction, the eyes move in the opposite direction with equal velocity (gain = eye velocity/head velocity = −1). This relationship of eye velocity to head velocity is expressed as the gain of the VOR. For example, when the head is moved down the anterior SCCs are excited. Excitation of the anterior SCC afferents rotates both eyes in the direction opposite the angular head movement, or up. VOR phase represents the timing relationship for the eye and head position, another useful measure of the vestibular system. Ideally, eye position should arrive at a point in time that is equal to the oppositely directed head position. By convention, this is described as zero phase shift.

The VOR has been tested across multiple frequencies and velocities and shows velocity-dependent nonlinearities (Minor et al., 1999) that may correlate with unique afferent physiology. The gain of the VOR remains constant (linear) across multiple frequencies of sinusoidal rotations, with peak velocities of 20 degrees per second (Minor et al., 1999). For rotations at higher frequencies and velocities, the VOR gain rises with increases in stimulus velocity (here we mean velocity as having both a magnitude and direction; nonlinear). Similar effects of stimulus frequency and velocity are seen in responses to steps of acceleration (change in velocity over time). Therefore, it may be that the output of the VOR is the combined result of linear and nonlinear components (Minor et al., 1999). This VOR gain dependence on velocity and acceleration may explain the incongruence of vestibular function tests in patients with Ménière's disease, who have been shown to have abnormal caloric tests yet healthy head impulse test results (Park, Migliaccio, Della Santina, Minor, & Carey, 2005), implying the linear component of the VOR is abnormal.

VOR gain and phase are among the important measures of vestibular function that laboratory tests, such as the rotational chair, use to objectify function.

The rotational chair test is a laboratory test that is useful to determine function of the velocity storage system (a grouping of cells in the brainstem that allow for storage of input from the peripheral vestibular, visual, and proprioceptive systems that allow further control of the eyes at extended low-frequency angular motion). This test stimulates each vestibular system by rotating subjects in the dark. Nystagmus should be generated for rotations in subjects with normal vestibular function. The extent of pathology is determined by comparing VOR gain, phase, and duration of the nystagmus (time constant) from rotations toward one ear with rotations toward the opposite ear. In addition, VOR gain and phase from persons with normal vestibular function can be compared with those of persons with suspected vestibular dysfunction. See Chapters 14 and 15 for further discussion of rotational chair testing.

The cervico-ocular reflex (COR) parallels the VOR and is thought to generate a slow phase eye movement in the direction opposite head movement. The difference, however, is that the eye motion is generated from receptors in the joints and ligaments of the upper cervical vertebrae (Hikosaka & Maeda, 1973). The COR has been proposed as a mechanism of gaze stability for subjects with bilateral hypofunction (Barnes, 1979; Bles & de Jong, 1982; Bronstein & Hood, 1987; Bronstein, Morland, Ruddock, & Gresty, 1995; Huygen, Verhagen & Nicolasen, 1991; Kasai & Zee, 1978; Mergner, Schweigart, Botti, & Lehmann, 1998) and unilateral vestibular hypofunction (Barnes, 1979; Schubert, Das, Tusa, & Herdman, 2004). In general, it appears that the gain of the COR (eye velocity/trunk velocity) is insignificant for individuals with healthy vestibular function but may be a mechanism of gaze stability in vestibular hypofunction.

Vestibulospinal Reflex

Not only does acceleration of the head cause a specific oculomotor response as detected by the sensory epithelia of the vestibular labyrinth, but it also causes an upper and lower limb response. The limbs ipsilateral to the direction of acceleration are extended, whereas those contralateral to the acceleration are contracted (Pompeiano & Allum, 1988). The purpose of the vestibulospinal reflex (VSR) is to maintain posture and center of mass over one's base of support. Chapter 17 provides greater detail of the VSR.

Vestibulocolic Reflex

The vestibulocolic reflex can be thought of as a righting reflex. This reflex assists in maintaining the head in horizontal gaze orientation relative to gravity, independent of trunk movement, and within the limits of range of motion of the neck in the sagittal and lateral planes. For example, an individual walking on a grass field trips over a rock and has his weight displaced to the side. The otolithic organs detect the changing gravitational vector and move the head toward the opposite direction, in order to maintain upright gaze. Experimental data suggest this reflex is mediated through the otolithic organs and the medial vestibulospinal tract (Pozzo, Berthoz, & Popov, 1994).

CENTRAL VESTIBULAR ANATOMY

Secondary vestibular afferents relay signals from the vestibular nuclei to the extraocular motor nuclei, the spinal cord, or the flocculus of the cerebellum (Highstein, Goldberg, Moschovakis, & Fernandez, 1987). Many vestibular reflexes are controlled by processes that exist primarily within the brainstem. Tracing techniques, however, have identified extensive connections between the vestibular nuclei and the reticular formation (Troiani, Petrosini, & Zannoni, 1976), thalamus (Buttner & Henn, 1976), and cerebellum (Brodal & Brodal, 1985). Vestibular pathways appear to terminate in a unique cortical area. In studies of primates, fibers terminating in the junction of the parietal and insular lobes have been identified and considered the location for a vestibular cortex (Buttner & Buettner, 1978; Grusser et al., 1990; Thier & Erickson, 1992). Recent evidence in studies of humans using functional magnetic resonance imaging appears to confirm the parietal and insular regions as the cortical location for processing vestibular information (Brandt et al., 2002). Connections with the vestibular cortex, thalamus, and reticular formation enable the vestibular system to contribute to the integration of arousal and conscious awareness of the body and to discriminate

between movement of self and the environment (Brandt & Dieterich, 1994; Dieterich, Bense, Stephan, Yousry, & Brandt, 2003). The cerebellar connections help maintain calibration of the VOR, contribute to posture during static and dynamic activities, and influence the coordination of limb movements.

One could question if the gain of the VOR for compensatory eye movements is a fixed value. If this were case, then when a person makes a gaze shift to the right (i.e., due to hearing their name being called), the foveae of their eyes would not be able to stay on the target of interest. Instead, the initial rightward eye rotation followed by a rightward head rotation toward the target of interest would be countered from the rigidly fixed VOR. Hence, it must be that the gain of the VOR is modulated for voluntary head movements in response to refixating gaze to the target of interest (i.e., reduced). A reduction in VOR gain between 20% and 50% has been shown to occur for saccadic eye movements with head movements in the same direction (Tabak, Smeets, & Collewijn, 1996). This is one example of the adaptive properties of the VOR. Other examples include the ability to alter the gain and phase of the VOR with changes in the visual input over time. This can be dramatic to the point of causing a full reversal of the direction of the compensatory eye movement during rotation in the dark by having an individual wear reversing lenses for multiple hours (the lenses reverse the direction of the visual world movement with a head turn, e.g., head turn to the right the world moves to the right) (Melvill Jones & Gonshor, 1982).

PRACTICAL NEUROPHYSIOLOGY

Recall that during angular head rotations, ipsilateral vestibular afferents can be excited up to 400 spikes per second with a concomitant hyperpolarization of the contralateral afferents also occurring (Goldberg & Fernandez, 1971). The hyperpolarization of the contralateral hair cells can only decrease the firing rate to zero spikes per second, at which point the inhibition is cut off (inhibitory cutoff). Inhibitory cutoff, coupled with the orthogonal orientation of the SCCs within the skull provides the clinician a powerful platform to assess individual SCC function. The head impulse test is a widely accepted clinical tool that is used to assess semicircular canal function (Cremer et al., 1998; Halmagyi & Curthoys, 1988). The head impulse test is performed by having the patient first fixate on a near target (e.g., the clinician's nose). Patients are asked to keep their eyes focused on a target while their head is manually rotated in an unpredictable direction using a small amplitude (5–15 degrees), high-acceleration (3000–4000 deg/sec^2) angular thrust (see Video 1–1). When the VOR is functioning normally, the eyes move in the direction opposite to the head movement and gaze will remain on the target. In a patient with a loss of vestibular function, the VOR will not move the eyes as quickly as the head rotation and the eyes move off the target. The patient will make a corrective saccade to reposition the eyes (fovea) on the target. The appearance of corrective saccades indicates vestibular hypofunction as evaluated by the head impulse test and occurs because inhibition of vestibular afferents and central vestibular neurons on the intact side (persons with unilateral vestibular hypofunction) is less effective (inhibitory cutoff) in encoding the amplitude of a head movement than excitation. A patient who has a unilateral peripheral lesion or pathology of the central vestibular neurons will not be able to maintain gaze when the head is rotated quickly toward the side of the lesion. A patient with a bilateral loss of vestibular function will make corrective saccades after a head impulse to either side. The head impulse test provides a sensitive indication of vestibular hypofunction in patients with complete loss of function in the affected labyrinth that occurs following ablative surgical procedures, such as labyrinthectomy (Aw, Halmagyi, Curthoys, Todd, & Yavor, 1994; Cremer et al., 1998; Foster, Foster, Spindler, & Harris, 1994; Halmagyi & Curthoys, 1988). The test is less sensitive in detecting hypofunction in patients with incomplete loss of function (Beynon, Jani, & Baguley, 1998; Harvey & Wood, 1996; Harvey, Wood, & Feroah, 1997; Schubert, Tusa, Grine, & Herdman, 2004). The head impulse test appears useful for identifying individual SCC lesions (Cremer et al., 1998).

Positional Testing

Knowledge of the SCC orientation and differences in excitation polarity among the vertical and horizontal canals is essential for identifying and treating the most common pathology affecting the vestibular labyrinth. Benign paroxysmal positional vertigo (BPPV) occurs when otoconia have been displaced into the semicircular canals, rendering the canals sensitive to changes in head position. Recall that normal specific gravity of the endolymph and cupula are similar and therefore independent of any gravitational vector. In the case of cupulolithiasis, however, the otoconial debris becomes adherent to the cupula—changing its specific gravity such that the cupula becomes a linear accelerometer, dependent on changing head position (changing gravitational vector)—which creates an abnormal cupular deflection. In the case of canalithiasis, the displaced otoconia are floating free within the canal. Although the specific gravity of the endolymph is unchanged, the otoconial motion provides a transcupular pressure differential with the endolymph and creates cupular deflection. In both cases, the abnormal signal results in nystagmus and vertigo, nausea with or without vomiting, and disequilibrium. Various clinical tests position patients' heads to align the gravitational vector with the SCC, which causes nystagmus. The nystagmus generated is essential to identify which semicircular canal is involved.

Head Shaking

The signal generated by movement of the cupula is brief, lasting only as long as the cupula is deflected (Dai, Klein, Cohen, & Raphan, 1999). The response is sustained, however, by a circuit of neurons in the medial vestibular nucleus and lasts longer than 10 s in people with normal vestibular function (Raphan, Matsuo, & Cohen, 1979). This is termed velocity storage, believed to sustain the vestibular input to assist the brain in detecting low-frequency head rotation. Clinical and laboratory examinations exist that enable the clinician information regarding the integrity of the velocity storage system.

The head-shaking induced nystagmus (HSN) test is a useful aid in the diagnosis of a unilateral peripheral vestibular defect. Patients undergoing the HSN test must have their vision blocked (i.e., video infrared goggles). The patient is instructed to close his or her eyes. The clinician then oscillates the head horizontally for 20 cycles at a frequency of two repetitions per second (2 Hz). Upon stopping the oscillation, the patient opens the eyes and the clinician checks for nystagmus. In subjects with normal vestibular function, nystagmus will not be present. An asymmetry between the peripheral vestibular inputs to central vestibular nuclei, however, may result in HSN. Typically, a person with unilateral vestibular hypofunction (UVH) will manifest a horizontal HSN, with the quick phases of the nystagmus directed toward the healthy ear and the slow phases directed toward the lesioned ear (Hain, Fetter, & Zee, 1987). Not all patients with UVH will have HSN. Patients with a complete loss of vestibular function bilaterally will not have HSN because neither system is functioning; therefore, the central neurons do not receive asymmetric input. The presence of vertical nystagmus after either horizontal or vertical head shaking suggests a lesion affecting the central vestibular pathways.

SUMMARY

The vestibular system is uniquely designed not only to detect head motion across velocity and acceleration ranges that encompass a broad activity spectra in which human activity typically encompasses, but also generates a motor output to address the challenges inherent with that motion. The unique characteristics of the VOR provide amazing precision in the representation of head motion in three dimensions. Knowledge of this information is critical to help the clinician better develop evaluation and treatment strategies to address disorders of the system.

VIDEO ASSOCIATED WITH THIS CHAPTER

Video 1–1. Shown is the clinical head impulse test of the horizontal and posterior semicircular canals. The horizontal test occurs first, with two thrusts in each direction. Each of these four tests is normal. Next you will see a thrust in the plane of the left posterior canal with a catch-up saccade indicating vestibular hypofunction of the left inferior vestibular nerve. Note the second time this canal is tested, a saccade does not occur—illustrating the importance of ran-

domizing the timing and direction of clinical head thrust testing. Normal head impulses in the right posterior canal are presented at the end of the video.

REFERENCES

Arbusow, V., Schulz, P., Strupp, M., Dieterich, M., von Reinhardstoettner, A., Rauch, E., & Brandt, T. (1999). Distribution of herpes simplex virus type 1 in human geniculate and vestibular ganglia: Implications for vestibular neuritis. *Annals of Neurology, 46,* 416–419.

Aw, S. T., Halmagyi, G. M., Curthoys, I. S., Todd, M. J., & Yavor, R. A. (1994). Unilateral vestibular deafferentation causes permanent impairment of the human vertical vestibulo-ocular reflex in the pitch plane. *Experimental Brain Research, 102,* 121–130.

Baloh, R. W., & Honrubia, V. (1990). *Clinical neurophysiology of the vestibular system* (2nd ed.). Philadelphia, PA: F. A. Davis.

Barnes, G. R. (1979). Head-eye coordination in normals and in patients with vestibular disorders. *Advances in Oto-Rhino-Laryngology, 25,* 197–201.

Beynon, G. J., Jani, P., & Baguley, D. M. (1998). A clinical evaluation of head impulse testing. *Clinical Otolaryngology, 23,* 117–122.

Bles, W., & De Jong, J. M. B. (1982). Cervico-vestibular and visuo-vestibular interaction: Self-motion perception, nystagmus, and gaze shift. *Acta Otolaryngolica, 64,* 61–72.

Bradshaw, A. D., Curthoys, I. S., Todd, M. J., Magussen, J. S., Taubman, D. S., Aw, S. T., & Halmagyi, G. M. (2010). A mathematical model of human semicircular canal geometry: A new basis for interpreting vestibular physiology. *Journal of Association for Research in Otolaryngology, 11,* 145–159.

Brandt, T., & Dieterich, M. (1994). Vestibular syndromes in the roll plane: Topographic diagnosis from brainstem to cortex. *Annals of Neurology, 36,* 337–347.

Brandt, T., Glasauer, S., Stephan, T., Bense, S., Yousry, T. A., Deutschlander, A., & Dieterich, M. (2002). Visual-vestibular and visuovisual cortical interaction: New insights from fMRI and PET. *Annals of the New York Academy of Science, 956,* 230–241.

Brodal, A. (1981). The cranial nerves. In A. Brodal (Ed.), *Neurological anatomy in relation to clinical medicine* (3rd ed., pp. 471–472). New York, NY: Oxford University Press.

Brodal, A., & Brodal, P. (1985). Observations on the secondary vestibulocerebellar projections in the macaque monkey. *Experimental Brain Research, 58,* 62–74.

Bronstein, A. M., & Hood, J. D. (1987). Oscillopsia of peripheral vestibular origin. Central and cervical compensatory mechanisms. *Acta Otolaryngolica, 104*(3–4), 307–314.

Bronstein, A. M., Morland, A. B., Ruddock, K. H., & Gresty, M. A. (1995). Recovery from bilateral vestibular failure: Implications for visual and cervico-ocular function. *Acta Otolaryngolica (Stockholm)*, (Suppl. 520), 405–407.

Buttner, U., & Buettner, U. W. (1978). Parietal cortex (2v) neuronal activity in the alert monkey during natural vestibular and optokinetic stimulation. *Brain Research, 153*, 392–397.

Buttner, U., & Henn, V. (1976). Thalamic unit activity in the alert monkey during natural vestibular stimulation. *Brain Research, 103*, 127–132.

Chen-Huang, C., & McCrea, R. A. (1998). Contribution of vestibular nerve irregular afferents to viewing distance-related changes in the vestibulo-ocular reflex. *Experimental Brain Research, 119*(1), 116–130.

Cohen, B., & Raphan, T. (2004). The physiology of the vestibuloocular reflex (VOR). In S. M. Higstein, R. R. Fay, & A. N. Popper (Eds.), *The Vestibular System.* New York, NY: Springer-Verlag.

Cremer, P. D., Halmagyi, G. M., Aw, S. T., Curthoys, I. S., McGarvie, L. A., Todd, M. J., . . . Hannigan, I. P. (1998). Semicircular canal plane head impulses detect absent function of individual semicircular canals. *Brain, 121*, 699–716.

Dai, M., Klein, A., Cohen, B., & Raphan, T. (1999). Model-based study of the human cupular time constant. *Journal of Vestibular Research, 9*(4), 293–301.

Das, V. E., Zivotofsky, A. Z., DiScenna, A. O., & Leigh, R. J. (1995). Head perturbations during walking while viewing a head-fixed target. *Aviation and Space Environmental Medicine, 66*, 728–732.

Della Santina, C. C., Potyagaylo, V., Migliaccio, A. A., Minor, L. B., & Carey, J. P. (2005). Orientation of human semicircular canals measured by three-dimensional multiplanar CT reconstruction. *Journal of the Association for Research in Otolaryngology, 6*(3), 191–206.

Dieterich, M., Bense, S., Stephan, T., Yousry, T. A., & Brandt, T. (2003). fMRI signal increases and decreases in cortical areas during small-field optokinetic stimulation and central fixation. *Experimental Brain Research, 148*, 117–127.

Ewald, J. (1892). *Physiolgische untersuchunge uber das endorgan des nervus octavus.* Wiesbaden, Germany: Bergmann.

Foster, C. A., Foster, B. D., Spindler, J., & Harris, J. P. (1994). Functional loss of the horizontal doll's eye reflex following unilateral vestibular lesions. *Laryngoscope, 104*, 473–478.

Furuya, N., Kawano, K., & Shimazu, H. (1975). Functional organization of vestibulofastigial projection in the horizontal semicircular canal system in the cat. *Experimental Brain Research, 24*, 75–87.

Goldberg, J. M. (2000). Afferent diversity and the organization of central vestibular pathways. *Experimental Brain Research, 130*, 277–297.

Goldberg, J. M., & Fernandez, C. (1971). Physiology of peripheral neurons innervating semicircular canals of the squirrel monkey, I: Resting discharge and response to constant angular accelerations. *Journal of Neurophysiology, 34*, 635–660.

Grossman, G. E., Leigh, R. J., Abel, L. A., Lanska, D. J., & Thurston, S. E. (1988). Frequency and velocity of rotational head perturbations during locomotion. *Experimental Brain Research, 70*, 470–476.

Grusser, O. J., Pause, M., & Schreiter, U. (1990). Localization and responses of neurones in the parieto-insular vestibular cortex of awake monkeys (*Macaca fascicularis*). *Journal of Physiology, 430*, 537–557.

Hain, T. C., Fetter, M., & Zee, D. S. (1987). Head-shaking nystagmus in patients with unilateral peripheral vestibular lesions. *American Journal of Otolaryngology, 8*, 36–47.

Halmagyi, G. M., & Curthoys, I. S. (1988). A clinical sign of canal paresis. *Archives of Neurology, 45*, 737–739.

Harada, Y. (1988). *The vestibular organs: S.E.M. atlas of the inner ear.* Niigata, Japan: Nishimura. Amsterdam, the Netherlands: Kugler & Ghedini.

Harvey, S. A., & Wood, D. J. (1996). The oculocephalic response in the evaluation of the dizzy patient. *Laryngoscope, 106*, 6–9.

Harvey, S. A., Wood, D. J., & Feroah, T. R. (1997). Relationship of the head impulse test and head-shake nystagmus in reference to caloric testing. *American Journal of Otology, 18*, 207–213.

Highstein, S. M., Goldberg, J. M., Moschovakis, A. K., & Fernandez, C. (1987). Inputs from regularly and irregularly discharging vestibular nerve afferents to secondary neurons in the vestibular nuclei of the squirrel monkey, II: Correlation with output pathways of secondary neurons. *Journal of Neurophysiology, 58*, 719–738.

Hikosaka, O., & Maeda, M. (1973). Cervical effects on abducens motor neurons and their interaction with vestibulo-ocular reflex. *Experimental Brain Research, 18*, 512–530.

Hillman, D. E., & McLaren, J. W. (1979). Displacement configuration of semicircular canal cupulae. *Neuroscience, 4*(12), 1989–2000.

Holman, H. A., Nguyen, L. N., Tran, V. M., Arungundram, S., Kuberan, B., & Rabbitt, R. D. (2013). *Remodeling and biosynthesis of glycosaminoglycans revealed using a*

BODIPY-xyloside conjugate in the vestibular system. Association for Research in Otolaryngology, Baltimore, MD, February, Abs., 163.

Holman, H. A., Tran, V. M., Arungundram, S., Balagururnathan, K., & Rabbitt, R. D. (2012). *BODIPY conjugated xylosides reveal repair and regeneration of the semicircular canal cupula.* Association for Research in Otolaryngology, Baltimore, MD, February, Abs., 155.

Huterer, M., & Cullen, K. E. (2002). Vestibuloocular reflex dynamics during high-frequency and high-acceleration rotations of the head on body in rhesus monkey. *Journal of Neurophysiology, 88,* 13–28.

Huygen, P. L. M., Verhagen, W. I. M., & Nicolasen, M. G. M. (1991). Cervico-ocular reflex enhancement in labyrinthine-defective and normal subjects. *Experimental Brain Research, 87,* 457–464.

Kasai, T., & Zee, D. S. (1978). Eye-head coordination in labyrinthine-defective human beings. *Brain Research, 144*(1), 123–141.

Korte, G. E., & Mugnaini, E. (1979). The cerebellar projection of the vestibular nerve in the cat. *Journal of Comparative Neurology, 184,* 265–278.

Lasker, D. M., Hullar, T. E., & Minor, L. B. (2000). Horizontal vestibuloocular reflex evoked by high acceleration rotation in the squirrel monkey. III. Responses after labyrinthectomy. *Journal of Neurophysiology, 83,* 1–15.

Lim, D. J., & Anniko, M. (1985). Developmental morphology of the mouse inner ear. A scanning electron microscopic observation. *Acta Oto-Laryngologica, 422*(Suppl.), 1–69.

Lopez, I., Honrubia, V., & Baloh, R. W. (1997). Aging and the human vestibular nucleus. *Journal of Vestibular Research, 7,* 77–85.

Lysakowski, A., Minor, L. B., Fernandez, C., & Goldberg, J. M. (1995). Physiological identification of morphologically distinct afferent classes innervating the cristae ampullares of the squirrel monkey. *Journal of Neurophysiology, 73,* 1270–1281.

Melvill, J. G., & Gonshor, A. (1982). Oculomotor response to rapid head oscillation (0.5–5.0 Hz) after prolonged adaptation to vision-reversal. "Simple" and "complex" effects. *Experimental Brain Research, 45,* 45–58.

Mergner, T., Schweigart, G., Botti, F., & Lehmann, A. (1998). Eye movements evoked by proprioceptive stimulation along the body axis in humans. *Experimental Brain Research, 120*(4), 450–460.

Minor, L. B., Lasker, D. M., Backous, D. D., & Hullar, T. E. (1999). Horizontal vestibuloocular reflex evoked by high-acceleration rotations in the squirrel monkey, I: Normal responses. *Journal of Neurophysiology, 82,* 1254 1270.

Naito, Y., Newman, A., Lee, W. S., Beykirch, K., & Honrunbia, V. (1995). Projections of the individual vestibular end-organs in the brain stem of the squirrel monkey. *Hearing and Research, 87,* 141–155.

Park, H. J., Migliaccio, A. A., Della Santina, C. C., Minor, L. B., & Carey, J. P. (2005). Search-coil head-thrust and caloric tests in Ménière's disease. *Acta Oto-Laryngologica, 125*(8), 852–857.

Park, J. J., Tang, Y., Lopez, I., & Ishiyama, A. (2001). Unbiased estimation of human vestibular ganglion neurons. *Annals of the New York Academy of Science, 942,* 475–478.

Pompeiano, O., & Allum, J. H. J. (Eds.). (1988). *Vestibulospinal control of posture and locomotion.* Amsterdam, the Netherlands: Elsevier.

Pozzo, T., Berthoz, A., & Popov, C. (1994). The effect of gravity on the coordination between posture and movement. In K. Taguchi, M. Igarashi, & S. Mori (Eds.), *Vestibular and neural front,* Proceedings of the 12th International Symposium on Posture and Gait. Amsterdam, the Netherlands: Elsevier.

Rabbitt, R. D., Damiano, E. R., & Grant, J. W. (2004). Biomechanics of the semicircular canals and otolith organs. In S. M. Higstein, R. R. Fay, & A. N. Popper (Eds.), *The vestibular system.* New York, NY: Springer-Verlag.

Raphan, T., Matsuo, V., & Cohen, B. (1979). Velocity storage in the vestibulo-ocular reflex arc (VOR). *Experimental Brain Research, 35*(2), 229–248.

Richter, E. (1980). Quantitative study of human Scarpa's ganglion and vestibular sensory epithelia. *Acta Oto-Laryngologica, 90,* 199–208.

Scherer, R. (2001). On the role of the ampulla in disturbances of vestibular function. *Biological Sciences in Space, 15*(4), 350–352.

Schubert, M. C., Das, V., Tusa, R. J., & Herdman, S. J. (2004). Cervico-ocular reflex in normal subjects and patients with unilateral vestibular hypofunction. *Otology and Neurotology, 25*(1), 65–71.

Schubert, M. C., Tusa, R. J., Grine, L. E., & Herdman, S. J. (2004). Optimizing the sensitivity of the head thrust test for identifying vestibular hypofunction. *Physical Therapy, 84*(2), 151–158.

Smith, C. A., Lowry, O. H, & Wu, M. L. (1965). The electrolytes of the labyrinthine fluids. *Laryngoscope, 64,* 141–153.

Tabak, S., Smeets, J. B. J., & Collewijn, H. (1996). Modulation of the human vestibuloocular reflex during saccades: Probing by high-frequency oscillation and torque pulses of the head. *Journal of Neurophysiology, 76*(5), 3249–3263.

Thier, P., & Erickson, R. G. (1992). Vestibular input to visual-tracking neurons in area MST of awake rhesus monkeys. *Annals of the New York Academy of Science, 656,* 960–963.

Troiani, D., Petrosini, L., & Zannoni, B. (1976). Relations of single semicircular canals to the pontine reticular formation. *Archives in Italian Biology, 11,* 337–375.

Uchino, Y., Hirai, N., & Suzuki, S. (1982). Branching pattern and properties of vertical-and horizontal-related excitatory vestibuloocular neurons in the cat. *Journal of Neurophysiology, 48*, 891–903.

Waespe, W., & Henn, V. (1987). Gaze stabilization in the primate: the interaction of the vestibulo-ocular reflex, optokinetic nystagmus, and smooth pursuit. *Reviews in Physiology and Biochemical Pharmacology, 106*, 37–125.

Yamauchi, A. M. (2002). *Cupular micromechanis and motion sensation in the toadfish vestibular semicircular canals.* Oral presentation at the University of Utah, Salt Lake City, UT.

Practical Anatomy and Physiology of the Ocular Motor System

Scott D. Z. Eggers

ABBREVIATIONS

aVOR angular vestibulo-ocular reflex	NPH nucleus propositus hypoglossi
CN cranial nerve	NRTP nucleus reticularis tegmenti pontis
DLPC dorsolateral prefrontal cortex	OMN ocular motor neurons
DLPN dorsolateral pontine nuclei	OPN omnipause neurons
EBN excitatory burst neurons	OTR ocular tilt reaction
FEF frontal eye fields	PAN periodic alternating nystagmus
IBN inhibitory burst neurons	PEF parietal eye fields
INC interstitial nucleus of Cajal	PPRF paramedian pontine reticular formation
INO internuclear ophthalmoplegia	riMLF rostral interstitial nucleus of the MLF
LGN lateral geniculate nucleus	SC superior colliculus
LLBN long-lead burst neurons	SCC semicircular canal
MLF medial longitudinal fasciculus	SEF supplementary eye fields
MST medial superior temporal visual cortex	tVOR translational vestibulo-ocular reflex
MVN medial vestibular nucleus	VOR vestibulo-ocular reflex

FUNCTIONAL CLASSES OF EYE MOVEMENTS

The common goal of all eye movements is to facilitate a clear and stable view of the environment (Leigh & Zee, 2006). Lateral-eyed animals like rabbits have a large field of view to survey the environment and avoid predators. But the brain cannot manage the data processing requirements of a visual system with high resolution across the entire visual field. Thus, lateral-eyed animals generally have the trade-off of poor visual acuity. Birds of prey have evolved a visual compromise by restricting their visual field in return for superior visual acuity within that narrow field. Other frontal-eyed animals like humans have developed a small area of very high spatial resolution at the center of the retina (the fovea) while maintaining lower resolution in the periphery. This "foveal compromise" (Wong, 2008) solves the problem of information overload but also requires that the image of an object of interest fall on the fovea for maximal visual acuity.

Mechanisms have evolved to complement this foveal compromise strategy by ensuring that images of interest are brought to and maintained on the foveae of both eyes. Image stability on the retina must be maintained despite object or head motion, because image "slip" across the retina or movement away from the fovea leads to blur or degrades visual acuity. Thus, one category of eye movements helps hold target images steady on the retina. These include (1) active processes of the visual fixation system to hold the image of stationary objects on the fovea when the head is still; (2) the vestibular system to hold target images steady on the retina during brief head movements; and (3) the optokinetic system to hold target images steady on the retina during sustained head rotation. A second category of eye movements has evolved to direct the high-resolution fovea to objects of interest. These include (1) the saccadic system to bring a target image rapidly onto the fovea; (2) the smooth pursuit system to hold the image of a small moving target on the fovea; and (3) the vergence system to move both eyes in opposite directions (i.e., convergence or divergence) in order to simultaneously place the target image onto both foveae regardless of target distance or eccentricity (Table 2–1). To fulfill these visual requirements, the ocular motor system requires complex anatomy and physiology at every level, from the extraocular muscles to cortical ocular motor regions.

Visual Fixation

The fixation system holds the image of a stationary target on the fovea while the head is still. Fixation may be a special type of smooth pursuit (suppressing unwanted drift of the eyes) or due to an independent fixation system. Rather than simply the absence of

Table 2–1. Functional Classes of Human Eye Movements

Class of Eye Movement	Main Function
Movements holding images steady on the retina	
Visual fixation	Holds the image of a stationary object on the fovea when the head is still
Vestibular	Holds images steady on the retina during brief head rotations or translations
Optokinetic	Holds images steady on the retina during sustained head rotation
Movements directing the fovea to an object of interest	
Saccades	Bring images of objects of interest rapidly onto the fovea
Nystagmus quick phases	Reset the eyes during prolonged rotation and direct gaze toward the oncoming visual scene
Smooth pursuit	Hold the image of a small moving target on the fovea; aids optokinetic responses to stabilize gaze during sustained head rotation
Vergence	Move both eyes in opposite directions so that images of a single object are simultaneously placed on the fovea of each eye

visible eye movements, visual fixation actually consists of constant miniature movements not detectable to the naked eye, with the illusion of steady fixation. Normal fixation includes (1) microtremor (<0.01 degree, up to 150 Hz); (2) microsaccades (average 0.1 degrees, 120 Hz); and (3) microdrift (<0.3 deg/sec). The role of these movements in visual fixation is unclear, though they may be important for preventing peripheral vision fade of stable objects due to habituation of a persistent stimulus.

Vestibular

The vestibulo-ocular reflex holds images of the seen world steady on the retina by producing compensatory eye movements during brief head rotations or translations. These phylogenetically old reflexes are generated with a much shorter latency than visually mediated eye movements and are critical for maintaining stable vision during natural activities such as walking and running.

Optokinetic

Optokinetic eye movements are those generated by movement of a large visual scene and serve to hold images of the world steady on the retina during sustained head rotation. They supplement the vestibular-induced eye movements that begin to decline during prolonged rotation. Optokinetic eye movements consist of a slow phase in the direction of visual scene motion and a nystagmus quick phase to reset the eye in the opposite direction.

Saccades

Saccades are rapid, brief, conjugate eye movements that shift the line of sight to bring target images onto the fovea. They may be volitional (elective and purposeful), reflexive (generated to novel stimuli occurring unexpectedly in the environment), predictive (in anticipation of or in search of the appearance of a target at a particular location), memory guided (to the location of a previous target), to command (generated on cue), or spontaneous (seemingly random in the absence of any specific task). Saccades are critical for exploring a visual scene and reading, among other things.

Nystagmus Quick Phases

The quick phases of nystagmus generated during vestibular and optokinetic stimulation are a form of saccades. The evolutionary forerunner of volitional saccades, they serve to reset the eyes during prolonged rotation and direct gaze toward the oncoming visual scene.

Smooth Pursuit

Smooth pursuit allows the image of a small, slowly moving target to be held on the fovea while the head is still. Smooth pursuit is primarily voluntary, driven by retinal slip from visual motion and modulated by attention and motivation. The pursuit system is also required to track an object on a complex moving background and to suppress reflexive vestibular and optokinetic responses during combined head and eye tracking.

Vergence

As opposed to versional eye movements, which conjugately move both eyes in the same direction by the same amount, vergence eye movements move the eyes in opposite directions (convergence or divergence) so that images of a single object are placed or held simultaneously on the fovea of each eye. Vergence is provoked by either the retinal blur (loss of image sharpness) or retinal disparity (image separation when images fall on noncorresponding areas of each retina) that occur with changes of target image distance during binocular fixation, such as when shifting gaze from a distant to a very near object.

THE FINAL COMMON PATHWAY FOR EYE MOVEMENTS

Orbital Muscle Gross Anatomy

The extraocular muscles reside within the bony confines of the cone-shaped orbit. At the orbital apex, the four rectus muscles and superior oblique originate from the dense fibrous annulus of Zinn through which the optic nerve passes. The four rectus muscles course anteriorly through orbital fat and terminate as tendinous tissue on the sclera. The superior oblique passes through a ring of connective tissue called the trochlea at the upper nasal portion of the orbital frontal bone to terminate on the lateral posterior portion of the sclera. The inferior oblique originates in the inferior nasal orbital wall, laterally crosses the orbital floor, and inserts on the lateral posterior globe. The globe is suspended and supported in the orbit by a fibrous sac of fascia called Tenon's capsule.

Extraocular Muscle Actions and Innervation

Six extraocular muscles control the movements of each eye: medial rectus, lateral rectus, superior rectus, inferior rectus, superior oblique, and inferior oblique (Figure 2–1). The medial rectus, superior rectus, inferior rectus, and inferior oblique are innervated by the oculomotor nerve (cranial nerve III).

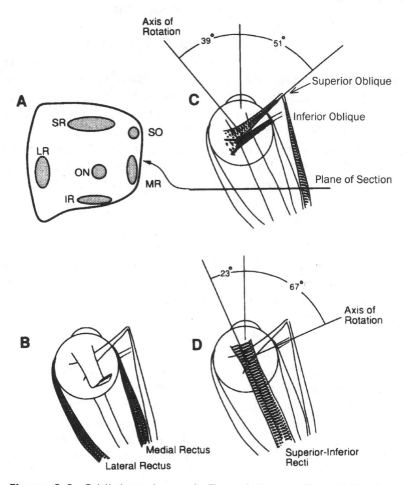

Figure 2-1. Orbital anatomy. **A.** The relative position of the five muscles just behind the eyeball. *SR*, superior rectus; *SO*, superior oblique; *LR*, lateral rectus; *MR*, medial rectus; *IR*, inferior rectus; *ON*, optic nerve. The plane of this section is shown in (C). **B.** Top view with the medial rectus and lateral rectus (*shown in the shaded area*), which are responsible for horizontal eye movements. Only a small segment of the superior rectus is shown in order to show the optic nerve beneath it. **C.** Similar view with the superior oblique, showing the pulling direction and axis of rotation. The axis of rotation and pulling direction are similar for the inferior oblique. **D.** Axis of rotation of the superior rectus (*shaded region*) and the inferior rectus located directly beneath it. The superior and inferior recti mainly move the eye vertically. From *Handbook of Balance Function Testing*, Jacobson et al., 1997. Reprinted with permission of Delmar Learning, a division of Thomson Learning: http://www.thomsonrights.com.

The lateral rectus is innervated by the abducens nerve (cranial nerve VI). The superior oblique is innervated by the trochlear nerve (cranial nerve IV).

Coordinated extraocular muscle action facilitates movement of the eyes in three directional planes (horizontal, vertical, and torsional) about three axes (craniocaudal, interaural, and naso-occipital). Nomenclature for these directions is described in Table 2–2. The actions of each muscle are dependent on the muscle's origin and terminal insertion, the center of rotation of the eye, and the optical axis of the eye. Growing evidence also suggests that connective tissue pulleys in the extraocular muscles contribute to their kinematic properties (Demer, 2006). The muscles of each eye work in agonist/antagonist pairs. In order to facilitate rotation of the eye, increased innervation to the agonist results in an equal amount of decreased innervation to the antagonist (Sherrington's law of reciprocal innervation). Muscle actions may vary depending on the position of the globe in the orbit. Each extraocular muscle has a primary action, and all but the medial and lateral recti also have secondary and tertiary actions. Horizontal eye movements are controlled by the antagonistic medial rectus and lateral rectus muscles. The primary and only action of the medial rectus is adduction, and the primary and only action of the lateral rectus is abduction. Vertical and torsional eye movements are controlled by two antagonist pairs: the superior and inferior recti and the superior and inferior oblique muscles. The contribution of a given muscle to vertical eye movement

Table 2–2. Nomenclature for Eye Movement Direction

Eye Movement Type	Directional Definition
Ductions: Monocular movements of each eye	**Abduction:** horizontal movement about the craniocaudal axis away from the median plane
	Adduction: horizontal movement about the craniocaudal axis toward the median plane
	Elevation: upward rotation about the interaural axis
	Depression: downward rotation about the interaural axis
	Intorsion (incycloduction): rotation about the naso-occipital axis so that the top pole of the eye rotates toward the median plane
	Extorsion (excycloduction): rotation about the naso-occipital axis so that the top pole of the eye rotates away from the median plane
Versions: Conjugate eye movements, rotating both eyes in the same direction by the same amount	**Dextroversion:** both eyes rotating to the right about the craniocaudal axis
	Levoversion: both eyes rotating to the left about the craniocaudal axis
	Elevation: both eyes rotating upward about the interaural axis
	Depression: both eyes rotating downward about the interaural axis
	Dextrocycloversion: both eyes rotating about the naso-occipital axis so that the top pole of the eyes rotates toward the subject's right
	Levocycloversion: both eyes rotating about the naso-occipital axis so that the top pole of the eyes rotates toward the subject's left
Vergence: Disjunctive eye movements, rotating the two eyes in opposite directions	**Convergence:** both eyes rotating horizontally about the craniocaudal axis toward the median plane
	Divergence: both eyes rotating horizontally about the craniocaudal axis away from the median plane
	Incyclovergence: both eyes rotating about the naso-occipital axis so that the top pole of both eyes rotates toward the median plane
	Excyclovergence: both eyes rotating about the naso-occipital axis so that the top pole of both eyes rotates toward the median plane

depends on the horizontal position of the eye. When the eye is in an abducted position, the superior and inferior rectus muscles are the principal elevator and depressor muscles, respectively. When the eye is in an adducted position, inferior oblique action causes elevation, and superior oblique action causes depression. The superior oblique and superior rectus muscles are intorters of the eye, and the inferior oblique and inferior rectus are extorters. The primary, secondary, and tertiary actions of each muscle are shown in Table 2–3.

In addition to each eye's antagonistic pairs with opposite directions of action, the extraocular muscles exist as "yoked" pairs between eyes to generate conjugate eye movements. The three yoked pairs include (1) the medial rectus in one eye and the lateral rectus in the other eye, (2) the superior rectus in one eye and the inferior oblique in the other eye, and (3) the inferior rectus in one eye and the superior oblique in the other eye. "Yoked" muscle pairs receive equal and simultaneous innervation generated from premotor control systems, stimulating the cranial nerve nuclei to elicit the conjugate eye movement (Hering's law of equal innervation).

Ocular Motor Nuclei and Nerves

Abducens Nerve (Cranial Nerve VI)

Paired abducens nuclei are located in the dorsomedial pons at the floor of the fourth ventricle, in close proximity to the fascicle of the facial nerve (Figure 2–2). Each nucleus contains abducens motor neurons that form the abducens nerve and interneurons that decussate at the level of the nucleus and ascend in the contralateral medial longitudinal fasciculus (MLF) to the oculomotor medial rectus subnucleus to facilitate conjugate horizontal gaze in the direction ipsilateral to the abducens nucleus of origin. The abducens fascicles arise from the ventral surface of the nucleus, traverse the brainstem, emerge from the ventral pontomedullary sulcus, and travel as the abducens nerve in the subarachnoid space where it ascends along the clivus. It pierces the dura, travels through the cavernous sinus lateral to the internal carotid artery, and enters the superior orbital fissure to innervate the ipsilateral lateral rectus muscle.

Clinical Correlation: Abducens Nucleus and Nerve Palsies

A lesion of the peripheral abducens nerve or its fascicles within the lower pons will both produce an isolated ipsilateral lateral rectus muscle weakness. The two may often be distinguished by the presence of additional central neurological signs in a pontine lesion, such as contralateral arm and leg weakness from involvement of the corticospinal tract. In either case, the lateral rectus is weak for all classes of eye movements (saccades, pursuit, vestibular), and thus ipsilateral eye movements will be slow, of limited range, or absent. However, if the abducens nucleus is intact, interneurons innervating the contralateral medial rectus subnucleus of III will still produce adduction upon attempted lateral gaze. If, on the other hand, the lesion affects the abducens nucleus (including the abducens motor neurons and interneurons), the result is a complete ipsilesional horizontal gaze paralysis of all eye movement classes, often producing a contralateral gaze deviation. In this case, the eyes cannot be brought past the midline even by the vestibulo-ocular reflex.

Table 2–3. Extraocular Muscle Actions With the Eye in Central Position

Muscle	Primary Action	Secondary Action	Tertiary Action
Medial rectus	Adduction		
Lateral rectus	Abduction		
Superior rectus	Elevation	Intorsion	Adduction
Inferior rectus	Depression	Extorsion	Adduction
Superior oblique	Intorsion	Depression	Abduction
Inferior oblique	Extorsion	Elevation	Abduction

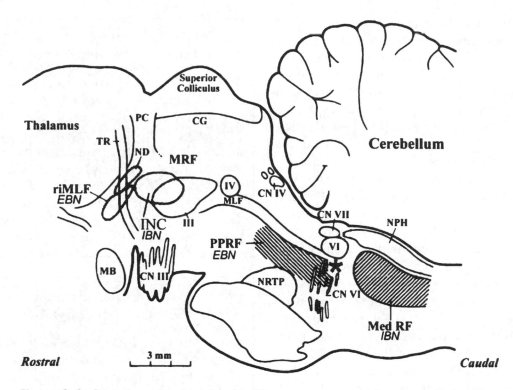

Figure 2-2. Brainstem structures involved in eye movements. A parasagittal section of the monkey brainstem shows the location of key structures responsible for saccadic eye movements. Excitatory burst neurons (*EBN*) for horizontal saccades lie in the parmedian pontine reticular formation (*PPRF*). Inhibitory burst neurons (*IBN*) for horizontal saccades lie in the medullary reticular formation (*MedRF*). EBN for vertical and torsional saccades lie in the rostral interstitial nucleus of the medial longitudinal fasciculus (*riMLF*). Some vertical *IBN* may reside in or close to the interstitial nucleus of Cajal (*INC*). *EBN* and *IBN* project to ocular motor neurons lying in the abducens nucleus (VI), trochlear nucleus (IV), and oculomotor nucleus (III). Omnipause neurons (*OPN*, indicated by an asterisk) lie in the nucleus raphe interpositus in the midline of the pons between the rootlets of the abducens nerve (CN VI) and influence the activity of *EBN* and *IBN*. The mesencephalic reticular formation (*MRF*) may help keep the *OPN* inhibited until a saccade is complete and the eye is on target. *CG*: central grey; *MB*: mammillary body; CN III: rootlets of the oculomotor nerve; CN IV: trochlear nerve; CN VII: genu of facial nerve; *ND*: nucleus of Darkschewitsch; *NRTP*: nucleus reticularis tegmenti pontis; *NPH*: nucleus prepositus hypoglossi: *PC*: posterior commissure; *TR*: tractus retroflexus. Reproduced from Ramat et al (2007) with permission from Dr. Jean Büttner-Ennever and Oxford University Press.

Trochlear Nerve (Cranial Nerve IV)

Paired trochlear nuclei lie very close to the dorsomedial surface of the midbrain just below the inferior colliculus. The fascicles emerge from the nuclei and briefly course dorsally before exiting the dorsal midbrain. The trochlear nerves are the only cranial nerves to emerge from the dorsal brainstem surface. After emerging, the nerves decussate within the anterior medullary velum and wrap around the surface of the midbrain to travel ventrally within the subarachnoid space toward the cavernous sinus. In the cavernous sinus, the trochlear nerve is located in the lateral dural wall, inferior to the oculomotor nerve. From the cavernous sinus, the nerve passes into the superior orbital fissure and ultimately innervates the superior oblique muscle contralateral to the nucleus of origin.

Oculomotor Nerve (Cranial Nerve III)

Paired oculomotor nuclei are located in the dorsal midbrain ventral to the periaqueductal gray matter at the level of the superior colliculus. Each nuclear complex includes individual subnuclei innervating the ipsilateral inferior rectus, medial rectus, and inferior oblique; a superior rectus subnucleus that innervates the contralateral superior rectus muscle; and an Edinger-Westphal nucleus supplying preganglionic parasympathetic output to the iris sphincter and ciliary muscles. A single midline caudal central subnucleus provides innervation to both levator palpebrae superioris muscles.

Third-nerve fascicles originate from the ventral surface of each nucleus and traverse the midbrain, passing through the red nucleus and in close proximity to the cerebral peduncles before emerging as ventral rootlets in the interpeduncular fossa. The rootlets converge into a third-nerve trunk that continues ventrally through the subarachnoid space toward the cavernous sinus, passing between the superior cerebellar artery and the posterior cerebral artery. In the cavernous sinus, the third nerve is located in the dural sinus wall, just lateral to the pituitary gland. From the cavernous sinus, the third nerve enters the superior orbital fissure. Just prior to entry, the nerve anatomically divides into superior and inferior divisions. The superior division innervates the superior rectus and the levator palpebrae superioris, and the inferior division innervates the inferior and medial recti, the inferior oblique, and the iris sphincter and ciliary muscles. Prior to innervating the ciliary and sphincter muscles, parasympathetic third-nerve fibers synapse in the ciliary ganglion within the orbit.

Internuclear Connections

The medial longitudinal fasciculus (MLF) is a paramedian pathway that lies in the dorsal brainstem and carries ocular motor and vestibular signals between the medulla and midbrain. As noted above, the MLF carries signals from the abducens nucleus to the contralateral medial rectus portion of the oculomotor nucleus. These signals allow conjugate horizontal eye movements with synchronous contraction of the ipsilateral lateral rectus and contralateral medial rectus muscles (Figure 2–3). The MLF also carries signals for vertical gaze from the vestibular nuclei in the medulla to the midbrain vertical gaze control centers important for vertical smooth pursuit and vestibular eye movements.

**Clinical Correlation:
Internuclear Ophthalmoplegia**

Unilateral inactivation of the MLF results in ipsilaterally slowed or absent adduction with abducting nystagmus in the contralateral eye during attempted contralateral gaze (internuclear ophthalmoplegia, INO), in combination with a skew deviation with ipsilateral hypertropia. Bilateral MLF inactivation results in bilateral impairment of adduction with bilateral dissociated abducting nystagmus (bilateral INO), impaired vertical smooth pursuit, and reduced vertical VOR gain.

**Clinical Correlation:
One-and-a-Half Syndrome**

Occasionally a lesion affects the abducens nucleus on one side and the ipsilateral MLF containing interneurons from the contralateral abducens nucleus that have already crossed and are destined for the ipsilateral oculomotor nucleus. The result is a complete conjugate horizontal gaze paralysis toward the side of the lesion as described earlier, plus an INO for gaze in the opposite direction. Thus, the patient loses all conjugate gaze ipsilesionally (the "one") and can only abduct the contralateral eye with attempted contralateral gaze (the "half").

CENTRAL VESTIBULAR STRUCTURES AND PATHWAYS

The basic three-neuron arc of the vestibulo-ocular reflex (VOR) consists of the vestibular ganglion and nerve, vestibular nuclei, and ocular motor nuclei (Figure 2–4). The VOR serves to maintain stable gaze direction by compensating for head movement. The drive for the VOR is vestibular rather than visual and thus can operate at a much shorter latency than could occur if visual information had to reach the visual cortex and then be relayed to the brainstem. However, the cerebellum has important connections that fine tune the VOR to changing visual requirements.

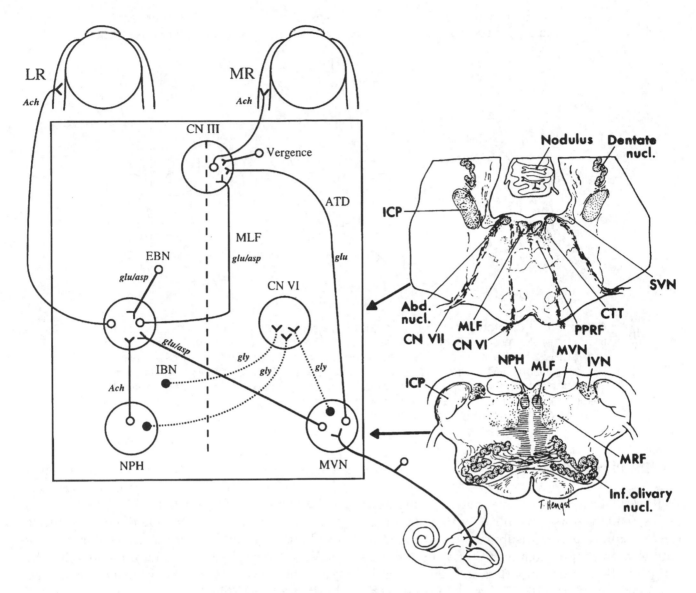

Figure 2-3. Anatomic scheme for the synthesis of signals for horizontal eye movements. The abducens nucleus (CN VI) contains abducens motor neurons that innervate the ipsilateral lateral rectus muscle (*LR*) and abducens internuclear neurons that send an ascending projection up the contralateral medial longitudinal fasciculus (*MLF*) to reach the medial rectus (*MR*) motor neurons in the contralateral oculomotor nucleus (CN III). From the horizontal semicircular canal, primary vestibular nerve afferents project mainly to the medial vestibular nucleus (*MVN*), where they synapse and then send an excitatory connection to the contralateral abducens nucleus and an inhibitory projection to the ipsilateral abducens nucleus. Saccadic inputs reach the abducens nucleus from the ipsilateral excitatory burst neurons (*EBN*) and contralateral inhibitory burst neurons (*IBN*). The neural integrator within the nucleus prepositus hypoglossi (*NPH*) and adjacent *MVN* send eye position information to the abducens nucleus. The medial rectus motor neurons in CN III also receive commands for vergence eye movements. Putative neurotransmitters for each pathway are shown: *Ach*: acetylcholine; *asp*: aspartate; *glu*: glutamate; *gly*: glycine. The anatomic sections on the right correspond to the level of the arrow heads on the schematic on the left. *Abd. nucl.*: abducens nucleus; CN VI: abducens nerve; CN VII: facial nerve; *CTT*: central tegmental tract; *ICP*: inferior cerebellar peduncle; *IVN*: inferior vestibular nucleus; *Inf. olivary nucl.*: inferior olivary nucleus; *MRF*: medullary reticular formation; *SVN*: superior vestibular nucleus. Reproduced from Leigh and Zee (2006) with permission from Oxford University Press.

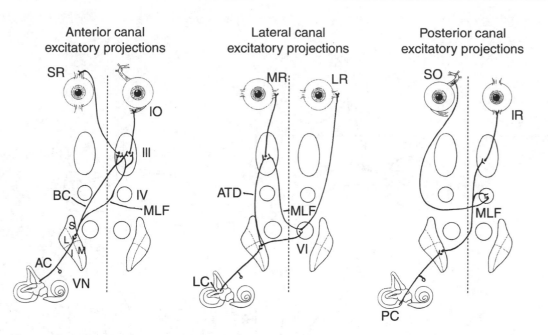

Figure 2–4. Excitatory projections from individual semicircular canals on the right side to the extraocular muscles. *SO*: superior oblique; *IO*: inferior oblique; *IR*: inferior rectus; *LR*: lateral rectus; *SR*: superior rectus; *MR*: medial rectus; *AC*: anterior canal; *PC:* posterior canal; *LC*: lateral canal; *MLF*: medial longitudinal fasciculus; *ATD*: ascending tract of Deiters; *BC*: brachium conjunctivum; *VN*: vestibular nuclei (*S* = superior; *I* = inferior; *L* = lateral; *M* = medial); III: oculomotor nucleus; IV: trochlear nucleus; VI: abducens nucleus. Reproduced from Fife (2010) with permission from Elsevier.

Vestibular Nuclei

Four nuclei form the vestibular nuclear complex on each side in the dorsal medulla: The rostral portions (medial and superior vestibular nuclei) predominantly receive input from the SCCs, with their central projections most important for generating the rotational (angular) VOR. The caudal portions (lateral and inferior nuclei) mainly receive projections from the otolith organs, affecting the linear (translational) VOR, vertical ocular alignment, and vestibulospinal reflexes.

Cerebellum

The cerebellum receives input from the vestibular nuclei as well as directly from vestibular nerve afferents that bypass the vestibular nuclei. These inputs travel in the juxtarestiform body of the inferior cerebellar peduncle to the ipsilateral vestibulocerebellum (flocculonodular lobe, consisting of the flocculus, adjacent paraflocculus, nodulus, and

ventral uvula). Additionally, the cerebellum receives visual and ocular motor signals from regions such as the pontine nuclei, nucleus reticularis tegmenti pontis, paramedian tract, and inferior olivary nuclei. Thus, although not part of the three-neuron arc of the VOR, the cerebellum is critical for adapting the gain (ratio of eye movement to head movement) and direction of the VOR to new visual requirements, as occurs in disease states like unilateral vestibular loss or even when changing spectacle prescriptions (Versino, Hurko, & Zee, 1996; Walker & Zee, 1999).

Central Organization of the Vestibulo-Ocular Reflex

The function of the VOR is to generate compensatory conjugate eye movements in the opposite direction of brief head movement and thereby maintain a stable angle of gaze and clear vision. The VOR can be subdivided into canal-ocular reflexes, with input from the semicircular canals driving the angular VOR (aVOR), and otolith-ocular reflexes driving the translational VOR (tVOR). An additional otolith-mediated VOR, ocular counterrolling, occurs in response to change in the static orientation of the head with respect to gravity in the roll (frontal) plane; a small change in the static torsion (counterrolling) of the eyes occurs in the opposite direction with sustained head tilt.

Canal-Ocular Reflexes

Stimulation or inhibition of a single SCC leads to slow-phase eye movements that rotate the eye in a plane parallel to the canal. Thus, the affected canal can be inferred from the pattern of nystagmus, such as the mixed vertical-torsional nystagmus of benign paroxysmal positioning vertigo occurring from inappropriate stimulation of the posterior SCC. Central mechanisms are used to suppress the effect of persistent vestibular imbalance and thereby compensate for vestibular lesions. The brisk nystagmus seen in acute peripheral vestibular lesions will gradually decrease in intensity as the central vestibular system compensates for the imbalance. In addition, visual fixation may significantly suppress the spontaneous nystagmus of an acute vestibular lesion, necessitating the use of examination techniques that eliminate fixation.

To generate the aVOR, the vestibular nuclei send excitatory and inhibitory signals to specific ocular motor nuclei in order to activate yoked pairs of extraocular muscles (and inhibit their antagonists) (Fife, 2010). This reflex leads to activation of specific muscles that move the eyes in the same plane but in the opposite direction as the semicircular canal being stimulated, regardless of the initial position of the eye in the orbit. The horizontal aVOR is the simplest and most commonly tested. Activation of the lateral semicircular canal by ipsilateral head rotation leads to vestibular nerve excitation synapsing on the vestibular nuclei. From there, second-order excitatory projections course rostromedially and then cross the midline to synapse on the contralateral abducens nucleus. As with generation of other conjugate eye movements, abducens motor neurons and interneurons are activated within the abducens nucleus, leading to activation of the ipsilateral lateral rectus (contralateral to the vestibular stimulus) and via the MLF to the oculomotor nucleus, activation of the opposite medial rectus (ipsilateral to the

vestibular stimulus). Some neurons also connect directly from the vestibular nuclei to the ipsilateral medial rectus subnucleus in the ascending tract of Deiters, but its functional significance is uncertain. For each extraocular muscle activated, its antagonist must be inhibited to permit rotation of the eye in the orbit. Thus, for each excitatory pathway, the vestibular nuclei send inhibitory projections to antagonist muscles (for the horizontal aVOR this is the ipsilateral lateral rectus and contralateral medial rectus). In addition, during head rotation, the semicircular canal being inhibited (such as the right horizontal canal during leftward head rotation) reduces its tonic firing rate, thereby facilitating relaxation of the antagonist muscles. The eye movements elicited by vestibular stimulation constitute the vestibular slow phase eye movements. However, sustained vestibular stimulation in an awake person leads to nystagmus quick phases opposite the slow phase direction (toward the side of vestibular stimulation). The nystagmus direction is named based on quick phase direction.

The vertical semicircular canal projections are more complicated but follow the same principles. Each anterior (superior) SCC sits in the same plane as the contralateral posterior SCC. Thus, in natural states of movement, one canal is activated while its contralateral functional pair is inhibited. The anterior semicircular canal is oriented along the same axis of rotation as that produced by activation of the ipsilateral vertical recti and contralateral obliques. Stimulation of the anterior canal leads to excitation of the ipsilateral superior rectus and contralateral inferior oblique via brainstem connections between the vestibular nuclei and the two oculomotor subnuclei. Activation of the posterior canal produces excitation of the contralateral inferior rectus and ipsilateral superior oblique. Thus, with the eyes in the straight ahead position, stimulation of an individual vertical SCC will produce a combination of vertical and torsional eye movement based on the actions of the muscles activated. For example, excitation of the right posterior SCC produces vestibular slow phases that are downward and with torsion where the top poles of the eyes roll toward the subject's left (extorsion of the left eye and intorsion of the right eye), with nystagmus quick phases that are upward and with oppositely directed torsion. Because of the fact that the trochlear nucleus and superior rectus subnucleus of III innervate contralateral muscles, vertical excitatory projections from the vestibular nuclei to ocular motor nuclei cross the midline, but vertical inhibitory connections do not.

During dynamic head roll in the frontal plane (tilting the head alternately to the right and left shoulder), the dynamic torsional VOR generates compensatory slow-phase torsional eye movements in the opposite direction predominantly by the vertical semicircular canals. Rolling to the right stimulates the right anterior and posterior canals while inhibiting the left anterior and posterior canals. Provided that brainstem saccade networks are intact, torsional nystagmus quick phases occur opposite the slow phases. The gain of the dynamic torsional VOR is between 0.4 and 0.7, lower than that of the horizontal or vertical VOR.

Otolith-Ocular Reflexes

The otolith-ocular reflexes refer to compensatory eye movements evoked by stimulation of the utricle or saccule. The two types include (1) the translational VOR (tVOR) in response to linear head acceleration, and (2) ocular counterrolling (or static torsional VOR) in response to static head tilt in the roll plane.

The central otolith projections for the tVOR are less studied than for the aVOR but must take into account target distance and eccentricity. It appears that the horizontal tVOR may arise from stimulation of the lateral portion of the utricle during ipsilateral linear head translation, with polysynaptic connections to the lateral vestibular nuclei then projecting (possibly via the cerebellum) contralaterally to the abducens nucleus and driving oppositely directed conjugate slow phase eye movements.

Projections from the medial portion of the utricle may be more important for signaling head tilt and generating compensatory counterrolling using vertical torsional eye muscles. The medial portion of the utricle would be excited by sustained ipsilateral head tilt, synapsing on the lateral vestibular nucleus, with connections via the MLF to the midbrain ocular motor nuclei, producing counterrolling of the eyes in the opposite direction via excitation of the ipsilateral superior oblique and superior rectus and contralateral inferior oblique and inferior rectus.

The brain is evidently able to use contextual cues to resolve the ambiguity of whether the head is being linearly translated or tilted relative to gravity despite the fact that the shear forces on the utricular macula would be the same for each. This may be based upon the frequency of linear acceleration input, with low-frequency input interpreted as tilt and high-frequency input as translation. The brainstem velocity storage mechanism may also contribute by computing an internal estimate of gravity by integrating angular head velocity signals from the SCCs.

Clinical Correlation: Ocular Tilt Reaction

A lesion anywhere along the otolith ocular pathway between the utricle and vertical/torsional ocular motor nuclei in the midbrain (including in the MLF) can lead to the ocular tilt reaction (OTR) (Brodsky, Donahue, Vaphiades, & Brandt, 2006). For example, a lesion of the left utricle or its peripheral or central connections disrupts the normally symmetric utricular input and leads to a shift in the patient's internal estimate of absolute vertical (gravity) in the roll plane to the left. Thus, the brain erroneously registers that the head is tilted to the right with respect to gravity. This results in an OTR to the left with the pathologic triad of (1) head tilt to the left to realign the head's vertical axis with the perceived but incorrect vertical gravitational axis, (2) torsional ocular counterrolling of the top pole of the eyes to the left to realign the eyes' vertical meridian with the perceived but incorrect vertical gravitational axis, and (3) skew deviation (the left eye depresses and right eye elevates) to realign the eyes' horizontal meridian with the perceived but incorrect internal estimate of the earth-horizontal (Figure 2–5). Because central utricular pathways cross at the pontomedullary junction to enter the MLF, a lesion of the utricular nerve or medulla will cause an ipsilesional OTR, while a lesion in the pons or midbrain after the projections have crossed will cause a contralesional OTR.

Velocity Storage Mechanism

The velocity storage mechanism is a central phenomenon by which the raw rotational vestibular signal

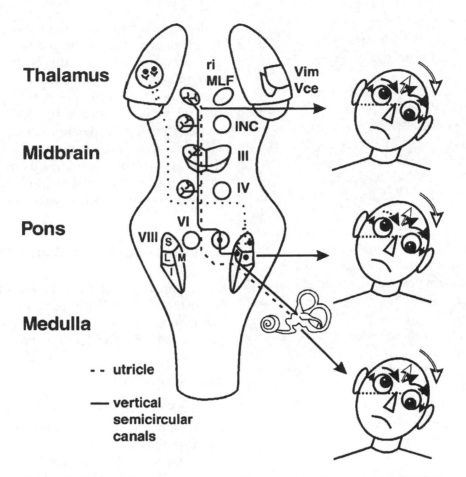

Figure 2–5. Graviceptive pathways from the otoliths and vertical semicircular canals mediating the vestibular reactions in the roll plane. The projections from the otoliths and the vertical semicircular canals to the ocular motor nuclei (trochlear nucleus IV, oculomotor nucleus III, abducens nucleus VI), and the supranuclear centers of the interstitial nucleus of Cajal (*INC*) and the rostral interstitial nucleus of the medial longitudinal fasciculus (*riMLF*), are shown. They subserve the vestibulo-ocular reflex (*VOR*) in three planes. The *VOR* is part of a more complex vestibular reaction that also involves vestibulospinal connections via the medial and lateral vestibulospinal tracts for head and body posture control. Ocular tilt reaction is depicted on the right in relation to the level of the lesion (i.e., ipsiversive with peripheral and pontomedullary lesions and contraversive with pontomesencephalic lesions). Reproduced from Brodsky et al. (2006) with permission from Elsevier.

from the cristae ampullaris is prolonged or perseverated in order to improve the ability of the aVOR to transduce the low-frequency components of sustained head rotation. The result is that the time constant (the time for an exponential function to decay to 37% of its initial value) of the aVOR is improved from 6 to 7 s (based on the physical properties of the cupula) to about 15 to 20 s (based on the nystagmus response to sustained rotation). Optokinetic afternystagmus is attributed to the vestibular velocity storage mechanism. The velocity storage mechanism may also be important for helping distinguishing tilt from translation. The vestibular commissure connects the two vestibular nuclear complexes and appears to be important for velocity storage, as if it is sectioned, velocity storage is abolished.

Clinical Correlation: Periodic Alternating Nystagmus

Acquired periodic alternating nystagmus (PAN) is a spontaneous horizontal jerk nystagmus present in straight-ahead gaze that reverses directions about every 2 min. It reflects instability of the velocity storage mechanism (Furman, Wall, & Pang, 1990; Leigh, Robinson, & Zee, 1981). Normally, GABAergic inhibitory inputs from the cerebellar nodulus and ventral uvula help control vestibular rotational responses. In the setting of a nodulus or ventral uvula lesion, the velocity-storage mechanism becomes unstable, and short-term vestibular adaptation leads to sustained horizontal nystagmus that reverses directions every 2 min as PAN. Although in pure form PAN is only present in darkness, it may be present during attempted visual fixation if the adjacent flocculus and paraflocculus are also involved (because of the floccular role in VOR suppression).

CONTROL OF SACCADIC EYE MOVEMENTS

In order to properly execute a saccadic eye movement to bring an image detected in the visual periphery to the fovea (for the purpose of visual search, reading, or to view a specific target), the brain must simultaneously carry out several complex tasks. The location of a visual stimulus is represented on the surface of the visual cortex, with different parts of this two-dimensional cortical map corresponding to different locations on the retina. However, the final effectors of the ocular motor system, the ocular motor neurons (OMN), encode the characteristics for saccades in terms of their temporal discharge, with the size of a saccade proportional to the total number of discharge spikes. Furthermore, the OMN cause the extraocular muscles to move the eyes with respect to the head, not to the environment. Thus, the brain must transform the visual stimulus that is two-dimensionally "place-coded" in terms of the location of active neurons in the visual cortex, into a saccadic command to the OMN that is "temporally

coded" in terms of discharge frequency and duration, further taking into account the three-axis nature of eye rotation. Once the trajectory for the saccade is determined, this vector must be separated into horizontal and vertical components to stimulate specific premotor burst neurons for oblique saccades. To ensure accuracy, the desired size of the saccade must take into account overcoming the elastic inertia of the extraocular orbital tissues, as well as whether the gaze change will consist of combined head and eye movements or eye movements alone (Sparks, 2002).

Brainstem Control of Saccades

Two main types of neurons are important in the brainstem network for generating the premotor commands for saccades, burst neurons and omnipause neurons (Scudder, Kaneko, & Fuchs, 2002).

Excitatory Burst Neurons

Brainstem excitatory burst neurons (EBN, sometimes referred to as short- or medium-lead or premotor burst neurons) carry the immediate supranuclear premotor saccadic command and project monosynaptically to OMN. They begin firing 8 to 12 ms before a saccade and fire throughout the duration of the saccade. They are silent during fixation and slow eye movements. The discharge characteristics of EBN are tightly correlated with saccade properties when the head is in a fixed position during the saccade. For example, the number of spikes in the burst discharge is correlated to the size of the saccade, the duration of the burst discharge is correlated with the duration of the saccade, and the peak frequency of the burst discharge is correlated with the peak velocity of the saccade. These relationships between neuronal discharge and saccade properties may be uncoupled when the head is not fixed during the saccade because small head movements also contribute to gaze changes and stabilization.

Excitatory burst neurons for horizontal saccades are located in the paramedian pontine reticular formation (PPRF) in the pons just rostral to the abducens nucleus. EBN for vertical and torsional saccades lie in the rostral interstitial nucleus of the medial longitudinal fasciculus (riMLF) rostral to the oculomotor nucleus and ventral to the periaqueductal gray in the mesencephalic reticular formation (Bhidayasiri, Plant, & Leigh, 2000). For horizontal saccades, premotor burst signals project to the ipsilateral abducens nucleus, contacting both abducens motor neurons and internuclear neurons, to generate a conjugate ipsilateral saccade (Figure 2–6). For vertical saccades, EBN for upward and downward saccades are intermingled in the riMLF. Upward EBN project bilaterally to elevator OMN, while downward EBN project only ipsilaterally to depressor OMN. EBN discharge most vigorously for saccades that rotate the eyes in a plane parallel to that of a pair of reciprocally acting vertical semicircular canals, which creates a torsional component. For example, EBN in the right riMLF discharge to extort the right eye and intort the left eye. Therefore, ipsilateral riMLF lesions abolish ipsilesional torsional quick phases of nystagmus and impair downward more than upward saccades.

Clinical Correlation: Supranuclear Saccadic Palsies

Disorders affecting excitatory burst neurons will impair saccades (rendering them slow or absent) but may leave smooth pursuit and the vestibulo-ocular reflex intact. Progressive conditions like spinocerebellar ataxia type 2 may gradually affect saccades, whereas acute saccadic palsy may occur with an infarction or demyelinating plaque in the EBN, such as the PPRF. Conditions may preferentially affect the pontine horizontal or midbrain vertical EBN. Progressive supranuclear palsy affects the riMLF early in its course, leading to slowing of vertical saccades. Pontine gliomas may affect the PPRF and lead to loss of horizontal saccades and quick phases, with preserved horizontal vestibular and vertical saccadic eye movements. Rarely after cardiopulmonary bypass, patients can awaken with permanent loss of all saccades and quick phases in all directions, with other functional classes of eye movements preserved, apparently from a lesion of the brainstem saccadic generating system (Baloh, Furman, & Yee, 1985; Bhidayasiri et al., 2001; Eggers, Moster, & Cranmer, 2008).

Inhibitory Burst Neurons

In addition to the EBN described above, inhibitory burst neurons (IBN) are another type of premotor burst neuron that project monosynaptically to in-hibit antagonist OMN and their extraocular muscles during a saccade. The IBN are located caudal to the abducens nucleus in the medullary reticular formation for horizontal eye movements and are intermingled with neurons in the interstitial nucleus of Cajal (INC) for vertical eye movements. For horizontal eye movements, IBN project to the contralateral abducens nucleus to inhibit it during ipsilateral saccades, in addition to inhibiting the contralateral EBN and IBN. IBN receive excitatory input from the contralateral superior colliculus and inhibitory inputs from omnipause neurons and contralateral IBN.

Omnipause Neurons

In order to maintain stable fixation, EBN require constant inhibition except when a saccade is called for. This inhibition is mediated by tonically discharging glycinergic omnipause neurons (OPN) located in the nucleus raphe interpositus, medial to the abducens nerve fascicles. OPN firing ceases just prior to saccades in any direction and resumes immediately at saccade end. Microstimulation of OPN in the middle of a saccade will stall the saccade midflight. The mechanism by which omnipause neurons are inhibited to allow a saccade to occur appears complicated. The initial inactivation of the OPN may result from activity in trigger-latch long-lead burst neurons (LLBN) in the rostral pons and midbrain, from the "fixation zone" of the superior colliculus, and from the frontal eye fields, supplementary eye fields, and fastigial nucleus of the cerebellum.

Long-Lead Burst Neurons

Long-lead burst neurons (LLBN) exhibit activity 40 to 100 ms prior to saccade onset. They are located throughout the midbrain and pontine reticular formations and likely consist of several types: relay LLBN, trigger-latch LLBN, and precerebellar LLBN. Relay LLBN may form a connection between the superior colliculus and excitatory burst neurons, synchronizing the onset and end of saccades. The

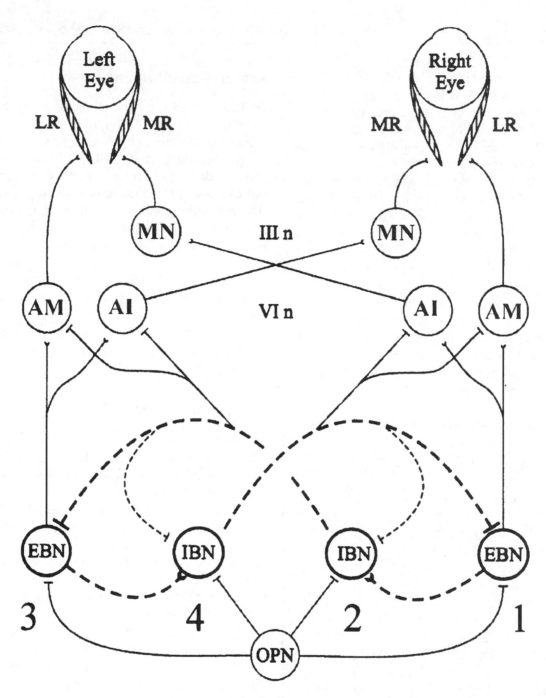

Figure 2-6. A brainstem neural network model for generating horizontal saccades. Projections with flat ending are inhibitory; the others are excitatory. Saccades require reciprocal innervation to the medial rectus (*MR*) and lateral rectus (*LR*) of both eyes. The *LR* is driven by the ipsilateral abducens nucleus (VI n) motoneurons (*AM*). The VI n also contains abducens internuclear neurons (*AI*) that send axons to the contralateral oculomotor nucleus (III n), which drive the *MR* of the other eye. Excitatory burst neurons (*EBN*) provide the saccadic drive to ipsilateral *AM* and *AI*. *EBN* also project to inhibitory burst neurons (*IBN*). *IBN* provide inhibition to the contralateral *AM* and *AI*. Thus, an *EBN/IBN* pair provides reciprocal innervation. *IBN* also provide inhibition to the contralateral *EBN* and *IBN*. A consequence of this cross-coupling is that the *EBN/IBN* pairs form a short-latency, positive feedback loop. When omnipause neurons (*OPN*) are active, they prevent this loop from oscillating. At the beginning of a saccade, *OPN* cease discharge, allowing one set of *EBN* (1) to start firing and activate ipsilateral *IBN* (2). During *IBN* (2) firing, contralateral *EBN* (3) receive a hyperpolarizing input that keeps them silent. At the end of the saccade, when the *IBN* (2) cease firing, the *EBN* (3) start to discharge because of rebound depolarization, which stimulates ipsilateral *IBN* (4), which in turn, inhibit original *EBN* (1) that fired. Thus, the *EBN/ IBN* pairs tend to spontaneously oscillate whenever the *OPN* are inhibited and there is no specified saccadic command. Reproduced from Leigh and Zee (2006) with permission from Oxford University Press.

role of trigger-latch LLBN is unclear, but they may function to inhibit omnipause neurons and to hold omnipause neurons off for the duration of the saccade. Precerebellar LLBN receive input from the superior colliculus and project to the nucleus reticularis tegmenti pontis (NRTP) which, in turn, projects primarily to the cerebellar saccadic areas (the oculomotor vermis and the fastigial oculomotor region) via the middle cerebellar peduncle.

Clinical Correlation: Opsoclonus and Ocular Flutter

A striking eye movement disorder occurs in which patients make involuntary bursts of high-frequency conjugate oscillations of the eyes, each consisting of a series of back-to-back saccades that lack an intersaccadic interval. When confined to the horizontal plane it is termed *ocular flutter*, and when it also includes vertical and torsional movements it is termed *opsoclonus* (Wong, 2007). Patients complain of oscillopsia and vertigo. Ataxia is a commonly accompanying feature. Diseases causing this include brainstem encephalitis and paraneoplastic syndromes (neuroblastoma in infants, breast or small cell lung cancer in adults). The pathophysiological basis for opsoclonus and flutter remains unclear. Since saccadic in origin, initially it was thought that dysfunction of the OPN was responsible, but neuropathological evidence for this is lacking. Abnormal feedback through a cerebellar loop also seems increasingly unlikely. A hypothesis based on brainstem models suggests the membrane properties of IBN may control the frequency and amplitude of these saccadic oscillations (Ramat, Leigh, Zee, & Optican, 2007).

Superior Colliculus

The superior colliculus (SC) is a multilayered structure that lies in the midbrain tectum as the upper portion of the quadrigeminal plate. It is the primary source of commands to the brainstem immediate premotor structures for generating saccadic eye movements. It receives signals from many cortical and subcortical areas and sends output, at least indirectly, to all of the premotor areas involved with controlling eye and head movements, including EBN, OMN, LLBN, and the vestibular nuclei. Inputs descend to the SC from frontal and parietal eye fields (directly and through the basal ganglia), as well as from visual cortex containing retinotopically coded information regarding target location. The SC contains a "motor map" where information about saccade direction and amplitude is represented as a "place code." The location of a SC neuron, not its discharge characteristics, determines the direction and amplitude of the saccade for which it encodes. This map is two dimensional, and downstream modifications (possibly in the NRTP) must convert collicular commands to three-dimensional displacement vectors for eye and head movements.

The rostral pole of this motor map seems important for maintaining steady fixation (suppressing saccades), and this "fixation zone" sends tonic excitatory projections directly to OPN. The more caudal portions are important for target selection (size and direction of movement) and initiation of eye and eye-head gaze shifts. Deeper layers of the caudal SC are important for coordinated movements of the head and eyes, including projections as the tectospinal tract. Discrete lesions of the SC are rare but may cause increased latency and slowing of saccades, although redundant pathways from the frontal eye fields prevent loss of saccade generation altogether.

Cortical Control of Saccades

Lesional and stimulation experiments in animals as well as functional neuroimaging studies in humans show that widespread areas of the frontal and parietal cortex are important for saccadic control. These cortical structures are integral for attention, motivation, target selection, and programming of eye movements. Rather than a top-down arrangement, these regions probably form a vast network with many reciprocal connections (Figure 2–7). The frontal regions include the frontal eye fields (FEFs), supplementary eye fields (SEFs), dorsolateral prefrontal cortex (DLPC), and cingulate cortex. The primary parietal region is the parietal eye fields (PEFs) within the posterior parietal cortex (Pierrot-Deseilligny, Milea, & Muri, 2004).

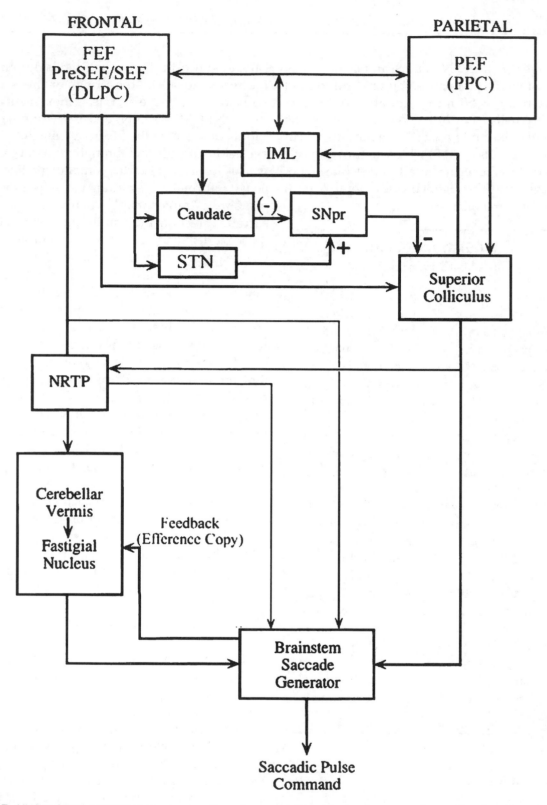

Figure 2–7. Higher-level control of the saccadic pulse generator. Shown here are the major structures that project to the brainstem saccade generator (premotor burst neurons in *PPRF* and *riMLF*). Also shown are projections from cortical eye fields to superior colliculus. *DLPC*, dorsolateral prefrontal cortex; *FEF*, frontal eye fields; *IML*, intramedullary lamina of thalamus; *NRTP*, nucleus reticularis tegmenti pontis; *PEF*, parietal eye field; *PPC*, posterior parietal cortex; *SEF*, supplementary eye field; *SNpr*, substantia nigra pars reticulata; *STN*, subthalamic nucleus. –, inhibition; +, excitation. Reproduced from Leigh and Zee (2006) with permission from Oxford University Press.

The FEF dispatch contralateral voluntary and visually guided saccades to targets. They project to the ipsilateral SC both directly and indirectly through the basal ganglia (caudate and substantia nigra pars reticulata). FEF also project directly to the contralateral NRTP and omnipause neurons of the pontine tegmentum. The SEF lie anterior to the supplementary motor cortex. They are important for programming saccades as part of a learned or complex behavior. DLPC facilitates memory-guided saccades, antisaccades, and advanced planning of environmental scanning using memory of target location. PEF receives input from secondary visual areas and the thalamic pulvinar nucleus. Projections go to the FEF and to the SC directly. The PEF are important for directing visual attention in extrapersonal space and initiating visually guided reflexive saccades. Inhibitory projections from the basal ganglia to SC inhibit extraneous reflexive saccades during attempted fixation and facilitate volitional saccades in the context of remembered and learned behavior.

Clinical Correlation: Cortical Saccadic Abnormalities

Frontal lobe lesions produce various saccade abnormalities based on the location of the lesion. Unilateral FEF lesions increase the reaction time of saccades, impair contralateral anticipatory saccades, and impair ability to inhibit inappropriate saccades to visual stimuli, as well as impair pursuit and optokinetic following toward the side of the lesion (Thurtell, Tomsak, & Leigh, 2007). SEF lesions impair memory-guided saccades after gaze shifts and affect ability to make a remembered sequence of saccades to an array of visible targets. DLPC lesions produce inaccurate contralateral memory-guided saccades and impair predictive saccades and antisaccades.

Larger acute destructive hemispheric lesions such as infarctions, especially right posterior lesions, may cause ipsilateral sustained horizontal conjugate gaze deviation (where patients may "look away from the hemiparesis" as opposed to gaze directed toward the hemiparesis in an acute pontine lesion). In a hemispheric lesion, it is usually possible to drive the eyes across the midline with head rotation or caloric stimulation. If able to make contralateral saccades, patients with parietal lobe lesions may have contralateral inattention (with or without homonymous hemianopia), ipsilateral gaze preference, increased latency for visually guided saccades, and impaired smooth pursuit ipsilaterally. Intermittent horizontal conjugate gaze deviation suggests seizures from the contralateral hemisphere.

Clinical Correlation: Ocular Motor Apraxia and Balint's Syndrome

Acute bilateral frontal or frontoparietal lesions such as infarctions may cause a striking disorder called acquired ocular motor apraxia, characterized by loss of voluntary control of saccades and pursuit but preservation of reflexive eye movements such as slow and quick phases of the VOR. Patients struggle to make saccades to command and to follow a pointer, often using blinks and head movements to facilitate gaze shifts.

When ocular motor apraxia is accompanied by disturbances of peripheral visual attention (simultagnosia) and inaccurate arm pointing (optic ataxia), the term *Balint's syndrome* is applied. Lesions are typically bilateral parieto-occipital. Voluntary saccades may be made more easily than in response to visual stimuli, reflecting defects in the visual guidance of saccades and impaired visual search. Smooth pursuit is also impaired.

GAZE HOLDING AND THE NEURAL INTEGRATOR

Once a visual target is acquired, the eyes must be held steady in an eccentric position to maintain fixation. To counteract the orbital elastic restoring forces that would tend to pull the eyes back to central position, tonic contraction of the extraocular muscles is achieved by an increase in the sustained rate of discharge of the OMN. This gaze-holding function is achieved by networks of neurons that mathematically integrate saccadic velocity "pulse" signals into position "step" commands, collectively referred to as the *neural integrator* (Figure 2–8).

The basic scheme for the neural integrator begins with the EBN. A pulse discharge from the EBN projects a velocity command signal to the OMN to cause phasic contraction of the extraocular muscle and overcome viscous drag of the orbit to generate a saccadic eye movement. Abnormalities of the pulse can result in hypometric or slow saccades (Figure 2–9). The same pulse signal from EBN is also sent through the neural integrator to generate a step of innervation, that is, a position command to the OMN that changes the tonic contraction of the extraocular muscle appropriate to hold the eye in the new position. If the performance of the neural integrator is perfect, the eye will be held perfectly on the eccentric target.

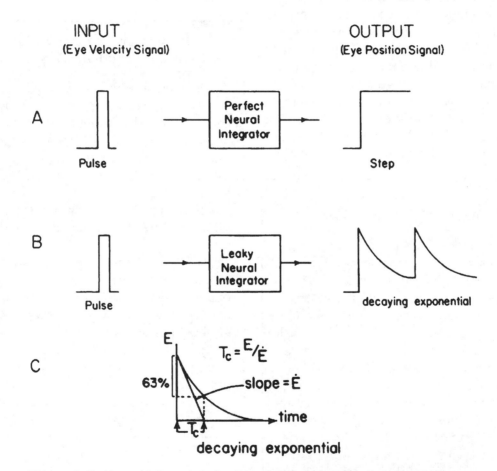

Figure 2–8. Neural integrator physiology. For saccades, a pulse of innervation is the input to the neural integrator that generates a step. If the system is perfect, the pulse (an eye velocity command) becomes a step (eye position command), as seen in **A.** If the neural integrator is leaky or imperfect (**B**), the eye position signal decays with time. In this case, the eye will drift toward the midline until a corrective saccade repositions the eye on target, creating gaze-evoked nystagmus. **C.** The centripetal drift of the eyes that occurs with a leaky integrator can be described by its time constant (*Tc*), given by the time at which the eye has drifted 63% of the way back to the midline. From *The Neurology of Eye Movements*, by R. J. Leigh. and D. S. Zee, 2006, p. 246, Figure 5–4. Reprinted by permission of Oxford University Press, Inc.

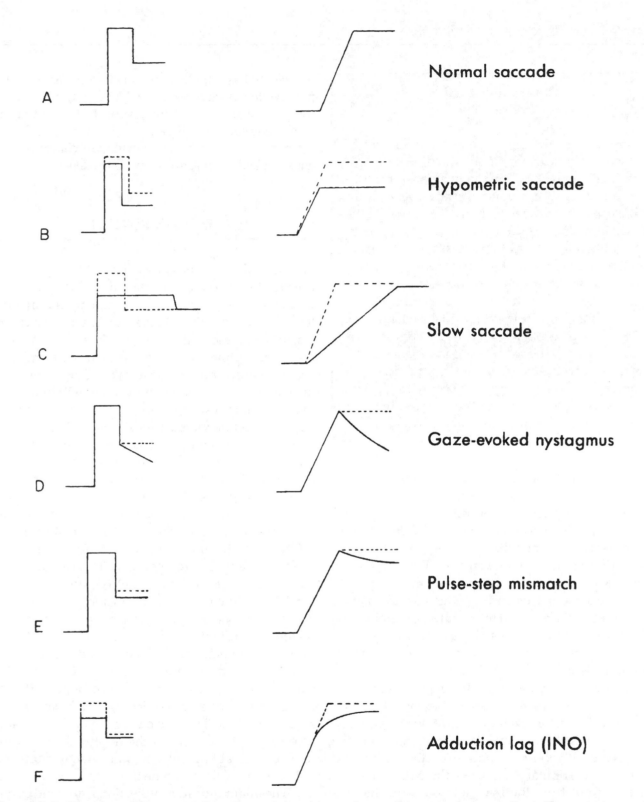

Figure 2-9. Disorders of the saccadic pulse and step. Innervation patterns are shown on the left, eye movements on the right. Dashed lines indicate the normal response. **A.** Normal saccade. **B.** Hypometric saccade: pulse amplitude (width × height) is too small but pulse and step are matched appropriately. **C.** Slow saccade: decreased pulse height with normal pulse amplitude and normal pulse-step match. **D.** Gaze-evoked nystagmus: normal pulse, poorly sustained step. **E.** Pulse-step mismatch (glissade): step is relatively smaller than pulse. **F.** Pulse-step mismatch due to internuclear ophthalmoplegia (*INO*: the step is larger than the pulse, and so the eye drifts onward after the initial rapid movement. Reproduced from Leigh and Zee (2006) with permission from Oxford University Press.

The neural substrate for gaze holding consists of cell groups throughout the brainstem and cerebellum. The nucleus propositus hypoglossi and adjacent medial vestibular nucleus (NPH-MVN) in the dorsal rostral medulla play a key role in integration of horizontal eye movements. The NPH-MVN receives inputs from every structure that projects to the abducens nucleus and encodes position signals to abducens neurons and interneurons, mainly those innervating fatigue-resistant extraocular muscle fibers capable of sustained contraction. The interstitial nucleus of Cajal (INC), located just caudal to the riMLF in the mesencephalic reticular formation, is the primary structure responsible for integration of vertical and torsional eye movements (and also appears important for eye-head coordination in the roll plane). It receives inputs from the riMLF and from the vestibular nuclei via the MLF. The primary output from the INC decussates in the posterior commissure to project position commands to the contralateral INC and CN III and IV nuclei. The cerebellum, particularly the paraflocculi (tonsils) and flocculi (collectively part of the "vestibulocerebellum"), appears critical for improving the performance of an inherently leaky neural integrator. For example, the NPH-MVN has connections with

the vestibulocerebellum that likely serve as part of a positive feedback loop to OMN, helping to increase the gain of the neural integrator. In the setting of conditions such as cerebellar degeneration or Chiari malformation (where the tonsils are compressed), gaze-evoked nystagmus commonly develops.

SMOOTH PURSUIT

The smooth pursuit system probably evolved to keep the fovea pointed at a stationary target ahead as we navigate through our environment. Minimizing foveal "slip" of a visual object of interest improves vision, while the "optic flow" of images across the rest of our retina as we walk provides information about the three-dimensional layout of our environment and our direction of movement within it. Subsequently, this system could be harnessed to pursue a small object moving across a complex background (without inducing a perception of motion of self or the stationary world) as well as assist with visual fixation (holding the image of a stationary object on the fovea while the observer is stationary).

Signals encoding speed and direction of retinal image motion pass via the lateral geniculate nucleus (LGN) to striate and extrastriate (middle temporal and medial superior temporal, MST) cortex and posterior parietal cortex (i.e., PEF) (Figure 2–10). The MST seems to contain visual tracking neurons that encode representations of object motion in world-centered coordinates, being sensitive to retinal slip, slow eye movements, and slow head movements. From there, further projections to the FEF and SEF may contribute to predictive aspects of pursuit, utilizing some of the same corticofugal pathways as the saccadic system. The nucleus of the optic tract and accessory optic system in the midbrain pretectum receives retinal slip information directly from the retina and may help initiate pursuit.

The main pursuit projections descend from parieto-temporo-occipital cortex to the pons, particularly the DLPN and NRTP, encoding various visual and ocular motor signals including eye velocity. The DLPN projects contralaterally to the cerebellar flocculus and paraflocculus via the middle cerebellar peduncle, whereas the NRTP projects to the dorsal vermis and then to the caudal fastigial nucleus. From

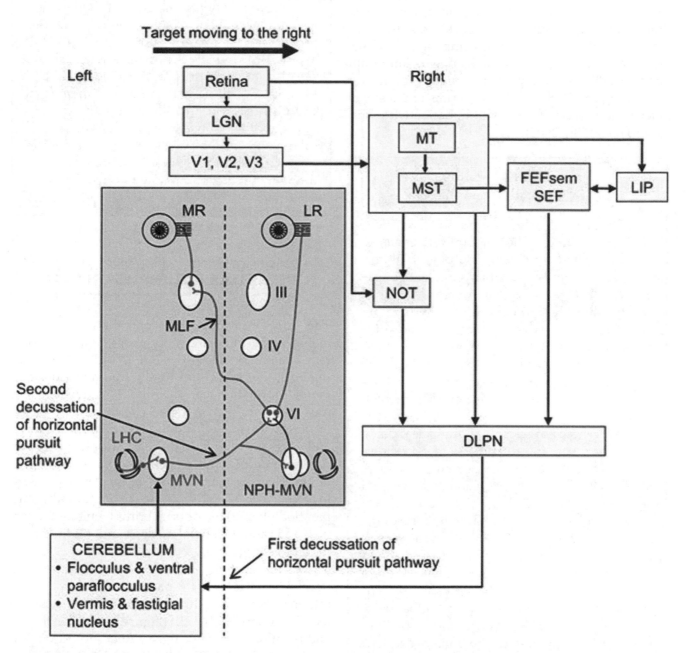

Figure 2–10. Smooth pursuit pathways. Shaded area represents common pathway shared by horizontal *VOR* and smooth pursuit. *LGN*, lateral geniculate nucleus; V1, striate cortex; V2 and V3, extrastriate cortex; *MT*, middle temporal visual area; *MST*, medial superior temporal visual area; *FEFsem*, pursuit subregion of the frontal eye field; *SEF*, supplemental eye field; *LIP*, lateral intraparietal area; *NOT*, nucleus of the optic tract; *DLPN*, dorsolateral pontine nuclei; *MVN*, medial vestibular nucleus; *LHC*, left horizontal canal; *NPH*, nucleus prepositus hypoglossi; *MLF*, medial longitudinal fasciculus; III, oculomotor nucleus; IV, trochlear nucleus; VI, abducens nucleus; *MR*, medial rectus; *LR*, lateral rectus. Reproduced from Wong (2008) with permission from Oxford University Press.

these cerebellar structures, fibers then reach the superior and medial vestibular nuclei, which then (for horizontal pursuit) project back across the midline to the abducens nucleus (completing a double decussation). The paraflocculus appears important for controlling smooth pursuit and the flocculus for calibrating the VOR, while the vermis and fastigial nucleus are critical for pursuit initiation (Krauzlis, 2004; Thier & Ilg, 2005).

Clinical Correlation: Smooth Pursuit Abnormalities

Pathways serving smooth pursuit are widespread throughout the cerebral hemispheres, brainstem, and cerebellum, so pursuit abnormalities commonly accompany lesions throughout the central nervous system. Reduced pursuit gain (the ratio of eye velocity to target velocity) manifests as "choppy" or "saccadic" pursuit, as small saccades are made to catch up with the moving target as the eyes fall behind. One must recognize that pursuit gain declines normally with advancing age, especially at high velocities, but also becomes impaired in Parkinson disease, progressive supranuclear palsy, cerebellar disorders, and large cerebral lesions. While diffuse disorders cause omnidirectional pursuit abnormalities, large unilateral cerebral lesions (especially of the parieto-occipital cortex and underlying white matter but also of the MST visual cortex and the FEF) cause pursuit tracking deficits predominantly to the side of the lesion, independent of homonymous hemianopia or visual neglect. This asymmetric pursuit can be demonstrated with an "optokinetic" tape or drum. Directional pursuit abnormalities may also be encountered with unilateral lesions of the descending pursuit pathways, including the midbrain tegmentum, DLPN, and cerebellum. Because of the double decussation of the pursuit pathway, lesions of the pontocerebellar projections and vestibular nuclei may impair either ipsilateral or contralateral smooth pursuit. Unless the VOR is also impaired by a disease process, smooth pursuit deficits are generally accompanied by impairment of VOR suppression during combined eye-head tracking.

Isolated defects of vertical pursuit are less common. Bilateral INO from MLF lesions impairs vertical pursuit (and the vertical VOR), as the MLF transmits pursuit and vestibular signals from the vestibular nuclei to CN III and IV serving vertical eye movements. An unusual disturbance can occur with cavernous angiomas of the middle cerebellar peduncle, where vertical pursuit is accompanied by torsional nystagmus, suggesting that pursuit signals processed through the cerebellum may be encoded in the same reference planes as the semicircular canals.

CEREBELLAR INFLUENCES ON GAZE

The cerebellum optimizes or refines eye movements so that they are calibrated to improve accuracy and ensure clearest vision. In order to perform this role, the cerebellum receives both sensory and motor information regarding the eye movement and must compare the predicted eye movement based on the command with the desired eye movement and generate a signal to decrease the error between predicted and desired to get the eyes accurately on target. Three primary regions of the cerebellum are involved with ocular motility: (1) the flocculus and paraflocculus; (2) the dorsal vermis (oculomotor vermis) and caudal fastigial nucleus; and (3) the nodulus and ventral uvula.

As part of the vestibulocerebellum, the paired flocculi lie adjacent to the paraflocculi, ventral to the inferior cerebellar peduncle and next to the vestibulocochlear nerve (CN VIII) (Figure 2–11). The flocculi and paraflocculi receive mossy fiber input from the vestibular nuclei, NPH, NRTP, DLPN, and paramedian tract cell group and climbing fiber input from the contralateral inferior olivary nucleus. The main output from the floccular and parafloccular Purkinje cells is to the ipsilateral superior and medial vestibular nuclei. Studies suggest that the flocculus is more important for calibrating the VOR, while the paraflocculus mainly contributes to smooth pursuit. The flocculus and paraflocculus also appear to contribute inhibitory influence to counteract the inherent tonic upward VOR bias otherwise favoring the

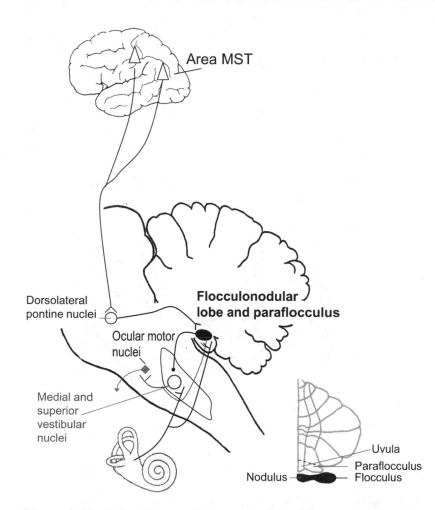

Figure 2–11. Role of the vestibulocerebellum (flocculonodular lobe and paraflocculus) in the control of eye movements. The main role of the flocculonodular lobe, adjacent uvula and ventral parafloc-culus (vestibulocerebellum) is the control of certain eye movements. The nodulus and uvula receive vestibular inputs both directly from the labyrinth and via the vestibular nuclei; inputs from the frontal eye fields and the middle superior temporal (*MST*) area via the dorsolateral pon-tine nuclei; and inputs from the ocular motor control network via the nucleus prepositus hypoglossi and the nuclei of the paramedian tracts (*not shown*). The flocculus and paraflocculus project to the medial and superior vestibular nuclei predominantly for control of the horizon-tal and vertical vestibulo-ocular reflexes and smooth pursuit. Reprinted with permission from Dr. Eduardo Benarroch (Benarroch, 2006) and Mayo Foundation for Medical Education and Research.

anterior over posterior SCC pathways, as lesions of these cerebellar structures often leads to upward slow phases and downbeat nystagmus as would be seen with unopposed anterior canal activation.

Lobules VI and VII of the dorsal vermis (Fig-ure 2–12) receive mossy fiber inputs from the PPRF, NRTP, DLPN, NPH, and vestibular nuclei as well as

climbing fiber input from the contralateral inferior olivary nucleus. Projections coming from the NRTP relay information necessary for planning saccades, whereas those from the DLPN are more important for smooth pursuit. Dorsal vermis Purkinje cells discharge prior to contralateral saccades as well as encode target velocity during pursuit and combined

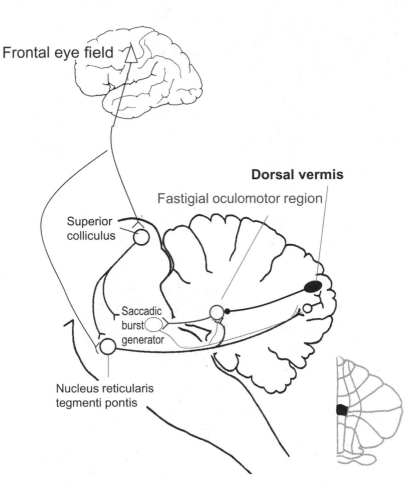

Figure 2-12. Role of the dorsal vermis and fastigial oculomotor region for control of saccades. The posterior or dorsal vermis, via the fastigial oculomotor region, controls the amplitude and direction of saccadic eye movements. These structures receive inputs from the paramedian pontine reticular formation, which contains the excitatory burst neurons for horizontal saccades, and from the nucleus reticularis tegmenti pontis, which relays saccadic signals from the frontal eye fields and superior colliculus. The fastigial nucleus projects to the saccadic burst generator of the brainstem via the uncinate fasciculus to control the amplitude of ipsilateral and contralateral saccades. Reprinted with permission from Dr. Eduardo Benarroch (Benarroch, 2006) and Mayo Foundation for Medical Education and Research.

eye-head tracking. Dorsal vermis Purkinje cells project to the caudal part of the deep cerebellar fastigial nucleus, coined the *fastigial oculomotor region*, which also receives collaterals from the same climbing and mossy fiber inputs destined for the dorsal vermis. The main projection from the fastigial nucleus crosses through the other fastigial nucleus and enters the uncinate fasciculus in the border of the superior cerebellar peduncle to reach the premotor burst neurons and OPN in the brainstem. Fastigial neurons discharge prior to and during contralateral saccades (facilitating them) and discharge late for ipsilateral saccades (perhaps serving as a stop signal to end a saccade on target).

The nodulus, which is the midline portion of the flocculonodular lobe, and the adjacent ventral uvula control the velocity-storage mechanism of the VOR. This central vestibular mechanism functions to enhance the responsiveness of the VOR to low-frequency stimuli such as sustained rotation. Without a velocity-storage mechanism, the discharge from vestibular nuclei driving the VOR would quickly decay during sustained rotation, based on the mechanical properties of cupular deflection in the semicircular canals. Velocity storage prolongs the raw vestibular signal so that the angular VOR can better transduce the low-frequency components of head rotation. The neural substrate for velocity storage may be the medial vestibular nuclei and their interconnections, since sectioning the vestibular commissure abolishes velocity storage. Purkinje cells of the nodulus send GABAergic projections to the vestibular nuclei to control the velocity-storage mechanism of the VOR.

Clinical Correlation: Cerebellar Syndromes

Three principal ocular motor syndromes may occur in the setting of cerebellar disease depending on the location of dysfunction, with overlap being common due to more widespread cerebellar dysfunction (Versino et al., 1996).

Lesions of the Flocculus and Paraflocculus

Focal dysfunction of the flocculi and parafloccculi, such as may be seen in Chiari malformation, produces several abnormalities. Gaze-evoked nystagmus results from loss of the cerebellar contribution to the fidelity of the brainstem neural integrator. Downbeat nystagmus and rebound nystagmus are other common sequelae. Smooth pursuit is impaired (choppy or saccadic), as is the ability to suppress the VOR during combined eye-head tracking or during caloric irrigation by fixating on a stationary target. Finally, patients cannot adapt the VOR to changing visual needs, such as new spectacle correction.

Lesions of the Dorsal Vermis and Fastigial Nucleus

Dorsal vermis and fastigial nucleus lesions cause saccadic dysmetria (inaccurate saccades), typically hypometria if the vermis alone is involved and hypermetria if the fastigial nuclei are involved. Unilateral lesions of the dorsal vermis would cause ipsilateral hypometria and mild contralateral hypermetria of saccades. A unilateral lesion of the fastigial nucleus would cause ipsilat-eral hypermetria and contralateral hypometria of saccades as well as cause the eyes to tonically deviate ipsilaterally (ipsipulsion). While such asymmetric dysfunction is rarely seen clinically since the fastigial projections cross within the opposite nucleus, the same functional effect occurs in Wallenberg syndrome (below). Because those crossed projections ascend in the contralateral uncinate fasciculus of the superior cerebellar peduncle, a lesion in the uncinate fasciculus can cause contrapulsion of saccades. Finally, dorsal vermis and fastigial lesions can impair smooth pursuit initiation.

Lesions of the Nodulus and Ventral Uvula

Nodulus and ventral uvula lesions lead to loss of the GABAergic inhibition of the velocity-storage mechanism, thus maximizing the velocity-storage effect in circumstances that would usually reduce it, such as pitching the head forward during post-rotatory nystagmus. The most clinically important result of a nodulus lesion is periodic alternating nystagmus (PAN), where the velocity-storage mechanism becomes unstable, and short-term vestibular adaptation leads to sustained horizontal nystagmus that reverses directions every 2 min. Although in pure form, PAN is only present in darkness, it may be present during attempted visual fixation if the adjacent flocculus and paraflocculus are also involved (because of their role in VOR suppression).

Clinical Correlation: Wallenberg Syndrome

Infarction of the dorsolateral medulla (generally from occlusion of the ipsilateral vertebral or posterior inferior cerebellar arteries or vertebral dissection) causes Wallenberg syndrome, consisting of ipsilateral impairment of facial pain and temperature sensation, Horner's syndrome, limb ataxia, and bulbar disturbances leading to dysarthria and dysphagia. Contralaterally, pain and temperature sensation are impaired in the trunk and limbs. Patients commonly report vertigo and a variety of unusual sensations of body and environmental tilt, including the room being tilted on its side or upside down. Lateropulsion, a compelling sensation of being pulled to one side (in this case toward the side of the lesion), is a common complaint.

Several ocular motor abnormalities are characteristic of Wallenberg syndrome and may be the main or sole manifestation (Baloh, Yee, & Honrubia, 1981; Brazis, 1992). Lateropulsion of saccades develops because the lesion affects the inferior cerebellar peduncle carrying climbing fibers from the inferior olivary nucleus to the dorsal cerebellar vermis, leading to the functional equivalent of a fastigial nucleus lesion. Lateropulsion of the eyes is easy to detect at the bedside. If the patient is asked to fixate straight ahead and gently close the eyes, the eyes will conjugately deviate toward the side of the lesion, requiring a refixation saccade back to the straight-ahead position after opening the eyes again. Horizontal saccades are hypermetric toward the side of the lesion (ipsipulsion) and hypometric contralateral to the lesion. Vertical saccades take an oblique trajectory, with an inappropriate horizontal component toward the side of the lesion (requiring a horizontal corrective saccade once the vertical saccade is complete).

The lesion's involvement of the vestibular nuclei can produce spontaneous nystagmus (often mixed horizontal-torsional), with slow phases usually directed toward the side of the lesion. Smooth pursuit is impaired for targets moving away from the side of the lesion. The ocular tilt reaction also occurs because of imbalance of the otolith-ocular pathway from the vestibular nucleus lesion. The result is skew deviation with the ipsilateral eye lower (with corresponding vertical diplopia), cylcodeviation where the top poles of the eyes roll toward the side of the lesion, and ipsilateral head tilt.

REFERENCES

Baloh, R. W., Furman, J., & Yee, R. D. (1985). Eye movements in patients with absent voluntary horizontal gaze. *Annals of Neurology, 17*(3), 283–286.

Baloh, R. W., Yee, R. D., & Honrubia, V. (1981). Eye movements in patients with Wallenberg's syndrome. *Annals of the New York Academy of Sciences, 374*, 600–613.

Benarroch, E. E. (2006). *Basic neurosciences with clinical applications*. Philadelphia, PA: Butterworth Heinemann/Elsevier.

Bhidayasiri, R., Plant, G. T., & Leigh, R. J. (2000). A hypothetical scheme for the brainstem control of vertical gaze. *Neurology, 54*(10), 1985–1993.

Bhidayasiri, R., Riley, D. E., Somers, J. T., Lerner, A. J., Buttner-Ennever, J. A., & Leigh, R. J. (2001). Pathophysiology of slow vertical saccades in progressive supranuclear palsy. *Neurology, 57*(11), 2070–2077.

Brazis, P. W. (1992). Ocular motor abnormalities in Wallenberg's lateral medullary syndrome. *Mayo Clinic Proceedings, 67*(4), 365–368.

Brodsky, M. C., Donahue, S. P., Vaphiades, M., & Brandt, T. (2006). Skew deviation revisited. *Survey of Ophthalmology, 51*(2), 105–128.

Demer, J. L. (2006). Current concepts of mechanical and neural factors in ocular motility. *Current Opinion in Neurology, 19*(1), 4–13.

Eggers, S. D., Moster, M. L., & Cranmer, K. (2008). Selective saccadic palsy after cardiac surgery. *Neurology, 70*(4), 318–320.

Fife, T. D. (2010). Overview of anatomy and physiology of the vestibular system. In S. D. Z. Eggers & D. S. Zee (Eds.), *Vertigo and imbalance: Clinical neurophysiology of the vestibular system* (pp. 575). Amsterdam, the Netherlands: Elsevier.

Furman, J. M., Wall, C., 3rd, & Pang, D. L. (1990). Vestibular function in periodic alternating nystagmus. *Brain, 113*(Pt 5), 1425–1439.

Krauzlis, R. J. (2004). Recasting the smooth pursuit eye movement system. *Journal of Neurophysiology, 91*(2), 591–603. doi:10.1152/jn.00801.2003

Leigh, R. J., Robinson, D. A., & Zee, D. S. (1981). A hypothetical explanation for periodic alternating nystagmus: Instability in the optokinetic-vestibular system. *Annals of the New York Academy of Sciences, 374,* 619–635.

Leigh, R. J., & Zee, D. S. (2006). *The neurology of eye movements.* New York, NY: Oxford University Press.

Pierrot-Deseilligny, C., Milea, D., & Muri, R. M. (2004). Eye movement control by the cerebral cortex. *Current Opinion in Neurology, 17*(1), 17–25.

Ramat, S., Leigh, R. J., Zee, D. S., & Optican, L. M. (2007). What clinical disorders tell us about the neural control of saccadic eye movements. *Brain, 130*(Pt. 1), 10–35.

Scudder, C. A., Kaneko, C. S., & Fuchs, A. F. (2002). The brainstem burst generator for saccadic eye movements: A modern synthesis. *Experimental Brain Research, 142*(4), 439–462.

Sparks, D. L. (2002). The brainstem control of saccadic eye movements. *Nature Reviews Neuroscience, 3*(12), 952–964.

Thier, P., & Ilg, U. J. (2005). The neural basis of smooth-pursuit eye movements. *Current Opinion in Neurobiology, 15*(6), 645–652.

Thurtell, M. J., Tomsak, R. L., & Leigh, R. J. (2007). Disorders of saccades. *Current Neurology and Neuroscience Reports, 7*(5), 407–416.

Versino, M., Hurko, O., & Zee, D. S. (1996). Disorders of binocular control of eye movements in patients with cerebellar dysfunction. *Brain, 119*(Pt. 6), 1933–1950.

Walker, M. F., & Zee, D. S. (1999). Directional abnormalities of vestibular and optokinetic responses in cerebellar disease. *Annals of the New York Academy of Sciences, 871,* 205–220.

Wong, A. (2007). An update on opsoclonus. *Current Opinion in Neurology, 20*(1), 25–31.

Wong, A. M. F. (2008). *Eye movement disorders.* New York, NY: Oxford University Press.

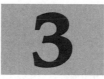

Ontogeny of the Vestibular System and Balance

Timothy A. Jones and Sherri M. Jones

INTRODUCTION AND BACKGROUND

In the human, embryonic development begins at fertilization of the ovum and lasts until the end of the eighth week after fertilization. The fetal period then extends from the ninth week until birth (36 to 40 weeks after fertilization). There are a number of major events occurring during weeks 3 and 4 of embryonic development that are critical for normal formation of the head and neck including the ear. This period includes the appearance of the cranial placodes and development of the pharyngeal apparatus. Disturbances in these and other important early processes, as may be produced by genetic variation or exposure to physiological stressors, teratogens, or other factors, can lead to serious head and neck developmental abnormalities including deafness and vestibular dysgenesis. Our purpose here is to present the normal ontogeny of vestibular sensors. Detailed consideration of the ontogeny of the auditory system as well as the consequences of genetic variation on vestibular and auditory development is available elsewhere (Jones & Jones, 2011). Considered here are developmental events common to both modalities during the early formation of the inner ear and important differences in developmental programs where appropriate. We begin during embryonic development and in particular emphasize the appearance of the first outward structural

sign of the emerging inner ear, the otic placode. The chapter concludes with vestibular functional maturation and subsequent acquisition of postural control and balance.

Detailed knowledge regarding the development of vestibular and auditory function comes primarily from the study of animals. Most of the information presented below is based on studies using chick or mouse models, and the developmental ages reflect mouse/chick embryonic age in days. Human developmental ages in weeks post fertilization are presented in parentheses (e.g., week 5) based on Bredberg (1968), Dechesne (1992), Pujol, Lavigne-Rebillard, and Lenoir (1998), Jeffery and Spoor (2004), Sans and Dechesne (1985), and Sulik and Cotanche (2004). Much, if not all, of the postnatal developmental changes observed in mammalian models occur prior to birth in the human. We indicate human ages estimated or found to correspond to those of animal models. For the chicken, equivalent days of incubation (E) are given based on Hamburger and Hamilton (1951) staging. For the mouse embryonic (E) days of gestation are equivalent to days postconception (dpc) where day E0.5 is the morning that the vaginal plug is found (Kaufman, 1992). Days postnatal are designated with a "P" where P0 is the day of birth or hatch.

Much of the research on early development is done in vitro, that is, conducted on cells or tissues that are removed from the animal and placed in artificial physiological solutions. In many cases, we must assume that the processes described from in vitro studies are similar to those that function in vivo, or in the intact animal.

During the first week of human development, the zygote undergoes cleavage to form a blastocyst which then attaches to the uterine wall (i.e., endometrium). By the end of the second week the blastocyst is fully implanted within the endometrium and has formed the bilaminar embryonic disk (Figure 3–1A and D). The lamina are termed *epiblast* and *hypoblast*.

The cells of the epiblast will give rise to all the cells of the adult. Cells of the hypoblast will form extra-embryonic structures. The basic anatomical axes and planes illustrated are already established by this stage prior to morphogenesis, which is initiated during gastrulation (week 3). The orientation of axes and planes shown are standard conventions and are referenced throughout the chapter.

The horizontal plane is formed by the lateral axis (Figure 3–1A and D, left (L) and right (R), line joining labels L and R) and the anterior-posterior axis

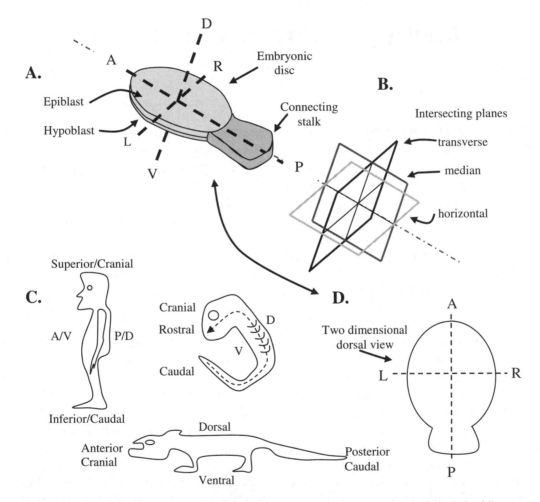

Figure 3–1. Anatomical axes and planes in the developing embryo. **A.** Isolated three-dimensional bilaminar embryonic disk with connecting stalk. **B.** Intersecting planes: transverse (*black*), median (*dark gray*, also called sagittal plane), and horizontal (*light gray*). The transverse or lateral plane contains the left-right (*LR*) and dorsal-ventral (*DV*) axes. The medial plane contains the anterior-posterior (*AP*) and dorsal-ventral axes. The horizontal plane contains the anterior-posterior and left-right axes. **C.** Anatomical directions in the adult human, embryo, and one amphibian species. **D.** Isolated bilaminar embryonic disk as seen from the dorsal view. Anterior-posterior and left-right axes are shown as dashed lines. From *Genetics, Embryology, and Development of Auditory and Vestibular Systems* (2011) (p. 98) by Sherri M. Jones and Timothy A. Jones.

(AP, Figure 3–1A and D, line joining labels A and P, also called cranial-caudal axis). The AP and dorso-ventral (DV) axes are perpendicular to one another and they form the median or sagittal plane of the embryo at its midline (Figure 3–1A and B). Points laying to the left or right of the median plane are said to be lateral to it. The lateral axis is perpendicular to the median plane and it identifies lateral distances from the midline. The lateral axis and the dorsoven-tral axis form the transverse plane (Figure 3–1A and B). A transverse section through the embryonic disc reveals structures in cross section showing the left and right lateral extent of the tissue. Sagittal sections also produce cross sections, but the view reveals the anterior-posterior extent of the tissue. The caudal pole of the embryonic disc is easily identified as the site of attachment for the connecting stalk.

FORMATION OF THE OTIC PLACODE AND OTIC VESICLE

The inner ear is formed from primordial ectodermal cells near rhombomeres five and six in the embryonic hindbrain. These cells form a flat, thickened patch of ectoderm called the otic placode (Figure 3–2) on embryonic day 8.5 (E8.5) for the mouse and dur-ing week 3 for humans. The otic placode appears morphologically as the first step in the formation of the inner ear. A variety of genetic signals define a region of tissue committed to form the otic placode, and subsequent molecular signaling leads to the separation of the otic placode from epidermal tis-sue (reviewed by Ohyama, Groves, & Martin, 2007). According to Groves (2005), the cells ultimately forming the placode are not simply gathered from adjacent cells, but rather it appears likely that the cells migrate from a wide area and somehow collect to form the placode.

Cells of the otic placode give rise to the otic vesicle (also called otocyst) at E10.5 for the mouse (week 4 for human) from which sensory, nonsen-sory, and most neural cells of the inner ear will be derived (see Figure 3–2). The otic vesicle, however, does not give rise to olivocochlear and vestibular efferents or to autonomic innervation of blood ves-sels. Shortly after forming, the otic placode begins to bend and fold inward producing a shallow dimple.

This invagination of ectoderm continues until a deep pit is formed, which is called the otic pit or otic cup (see Figure 3–2). The dorsal edge of the otic tissue remains in close approximation to the hindbrain/neural plate during this process. This association favors molecular signaling and formation of asym-metric molecular signal fields. Ultimately, the otic cup closes to form the otic vesicle. Closure of the otic cup and the proximal neural groove (thus form-ing the neural tube locally) occurs at about the same time during week 4 in humans.

During and after its formation, the otic vesicle is influenced by signals from the hindbrain as well as the mesenchyme surrounding the otic vesicle (known as the periotic mesenchyme or mesoderm) that becomes the bony labyrinth of the inner ear. Sev-eral important signaling molecules play a dominant role in establishing the dorsal-ventral morphological axis within the otocyst. The dorsal-ventral boundary of the otic vesicle (a line midway between the bottom and top of the otic vesicle) distinguishes the dorsal vestibular sensors from the ventral cochlear sensors. Molecular signals are thought to form gradients of influence along the dorsal-ventral extent of otic tis-sue (Schneider-Maunoury & Pujades, 2007). Tissue elements at any given position experience a unique combination of signal levels, and each combination of signals has the potential to favor one program of development or another. Molecular signals within the otocyst and in the surrounding regions are also responsible for the order and layout of structures along the anteroposterior and mediolateral dimen-sions of the otic vesicle.

DELAMINATION AND FORMATION OF THE STATOACOUSTIC GANGLION

Under the influence of particular proteins, proneu-ral cells (neuroblasts, cells that will become afferent neurons) detach from and leave the epithelium of the otic cup and vesicle and then migrate medially and ventrally into the mesenchyme ultimately to form the statoacoustic ganglion (Figures 3–2 and 3–3). This process is called *delamination*; it begins in epithelial regions of the presumptive utricle and cristae as early as E10.5 (week 4 in humans), and rep-resents the beginning of neurogenesis. The epithelial

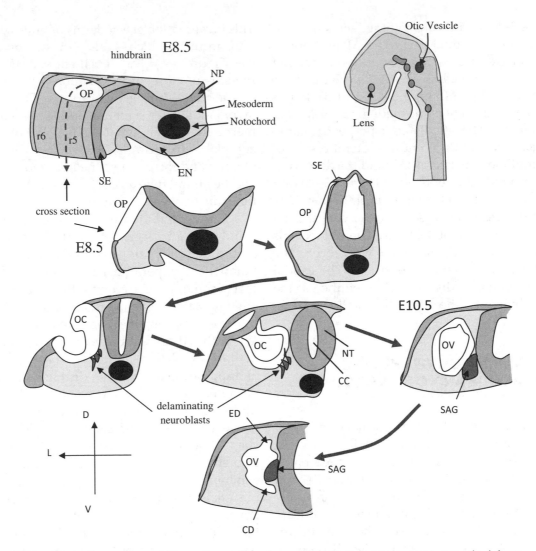

Figure 3–2. Formation of the otic vesicle from the otic placode over a period from approximately E8.5 to just beyond E10.5 in mouse (*follow gray arrows*). *ED* = endolymphatic duct; *EN* = endoderm; *CC* = central canal; *CD* = cochlear duct; *D* = dorsal; *L* = lateral; Mesoderm = mesenchyme presumptive mesoderm; *NP* = neural plate; *NT* = neural tube; *OC* = otic cup; *OP* = otic placode; *OV* = otic vesicle; *r5-r6* = rhombomeres 5 and 6; *SAG* = statoacoustic ganglion; *SE* = surface ectoderm (epidermis); *V* = ventral. From *Genetics, Embryology, and Development of Auditory and Vestibular Systems* (2011) (p.158) by Sherri M. Jones and Timothy A. Jones.

neuroblasts divide and ultimately differentiate into auditory and vestibular neurons. Delamination expands to include prosensory regions (i.e., regions containing cells that will become sensory hair cells) within or adjacent to the sacculus and eventually the cochlea. Delamination continues through periods as late as E17 (week 9 in humans). We consider the formation of the statoacoustic ganglion in more detail later in the chapter.

FORMATION OF PROSENSORY PATCHES

For warm-blooded vertebrates, there are six or seven sensory patches in the mature inner ear (utricle, saccule, cochlea, three cristae, and the macula lagena in birds). This list does not include the very small sensory patch called the crista neglecta, about which little is known (Montandon, Gacek, & Kimura, 1970).

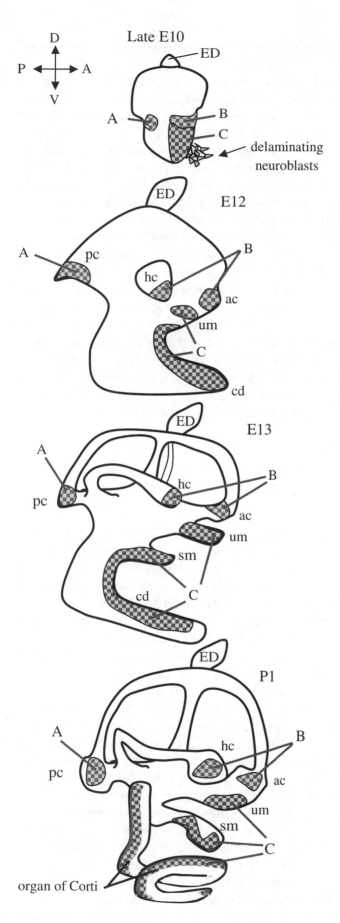

Figure 3–3. Lateral views of locations for important markers of prosensory and sensory domains during development. Regions forming the most dorsal sensory epithelia (cristae of semicircular canals) are distinguished early by the expression of particular genes (labels *A* and *B*), whereas the more ventral regions are marked with a different combination of signals (labeled *C*). The ventral prosensory domains elaborate the sensory epithelia of the utricular macula (*um*), sacular macula (*sm*) and cochlear duct (*cd*) in that order. *ac* = anterior crista. *hc* = horizontal (lateral) crista. *pc* = posterior crista. E days are equivalent to days post coitum (dpc). *P1* = postnatal day 1. Adapted from Bok, Chang, and Wu, 2007, with permission from *The International Journal of Developmental Biology, 51,* 526.

The sensory epithelia form in close association with the nonsensory components (i.e., cristae with canals, maculae with vestibule, and cochlea with cochlear duct). There is evidence that molecular signals from the sensory patches guide surrounding nonsensory structures in morphogenesis (reviewed by Bok, Chang, & Wu, 2007).

Before such cooperative signaling can occur, the proneural and prosensory cells must be specified and distinguished from the surrounding epithelium. These precursor "neurosensory" cells (cells that yet may take on a neural or sensory cell fate) are specified early in the development of the otocyst. A neurosensory domain (i.e., region of cells that will become hair cells or neurons) can be identified at late E10 (week 4) with the expression of genes that may be viewed as markers for cells destined to become neurons or sensory cells (Bok et al., 2007; Morsli, Choo, Ryan, Johnson, & Wu, 1998). Inactivation of these genes or of corresponding pathways interferes with the formation of the statoacoustic ganglion and sensory organs. Those cells destined to become neural cells will soon delaminate as described above while the remaining cells will become the sensory epithelia.

Sensory Patches

At late E10 (week 4), certain regions of the otic vesicle (see regions A, B, and C of Figure 3–3) express specific genes that outline the neurosensory domain including presumptive cristae, maculae, and cochlear prosensory fields as well as the proneural fields where neuroblasts delaminate. The dorsal fields (see A and B of Figure 3–3) are distinguished from ventral prosensory regions (see C of Figure 3–3) by being marked with different combinations of gene signals. The patterns mark and distinguish which domains become cristae and which become macular and cochlear sensors. One gene is expressed only in the presumptive lateral (horizontal) canal and in its absence, the lateral canal fails to form (Morsli et al., 1999).

Anteroventral regions of the otocyst form in sequence the utricle, then the saccule, and finally the cochlea. As noted above, neuroblasts delaminate from this region and migrate anteriorly to form the statoacoustic ganglion over the period from E10.5 to E17 (weeks 4 to 9). Initially, there is no distinc-

tion between presumptive macular and cochlear regions (see Figure 3–3, E10); however, development proceeds from dorsal to ventral revealing first the more dorsal utricular maculae (see Figure 3–3, E12 and E13) and then later the saccular macula and cochlea (see Figure 3–3, P1). By E12 (week 5), the utricle is clearly segregated and by E13 (late week 5) the saccule is easily recognized, but a clear segregation from cochlear fields is evident only after E13.5 (week 6) (Morsli et al., 1998). Segregation of these macular and cochlear sensory patches requires signals from nonsensory regions of the otic vesicle after E10.5 (week 4) (Nichols et al., 2008). In the absence of such signaling, the utricle, saccule, and cochlea form a combined malformed single mosaic sensory epithelium. The progressive segregation of sensory epithelia also appears to be linked to the simultaneous delamination process as cells migrate from the prosensory regions to become neurons of the statoacoustic ganglion (Fritzsch et al., 2002).

FORMATION OF THE COCHLEA AND ZONE OF NONPROLIFERATION (ZNP)

The emerging cochlear duct can be seen initially as a lengthening of the ventral pole of the otocyst beginning at about E11 in the mouse (week 5 in humans) (see Figure 3–3). The duct continues to extend first ventromedially, then it turns abruptly, anteriorly forming a curved hook by late E12 (late week 5) (Morsli et al., 1998). This represents initiation of the cochlear coil, and by E13 (week 6) a full half turn is achieved (see Figure 3–3). The cochlea will continue to elongate and increase the number of coils.

At the early stages of cochlea formation (week 5), the cochlear duct (see Figures 3–3 and 3–4B) houses a thick (four to five cells thick) undifferentiated epithelium that forms a ridge or sheet extending from the base to apex. This ridge of cells contains prosensory cells that have segregated ventrally from the sacculus (approximately E13.5 for mouse, week 6 for human). The ridge contains the presumptive organ of Corti. All cochlear hair cells and supporting cells will arise from this epithelial ridge.

Elongation and coiling of the cochlea continues with the leading edge of extension represented at the apical tip. Beginning at about E12.5 (late week 5), a

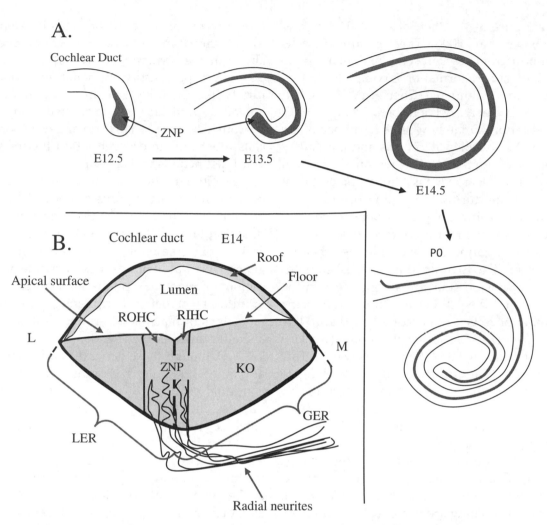

Figure 3–4. A. Formation of the zone of nonproliferation (ZNP, *marked gray*) in the cochlear duct at four stages of development. The ZNP appears first in the apex and then sweeps toward the base over the next 48 hr. The formation of ZNP is completed by approximately E14 (Chen et al., 2002; Lee et al., 2006); however, the cochlea continues to elongate and coil until P0. During this latter period of elongation the sensory epithelium thins and narrows. **B.** Schematic of the cochlear duct circa E14. According to Lim and Rueda (1992), the greater epithelial ridge (*GER*) incorporates the region of inner hair cells, whereas the lesser epithelial ridge (*LER*) incorporates the region where outer hair cells will form. Together they form the floor of the early cochlear duct also called generally the epithelial ridge. The zone of nonproliferation identifies the epithelial region of prospective inner and outer hair cells. Kolliker's organ (*KO*) has been defined a number of ways. Here, Kolliker's organ includes only that portion of the *a* that does not include prospective sensory hair cells. *RIHC* = region of inner hair cells. *ROHC* = region of outer hair cells. From *Genetics, Embryology, and Development of Auditory and Vestibular Systems* (2011) (p. 164 and 166) by Sherri M. Jones and Timothy A. Jones.

central strip of the apical epithelial ridge begins to exit the cell cycle and terminate mitosis (Figure 3–4) (Chen, Johnson, Zoghbi, & Segil, 2002; Chen & Segil, 1999; Lee, Liu, & Segil, 2006). Over a period of about a day in mice (E12.5 to E13.5), equivalent to a week in humans (late week 5 to week 6), a wave of termi-

nal mitosis sweeps along a central strip of the epithelial ridge from the cochlear apex to base. This is followed shortly afterward by a wave of cells exiting the cell cycle, which also moves along the central strip from the cochlear apex to base forming a cellular zone of nonproliferation (ZNP) along the epithelial ridge (see Figure 3–4) (Chen et al., 2002; Chen & Segil, 1999; Lee et al., 2006). These postmitotic cells form the undifferentiated prosensory domain of the organ of Corti, and its formation is completed before E14 (weeks 7 to 8 in humans) (Chen et al., 2002; Chen & Segil, 1999; Lee et al., 2006; Ruben, 1967).

By E14 (approximately week 8 in humans), the cochlear coil has reached 1.25 turns and the ZNP is in place (Chen & Segil, 1999). The region of the initial ventromedial cochlear extension in the otocyst continues to elongate during the coiling process, thus importantly, increasing the distance between the saccular macula and the first turn of the cochlea (Morsli et al., 1998). Elongation of the cochlear epithelium after E14 (weeks 7 to 8) must be accomplished without ZNP cell division since prosensory cells in the ZNP have exited the cell cycle. Completion of the adult number of coils is not accomplished until late embryonic ages (E17 to E19) for the mouse (weeks 9 to 10 for the human) (Chen & Segil, 1999; Morsli et al., 1998; Sher, 1971). The cochlea continues to elongate in the human from 20 mm to 35 mm between 10 and 16 weeks (Bredberg, 1968; Sulik & Cotanche, 2004).

Coiling and elongation of the ZNP is thought to be accomplished largely through the process of convergent extension. For this reason, the cochlea is subject to abnormal morphogenesis (short, thickened organ of Corti) when alterations in planar cell polarity (PCP) signaling are present (Jones & Chen, 2007; Kelley & Chen, 2007; McKenzie, Krupin, & Kelley, 2004; Montcouquiol et al., 2003; Wang et al., 2005; Wang, Guo, & Nathans, 2006). Mutations in, or knockouts of, core PCP genes or related signaling pathways prevent elongation and result in a shortened cochlea. The extent to which vestibular sensors depend on the convergent extension process is not clear. However, like the cochlea the vestibular epithelia start out as a layered partition of four to five epithelial cells and at maturity are reduced to an apical layer of sensory cells supported by one or two nonsensory cells (Dechesne, 1992). Whether the thinning process involves convergent extension to our knowledge has not been clarified.

HAIR CELL DIFFERENTIATION

Before differentiation can begin, vestibular and auditory prosensory epithelial cells must complete the last or terminal cell division. This is often referred to as terminal mitosis and this was an event noted above in the formation of the cochlear ZNP. The postmitotic prosensory epithelial cells appear structurally like any other cells in the epithelium. There are no superficial structural distinctions and no obvious evidence of axial polarization. Prosensory cells must initiate differentiation before such outward distinctions will appear.

Vestibular afferent and efferent neurons are present in sensory regions at about E12 (week 6). Prosensory cells evidence ongoing mitosis at this time. Within vestibular epithelia there are temporal and spatial gradients for the course of mitosis. In general, central regions (apex of cristae and striolar regions of maculae) initiate and reach peak levels of mitosis well before peripheral regions (base cristae, edges of maculae). Terminal mitosis occurs in a similar order (Mbiene & Sans, 1986; Sans & Chat, 1982). Although these general trends may hold, for any given vestibular region there is a more or less continual eruption of new immature stereociliary bundles until late fetal periods thus suggesting that some cells do not complete terminal cell division until very late.

Differentiation of prosensory cells of the cristae, maculae, and cochlea all require the induction of the gene atonal homolog 1 (*Atoh1*) (also known as mouse atonal homolog 1, *Math1*) (Bermingham et al., 1999). Prosensory cells exit the cell cycle and ultimately must express *Atoh1* before differentiating into hair cells. *Atoh1* expression and differentiation of hair cells begins in the cristae and maculae at E12, about 1 day (approximately 1 week in humans) before similar levels are expressed in the cochlea (approximately E13, week 7) (Bermingham et al., 1999; Chen et al., 2002; Lanford, Shailam, Norton, Gridley, & Kelley, 2000; Woods, Montcouquiol, & Kelley, 2004). Atoh1 expression is present throughout the sensory epithelium by E14.5 (weeks 8 to 10) and then is downregulated in the neonate (Driver et al., 2013; Lanford et al., 2000; Shailam et al., 1999).

During differentiation of the sensory epithelium, a remarkable pattern of hair cells and supporting cells emerges. Our understanding of the molecular signals orchestrating these events is more detailed for the cochlea than vestibular sensors, but in either case, there are many more questions to answer. One feature of both auditory and vestibular epithelia suggests a common organizing mechanism. The presence of orderly patterned mosaics of hair cells and supporting cells in all inner ear sensory epithelia implies a role for notch-mediated lateral inhibition (Lanford et al., 1999, 2000). In particular, all epithelia are arranged such that every hair cell is isolated from other hair cells by a ring of supporting cells or their processes. Lateral inhibition is one strategy that produces a "center on, surround off" pattern, where "on" refers to a hair cell and "off" to a nonsensory supporting cell.

In due course across the entire postmitotic sensory epithelium, a molecular scheme can be imagined to produce a mosaic of patches, where each patch is composed of a hair cell surrounded by supporting cells. This scheme is simplistic and incomplete, but it provides a basis for us to begin to understand how such mosaics can be shaped by molecular signaling and how the remarkable structures of the vestibular system and cochlea may be formed.

Prior to differentiation, prosensory cells appear as homogenous epithelial cells interconnected to each other by gap junctions (Ginzberg & Gilula, 1979). Gap junctions are subsequently lost only in cells committed to a hair cell fate. This occurs during the earliest period of hair cell differentiation (Bryant, Forge, & Richardson, 2005; Forge, Souter, & Denman-Johnson, 1997). Thus, one of the earliest events of hair cell differentiation includes the isolation of hair cells from surrounding supporting cells by eliminating direct electrochemical coupling between them.

VESTIBULAR STEREOCILIARY BUNDLES

The traditional definitive structural sign of hair cell differentiation is the elaboration of microvilli and formation of stereociliary bundles. Using scanning electron microscopy, vestibular hair cells can be definitively identified with the appearance of stereociliary bundles by E13.5 (week 7) (Bryant et al., 2005; Dechesne, 1992; Denman-Johnson & Forge, 1999; Mbiene & Sans, 1986). In contrast, the first morphological evidence of cochlear stereocilia begins to emerge between E14 and E15 (weeks 8 to 10) (Anniko, 1983b; Lim & Anniko, 1985; Pujol et al., 1998).

The earliest hair cells appear with microvilli or stereocilia encircling a single kinocilium in the center of the cell (Figure 3–5). The first sign of intrin-

sic hair cell polarization begins almost immediately with a movement of the kinocilium toward the lateral edge of the cell, thus taking an eccentric position in each hair cell. The direction of the movement reflects the emergence of the preferred direction of stimulation for each hair cell and hence the incipient morphological polarization vector (MPV). As noted above, the process associated with cilia formation and its direction of initial migration reflects the intrinsic cell polarization. Preventing the formation of the primary cilium (kinocilium) prevents proper planar orientation of outer hair cells (OHCs) (Jones, Roper et al., 2008). Disruption of PCP signaling pathways has similar effects. In looptail mouse mutants, auditory and vestibular hair cells are disoriented, indicating a role for PCP signaling in establishing vestibular hair cell orientation (Montcouquiol et al., 2003, 2006; reviewed by Jones & Chen, 2007; Kelley & Chen, 2007; Rida & Chen, 2009).

There are also a number of important structures that serve to mechanically couple stereocilia together as well as link the stereocilia to the kinocilium mechanically. There is of course the protein linkage to hair cell transduction channels called "tip links" that are critical to sensory transduction. Cadherin 23 (Cdh23) and protocadherin 15 (Pcdh15) make up the tip links (Kazmierczak et al., 2007). Given the complex architecture of the stereociliary bundle (see Chapter 1), much more remains to be learned about its molecular and functional development.

Like the cochlea, each vestibular hair cell is surrounded by supporting cells. However, there is an additional layer of organization in the vestibular system. In the cochlea, the direction of polarization for the hair bundle is the same for all hair cells with respect to the axis of the cochlea (all point laterally from the central axis). In vestibular maculae, hair bundle orientation is a function of the particular sensory organ examined. Intrinsic vestibular hair cell polarization is marked by the cells MPV. In each crista, MPVs of hair cells are oriented in the same direction. However, in the maculae, MPV orientation depends on the position of the hair cell on the epithelial surface. Recall from Chapter 1 that MPVs of hair cells are arranged systematically over the surface of the macular epithelium and in the adult, both maculae show a line coursing through the middle regions of the epithelium (striolar regions), where MPV directions abruptly reverse. Across this line of polarity reversal, MPVs point in opposite directions.

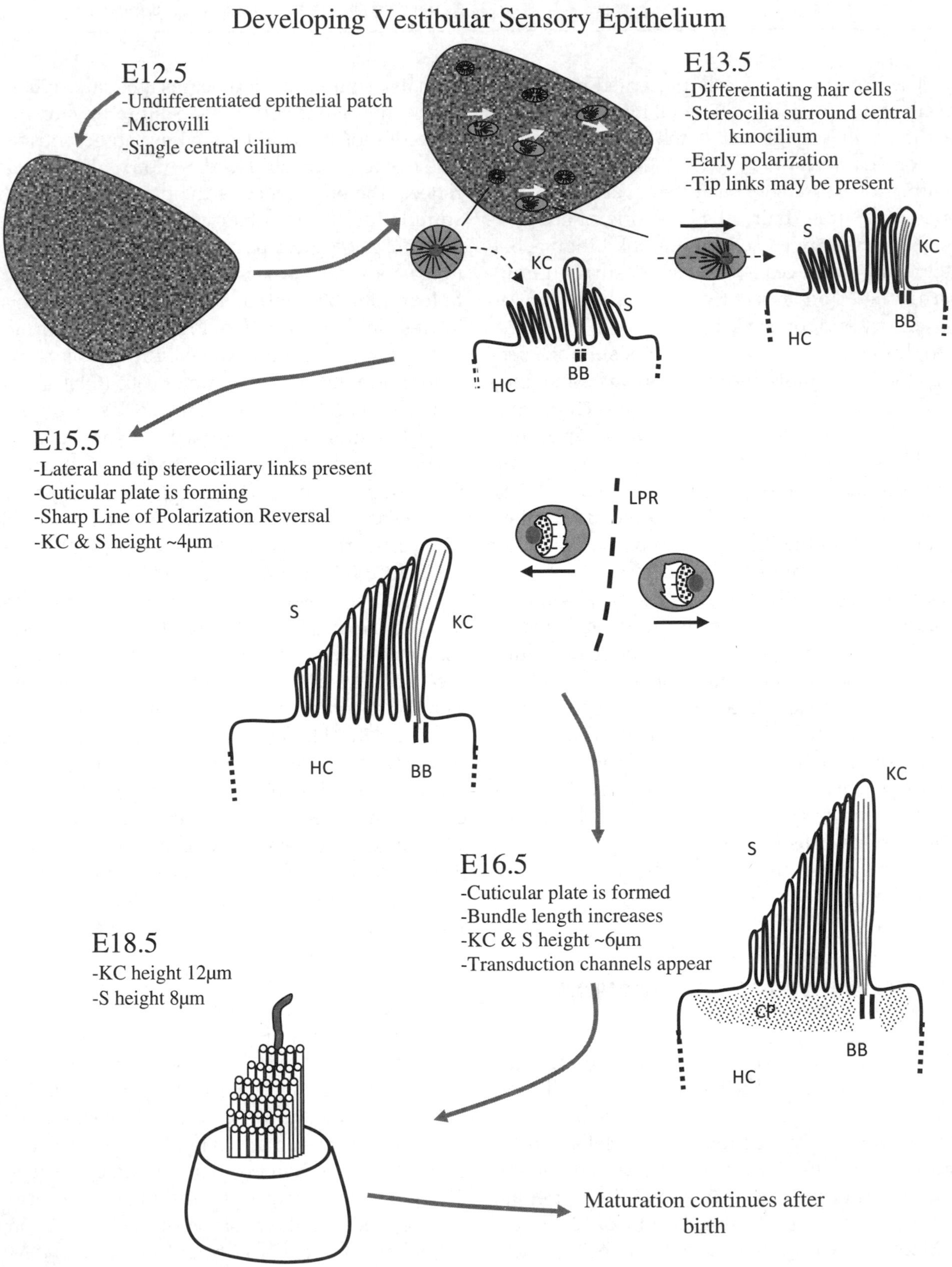
Developing Vestibular Sensory Epithelium
E12.5
-Undifferentiated epithelial patch
-Microvilli
-Single central cilium
E13.5
-Differentiating hair cells
-Stereocilia surround central kinocilium
-Early polarization
-Tip links may be present
KC
S
BB
HC
S
KC
BB
HC
E15.5
-Lateral and tip stereociliary links present
-Cuticular plate is forming
-Sharp Line of Polarization Reversal
-KC & S height ~4μm
LPR
S
KC
HC
BB
E16.5
-Cuticular plate is formed
-Bundle length increases
-KC & S height ~6μm
-Transduction channels appear
KC
S
CP
BB
HC
E18.5
-KC height 12μm
-S height 8μm
Maturation continues after birth

Figure 3–5. Development of vestibular stereociliary bundles. Ages and sizes represent mouse development. Early stages of development are similar for both auditory and vestibular hair cells although vestibular hair bundles begin appearing earlier than cochlear bundles. *KC* = kinocilium; *S* = stereocilia; *HC* = hair cell; *BB* = basal body; *LPR* = line of polarity reversal; *CP* = cuticular plate. From *Genetics, Embryology, and Development of Auditory and Vestibular Systems* (2011) (p.174) by Sherri M. Jones and Timothy A. Jones.

These MPV patterns arise during development and are thought to depend critically both on PCP signaling pathways and on intrinsic cell polarity.

Stereociliary bundles are not readily identified in vestibular hair cells before E13 (week 7), but as noted above they do begin to appear earlier than auditory hair cells (Bryant et al., 2005; Dechesne, 1992; Denman-Johnson & Forge, 1999; Forge et al., 1997; Mbiene, Favre, & Sans, 1984; Mbiene & Sans, 1986). Similar to the cochlea, the hair bundle is generally not polarized with its first appearance in a newly formed vestibular hair cell. The kinocilium is centrally located and surrounded by emerging stereocilia (see Figure 3–5). Although outward signs of polarization may not be apparent at this time, intracellular changes have already begun that clearly indicate proteins are being organized asymmetrically in the cell. The progressive development of selected features of vestibular hair cell bundles over the period E12 to E18.5 in the mouse (weeks 7 to 15) is illustrated in Figure 3–5. Morphological polarization occurs rapidly as the kinocilium assumes an eccentric position on the apical surface of hair cells. By E13.5 (week 8), signs of morphological polarization are seen in large numbers of cells (see Figure 3–5; E13.5). Moreover, already at this stage there is evidence of a planar organization of MPVs. MPV angles shift systematically as a function of position over the macular surface. A clear line of MPV reversal however is not seen. Thus, like auditory hair cells, planar organization of vestibular MPVs does not precisely match the mature organization initially. Reorientation of incipient MPVs is required. This happens quickly. By E15.5 (week 10) the striolar line of MPV reversal is sharp and clearly established (Denman-Johnson & Forge, 1999). The cuticular plate is first apparent in some macular hair cells using electron microscopy at about this time (E15.5, week 10), although traces of the cuticular plate are seen earlier using specific immunological markers (E13-E14) (Nishida, Rivolta, & Holley, 1998). Once bundles appear in vestibular hair cells, development of the normal staircase form and maturation occurs rapidly (see Figure 3–5). By E15.5 (week 11), typical staircase shapes and numerous lateral and tip stereocilia links can be found (Anniko, 1983a; Forge et al., 1997; Mbiene & Sans, 1986). Bundle height increases progressively from E15 (e.g., utricle on average ~4 μm) until maturation after birth (e.g., ste-

reocilia utricle ~12 μm) (Denman-Johnson & Forge, 1999). In the human, bundle height increases dramatically between weeks 10 and 11, and the bundles have achieved adult size by week 15 (Dechesne, 1992). Functional transduction channels make their appearance in the tips of stereocilia at about E16 (Géléoc & Holt, 2003), estimated to be week 12 for the human. Nascent hair cells continue to appear at the vestibular epithelial surface. Discrete samples in time give the impression of successive waves of new immature bundles. Hair bundles at various stages of development continue to mature, and the overlying otoconial membrane continues to elaborate until relatively mature hair bundle forms dominate the surface at E18 (weeks 11 to 12) (Denman-Johnson & Forge, 1999).

INNERVATION OF THE VESTIBULAR END ORGANS

There are three types of innervation to the inner ear. First, vestibular receptors communicate information about head motion to the brain via primary sensory afferent neurons having cell bodies in the peripheral statoacoustic ganglion. Statoacoustic ganglion neurons arise from within the otocyst during development as noted above. Second, the brain can also modify peripheral sensory receptors by adjusting activity in efferent neurons that have cell bodies in the brainstem and axon terminals on the inner ear hair cell sensors or on primary afferent terminals. Efferent neurons arise from rhombomere 4 during development (see below). Third, blood vessels of the inner ear are under the control of sympathetic neurons. These autonomic neurons originate from neural crest cells during development.

Development of Afferent Innervation

The statoacoustic ganglion and its neural projections form over the period from E10.5 to E17 (weeks 4 to 9) as progenitor cells delaminate from the anteroventral wall of the otocyst. By E13 (week 7), cochlear and vestibular anlagen can be distinguished histologically as medial and lateral portions of the statoacoustic ganglion, respectively (Figure 3–6). Although distinguishable, these two portions remain

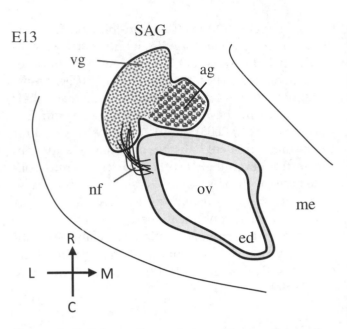

Figure 3–6. Schematic rendering of horizontal section through the otic vesicle (*ov*), statoacoustic ganglion (vestibular ganglion, *vg*, and acoustic ganglion, *ag*) at E13 in the mouse. Neural fibers (*nf*) projecting into the lateral wall of the otic vesicle. Arrows designate orientations for rostro-caudal axis (R, C, respectively) and medio-lateral axis (M, L, respectively). *ed* = endolymphatic duct, *me* = mesenchyme. From *Genetics, Embryology, and Development of Auditory and Vestibular Systems* (2011) (p.181) by Sherri M. Jones and Timothy A. Jones.

as a contiguous collection of cells until about E18 (by week 9) when they actually separate physically into the spiral and vestibular ganglia (Sher, 1971; Sulik & Cotanche, 2004). The geniculate ganglion (seventh or facial cranial nerve) separates completely from the vestibular ganglion finally on P1 in mouse.

Most sensory neurons are born between E11 and E14 (weeks 4 and 8). On E12 (week 6), fibers from the statoacoustic ganglion can be seen entering the rostrolateral wall and projecting well into the epithelium near the luminal surface of the otocyst (see Figure 3–6) (Sher, 1971; Van de Water, 1984). Efferent neurites arrive at about the same time (Bruce, Kingsley, Nichols & Fritzsch, 1997). The presence of auditory and vestibular afferents in epithelia is thought to precede slightly the arrival of efferent terminals and efferent neurites appear to follow afferent tracts during their growth (Bruce et al., 1997).

Neurotrophins regulate primary afferent innervation density. Neurotrophins are proteins secreted by target tissues that serve to prevent the natural cell

death of path finding neurons (Davies, 1996; Lewin & Barde, 1996; Levi-Montalcini, 1987; Levi-Montalcini & Angeletti, 1968). Hypothetically, the amount of neurotrophin present ultimately determines the number of neural cells that survive to innervate target cells. This ability to determine whether developing neurons survive is known as a neurotrophic effect. Elevated amounts of neurotrophin can cause excessive growth of neurites, whereas reduced levels of neurotrophin decrease neurite outgrowth and decrease survival of cells. The absence of neurotrophins can result in the loss of innervation entirely. Neurotrophins also have neurotropic effects, that is, they may serve to guide neurites along their growth paths (Fekete & Camparo, 2007; Fritzsch, Silas-Santiago, Bianchi, & Farinas, 1997; Levi-Montalcini, 1987).

The elaboration of afferent neurites appears to occur simultaneously with the delamination process in the otocyst. Two processes underlying afferent innervation of sensors have been emphasized (Fekete & Camparo, 2007; Fritzsch et al., 1997). In one model, neuroblasts send neurites back into sensory epithelia after delaminating and migrating out of the otocyst. This model requires a major guidance signal to aid neurites in their pathfinding. In the second model, the dendritic terminal endings of afferent neurites remain in the region of the original site of delamination, whereas the cell bodies migrate (translocate) to the mesenchyme rostromedial to the otocyst (see Figure 3–6). This leaves a ready-made dendritic path to target sensory regions. In this case, even though neurites are initially in the proximity of target sensory regions they must yet grow extensively and find their specific final sensory destinations. This second model provides an early formed path for arriving efferent neurites to follow on their way to the vestibular epithelium. There is evidence for both models, and it is conceivable that both models operate to some extent depending on the sensory organ involved. The importance of each model may depend on the species in question (e.g., bird versus mammal). The molecular cues operating to guide neurite growth are not clear in the inner ear, although several candidates have been entertained (Fekete & Camparo, 2007; Fritzsch et al., 1997; Pauley, Matei, Beisel, & Fritzsch, 2005). The candidates include neurotrophins that may be involved in both guidance and survival of primary afferent dendrites. The neurotrophins' brain-derived neurotrophic factor (BDNF) and neurotrophin-3 (NT-3) are required for proper innervation patterns and maintenance of all inner ear ganglion cells. In the absence of BDNF and NT-3, all ganglion cells die before birth (Ernfors, Van de Water, Loring, & Jaenisch, 1995; Liebl, Tessarollo, Palko, & Parada, 1997; Silos-Santiago, Fagan, Garber, Fritzsch, & Barbacid, 1997).

Statoacoustic ganglion neurons must also form central projections. Neurites of the central axon must grow and terminate on cells within the vestibular nuclei of the brainstem and cerebellum. Guidance mechanisms for axons projecting to the CNS are independent of those responsible for peripheral afferent terminations (Pauley et al., 2005). The signals guiding central afferent projections are unknown.

By E13 (week 7), peripheral afferent projections extend to all presumptive vestibular sensory epithelia (cristae and maculae) as well as to the wall of the cochlear duct (Dechesne, 1992; Sher, 1971). Terminals for vestibular afferent neurons at this stage are immature, and the final differentiation and refinement of these projections takes place over a prolonged period. In the mouse, final refinements in vestibular dendrites are made during postnatal periods. In the human, final refinements occur during the last trimester.

Vestibular afferent neurite terminals are present in the undifferentiated prosensory epithelium of the otocyst (see above). Specialized synaptic contacts have been reported for the mouse vestibular epithelium as early as E15 (Mbiene, Favre, & Sans, 1988). Early vestibular synaptic contacts form on postmitotic prosensory cells before, or coincident with, the onset of hair cell differentiation (~E12). Development of primary afferents in the human parallels events characterized in other mammals. Unmyelinated vestibular primary afferents in humans arrive in the undifferentiated epithelium during weeks 6 to 7 (Dechesne, 1992; Desmadryl, Dechesne, & Raymond, 1992). Apical tight junctions are present in nascent hair cells and prosensory epithelia in the human during this early period. Afferent neurites form numerous synaptic contacts on hair cells displaying emerging kinocilia by week 8. By 14 to 15 weeks, most hair bundles are relatively mature with only a few immature bundles appearing on the surface (Dechesne, 1992). Thus, given an early presence, it is likely that the earliest primary afferent contacts are made with immature "nonpolarized" hair cells.

Through collateralization, contacts may be made with a mixture of nonpolarized and polarized hair cells. Descriptions of the surface of the vestibular epithelium at E13 to E15 (weeks 8 to 10) suggest that, at any given time, despite a clearly established striolar boundary, there are a wide variety of hair cell developmental stages coexisting in the same vicinity. Moreover, this developmental mosaic is generalized across the macula (Denman-Johnson & Forge, 1999). Hair cells with immature bundles appear between relatively more mature hair cells forming a complex mosaic of hair cell stages. It is reasonable to imagine that a sensory unit, defined as one primary afferent and all hair cells it innervates, at this stage also incorporates a mosaic of hair cell polarization stages and directions. Thus, nascent sensory units are likely composed of hair cells that do not have a uniform hair bundle polarization status. It would appear that hair cells at this stage may take on a wide range of immature features including hair cells with varying and just emerging polarization vectors, particularly those innervating regions of the line of polarity reversal.

It is important to note that during the period from E14 to E16 (weeks 7 to 8), otoconial growth begins and calcification rates are at their highest levels (Lim, 1984; Nakahara & Bevelander, 1979; Salamat, Ross, & Peacor, 1980; Veenhof, 1969). Presumably, therefore, stimulus-dependent developmental processes in macular organs could become effective only during and after this period of otoconial formation. Although initial contacts may form early (~E12, ~week 7 in humans), they may not be functional synaptic contacts as most of the differentiation of vestibular neural dendrites occurs relatively late, from E18 to P9 (weeks 11 to 23) (Van de Water, Anniko, Nordemar, & Wersall, 1977; Dechesne, Rabejac, & Desmadryl, 1994; Rüsch, Lysakowski, & Eatock, 1998). Similarly the final maturation of vestibular hair cells (particularly membrane conductances), especially type I hair cells, occurs during the first and second postnatal weeks for mice (week 23+ for humans) (Dechesne, 1992).

By E17 in the mouse crista (week 8), primary afferent dendrites penetrate the basal lamina and send a single process passing through lower layers to the superficial apical layer where they branch to produce several undifferentiated collaterals (Desmadryl et al., 1992). The terminals are initially restricted in their extent and density but by E20 (week 12) they begin to ramify considerably, covering distances of 30 to 50 microns in diameter. At E18 (week 8), clear evidence of synaptic contacts between afferents and hair cells is present. Synaptic bodies and coated vesicles can be recognized in hair cell synaptic regions at 8 to 10 weeks (Dechesne, 1992). At these early stages the afferent terminals are still immature. Soon thereafter (E18 to E20) (week 12), the first evidence of incomplete calyces as well as bouton terminals can be seen (Dechesne, 1992; Dechesne et al., 1994; Rüsch et al., 1998; Van De Water et al., 1977). On P0 (weeks 12 to 13), there is a slight improvement where incomplete calyces, boutons, and type I and type II hair cells can be distinguished but are not mature. Numerous tethered dense core vesicles associated with well-formed synaptic ribbons can be identified between weeks 13 and 15 in the human (Dechesne, 1992). By approximately P5 (week 20), all three dendritic types are present and are distributed in their normal proportions over the crista. Although most features of the mature cristae are present, fine structure and function of the vestibular system in general continues to mature over several weeks after birth in the mouse. Development of these late features is discussed in more detail below.

Development of Efferent Innervation

The first efferent axons arrive in the prosensory regions of the mouse otocyst at about E12 (week 6) (Fritzsch & Nichols, 1993; Pujol et al., 1998). These neural processes have origins (cell bodies) in rhombomere 4 of the hindbrain (future brainstem; see Simmons, Duncan, Craponde Caprona, & Fritzsch, 2011, for review) and appear in the otocyst before hair cell differentiation (Bruce et al., 1997). Initially, vestibular efferent cell bodies form a single nucleus on each side of the brainstem (medial to vestibular nuclei, lateral to cranial nerve motor nucleus VI). Both ipsilateral and contralateral cell bodies give rise to early projections to each end organ. On either side of the cochlear and vestibular ganglia, efferent fibers tend to grow along the afferent tracts, and their appearance in time follows that of afferent projections (Bruce, Christensen, & Warr, 2000; Bruce et al., 1997). In the absence of afferent projections, efferent neurites do not reach the end organs (Ma, Anderson,

& Fritzsch, 2000). Efferents travel in the vestibular nerve until they reach the vestibulocochlear anastomosis, at which point cochlear efferents segregate from vestibular efferents and enter the spiral ganglion (by E12), initiating the intraganglionic spiral bundle (IGSB) by E14.5 (weeks 8 to 9). The IGSB follows the spiral ganglion through the course of the cochlear coil. There is some evidence that the earliest arrivals in the cochlea are medial olivocochlear fibers with cell body origins distinct from vestibular efferents (reviewed by Simmons, 2002).

As noted, vestibular efferents reach prosensory regions of the otocyst by E12, presumably having followed projections of post mitotic delaminating vestibular ganglion cells. Ultimately, efferent neurites follow afferent projections in the inferior and superior vestibular nerves to reach respective end organs. Little is known about the nature of terminal contacts made by efferents during these very early embryonic periods. It is likely that early efferent arrivals contact precursors to both Type I and Type II hair cells directly. Ultimately, efferents undergo extensive branching in all end organs and form bouton-type axosomatic endings on Type II hair cells and at later stages form axodendritic endings on calyx dendrites innervating Type I vestibular hair cells. Axodendritic efferent contacts appear relatively late since calyces begin forming late E18 to P0. It is likely that efferent contacts are made on the progenitors of Type I hair cells prior to calyx formation (Favre & Sans, 1978). However, what role, if any, these terminals play in the differentiation and maturation of the Type I hair cell is unknown. In his pioneering work, Van De Water (1976) concluded there was no influence of innervation on cytodifferentiation in explanted otocysts. Inasmuch as there was no ultrastructural evaluation of the explants, it may be worth reexamining this issue.

LATE DEVELOPMENT AND MATURATION OF VESTIBULAR SENSORS

Although still immature, the human can hear and respond to head movement at birth. Therefore, a functional inner ear emerges in the human fetus and, for this reason, the human is considered to be precocial. In contrast, many nonhuman mammals (e.g., mice, rats, cats, dogs, ferrets) (Rüsch et al., 1998; Curthoys, 1983; Heywood, Pujol, & Hilding, 1976; Van Cleave & Shall, 2006) are relatively unresponsive to head movement and deaf at birth and thus are considered altricial (or altricous). Vestibular function in these neonatal, nonhuman mammals matures during subsequent weeks.

In order to perceive head motion, the forces associated with head movement must reach the vestibular sensory apparatus, hair cells must transduce the mechanical stimulus into membrane currents and release neurotransmitter, and postsynaptic vestibular ganglion neurons must respond to the neurotransmitter and transmit discharges to the central nervous system (CNS). Once in the CNS, the signals must be processed and relayed via the brainstem nuclei and thalamus to vestibular sensory regions of the cortex (e.g., Lopez & Blanke, 2011; Shiroyama, Kayahara, Yasui, Nomura, & Nakano, 1999) where perception can take place. We focus here on the emergence of peripheral vestibular function, which covers adequate stimulation, stimulus transduction, and encoding of information in the primary afferents of the vestibular nerve.

Adequate Stimulation

The vestibular system is an example of a special sense that relies on elaborate ancillary structures to preferentially select, from among numerous potential environmental stimuli, only a few particular mechanical events that serve as adequate stimuli. For example, both vestibular and auditory hair cells are mechanoreceptors responding to displacement of the hair bundle along the axis of polarization. However, the most effective stimulus causing such shearing motion naturally is considerably different for the two sensors. In the vestibular system, normal head motion is effective in stimulating vestibular hair cells but not cochlear hair cells. Low levels of airborne sound effectively stimulate cochlear but not vestibular hair cells. Special structures are largely responsible for these functional attributes rather than substantial differences in the receptors (although there are differences to be sure).

In the vestibular system, there are dense otoconia that are packed into the otoconial membrane lying immediately over the stereociliary bundles in the maculae (utricle and saccule, see Chapter 1). These dense otoconial crystals, being fixed in the otoconial matrix, introduce a shearing force on macular hair cell bundles when placed under a linear acceleration field. Such a field occurs in association with head movement or in the presence of gravity, thus leading to the displacement of the otoconial membrane and stimulation of macular sensors. Without dense otoconia, macular hair cells are not stimulated (Jones, Erway, Bergstrom, Schimenti, & Jones, 1999; Jones, Jones, & Hoffman, 2008). Stimulation of ampullar organs depends on the semicircular canals and the inherent inertia of the endolymphatic fluids within the membranous labyrinth (see Chapter 1). During head rotation, pressure gradients develop across the cupula within the canal lumen due to the inertia of endolymphatic fluid. These pressure gradients distort the cupula and produce shearing forces at the surface of the sensory epithelium where hair cell bundles are displaced and hair cells are activated or inhibited. Without the canals and their fluid-filled patent lumen, the ampullae would be insensitive to head rotation.

Development of Vestibular Function

In mammals, movements of the mother or the fetus could serve as natural stimuli before birth. However, the actual time of onset for vestibular function (i.e., an adequate stimulus producing an appropriate neural response) during development in mammals and birds has not been determined. Nonetheless, we can estimate an earliest age based on known requirements for a functioning vestibular apparatus. In mice, the otoconial membrane and otoconia form from E14 to E16 and continue to elaborate at least until birth (Anniko, 1983a; Lim 1984; Nakahara & Bevelander, 1979; Salamat et al., 1980; Veenhof, 1969). In the human this occurs by week 10 (Dechesne, 1992). The semicircular canals form initially as epithelial tubes (semicircular ducts) beginning about E12.5 (Lim & Anniko, 1985; Sher, 1971). The ducts generally are well-formed and patent by about E15.5 (week 7). Between E12.5 and E14.5 (weeks 6 to 7), the cross-sectional shape of the ducts enlarges from a slit-like form to a much wider oval and the three ampullae are present by E13.5 (week 7). The cristae are emerging during this same period. The incipient cupula forms a thin membrane extending from the crista to the ampullar roof by E14.5 (Anniko, 1983a; Lim & Anniko, 1985). In the human the cupula is present by week 8 (Dechesne 1992). By birth in the mouse (weeks 10 to 12), the crista and cupula are well formed and semicircular ducts have the characteristic circular cross section (Lim & Anniko, 1985). Thus, it is conceivable that natural stimulation of ampullar and macular sensors could begin well before birth between E15.5 and P0 in rodents and at 9 to 12 weeks in the human (Dechesne, 1992).

Transduction Channels and Associated Membrane Currents

Although delivery of an adequate stimulus to the vestibular epithelium may be possible in the fetal human and mouse, are vestibular receptors capable of responding to natural stimulation prior to birth? Hair cell transduction channels are believed to be located in the tips of stereocilia (Beurg, Fettiplace, Nam, & Ricci, 2009; Hudspeth, 1982). The opening and closing of transduction channels are thought to be controlled by tip links tethered to adjacent stereocilia (Hudspeth, 1985; Pickles, Comis, & Osborne, 1984; Xu, Ricci, & Heller, 2009). Functional transduction channels appear first in vestibular hair cells. In the mouse, they appear suddenly over a period of approximately 24 hr between E16 and E17 (Géléoc & Holt, 2003) (estimated to be week 12 in the human). Tip links may appear 1 or 2 days earlier than transduction channels in the mouse (Denman-Johnson & Forge, 1999; Nayak, Ratnayaka, Goodyear, & Richardson, 2007). This timing parallels that of the appearance of otoconia in the maculae (Anniko, 1983a; Lim, 1984; Nakahara & Bevelander, 1979; Salamat et al., 1980; Veenhof, 1969) and the canal apparatus for the ampullae noted above. In the bird, hair cells are capable of responding to injected transduction currents very early (by E10) (Masetto, Perin, Malusà, Lucca, & Valli, 2000). However, it is not clear when transduction channels are actually functional in the bird. By E12, avian cochlear hair cells show evidence of open transduction channels (Si, Brodie, Gillespie, Vazquez, & Yamoah, 2003) and at E10 short hair cell bundles in the cochlea are present with tip links (Tilney, Tilney, Saunders, & DeRosier, 1986). Given that immature otoconia are present beginning at about E5 to E6 in the bird, it is likely that transduc-

tion channels appear sometime after the formation of otoconia (Dickman, Huss, & Lowe, 2004; Fermin & Igarashi, 1985, 1986; Kido et al., 1993; Kido, 1997). Thus, in the mammalian fetus, natural mechanical stimuli likely do reach vestibular hair cell receptors as they acquire the ability to transduce them into receptor potentials.

Hair Cell Response to Transduction Currents

The vestibular hair cell response (i.e., the receptor potential) to transduction currents depends on the nature of ionic channels located within basolateral portions of the hair cell membrane. When gated open, these basolateral ion channels permit the movement of particular ions across the membrane, thus contributing to current flow. Collectively, the ability to conduct currents (i.e., the property of conductance, symbolized as g) depends on the number of channels open for each type of channel. Each channel type is named according to the dominant ion species it conducts. Currents associated with particular channels are designated with an I and a subscript indicating the specific ion channel (e.g., potassium current, I_K). Conductance associated with the current I_K for example is designated as g_K. There are a variety of voltage-gated channels that are important in shaping the receptor potential. These include K^+, Na^+, and Ca^{2+} channels (Eatock & Hurley, 2003).

The mature hair cell receptor potential reproduces the shape of an applied depolarizing current. The receptor potential follows the input signal reliably so that the gating of channels at the basolateral surface and the release of neurotransmitter is synchronized to the stimulus input. The first hair cells born are not equipped with the adult complement of channels. Undifferentiated otocyst cells and new hair cells have few if any voltage-gated K^+ membrane channels (Correia, Rennie, &Koo, 2001; Eatock & Hurley, 2003; Sokolowski, Stahl, & Fuchs, 1993). Specific channels appear at different developmental stages in hair cells and each channel can impart different characteristics to the hair cells' response to transduction currents. By E10 in the chick, hair cell responses to simulated transduction currents show that early responses are slow and follow current profiles poorly. With the acquisition of new conductances, the hair cell's ability to follow stimuli improves. In the bird, mature-like vestibular hair cell membrane responses and a full complement of channels are present just before hatching (Masetto et al., 2000), whereas in the altricial mammal the mature configurations of channels and more mature responses emerge in the late embryo and neonate (E18 to P4) (Géléoc, Risner, & Holt, 2004; Masetto et al., 2000; Rüsch & Eatock, 1996; Rüsch, Lysakowski, & Eatock, 1998). Figure 3–7 illustrates how a vestibular hair cell receptor response to a depolarizing current step changes with the acquisition of new channels during development. The imposed depolarizing current is used to simulate depolarizing transduction currents. A relatively mature response (bottom trace) does not appear until the $g_{K,L}$ channels are present. The voltage response of the hair cell is the resulting receptor potential, which modulates transmitter release from the hair cell. Note the changes in the shape of the receptor potential as new ion channels are added at different ages of development.

A number of studies have examined the temporal sequence of channel acquisition (Eatock & Rüsch, 1997; Géléoc & Holt 2003; Géléoc et al., 2004; Hurley et al., 2006; Li, Meredith, & Rennie, 2010; Masetto et al., 2003; Rüsch et al., 1998; Sokolowski et al., 1993). We have tabulated the sequence of acquisition of several membrane ion channels for the chick and mouse

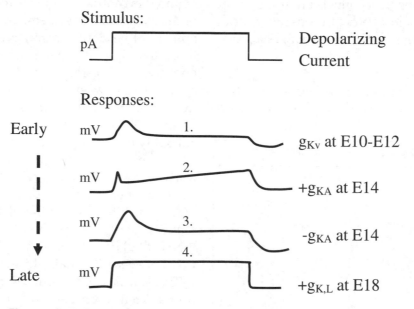

Figure 3–7. The effects of acquiring selected K⁺ channels on the hair cell receptor response. Top tracing shows the hypothetical step depolarizing current applied. This stimulus (levels reflected in picoamps, pA) simulates transduction currents. The four traces below the stimulus *trace (1–4)* are schematic representations of the receptor potential response. During development, the shape of the receptor potential changes with the addition or removal of each channel. The first response tracing represents a young age where the hair cell has acquired only the early delayed rectifier, g_{Kv} (*trace 1*). Additional channels appear successively over time (e.g., g_{KA}, $g_{K(Ca)}$, and $g_{K,L}$ *traces 2 and 4*). *Traces 2 and 3* illustrate the kind of change in membrane response produced by electrically inactivating g_{KA} (−g_{KA}) before presenting the stimulus (*trace 3*). Corresponding ages in the chick are shown to the right of traces. Note how ultimately the response follows the step depolarizing currents closely as the cell acquires $g_{K,L}$ (*trace 4*) and matures. Hair cell membrane voltage responses (mV) are schematic representations of data reported by Masetto et al. (2000) and Chen and Eatock (2000) with permission. From *Genetics, Embryology, and Development of Auditory and Vestibular Systems* (2011) (p. 216) by Sherri M. Jones and Timothy A. Jones.

(Table 3–1) based on the work of several laboratories (i.e., Géléoc et al., 2004; Masetto et al., 2000; Rüsch, Lysakowski et al., 1998). One striking difference to be noted regarding the acquisition sequence in vestibular hair cells versus that for auditory hair cells is the fact that there are no descriptions of Ca^{2+}-based hair cell action potentials (spikes) during vestibular development. Although the reason for this has not been explored, one might speculate that the early appearance of the fast I_{KA} and $I_{K(Ca)}$ (BK) channels in vestibular hair cells may prevent the development of hair cell spiking. In the cochlea, BK channels appear late in the maturation of inner hair cells (IHCs), and prior to their appearance, the IHCs generate spontaneous Ca^{2+}-based action potentials. Cochlear IHC spiking disappears as BK channels are upregulated during development just before the onset of hearing (Brandt et al., 2007; Fuchs & Sokolowski, 1990; Kros, Ruppersberg, & Rüsch, 1998; Marcotti, Johnson, Holley, & Kros, 2003a; Schweizer, Savis, Suu, Sultemeier, & Hoffman, 2009).

Table 3–1. Age of Appearance for Various Currents Recorded From Vestibular Hair Cells or Primary Afferent Neurons: Chicken and Mouse

Current	Chick	Mouse
I_{Kv}	E10	E14
I_{Ca}	E10	E15–birth*
I_{KA}	E12	?
$I_{K(Ca)}$	E14	P12–P23**
I_h	E16	P3
$I_{K,L}$	E17	E18
I_{Kir}	E19	E15

Note. The appearance and distribution of different ion channels throughout development contributes to the developing hair cell's response to stimulation, release of neurotransmitter, and developing neural discharge patterns. E = Chick: equivalent day of incubation; Mouse: Embryonic day or days postconception. P = postnatal day. ? = not reported. Information from Masetto et al. (2000) and Géléoc et al. (2004) unless otherwise noted.
Source: Genetics, Embryology, and Development of Auditory and Vestibular Systems (2011) (p. 217) by Sherri M. Jones and Timothy A. Jones.

*Expression in vestibular primary afferents beginning at E15 and decreasing by birth. Changes in the density of the different I_{Ca} types (L, P/Q, N, R, T) also occurred from E15 to birth (Chambard, Chabbert, Sans, & Desmadryl, 1999).

**Based on expression of BK channels in the rat (Schweizer, Savin, Luu, Sultemeier, & Hoffman, 2009), which first appear at P12 and diminish by P23.

BEHAVIORAL RESPONSE TO HEAD MOTION

In the precocial chicken, there is no question that the vestibular system is virtually mature at hatch inasmuch as hatchlings quickly learn to walk bipedally within minutes to hours. In the human, it also is likely that the peripheral vestibular system is mature at birth. However, it will be at least a year before any walking is done. Considerable maturation is required in central motor control circuitry as well as in the skeletomotor system. To evaluate the development of vestibular responses to head motion, it is useful to study the behavior of altricial mammals (rats, cats, mice, gerbils, etc.). In such animals, during a span of 2 or 3 weeks, the vestibular apparatus goes from nonfunctional to functionally mature and this occurs with observable behaviors. When a mature animal lying face up is dropped from a reasonable height onto a soft sponge base, it will turn quickly to right itself and land on its feet. This is the airrighting reflex and it can be used to assess the combined maturity of the vestibular and motor control systems. This reflex is absent at birth in rats when the vestibular system is still immature. It appears first between P10 and P15 (e.g., Hard & Larsson 1975; Laouris, Kalli-Laouri, & Schwartze, 1990). In contrast, reflex compensation to maintain gaze during rotation on a turntable appears as early as P4 in the rat (Parrad & Cottereau, 1977). Thus, despite immature peripheral receptors (noted above), it is clear that some behavioral responses can be elicited in the neonatal rodent. Of course behavioral testing alone leaves open to question whether the behavioral immaturities reflect the functional status of peripheral or central components or both. Human studies evaluating eye movements in response to rotational stimuli suggest some aspects of compensatory eye movements are mature at 6 to 10 months of age (e.g., Cioni, Favilla, Ghelarducci, & La Noce, 1984; Cyr, Brookhouser, Valente, & Grossman, 1985; Wiener-Vacher, Toupet, & Narcy, 1996) although other aspects continue to mature up to late childhood or adolescence (e.g., Cyr et al., 1985; Herman, Maulucci,

& Stuyck, 1982; Wiener-Vacher et al., 1996; Valente, 2007). Studies of standing balance function generally demonstrate continued maturation of balance into late childhood and adolescence (e.g., Casselbrant et al., 2010; Charpiot, Tringali, Ionescu, Vital-Durand, & Ferber-Viart, 2010; Hirabayashi & Iwasaki 1995; Valente, 2007). It is likely that behavioral maturation in the human is due to central myelination and circuit refinements after birth. Recent work in this area is summarized at the end of this section.

PRIMARY AFFERENT FUNCTION

When recording normal mature individual vestibular primary afferent neurons in the absence of head movement, the neurons are not silent but rather discharge spontaneously and continuously (Figure 3–8). This is true for afferent neurons innervating both ampullar (semicircular canal) and macular (otoconial or gravity) receptors. Discharge rate (action

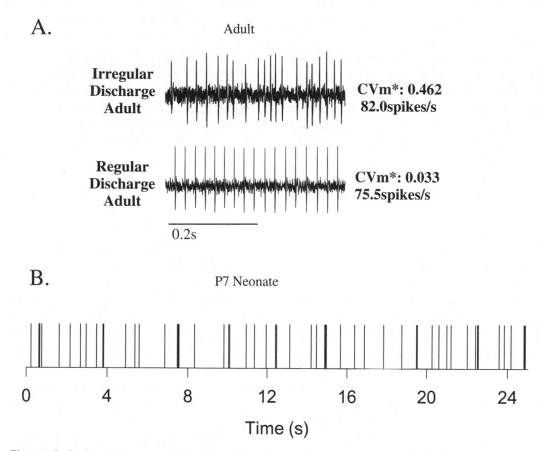

Figure 3–8. Spontaneous discharge activity of vestibular primary afferent neurons in mice. **A.** Adult mice: Each voltage spike represents an individual action potential. No stimulus is presented. These cells were chosen for illustration because they have similar high discharge rates. Two types of activity patterns are recognized. Irregular discharge (*top tracing*) is characterized by irregular spacing between spikes. A regular spike discharge pattern tends to show regular spacing between spikes and a low CV. Modified from Jones, Jones et al. (2008). **B.** Spontaneous spike train of primary afferent neuron recorded from the superior vestibular nerve in the neonatal mouse at P7. Note the time scale difference in B. This record was made over a period of approximately 24 s. Each vertical "spike" represents the onset time of the neural spike discharge during this portion of the recording. Discharge rate is slow and an irregular firing pattern (with high CV) typical for neonatal vestibular neurons is apparent. CVm* = indicates that CV values were normalized for spontaneous rate based on mouse data. From *Genetics, Embryology, and Development of Auditory and Vestibular Systems* (2011) (p. 219) by Sherri M. Jones and Timothy A. Jones.

potentials/sec, also called spikes/sec) remains relatively constant unless the head is moved thus stimulating or inhibiting hair cells and neurons innervating them. At first thought, in the absence of head movement one might suppose that such tonic activity is due to the constant stimulation of gravity receptors (utricle and saccule) by the ever-present gravitation field of Earth. However, tonic spontaneous vestibular afferent discharge is present in animals that have no otoconia and thus animals that cannot sense gravity (Jones, Jones et al., 2008). Continuous (tonic) activity arising from the vestibular sensors normally provides a profound influence on central nervous system circuitry throughout most of the neuraxis including brainstem, hypothalamic, and limbic systems (e.g., Balaban, 2002; Balaban & Porter, 1998; Porter & Balaban 1997; Yates, 1996; Yates & Miller, 1998). These afferent signals assert a powerful influence on descending skeletomotor and autonomic systems as well as provide input for compensatory eye movements, perceptual tracking of position and orientation in space. Tonic vestibular activity constantly adjusts alpha and gamma motor neuron outflow thus controlling background antigravity muscle tone and posture under an imposing gravitational force field. Thus, spontaneous as well as sensory-induced tonic activity arising from vestibular sensors plays an important role in nervous system function generally.

Spontaneous vestibular discharge patterns are of two types in mammals and birds: regular and irregular. Just how regular or irregular the neural discharge is depends in part on the nature of the dendritic synaptic termination and on the nature of the membrane channels resident in the neuron (Eatock, Xue, & Kalluri, 2008; Iwasaki, Chihara, Komuta, Ito, & Sahara, 2008; Kalluri, Xue, & Eatock, 2010). The regularity can vary widely and this variety can be quantified using a single number called the coefficient of variation (CV = standard deviation/mean spike interval). The value of the CV varies generally between 0 and 1. The CV approaches 1.0 as the discharge pattern becomes more irregular (more stochastic to be precise), whereas CV approaches 0.0 as the discharge becomes more regular. Figure 3–8 illustrates the discharge patterns of regular and irregular vestibular afferents in mature (see Figure 3–8A) and developing (see Figure 3–8B, P7 neonate) mice. Discharge rates in mature mice range from less

than 10 to over 140 spikes/sec with most between 55 and 110 spikes/sec (e.g., Jones, Jones et al., 2008). The recordings of Figure 3–8B were made in vivo from primary afferent neurons of the superior vestibular nerve (Jones & Jones, 2011). The discharge pattern of the neonate reflects a relatively low discharge rate (~8 spikes/sec) with irregular discharge timing (CV = 0.66).

Recording the activity patterns of individual vestibular primary afferent neurons in intact animals (i.e., in vivo) is challenging. Some investigators have instead explored the use of vestibular explant preparations. In this case, the labyrinth with the ganglia are removed and maintained in a physiological solution. Vestibular primary afferents recorded in a mouse inner ear explant preparation are also spontaneously active (Desmadryl, Raymond, & Sans, 1986). Afferent discharge patterns in explants have been measured on different postnatal days. Mean spontaneous discharge rates were low initially (P0: 5 to 10 spikes/sec) and all neurons displayed irregular activity. Remarkably, regular discharge patterns were found at P1 and older. Beginning between P6 and P8 discharge rates increased dramatically (>80 spikes/sec), and the proportion of regular fibers increased as well. In a similar preparation in the chicken, Galicia, Cotes, and Galindo (2010) reported irregular spontaneous discharge rates on the order of 40 spikes/sec and CVs above 1.0 in recordings as early as E15. Many of the patterns found in the in vitro preparation were similar to those reported for in vivo studies (discussed below). In vitro studies provide many practical advantages while at the same time raising the question of whether neurons behave the same when studied in their natural environment, that is, in vivo.

Spontaneous discharge patterns of horizontal canal neurons have also been recorded in vivo in the neonatal rat from ages P1 to P20 (Curthoys, 1983). Discharge rates were low at the youngest ages (<10 spikes/sec, P1 to P3), and all neurons exhibited irregular spontaneous discharge patterns. The first regular fibers were seen on P4. Discharge rates and the proportion of regular fibers increased substantially after P10 (30 to 40 spikes/sec). Nonetheless, rates for regular cells were still somewhat below the adult values at P20. Romand and Dauzat (1982) reported similar findings in the cat except that regular spontaneous discharge patterns were seen as early as P1. An example of an irregularly discharging macular primary afferent at P7 is shown in Figure 3–8B (mouse in vivo recording). In vivo recordings in the chick embryo at E19 showed that regular discharge patterns were present, and on average the rate for embryos was 22 spikes/sec versus 60 spikes/sec for posthatch animals (Jones & Jones, 2000b). Note that discharge rates were somewhat lower in the in vivo recordings compared to explants. This may reflect the effects of anesthesia used in in vivo preparations or conditions associated with in vitro preparations. In summary, in the rodent at birth, spontaneous activity is immature evidencing low discharge rates and dominated by irregular firing patterns. Maturation of discharge patterns progresses over a period of weeks.

One role of the horizontal canal is to detect head turning and to activate vestibular neurons to send a signal to the brainstem that produces eye movements that compensate for head motion and maintain gaze on a stationary visual target. This is known as the vestibulo-ocular reflex (VOR). One question to ask is when primary afferents are capable of delivering a compensatory signal comparable to that of the mature system. Curthoys (1983) evaluated this question by measuring the response of horizontal canal primary afferent neurons to head rotation in rats at ages from P1 to P20. At P1 neural responses were sluggish and highly variable. By P6 to P8, the neural response gain approached that of the adult. This suggests that, for some stimuli, the neuroepithelium at P8 is capable of generating signals comparable to those of an adult. These findings are consistent with results noted above showing that morphological and electrophysiological features of hair cell function (e.g., calyx, membrane channels, vestibular efferents, etc.) emerge during the first 2 to 3 postnatal weeks in rodents (weeks 13 to 23). Indeed, VOR gains in juvenile mice (P21 to P26) are slightly, but significantly, lower than mature animals at 3 to 4 months old (Faulstich, Onori, & du Lac, 2004). Central improvements likely mediate the final maturation changes. Similar maturational changes are reported for children (Casselbrant et al., 2010).

The basic structural elements of the macula are in place in the chick before hatch (by E16). The question is, when does macular function emerge? Little information is available regarding macular

functional development in any species. Recordings of vestibular macular compound action potentials (VsEPs) have been made in embryos and hatchling chicks (E18 to P22) (Jones & Jones, 2000a). Responses were obtained as early as E19 (1 to 2 days before hatch). Therefore, the onset of macular function occurs at least by E19 in the chick and likely earlier. Macular response thresholds decreased rapidly to approach adult values within days of hatch. Other response characteristics also matured systematically over similar periods (response latency shortened and amplitudes increase). These findings and the fact that chicks are able to walk and run within hours of hatching show that in the chick the vestibular periphery matures early and is functional even before hatch.

DEVELOPMENTAL MILESTONES OF VESTIBULAR FUNCTION AND BALANCE BEHAVIORS IN THE HUMAN

By the 12th to 14th week of gestation, the human vestibular epithelium appears almost mature and contains Type I and II hair cells, myelinated calyx-bearing and bouton terminated afferent neurons as well as efferent axon terminals (Dechesne, 1992). Ten weeks later (week 24) they are considered adult-like and at birth, some 10 to 16 weeks later (weeks 36 to 40), the periphery is considered mature. Although the vestibular periphery may be mature at birth in the human, this is not readily apparent from human behavior (unlike the case in the chick above). The human neonate requires a substantial period of time (years, see below) to acquire a mature vestibular-linked behavioral repertoire. It is clear that central myelination and circuit refinements must take place in order to fully equip the otherwise largely immature cortical, cerebellar, extrapyramidal, and brainstem descending motor control systems for the support of mature behavioral motor programs and postures. Behaviors such as walking and running as well as mature posturing must develop after birth in the human (e.g., sitting up, rolling over, even holding one's head up, see Table 3–2) (Eviatar & Eviatar 1978; Frankenburg & Dodds, 1967). Table 3–2 summarizes well-known developmental milestones for

Table 3–2. Familiar Developmental Milestones for Motor Skills in the Human Infant

Motor Skill	25% (months)	50% (months)	75% (months)	90% (months)
Lifts head (prone)				0.7
Lifts head 90 degrees (prone)	1.3	2.2	2.6	3.2
Chest up, arm support (prone)	2.0	3.0	3.5	4.3
Sits (head steady)	4.8	5.5	6.5	7.8
Rolls over	2.3	2.8	3.8	4.7
Stands holding on	5.0	5.8	8.5	10.0
Walks well	11.3	12.1	13.5	14.3

Note. Selected data from Frankenberg and Dodds (1967). Age (months) at which the respective fraction (25%, 50%, 75%, and 90%) of infants successfully completed motor tasks listed.

motor skills in the human infant. Central immaturities therefore can obscure or mask true vestibular functional capability as well as deficits in neonates and children. Moreover, failure to recognize vestibular deficits may, in the absence of intervention, put individuals at risk for developing abnormal postural, dynamic motor control and/or motor effector systems (e.g., De Kegel, Maes, Baetens, Dhooge, & Van Waelyelde, 2012; Fife, Tusa, & Furman, 2000; Shall, 2009; Van Cleave & Shall, 2006).

A functional vestibular periphery is evident in the human neonate. Full-term normal infants generally evidence vestibular mediated ocular compensation induced by head rotation (Cyr et al., 1985; Donat, Donat, & Lay, 1980; Eviatar & Eviatar, 1978, 1979; Eviatar, Eviatar, & Naray, 1974; Ornitz, Atwell, Walter, Hartmann, & Kaplan, 1979; Staller, Goin, & Hildebrandt, 1986; Tibbling, 1969; Wiener-Vacher et al., 1996). Head rotation elicits a bilateral response from the vestibular periphery. VOR measurements at the youngest ages generally show tonic conjugate deviation of the eyes in a direction opposite that of rotation, and may include occasional rapid saccades. The slow compensatory movement is dependent on the vestibular periphery, whereas saccades depend on brainstem circuitry (see Chapter 2). A reduced number or frequency of saccades reflects the immature state of brainstem neural circuits. The presence of saccades in the neonate is in part dependent on frequency of rotation. Saccades may be absent in very young or premature infants but are found consistently in normal 1- to 3-month-old babies.

Caloric testing in the neonate evaluates each ear separately and has often provided evidence of central immaturity especially in premature infants (Donat et al., 1980; Eviatar et al., 1974; Eviatar & Eviatar, 1979). VOR responses to calorics are variable and may be absent in infants less than 6 months. By 3 to 6 months a consistent VOR is generally present (Cyr et al., 1985; Donat et al., 1980; Eviatar et al., 1974; Eviatar & Eviatar, 1979). The absence of a VOR at 10 months or older is considered abnormal (Fife et al., 2000). Most abnormal responses (e.g., disconjugate eye movements, tonic ocular deviation, absent saccades) were found in premature or very young normal-term babies (Donat et al., 1980; Tibbling, 1969, rotary chair Bárány test), but such abnormalities generally reflected central immaturities which disappeared with maturation. Thus, improvements in vestibular responses largely represent central maturational processes which ultimately occur over several years.

Vestibular reflex testing and posturography also have been used to provide insight regarding the time course of maturation in children and demonstrate that the process begins very early in the neonate and continues into adolescence. There is considerable variation in the VOR findings for some parameters in growing children. Results depend on the particular metric used to characterize eye movements and range of subject ages represented. Measurements can also be affected by the subjects' state of alertness. The ability to arouse and maintain alertness throughout testing is itself a function of age and this can influence results.

Using Bárány rotary chair testing, a number of investigators have reported a decrease in velocity of the VOR slow component with maturation (Ornitz et al., 1979; Tibbling, 1969; Wiener-Vacher et al., 1996). Maturational changes appeared to be larger during the first year after birth, and change more slowly thereafter into adolescence. Although these results outline a temporal profile, it is difficult to relate the findings to specific components of the vestibular ocular reflex.

VOR gain provides better insight regarding the effectiveness of vestibular reflex compensation for head motion. VOR gain reportedly increased linearly in a group of 120 children studied longitudinally over the period from 3 to 9 years of age (e.g., mean gains: 3 years: 0.58 to 9 years: 0.82, for 0.5 Hz) (Casselbrant et al., 2010), whereas thereafter from young adolescence to the adult, gain reportedly may decrease slightly at some frequencies (Herman et al., 1982; Valente, 2007). The findings of Charpiotet et al. (2010) also indicated a decreasing gain for a slightly older group of children (6 to 12 years old). Others found little difference in VOR gain over ages studied (7 to 12 years old: Horak, Schumway-Cook, Crowe, & Black, 1988; 3 months to 6 years: Cyr et al., 1985). However, the range of ages and frequencies studied were somewhat different and sample sizes were smaller in the latter cases, which may in part account for differences in findings. At any given age the variance for VOR gain in humans is quite large (e.g., Peterka, Black, & Schoenhoff, 1990a, 1990b). Nonetheless, there is support for the hypothesis that a slow systematic maturation of VOR gain (increasing mean) occurs in the young child through preadolescence and small reductions in mean gain from the second to third decade of life. In addition to evidence cited above, evidence for this comes from a large cross-sectional study of 261 individuals, ages 7 to 81 years old, which indicates a similar temporal profile where VOR gains appear highest for ages 7 to 20 years old and then decrease somewhat and remain relatively stable over the ages from 30 to 81 years old (Peterka et al., 1990a, 1990b). Changes in VOR gain are small relative to the variance in any

case. Controversy persists in the literature regarding maturation over ages from approximately 10 to 30 years old. In the future, it will be important to use standardized methods and metrics including standard frequencies and rotational velocities to minimize variability across studies. It would be helpful to see large longitudinal studies providing normative data for VOR in children and adults through the third decade of life. Such studies, although difficult to achieve, would serve to clarify the profile of change in the VOR over the human lifetime.

Computerized dynamic posturography (CDP) includes a sensory organization test (SOT), which provides a measure of how effectively sensory information is used by an individual to maintain balance and stability under dynamic postural challenge. SOT examines how one uses visual, somatosensory, and vestibular information to maintain balance and quantifies, among other things, the amount of sway exhibited. Several investigators have used the SOT in children between the ages of 3 and 15 years old to characterize changes in balance skills with maturation and to develop normative data on sensory weighting strategies (e.g., Casselbrant et al., 2010; Charpiot et al., 2010; Hirabayashi & Iwasaki, 1995; Peterka & Black, 1990; Peterson, Christou, & Rosengren, 2006; Valente, 2007). The evidence suggests a steady improvement on vestibular tasks that continues into late childhood and by some reports into adolescent years when scores approached those of adults. In general, skills in the use of vestibular sensory input were the last to mature relative to use of somatosensory and visual cues for maintaining balance.

In summary, whereas the peripheral vestibular apparatus is essentially mature at birth, central maturation continues into adolescence. The VOR can be elicited in the neonate and it matures substantially over the first 3 years. Improvement generally continues into adolescence when adult balance skills are achieved. Although progress in our understanding has been made, it should be clear that we are only meagerly informed about the complex multisensory process of maturation in human postural balance and vestibular reflex systems. Our understanding of human vestibular development would benefit substantially from additional research aimed at establishing normative data over wider age ranges and improving our ability to make functional assessments at all ages.

REFERENCES

Anniko, M. (1983a). Embryonic development of vestibular sense organs and their innervation. In R. Romand (Ed.), *Development of auditory and vestibular systems* (pp. 375–423). New York, NY: Guilford Press.

Anniko, M. (1983b). Cytodifferentiation of cochlear hair cells. *American Journal of Otolaryngology, 4*, 375–388.

Balaban, C. D. (2002). Neural substrates linking balance control and anxiety. *Physiology & Behavior, 77*, 469–475.

Balaban, C. D., & Porter, J. D. (1998). Neuroanatomic substrates for vestibulo-autonomic interatctions, *Journal of Vestibular Research, 8*, 7–16.

Bermingham, N. A., Hassan, B. A., Price, S. D., Vollrath, M. A., Ben-Arie, N., Eatock, R. A., . . . Zoghbi, H. Y. (1999). Math1: An essential gene for the generation of inner ear hair cells. *Science, 284*, 1837–1841.

Beurg, M., Fettiplace, R., Nam, J. -H., & Ricci, A. J. (2009). Localization of inner hair cell mechanotransducer channels using high-speed calcium imaging. *Nature Neuroscience, 12*, 553–558.

Bok, J., Chang, W., & Wu, D. K. (2007). Patterning and morphogenesis of the vertebrate inner ear. *International Journal of Developmental Biology, 51*, 521–533.

Brandt, N., Kuhn, S., Münker, S., Braig, C., Winter, H., Blin, N., . . . Engel, J. (2007). Thyroid hormone deficiency affects postnatal spiking activity and expression of Ca^{2+} and K^+ channels in rodent inner hair cells. *Journal of Neuroscience, 27*(12), 3174–3186.

Bredberg, G. (1968). Cellular pattern and nerve supply of the human organ of Corti [Supplemental material]. *Acta Oto-Laryngologica, 236*, 1–135.

Bruce, L. L., Christensen, M. A., & Warr, B. (2000). Postnatal development of efferent synapses in the rat cochlea. *Journal of Comparative Neurology, 423*, 532–548.

Bruce, L. L., Kingsley, J., Nichols, D. H., & Fritzsch, B. (1997). The development of vestibulocochlear efferents and cochlear afferents in mice. *International Journal of Developmental Neuroscience, 15*(4–5), 671–692.

Bryant, J. E., Forge, A., & Richardson, G. P. (2005). The differentiation of hair cells. In M.W. Kelley, D. Wu, A. A. Popper, & R. R. Fay (Eds.), *Development of the inner ear* (pp. 158–203). New York, NY: Springer-Verlag.

Casselbrant, M. L., Mandel, E. M., Sparto, P. J., Perera, S., Redfern, M. S., Fall, P.A., . . . Furman, J. (2010). Longitudinal posturography and rotational testing in children three to nine years of age: Normative data. *Otolaryngology-Head and Neck Surgery, 142*, 708–714.

Charpiot, A., Tringali, S., Ionescu, E., Vital-Durand, F., & Ferber-Viart, C. (2010). Vestibulo-ocular reflex and balance maturation in healthy children aged from six to twelve years. *Audiology and Neurotology, 15*, 203–210.

Chen, P., Johnson, J. E., Zoghbi, H. Y., & Segil, N. (2002). The role of Math1 in inner ear development: Uncoupling the establishment of the sensory primordium from hair cell fate determination. *Development, 129*, 2495–2505.

Chen, P., & Segil, N. (1999). P27kip1 links cell proliferation to morphogenesis in the organ of Corti. *Development, 126*, 1581–1590.

Cioni, G., Favilla, M., Ghelarducci, B., & La Noce, A. (1984). Development of the dynamic characteristics of the horizontal vestibulo-ocular reflex in infancy. *Neuropediatrics, 15*(3), 125–130.

Correia, M. J., Rennie, K. J., & Koo, P. (2001). Return of potassium ion channels in regenerated hair cells. Possible pathways and the role of intracellular calcium signaling. *Annals of the New York Academy of Sciences, 942*, 228–240.

Curthoys, I. S. (1983). Development of function of primary vestibular neurons. In R. Romand (Ed.), *Development of auditory and vestibular systems* (pp. 425–461). New York, NY: Academic Press.

Cyr, D. G., Brookhouser, P. E., Valente, M., & Grossman, A. (1985). Vestibular evaluation of infants and preschool children. *Journal of Otolaryngology-Head and Neck Surgery, 93*, 463–468.

Davies, A. M. (1996). The neurotrophic hypothesis: Where does it stand? *Philosophical Transactions of the Royal Society of London B, 351*, 389–394.

Dechesne, C. J. (1992). The development of vestibular sensory organs in human. In R. Romand (Ed.), *Development of auditory and vestibular systems 2* (pp. 419–447). Amsterdam, the Netherlands: Elsevier.

Dechesne, C. J., Rabejac, D., & Desmadryl, G. (1994). Development of calretinin immunoreactivity in the mouse inner ear. *Journal of Comparative Neurology, 346*, 517–529.

De Kegel, A., Maes, L., Baetens, T., Dhooge, I., & Van Waelvelde H. (2012). The influence of a vestibular dysfunction on the motor development of hearing-impaired children. *Laryngoscope, 122*, 2837–2843.

Denman-Johnson, K., & Forge, A. (1999). Establishment of hair bundle polarity and orientation in the developing vestibular system of the mouse. *Journal of Neurocytology, 28*, 821–835.

Desmadryl, G., Dechesne, C., & Raymond, J. (1992). Recent aspects of development of the vestibular sense organs and their innervation. In R. Romand (Ed.), *Development of auditory and vestibular systems 2* (pp. 461–487). Amsterdam, the Netherlands: Elsevier.

Desmadryl, G., Raymond, J., & Sans, A. (1986). In vitro electrophysiological study of spontaneous activity in neonatal mouse vestibular ganglion neurons during development. *Developmental Brain Research, 25*, 133–136.

Dickman, J. D., Huss, D., & Lowe, M. (2004). Morphometry of otoconia in the utricle and saccule of developing Japanese quail. *Hearing Research, 188,* 89–103.

Donat, J. F. G., Donat, J. R., & Lay, K. S. (1980). Changing response to caloric stimulation with gestational age in infants. *Neurology, 30,* 776–778.

Driver, E. C., Sillers, L., Coate, T. M., Rose, M. F., & Kelley, M. W. (2013). The Atoh1-lineage gives rise to hair cells and supporting cells within the mammalian cochlea. *Developmental Biology, 376,* 86–98.

Eatock, R. A., & Hurley, K. M. (2003). Functional development of hair cells. In R. Romand & I. Vareal-Nieto (Eds.), *Development of auditory and vestibular systems 3* (pp. 389–448). Amsterdam, the Netherlands: Elsevier.

Eatock, R. A., & Rüsch, A. (1997). Developmental changes in the physiology of hair cells. *Seminars in Cell & Developmental Biology, 8,* 265–275.

Eatock, R. A., Xue, J., & Kalluri, R. (2008). Ion channels in mammalian vestibular afferents may set regularity of firing. *Journal of Experimental Biology, 211,* 1764–1774.

Ernfors, P., Van de Water, T., Loring, J., & Jaenisch, R. (1995). Complementary roles of BDNF and NT-3 in vestibular and auditory development. *Neuron, 14,* 1153–1164.

Eviatar, L., & Eviatar, A. (1978). Neurovestibular examination of infants and children. *Advanced Oto-Rhino-Laryngology, 23,* 169–191.

Eviatar, L., & Eviatar, A. (1979). The normal nystagmic response of infants to caloric and perrotatory stimulation. *Laryngoscope, 89,* 1036–1045.

Eviatar, L., Eviatar, A., & Naray, I. (1974). Maturation of neurovestibular responses in infants. *Developmental Medicine and Child Neurology, 16,* 435–446.

Faulstich, B. M., Onori, K. A., & du Lac, S. (2004). Comparison of plasticity and development of mouse optokinetic and vestibulo-ocular reflexes suggests differential gain control mechanisms. *Vision Research, 44,* 3419–3427.

Favre, D., & Sans, A. (1978). The development of vestibular efferent nerve endings during cat maturation: Ultrastructural study. *Brain Research, 142,* 333–337.

Fekete, D. M., & Camparo, A. M. (2007). Axon guidance in the inner ear. *International Journal of Developmental Biology, 51,* 549–556.

Fermin, C. D., & Igarashi, M. (1985). Development of otoconia in the embryonic chick. *Acta Anatomica, 123,* 148–152.

Fermin, C. D., & Igarashi, M. (1986). Review of statoconia formation in birds and original research in chick. *Scanning Electron Microscopy, 4,* 1649–1655.

Fife, T. D., Tusa, R. J., & Furman, J. M. (2000). Assessment: Vestibular testing techniques in adults and children: Report of the Therapeutics and Technology Assessment Subcommittee of the American Academy of Neurology. *Neurology, 55,* 1431–1441.

Forge, A., Souter, M., & Denman-Johnson, K. (1997). Structural development of sensory cells in the ear. *Seminars in Cell & Developmental Biology, 8,* 225–237.

Frankenburg, W. K., & Dodds, J. B. (1967). The Denver Developmental Screening test. *Journal of Pediatrics, 71,* 181–191.

Fritzsch, B., Beisel, K. W., Jones, K., Farinas, I., Maklad, A., Lee, J., & Reichardt, L. F. (2002). Development and evolution of inner ear sensory epithelia and their innervations. *Journal of Neurobiology, 53,* 143–156.

Fritzsch, B., & Nichols, D. H. (1993). DiI reveals a prenatal arrival of efferents at the differentiating otocyst of mice. *Hearing Research, 65,* 51–60.

Fritzsch, B., Silas-Santiago, I., Bianchi, L. M., & Farinas, I. (1997). The role of neurotrophic factors in regulating the development of inner ear innervation. *Trends in Neuroscience, 20*(4), 159–164.

Fuchs, P. A., & Sokolowski, B. H. A. (1990). The acquisition during development of Ca++ activated potassium currents by cochlear hair cells of the chick. *Proceedings of the Royal Society of London B, 241,* 122–126.

Galicia, S., Cotes, C., & Galindo, F. (2010) Development of spontaneous activity and response properties of primary lagenar neurons in the chick. *Cell and Molecular Neurobiology, 30,* 327–331.

Géléoc, G. S. G., & Holt, J. R. (2003). Developmental acquisition of sensory transduction in hair cells of the mouse inner ear. *Nature Neuroscience, 6*(10), 1019–1020.

Géléoc, G. S. G., Risner, J. R., & Holt, J. R. (2004). Developmental acquisition of voltage-dependent conductances and sensory signaling in hair cells of the embryonic mouse inner ear. *Journal of Neuroscience, 24*(49), 11148–11159.

Ginzberg, R. D., & Gilula, N. B. (1979). Modulation of cell junctions during differentiation of the chicken otocyst sensory epithelium. *Developmental Biology, 68,* 110–129.

Groves, A. K. (2005). The induction of the otic placode. In M. W. Kelley, D. K. Wu, A. N. Popper, & R. R. Fay (Eds.), *Development of the ear* (pp. 10–42). New York, NY: Springer-Verlag.

Hamburger, V., & Hamilton, H. L. (1951). A series of normal stages in the development of the chick embryo. *Journal of Morphology, 88,* 49092.

Hard, E., & Larsson, K. (1975). Development of righting in rats. *Brain and Behavioral Evolution, 11,* 53–59.

Herman, R., Maulucci, R., & Stuyck, J. (1982). Development and plasticity of visual and vestibular generated eye movements. *Experimental Brain Research, 47,* 69–78.

Heywood, P., Pujol, R., & Hilding, D. A. (1976). Development of the labyrinthine receptors in the guinea pig, cat and dog. *Acta Oto-Laryngologica, 82,* 359–367.

Hirabayashi, S., & Iwasaki, Y. (1995). Developmental perspective of sensory organization on postural control. *Brain & Development, 17,* 111–113.

Horak, F. B., Schumway-Cook, A., Crowe, T. K., & Black, F. O. (1988). Vestibular function and motor proficiency of children with impaired hearing, or with learning disability and motor impairments. *Developmental Medicine and Child Neurology, 30,* 64–79.

Hudspeth, A. J. (1982). Extracellular current flow and the site of transduction by vertebrate hair cells. *Journal of Neuroscience, 2*(1), 1–10.

Hudspeth, A. J. (1985). The cellular basis of hearing: The biophysics of hair cells. *Science, 230,* 745–752.

Hurley, K. M., Gaboyard, S., Zhong, M., Price, S. D., Wooltorton, J. R. A., Lysakowski, A., . . . Eatock, R. K. (2006). M-like K+ currents in type I hair cells and calyx afferent endings of the developing rat utricle. *Journal of Neuroscience, 26*(40), 10253–10269.

Iwasaki, S., Chihara, Y., Komuta, Y., Ito, K., & Sahara, Y. (2008). Low-voltage-activated potassium channels underlie the regulation of intrinsic firing properties of rat vestibular ganglion cells. *Journal of Neurophysiology, 100,* 2192–2204.

Jeffery, N., & Spoor, F. (2004). Prenatal growth and development of the modern human labyrinth. *Journal of Anatomy, 204,* 71–92.

Jones, C., & Chen, P. (2007). Planar cell polarity signaling in vertebrates. *BioEssays, 29,* 120–132.

Jones, C., Roper, V., Foucher, I., Qian, D., Banizs, B., Petit, C., . . . Chen, P. (2008). Ciliary proteins link basal body polarization to planar cell polarity regulation. *Nature Genetics, 40*(1), 69–77.

Jones, S. M., Erway, L. C., Bergstrom, R. A., Schimenti, J. C., & Jones, T. A. (1999). Vestibular responses to linear acceleration are absent in otoconia-deficient C57BL/6JEi-het mice. *Hearing Research, 135,* 56–60.

Jones, S. M., & Jones, T. A. (2000a). Ontogeny of vestibular compound action potentials in the domestic chicken. *Journal of the Association for Research in Otolaryngology, 1,* 232–242.

Jones, S. M., & Jones, T. A. (2011). *Genetics, embryology and development of auditory and vestibular systems.* San Diego, CA: Plural.

Jones, T. A., & Jones, S. M. (2000b). Spontaneous activity in the statoacoustic ganglion of the chicken embryo. *Journal of Neurophysiology, 83,* 1452–1468.

Jones, T. A., Jones, S. M., & Hoffman, L. F. (2008). Resting discharge patterns of macular primary afferents in otoconia-deficient mice. *Journal of the Association for Research in Otolaryngology, 9,* 490–505.

Kalluri, R., Xue, J., & Eatock, R. A. (2010). Ion channels set spike timing regularity of mammalian vestibular afferent neurons. *Journal of Neurophysiology, 104,* 2034–2051.

Kaufman, M. H. (1992). *The atlas of mouse development.* Amsterdam, the Netherlands: Elsevier Academic Press.

Kazmierczak, P., Sakaguchi, H., Tokita, J., Wilson-Kubalek, E. M., Milligan, R. A., Müller, U., & Kachar, B. (2007). Cadherin 23 and protocadherin 15 interact to form tip link filaments in sensory hair cells. *Nature, 449*(7158), 87–91.

Kelley, M. W., & Chen, P. (2007). Shaping the mammalian sensory organ by the planar cell polarity pathway. *International Journal of Developmental Biology, 51,* 535–547.

Kido, T. (1997). Otoconial formation in the chick: Changing patterns of tetracycline incorporation during embryonic development and after hatching. *Hearing Research, 105,* 191–201.

Kido, T., Sekitani, T., Yamashita, H., Endo, S., Okami, K., Ogata, Y., & Hara, H. (1993). The otolithic organ in the developing chick embryo. *Acta Oto-Laryngologica, 113,* 128–136.

Kros, C. J., Ruppersberg, J. P., & Rüsch, A. (1998). Expression of a potassium current in inner hair cells during development of hearing in mice. *Nature, 394,* 281–284.

Lanford, P. J., Lan, Y., Jiang, R., Lindsell, C., Weinmaster, G., Gridley, T, & Kelley, M. W. (1999). Notch signaling pathway mediates hair cell development in mammalian cochlea. *Nature Genetics, 21,* 289–292.

Lanford, P. J., Shailam, R., Norton, C. R., Gridley, T., & Kelley, M. W. (2000). Expression of Math1 and HES5 in the cochlea of wildtype and Jag2 mutant mice. *Journal of the Association for Research in Otolaryngology, 1,* 161–171.

Laouris, Y., Kalli-Laouri, J., & Schwartze, P. (1990). The postnatal development of the air-righting reaction in albino rats. Quantitative analysis of normal development and the effect of preventing nec-torso and torso-pelvis rotations. *Behavioural Brain Research, 37,* 37–44.

Lee, Y. S., Liu, F., & Segil, N. (2006). A morphogenetic wave of p27kip1 transcription directs cell cycle exit during organ of Corti development. *Development, 133,* 2817–2826.

Levi-Montalcini, R. (1987). The nerve growth factor: 35 years later. *Science, 237,* 1154–1162.

Levi-Montalcini, R., & Angeletti, P. U. (1968). Nerve growth factor. *Physiological Reviews, 48*(3), 534–569.

Lewin, G. R., & Barde, Y. A. (1996). Physiology of the neurotrophins. *Annual Review of Neuroscience, 19,* 289–317.

Li, G. Q., Meredith, F. L., & Rennie, K. J. (2010). Development of K+ and Na+ conductances in rodent postnatal semicircular canal type I hair cells. *American Journal of Physiology-Regulatory Integrative and Comparative Physiology, 298,* R351–R358.

Liebl, D. J., Tessarollo, L., Palko, M. E., & Parada, L. F. (1997). Absence of sensory neurons before target innervation in brain derived neurotrophic factor-, neurotrophin 3-, and Trk-C deficient embryonic mice. *Journal of Neuroscience, 17*(23), 9113–9121.

Lim, D. J. (1984). The development and structure of otoconia. In I. Friedman & J. Ballantyne (Eds.), *Ultrastructural atlas of the inner ear* (pp. 245–269). London, UK: Butterworth.

Lim, D. J., & Anniko, M. (1985). Developmental morphology of the mouse inner ear. *Acta Oto-Laryngologica, Supplement 422,* 1–69.

Lim, D. J., & Rueda, J. (1992). Structural development of the cochlea. In R. Romand (Ed.), *Development of the auditory and vestibular systems 2* (pp. 33–58). Amsterdam, the Netherlands: Elsevier.

Lopez, C., & Blanke, O. (2011). The thalamocortical vestibular system in animals and humans. *Brain Research Reviews, 67,* 119–146.

Ma, Q., Anderson, D. J., & Fritzsch, B. (2000). Neurogenin 1 null mutant ears develop fewer, morphologically normal hair cells in smaller sensory epithelia devoid of innervation. *Journal of the Association for Research in Otolaryngology, 1,* 129–143.

Marcotti, W., Johnson, S. J., Holley, M. C., & Kros, C. J. (2003a). Developmental changes in the expression of potassium currents of embryonic, neonatal, and mature mouse inner hair cells. *Journal of Physiology, 548,* 383–400.

Masetto, S., Bosica, M., Correia, M. J., Ottersen, O. P., Zucca, G., Perin, P., . . . Valli, P. (2003). Na⁺ currents in vestibular type I and type II hair cells of the embryo and adult chicken. *Journal of Neurophysiology, 90,* 1266–1278.

Masetto, S., Perin, P., Malusà, A., Lucca, G., & Valli, P. (2000). Membrane properties of chick semicircular canal hair cells in situ during embryonic development. *Journal of Neurophysiology, 83,* 2740–2756.

Mbiene, J. P., Favre, D., & Sans, A. (1984). The pattern of ciliary development in fetal mouse vestibular receptors. *Anatomy and Embryology, 170,* 229–238.

Mbiene, J. P., Favre, D., & Sans, A. (1988). Early innervation of hair cells in the vestibular epithelia of mouse embryos: SEM and TEM study. *Anatomy and Embryology, 177,* 331–340.

Mbiene, J. P., & Sans, A. (1986). Differentiation and maturation of the sensory hair bundles in the fetal and postnatal vestibular receptors of the mouse: A scanning microscopy study. *Journal of Comparative Neurology, 254,* 271–278.

McKenzie, E., Krupin, A., & Kelley, M. W. (2004). Cellular growth and rearrangement during the development of the mammalian organ of Corti. *Developmental Dynamics, 229,* 802–812.

Montandon, P., Gacek, R. R., & Kimura, R. S. (1970). Crista neglecta in the cat and human. *Annals of Otology Rhinology and Laryngology, 79,* 105–112.

Montcouquiol, M., Rachel, R. A., Lanford, P. J., Copeland, N. G., Jenkins, N. A., & Kelley, M. W. (2003). Identification of Vangl2 and Scrb1 as planar polarity genes in mammals. *Nature, 423,* 173–177.

Montcouquiol, M., Sans, N., Huss, D., Kach, J., Dickman, J. D., Forge, A., . . . Kelley, M. W. (2006). Asymmetric localization of Vangl2 and Fz3 indicate novel mechanisms for planar cell polarity in mammals. *Journal of Neuroscience, 26*(19), 5265–5275.

Morsli, H., Choo, D., Ryan, A., Johnson, R., & Wu, D. K. (1998). Development of the mouse inner ear and origin of its sensory organs. *Journal of Neuroscience, 18*(9), 3327–3335.

Morsli, H., Tuorto, F., Choo, D., Postiglione, M. P., Simeone, A., & Wu, D. K. (1999). Otx1 and Otx2 activities are required for the normal development of the mouse inner ear. *Development, 126,* 2335–2343.

Nakahara, H., & Bevelander, G. (1979). An electron microscope study of crystal calcium carbonate formation in the mouse otolith. *Anatomical Record, 193,* 233–242.

Nayak, G. D., Ratnayaka, H. S. K., Goodyear, R. J., & Richardson, G. P. (2007). Development of the hair bundle and mechanotransduction. *International Journal of Developmental Biology, 51,* 597–608.

Nichols, D. H., Pauley, S., Jahan, I., Beisel, K. W., Millen, K. J., & Fritzsch, B. (2008). Lmx1a is required for segregation of sensory epithelia and normal ear histogenesis and morphogenesis. *Cell and Tissue Research, 334*(3), 339–358.

Nishida, Y., Rivolta, M. N., & Holley, M. C. (1998). Timed markers for the differentiation of the cuticular plate and stereocilia in hair cells from the mouse inner ear. *Journal of Comparative Neurology, 395,* 18–28.

Ohyama, T., Groves, A. K., & Martin, K. (2007). The first steps toward hearing: Mechanisms of otic placode induction. *International Journal of Developmental Biology, 51,* 463–472.

Ornitz, O. M., Atwell, C. W., Walter, D. O., Hartmann, E. E., & Kaplan, A. R. (1979). The maturation of vestibular nystagmus in infancy and childhood. *Acta Oto-Laryngologica, 88,* 244–256.

Parrad, P. J., & Cottereau, P. (1977). Apparition des réactions rotatoires chez le rat nouveau-né. *Physiology and Behavior, 18,* 1017–1020.

Pauley, S., Matei, V., Beisel, K. W., & Fritzsch, B. (2005). Wiring the ear to the brain: The molecular basis of neurosensory development, differentiation, and survival. In M. W. Kelley, D. K. Wu, A. N. Popper, & R. R. Fay (Eds.), *Development of the inner ear* (pp. 85–121). New York, NY: Springer-Verlag.

Peterka, R. J., & Black, F. O. (1990). Age-related changes in human posture control: Sensory organization tests. *Journal of Vestibular Research, 1,* 73–85.

Peterka, R. J., Black, F. O., & Schoenhoff, M. B. (1990a). Age-related changes in human vestibulo-ocular reflexes: Sinusoidal rotation and caloric tests. *Journal of Vestibular Research, 1,* 49–59.

Peterka, R. J., Black, F. O., & Schoenhoff, M. B. (1990b). Age-related changes in human vesitbulo-ocular and optokinetic reflexes: Pseudorandom rotation tests. *Journal of Vestibular Research, 1,* 61–71.

Peterson, M. L., Christou, E., & Rosengren, K. S. (2006). Children achieve adult-like sensory integration during stance at 12-years-old. *Gait & Posture, 23,* 455–463.

Pickles, J. O., Comis, S. D., & Osborne, M. E. (1984). Cross links between stereocilia in the guinea pig organ of Corti, and their possible relation to sensory transduction. *Hearing Research, 15*(2), 103–112.

Porter, J. D., & Balaban, C. D. (1997). Connections between the vestibular nuclei and brain stem regions that mediate autonomic function in the rat. *Journal of Vestibular Research, 7,* 63–76.

Pujol, R., Lavigne-Rebillard, M., & Lenoir, M. (1998). Development of sensory and neural structures in the mammalian cochlea. In E. W. Rubel, A. N. Popper, & R. R. Fay (Eds.), *Development of the auditory system* (pp. 146–192). New York, NY: Springer-Verlag.

Rida, P. C. G., & Chen, P. (2009). Line up and listen: Planar cell polarity regulation in the mammalian inner ear. *Seminars in Cell & Developmental Biology, 20,* 978–985.

Romand, R., & Dauzat, M. (1982). Modification of spontaneous activity in primary vestibular neurons during development in the cat. *Experimental Brain Research, 45,* 265–268.

Ruben, R. J. (1967). Development of the inner ear of the mouse: A radioautographic study of terminal mitoses [Supplemental material]. *Acta Oto-Laryngologica, 220,* 5–44.

Rüsch, A., & Eatock, R. A. (1996). A delayed rectifier conductance in Type I hair cells of the mouse utricle. *Journal of Neurophysiology, 76,* 995–1004.

Rüsch, A., Lysakowski, A., & Eatock, R. A. (1998). Postnatal development of Type I and Type II hair cells in the mouse utricle: Acquisition of voltage-gated conductances and differentiated morphology. *Journal of Neuroscience, 18,* 7487–7501.

Salamat, M. S., Ross, M. D., & Peacor, D. R. (1980). Otoconia formation in the fetal rat. *Annals of Otology, Rhinology, and Laryngology, 89,* 229–238.

Sans, A., & Chat, M. (1982). Analysis of temporal and spatial patterns of rat vestibular hair cell differentiation by tritiated thymidine radiography. *Journal of Comparative Neurology, 206,* 1–8.

Sans, A., & Deschesne, C. (1985). Early development of vestibular receptors in human embryos: An electron microscopic study [Supplemental material]. *Acta Oto-Laryngologica, 423,* 51–58.

Schneider-Maunoury, S., & Pujades, C. (2007). Hindbrain signals in otic regionalization: Walk on the wild side. *International Journal of Developmental Biology, 51,* 495–506.

Schweizer, F. E., Savin, D., Suu, C., Sultemeier, E. R., & Hoffman, L. F. (2009). Distribution of high-conductance calcium-activated potassium channels in rat vestibular epithelia. *Journal of Comparative Neurology, 517,* 134–145.

Shailam, R., Lanford, P. J., Dolinsky, C. M., Norton, C. R., Gridley, T., & Kelley, M. W. (1999). Expression of proneural and neurogenic genes in the embryonic mammalian vestibular system. *Journal of Neurocytology, 28,* 809–819.

Shall, M. S. (2009). The importance of saccular function to motor development in children with hearing impairments. *International Journal of Otolaryngology, 10,* 1–5.

Sher, A. E. (1971). The embryonic and postnatal development of the inner ear of the mouse. *Acta Oto-Laryngologica Supplement, 285,* 1–77.

Shiroyama, T., Kayahara, T., Yasui, Y., Nomura, J., & Nakano, K. (1999). Projections of the vestibular nuclei to the thalamus in the rat: A Phaseolus vulgaris leucoagglutinin study. *Journal of Comparative Neurology, 407,* 318–332.

Si, F., Brodie, H., Gillespie, P., Vazquez, A., & Yamoah, E. (2003). Developmental assembly of transduction apparatus in chick basilar papilla. *Journal of Neuroscience, 23*(34), 10815–10826.

Silos-Santiago, I., Fagan, A. M., Garber, M., Fritzsch, B., & Barbacid, M. (1997). Severe sensory deficits but normal CNS development in newborn mice lacking TrkB and TrkC tyrosine protein kinase receptors. *European Journal of Neuroscience, 9,* 2045–2056.

Simmons, D. D. (2002). Development of the inner ear efferent system across vertebrate species. *Journal of Neurobiology, 53,* 228–250.

Simmons, D., Duncan, J., Craponde Caprona, D., & Fritzsch, B. (2011). Development of the inner ear efferent system. In D. K. Ryugo, R. R. Fay, & A. N. Popper (Eds.), *Auditory and vestibular efferents* (pp. 187–216). New York, NY: Springer.

Sokolowski, B. H. M., Stahl, L. M., & Fuchs, P. A. (1993). Morphological and physiological development of vestibular hair cells in the organ-cultured otocyst of the chick. *Developmental Biology, 155,* 134–146.

Staller, S. J., Goin, D. W., & Hildebrandt, M. (1986). Pediatric vestibular evaluation with harmonic acceleration. *Otolaryngology and Head and Neck Surgery, 95,* 471–476.

Sulik, K. K., & Cotanche, D. A. (2004). Embryology of the ear. In H. V. Toriello, W. Reardon, & R. J. Gorlin (Eds.), *Hereditary hearing loss and its syndromes* (2nd ed., pp. 17–36). New York, NY: Oxford University Press.

Tibbling, L. (1969). The rotatory nystagmus response in children. *Acta Oto-Laryngologica, 68,* 459–467.

Tilney, L. G., Tilney, M. S., Saunders, J. S., & DeRosier, D. J. (1986). Actin filaments, stereocilia, and hair cells of the bird cochlea. III. The development and differentiation of hair cells and stereocilia. *Developmental Biology, 116,* 100–118.

Valente, M. (2007). Maturational effects of the vestibular system: A study of rotary chair, computerized dynamic posturography, and vestibular evoked myogenic potentials with children. *Journal of the American Academy of Audiology, 18,* 461–481.

Van Cleave, S., & Shall, M. S. (2006). A critical period for the impact of vestibular sensation on ferret motor development. *Journal of Vestibular Research, 16,* 179–186.

Van de Water, T. R. (1976). Effects of removal of the statoacoustic ganglion complex upon the growing otosysts. *Annals of Otology, Rhinology, and Laryngology, 85,* 2–31.

Van de Water, T. R. (1984). Developmental mechanisms of mammalian inner ear formation. In C. Berlin (Ed.), *Hearing science* (pp. 49–170). San Diego, CA: College-Hill Press.

Van de Water, T. R., Anniko, M., Nordemar, H., & Wersall, J. (1977). Embryonic development of the sensory cells in macula utriculae of mouse. *I'Institut National de la Sante et de la Recherche Medicale, 68,* 25–35.

Veenhof, V. B. (1969). *The development of statoconia in mice.* Amsterdam-London, UK: N.V. North-Holland.

Wang, J., Mark, S., Zhang, X., Qian, D., Yoo, S. J., Radde-Gallwitz, K., . . . Chen, P. (2005). Regulation of polarized extension and planar cell polarity in the cochlea by the vertebrate PCP pathway. *Nature Genetics, 37*(9), 980–985.

Wang, Y., Guo, N., & Nathans, J. (2006). The role of *Frizzled3* and *Frizzled6* in neural tube closure and in the planar polarity of inner-ear sensory hair cells. *Journal of Neuroscience, 26*(8), 2147–2156.

Wiener-Vacher, S. R., Toupet, F., & Narcy, P. (1996). Canal and otolith vestibule-ocular reflexes to vertical and off vertical axis rotations in children learning to walk. *Acta Oto-Laryngologica, 116,* 657–665.

Woods, C., Moncouquiol, M., & Kelley, M. W. (2004). Math1 regulates the development of the sensory epithelium in the mammalian cochlea. *Nature Neuroscience, 7,* 1310–1318.

Xu, Z., Ricci, A. J., & Heller, S. (2009). Rethinking how hearing happens. *Neuron, 62,* 305–307.

Yates, B. J. (1996). Vestibular influences on the autonomic nervous system. *Annals of the New York Academy of Sciences, 781,* 458–473.

Yates, B. J., & Miller, A. D. (1998). Physiological evidence that the vestibular system participates in autonomic and respiratory control. *Journal of Vestibular Research, 8,* 17–25.

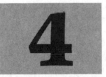

Clinical Neurophysiology of Vestibular Compensation

Kamran Barin

OVERVIEW

Peripheral vestibular abnormalities affect the function of both sensory and motor mechanisms and result in a number of symptoms. These symptoms can be divided into two distinct types (Halmagyi, Weber, & Curthoys, 2010). First, *static symptoms* are those that are present in the absence of head movements. These symptoms are commonly associated with a sudden unilateral loss of vestibular function and include vertigo, imbalance, nausea, and vomiting. Second, *dynamic symptoms* are those that are present only during head movements. These symptoms often become apparent shortly after the onset of the vestibular loss and include blurry vision, loss of visual acuity, and disorientation in complex sensory environments when the head is moving.

The vestibular symptoms become less intense over several days and eventually disappear in many patients even when the vestibular loss is persistent. This process of functional recovery after a peripheral vestibular lesion is called *vestibular compensation* and is related to the high degree of plasticity within the central vestibular pathways (Curthoys & Halmagyi, 1995). Vestibular compensation should not be mistaken for the full recovery that sometimes occurs due to the resolution of the lesion and restoration of normal vestibular function (Manzari, Burgess, MacDougall, & Curthoys, 2013).

Cellular, neural, and behavioral aspects of vestibular compensation have been studied extensively in recent years in both humans and animals (Curthoys, 2000; Darlington, Flohr, & Smith, 1991; Dutia, 2010). These studies have provided a better understanding of the time course of vestibular disorders and a basis for devising effective rehabilitation protocols to expedite recovery after a vestibular lesion. However, significant gaps remain in our understanding of the vestibular compensation process. For example, most of the studies on vestibular compensation so far have focused on the functional recovery of the vestibulo-ocular reflex (VOR) and primarily on the recovery of the horizontal VOR. There are very few studies that address vestibular compensation following isolated lesions in the vertical canal or the otolith pathways. Similarly, the compensation process for the human postural control deficits has been studied mainly from the behavioral point of view with little consideration for the neural or cellular aspects of recovery.

This chapter is a selective review of the neurophysiology of vestibular compensation following a vestibular lesion. The focus of this review is on the clinical findings during various stages after the onset of the lesion. Disorders that cause transient effects such as benign paroxysmal positional vertigo (BPPV) are discussed elsewhere in this book and are not considered here.

EFFECTS OF VESTIBULAR LESIONS

A general description of peripheral vestibular lesions is provided in this section. There are several different disorders that can cause vestibular abnormalities (Strupp & Brandt, 2013). However, they all produce peripheral vestibular lesions by one of two ways: either by damaging the hair cells within the labyrinth or by damaging the nerve fibers that originate from those hair cells.

Some of the more obvious causes of damage to the hair cells include infections such as in labyrinthitis, trauma such as in labyrinthine concussion, or exposure to toxic agents such as in gentamycin vestibulotoxicity (Magnusson & Karlberg, 2002; Strupp & Brandt, 2013). The mechanism of damage to the hair cells is less obvious in conditions such as Ménière's disease (Carey, 2010). In a normal inner ear, there is no contact between the endolymph, the fluid that fills the labyrinth, and the perilymph, the fluid that surrounds the labyrinth. It is believed that in patients with Ménière's disease, for reasons that are still unknown, the endolymph absorption becomes impaired and leads to increased pressure in the inner ear. This condition, known as *endolymphatic hydrops*, leads to the rupture of the labyrinthine membrane and exposure of the hair cells to perilymph. Mixing of the inner ear fluids apparently has a toxic effect on the hair cells and causes them to briefly become hyperactive followed by a much longer period of deactivation. Once the rupture closes and the perilymph is flushed out of the labyrinthine space, most but not all of the hair cells regain function. As the cycle of increase in the inner ear pressure followed by the rupture of the membrane continues during the Ménière's attacks, more and more hair cells may fail to regain normal function. This explains both the fluctuating and progressive nature of the Ménière's disease (Li & Lorenzo, 2013).

Another mechanism of damage to the hair cells is the disruption of the blood supply to the labyrinth (Lee, Park, Kim, Kim, Park, & Kim, 2014). The arteries that serve the inner ear have no collateral connections, and therefore, the inner ear hair cells are highly sensitive to ischemic events that interrupt the blood flow to the labyrinth. Brief interruptions can cause reversible deactivation of the hair cells, but if the ischemia persists for more than a few minutes, the damage will become permanent. Depending on which branch of the labyrinthine artery is involved, the hair cell damage may be confined to specific structures within the labyrinth or may include the entire labyrinth as well as the cochlea. Examples of diseases that can permanently affect the labyrinthine blood supply are infarcts and transient ischemic attacks (Cloutier & Saliba, 2008). Brief changes in the blood flow, such as the type commonly associated with migraine-associated vertigo, can modulate the activity of the hair cells and result in fluctuating auditory and vestibular symptoms (Karatas, 2011).

The most common cause of damage to the vestibular nerve fibers is infection such as in vestibular neuritis (Halmagyi et al., 2010). It is now clear that there are different types of vestibular neuritis (Manzari et al., 2013). For example, the infection can cause inflammation of the vestibular nerve, which results in a temporary loss of vestibular function. The function is restored once the inflammation goes away. However, the infection can also cause degeneration of the nerve fibers, which results in a permanent and irreversible damage to the vestibular nerve. In addition, vestibular neuritis can affect the superior branch, the inferior branch, or both branches of the vestibular nerve (Kim & Kim, 2012; Manzari, Burgess, & Curthoys, 2012). The symptoms and the clinical presentation of the disease will depend on which branch or branches of the vestibular nerve are affected.

Another cause of vestibular nerve damage is compression of the nerve fibers by tumors such as vestibular schwannoma (i.e., acoustic neuroma), which blocks the transmission of neural signals to the vestibular nuclei (Kutz, Roland, & Isaacson, 2012). If the tumor becomes large, it can also compress the brainstem or the cerebellum and generate both peripheral and central vestibular findings.

Finally, neurotoxic agents can also damage the vestibular nerve fibers. However, the incidence of such damage is thought to be far less than that of the toxic agents that damage the hair cells.

Regardless of the underlying cause of damage to the peripheral vestibular system, the compensation process appears to be the same. In the remainder of this section, first a brief review of the normal vestibular function in humans is presented. Then, the effects of different types of lesions immediately after the onset of the lesion are discussed. The process of compensation for each type is discussed in the next section. As noted earlier, the focus of this chapter is on the compensation of the VOR pathways because of the limited knowledge about the other aspects of compensation.

Vestibular Responses to Different Types of Head Movements

The role of the VOR is to provide clear vision by stabilizing images on the retina during head movements. This task requires moving the eyes such that the eye velocity matches the head velocity but in the opposite direction. Figure 4–1 shows the neural activities of one hair cell from the right lateral semicircular canal and one hair cell from the left lateral semicircular canal in response to different types of head movements. When the head is at rest, each hair cell generates tonic neural activity of approximately 80 to 100 spikes per second. Because there are several thousand hair cells in each canal, the primary vestibular neurons transmit a large amount of neural activity to the vestibular nuclei. In the absence of head movements, the neural activities received from the right and left labyrinths are approximately equal (see Figure 4–1A).

When the head moves to one side in a manner that resembles natural head movements, neural activities from both labyrinths are modulated from their baseline level (Barin, 2009). The leading ear generates excitation, whereas the lagging ear generates inhibition of neural activity. However, the change of neural activity from the baseline is approximately proportional to the head velocity (see Figure 4–1B). The secondary vestibular neurons within the vestibular nuclei relay the difference between the right and left neural activities to the oculomotor nuclei, which generates eye movements that are also proportional to the head velocity except that they are in the opposite direction. It is important to note that the entire process takes place at the brainstem level without the need for higher cortical level involvement. As a result, VOR-generated eye movements have a very short latency and are much faster than other types of eye movements.

If the head moves sinusoidally side to side similar to the type of head movements that occur during low-frequency rotation chair testing, the change in the neural firing is also sinusoidal but differs from the head velocity in two characteristics (see Figure 4–1C). First, the amplitude of the change is much less than the head velocity, which results in a gain of lower than 1.0 in the rotation test. Second, there is a time difference between the change in the neural firing and the head velocity, which results in a phase shift in the rotation test. The reason for these differences is related to two factors (Barin, 2009). The first factor is the physical characteristics of the cupula and the endolymph. That is, the inertia of the cupula and the viscosity of the endolymph cause the hair cell responses to differ from the head movements in the low-frequency range. The second factor is related to a neural integrator within the vestibular nuclei, called the *velocity storage mechanism*. The purpose of the velocity storage mechanism is to improve the low-frequency performance of the cupula. The best analogy for its function is a storage tank that has a large inlet but a small outlet. As a result, the neural firing builds up within the velocity storage mechanism and continues to discharge slowly even after the stimulus has stopped. The combination of the cupular dynamics and the velocity storage mechanism allows the VOR to work well for natural head movements that are in the mid- to high-frequency range but not so well for very low-frequency head movements as in Figure 4–1C. As the frequency increases, the gain increases and the phase shift decreases until the change in neural firing becomes proportional to the head velocity during natural head movements.

The behavior of the cupula and the velocity storage mechanism is also apparent when the head is accelerated rapidly and then rotated at a constant velocity for a long time (Barin, 2009). This type of stimulus is similar to the velocity step test in the rotation chair testing. During the acceleration phase, the change in the neural firing is proportional to the head velocity (see Figure 4–1D). After reaching the final velocity and during the constant velocity rotation phase, the cupula begins to return to its resting position and the neural firing declines toward the baseline accordingly. In humans, it takes approximately 20 s for the cupula to return to its resting

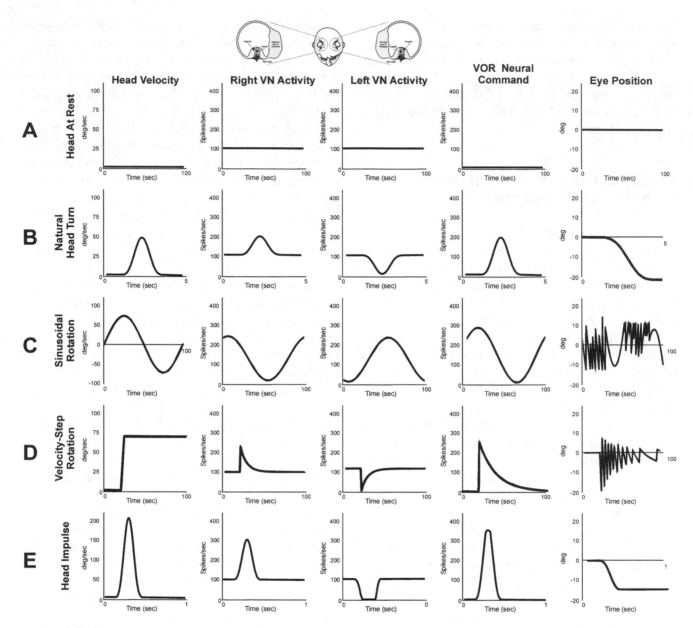

Figure 4-1. Responses of a normal individual to different types of head movements. Right and left vestibular nerve (*VN*) activities, *VOR* neural command, and the final eye position are shown. The *VOR* neural command is the difference between the right and left *VN* activities that is further processed within the vestibular nuclei. Ideally, the *VOR* command should be proportional to the head velocity. **A.** Head at rest. **B.** Rightward natural head movement. **C.** Sinusoidal head movements in the rotation chair testing. **D.** Rightward velocity-step head movement in the rotation chair testing. **E.** Rightward head movement in the head impulse test. All responses are obtained in the absence of fixation except for **E.** Note that time and amplitude scales are different for different stimuli. Also note that the responses are approximate and are not intended to exactly match actual responses. Based on Barin, K. (2014). VNG/ENG Course Handout. *GN Otometrics.*

position but the change in the neural firing persists for up to 60 s because of the influence of the velocity storage mechanism.

If the head is moved very rapidly to one side similar to the type of head movements that occur during the head impulse test, the excitatory change in the neural firing from the leading ear resembles the head velocity (see Figure 4–1E). However, the inhibitory change in the neural firing from the opposite ear saturates and the response is clipped at 0 spikes per second. During the saturation phase, the labyrinth no longer provides an accurate measure of the head movement. As a result of this nonlinearity, the input to the oculomotor system is not proportional to the head velocity. Nonetheless, the adjustments in the central vestibular pathways allow the VOR to function fairly effectively as long as one labyrinth can provide an accurate measure of the head velocity (Weber, MacDougall, Halmagyi, & Curthoys, 2009).

The above examples demonstrate that head movements generate an asymmetry between the right and left neural activities. Determining which side is generating excitation and which side is generating inhibition identifies the direction of head movements. The degree and the type of neural asymmetry determine the amplitude and the type of head movements. For example, the neural asymmetry for natural head movements mimics the head velocity, which can be relayed to the oculomotor nuclei to generate compensatory eye movements.

The question of how the central nervous system (CNS) can determine the properties of the head movement from different patterns of neural firing is an important one and has a profound implication regarding vestibular compensation. One hypothesis is the existence of a lookup table or a database that for every pattern of head movement contains a corresponding neural firing pattern (Borel, Lopez, Péruch, & Lacour, 2008). It is possible that this database is formed early in life and may explain why children and young adults engage in the type of movements that may not be easily tolerated in older ages. In fact, part of the play activities in childhood may be related to the formation of this database. The support for this hypothesis comes from the fact that the morphological development of the labyrinthine structures seems to be complete within a few months after birth but the central vestibular pathways continue to mature for several years.

It should be noted that other oculomotor systems interact with the vestibular system and participate in controlling the eye movements. For instance, in some of the above examples, if the VOR drives the eyes close to the orbital limit, the saccadic sys-

tem moves the eyes quickly in the opposite direction (Abadi, 2002). This is the mechanism of generating nystagmus with the slow phase mediated by the vestibular system and the fast phase mediated by the saccadic system.

Effects of Acute Unilateral Vestibular Lesions

Unilateral lesions are by far the most common type of peripheral vestibular abnormalities. This type of lesion generates asymmetries in the vestibular pathways that mimic head movements. Figure 4–2 shows what happens when the hair cells or their afferent nerve fibers are damaged in one of the lateral semicircular canals. Of course, the loss of a small number of hair cells or nerve fibers will not cause significant consequences, but if the damage is substantial, the neural activity present at the vestibular nuclei of the damaged side will be reduced proportional to the number of lost hair cells or nerve fibers (see Figure 4–2A). The resulting neural asymmetry is perceived as the head moving away from the damaged ear in the plane of the affected semicircular canal (Barin, 2009). Accordingly, spontaneous nystagmus is generated because the VOR moves the eyes slowly toward the damaged ear followed by the saccadic system resetting the eyes in the opposite direction. The slow-phase velocity (SPV) of spontaneous nystagmus is an important parameter because it reflects the velocity of the perceived head movements. At the onset of the lesion, the intensity of spontaneous nystagmus is directly related to the number of hair cells or nerve fibers that are damaged. However, as we will see, the intensity of spontaneous nystagmus changes quickly due to the vestibular compensation process.

Because the perception of motion after a unilateral vestibular lesion is contradicted by other sensory mechanisms, namely vision and proprioception, the patient experiences vertigo and the associated autonomic symptoms in the absence of head movements. Other static symptoms following a unilateral vestibular lesion often include imbalance and tilting of the head and body to one side.

When the patient moves his or her head following a unilateral vestibular lesion, the asymmetry

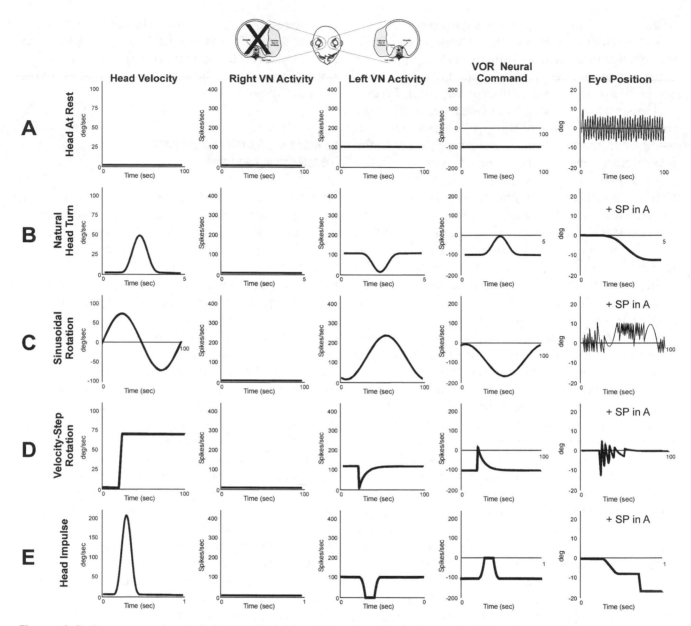

Figure 4-2. Responses of an individual with right peripheral vestibular lesion to different types of head movements. See Figure 4–1 for other details. The negative values for the *VOR* neural command indicate that the activity from the left side is greater than the activity from the right side. Also, note that the spontaneous nystagmus (*SP*) in **A** is superimposed on all of the other eye movements but they are not shown in the figure. Based on Barin, K. (2014). VNG/ENG Course Handout. *GN Otometrics.*

in the neural firing is not as large as that before the onset of the lesion (see Figure 4–2B). Therefore, the resulting eye movements are not completely compensatory, which causes the images not to be stationary on the retina. The lack of coordination between head and eye movements leads to dynamic symptoms such as blurry vision and the loss of visual acuity during head movements.

Figure 4–2 shows the neural firing for different types of head movements following an acute unilateral lesion. As noted for natural head movements, the neural firing does not match the head velocity and the resulting eye movements are smaller than the head movements (see Figure 4–2B). For low-frequency sinusoidal head movements, the gain of the VOR (amplitude) decreases and the phase shift (timing) increases (see Figure 4–2C). Similarly, for step-velocity movements, the amplitude of neural responses immediately after the acceleration phase is smaller and the decline of the response toward the baseline (time constant) is faster (see Figure 4–2D). The effect is more noticeable for head movements toward the side of the lesion. Finally, the nonlinearity in the VOR pathways causes the neural firing from the intact side to saturate during head impulses toward the damaged ear and the eyes fall well-short of the head movements (see Figure 4–2E). In this case, the patient usually uses saccadic eye movements to refixate on the target (catch-up saccades). The effect is present for movements

toward and away from the side of lesion but it is far more noticeable for the movements toward the side of lesion.

In addition to the lateral semicircular canals, damage to the other structures within the peripheral vestibular system also causes asymmetries in the neural firings that mimic head movements in different planes. The eye movements following a focal lesion in different vestibular structures are shown in Figure 4–3 (Barin, 2009). As noted, damage to one of the lateral canals is perceived as the head moving toward the intact ear and results in horizontal spontaneous nystagmus with the fast phases beating away from the side of lesion (see Figure 4–3A).

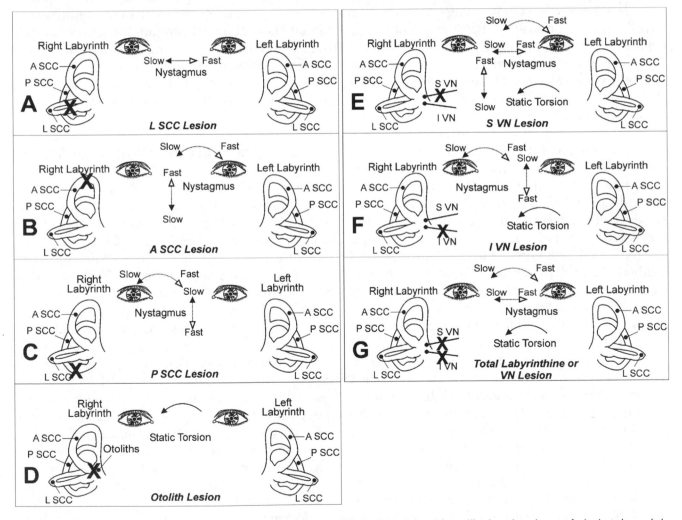

Figure 4–3. Eye movements following a focal lesion in different peripheral vestibular structures. **A.** Lateral semicircular canal (*L SCC*). **B.** Anterior semicircular canal (*A SCC*). **C.** Posterior semicircular canal (*P SCC*). **D.** Otoliths. **E.** Superior branch of the vestibular nerve (*S VN*). **F.** Inferior branch of the vestibular nerve (*I VN*). **G.** Total labyrinthine or vestibular nerve. Based on Barin, K. (2014). VNG/ENG Course Handout. *GN Otometrics.*

A focal lesion of the anterior canal is perceived as the head moving backward in the plane of anterior-posterior canal pairs and results in vertical nystagmus beating up and torsional nystagmus beating away from the side of lesion (see Figure 4–3B). Because of the synergistic pairing of the canals, the same type of nystagmus can be seen for excitation of the opposite posterior canal. Such an excitation can happen for BPPV of the posterior canal but unlike the BPPV-type nystagmus, the nystagmus following damage to the anterior canal is persistent.

A focal lesion of the posterior canal is perceived as the head moving downward in the plane of anterior-posterior canal pairs and results in vertical nystagmus beating down and torsional nystagmus again beating away from the side of lesion (see Figure 4–3C). The same type of nystagmus can be seen for BPPV of the opposite anterior canal, but again the resulting nystagmus is transient.

Focal lesions of the utricle or saccule are not as well understood as those of the semicircular canals. One can assume that damage to one of the otolith organs will cause loss of orientation with respect to gravity and will be perceived as the head tilting away from the damaged side (see Figure 4–3D). Consistent with that hypothesis, it has been demonstrated that in humans, such a lesion will result in a tonic torsion of the eyes toward the side of lesion. This type of torsion can be tested with the subjective visual vertical test. It is not clear how common it is to have a focal lesion of the otoliths. However, mild residual symptoms after a successful repositioning maneuver in BPPV patients may represent one form of otolith abnormalities. After all, a substantial loss of otoconia from the utricle in these patients can disrupt normal otolith function.

The manifestation of a lesion in different branches of the vestibular nerve can be determined by combining the effects of lesions in different semicircular canals or the otolith organs that are mediated through that branch. For example, the superior portion of the vestibular nerve transmits information from the lateral and anterior semicircular canals as well as the utricle. A few nerve fibers from the saccule also travel through the superior portion of the vestibular nerve but the effect is usually considered to be insignificant. As a result, damage to this branch of the vestibular nerve results in horizontal nystagmus beating away from the side of the lesion, vertical nystagmus beating up, torsional nystagmus beating away from the side of the lesion, and tonic torsion of the eyes toward the side of the lesion (see Figure 4–3E). Similarly, the inferior portion of the vestibular nerve is supplied by the posterior canal and the saccule. Damage to this branch of the vestibular nerve results in vertical nystagmus beating down, torsional nystagmus beating away from the side of the lesion, and tonic torsion of the eyes toward the side of the lesion (see Figure 4–3F). Finally, damage to both branches of the vestibular nerve or a total labyrinthine lesion results in combination of all lesions for individual structures within the labyrinth. However, the vertical components of the nystagmus are in opposite directions and cancel out. As a result, damage to both branches of the vestibular nerve or a total labyrinthine lesion results in horizontal nystagmus beating away from the side of the lesion, torsional nystagmus beating away from the side of the lesion, and tonic torsion of the eyes toward the side of the lesion (see Figure 4–3G).

Effects of Acute Bilateral Vestibular Lesions

Bilateral vestibular lesions are rare compared to unilateral lesions. They can be present in one of two ways. When the loss of function is approximately equal in both peripheral vestibular systems, the patient exhibits very few of the static symptoms described in the previous section. That is, vertigo and spontaneous nystagmus that are typical of unilateral vestibular lesions are not present because of the absence of neural asymmetries. Instead, these patients usually experience dynamic symptoms such as unsteadiness, oscillopsia (sensation of stationary objects moving during head movements), loss of visual acuity, and blurry vision during head movements (Jen, 2009). Although the acute symptoms may not appear to be as troublesome as those resulting from unilateral lesions, long-term functional consequences of bilateral lesions are far more serious and more difficult to overcome (Kim, Oh, Koo, & Kim, 2011).

When bilateral loss of function is present but it is more significant on one side, the patient exhibits both symptoms associated with the unilateral vestibular lesions described in the previous section as well as symptoms associated with the bilateral vestibular loss described above (Fujimoto et al., 2013). Again, the consequences of this type of lesion both in the acute and chronic phases of the lesion are very serious (Guinand, Boselie, Guyot, & Kingma, 2012).

Effects of Acute Central Vestibular Lesions

Very little is known about focal lesions affecting the vestibular nuclei (Shepard, 2009). If damage to the vestibular nuclei affects the tonic neural activity of the secondary vestibular neurons on one side, then the symptoms and presentation are expected to be similar to those for unilateral peripheral vestibular lesions. However, the clinical picture is more complicated. In humans, the majority of the conditions that damage the vestibular nuclei are due to vascular diseases, tumors, or trauma (Furman & Whitney, 2000). As a result, the effects are not necessarily confined to the vestibular nuclei and often involve other structures within the brainstem, cerebellum, or cerebellar cortex. Animal studies have demonstrated spontaneous nystagmus following focal lesions within the vestibular nuclei. However, unlike peripheral vestibular lesions, focal lesions of the vestibular nuclei did not produce a caloric weakness. Instead, the caloric findings included perverted nystagmus and other central findings.

It is clear that our understanding of central vestibular lesions is still emerging. Although compensation following central vestibular lesions will be mentioned briefly, a better understanding of the underlying pathophysiology of these disorders is needed before effective rehabilitation methods can be devised.

VESTIBULAR COMPENSATION

The vestibular pathways possess a high degree of plasticity, which is essential to overcome the effects of environmental and developmental changes, such as aging (Zee, 2000). The adaptation of the VOR behavior after wearing special prisms that reverse the visual field is a remarkable demonstration of this plasticity (Melvill Jones, Guitton, & Berthoz, 1988). The same adaptive mechanisms participate in the vestibular compensation process so that the patients can recover functionally after a vestibular lesion. However, vestibular compensation is not limited to the adaptation of the vestibular pathways and may include substitution by other oculomotor and postural control mechanisms such as the saccadic system (Curthoys, 2000).

Figure 4–4 shows a highly simplified view of the vestibular compensation mechanisms. The head movements are transduced into neural activity by the hair cells within the labyrinth. The changes in the neural activity are transmitted to the vestibular nuclei via the primary vestibular neurons within the vestibular nerve. The secondary vestibular neurons usually relay the neural activity to the motor centers such as the oculomotor nuclei or the spinal cord. The cerebellum constantly monitors the changes in the neural activity within the vestibular nuclei but does not intervene as long as they are within the expected response of the system. However, when changes in the neural activity do not match the expected responses of the vestibular system, vestibular compensation mechanisms alter the behavior of the secondary vestibular neurons so that the motor centers receive a modified representation of the activity of the primary vestibular neurons. The alteration at

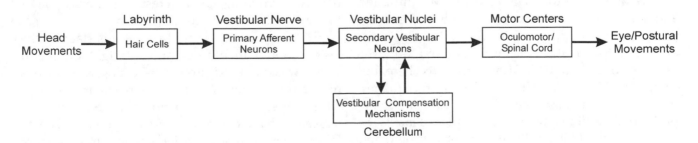

Figure 4–4. A simplified representation of the vestibular compensation process.

the vestibular nuclei level may include reduction in gain, increase in gain, change in the timing, or other modification of the neural activity. In this view of the vestibular compensation process, the cerebellum, namely the cerebellar flocculus, plays an important role in initiating the compensation process (Courjon, Flandrin, Jeannerod, & Schmid, 1982; Johnston, Seckl, & Dutia, 2002).

It is now clear that vestibular compensation occurs in different steps (Lacour, 2006). *Static compensation* begins almost immediately after the onset of the lesion in order to reduce the more distressing symptoms that are present in the absence of head movements. *Dynamic compensation* occurs later to reduce the longer term negative effects of damage to the vestibular system. Dynamic compensation appears to be a more complex process that may never fully resolve the symptoms in some patients.

Compensation After Unilateral Vestibular Lesion

It is well known that most patient complaints after a sudden unilateral peripheral vestibular lesion follow a typical pattern. The patients usually exhibit a few days of severe and often disabling symptoms, a few weeks of moderate and improving symptoms, followed by a few months of mild and manageable symptoms (Halmagyi et al., 2010). Of course, there are individual differences depending on the age, activity levels, and presence of other confounding conditions. Nonetheless, this relatively universal pattern of recovery corresponds to the various stages of compensation that are discussed in this section.

Figure 4–5 shows various steps of the static compensation process after the onset of a peripheral vestibular lesion. This is a highly simplified and somewhat speculative presentation of the vestibular compensation process. Several assumptions are made for illustrative purposes. First, only the recovery of horizontal VOR is considered here, but the process is similar for the VOR in other planes. Furthermore, it is assumed that the damage to the peripheral vestibular system is complete. Finally, the neural activity of a single nerve fiber is shown and it is assumed arbitrarily that its tonic neural firing is 100 spikes/second.

Prior to the Onset of Lesion

Figure 4–5A shows the neural activity at the vestibular nuclei of a normal individual immediately following a sudden horizontal head rotation toward the left ear. It is assumed, again arbitrarily, that for the given change in the head velocity, the momentary change in the neural firing is 50 spikes/second. The difference between the excitatory response from the left side and the inhibitory response from the right side immediately after the onset of rotation is 100 spikes/second (2 × 50 spikes/second). As the VOR is functioning normally in this individual, head movements are extrapolated accurately from the pattern of neural activities and compensatory eye movements are generated in the opposite direction of head movements with the SPV matching the head velocity. As the rotation continues, the saccadic system resets the eyes when they approach the orbital limit and generates nystagmus with fast phases toward the direction of head acceleration (left-beating for this example).

Immediately After the Onset of Lesion

Figure 4–5B shows the neural activity at the vestibular nuclei immediately following a lesion in the right lateral semicircular canal or its afferent neural pathway. The neural asymmetry is perceived as the head rotation to the left, and spontaneous nystagmus is generated with the fast phases directed toward the direction of the perceived head motion and away from the side of lesion (Fetter & Zee, 1988). Furthermore, the SPV of the nystagmus is the same as that of Figure 4–5A because the neural asymmetry of 100 spikes/second is the same in both conditions. It is important to note that the SPV of spontaneous nystagmus reflects how fast the patient perceives his or her head is rotating, and as a result, it directly relates to the severity of symptoms.

The vestibular test findings at this stage of the lesion should include significant right unilateral caloric weakness and strong left-beating spontaneous nystagmus without fixation. The nystagmus is usually strong enough that is not fully suppressed and can be seen with fixation also. This nystagmus is likely to follow Alexander's law (Hegemann, Straumann, & Bockisch, 2007), which means it is stronger with the gaze toward the fast phases (left gaze in this case).

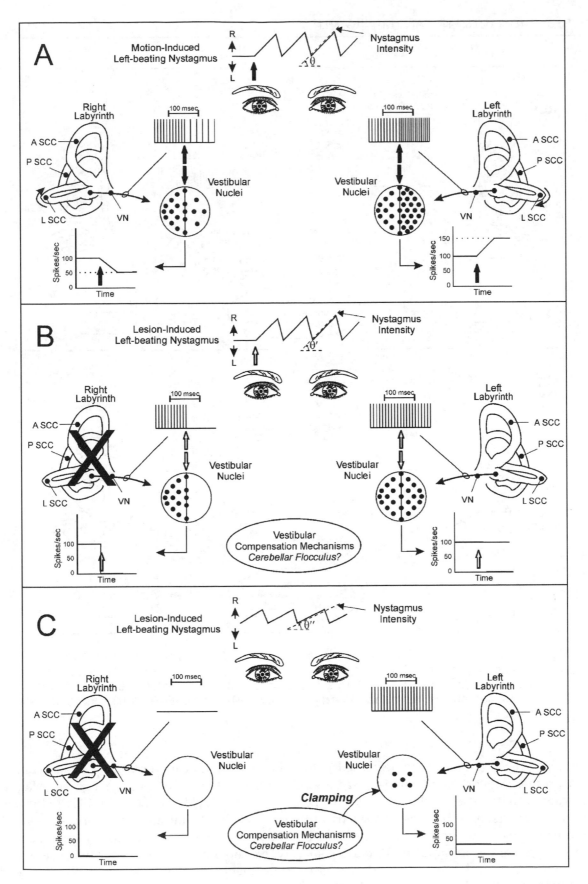

Figure 4-5. Static compensation following a right peripheral vestibular lesion. See the text for the description of each step. Solid arrows identify the onset of head acceleration. *continues*

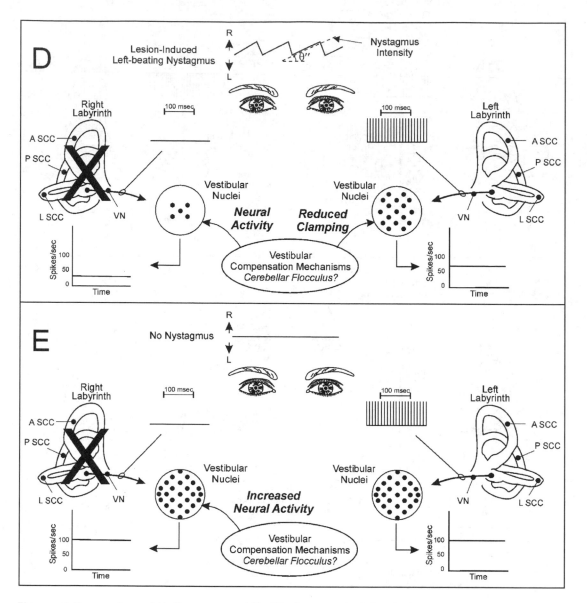

Figure 4–5. *continued* Hollow arrows identify the onset of the lesion. θ, θ′, and θ″ represent slow-phase nystagmus intensities. The density of the dots represents the level of neural activity within the vestibular nuclei. *L SCC*, lateral semicircular canal; *A SCC*, anterior semicircular canal; *P SCC*, posterior semicircular canal. Based on Barin, K. (2014). VNG/ENG Course Handout. *GN Otometrics.*

The head impulse test should show decreased VOR gain and presence of consistent catch-up saccades for rightward head impulses (Weber et al., 2008). The same findings are likely to be present for leftward head impulses as well, but they are not as prominent as those for rightward head impulses. Rotation chair testing should show decreased gain and increased phase at very low frequencies (Baloh, Jacobson, Beykirch, & Honrubia, 1989). Also, the asymmetry should be significant for all frequencies reflecting the presence of spontaneous nystagmus (Magnusson, Brantberg, Pyykkö, & Schalén, 1989). However, the rotation chair findings at the early stages of lesion should be interpreted cautiously because the same type of nonlinearity that occurs with very fast head movements (see Figure 4–1E) can also happen in the rotation testing at the onset of the lesion. As a result, eye velocities resemble a rectified sinusoid instead of a full sinusoid. Most of the commercial rotation chair systems use a curve-fitting technique to estimate the gain, phase, and asymmetry parameters of the VOR eye movements. However, the results at the early stages of lesion may be contaminated because the VOR eye velocities resemble a half sinusoid instead of a full sinusoid. In fact, what is assumed to be a reflection of vestibular compensation in rotation testing may simply be due to the way the test parameters are calculated. Finally, the responses in vestibular-evoked myogenic potential (VEMP) testing are assumed to originate from the otolith organs. Therefore, the findings will depend on whether or not the damage involves the vestibular nerve. Regardless, VEMP testing will not be discussed here further because the findings are lesion-dependent similar to the caloric test and are unlikely to change with compensation.

Cerebellar Clamping Stage

The neural asymmetry caused by the peripheral vestibular lesion (see Figure 4–5B) is similar to the asymmetry caused by the head movement (see Figure 4–5A) with one notable exception. The neural asymmetries between the right and left neural firings that are induced by head movements are temporary and do not persist for an extended period of time. The asymmetries caused by a lesion are persistent. Therefore, any prolonged and constant asymmetry is interpreted as a sign of a malfunction within the VOR pathways and results in the activation of the vestibular compensation process.

The first step in the vestibular compensation process is *cerebellar clamping* in which the neural activity from the intact side is reduced at the vestibular nuclei level before it is relayed to the motor centers. This step begins within hours if not minutes after the onset of the lesion and its effect is to reduce the asymmetry and ease the patient's symptoms. This is essentially the same role that vestibular suppressants play when they are prescribed during the early stages of a lesion when the symptoms are likely to be severe. It should be noted that although cerebellar clamping reduces the static symptoms, it may have a short-term adverse effect on the dynamic symptoms. The reason is that cerebellar clamping reduces the neural activity from the intact side during head movements and further impairs the VOR function.

The evidence for the cerebellar clamping stage comes from the studies by Vibert and his colleagues (Vibert et al., 1999). They studied guinea pigs that had undergone a unilateral labyrinthectomy. If a secondary vestibular nerve section was performed on the opposite side within the first 3 days after the first labyrinthectomy, the impact was minimal. This suggests that the neural activities were already reduced on the initially intact side due to cerebellar clamping and that is why the effects of the subsequent deafferentation were marginal.

The vestibular test findings at the cerebellar clamping stage should include significant spontaneous nystagmus without fixation. However, the intensity should be reduced compared to the intensity at the onset of the lesion. This reflects the decrease in neural asymmetry and accompanies improvement in the patient's symptoms. The caloric test should continue to show a significant right weakness, but at times, the responses can be bilaterally weak because of the strong clamping effect. The rotation test results should be similar to those at the onset of the lesion although the gain may again be reduced because of the clamping effect. The rotation asymmetry should also decrease because of the reduction of the spontaneous nystagmus intensity. Similarly, the head impulse test should be similar to those at the onset of the lesion.

Appearance of Neural Activity at the Vestibular Nuclei of the Damaged Side

Shortly after the cerebellar clamping stage, the tonic neural activity of the secondary vestibular neurons begins to increase at the vestibular nuclei of the damaged side. Assuming that the peripheral vestibular lesion is permanent, this neural activity cannot be originating from the primary vestibular neurons. Instead, the most likely source for the increased neural activity is the vestibular nuclei of the intact side that communicates with the other side through the commissural fibers (Olabi, Bergquist, & Dutia, 2009). Simultaneous with the increase of neural activity on the damaged side, the clamping effect on the intact side is reduced (Beraneck et al., 2004). The neural asymmetry is still present, but it is not as severe compared to the onset of the lesion. Furthermore, the reduction in the clamping allows for the neural activity on the intact side to be more representative of the head movements. In short, the patient still suffers from both static and dynamic symptoms, but the severity of both is reduced.

The evidence for this stage of the compensation also comes from the same series of studies by Vibert et al. (1999). They demonstrated that if the secondary vestibular nerve section was performed more than 3 days after the first labyrinthectomy, the guinea pigs again experienced increase in the symptoms and showed spontaneous nystagmus, but this time, the nystagmus was in the opposite direction of the initial spontaneous nystagmus immediately after the labyrinthectomy. This suggests an increase in the neural activity of the vestibular nuclei on the damaged side so that the subsequent nerve section created a secondary asymmetry in the opposite direction. As the animals were labyrinthectomized, the increase in the neural activity must have been generated centrally.

Again, the intensity of spontaneous nystagmus continues to decline in the vestibular tests even though the caloric weakness persists. In the rotation chair test, the phase and gain parameters should improve, especially for low frequencies, and the asymmetry parameter should decrease as the spontaneous nystagmus intensity declines (Allum & Honegger, 2013). As noted before, it is not clear how much of the changes in the rotation test findings are directly related to compensation and how much to the way these parameters are calculated. Finally, the head impulse test findings remain essentially unchanged with one possible exception. It is suggested that the latency of catch-up saccades decrease with compensation so that they occur during head impulses (MacDougall, Weber, McGarvie, Halmagyi, & Curthoys, 2009). These catch-up saccades are called covert saccades as opposed to the overt saccades that occur after the head impulse. Coverts saccades are assumed to be more efficient because they place the eyes on the target and stabilize the vision more quickly (MacDougall & Curthoys, 2012). More on this topic can be found in Chapter 16.

Static Compensation

The process of increase in the neural activity of the damaged side continues until it returns to its prelesion level. At the same time, cerebellar clamping on the intact side continues to decrease until it is completely lifted. At this point, the patient has achieved static compensation because the neural asymmetry has disappeared and the patient is no longer symptomatic as long as the head remains stationary (Halmagyi et al., 2010).

Vestibular test findings continue the trend from the previous step. Spontaneous nystagmus should disappear completely or its intensity should decrease to an insignificant level. However, the caloric weakness should persist as before. For rotation testing, the phase parameter should stabilize at a level higher than its prelesion level and the gain parameter should stabilize at a level lower than its prelesion level (Baloh et al., 1989). Similarly, the asymmetry parameter should drop to an insignificant level along with the intensity of spontaneous nystagmus. The head impulse test findings should be similar to those in the previous step but perhaps exhibiting even more covert saccades than before.

Static compensation represents a significant milestone in the recovery from a peripheral vestibular lesion. Therefore, it is worthwhile to better understand the process:

1. In animals, if the mobility and visual stimulation are restricted, static compensation is delayed and recovery may never be complete (Zee, 2000). In humans, static compensation seems to occur spontaneously although head-eye coordination exercises may expedite the recovery.

2. Theoretically, static compensation requires complete resolution of the neural asymmetry and disappearance of spontaneous nystagmus. In practice, a small degree of asymmetry may persist indefinitely because the process of compensation continues until the asymmetry reaches a threshold that it is no longer perceived by the patient as head motion. The manifestation of this asymmetry is the continued presence of spontaneous nystagmus with the SPV that is below a certain threshold (typically 4 degrees/second).

3. Static compensation takes place regardless of whether the lesion occurs suddenly or gradually. For example, patients with a vestibular schwannoma usually do not experience many of the symptoms that are associated with the sudden loss of peripheral vestibular function (Parietti-Winkler, Gauchard, Simon, & Perrin, 2011). The reason is that static compensation takes place

incrementally and without obvious signs as the tumor grows gradually and impinges on the vestibular nerve (Uehara et al., 2011).

4. Static compensation is most effective when the lesion is stable. Patients with fluctuating lesions such as in Ménière's disease may not compensate as well as those with nonfluctuating lesions, especially if the attacks are frequent (Lacour, Dutheil, Tighilet, Lopez, & Borel, 2009). In fact, patients with fluctuating lesions may present an interesting pattern of response during the compensation process. After damage to the hair cells or nerve fibers, the compensation process is expect to proceed with the cerebellar clamping stage regardless of whether the lesion is stable or fluctuating (Figure 4–5C). However, if the function returns to the damaged labyrinth during the clamping stage, such as after healing of the ruptured membrane in Ménière's disease, suddenly the asymmetry will be reversed (Figure 4–6). The patient must now undergo another phase of compensation to reverse the effect of cerebellar clamping and restore neural symmetry. In effect, the compensation process extends the length of time that the patient suffers from symptoms. That is why one of the management options for Ménière's disease is to destroy the affected labyrinth and to make the damage permanent. If the attacks of fluctuating lesions are not frequent, the ineffectiveness of the compensation process may not have a long-term effect. However, in patients who suffer from frequent attacks, the compensation mechanisms may cease to respond because of their ineffectiveness and because they lengthen the symptoms.

The reversal of neural asymmetry in Figure 4–6 results in the reversal of spontaneous nystagmus direction (McClure, Copp, & Lycett, 1981). This type of nystagmus that beats toward the side of lesion is sometimes seen with fluctuating lesions. It is called *recovery* nystagmus because it is due to the recovery of vestibular function on the affected side. Significant recovery nystagmus is short lived because the neural activity on the clamped side is elevated rapidly until the asymmetry is resolved. However, residual mild spontaneous nystagmus beating toward the side of lesion may persist for the same reason that was discussed in item 2 above. That is, once the asymmetry decreases below a level that is no longer perceived as head motion, the change in neural activities stops. This discussion also provides a clear example that the direction of spontaneous nystagmus does not always identify the side of the lesion.

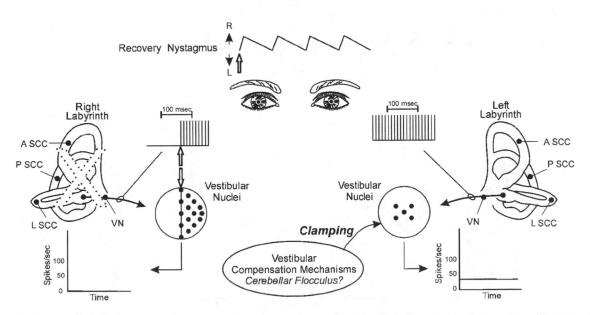

Figure 4–6. Mechanism of recovery nystagmus in fluctuating lesions. Hollow arrows identify the onset of restoration of neural activity after the lesion. Abbreviations are the same as in Figure 4–5. Based on Barin, K. (2014). VNG/ENG Course Handout. *GN Otometrics.*

Dynamic Compensation

After static compensation, the patient no longer suffers symptoms when the head is at rest, but as soon as the head moves, the patient may experience blurry vision and loss of visual acuity. Figure 4–7 shows the underlying reason. If the head moves exactly the same way that it did prior to the onset of the lesion (see Figure 4–5A), the resulting neural asymmetry after static compensation is only half as large as that before the onset of the lesion. There-fore, the head velocity is interpreted to be only half as large as it actually is, and the eyes are moved only half as fast as they should (see Figure 4–7A). The difference between the head and eye velocities is called *retinal slip*. When the retinal slip is not close to zero, images do not stay stationary on the retina, and the patient experiences blurry vision.

One possible method for improving the VOR performance and minimizing the retinal slip is to increase the neural activity of the secondary vestibular neurons from the prelesion level for the same

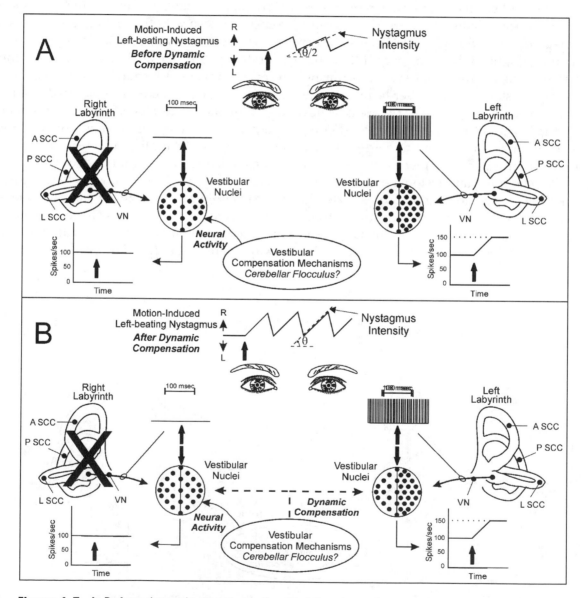

Figure 4–7. A. Before dynamic compensation. **B.** After dynamic compensation. See the text for the description of the process. Abbreviations are the same as in Figure 4–5. Based on Barin, K. (2014). VNG/ENG Course Handout. *GN Otometrics.*

head velocities. There is no direct evidence that such an increase in the VOR gain occurs but there are some compelling correlates. Recall the function of the velocity storage mechanism that behaves as a storage tank with a small outlet. Increasing the VOR gain can be accomplished by increasing the outflow of the neural activity from the velocity storage mechanism (see Figure 4–7B). Although this increases the VOR gain, it also degrades the performance of the VOR for low frequencies, which is the main function of the velocity storage mechanism (Laurens, Valko, & Straumann, 2011). The decline of VOR function in low frequencies is in fact evident in the rotation chair results in which the phase parameter increases and the gain parameters decreases in low frequencies (Baloh et al., 1989).

Understanding the cause of dynamic symptoms provides a clue as to why the compensation process for these symptoms is far more challenging than static compensation. As described before, the internal database that relates different patterns of neural activity to various types of head movements is developed over several years. After a unilateral vestibular lesion, the database no longer provides an accurate measure of the head movements and must be replaced. In addition to the length of time that seems to be required for reestablishing the relationship between neural firing patterns and head movements, one should also recall that the original database is developed during age periods in which the sensory and motor mechanisms are at their peak performance. Later in life when the incidence of vestibular abnormalities is higher, patients often have more difficulty with dynamic compensation because of other confounding issues common to aging such as decline of acuity in the sensory and motor pathways. This may also explain why some patients who successfully achieve dynamic compensation are susceptible to episodes of *decompensation* (Katsarkas & Segal, 1988). That is, a seemingly unrelated event may trigger a bout of symptoms because the compensation mechanisms seem to "forget" the new pattern of neural behavior and revert to the original database.

In addition to the conceptual difficulty in achieving dynamic compensation, there is also a clinical issue in assessing dynamic compensation. That is, the outcome of most vestibular function tests such as the caloric test are the same before and after dynamic compensation and give very little

information about the state and level of compensation (Slattery, Sinks, & Goebel, 2011). Similar to the intensity of spontaneous nystagmus that is a measure of static compensation, retinal slip is the best measure of dynamic compensation. However, most of the existing vestibular function tests do not provide a direct measure of the retinal slip. One test that does provide an indirect measure of the retinal slip is dynamic visual acuity test (Mohammad et al., 2011). However, the test is prone to a number of artifacts, which reduces its effectiveness in assessing dynamic compensation. Dynamic posturography is another method for evaluating dynamic compensation, but postural control abnormalities after a unilateral vestibular lesion usually resolve very quickly and often do not correspond to the patient's dynamic symptoms (Furman, 1994).

If our understanding of the dynamic compensation process turns out to be accurate, the best method to facilitate it is for the patient to be exposed to a variety of head movements. The difference between the head and eye velocities serves as an error signal so that the retinal slip can be reduced gradually. However, some have questioned the neural basis of dynamic compensation. Instead, they propose that dynamic compensation is achieved by other oculomotor mechanisms, such as saccades, substituting for the VOR function (Curthoys, 2000). Although there is merit to the concept of substitution for vestibular compensation, it fails to explain some observations such as the change of gain and phase parameters in the rotation test. Perhaps a combination of neural changes and substitution is a better model for describing the process of dynamic compensation. Interestingly, regardless of whether the aim is adaptation or substitution, the same type of exercises can be used to promote dynamic compensation. More on this topic will follow.

Compensation After Vertical Canal and Otolith Lesions

After a unilateral loss of vestibular function, most patients exhibit imbalance and other postural control deficits. These deficits are likely to be related to the loss function in the vertical canals or the otolith organs. However, postural control deficits seem to resolve more quickly compared to the oculomotor deficits. Perhaps, incorporating the remaining function from the intact labyrinth into the postural control mechanisms is more efficient (Horak, 2010).

The oculomotor effects of vertical canal lesions are similar to those described here for the lateral canal lesions (Aw et al., 1995). The only difference is that the spontaneous nystagmus has both vertical and torsional components. Similarly, the static compensation process is also the same as that described here. In fact, static compensation for vertical and torsional nystagmus seems to require less time than the time required for the resolution of horizontal nystagmus. Although not much is known about the dynamic compensation process for vertical canal lesions, it is logical to expect that it is similar to the process described above as long as the head-eye coordination exercises are performed in the plane of vertical canals.

As noted earlier, very little is known about the effects of otolith lesions other than the fact there is a tonic torsion of the eyes toward the side of lesion (Curthoys, 2000). Over time, the degree of torsion is reduced indicating some level of compensation similar to the disappearance of spontaneous nystagmus (Furman, Hsu, Whitney, & Redfern, 2003). However, the torsion does not resolve completely, which indicates the necessity of some form of dynamic compensation (Curthoys, Dai, & Halmagyi, 1990). If one accepts that view, then exercises that stimulate the otoliths such as translational head movements or eccentric rotation may be needed for compensation (Akin, Hall, & Murnane, 2013).

Compensation After Bilateral Vestibular Lesions

Complete bilateral loss of peripheral vestibular function usually does not result in static symptoms because of the absence of neural asymmetries. At the same time, dynamic compensation based on the changes of neural behavior similar to those described for unilateral lesions is not possible because of the complete loss of vestibular input (McCall & Yates, 2011). Instead, the compensation process involves substitution of other sensorimotor mechanisms for the missing vestibular system. However, compensation is usually incomplete and sometimes ineffective because of the differences in the operating frequency ranges of different sensory mechanisms

(Guinand et al., 2012). For example, the neck receptors can provide information about head movements but the frequency range is considerably lower than the vestibular system. Interestingly, individuals with congenital loss of vestibular function often can function at a level that their impairments may not be obvious to casual observers. Obviously, these individuals have developed alternative strategies that do not rely on the vestibular system. Although it is possible, it is unlikely that most patients with acquired bilateral vestibular loss can reach that level of compensation.

The compensation process is more successful if there is residual vestibular function. A combination of substitution and reliance on the residual vestibular function can provide a moderate level of functional recovery.

When bilateral loss of function is present but it is more significant on one side, the patient undergoes the same type of static and dynamic compensation described for unilateral lesions. However, functional recovery is not likely to be as successful for the same reasons stated above.

Compensation After Central Vestibular Lesions

Central abnormalities can cause vertigo and other balance symptoms. Some of these abnormalities such as those caused by vascular lesions or head trauma can affect peripheral vestibular pathways as well as the central structures. For example, infarcts of some arteries are known to cause sudden hearing and vestibular loss. For those lesions, vestibular compensation for the peripheral component of the abnormality can proceed as described before. However, if there is a simultaneous or preexisting damage to the central compensation mechanisms, then functional recovery may be difficult or impossible to achieve. Animal studies have identified the cerebellar flocculus as an important site for vestibular compensation (Aleisa, Zeitouni, & Cullen, 2007). Therefore, damage to this or the surrounding areas in humans may have a similar adverse effect on the compensation process.

In general, vestibular compensation is not as successful for central vestibular lesions as compared to the peripheral vestibular lesions (Brown, Whitney,

Marchetti, Wrisley, & Furman, 2006). For one thing, it is not known what type of activities may be effective in promoting recovery in these patients. Also, patients with central lesions constitute a nonhomogenous group, and the outcome may depend on the type of lesion.

IMPLICATIONS FOR REHABILITATION

Most of the studies on rehabilitation and exercise therapy for vestibular lesions have focused on unilateral peripheral lesions. As discussed earlier, static compensation after a unilateral peripheral vestibular lesion takes place spontaneously in most patients. However, physical and exercise therapy can expedite the recovery. The most effective approach for promoting dynamic compensation appears to be exercises that are focused on head-eye coordination. These exercises provide the central compensation mechanisms with the error signal (retinal slip) that is necessary to either cause adaption or substitution of the vestibular pathways (Herdman, 2013). These exercises should cover different head velocities and different planes of motion. Furthermore, the exercises should involve visual, proprioceptive, and other sensorimotor mechanisms so that the vestibular input can be properly integrated within the balance control system.

A review of the literature shows that in fact the type of exercises described above is a common part of the rehabilitation protocol for unilateral vestibular lesions (Whitney & Sparto, 2011). These exercises are usually referred to as X1 and X2 viewing exercises. For a detailed discussion, see Chapter 31.

The same type of head-eye coordination exercises can be used for bilateral vestibular lesions (Telian, Shepard, Smith-Wheelock, & Hoberg, 1991). Although the adaptive effects may not be significant, these exercises can promote substitution of the missing or reduced vestibular function in these patients (Porciuncula, Johnson, & Glickman, 2012). For example, during X1 viewing exercises, the patient moves his or her head side to side while fixating on a stationary target. This type of exercise in patients with bilateral vestibular lesions can promote the use of neck receptors to control the eye movements. The success rate of exercise therapy in patients with bilateral lesions is not as high as that of patients with unilateral lesions and often depends on the residual vestibular function.

The rehabilitation protocols for other types of lesions are still evolving because of our limited knowledge of the underlying physiology. It is assumed that general conditioning exercises along with customized protocols may be beneficial, but so far very few studies have focused on these patients.

SUMMARY

Vestibular compensation is the process by which patients achieve functional recovery after a vestibular lesion. The process is most effective for unilateral lesions in which the tonic neural activity is restored at the vestibular nuclei to achieve static compensation and adaptive changes are made to the intact vestibular pathways to achieve dynamic compensation. Compensation for other types of lesions is possible but not as effective.

REFERENCES

Abadi, R. (2002). Mechanisms underlying nystagmus. *Journal of the Royal Society of Medicine, 95*(5), 231–234.

Akin, F., Hall, C., & Murnane, O. (2013). The role of rotational stimulation in vestibular compensation. *Otolaryngology-Head and Neck Surgery, 148*(1), 176–177.

Aleisa, M., Zeitouni, A., & Cullen, K. (2007). Vestibular compensation after unilateral labyrinthectomy: Normal versus cerebellar dysfunctional mice. *Journal of Otolaryngology, 36*(6), 315–321.

Allum, J., & Honegger, F. (2013). Relation between head impulse tests, rotating chair tests, and stance and gait posturography after an acute unilateral peripheral vestibular deficit. *Otology & Neurotology, 34*(6), 980–989.

Aw, S., Halmagyi, G., Pohl, D., Curthoys, I., Yavor, R., & Todd, M. (1995). Compensation of the human vertical vestibulo-ocular reflex following occlusion of one vertical semicircular canal is incomplete. *Experimental Brain Research, 103*(3), 471–475.

Baloh, R., Jacobson, K., Beykirch, K., & Honrubia, V. (1989). Horizontal vestibulo-ocular reflex after acute peripheral lesions. *Acta Oto-Laryngologica. Supplementum, 468*, 323–327.

Barin, K. (2009). Clinical neurophysiology of the vestibular system. In J. Katz, L. Medwetsky, R. Burkhart, & L. Hood, (Eds.), *Handbook of clinical audiology* (6th ed., pp. 431–466). Philadelphia, PA: Lippincott Williams & Wilkins.

Beraneck, M., Idoux, E., Uno, A., Vidal, P., Moore, L., & Vibert, N. (2004). Unilateral labyrinthectomy modifies the membrane properties of contralesional vestibular neurons. *Journal of Neurophysiology, 92*(3), 1668–1684.

Borel, L., Lopez, C., Péruch, P., & Lacour, M. (2008). Vestibular syndrome: A change in internal spatial representation. *Clinical Neurophysiology, 38*(6), 375–389.

Brown, K., Whitney, S., Marchetti, G., Wrisley, D., & Furman, J. (2006). Physical therapy for central vestibular dysfunction. *Archives of Physical Medicine and Rehabilitation, 87*(1), 76–81.

Carey, J. P. (2010). Meniere's disease. In S. D. Z. Eggers & D. S. Zee (Eds.), *Vertigo and imbalance: Clinical neurophysiology of the vestibular system* (pp. 371–381). Philadelphia, PA: Elsevier.

Cloutier, J., & Saliba, I. (2008). Isolated vertigo and dizziness of vascular origin. *Journal of Otolaryngology-Head and Neck Surgery, 37*(3), 331–339.

Courjon, J., Flandrin, J., Jeannerod, M., & Schmid, R. (1982). The role of the flocculus in vestibular compensation after hemilabyrinthectomy. *Brain Research, 239*(1), 251–257.

Curthoys, I. (2000). Vestibular compensation and substitution. *Current Opinion in Neurology, 13*(1), 27–30.

Curthoys, I., Dai, M., & Halmagyi, G. (1990). Human otolithic function before and after unilateral vestibular neurectomy. *Journal of Vestibular Research: Equilibrium & Orientation, 1*(2), 199–209.

Curthoys, I., & Halmagyi, G. (1995). Vestibular compensation: A review of the oculomotor, neural, and clinical consequences of unilateral vestibular loss. *Journal of Vestibular Research: Equilibrium & Orientation, 5*(2), 67–107.

Darlington, C., Flohr, H., & Smith, P. (1991). Molecular mechanisms of brainstem plasticity. The vestibular compensation model. *Molecular Neurobiology, 5*(2–4), 355–368.

Dutia, M. (2010). Mechanisms of vestibular compensation: Recent advances. *Current Opinion in Otolaryngology & Head and Neck Surgery, 18*(5), 420–424.

Fetter, M., & Zee, D. (1988). Recovery from unilateral labyrinthectomy in rhesus monkey. *Journal of Neurophysiology, 59*(2), 370–393.

Fujimoto, C., Murofushi, T., Chihara, Y., Ushio, M., Suzuki, M., Yamaguchi, T., & Iwasaki, S. (2013). Effect of severity of vestibular dysfunction on postural instability in idiopathic bilateral vestibulopathy. *Acta Oto-Laryngologica, 133*(5), 454–461.

Furman, J. (1994). Posturography: Uses and limitations. *Baillière's Clinical Neurology, 3*(3), 501–513.

Furman, J., Hsu, L., Whitney, S., & Redfern, M. (2003). Otolith-ocular responses in patients with surgically confirmed unilateral peripheral vestibular loss. *Journal of Vestibular Research: Equilibrium & Orientation, 13*(2–3), 143–151.

Furman, J., & Whitney, S. (2000). Central causes of dizziness. *Physical Therapy, 80*(2), 179–187.

Guinand, N., Boselie, F., Guyot, J., & Kingma, H. (2012). Quality of life of patients with bilateral vestibulopathy. *Annals of Otology, Rhinology, and Laryngology, 121*(7), 471–477.

Halmagyi, G., Weber, K., & Curthoys, I. (2010). Vestibular function after acute vestibular neuritis. *Restorative Neurology and Neuroscience, 28*(1), 37–46.

Hegemann, S., Straumann, D., & Bockisch, C. (2007). Alexander's law in patients with acute vestibular tone asymmetry—evidence for multiple horizontal neural integrators. *Journal of the Association for Research in Otolaryngology, 8*(4), 551–561.

Herdman, S. (2013). Vestibular rehabilitation. *Current Opinion in Neurology, 26*(1), 96–101.

Horak, F. (2010). Postural compensation for vestibular loss and implications for rehabilitation. *Restorative Neurology and Neuroscience, 28*(1), 57–68.

Jen, J. (2009). Bilateral vestibulopathy: Clinical, diagnostic, and genetic considerations. *Seminars in Neurology, 29*(5), 528–533.

Johnston, A., Seckl, J., & Dutia, M. (2002). Role of the flocculus in mediating vestibular nucleus neuron plasticity during vestibular compensation in the rat. *Journal of Physiology, 545*(Pt. 3), 903–911.

Karatas, M. (2011). Vascular vertigo: Epidemiology and clinical syndromes. *Neurologist, 17*(1), 1–10.

Katsarkas, A., & Segal, B. (1988). Unilateral loss of peripheral vestibular function in patients: Degree of compensation and factors causing decompensation. *Otolaryngology-Head and Neck Surgery, 98*(1), 45–47.

Kim, J., & Kim, H. (2012). Inferior vestibular neuritis. *Journal of Neurology, 259*(8), 1553–1560.

Kim, S., Oh, Y., Koo, J., & Kim, J. (2011). Bilateral vestibulopathy: Clinical characteristics and diagnostic criteria. *Otology & Neurotology, 32*(5), 812–817.

Kutz Jr, J. W., Roland, P. S., & Isaacson, B. (2012). *Acoustic neuroma.* Retrieved January 7, 2014, from http://emedicine.medscape.com/article/882876-overview

Lacour, M. (2006). Restoration of vestibular function: Basic aspects and practical advances for rehabilitation. *Current Medical Research and Opinion, 22*(9), 1651–1659.

Lacour, M., Dutheil, S., Tighilet, B., Lopez, C., & Borel, L. (2009). Tell me your vestibular deficit, and I'll tell you how you'll compensate. *Annals of the New York Academy of Sciences, 1164,* 268–278.

Laurens, J., Valko, Y., & Straumann, D. (2011). Experimental parameter estimation of a visuo-vestibular interaction model in humans. *Journal of Vestibular Research: Equilibrium & Orientation, 21*(5), 251–266.

Lee, J., Park, S., Kim, H., Kim, M., Park, B., & Kim, J. (2014). Vulnerability of the vestibular organs to transient ischemia: Implications for isolated vascular vertigo. *Neuroscience Letters, 558,* 180–185.

Li, J. C., & Lorenzo, N. (2013). *Meniere disease (idiopathic endolymphatic hydrops).* Retrieved January 7, 2014, from http://emedicine.medscape.com/article/1159069-overview

MacDougall, H., & Curthoys, I. (2012). Plasticity during vestibular compensation: The role of saccades. *Frontiers in Neurology, 3,* 1–21.

MacDougall, H., Weber, K., McGarvie, L., Halmagyi, G., & Curthoys, I. (2009). The video head impulse test: Diagnostic accuracy in peripheral vestibulopathy. *Neurology, 73*(14), 1134–1141.

Magnusson, M., Brantberg, K., Pyykkö, I., & Schalén, L. (1989). Reduction of the time constant in the VOR as a protective mechanism in acute vestibular lesions. *Acta Oto-Laryngologica. Supplementum, 468,* 329–332.

Magnusson, M., & Karlberg, M. (2002). Peripheral vestibular disorders with acute onset of vertigo. *Current Opinion in Neurology, 15*(1), 5–10.

Manzari, L., Burgess, A., & Curthoys, I. (2012). Ocular and cervical vestibular evoked myogenic potentials in response to bone-conducted vibration in patients with probable inferior vestibular neuritis. *Journal of Laryngology and Otology, 126*(7), 683–691.

Manzari, L., Burgess, A., MacDougall, H., & Curthoys, I. (2013). Vestibular function after vestibular neuritis. *International Journal of Audiology, 52*(10), 713–718.

McCall, A., & Yates, B. (2011). Compensation following bilateral vestibular damage. *Frontiers in Neurology, 2,* 88.

McClure, J., Copp, J., & Lycett, P. (1981). Recovery nystagmus in Ménière's disease. *Laryngoscope, 91*(10), 1727–1737.

Melvill Jones, G., Guitton, D., & Berthoz, A. (1988). Changing patterns of eye-head coordination during 6 h of optically reversed vision. *Experimental Brain Research, 69*(3), 531–544.

Mohammad, M., Whitney, S., Marchetti, G., Sparto, P., Ward, B., & Furman, J. (2011). The reliability and response stability of dynamic testing of the vestibulo-ocular reflex in patients with vestibular disease. *Journal of Vestibular Research: Equilibrium & Orientation, 21*(5), 277–288.

Olabi, B., Bergquist, F., & Dutia, M. (2009). Rebalancing the commissural system: Mechanisms of vestibular compensation. *Journal of Vestibular Research: Equilibrium & Orientation, 19*(5–6), 201–207.

Parietti-Winkler, C., Gauchard, G., Simon, C., & Perrin, P. (2011). Pre-operative vestibular pattern and balance compensation after vestibular schwannoma surgery. *Neuroscience, 172,* 285–292.

Porciuncula, F., Johnson, C., & Glickman, L. (2012). The effect of vestibular rehabilitation on adults with bilateral vestibular hypofunction: A systematic review. *Journal of Vestibular Research: Equilibrium & Orientation, 22*(5–6), 283–298.

Shepard, N. T. (2009). Signs and symptoms of central vestibular disorders. *American Speech-Language-Hearing Association Access Audiology e-Newsletter.* Retrieved January 7, 2014, from http://www.asha.org/aud/articles/CentralVestib/

Slattery, E., Sinks, B., & Goebel, J. (2011). Vestibular tests for rehabilitation: Applications and interpretation. *Neurorehabilitation, 29*(2), 143–151.

Strupp, M., & Brandt, T. (2013). Peripheral vestibular disorders. *Current Opinion in Neurology, 26*(1), 81–89.

Telian, S., Shepard, N., Smith-Wheelock, M., & Hoberg, M. (1991). Bilateral vestibular paresis: Diagnosis and treatment. *Otolaryngology-Head and Neck Surgery, 104*(1), 67–71.

Uehara, N., Tanimoto, H., Nishikawa, T., Doi, K., Katsunuma, S., Kimura, H., & Nibu, K. (2011). Vestibular dysfunction and compensation after removal of acoustic neuroma. *Journal of Vestibular Research: Equilibrium & Orientation, 21*(5), 289–295.

Vibert, N., Babalian, A., Serafin, M., Gasc, J., Mühlethaler, M., & Vidal, P. (1999). Plastic changes underlying vestibular compensation in the guinea-pig persist in isolated, *in vitro* whole brain preparations. *Neuroscience, 93*(2), 413–432.

Weber, K., Aw, S., Todd, M., McGarvie, L., Curthoys, I., & Halmagyi, G. (2008). Head impulse test in unilateral vestibular loss: Vestibulo-ocular reflex and catch-up saccades. *Neurology, 70*(6), 454–463.

Weber, K., MacDougall, H., Halmagyi, G., & Curthoys, I. (2009). Impulsive testing of semicircular-canal function using video-oculography. *Annals of the New York Academy of Sciences, 1164,* 486–491.

Whitney, S., & Sparto, P. (2011). Principles of vestibular physical therapy rehabilitation. *Neurorehabilitation, 29*(2), 157–166.

Zee, D. S. (2000). Vestibular adaptation. In S. J. Herdman, (Ed.), *Vestibular rehabilitation* (pp. 77–90). Philadelphia, PA: F. A. Davis.

Eye Movement Recording Techniques

Gary P. Jacobson, Neil T. Shepard, Devin L. McCaslin, Erin G. Piker, and J. Andrew Dundas

IMPORTANCE OF EYE MOVEMENT RECORDINGS FOR THE DIAGNOSIS OF VESTIBULAR SYSTEM IMPAIRMENT

The peripheral vestibular system is encased in the temporal bone; accordingly, it is impossible to assess it directly (i.e., as the retina of the eye can be evaluated directly through ophthalmoscopy). However, central nervous system connections exist between the origin of the vestibular second-order neurons in the vestibular nuclei and the central eye movement system. These connections make it possible for individuals with intact vestibular and eye movement systems to ambulate and view stationary objects in front of them with no difficulty. This eye movement function has been described earlier in this text as the vestibulo-ocular reflex (VOR). It is the measurement and quantification of this reflex that enables clinicians to infer indirectly the functional status of the peripheral and central vestibular systems. Additionally, these connections make it possible for clinicians to quantify the dynamics of the eye movement subsystems (e.g., the intactness of gaze maintenance, saccade, pursuit, and optokinetic subsystems).

EYE MOVEMENT RECORDING TECHNIQUES

The measurement of the VOR and ocular motility requires the use of sophisticated methods to transform the movements of the eyes into electrical sig-

nals that can be digitized, processed, and analyzed. There are at least three methods for accomplishing this, and they are described in this chapter. The methods include electro-oculography (EOG) (electronystagmography [ENG]), infrared videonystagmography (VNG) (i.e., video-oculography [VOG]) techniques and scleral search coil techniques. In this chapter we will constrain the discussion of eye movement recording techniques to those used in contemporary vestibular system assessment clinics. Those techniques include ENG and VNG.

Electro-Oculography (EOG)/ Electronystagmography (ENG)

Origin of the Corneoretinal Potential

The electrical transducer of the visual system is the retina which also serves as the source of the corneoretinal potential (CRP). The CRP is a bioelectrical signal that is measured during EOG which is the recording technique used in ENG. The eyeball has a dipolar orientation like a "battery" with the cornea being positively polarized and the retina negatively polarized. This standing potential is propagated through the eye by volume conduction where it is capable of being recorded with conventional surface electrodes.

The origin of the CRP is metabolic activity in the retina and primarily in the retinal pigment epithelium (RPE). This standing potential (i.e., the CRP) is generated by the transepithelial potential across the RPE (Carl, 1997; Marmor & Zrenner, 1993). The pigment epithelial cells located in the retina are spaced closely together, thereby allowing the RPE to maintain the positive and negative charges. When measured at the cornea, the strength of this potential may range from one to several millivolts (Carl, 1997; Marmor & Zrenner, 1993). In ophthalmology, the integrity of the RPE is assessed by recording the standing potential that exists between the cornea and the posterior pole of the eye. The EOG, which reflects RPE function, is the "gold standard" for evaluating vitelliform macular dystrophy (e.g., Best's disease). As metabolic activity in the retina is affected by light, it is not surprising that the CRP varies across levels of illumination. In fact, when the potential is measured in an individual who has been light adapted, there is a twofold increase compared to the dark-adapted measurement. Dark-adapting a patient (i.e., placing the patient in a darkened room) reduces metabolic activity in the RPE, thereby decreasing the CRP potential to its lowest magnitude. It is intuitive that retinal disease would also decrease the magnitude of the CRP because there are fewer functioning pigment epithelial cells to maintain the standing potential.

How Electrodes Are Used to Record the CRP

As the cornea is positively charged and the retina is negatively charged, two electrodes placed at the outer canthus of each eye and routed into a differential amplifier should "see" neither a positive nor a negative charge with the eyes in primary position (Figure 5–1A). If the eyes move conjugately to the right, the electrode at the right outer canthus should record a positive charge (i.e., as the positive pole of the right eye is pointed toward it) and the electrode at the left outer canthus should record a less positive charge (i.e., as less of that cornea is pointing toward that electrode). Thus, if the right electrode sees a +5 mV signal and the left electrode sees a +2 mV signal, the net output of a differential amplifier would be +5 mV minus +2 mV or +3 mV (Figure 5–1B).

A leftward conjugate eye movement of similar magnitude results in the left electrode recording a +5-mV signal and the right electrode recording a +2-mV signal. The net difference between these two inputs would be +2 minus +5 or −3 mV (Figure 5–1C). The convention in EOG recordings is for positive voltages to be represented by upward pen deflections (i.e., for rightward and upward eye devi-

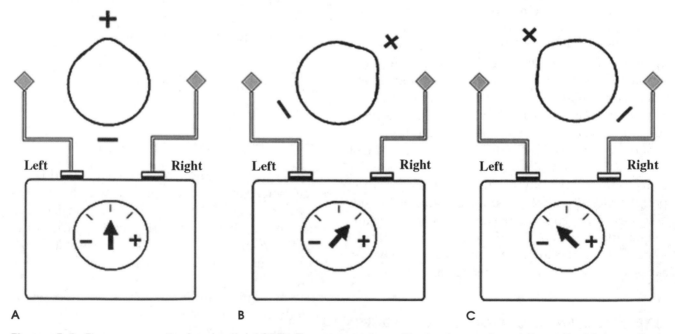

Figure 5-1. The corneoretinal potential (*CRP*). The cornea is positively charged and the retinal is negatively charged. **A.** When the eye is in midline position a pair of electrodes placed on either side of the eye will see neither a positive nor a negative voltage. **B.** When the eye turns to the right, a positive electrical potential is generated. **C.** When the eye turns to the left, a negative electrical potential is generated.

ations), and for negative voltages to be represented by downward pen deflections (i.e., for leftward or downward eye deviations).

Assuming the examiner observes a full, conjugate, range of movement of the eyes during informal testing, most clinicians record EOG using a "bitemporal" electrode array (Figure 5–2). For the detection of lateral eye movements, a pair of electrodes are placed with one located at the outer canthus of each eye. These electrodes should be placed in such a way that a line drawn laterally connecting the electrodes would pass through the center of each pupil when the patient is staring at a midline target. For detection of vertical eye movements, an electrode is placed above and below one eye (i.e., the left eye

in our laboratory for the sake of convenience and consistency) in such a way that the pupil will be bisected by a line connecting the centers of the two electrodes. As the magnitude of the electrical signal emitted by the eye is proportional to the distance separating the electrodes from the eye, the electrodes should be placed as close to the eye as possible without being so close that the electrode becomes an irritant to the patient.

It must be stated that for bitemporal recordings, electrical activity for the two eyes is "averaged." This means that disconjugate movements of the eyes will be missed and underscores the importance for the clinician to examine informally the movements of the eyes to detect gross or subtle ocular

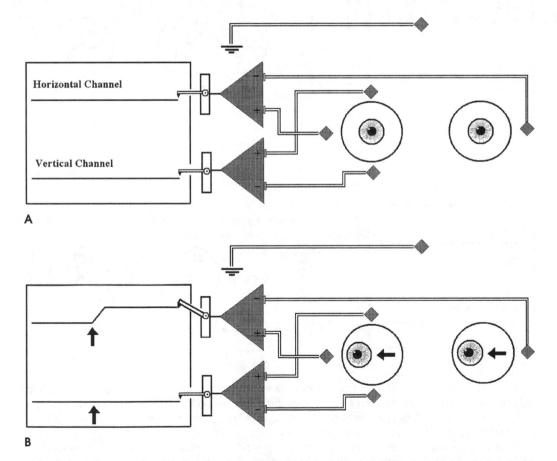

Figure 5–2. Bitemporal electrode montage and the connections to a two-channel differential amplifier (i.e., two channels permit the recording of horizontal and vertical eye deviations). **A.** The horizontal and vertical amplifier outputs to a printer when the eyes are at primary (central) gaze (i.e., there is no pen deflection). **B.** The horizontal and vertical amplifier outputs to a printer for a rightward eye deviation. Notice that a rightward eye movement results in an upward pen deflection in the horizontal channel (a leftward eye deviation would result in a downward pen deflection). *continues*

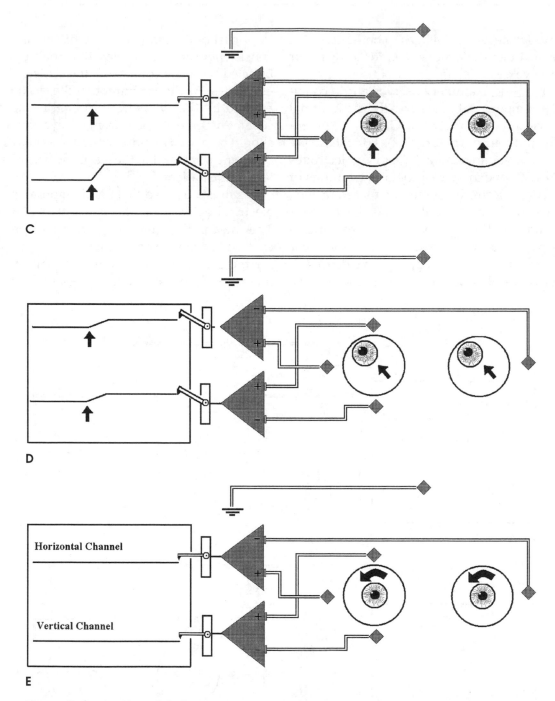

Figure 5–2. *continued* **C.** The horizontal and vertical amplifier outputs to a printer for an upward eye deviation. Notice that an upward eye deviation results in an upward pen deflection in the vertical channel (a downward eye movement would result in a downward pen deflection). **D.** The horizontal and vertical amplifier outputs to a printer for an oblique eye deviation (i.e., an up/right eye movement). Notice that the eye movement is represented by deflections in both the horizontal and vertical channels. **E.** The horizontal and vertical amplifier outputs to a printer for a torsional eye movement. Notice that as the eye is rotating about its anterior/posterior axis there is neither a deviation in the horizontal nor in the vertical channels. This figure was adapted from *An Introduction to ENG,* by C. W. Stockwell, 2004. Schaumburg, IL: GN Otometrics.

motility disorders such as disconjugate eye movements before electrodes are placed on the face or goggles are placed over the eyes. An alternative to the bitemporal electrode placement is the monocular technique (Figure 5–3). The monocular recording technique permits the recording of eye position for each eye separately. This technique is most appropriately used when there is a suspicion that a patient's eye movements may be disconjugate. In this case, for the left eye, one electrode (the "+" or noninverting input) is placed at the left outer canthus, and its mate (the "–" or inverting input) is placed on the lateral side of the nose (i.e., the inside of the bridge of the nose). The noninverting electrode input for the right eye is placed at the right outer canthus, and the inverting electrode input is placed at the inside of the right nasal bridge. The noninverting electrode input for the vertical recordings is placed above the eye and the inverting electrode input for the vertical recordings is placed below the eye. For both bitemporal and monocular recordings, a ground electrode is placed at the nasion, or high forehead (e.g., FPz).

For EOG recording techniques, our objective is to record electrical signals (i.e., the CRP) from the skin surface. However, skin oils, dead skin cells, and cosmetic residue creates an electrical resistance that must be removed to enable electrophysiologic recordings. Thus, prior to application of skin surface electrodes, the skin should be cleansed with a degreasing agent like rubbing alcohol (Figure 5–4A). Additionally, it is common to remove the squamous epithelium of the epidermis with a commercially available, medical-grade, mild liquid abrasive that is best applied to the skin with a cotton-tipped applicator (Figure 5–4B). Following this, the liquids are removed with a gauze pad (Figure 5–4C) and the disposable Ag/AgCl electrodes are applied (Figures 5–4D and 5–4E). Following this protocol will result in individual electrode impedances <10,000 ohms. The objective should be for individual electrode impedances to be <10,000 ohms and for interelectrode impedances to be no greater than 3000 ohms. Obtaining these targets will ensure full benefit of the common mode rejection in the differential amplifiers, resulting in a quiet signal with sensitivity in the 1-degree subtended arc range.

The electrode pairs are routed to a differential amplifier that literally subtracts the electrical signal

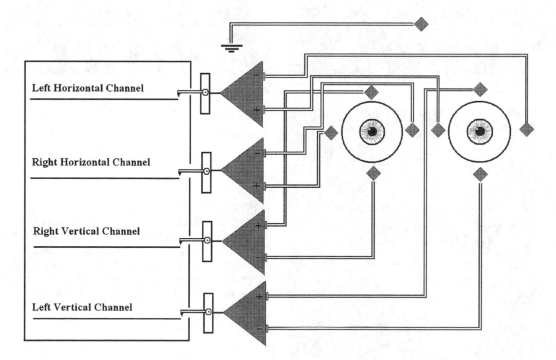

Figure 5–3. Electrode locations and four-channel amplifier connections for a monocular montage.

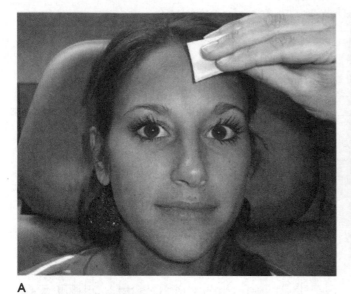

A

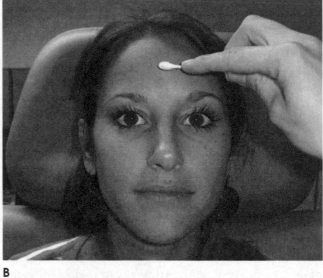

B

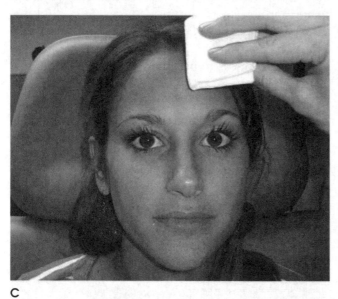

C

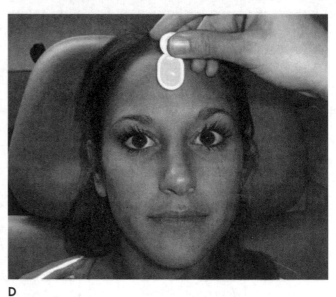

D

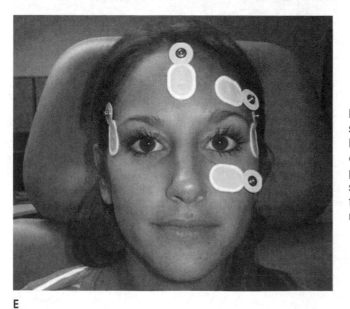

E

Figure 5-4. EOG skin preparation technique. **A.** The skin is rubbed lightly with an alcohol soaked gauze pad. **B.** The skin is then rubbed with a commercially available medical-grade mild abrasive preparation. **C.** The preparation is then wiped from the skin. **D.** A disposable silver/silver-chloride electrode is placed on the site. **E.** All five electrodes have been placed for a bitemporal recording.

recorded by the inverting electrode input from the electrical signal recorded by the noninverting electrode input (see Figures 5–2A through 5–2C). In doing this, electrical activity that is unrelated to the CRP (i.e., unwanted electrical interference) that is common to both the inverting and noninverting electrodes (e.g., stray 60-Hz electrical signals, EKG interference) will be subtracted out (and eliminated), a technique referred to as common mode rejection (CMR). This should result in a reduction in the noisiness of the EOG recordings.

Placement of the electrodes in these positions and routing the electrode wires to the amplifier inputs described above results in upward pen deviations for rightward eye movements and downward pen deviations for leftward eye movements for the horizontal recordings. For vertical recordings, upward eye deviations result in upward pen deflections, and downward eye deviations result in downward pen deflections.

The electrical signals resulting from conjugate horizontal eye deviations are approximately 20 µV per 1 degree of eye deviation in normal subjects with normal retinal function. These eye signals must be amplified by a factor of approximately 10,000 for the eye signals to be within an amplitude range that can be digitized and processed by most computerized data acquisition and processing systems.

How Ag/AgCl Electrodes Are Superior to Silver Electrodes for Near Direct Current (DC) Recordings

There are a number of types of electrodes that may be used to record the EOG. The most common types of electrodes are nondisposable disk or cup electrodes that are made of precious metals (e.g., silver, gold, or silver/silver chloride pellets), or disposable electrodes that usually are silver/silver chloride (i.e., Ag/AgCl) in composition. Of the most common types, the disposable Ag/AgCl electrodes are most often used in busy clinics. The attractiveness of the disposable Ag/AgCl electrodes is their consistency in quality (i.e., quality control during production) and their stability for recording eye movements over an extended period of time (i.e., over 1 to 2 h). The added benefit of the Ag/Ag/Cl electrode is its sensitivity to low-frequency eye signals that are at the DC level.

For most eye movement recording tasks, we attempt to record an eye position that is changing over time. Thus, for most applications, the clinician is attempting to record an alternating current, or AC signal. However, to test for gaze stabilization, the eyes move from one position to another and that position may be held for 20 to 30 s. Thus, for gaze system testing the eye signal is much closer to a direct current, or DC signal. Silver is an element that has an excess of positive ions (Ag+). As such, and in an effort to equilibrate this imbalance in ions, a silver electrode placed on the skin will draw from the skin to its face negative ions. Any attempt to record a steady DC signal with a conventional silver electrode may be contaminated with a steady, slow negative potential drift (i.e., until the positive charge of the silver electrode has been equilibrated with negative charges from the skin). The drift continues until the amplification system becomes unable to offset this DC drift and the amplifier becomes saturated. A solution to this problem is to deposit negative ions on the face of a silver electrode and in so doing equilibrate the positive charge. A simple method of doing this is depositing (or electroplating) chloride (Cl–) onto the face of the electrode. Recording a near DC eye signal with a "chlorided" silver electrode will offset the skin potential drift. However, chloriding a silver electrode is no small feat. If too many negative ions are placed on the electrode face an opposite situation can occur where the electrode may demonstrate a positive DC drift as once again the body attempts to equilibrate the charge. A much simpler method of obtaining an Ag/AgCl electrode is to purchase disposable electrodes from companies that manufacture instrumentation that is used in clinical electroneurodiagnostics (e.g., evoked potentials, electro-oculography).

Sensitivity of EOG/ENG Recordings in Degrees of Subtended Eye Movement

The naked eye of a skilled observer is capable of detecting an eye movement on the order of 0.5 degrees. The noise floor of most EOG recording systems is approximately 1 degree. EOG techniques are capable of detecting a 1-degree deviation of the eye. However, this sensitivity assumes no noise in the recording system. That is, if EMG activity is producing particularly high electrical noise in the recording, the eye deviation will have to be greater to overcome this noise and be visible. In a similar vein, if the CRP is extraordinarily low (i.e., due to retinal disease), the recording system will have to amplify the residual CRP to such a high level during calibration that a 1-degree eye movement will become embedded in the amplifier noise of the recording system. Finally, the range of movement that can be recorded with EOG techniques is approximately 40 degrees.

Advantages of EOG/ENG

There are a number of advantages to the use of EOG for recording eye position during ENG testing. EOG electrodes are inexpensive. The cost of VNG goggles is approximately $6,000 per set. EOG recording techniques enable us to record the position of the eye over a larger portion of its range of movement compared to VNG recording methods. EOG provides a method for indirectly assessing the intactness of retinal function (see section on retinal pathology and the CRP). Additionally, there are situations where VNG techniques cannot be used. Patients with ptosis of the eyelids (i.e., drooping eyelids that cover the pupil), children under the age of 5 who do not tolerate the occlusive goggle systems because their faces are too small, and patients with disease affecting the shape of the pupil and patients who, for various reasons, are unable to keep their eyes open constitute groups where attempts to use VNG techniques may be unsuccessful.

Disadvantages of EOG/ENG

For each of the advantages associated with EOG recordings, there also are disadvantages.

CRP Strength. The magnitude of the CRP is affected by nonpathologic variables such as the level of ambient room light as well as pathologies such as retinal degeneration, diabetic retinopathy, hypertensive retinopathy, and retinitis pigmentosa.

Ambient Illumination and the CRP. Ambient illumination has an impact on the strength of the CRP. In this regard, the magnitude of the CRP in the dark-adapted environment is twofold smaller than the CRP in a light-adapted environment. Darkness adaptation requires 7 to 12 min. That is, 7 to 12 min are required for the CRP to stabilize at its lowest level when moving from light to dark conditions. Conversely, 6 to 9 min are required for the CRP to stabilize when moving from dim light to bright light (Lightfoot, 2004). In many laboratories ocular motility testing and positional testing are conducted in lighted environments (i.e., to maximize CRP strength) and caloric testing is done in dimly lit environments. If patients are tested in a dimly lit room with the calibration obtained in normal room light, the magnitude of the nystagmus slow phase velocity may be spuriously low (i.e., as the CRP signal will be reduced in strength in the darkened room). Because of this, it is recommended that recalibration of eye movements occur frequently during the ENG examination, at least prior to each subset of tests (i.e., ocular motility testing, positional/positioning testing, and caloric testing).

Retinal Pathology and the CRP. On occasion we noticed that our ENG traces appeared "fuzzy." We were unsure at first whether the poor quality of the tracings represented overlaid EMG activity. In fact, it became apparent that during the automated calibration routine the acquisition computer was increasing the amplification of the eye signal to its maximum level as the CRP was inordinately small. What we were observing was system noise (i.e., the noise floor of the recording system) resulting as a byproduct of this amplification. When they were referred to an ophthalmologist these patients were found to have retinal disease. In this investigation, Jacobson and McCaslin (2004) reported that undiagnosed retinal disease could be identified by observing the magnitude of amplification provided by the EOG recording system for purposes of eye movement calibration in the dark-adapted condition. It is in this condition that the CRP should be the lowest. The same investigators reported first percentile values for men and women as 7.1 μV per degree and 9.0 μV per degree, respectively, and fifth percentile values for men and women as 8.2 μV per degree and 10.8 μV per degree, respectively. As a result of our observations we created a data pool and, from that, percentile values for CRP strength in a dark-adapted environment. These values are shown in Table 5–1 for both men and women. Examples of two patients with abnormally low CRPs are shown in Figures 5–5A and 5–5B and Figures 5–6A and 5–6B.

Table 5-1. Percentile Values Associated With CRP Values Corresponding to 1-Degree Eye Deviations From Midline

Gender	1st	5th	10th	15th	20th	50th	80th	85th	90th	95th	99th
Male	7.1	8.2	9.2	9.5	10.4	13.8	17.3	19.1	19.9	21.8	25.8
Female	9.0	10.8	11.4	13.0	13.2	17.2	21.7	22.2	24.5	27.3	28.2

Source: From G. P. Jacobson and D. L. McCaslin, 2004. Detection of ophthalmic impairments indirectly with electronystagmography. *Journal of the American Academy of Audiology, 15,* 258–263. Courtesy of the American Academy of Audiology.

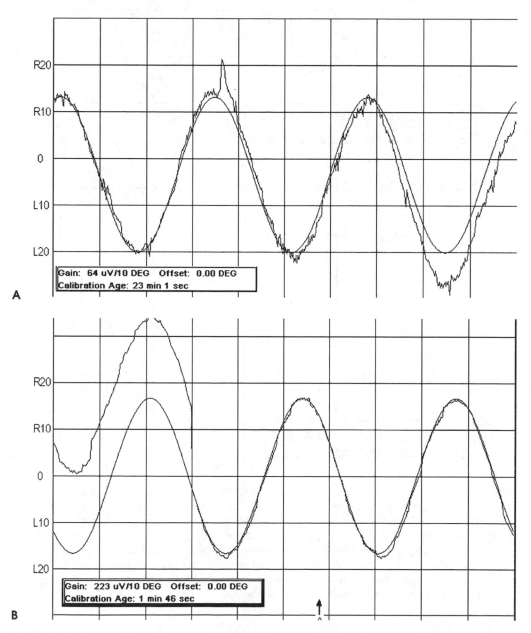

Figure 5-5. A. Horizontal (i.e., bitemporal electrode derivation) calibration tracing obtained from a 69-year-old male with diabetic retinopathy. Notice the noise superimposed on the eye movement recording. This patient's calibration values fell below the first percentile for a cohort of men. **B.** Horizontal calibration tracing obtained from a normal patient. From: G. P. Jacobson and D. L. McCaslin, 2004. Detection of ophthalmic impairments indirectly with electronystagmography. *Journal of the American Academy of Audiology, 15,* 258–263. Courtesy of the American Academy of Audiology.

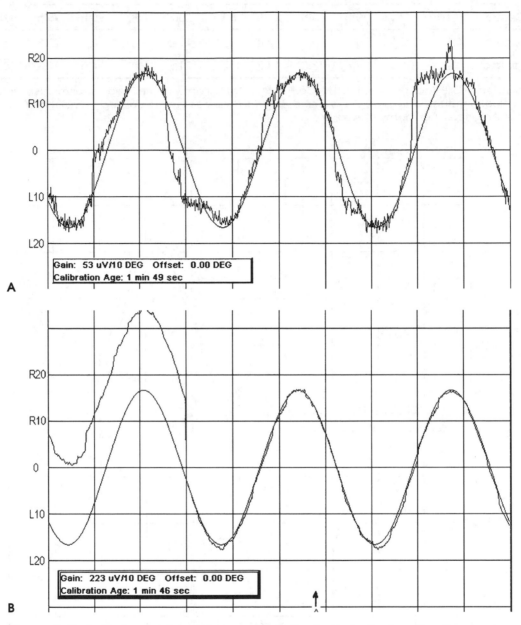

Figure 5-6. A. Horizontal (i.e., bitemporal electrode derivation) calibration tracing obtained from an 80-year-old female patient with advanced glaucoma and hypertensive retinopathy. Notice the noise superimposed on the eye movement recording. This patient's calibration values fell below the first percentile for a cohort of men. **B.** Horizontal calibration tracing obtained from the same normal patient as in Figure 3–5B. From: G. P. Jacobson and D. L. McCaslin, 2004. Detection of ophthalmic impairments indirectly with electronystagmography. *Journal of the American Academy of Audiology, 15,* 258–263. Courtesy of the American Academy of Audiology.

Eye-Blink Artifact. The most common contaminant in EOG recordings is eye-blink artifact. This artifact is a combination of contractions of both the levator palpebrae and orbicularis oculi muscles. Additionally, for bitemporal recordings, if one or both electrodes are placed above the outer canthus it is possible for vertical eye-blink artifact to be "injected" into the horizontal eye movement recording channel (i.e., because the electrodes are in the plane for recording vertical eye movements). An example of how eyeblink artifact can mimic horizontal nystagmus is shown in Figure 5–7.

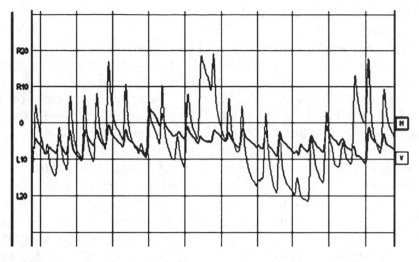

Figure 5-7. Bitemporal recordings of a patient with eye-blink artifacts throughout a center gaze recording. Notice how the eye-blink artifact "bleeds" into the horizontal channel. It is difficult to determine whether the deflections in the horizontal channel represent horizontal, right-beating nystagmus, or cross-talk from the vertical channel.

Insensitivity to the Recording of Torsional Eye Movements. EOG techniques are capable of recording horizontal eye movements with high fidelity but are less able to represent faithfully vertical eye movements due to the influence of eye-blink artifacts. EOG techniques are incapable of recording torsional eye movements. That is, if the eye moves in a circular direction about an anterior/posterior axis (i.e., a torsional eye movement, with the axis passing through the pupil), there will be no net change in the CRP as the eye will be moving neither right nor left, nor up nor down. Accordingly, the torsional eye movement will be missed by EOG recording techniques. Although not dominant as in benign paroxysmal positional vertigo (BPPV), torsional eye movements do occur with the majority of horizontal and vertical movement but are overshadowed by those movements. When torsional eye movements do occur likely secondary to pathology, the use of the EOG recording system will reflect the not pure torsional movements as a series of horizontal and vertical movements and hence misrepresent the positional of the eye in the orbit over time. This is typically represented as diagonal movements of the eye. Disorders like BPPV result in eye movements with a strong torsional component. The use of video-recording techniques provides a means for identifying visually these eye movements.

Bell's Phenomenon. Bell's phenomenon describes the reflexive and protective averting and adducting movement of the eyes that occurs during eye closure. The magnitude of the vertical component can be as great as 151 degrees (Goebel, Stroud, Levine, & Muntz, 1983). In these situations it has been reported that induced nystagmus may become dysrhythmic (Goebel et al., 1983). As positional and positioning tests are often conducted with eyes closed, it is possible for nystagmus to be distorted in patients who have unusually large Bell's phenomena.

DC Drift. The drawing of negative ions out of the skin to the face of a metal electrode (e.g., silver) results in DC drift (see above discussion). This can be offset by better skin preparation, more aggressive high-pass filtering (i.e. filtering out low-frequency DC-like signals) or connecting the patient to an AC-coupled amplifier with a sufficiently short time constant.

Infrared Videorecording Techniques

Infrared video eye tracking systems have recently been adopted by several manufacturers of vestibular testing equipment because of their reliability, precision, patient comfort, and ease of use. Video tracking systems make use of pupil localization technology and the reflective properties of the corneal surface to calculate pupil position and angle of gaze. Implementation of the system varies between manufacturers, but most make use of a goggle-type headpiece that contains infrared diodes to illuminate the eyes, dichroic glass "mirrors" that reflect the image of the eyes into a pair of cameras that record the image of the eye. A headband holds the assembly over the eyes (Figure 5–8). This setup fixes the camera in place relative to the head, ensuring that changes in observed pupil position are caused solely by eye movements rather than a combination of head and eye movements.

Although scleral search coils are still considered the gold standard for eye movement recordings, infrared video tracking systems have rapidly become the state-of-the-art technique for recording eye movements. A method for creating a vision-denied condition is the final component of the hardware.

The goggle set is best placed over the patient's eyes with the headband placed as low on the scalp as possible and then secured with the headband as tight as the patient will permit. The infrared diodes illuminate the eyes. The dichroic glass makes it possible for room light to pass through unaltered (so the

patient can follow the visual targets during ocular motility testing) but will reflect into the left and right eye cameras. Last, there are controls on the goggles that permit the eye image to be raised, lowered, converged, diverged, or focused.

The systems currently on the market can be grouped broadly into bright-pupil and dark-pupil systems. Bright-pupil systems utilize an infrared illumination source coaxial to (i.e., in line with) the camera. The reflection of light from the retina causes the pupil to appear bright relative to the surrounding iris and cornea similar to the "red-eye" effect commonly seen in flash photography. This contrast allows identification of the pupil with high accuracy. Dark-pupil tracking systems make use of off-axis illumination to generate contrast between the pupil and the iris. In this case, the pupil appears dark relative to the higher reflectivity of the iris and cornea tissues. In both cases, the video signal is analyzed by computer to locate the pupil/iris interface using a circle detection algorithm known as a Hough transform (Clarke, Ditterich, Druen, Schonfeld, & Steineke, 2002) (Figure 5–9). The center of the detected pupil circle is used as one point of reference for the calculation of eye position. The spatial coordinates of at least one additional reference point are required to allow calculation of eye position. Ideally, this point would be static regardless of eye movements. Such a reference point can be created by locating the position of a reflected light pattern on the cornea. Known as the first Purkinje image, this pattern is typically generated using an infrared light source or sources oriented in a distinct pattern. Infrared light is utilized as it is invisible to the human visual system and does not induce a contraction of the pupil or allow fixation in the dark.

To calculate eye position, two assumptions are necessary. First, it must be assumed that the surface of the cornea is essentially spherical. Thus, as eye position changes, the location of the reflected image remains static on the cornea, whereas the position of the pupil changes. Second, it must be assumed that the ray projected through the center of the cornea and the center of the pupil approximates the axis of gaze. The optic axis is approximately 5 degrees above the visual axis and, thus, the second assumption can be compensated with a constant addition of angle. As the distance between the eye and the camera is fixed, the vector (i.e., the distance and direc-

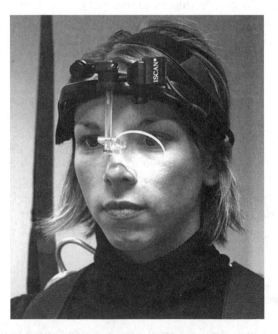

Figure 5-8. Model wearing a monocular, video eye movement recording system. The lens reflects the left eye image into a head-mounted video camera.

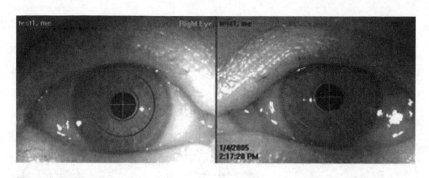

Figure 5–9. How software in a video eye-movement recording system permits the identification of the pupil and iris.

tion) between the reference reflection position and the ray through the center of the detected pupil can be computed, and the direction of gaze due to rotation of the eye about its axis interpolated. Rapidly repeated calculations of direction of gaze allow for the calculation of the position of the eye over time, and derivation of instantaneous eye velocity and acceleration.

Figures 5–10 and 5–11 illustrate the effect of eye movements on the length of the vector between the center of the pupil, (*P*), and the first Purkinje image, or "glint" (*G*) reflected from a light source to the camera. Figure 5–10 illustrates a dark-pupil system, whereas Figure 5–11 illustrates a bright-pupil system. Following calibration movements, the radius of curvature of the cornea can be approximated. When the eye rotates to the left, vector PG increases in length. As the distance between the camera focal point and the light source *L* is known, the magnitude of angle GCP can be calculated. As the target, camera focal point, and light source are collinear, subtending the ray (C*t*) (direction of gaze) through the pupil at angle GCP allows for calculation of the position of the target. Figure 3–10(i) illustrates the large vector produced between the center of the pupil and the first Purkinje image when gaze is directed away from the light source. Figure 3–10(iii) illustrates the small vector produced when gaze is directed toward the light source.

Advantages of Infrared Video-Oculography (VOG)

Video-oculography does not require the application of electrodes. Temporal resolution is sufficient for the documentation of all but the fastest eye move-

ments (i.e., those seen with large saccades, at 400 to 500 degrees per second; also see Chapters 9 and 10 for further discussion). Numerous authors have reported that with each successive revision of the technology, both angular and temporal resolution is improved (Ruetsche, Baumann, Jiang, & Mojon, 2003; van der Geest & Frens, 2002). Currently, temporal resolution is limited only by the frame rate of the camera (i.e. currently state of the art is 250 frames per second for each eye). Measurements can be performed with the patient in complete darkness by sealing the eyes inside a "light-tight" goggle. For most instruments vision is occluded with the use of a cover that is applied to the front of the goggle. Even though the patient is in complete darkness, lumination of the eye still is provided by the infrared LED array. These wavelengths of light are invisible to the subject but easily detectable by the measurement camera. Perhaps the greatest advantage of VOG is that video of the moving eye can be recorded and replayed for post hoc analysis in difficult to recognize eye movement, for the patient (i.e., for patient counseling), for the referring provider (i.e., to assist with the diagnosis), and for students (i.e., for educational purposes).

Disadvantages of Video-Oculography (VOG)

It is impossible to measure eye movements with the eyes closed as the system requires visualization of the pupil and cornea to perform the necessary calculations for localization of gaze. This means that patients with ptosis are poor candidates for VOG recordings. Angular range is lower than that which can be achieved with electro-oculography measurement techniques. This limitation is imposed by the

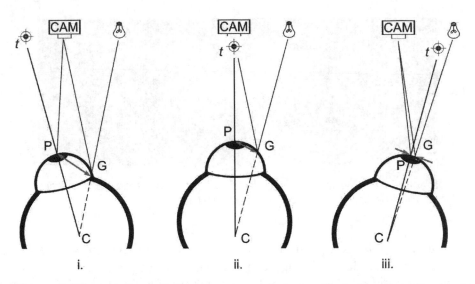

Figure 5–10. A dark-pupil video oculography setup illustrating the effects of eye movements on the magnitude of vector PG between the center of the pupil (*P*) and the center of the first Purkinje image (*G*) for (i) eye movement away from the light source, (ii) eyes in the primary position, and (iii) eye movement toward the light source.

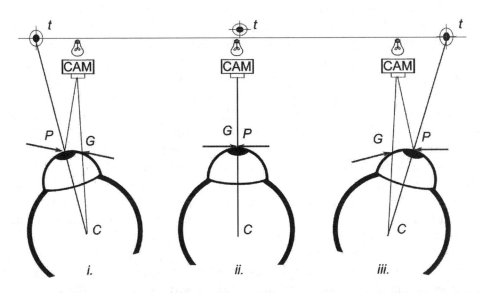

Figure 5–11. A bright-pupil video oculography setup illustrating the effects of eye movements on the magnitude of vector PG between the center of the pupil (*P*) and the center of the first Purkinje image (*G*) for (i) eye movement away from the light source, (ii) eyes in the primary position, and (iii) eye movement toward the light source.

requirement to maintain the first Purkinje reflection on the surface of the cornea to satisfy the requirements of angle of gaze calculation algorithm. Also, the goggle housing of most current goggles makes it difficult for patients to view visual targets at the extremes of gaze (i.e., 30 degrees). Most manufacturers have not created goggles specifically for use with pediatric patients. When vision is occluded (e.g., during VOR suppression testing, position or caloric testing) some claustrophobic patients may be frightened and indeed may panic. This problem does not occur with ENG recoding techniques. Last, VNG goggles are more costly than are electrodes. However, we feel that the cost difference is negligible when compared to the cost of purchasing disposable electrodes over, for example, a 5-year period.

A summary of the characteristics of the various eye movement recording techniques is presented in Table 5–2, including scleral search coil techniques which are not typically used for recording nystagmus in a clinical setting, and thus are not discussed in detail in this chapter.

RECORDING CONSIDERATIONS

In the world of the dizzy patient, all of the four techniques presented in Table 5–2 are used, but only two of the four are used on a regular basis by the vast majority of facilities evaluating this patient group. These are the electro-oculography and videorecording (video-oculography) techniques. As different as these techniques are, there are common requirements that are necessary to provide for accurate representation of the movements of the eye relative to the head reference. These issues deal with the bandwidth of the signal (the range of frequencies accepted into the recording), the rate of sampling of the eye movements (i.e., the digitization rate sets the limits on how fast an eye movement the recording system can resolve), and type and gain of the amplifiers. The majority of these parameters are specified in the American National Standards Institute's (ANSI) "Procedures for testing basic vestibular function" (ANSI, 1999). The following are the basic recommendations for eye movement recordings via either of the two principal methods.

Electro-Oculography (EOG/ENG)

- Maximum impedance of the electrode to the skin of 10,000 ohms is measured in a frequency range of 0.1 to 40 Hz.
- Routine use of EOG will involve a minimum of two channels for recording, one for horizontal and one for vertical movements.
- The accuracy of the analog to digital conversion will be a minimum of a 12-bit conversion.
- The sampling rate should be a minimum of 100 samples per second.

Table 5–2. Comparison of Characteristics of Four Techniques for Recording Eye Movements

Variable	EOG/ENG	VOG/VOG	Infrared	Scleral Coil
Spatial resolution	~0.1 degree	~0.5 degree	~0.1 degree	~0.01 degree
Temporal resolution	40 Hz	60 Hz	100 Hz	1000 Hz +
Vertical recording	Possible but confounded by eye-blink artefact	Good (can view/store video of torsional eye movements)	Possible but confounded by eye-blink artefact	Good, torsional recordings also are possible
Setup	Slow (requires electrode application) Calibration is required	Fast (calibration is required; however, there is no CRP to vary with illumination)	Fast (but requires calibration)	Slow (requires calibration)
Linearity	Good	Reasonable	Problematic; signal may reverse between +15 and +20 degrees	Good
Cost	Low	Expensive	Moderate	Expensive

Source: Adapted from http://www.tchain.com/otoneurology/practice/eyemove.html

- A differential, DC-coupled amplifier with at least a 100-dB common-mode rejection rating and a minimum gain of 60 dB with both coarse and fine adjustments.
- The input will incorporate a minimum band-pass filter between 0 and 40 Hz
- Resolution of eye movements with this technique should be at least ±1 degree in both the vertical and horizontal planes of movement.

Infrared Video-Oculography (VOG/VNG)

- Use two cameras, one per eye, with a minimum resolution of 400 TV lines per camera.
- Recordings will involve two channels of resolution, one for horizontal and one for vertical tracking.
- Frame rates for the cameras should be at least 30 frames per second sampling rate. These should be arranged in an interleaving method so that the resulting overall rate is 60 frames per second. It should be noted that although this is sufficient to handle most of the eye movements during a routine VNG examination, eye movements with frequencies greater than half the sample rate may not be represented accurately. For eye movement with speeds in the range of large saccades, this sampling rate may underestimate the peak velocity (i.e., see Chapter 9 for further discussion of this issue). The ANSI recommendation is to move the equipment to cameras with frame rates of 60 frames per second as soon as the technology is available at reasonable prices.
- The camera location with occlusive goggles or see-through systems should be adjustable so as to align with the primary (straight ahead gaze) line of vision of the eye to within ±10 degrees.
- The goggles should provide for clear visual field viewing when fixation is present in a minimum range of ±30 degrees horizontally and ±20 degrees vertically.
- When the goggle system is used to provide the "fixation-removed," or "vision-denied" condition for testing, it should not allow

any significant visible light. Additionally, the inferred light sources within the goggles should not be visible when the subject is fully dark adapted. The illumination in the fixation-removed condition should be uniformly distributed so as to allow for recording of the eye movement in the range of ±30 degrees horizontally and ±20 degrees vertically.

- Resolution of this technique should be at least 0.2 degrees of movement horizontally and 0.3 degrees of movement vertically.

Calibration

For either the EOG or VOG techniques, a method is needed by which a specified movement of the eye, in degrees of subtended arc, is associated with the parameter used by the computer system to record the eye (i.e., voltage in the use of EOG, and pixels in the use of VOG). ANSI recommends that the magnitude of the eye movement used to calibrate the system be ±20 degrees to either side of center horizontally and ±10 degrees vertically. It is also recommended that during the calibration process, a minimum of eight movements of the eye to each of the horizontal and vertical positions be used to establish the relationship between the degrees of eye movement and the recording parameter for the technique.

Various manufacturers use different target trajectories for calibration targets, saccades, or sinusoidal movements. The trajectory of the target is only a means by which to provoke the subject to move the eyes to a specific location. Therefore, the shape of the target movement is not important as long as the peak excursion meets the needs for the calibration procedure. For some patients one movement of the target may be more easily followed than another. Thus, having options for different target movements or being able to slow down the target movement is desirable.

A final consideration when comparing the two-dimensional EOG to the VOG techniques involves the information available in the recorded data. Even though the VOG technique provides a means for viewing the full three-dimensional movements of the eyes (i.e., horizontal-yaw, vertical pitch, and tor-sional-roll planes), the final recorded material is not different from the EOG. Both provide for only yaw and pitch movement recordings. One of the advantages to the VOG system is that videorecordings provide a means of documenting the presence of, and direction of, torsional eye movements. As torsional movements of the eye result in both yaw and pitch movements simultaneously, one must keep in mind that what may appear as a diagonal movement from the final recorded material could easily have involved torsional movement. The eye movements during posterior canal BPPV represent a classic example. In right-sided BPPV the right torsional beating (superior pole of the eye beating toward the right) is represented on a two-dimensional recording system (i.e., EOG/ENG) as up-beating and left-beating nystagmus.

SUMMARY

This chapter provides a basic foundation in the various eye movement recording techniques used both in assessment of eye movement abnormalities and the dizzy patient. Although these methods allow for archival information, one must not overlook the method of direct visualization. The well-trained and experienced examiner can obtain a thorough initial assessment of the dizzy patient with the use of little in the way of equipment (see Chapter 9 in this text for a complete discussion). As is the case in all aspects of the evaluation of the patient with complaints of dizziness and balance disorders, the patient's presenting signs and symptoms via the intake history constitute the paramount information for the diagnosis and decisions on management.

Therefore, the recorded movements of the eyes, no matter how abnormal, always need to be interpreted in the context of the patient's neuro-otologic history.

REFERENCES

ANSI. (1999). Procedures for testing basic vestibular function. *American National Standards Institute*, BSR S3.45-200X, revision of ANSI S3.45.

Carl, J. R. (1997). Principles and techniques of electrooculography. In G. P. Jacobson, C. W. Newman, & J. M. Kartush (Eds.), *Handbook of balance function testing* (pp. 69–82). San Diego, CA: Singular.

Clarke, A. H., Ditterich, J., Druen, K., Schonfeld, U., & Steineke, C. (2002). Using high frame-rate CMOS sensors for three-dimensional eye tracking. *Behavior Research Methods, Intruments, and Computers, 34*, 549–560.

Goebel, J. A., Stroud, M. H., Levine, L. A., & Muntz, H. R. (1983). Vertical eye deviation and nystagmus inhibition during mental tasking. *Laryngoscope, 93*, 1127–1132.

Jacobson, G. P., & McCaslin, D. L. (2004). Detection of opthalmic impairments indirectly with electronystagmography. *Journal of the American Academy of Audiology, 15*, 258–263.

Lightfoot, G. R. (2004). The origin of order effects in the results of the bi-thermal caloric test. *International Journal of Audiology, 43*, 276–282.

Marmor, M. F., & Zrenner, E. (1993). Standard for clinical electro-oculography. International Society for Clinical Electrophysiology of Vision (Abstract). *Archives in Ophthalmology, 111*, 601–604.

Ruetsche, A., Baumann, A., Jiang, X., & Mojon, D. S. (2003). Automated analysis of eye tracking movements. *Opthalmologica, 217*, 320–324.

van der Geest, J. N., & Frens, M. A. (2002). Recording eye movements with video-oculography and scleral search coils: A direct comparison of two methods. *Journal of Neuroscience Methods, 114*, 185–195.

6

The Vertigo Case History

Lauren T. Roland, Belinda C. Sinks, and Joel A. Goebel

This chapter focuses on the elements of the case history of the dizzy patient. The diagnosis is often revealed during the clinical interview.

MAGNITUDE OF THE PROBLEM

Dizziness is a common problem seen in primary care clinics and emergency departments and is one of the most common symptoms referred to neurology and otolaryngology practices (Kroenke, Hoffman, & Einstadter, 2000). Dizziness is prevalent in all adult populations and accounts for significant health care costs. The prevalence of dizziness in the elderly population is estimated at greater than 30% (Sloane, Coeytaux, Beck, & Dallara, 2001). A literature review reported that of patients presenting to primary-care offices, emergency rooms, and referral clinics, 44% of patients with dizziness complaints suffered from peripheral vestibulopathy, whereas only 11% of dizziness was attributed to central vestibulopathy (Kroenke et al, 2000). While life-threatening emergencies associated with dizziness complaints are rare, it is important to differentiate between disorders of dizziness to ensure that permanent impairments are avoided (Sloane et al., 2001).

IMPORTANCE OF TAKING A COMPLETE HISTORY

A complete history is crucial to the diagnosis and management of the dizzy patient. Diagnostic vestibular tests quantify function within the system, which is sometimes helpful for a differential diagnosis; however, an accurate diagnosis can often be made from the history alone if the appropriate questions are asked and time is taken to understand the patient's true experience.

For patients complaining of symptoms of disequilibrium, unsteadiness, or light-headedness, history taking is an important tool to evaluate for the possibility of a disorder originating outside of the inner ear. Many patients will present to the audiologist or otolaryngologist with complaints of vertigo but will actually be experiencing something very different. Additionally, true vertigo can be a sign of serious neurologic disease and there are red-flag symptoms that should not be overlooked. Some patients may have not yet discussed their symptoms in depth with any other specialist or health care worker; a detailed history will both elicit and identify these warning signs.

It is important and time efficient to have every new patient fill out a questionnaire regarding the nature and time course of their symptoms, past medical and surgical history, family history, medications and lifestyle prior to their first visit. When scheduling a new patient with a complaint of dizziness, the questionnaire can be mailed to the patient's home for review prior to coming to the office. Depending on the patient, the questionnaire may take up to 30 min to complete. If patients do not fill out the questionnaire prior to coming to the office, they may be rushed to complete the form and their answers will not be well thought out, complete, or accurate. This time spent may also interfere with the timely flow of clinic. Due to advances in technology and secure survey databases, it may also be possible to distribute the questionnaire electronically by e-mail, giving the physician and audiologist access to the electronic version of the form as soon as it is completed.

In order to remain effective and time efficient during the office visit, it is important for the examiner to review the questionnaire answers prior to evaluating the patient. A complete review of the patient's answers will allow the interviewer to direct the conversation toward relevant aspects of the questionnaire and better focus the specialist's evaluation. It is also important to clarify any questions that the patient may have found confusing, as a lack of understanding of the questions may affect the physician's review of the form. Even though the questionnaire is extremely helpful and time efficient, it is not a substitute for a thorough discussion with the patient regarding his or her symptoms. It is not uncommon for new information to arise from the face-to-face discussion that was not made clear in the questionnaire.

A structured written questionnaire serves to obtain a thorough history, and a systematically designed survey may also prove to be a powerful tool for predicting diagnoses. A recent study assessing over 600 patients presenting to the otolaryngology clinic with complaints of dizziness utilized a dizziness questionnaire (Appendix 6–A) to predict the ultimate clinical diagnosis (following complete history, physical exam, and vestibular testing, when appropriate). Results from this study demonstrated that when a subset of 47 questions was used, the model was correct in predicting the ultimate diagnosis 84% of the time (Zhao, Piccirillo, Spitznagel, Kallogieri, & Goebel, 2011).

KEY COMPONENTS OF THE HISTORY

There are several key components of the history that can give the examiner clues to the proper diagnosis (Table 6–1).

Characteristic of the Sensation

It is crucial to differentiate between true vertigo, light-headedness, presyncope/syncope, and disequilibrium. Patients may describe these sensations in a variety of ways, so it is important to take the time to fully understand their individual symptom experience.

Vertigo

The meaning of the word *vertigo* is often misunderstood and clinical experts will even disagree on the

Table 6–1. Key Components of the History

Key Components of the Interview	Possible Answers
Characteristic of the sensation	Vertigo Light-headedness Presyncope/syncope Disequilibrium
Time course of attacks	Seconds Minutes–hours Hours–days
Associated events and symptoms	Hearing loss Ear pressure Drop attacks Tinnitus Amplification of sound Headaches
Exacerbating factors	Movement Loud noises Atmospheric and weather changes Diet Medication

true definition of the word (Blakley & Goebel, 2001). True vertigo is the false sensation that the individual or environment is moving. This is commonly described as a "room spinning" sensation. The term *dizziness* can involve light-headedness, disorientation, or loss of balance. The term *vertigo* is more specific and is defined as the illusion of movement, which can be in the horizontal, vertical, or oblique axis (Waheeda & Davies, 2004). Balance is dependent on multiple sensory inputs including input from the visual, vestibular, and sensory systems. Vertigo results from mismatched information between these input systems (Waheeda & Davies, 2004). When a diagnosis of true vertigo is made, it is then important to differentiate between central and peripheral vertigo.

Peripheral Vertigo

The peripheral vestibular system consists of the semicircular canals, the utricle and saccule, and the vestibular nerve. Peripheral causes of vertigo are more likely than central causes of vertigo to present with an acute illusion of movement, nausea, and vomiting (Waheeda & Davies, 2004). Peripheral causes of vertigo are also more likely than central causes to produce auditory symptoms, such as ringing, aural fullness, or pressure or hearing changes. Additionally, while balance is impaired with peripheral vertigo, patients with central vertigo will often be unable to stand or walk without falling (Baloh, 1998). This symptom is a red flag that should not be overlooked. If a patient is unable to stand or take a step, this suggests significant central pathology. Although patients with acute peripheral vestibular pathology may feel too sick or imbalanced to walk, they are capable of enough posture control to stand and ambulate.

Central Vertigo

The central vestibular system consists of the vestibular nuclear system, the cerebellum, brainstem, spinal cord, and vestibular cortex. This chapter focuses on peripheral causes of vertigo, but it is important to note that central vertigo may be associated with potentially life-threatening conditions that require immediate medical attention, such as stroke, dissec-tion, or tumors. Central disorders will often involve other neurologic signs and symptoms such as facial weakness or difficulty talking or ambulating (Baloh, 1998).

Tumors. The possibility of a tumor must always appear on the differential diagnosis in a patient presenting with vertigo. Cerebellopontine angle tumors include vestibular schwannomas, meningioma, epidermoid cysts, facial nerve schwannomas, lipomas, trigeminal neuromas, and metastatic tumors (Karatas, 2008). Schwannomas of the eighth cranial nerve are the most common cerebellopontine angle tumors, accounting for 60% to 90% of cerebellar pontine angle (CPA) lesions (Swartz, 2004). Patients with cerebellopontine angle tumors can present with unilateral hearing loss, tinnitus, ataxia, vertigo, and facial numbness and weakness, all due to compression and displacement of nearby structures (Karatas, 2008).

Cerebellar tumors can produce similar symptoms to cerebellopontine angle tumors including ataxia, nystagmus, headache, and vertigo. Cerebellar tumors include astrocytomas, ependymomas, medulloblastomas and hemangioblastomas, and metastatic tumors (Karatas, 2008).

Ataxia. Ataxia presents as difficulty coordinating voluntary movements and unsteadiness. Some forms of ataxia can present with vertigo if there is involvement of the vestibular nerve. Multiple hereditary ataxias exist, but the most common is Friedreich ataxia (Karatas, 2008). Friedreich ataxia is a slowly progressive disease with deficits due to degeneration of the spinal cord and cerebellum. The disease process can also cause degeneration of the vestibular nerve, likely leading to symptoms of vertigo (Delatycki & Corben, 2012).

Multiple Sclerosis. Multiple sclerosis (MS) is an autoimmune demyelinating disorder that affects the central nervous system. Patients with MS can present with dizziness or vertigo as their initial complaint, or these symptoms can be experienced later during the course of this progressive disease. Symptoms can be acute or prolonged, making it difficult to differentiate from other diagnoses from the history alone. The dizziness of MS is caused by demyelination, similar to the mechanism of some forms of ataxia.

MS plaques, which represent areas of active demyelination, can be located on the vestibular nerve or near the vestibular nuclei (Pula, Newman-Toker, & Kattah, 2013).

Cerebrovascular. The vertebrobasilar system supplies the inner ear, brainstem, cerebellum, and occipital lobes. A disruption of blood flow to these areas can result in weakness, clumsiness, ataxia, disequilibrium, and vertigo. It is important to remember that transient symptoms, such as intermittent clumsiness, weakness, dysarthria, and even drop attacks can be a sign of transient brainstem ischemia (Troost, 1980).

Disequilibrium

Disequilibrium is another form of dizziness that is commonly encountered in the otolaryngology clinic. Disequilibrium is defined as imbalance or unsteadiness, with dizziness, and without the illusion of motion or vertigo. Patients usually report that symptoms are worse with standing or navigating within their environment due to uncoordinated movements. It can be caused by an abnormality in multiple organs including the vestibular system, musculoskeletal system, and cerebellum (Karatas, 2008). Usually this sensation is thought to be caused by neurological deficits; however, bilateral or uncompensated unilateral vestibular disorders can also present with disequilibrium.

Presyncope and Syncope

Presyncope is the feeling of light-headedness, blurred vision, and/or muscular weakness that is experienced immediately before fainting. Syncope is defined as a transient decrease in blood flow to the brain and temporary loss of consciousness, followed by full recovery (Hilz, Marthol, & Neundorfer, 2002). Patients report symptoms such as weakness, headache, changes in vision, nausea, and vomiting prior to fainting (Karatas, 2008).

Categories of syncope and presyncope include cardiovascular, neurologic, and neurocardiogenic. These disorders can be dangerous, and it is important to differentiate these potentially life-threatening causes of dizziness from inner ear causes. Because presyncope and syncope are normally not associated with true motion sensation, or vertigo, it is possible to make this distinction (Karatas, 2008).

Cardiovascular causes of presyncope and syncope include structural heart disease, coronary heart disease, and arrhythmias (Karatas, 2008). These conditions can be considered dangerous and can even precede sudden cardiac death.

Neurologic causes of presyncope/syncope include orthostatic hypotension and postural orthostatic tachycardia syndrome (POTS) (Karatas, 2008). Orthostatic hypotension is defined as an abnormal decrease in systolic blood pressure when standing. Although it can be asymptomatic in some people, it is also associated with increased mortality (Ong, Myint, Shepstone, & Potter, 2013). Postural orthostatic tachycardia is a more serious form of orthostatic hypotension caused by dysfunction of the autonomic system. The symptoms of presyncope occur in the upright position and are associated with a marked rise in heart rate. Symptoms will then decrease when lying flat. The disorder is most commonly seen in women and can be brought on by trauma, infection, stress, exertion, heat, or food ingestion. Behavioral changes as well as pharmacological treatments are offered for both orthostatic hypotension and POTS (Mathias et al., 2012).

Neurocardiogenic syncope is also known as vasovagal syncope. Vasovagal syncope is often seen with emotional, stressful situations or prolonged standing (Karatas, 2008). While the exact cause of vasovagal syncope remains uncertain, it is thought that venous pooling in the lower extremities contributes to the phenomenon. Symptoms include decreases in vision and hearing as well as nausea and a feeling of impending doom (Waheeda & Davies, 2004). Vasovagal syncope is the most common abnormal response to upright posture and has been known to occur in all age groups. For most patients, vasovagal syncope can be treated with increased intake of salt and fluids and education regarding the condition (Bloomfield, 2002).

Light-Headedness

The feeling of light-headedness, the sensation of faintness, without the illusion of motion, has many possible causes. The dizziness associated with psychiatric disorders is often reported as light-headedness, floating, or being removed from one's body (Karatas, 2008). While panic attacks with dizziness can be accompanied by fear, palpitations, chest pain, and sweating, anxious patients with dizziness usually describe their symptoms as fogginess, light-headedness, and motion sickness (Staab, 2008). Other psychiatric disorders, such as post-traumatic stress disorder (PTSD), obsessive compulsive disorder, and social and specific phobias have been found to be associated with somatic syndromes, such as unexplained dizziness (Gupta, 2013). Psychiatric disorders associated with dizziness do not present as ataxia or true vertigo and symptoms slowly decline over an hour. It is also important to note that anxiety and depression are more common in patients with neurotologic disease than in the general population, which can make diagnosis of dizziness more complicated. Psychiatric patients with vestibular dysfunction and true vertigo likely suffer from a coexisting neurotologic disorder (Staab, 2008).

Metabolic disorders, when untreated, can also lead to a feeling of light-headedness. Patients with glucose abnormalities from diabetes or diabetes-related treatment can experience light-headedness from hypoglycemia. Similarly, patients with electrolyte abnormalities or untreated hypertension can experience dizziness.

Time Course of Attacks

The time course of attacks of dizziness can give the clinician several clues toward the diagnosis. It is important to note that patients may exaggerate or fail to recall the exact time course of their dizziness due to the severity of their symptoms. Additionally, it is important to determine the time course of true vertigo. Attacks of vertigo may be followed by prolonged disequilibrium or unsteadiness.

Seconds

Vertigo with a short duration of less than a minute is most consistent with benign paroxysmal positional vertigo (BPPV). BPPV is the most frequent form of peripheral vestibular disorder (Strupp & Brandt, 2013) and is characterized by brief attacks of vertigo with nystagmus. BPPV is a mechanical disorder of the inner ear due to movement of free-floating otoconia and is elicited by the influence of gravity during

head movements (Parnes & McClure, 1992). A common history of patients with BPPV is sudden onset of short-duration vertigo with rapid head movements such as those elicited from rolling or turning over in bed, from turning one's head abruptly while driving, or from looking up or down to pick something up. The cause of BPPV is free-floating otoconia that settle most commonly in the posterior semicircular canal due to the effects of gravity. This phenomenon is known as *canalithiasis*. The term *cupulolithiasis* describes particles that become adherent to the cupula of the semicircular canal. BPPV can technically be caused by either of these conditions (Parnes, Agrawal, & Atlas, 2003). Movement of the head will then cause abnormal stimulation of the affected semicircular canal, resulting in vertigo and nystagmus. BPPV may be underestimated in the population due to the fact that many patients have spontaneous resolution. Primary or idiopathic BPPV is responsible for the majority of cases, approximately 50% to 70% (Parnes et al., 2003). However, trauma as well as other vestibular conditions have been found to be associated with BPPV.

Minutes to Hours

Vertigo attacks lasting minutes to hours frequently are seen with Ménière's disease. Ménière's disease is characterized by vertigo, ringing/roaring (tinnitus), fluctuating low-frequency sensorineural hearing loss, and the sensation of aural pressure or fullness. One theory of the pathophysiology of Ménière's disease is that impaired resorption of endolymph by the endolymphatic sac results in endolymphatic hydrops, which contributes to the symptoms of the disorder. Other possible hypotheses include infectious, vascular, or immunologic etiologies (Strupp & Arbusow, 2001). Although vertigo attacks are intermittent, over time, due to progressive loss of vestibular function from attacks, patients can experience general imbalance even between vertigo episodes (Wipperman, 2014).

Another cause of episodic vertigo with symptoms lasting between minutes and hours includes vertigo associated with perilymph fistulas. These abnormal connections allow leakage of perilymph and the abnormal transfer of pressure (Strupp & Arbusow, 2001). Fistulas may be caused by trauma, cholesteatoma, or idiopathic dehiscence in bone.

A specific variant of perilymph fistula is *superior semicircular canal dehiscence* (SSCD). As the name implies, this syndrome is caused by a defect of the bone overlying the superior semicircular canal, which can often be seen on high-resolution CT scan images. The dehiscence allows for formation of a movable third window. Stimuli that cause a change in middle ear or intracranial pressure can induce vertigo (Minor, Solomon, Zinreich, & Zee, 1998).

A concerning neurologic form of vertigo with an intermediate duration is transient ischemic attacks (TIAs). TIAs of the vertebrobasilar circulation can present with intermittent vertigo events. Symptoms can last for up to 20 minutes with complete resolution. If other neurologic changes occur with vertigo events, the diagnosis of TIA should be seriously considered.

Hours to Days

Peripheral causes of vertigo do not usually have attacks of long duration as compared to central disorders. However, vestibular neuritis, a common peripheral vestibular disorder, has a prolonged course without resolution for up to hours or days from the time of onset. Vestibular neuritis is described as an acute-onset vertigo with nausea/vomiting, which is described as very severe. Even after the acute phase has resolved, balance abnormalities may persist for weeks. Auditory symptoms are rare with the acute, initial attack (Goddard & Fayad, 2011). Patients will often report that they will lie completely still for hours in an attempt to decrease the vertigo. Due to the severity of symptoms, patients will often present to the emergency department.

The pathophysiology of vestibular neuritis is controversial. The two leading hypotheses for the disorder are an inflammatory or an ischemic cause (Strupp & Arbusow, 2001). Viral inflammation is a popular theory due to findings of herpes simplex virus DNA and anatomic observations (Goddard & Fayad, 2011). Anatomic studies have shown that the superior division of the vestibular nerve is more commonly involved in vestibular neuritis than the inferior division. This effect may be explained by anatomic differences in the nerve divisions, as the superior division has a longer and narrower bony channel than the inferior division, increasing the

risk for damage, entrapment, and ischemia following viral inflammation (Gianoli, Goebel, Mowry, & Poomipannit, 2005).

The vertigo experienced with vestibular migraine has a variable time course. Patients report symptoms of vertigo and dizziness for durations ranging from minutes to days (Reploeg & Goebel, 2002). The etiology of vertigo with migraine headaches is not well understood, as the pathophysiology of migraine disorder is still not well documented. Although this mechanism of this disorder is not well studied, vestibular migraines are thought to be central causes of vertigo (see detailed discussion of this in Chapter 29).

A concerning disorder presenting with acute vertigo lasting for hours to days is acute stroke or cerebrovascular event. Ischemic strokes of posterior circulation can cause central vertigo. Again, neurological deficits are clues toward a diagnosis of a cerebrovascular event.

Associated Events and Symptoms

Hearing Loss

Hearing loss in the setting of vertigo is commonly associated with Ménière's disease. In addition to fluctuating hearing loss and vertigo, Ménière's patients present with aural fullness and tinnitus. The diagnosis can be challenging as the symptoms are episodic. The hearing loss associated with Ménière's disease is initially a low-frequency hearing loss but can progress to hearing loss in all frequencies (Wipperman, 2014).

Sudden sensorineural hearing loss accompanied by acute vertigo can be associated with symptoms similar to vestibular neuritis. When hearing loss occurs with symptoms of vestibular neuritis, usually acute labyrinthitis is suspected. Patients will complain of acute-onset vertigo with sudden unilateral hearing loss and tinnitus. Patients may report a recent illness preceding the event.

Hearing loss is also a complaint in some patients presenting with signs and symptoms of SSCD (Yew, Zarinkhou, Spasic, Trang, Gopen, & Yang, 2012). Audiograms for these patients can show an air-bone gap, suggesting a conductive hearing loss (Brantberg,

Ishiyama, & Baloh, 2005), which is likely due to the third window effect where the air conduction signal is being shunted away from the extra mobile window.

It is also important to note that acute-onset vertigo accompanied by hearing loss can be present in patients with cerebrovascular events involving the posterior circulation, as the vertebrobasilar system provides blood supply to the inner ear. When weakness, dysarthria, confusion, or any neurological signs are present with acute onset of vertigo and hearing loss, a cerebrovascular event should be suspected and addressed immediately.

Ear Pressure

Ménière's disease is associated with feelings of increased aural pressure or fullness. Patients complain that this symptom often coincides with times of hearing loss. This symptom is episodic and may also correspond with weather and barometric pressure changes.

Drop Attacks

Drop attacks in Ménière's patients were first described in 1936 (Tumarkin, 1936). The attacks are thought to be otolithic crises due to sudden changes in endolymphatic fluid pressure. The fluctuation in pressure contributes to stimulation of inappropriate reflexes. Patients report feeling the sensation of being pulled down (Ozeki, Iwasaki, & Murofushi, 2008). Although patients do not lose consciousness from the drop attack alone, unexpected falls lead to increased risks of injury for these patients.

Drop attacks have also been seen in patients with SSCD. These attacks have reportedly improved after surgical correction (Brantberg et al., 2005). The exact process of these attacks in SSCD is unknown but may have a similar explanation to the etiology of drop attacks in Ménière's disorder, as SSCD patients can also experience sudden changes in endolymphatic pressure.

The above causes of drop attacks are peripheral causes of vertigo; central causes of dizziness and vertigo may also present with episodes similar to drop attacks. Orthostatic hypotension and vasovagal syncope can result in fainting with loss of consciousness. Syncopal events always require additional investigation to rule out dangerous cardiac abnormalities. Ataxia and disequilibrium may also result in frequent falls.

Tinnitus

As mentioned previously, tinnitus often coincides with Ménière's disease attacks. Interestingly, the tinnitus experienced by Ménière's patients can change in character during an actual vertigo attack and become louder, or change in pitch (Wipperman, 2014).

Patients with labyrinthitis will also complain of tinnitus associated with their hearing loss. Labyrinthitis is also thought to be caused by an infectious process and is associated with vertigo, sudden hearing loss, and tinnitus (Beyea, Agrawal, & Parnes, 2012).

Amplification of Sound

SSCD patients often complain of abnormal amplification of sounds such as their own heartbeat or eye movements. This amplification is thought to be due to abnormalities in pressure of the inner ear from the third window phenomenon (Yew et al., 2012).

Headaches

Vestibular migraine is a common diagnosis with a prevalence of 1% of the population affected by the disorder (Neuhauser et al., 2006). Patients with vestibular migraine are defined as those with current migraines or a history of diagnosed migraines and at least five episodes of vestibular symptoms lasting between 5 min and 72 hr. In order to meet criteria of the vestibular migraine diagnosis, at least half of the vestibular episodes must present with concurrent migraine features such as localization to one side, pulsations, photophobia, phonophobia, visual aura, moderate to severe pain, or worsening with physical activity. Patients will report variable time frames of symptoms, and the vertigo may be spontaneous or induced by movement or visual stimuli (Lempert et al., 2012). The International Headache Society has adopted these criteria for the diagnosis of vestibular migraine on a trial basis, as this disorder is still an area under investigation. Although the mechanism of vestibular migraine is still not well understood, the diagnosis is thought to be a central form of vertigo.

Exacerbating Factors

Movement

In BPPV patients, head movements are thought to stimulate movement of otoconia and stimulate an abnormal vestibular response. Patients will often describe their vertigo attacks as occurring when they roll over in bed, look up or down suddenly, or are driving and attempting to switch lanes. Patients may be able to identify the laterality of their disease based on the direction of head movements that stimulate a response for them. Due to this phenomenon, diagnosis can often be made by asking patients to recall the direction of head movements that preceded their attacks or reliving the experience through maneuvers in the office.

With peripheral pathology, uncompensated unilateral vestibular disorders will also present with symptoms during head movement. The incongruent output from each vestibular system can lead to instability.

Neurologic and neurocardiogenic dizziness can also be influenced by movement or positional factors. Orthostatic hypotension is often stimulated by standing up quickly from a seated position, and neurocardiogenic or vasovagal dizziness is often preceded by prolonged standing.

Loud Noises, Pressure Changes

Patients with SSCD often complain that loud sounds cause vertigo or disequilibrium. This phenomenon is known as the Tullio phenomenon. Activities that produce changes in middle ear or intracranial pressure, such as straining, nose blowing, or putting pressure on the external ear, can also cause vertigo (Minor, 2000). This is due to the abnormal communication between the middle fossa and vestibule, or the third window effect, resulting in sensitivity to sounds transmitted through bone and intracranial pressure changes (Yew et al., 2012).

Atmospheric, Weather, and Lifestyle Changes

Atmospheric and weather changes have been shown to be associated with the onset or worsening of Ménière's symptoms (Mizukoshi et al., 1995). Many patients will attribute variations in symptoms to sudden changes in the weather. Additionally, Ménière's disease is thought to be heavily influenced by dietary intake. This is due to the fact that episodes are often preceded by certain foods including salt, caffeine, alcohol, and nicotine. In fact, primary treatment for Ménière's disease includes dietary changes.

Similar to Ménière's disease, vestibular migraine can also be affected by weather and diet. Migraine headaches are commonly triggered by environmental, stress, and dietary changes (Fraga et al., 2013). Additionally, stress may play a role in psychiatric causes of dizziness.

Medication

It is always important to evaluate a patient's prescription medications, specifically any recent changes in medications or dosages that may have preceded a change in symptoms. Medications that affect blood pressure can cause light-headedness, presyncope, and syncope. Additionally, medications that affect the central nervous system can lead to dizziness or disequilibrium. Common medications causing dizziness include treatments for depression and pain. Polypharmacy, particularly in older patients and those on multiple medications for hypertension, has been found to be associated with an increased frequency of dizziness (Shoair, Nyandege, & Slattum, 2011). Polypharmacy can also occur with other classes of drugs including sedatives, antihistamines, and muscle relaxants. Additionally, there are multiple medications that are known to damage the inner ear organs and contribute to vertigo or disequilibrium. These medications include antibiotics used for aggressive treatment of infection as well as chemotherapy agents. These medications may have been taken in the distant past by patients, so it is important to inquire about prior hospitalizations and severe illnesses (Table 6–2).

PAST MEDICAL AND SURGICAL HISTORY

It is always important to elicit a complete past medical and surgical history during an interview. Even though the questionnaire can help focus the

Table 6–2. Common Peripheral Vertigo Disorders

	BPPV	Ménière's Disease	Vestibular Neuritis	Labyrinthitis	Superior Semicircular Canal Dehiscence
Time course					
Seconds	✓				
Minutes to hours		✓			✓
Hours to days			✓	✓	
Associated symptoms					
Hearing loss		✓		✓	✓
Ear pressure		✓			
Drop attacks		✓			✓
Tinnitus		✓		✓	
Amplification of sound					✓
Exacerbating factors					
Movement	✓				
Loud noises					✓
Atmospheric and weather changes		✓			
Diet		✓			

questions about the past medical and surgical history, the patient's responses to inquiries about the sensation, associated symptoms, and exacerbating factors may lead this portion of the interview in multiple directions. It is important to consider the patient's description of the sensation and rule out any concerning diagnoses. For example, if the patient reports presyncope or syncopal events, a thorough past medical and family history of cardiac disease must be taken. Similarly, if the patient reports any neurological signs at the time of vertigo attacks, stroke and risk factors for stroke should be considered.

As previously discussed, clues from the medical or surgical history may help in understanding the etiology of peripheral vertigo. Head trauma can predispose patients to BPPV and SSCD. Similarly, prior surgery or cholesteatoma can put patients at risk for perilymphatic fistulas. A recent illness or surgery may have complications related to the patient's vertigo. The past medical and surgical history can be very valuable in putting together such clues regarding a patient's dizziness.

VESTIBULAR CONTRIBUTIONS TO AUTONOMIC REGULATION

The diagnosis of dizziness can become complicated in many patients who present to the clinic. While we often see patients with neurologic or neurocardiogenic presyncope and dizziness that is unrelated to the inner ear, it is also possible for otolith organs to play a role in orthostasis, blood pressure, and pulse changes. The vestibular system contributes to respiratory and cardiovascular control, and studies of vestibular injuries in animals have resulted in an inability to control blood pressure and breathing during position changes. It is important to note that patients usually recover and compensate quickly after vestibular injury, making the pathophysiology of vestibular-autonomic reflexes difficult to study (Yates & Bronstein, 2005).

POSSIBILITY OF MULTIPLE DIAGNOSES

Significant effort can be put into making an accurate diagnosis of vertigo, but many patients may be difficult to classify into only one category. In fact, multiple diagnoses are often given to complicated patients.

Vestibular Migraine and BPPV

Vestibular migraine and BPPV are often diagnosed together in the clinical setting. A prospective study found that patients with migraines met criteria for BPPV more than any other diagnosis of vertigo (Neuhaser, Leopold, von Brevern, Arnold, & Lempert, 2001). Patients with migraines may become more susceptible to BPPV due to damage to inner ear structures from ischemia or vasomotor changes responsible for the migraine disorder (Ishiyama, Jacobson, & Baloh, 2000).

Vestibular Neuritis and BPPV

The association of vestibular neuritis and BPPV has been reported in the literature and is a common combination of diagnoses seen in the clinical setting. Vestibular neuritis may be an inciting event for the development of BPPV. Vestibular neuritis is thought to affect the superior vestibular nerve, which innervates the utricle. Following the damage of vestibular neuritis, otoconia from the utricle may be able to migrate to the semicircular canals and cause BPPV (Balatsouras et al., 2014).

Ménière's Disease and BPPV

Ménière's disease is another diagnosis that is often found in BPPV patients. Studies report variable rates of coinciding diagnoses but the pathophysiology of the relationship remains unclear. It is possible that similar to vestibular neuritis, Ménière's disease may cause damage to the utricle through the chronic disease process, rendering the inner ear more susceptible to displaced otoconia and BPPV (Balatsouras et al., 2012).

Vestibular Migraines and Ménière's Disease

Patients with Ménière's disease have a higher prevalence of migraines than the general population (Radtke et al., 2002). Multiple studies have shown that patients may often present with features of both vestibular migraines and Ménière's disease. During Ménière's attacks, patients have noted aura, photophobia, and migraines, and similarly, patients with vestibular migraine report aural fullness, hearing loss, and tinnitus (Lempert, 2013). These diagnoses commonly overlap and are difficult to differentiate; however, the cause of the relationship is not well understood.

CONCLUSION

There are several clinical clues that can help lead an astute clinician to a patient's diagnosis when presenting with symptoms of dizziness. In our experience, the history is an important component of the interaction as dizziness can often be a completely clinical diagnosis. Listening carefully to the description and timing of the sensation, associated symptoms, and exacerbating factors, it may be possible to arrive at an accurate differential diagnosis. Additionally, it is always important to remain cognizant of concerning signs of dangerous cardiac or neurologic disorders when taking the history. The dizziness questionnaire, specifically if it is completed prior to the clinic visit, can provide critical information about the patient's experience and can direct the interview, allowing for proper diagnosis and maximal time efficiency.

REFERENCES

Balatsouras, D. G., Ganelis, P., Aspris, A., Economou, N., Moukos, A., & Koukoutsis, G. (2012). Benign paroxysmal positional vertigo associated with Meniere's disease: Epidemiological, pathophysiologic, clinical, and therapeutic aspects. *Annals of Otology, Rhinology and Laryngology, 121*(10), 682–688.

Balatsouras, D. G., Koukoutsis, G., Ganelis, P., Economou, N. C., Moukos, A., Aspris, A., & Katotomichelakis, M. (2014). Benign paroxysmal positional vertigo secondary to vestibular neuritis. *European Archives of Otorhino-laryngology, 271*(5), 919–924.

Baloh, R. W. (1998). Vertigo. *Lancet, 352,* 1841–1846.

Beyea, J. A., Agrawal, S. K., & Parnes, L. S. (2012). Recent advances in viral inner ear disorders. *Current Opinion in Otolaryngology and Head and Neck Surgery, 20,* 404–408.

Blakley, B. W., & Goebel, J. (2001). The meaning of the word "vertigo." *Otolaryngology-Head and Neck Surgery, 125,* 147–150.

Bloomfield, D. M. (2002). Strategy for the management of vasovagal syncope. *Drugs and Aging, 19*(3), 179–202.

Brantberg, K., Ishiyama, A., & Baloh, R. W. (2005). Drop attacks secondary to superior canal dehiscence syndrome. *Neurology, 64*(12), 2126–2128.

Delatycki, M. B., & Corben, L. A. (2012). Clinical features of Friedreich ataxia. *Journal of Child Neurology, 27*(9), 1133–1137.

Fraga, M. D., Pinho, R. S., Andreoni, S., Vitalle, M. S., Fisberg, M., Peres, M. F., . . . Masruha, M. R. (2013). Trigger factors mainly from the environmental type are reported by adolescents with migraine. *Arguivos de Neuro-Psiquiatria, 5,* 290–293.

Gianoli, G., Goebel, J., Mowry, S., & Poomipannit, P. (2005). Anatomic differences in the lateral vestibular nerve channels and their implications in vestibular neuritis. *Otology & Neurotology, 26*(3), 489–494.

Goddard, J. C., & Fayad, J. N. (2011). Vestibular neuritis. *Otolaryngologic Clinics of North America, 44,* 361–365.

Gupta, M. A. (2013). Review of somatic symptoms in post-traumatic stress disorder. *International Review of Psychiatry, 25*(1), 86–99.

Hilz, M. J., Marthol, H., & Neundorfer, B. (2002). Syncope—a systematic overview of classification, pathogenesis, diagnosis and management. *Fortschritte der Neurologie-Psychiatrie, 70*(2), 95–107.

Ishiyama, A., Jacobson, K. M., & Baloh, R. W. (2000). Migraine and benign positional vertigo. *Annals of Otology, Rhinology, and Laryngology, 109*(4), 377–380.

Karatas, M. (2008). Central vertigo and dizziness: Epidemiology, differential diagnosis, and common causes. *Neurologist, 14,* 355–364.

Kroenke, K., Hoffman, R. M., & Einstadter, D. (2000). How common are various causes of dizziness? A critical review. *Southern Medical Journal, 93*(2), 160–167.

Lempert, T. (2013). Vestibular migraine. *Seminars in Neurology, 33,* 212–218.

Lempert, T., Olesen, J., Furman, J., Waterston, J., Seemungal, B., Carey, J., . . . Newman-Toker, D. (2012). Vestibular migraine: Diagnostic criteria. *Journal of Vestibular Research, 22,* 167–172.

Mathias, C. J., Low, D. A., Iodice, V., Owens, A. P., Kirbis, M., & Grahame, R. Postural tachycardia syndrome—current experience and concepts. *Nature Reviews Neurology, 8,* 22–34.

Minor, L. B. (2000). Superior canal dehiscence syndrome. *American Journal of Otology, 21*(1), 9–19.

Minor, L. B., Solomon, D., Zinreich, J. S., & Zee, D. S. (1998). Sound- and/or pressure-induced vertigo due to bone dehiscence of the superior semicircular canal. *Archives of Otolaryngology-Head and Neck Surgery, 124*(3), 249–258.

Mizukoshi, K., Watanabe, Y., Shojaku, H., Ito, M., Ishikawa, M., Aso, S., . . . Motoshima, H. (1995). Influence of a cold front upon the onset of Meniere's disease in Toyama, Japan. *Acta Oto-Laryngologica Supplementum, 520,* 412–414.

Neuhauser, H., Leopold, M., von Brevern, M., Arnold, G., & Lempert, T. (2001). The interrelations of migraine, vertigo, and migrainous vertigo. *Neurology, 56*(4), 436–441.

Neuhauser, H. K., Radtke, A., von Brevern, M., Feldmann, M., Lezius, F., Ziese, T., & Lempert, T. (2006). Migrainous vertigo: Prevalance and impact on quality of life. *Neurology, 67*(6), 1028–1033.

Ong, A. C., Myint, P. K., Shepstone, L., & Potter, J. F. (2013). A systematic review of the pharmacological management of orthostatic hypotension. *International Journal of Clinical Practice, 67*(7), 633–646.

Ozeki, H., Iwasaki, S., & Murofushi, T. (2008). Vestibular drop attack secondary to Meniere's disease results from unstable otolithic function. *Acta Oto-Laryngologica, 128,* 887–891.

Parnes, L. S., Agrawal, S. K., & Atlas, J. (2003). Diagnosis and management of benign paroxysmal positional vertigo (BPPV). *JAMC, 169*(7), 681–693.

Parnes, L. S., & McClure, J. A. (1992). Free-floating endolymph particles: A new operative finding during posterior semicircular canal occlusion. *Laryngoscope, 102*(9), 988–992.

Pula, J. H., Newman-Toker, D. E., & Kattah, J. C. Multiple sclerosis as the cause of the acute vestibular syndrome. *Journal of Neurology, 260,* 1649–1654.

Radtke, A., Lempert, T., Gresty, M. A., Brookes, G. B., Bronstein, A. M., & Neuhauser, H. (2002). Migraine and Meniere's disease: Is there a link? *Neurology, 59,* 1700–1704.

Reploeg, M. D., & Goebel, J. A. (2002). Migraine-associated dizziness: Patient characteristics and management options. *Otology and Neurotology, 23,* 364–371.

Shoair, O. A., Nyandege, A. N., & Slattum, P. W. (2011). Medication-related dizziness in the older adult. *Otolaryngologic Clinics of North America, 22*(2), 455–471.

Sloane, P. D., Coeytaux, R. R., Beck, R. S., & Dallara, J. (2001). Dizziness: State of the science. *Annals of Internal Medicine, 134,* 823–832.

Staab, J. P. (2008). Psychiatric origins of dizziness and vertigo. In G. P. Jacobson, & N. T. Shepard (Eds.), *Balance function assessment and management* (pp. 517–541). San Diego, CA: Plural.

Strupp, M., & Arbusow, V. (2001). Acute vestibulopathy. *Current Opinion in Neurology, 14,* 11–20.

Strupp, M., & Brandt, T. (2013). Peripheral vestibular disorders. *Current Opinion in Neurology, 26,* 81–89.

Swartz, J. D. (2004). Lesions of the cerebellopontine angle and internal auditory canal: Diagnosis and differential diagnosis. *Seminars in Ultrasound, CT and MRI, 25*(4), 332–352.

Troost, B. T. (1980). Dizziness and vertigo in vertebrobasilar disease. Part II. Central causes and vertebrobasilar disease. *Stroke, 11,* 413–415.

Tumarkin, A. (1936). The otolithic catastrophe: A new syndrome. *BMJ, 2,* 175–177.

Waheeda, P., & Davies, R. (2004). Dizziness. *Medicine, 32*(9), 18–23.

Wipperman, J. (2014). Dizziness and vertigo. *Primary Care, 41*(1), 115–131.

Yates, B. J., & Bronstein, A. M. (2005). The effects of vestibular system lesions on autonomic regulation: Observations, mechanisms, and clinical implications. *Journal of Vestibular Research, 15,* 119–129.

Yew, A., Zarinkhou, G., Spasic, M., Trang, A., Gopen, Q., & Yang, I. (2012). Characteristics and management of superior semicircular canal dehiscence. *Journal of Neurological Surgery, 73,* 365–370.

Zhao, J. G., Piccirillo, J. F., Spitznagel, E. L., Jr., Kallogjeri, D., & Goebel, J. A. (2011). Predictive capability of historical data for diagnosis of dizziness. *Otology and Neurotology, 32,* 284–290.

Washington University School of Medicine
Department of Otolaryngology-Head and Neck Surgery
Dizziness and Balance Center

Patient Name: _____ D.O.B: __/__/__ Sex: M__ F__ Date: __/__/__

The following questions refer to your feeling of dizziness. Please answer them as "yes" or "no" and fill in all of the blanks.

Please describe in your own words the sensation you feel without using the word "dizzy":

_____

_____

_____

I. Do you ever have any of the following sensations?

Yes	Spinning in circles	No
Yes	Falling to one side	No
Yes	World spinning around you	No

II. The following refer to typical dizzy spells:

Yes	Do your dizzy spells come in attacks?	No
	How often? _____	
	How long is the attack? _____	
	Date of first spell? _____	
Yes	Are you free from dizziness between attacks?	No
Yes	Does your hearing change with an attack?	No
Yes	Are you dizzy mainly when you sit or stand up quickly?	No
Yes	Are you dizzier in certain positions?	No
	Which position? _____	
Yes	Are you nauseated during an attack?	No
Yes	Are you dizzy even when lying down?	No
Yes	Have you had a recent cold or flu preceding recent dizzy spells?	No

continues

Yes	Have you had fullness, pressure, or ringing in your ears?	No
Yes	Have you had pain or discharge in your ear of recent onset?	No
Yes	Have you had trouble walking in the dark?	No
Yes	Are you better if you sit or lie perfectly still?	No
Yes	Do loud sounds make you dizzy?	No

III. The following refer to other sensations you may have:

Yes	Do you black out or faint when dizzy?	No

Have you had:

Yes	Severe or recurrent headaches?	No
Yes	Light sensitivity with your headaches or dizziness?	No
Yes	Any double or blurry vision?	No
Yes	Numbness in your face or extremities?	No
Yes	Weakness or clumsiness in arms, legs?	No
Yes	Slurred or difficult speech?	No
Yes	Difficulty swallowing?	No
Yes	Tingling around your mouth?	No
Yes	Spots before your eyes?	No
Yes	Jerking of arms or legs?	No
Yes	Seizures?	No
Yes	Confusion or memory loss?	No
Yes	Recent head trauma? (If yes, please explain)	No

_____

_____

_____

IV. The following refer to your hearing. Indicate which side has been affected:

Yes	Difficulty hearing in one ear?	Left	Right	Both	No
Yes	Ringing in one ear?	Left	Right	Both	No
Yes	Fullness in one ear?	Left	Right	Both	No
Yes	Change in hearing when dizzy?				No

Have you had any of the following?

Yes	Pain in ears?	Left	Right	Both	No
Yes	Discharge from ears?	Left	Right	Both	No
Yes	Hearing change?				No
Yes	Better?	Left	Right	Both	No
Yes	Worse?	Left	Right	Both	No
Yes	Exposure to loud noises?				No
Yes	Previous ear infections?				No
Yes	Trauma to your ear(s)?				No
Yes	Previous ear surgery?				No

What? _____

Yes	Family history of deafness?		No

V. The following refer to habits and lifestyle:

Yes	Is there added stress to your life recently?	No
Yes	Are you dizzy or unsteady constantly?	No

Is your dizziness related to:

Yes	Moments of stress?	No
Yes	Menstrual period?	No
Yes	Overwork or exertion?	No
Yes	Do you feel lightheaded or have a swimming sensation when you are dizzy?	No
Yes	Do you find yourself breathing faster or deeper when excited or dizzy?	No
Yes	Did you recently change eyeglasses?	No
Yes	Have you ever had weakness or faintness a few hours after eating?	No
Yes	Do you drink coffee? How much? _____	No
Yes	Do you drink tea? How much? _____	No
Yes	Do you drink soft drinks? How much? _____	No
Yes	Do you drink alcohol? How much? _____	No
Yes	Do you smoke? What? _____ How much? _____	No

continues

Past Medical History:

Please list your current medical problems and length of illness:

_____

_____

_____

_____

Please list all surgery performed and approximate dates:

_____

_____

_____

_____

Please list all allergies (including drugs) and reaction:

_____

_____

_____

_____

Please list all medicines you currently take (including pain medicine, nonprescription medicine, nerve pills, sleeping pills, or birth control pills).

_____

_____

_____

_____

Have you had any previous testing (hearing, x-rays, head scans, etc.)?

_____

_____

_____

Family History:

Any family history of:

Yes	Migraine?	No
Yes	High blood pressure?	No
Yes	Low blood pressure?	No
Yes	Diabetes?	No
Yes	Low blood sugar?	No
Yes	Thyroid disease?	No
Yes	Asthma?	No

Please list any other diseases that run in your immediate family:

_____

_____

_____

System Review:

Check all applicable symptoms:

Constitutional:			
☐ Recent weight change	☐ Fever	☐ Fatigue	☐ N/A

Eyes:			
☐ Loss of Vision	☐ Pain	☐ Discharge/Tearing	☐ N/A
☐ Left ☐ Right ☐ Both	☐ Left ☐ Right ☐ Both	☐ Left ☐ Right ☐ Both	

Ear, Nose, Mouth, Throat:			
☐ Itchy ears	☐ Facial weakness	☐ Nasal obstruction	☐ Nasal discharge
☐ Nosebleed	☐ Sneezing	☐ "Stuffy" nose	☐ Snoring
☐ Loss of sense of smell	☐ Growth in nose	☐ Nasal bleeding	☐ Drooling
☐ Mouth growth, ulcer	☐ Chewing difficulty	☐ Lump in neck	☐ Dental problems/ Poorly fitting dentures
☐ Pain on swallowing	☐ Heartburn	☐ Sore throat	☐ Bleeding from throat
☐ Voice changes	☐ Breathing difficulty	☐ N/A	

Cardiovascular:			
☐ Chest pain	☐ Irregular Heart Beat	☐ Swelling of legs	☐ Leg pain with walking
☐ Leg pain with rest	☐ N/A		

Respiratory:			
☐ Wheezing	☐ Cough	☐ Shortness of breath	☐ Mucous
☐ Coughing up blood	☐ N/A		

continues

Gastrointestinal:			
☐ Decrease in appetite	☐ Nausea/vomiting	☐ Blood in stool	☐ Difficulty swallowing (food sticks)
☐ Diarrhea/constipation	☐ Indigestion	☐ Food intolerance	☐ N/A

Musculoskeletal:			
☐ Neck pain	☐ Joint pain/stiffness	☐ Arthritis Name joint:	☐ N/A

Skin:			
☐ Rash	☐ Jaundice	☐ Recent baldness	☐ N/A

Neurological:			
☐ Headache	☐ Blackout	☐ Seizures	☐ Paralysis
☐ Tremor	☐ N/A		

Psychiatric:			
☐ Insomnia	☐ Depression	On Medication: ☐ Yes ☐ No	☐ N/A

Endocrine:			
☐ Thyroid trouble ☐ N/A	☐ Heat or cold intolerance	☐ Excessive sweating	☐ Excessive thirst, hunger, urination

Genitourinary:			
☐ Painful urination	☐ Venereal disease	☐ Blood in urine	☐ Frequent urination at night
☐ Difficulty passing urine	☐ Incontinence	☐ N/A	

Hematologic/ Lymphatic:			
☐ Anemia	☐ Bleeding problems	☐ Blood disorder (e.g., Sickle cell)	☐ N/A
	☐ Easy bruising		

Do you have anything else to tell us about your particular problem that we have not asked you on this questionnaire?

_____

_____

_____

_____

_____

Physician Review With Patient:

_____

_____

_____

_____

_____

_____   _____

Physician Signature   Date

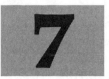

Bedside Assessment of the Vestibular System

Devin L. McCaslin, J. Andrew Dundas, and Gary P. Jacobson

INTRODUCTION AND HISTORY

"Bedside tests" of vestibular function are brief, informal assessments designed to help clinical neurophysiologists form hypotheses of what they will observe during more formal quantitative testing. Alone these tests are capable of identifying relatively large asymmetries in unilateral vestibular impairments. They also are valuable for quickly identifying patients with bilateral peripheral vestibular system impairments. As a general statement, bedside tests can identify unilateral vestibular impairments when caloric asymmetries are ~40% to 50%. We describe in this chapter several of the most common and useful "bedside" tests and present a brief description of their administration and interpretation. The majority of the chapter describes what is currently known about the bedside tests of the vestibular system but does not extend this discussion to the evaluation of the oculomotor system, as this topic is covered elsewhere in this text (see Chapters 9 and 10). Additionally, the sensitivity and specificity of each test is described along with the mechanism of action of each test. Sensitivity is defined as the percentage of subjects known to be abnormal that produce an abnormal test result. Specificity is defined as the percentage of subjects known to be normal who produce a normal or negative test result.

EXAMINATION TO IDENTIFY SPONTANEOUS VESTIBULAR NYSTAGMUS (SN)

Introduction

The origin of the word *nystagmus* is derived from the Greek word "nystazein" which translates to the type of "nod" that occurs when we sit in class and start to fall asleep. The head drops down slowly and then as we wake up the head jerks quickly upward (i.e., mirroring the slow phase/fast phase of a beat of nystagmus). Decades of research into this phenomenon has provided investigators with a clear understanding of most types of nystagmus. This chapter discusses vestibular nystagmus only. This type of nystagmus is a cardinal sign indicating that a static imbalance exists between the resting outputs of the two peripheral vestibular systems.

Technique

Prior to beginning the search for spontaneous nystagmus (SN), a thorough history should be taken to determine whether the patient has any visual symptoms and what, if any, other neurologic symptoms exist (Serra & Leigh, 2002). It is also advisable to compile and review a list of the patient's medications as some can cause nystagmus. Next, an evaluation of gross eye movements is suggested. Specifically, check that the patient has full range of movement for each eye and record any evidence of strabismus. This can be performed by simply having the patient follow the examiner's finger 30 degrees to the right and the left. Following this step, have the patient fixate on a target that is approximately 4 feet away. Again, the examiner can use a finger as the target. Similarly, the center gaze subtest on an ENG/VNG test system light-bar provides a suitable target. If nystagmus is noted while the patient is fixating on the target directly in front of him or her, the amplitude and direction of nystagmus (vertical or horizontal) should be recorded, as should the presence of any differences in the nystagmus between eyes. Once the search for SN has been completed with vision, videonystagmography (VNG) goggles should be applied and the search continued with vision denied. The reason that a SN examination must be performed in light as well as with vision denied, is that when a patient has access to vision, visual fixation mechanisms activate subcortical inhibitory pathways connected to the vestibular nuclei (VN). This inhibitory action on the VN will act significantly to suppress any vestibular-generated SN. VNG goggles have been available for several years and should be used whenever possible to help identify nystagmus when vision is denied. Two primary advantages of infrared VNG goggles over traditional Frenzel lenses are the following: (1) the patient cannot fixate on anything inside the goggles as it is completely dark, and (2) most systems allow the option to record so that the eye movements can be further examined offline. With vision denied and the patient sitting upright, begin mental alerting tasks while examining the eyes for any SN. If SN is noted with vision denied, again, record the amplitude and direction of eye movements, as well as any other characteristics (e.g., torsional components or whether right- or left-beating).

Results

Normal Result

No nystagmus is visible with vision denied.

Abnormal Result

Nystagmus is observed (Video 7–1). The direction of the fast phase and velocity (deg/s) of the nystagmus should be documented as well as any changes in these two parameters that occur with visual fixation. Acute peripheral disorders of the labyrinth and vestibular portion of the VIIIth nerve commonly result in a direction-fixed horizontal-rotary nystagmus that increases in amplitude when vision is denied.

For peripheral vestibular system impairments, this nystagmus should increase in velocity when the patient deviates gaze in the direction of the fast phase, become smaller in velocity when the patient stares at midline, and become smallest when the patient stares in the direction of the slow phase. Those characteristics follow what is has been called *Alexander's law* (Alexander, 1912). It is important that a comparison be made between nystagmus velocity with visual fixation and nystagmus velocity without visual fixation, as central nervous system disorders often produce nystagmus that is not suppressed by fixation.

Mechanism

A primary function of the semicircular canals is to transduce angular acceleration of the head into a neural pattern that is routed through the vestibulo-ocular reflex (VOR). The VOR permits the maintenance of clear vision during head movements. The SCCs are organized in orthogonal planes allowing for a synergistic pairing between them. The vestibular nerves that run from the semicircular canals to the vestibular nuclei maintain an average baseline tonic firing rate of approximately 70 to 90 spikes per second (Goldberg & Fernandez, 1971). When the head is accelerated in the plane of a particular canal, the neurons connected to the canal of the leading ear will assume a level of increased neural activity over their resting rate. This is accompanied by a corresponding decrease in firing rate in the nerve associated with the paired canal on the opposite side. This neural pattern is relayed rostrally through the central vestibular system to the oculomotor nuclei which provide tonus to the oculomotor muscles. When an insult is incurred by the peripheral vestibular system, specifically, to the hair cells in the labyrinth or to the vestibular portion of the VIIIth nerve, the tonic rate of firing is reduced on the affected side. This unilateral loss of peripheral function creates an asymmetry in the tonic resting activity of the two peripheral vestibular systems similar to that which normally occurs during movement of the head. This asymmetry routed thought the VOR results in *spontaneous nystagmus* (SN) as the system attempts to visually track perceived rotation away from the side of lesion. This pathologic eye movement consists of a slow conjugate deviation of the eyes away from the intact side followed by a quick corrective movement toward the impaired side. SN is described by noting the direction of the fast phase, even though it is the slow component that is generated by the vestibular system. SN due to an asymmetry in the neural resting rate between the two end organs generates the illusion of rotary motion in the absence of any head movement. Specifically, patients describe that they feel as though they are rotating toward the intact side. SN due to an acute loss of peripheral vestibular function is primarily horizontal with a torsional component.

Test Performance

The ability to identify SN following a unilateral vestibular system impairment is greatest within the first 3 to 7 days (Fetter & Dichgans, 1990). However, a phenomenon known as *vestibular compensation* uses a centrally mediated adaptive mechanism to restore neural activity to the impaired side, which results in a reduction in the amplitude of the SN and a cessation of the patient's perception of vertigo. Depending on the integrity of the neural structures responsible for vestibular compensation, resolution of the SN may take much longer (Cass, Kartush, & Graham, 1992; Furman, Balaban, & Pollack, 1997). Using SN to diagnose an end-organ disorder is also complicated by the fact that the damaged peripheral system can spontaneously regain function and produce a paradoxical SN known as *recovery nystagmus* that beats toward the affected ear (Jacobson, Pearlstein, Henderson, Calder, & Rock, 1998; McClure & Lycett, 1978). Vestibular compensation is dependent on factors such as the patient's age and activity level, the

presence of one functioning end organ, the patient's use of vestibular suppressants, and the presence of intact vestibular nuclei, posterior and anterior vermis, flocculonodular lobe, and the inferior olive (Igarashi & Ishikawa, 1985; Kaufman, Anderson, & Beitz, 1992). Due to the efficiency of vestibular compensation, in most cases, unless a patient is seen directly after the insult there is a good chance there will be no evidence of SN. Using the presence of SN as a bedside test to diagnose unilateral vestibular dysfunction therefore is not recommended without quantitative testing. The presence of SN demonstrating the characteristics described above is a good sign that a peripheral asymmetry exists. However, due to the intersubject variability and quality of central compensation mechanisms, it is impossible to determine the degree and side of the impairment from the direction of SN. There have been a few studies that have examined the sensitivity and specificity of spontaneous nystagmus for identifying peripheral end-organ dysfunction (Table 7–1). Dayal, Tarantino, Farkashidy, and Paradisgarten (1974) presented data from 302 patients with spontaneous, positional, or paroxysmal positional nystagmus. All of the cases had a clinical diagnosis and there was no control group. When only the peripheral disorders were examined the presence of spontaneous activity was very low. Specifically, the sensitivity of SN for Ménière's disease was 52%, for labyrinthectomy 71%, for acoustic neuroma 75%, and for vestibular neuritis 49%.

In a recent study by Guidetti, Monzani, and Rovatti (2006), the sensitivity and specificity of spontaneous nystagmus to peripheral vestibular system hypofunction in 528 outpatients and 133 control subjects was examined using three methods. SN was identified using direct observation in light, Frenzel lenses, and videonystagmography. When labyrinthine-defective patients were examined for SN using direct observation in light and Frenzel lenses the sensitivity was low and there was no significant difference between the two methods. Specifically, direct observation in light had a sensitivity of 19%, whereas Frenzel lenses had a sensitivity of 20%. Both techniques had a specificity of 96%. VNG, although better, still only had a sensitivity of 48% and a specificity of 92%. These findings suggest that using only the presence or absence of spontaneous nystagmus

Table 7–1. Comparison of Studies Evaluating Spontaneous Nystagmus

Study	n	Controls	Disorder	Condition	Sensitivity	Specificity
Dayal, Tarantino, Farkashidy, & Paradisgarten (1974)	302	0	Ménière's		52%	Could not calculate
			Labyrinthectomy		71%	Could not calculate
			Acoustic neuroma		75%	Could not calculate
			Vestibular neuritis		49%	Could not calculate
Guidetti, Monzani, & Rovatti (2006)	661		Peripheral	Direct observation	19%	96%
			Vestibular	Frenzel goggles	20%	96%
			hypofunction	VNG	48%	92%
Totals	963				48%	95%

to diagnose unilateral peripheral vestibular system hypofunction (UVH) is unacceptable. Although the presence of SN may lead an examiner to suspect UVH, the sensitivity using the best techniques is less than 50%. As discussed above, central compensation mechanisms among other factors greatly influence whether SN will be observed. Thus, when an organic vestibular disorder is suspected, quantitative testing should always be completed to confirm or refute its existence.

HEAD-IMPULSE TEST (HIT)

Introduction

The head-impulse test (HIT) is a screening test that utilizes the oculocephalic response, or doll's eye reflex, to identify unilateral and bilateral peripheral vestibular system impairment. This reflex was originally employed to identify vestibular function in comatose or unresponsive patients (Fisher, 1969). In 1988, Halmagyi and Curthoys expanded the clinical utility of the test with their description of its application in patients with complete loss of labyrinth function. The ability, or inability, of the patient to maintain fixation on a target during an extremely fast angular excursion of the head can give the exam-

iner some insight into the integrity of the lateral semicircular canal ipsilateral to the direction of the head turn. As described in the initial paper by Halmagyi and Curthoys (1988), a patient will demonstrate an abnormal catch-up saccade when the head is thrust in the direction of the impaired system. It follows that a patient with bilateral peripheral vestibular losses will exhibit abnormal catch-up saccades opposite to the direction of head turn in either direction. The HIT is now a routine component in the bedside assessment of vestibular function that is quickly and easily administered and interpreted. This chapter addresses only the bedside version of the HIT test and not the video HIT (vHIT) that is described in depth in Chapter 16.

Technique

The test is composed of the examiner gently grasping the patient's head and passively moving it through a quick head turn (Figure 7–1). Before the head is turned, the patient is instructed to fixate on a target (often the examiner's nose) and maintain fixation on it throughout the head turn. The patient's head should be tilted forward 30 degrees in order to position the lateral semicircular canals coplanar to the ground (Schubert, Tusa, Grine, & Herdman, 2004). The examiner then gently grasps the patients head on

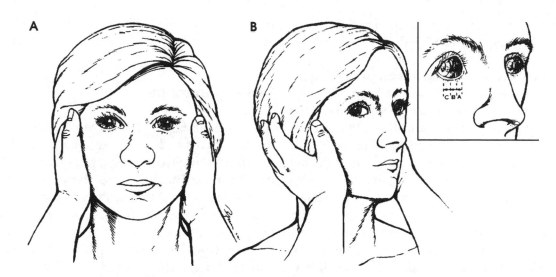

Figure 7–1. A. The patient is instructed to fixate on a target directly in front of him or her and the head is tilted forward 30 degrees. **B.** When the patient's head is rotated abruptly 15 to 20 degrees to one side the eyes should deviate 180 degrees out of phase with the head thrust and remain fixed on the target. The inset in the right-hand corner details what happens when the eyes cannot maintain fixation on the target due to an impaired vestibular system ipsilateral to the head thrust. As illustrated, the eyes initially move with the head in the direction of thrust toward the lesioned ear (from position C to position A). In order to reacquire the target, saccades are generated to bring the eyes back to the point of visual fixation (from position A to position C). From *Laryngoscope*, 1996, *106*, 6–9. Reprinted with permission.

both sides and rapidly and abruptly (>2000 deg/s²) rotates the patient's head approximately 15 to 20 degrees to one side, then the other. While the head is being rapidly turned the examiner observes the patient's eyes to confirm that they remain stationary on the target. The examiner should be vigilant for the appearance of any movement of the pupil during the head thrust, and for a catch-up saccade to refixate the target after the head movement is complete.

Results

Normal Result

A quick translation of a patient's head to the patient's left (Video 7–2) should invoke a corresponding compensatory eye movement to the right due to stimulation of the left lateral semicircular canal, and inhibition of the right lateral semicircular canal. This compensatory eye movement should be very close to 180 degrees out of phase from the movement of the head. Thus, translation to the right will stimu-

late the right lateral semicircular canal and inhibit the left lateral semicircular canal, resulting in a compensatory leftward eye movement to maintain the target on the fovea (Kelly, 1985). When this occurs fixation is maintained on the target throughout the head acceleration.

Abnormal Result

Damage to the left peripheral vestibular system (Video 7–3) will result in a catch-up saccade to the right on left head turn, and the maintenance of normal fixation through a normal vestibular ocular reflex with right head turn.

Mechanism

Whereas the horizontal VOR has been described in detail in Chapter 1, this chapter describes the neural mechanism of the HIT using an adaptation of Halmagyi and Curthoy's (1988) description. It is important to remember that the two lateral semicircular canals are working in tandem in a push-pull fashion and that the contribution and integrity of both canals must be considered when describing the mechanism of the HIT.

Gain is classically defined as output divided by input. The purpose of the VOR is to keep an image centered on the retina when the head is moved. In order to keep the eye stable and the retina on the target, output would have to be equal to the input. If the input (head impulse) matched output (VOR) perfectly it would be said to have gain of 1.

According to Halmagyi, Curthoys, and Cremer (1990), when a high-frequency stimulus such as the head impulse is applied to subjects with intact end organs, the gain of the VOR in the yaw plane is very close to 1 (0.94 ± 0.08 SD) at 122 deg/s head velocity. Because the head movement is rapid (greater than 0.10 Hz) the VOR is evoked rather than the opto-kinetic subsystem resulting in a vestibular driven compensatory eye movement that is close to 180 degrees out of phase with the head movement. This has the effect of keeping the retinas stable and on the target while the head rotates around the eye.

Halmagyi et al. (1990) have investigated the effect of complete UVH on the HIT. When patients with a complete loss of function of one end organ are subjected to the same head impulse as described above (122 deg/s head movement), the gain of the VOR has been shown to drop to 0.20 (Halmagyi et al., 1990). Thus, the electrical drive to the VOR is less than what is necessary to maintain the 180-degree opposite phase compensatory eye movement. Accordingly, a catch-up saccade is required to bring the eye to the target. It would be reasonable to expect with complete vestibular hypofunction that gain would decrease to "0" during ipsilesional accelerations as the VOR output from the affected side would be miniscule relative to the magnitude of the head impulse input. The reason the drop in gain is not 0 is that there is believed to be a small neural contribution from the contralateral end organ. Although the exact neural mechanism is not completely understood, if the head is turned toward the ipsilesional side, which in this example is the right, utriculofugal endolymph flow in the left lateral SCC will result in inhibition of the intact lateral SCC and become the primary (although inefficient) source of drive toward the impaired side. Halmagyi et al. (1990) suggest that as this utriculofugal response

from the intact side is so small, it is unlikely to be an integral part of the bilaterally generated VOR.

Test Performance

An extensive body of literature exists concerning the sensitivity and specificity of the bedside head-impulse test for identifying lateral semicircular canal (SCC) paresis. The function of the lateral canal can be assessed easily in the laboratory using caloric testing and/or rotational testing. As such, most investigations have been designed using the bithermal caloric test as the gold standard against which the performance characteristics of the HIT are compared. What must be kept in mind when reviewing the relationship between caloric responses and the HIT is that the two tests employ stimuli that are at opposite ends of the frequency spectrum. The caloric response is analogous to a rotational stimulus of 0.003 Hz (i.e., 1 cycle every 5 1/2 min), whereas the HIT represents a high-frequency movement characteristic of those occurring in everyday life. This is important to know as peripheral vestibular system disorders affect the low-frequency spectrum earlier, and more severely, than the high-frequency spectrum (Angelaki & Perachio, 1993). This phenomenon greatly favors the caloric response being more sensitive than the HIT to peripheral vestibular impairment.

In the original description of the HIT test by Halmagyi and Curthoys (1998), 12 experimental subjects who had undergone unilateral vestibular neurectomy were compared to a control group of 12 neurologically intact patients. Patients who have undergone a nerve section surgical procedure usually have a complete loss of vestibular function on the affected side. The initial report described the HIT test as having 100% sensitivity and specificity. Subsequent studies examining the HIT in patients with nerve sections also demonstrated high degrees of sensitivity and specificity (Cremer et al., 1998; Foster, Foster, Spindler, & Harris, 1994; Halmagyi, Black, Thurtell, & Curthoys, 2003; Lehnen, Aw, Todd, & Halmagyi, 1994). However, for any bedside test to be considered useful to the clinician, it must have a high sensitivity and specificity in a broader population. Although the previous studies demonstrated the HIT to be highly sensitive and specific in subjects with complete vestibular end-organ damage, the majority of patients that present to a dizziness clinic will have unilateral vestibular impairments of varying magnitudes. Studies in Table 7–2 illustrate how the magnitude of unilateral peripheral vestibular system hypofunction as represented by unilateral caloric weakness is highly predictive of whether an abnormal HIT will be observed. Whereas the majority of the literature suggests that the sensitivity of the HIT test increases as degree of peripheral vestibular system hypofunction increases, it can be observed

from the studies illustrated in Table 7–2 that if a patient demonstrates a caloric asymmetry exceeding 40% there is a high probability that the patient will exhibit an abnormal HIT test result regardless of the technique used (Beynon, Jani, & Baguley, 1998; Harvey, Wood, & Feroah, 1997; Perez & Rama-Lopez, 2003; Shepard, 1998). However, the fact remains that when only the studies utilizing patients with partial vestibular hypofunction are considered, the mean sensitivity of the HIT test is approximately 46% and the specificity is approximately 94%. This suggests

Table 7–2. Comparison of Studies Evaluating the Head Impulse Test

Study	n	Controls	Disorder	Condition	Sensitivity	Specificity
Halmagyi & Curthoys (1988)	12	12	Unilateral vestibular neurectomy		100%	100%
Cremer et al. (1998)	10	9	Unilateral vestibular deafferentation (7), Unilateral posterior SCC occluded (3)	100%	100%	Could not calculate
Halmagyi, Black, Thurtell, & Curthoys (2003)	4	0	Postvestibular neurectomy	Active and Passive head movements	100%	Could not calculate
Foster, Foster, Spindler, & Harris (1994)	6	6	Complete surgical lesions or canal paresis		100%	97%
Lehnen, Aw, Todd, & Halmagyi (1994)	16		Vestibular neurectomy (9), Vestibulocochlear neurectomy (7)		100%	Could not calculate
Harvey & Wood (1996)	112		Complaints of dizziness	≤30% >30% UW	<39% 68%	97%
Harvey, Wood, & Feroah (1997)	105		Dizziness		35%	95%
Beynon, Jani, & Baguley (1998)	150		Dizziness		34%	Could not calculate
Perez & Rama-Lopez (2003)	265		Vertigo		45%	91%
Schubert, Tusa, Grine, & Herdman (2004)	111	65	UVH (79) BVH (32) Nonvestibular dizziness (65)		71% 84%	82%
Total	791				76%	94%

that the HIT test is clearly less sensitive than a full electrodiagnostic balance examination and thus should only be used in conjunction with and never in lieu of an electrophysiologic balance test battery. The reader is directed to Chapter 16 where the computerized and video version of the bedside test (i.e., the video HIT or vHIT) is described.

HEAD SHAKE

Introduction

When the head is shaken vigorously for 10 to 30 cycles and then stopped, a transient vestibular nystagmus may emerge in patients with peripheral and central vestibular system disorders. Originally described by Bárány (1907), this aberrant response has been termed head-shaking nystagmus (HSN). The appearance of spontaneous nystagmus following repetitive shaking of the head has led to the development of a large body of literature referring to what is today known as the head-shake test. The head-shake test evolved from an early test described by Borries (1923) where the investigators described how head shaking could change the nature of spontaneous nystagmus. Vogel (1929) expanded this work and described how shaking the head could elicit spontaneous nystagmus from patients who were in the process of central compensation. The contemporary head-shake test was described by Kamei and Kornhuber (1964). In this original report the patient was fitted with Frenzel lenses and instructed to shake the head back and forth 30 times in four different conditions after which the clinician observed the eyes for spontaneous nystagmus. The four conditions varied in terms of plane and direction of head shake in an effort to elicit responses from each of the semicircular canals. They included shaking the head when it was tilted 30 degrees forward, positioned normally, in the coronal plane, and in the sagittal plane.

Technique

The optimal situation to evaluate the head-shake test is with the patient wearing videonystagmog-

raphy (VNG) goggles and with vision denied. This eliminates the possibility that the patient will visually fixate on an object and reduce the intensity and duration of HSN, thereby making it more difficult to identify. Most VNG systems provide a digital videorecording option, which allows for the examiner to review the results without having the patient repeat the test. In the absence of VNG equipment, a patient can also be evaluated while wearing Frenzel lenses. Although Frenzel lenses will help the examiner observe the eyes, patients may still fixate on the inside of the goggles. When this occurs HSN may be attenuated or eliminated because of VOR cancellation mechanisms. The test can be performed as an active or passive procedure. To begin, the patient's head is tilted forward 30 degrees to position the lateral semicircular canals parallel to the ground. If an active procedure is being performed, the patient is instructed to oscillate the head from side to side approximately 30 to 45 degrees from center for 25 cycles at a frequency of 2 Hz. If a passive procedure is being employed, the same procedures described for the active test should be undertaken; however, in this case the examiner vigorously rotates the subject's head at the same frequency.

A positive head-shake test can produce HSN with three different qualitative characteristics (Hain & Spindler, 1993). First, the HSN can be monophasic or biphasic (i.e., it changes direction as it decays). Second, the HSN can beat toward or away from the impaired side. Finally, there can be a vertical component to the HSN, which is referred to as cross-coupled nystagmus.

Results

Normal Result

Following head shaking (Video 7–4), there is no identifiable post-head-shake nystagmus.

Abnormal Result

The presence of post-head-shake nystagmus (Video 7–5) is considered a pathologic sign of imbalance in the vestibular inputs in the plane of rotation. In most instances, a peripheral cause is identified with the fast phase of the nystagmus directed toward the contralesional ear (Video 7–6). A small reversal phase is sometimes observed. Signs of central etiology include prolonged, vertical, or disconjugate nystagmus.

Mechanisms of HSN

A popular and accepted theory regarding the mechanism for the peripheral pattern of HSN has been set forth by Hain, Fetter, and Zee (1987). This theory combines Ewald's second law of canal function and the concept of an asymmetrically charged velocity storage system. Ewald's second law states that ampulopetal endolymph flow in the horizontal canal results in a greater electrical output than ampullofugal endolymph flow.

HSN cannot be explained by Ewald's law alone because the law does not account for any nystagmus that may persist after completion of the head shake. The nystagmus that occurs when the head is abruptly stopped after oscillating is thought to be due to a central phenomenon known as velocity storage (VS) (Raphan, Matsuo, & Cohen, 1979). When the head is rotated at a constant velocity during earth-axis rotation in a single direction, there is an initial increase in neural activity from vestibular afferents corresponding to the initial deflection of the horizontal semicircular canal cupula due to angular acceleration. As the rotation is maintained but acceleration drops to zero, the cupula slowly returns to its neutral position due to the elasticity of the organ. At this point, afferent activity in the nerve decreases (Goldberg & Fernandez, 1971). These neural responses are often described in terms of their time constant (TC). Time constant is defined as the interval after the onset of a stimulus for the response to decline to 37% of the initial value (Leigh & Zee, 1999). The time constant of vestibular nerve fibers innervating the horizontal semicircular canal is approximately 6 s. However, the time constant of the VOR (i.e., the compensatory eye movement generated in response to stimulation of the horizontal semicircular canals) is approximately 16 s. VS causes the VOR to persist two to three times longer than the neural "drive" from the periphery. Several groups have attributed a central vestibular system construct called the "neural integrator" to account for this dif-

ference in the response times between the VOR and peripheral neural activity (Cohen, Henn, Raphan, & Dennett, 1981; Cohen, Matsuo, & Raphan, 1977; Raphan et al., 1979).

In patients with a unilateral peripheral vestibular weakness, Hain et al. (1987) suggests that as the head is oscillated side to side, there is an asymmetry in the magnitude of peripheral neural input that results in an asymmetric "charging" up of the neural integrator system. During each half-cycle of head movement toward the impaired side, there is a lower level of neural activity transmitted to the central vestibular system than when the head is rotated toward the intact side. Once the head is stopped, the stored activity in the VS system will discharge slowly through the VOR pathway and produce HSN.

Test Performance

It is well known that HSN can occur in patients with both peripheral and central vestibular system disorders. What is disputed is the sensitivity of the head-shaking test to UVH, and how large of an asymmetry must there be to observe HSN.

In this regard, Hain et al. (1987) examined patients with complete unilateral losses of peripheral vestibular function. This group of patients exhibited HSN with a velocity of approximately 20 deg/s and a time course lasting approximately 20 s with a small reversal lasting an additional 100 s. The addition of a vertical component or "cross-coupling" was occasionally observed, but was usually small if seen at all. Vertical head shaking has also been reported to elicit horizontal nystagmus that beats toward the impaired side (Hain et al., 1987; Moritz, 1951). In peripheral disorders, it has been shown that the amplitude of the nystagmus will increase with an increased number of oscillations of the head up to 30 cycles.

For the HSN test to be useful in a dizziness clinic it must have a high specificity and sensitivity. The number of patients reporting to a dizziness clinic who will have complete unilateral loss of vestibular system function will be rare in comparison to those presenting with varying degrees of loss. Research pertinent to the sensitivity and specificity of the head-shake test in groups of patients that have different degrees of peripheral dysfunction is presented (Table 7–3).

The studies in Table 7–3 demonstrate the variability and sensitivity of the HSN test in groups of patients with different degrees of vestibular weakness. Although the research supports the notion that with increasing peripheral vestibular system loss the sensitivity of the HSN test increases, there is no agreed on criterion of how much loss is needed to observe a positive HSN test. When utilizing the HSN as a screening tool for unilateral vestibular dysfunction, the presence of HSN is a good indicator that the patient should be referred for quantitative testing. The absence of HSN but a case history positive for

Table 7–3. Comparison of Studies Evaluating the Head-Shake Test

Study	*n*	Controls	Disorder	Condition	Sensitivity	Specificity
Hain, Fetter, & Zee (1987)	6	7	Complete UVH	Peripheral vestibular lesion	100%	43%
Wei, Hain, & Proctor (1989)	108		Dizziness	No bilateral weaknesses	40%	60%
Vicini, Casani, & Ghilardi (1989)	277	73	Patients referred for ENG		29%	90%
Takahashi, Fetter, Koenig, & Dichgans (1990)	16		UVH		90%	64%
Hall & Laird (1992)	340	20	Dizziness			50%
Jacobson, Newman, & Safadi (1990)	116		Dizziness		27%	85%
Burgio, Blakley & Myers (1991)	115	17	Dizziness		44%	65%
Goebel & Garcia (1992)	214		Dizziness	UVH BVH	42% 18%	85% 85%
Fujimoto, Rutka, & Mai (1993)	259		Vestibular weakness	>20% UVH >40% UVH >60% UVH >80% UVH Overall	50.21% 64.36% 68.33% 77.14% 49.28%	73.18% 71.69% 70.68% 70.14%
Harvey, Wood, & Feroah (1997)	105		Dizziness		35%	92%
Tseng & Chao (1997)	258		Canal paresis		90%	53%
Guidetti, Monzani, & Civiero (2002)	273		Confirmed peripheral weakness	Initial visit	74%	Could not calculate
Iwasaki, Ito, Abbey, & Murofushi (2004)	132		Dizziness	Six months of recovery	66	Could not calculate
Totals	2219	117		UVH >20%	56%	70.92%

dizziness would also warrant a referral for a complete balance function assessment. However, the HSN test in isolation appears to be a poor predictor of low and moderate levels of vestibular hypofunction. The body of research (see Table 7–3) suggests that the HSN test therefore should be used in conjunction with other bedside tests or formal balance function testing.

DYNAMIC VISUAL ACUITY

Introduction

Head movements may evoke dizziness or visual blurring in patients with either unilateral or bilateral vestibular hypofunction. This perception of objects "bouncing" or "blurring" when the head is moving has been termed *oscillopsia*, meaning "oscillating vision" (Brickner, 1936). It can be attributed to a defect in the VOR. One of the primary functions of the VOR is to keep the retina stable on an object of interest when the head is moving. When the vestibular labyrinths sense head movement they produce, by way of the VOR, an equal and opposite compensatory eye movement that keeps the eyes steady. This vestibular-driven reflexive process allows the observer to retain visual acuity with head movement and is known as dynamic visual acuity (DVA) (Miller & Ludvigh, 1962). The VOR is extremely precise and requires only a few degrees of error per second between the retina and the target to significantly degrade visual acuity and result in oscillopsia (Westheimer & McKee, 1975). Barber (1984) suggested that an examiner may be able to identify an underlying vestibular disorder if DVA was found to abnormal. The "oscillopsia test" was his initial description of a method to quantify the performance of a patient's DVA. This very simple test permitted the quantification of a patient's visual acuity with and without oscillation of the head. The premise was that if there was damage to the VOR then a patient's visual acuity would be poorer with head movement than without. Throughout the years there have been many variations on the original oscillopsia test or, as it is often termed, DVA test. For the purposes of this chapter it is referred to as DVA.

Technique

Recent reports have suggested that commercially available computerized DVA systems greatly increase the sensitivity of the test to vestibular dysfunction (Herdman, Tusa, Blatt, Suzuki, Venuto, & Roberts, 1998). However, as these systems are not yet widely available, a standard protocol that can be performed in most clinics is described. The patient should perform the following test with best corrected vision (i.e., while wearing glasses or contacts). First, position a standard Snellen eye chart at a distance where the patient is able to read at least the line second from the bottom. The threshold is defined as the lowest line read with three or fewer errors. Gently grasp the patient below the malar eminences and over the parietal region and oscillate the head in a random fashion at a frequency between 2 to 7 Hz and less than 20 degrees of arc displacement in the yaw plane. The direction of line reading should be alternated to control for memorization and the examiner much be careful not to pause when direction of head rotation is changed.

Results

Normal Result

A drop in best-corrected vision of no more than one line from baseline acuity with head rotation is obtained.

Abnormal Result

A drop in best-corrected vision of two or more lines from baseline acuity with head rotation is obtained.

Mechanism

When the head is moved, the orbit of the eye moves as well. To adjust the eye in the orbit so that clear vision can be maintained by retaining the image of the target on the fovea, the VOR provides a precisely calculated neural input to contract or relax the appropriate oculomotor muscles. The oscillation of the head back and forth during the DVA test stimulates the lateral semicircular canals. The hair cells in the lateral SCCs are oriented in such a way as to provide information regarding rotational acceleration of the head in the yaw plane. When the head is turned toward the right in the yaw plane, there is an increase in neural firing rate in the vestibular nerves on the right side and a slow deviation of the eye in the opposite direction. Simultaneously, there is a corresponding decrease in firing rate in the afferent nerves on the left side. This asymmetry in firing rates between the corresponding lateral SCCs is proportionate to the acceleration of the head. The vestibular end organs transduce the acceleration into a neural code that the central vestibular system uses to adjust the oculomotor muscles and move the eye in the opposite direction of the head movement.

For the VOR to generate an appropriate compensatory eye movement, gain (the *ratio* of slow phase eye velocity to head velocity) and phase (the *temporal difference* of slow-phase eye velocity to head velocity) must be accurate. When a vestibular end organ loses sensory cells, the frequency response of the peripheral system is reduced.

Take, for example, the case where one vestibular end organ has been severely impaired and a large number of sensory hair cells in the lateral SCCs are damaged. With a quick head movement in the yaw plane, fewer sensory cells respond in the damaged ear than in the intact ear for the same frequency. The leading ear will produce a lesser amount of neural activity. The ratio of the vestibular-driven compensatory slow-phase eye velocity would be smaller than normal for the given head velocity. This would result in the eye moving to some degree with the head instead of the normal compensatory eye deviation (via the VOR) away from the direction of rotation of the head. The ultimate result would be a reduction in visual acuity due to the slippage of the target from the fovea of the retina.

This relationship between the VOR and DVA enables the clinician to make inferences regarding the status of the vestibular system. For head movements at frequencies above 2 Hz, or those that are associated with normal everyday movements, even a small amount of retinal slippage during head movement can be an indication of vestibular dysfunction. The effect of oscillopsia is most often encountered in those patients with bilateral vestibular system hypofunction due to ototoxicity, bilateral end-organ disease (e.g., bilateral Ménière's disease), or aging (Longridge

& Mallinson, 1984). Patients with poorly compensated unilateral hypofunction or who have severe UVH can also have impaired dynamic visual acuity.

Test Performance

Findings of investigations describing the ability of the DVA test to differentiate between normal individuals and those with vestibular disorders are mixed. When the complete body of literature describing the use of the DVA test to identify and quantify vestibular deficits is examined, it becomes apparent that there are many factors that can explain the differences in specificity and sensitivity found between studies.

Several groups have described a positive relationship between peripheral vestibular dysfunction and DVA performance (Demer, Honrubia, & Baloh, 1994; Herdman et al., 1998; Longridge & Mallinson, 1984, 1987a, 1987b). In one of the first series of studies, Longridge and Mallinson (1984, 1987a, 1987b) described a customized eye chart called the *dynamic illegible E* (DIE) to assist in the detection of vestibular hypofunction. The authors designed a chart using only the "E" from the Snellen chart oriented in different directions. This was to control for some of the letters in the standard Snellen chart being more readily identifiable than others. Each orientation was referred to as an optotype. The DIE test procedure consisted of the patient indicating the direction in which the optotypes were pointing in each column with the head still. This procedure was then repeated while the patient's head was oscillated back and forth at a frequency of 1 Hz. The examiner then observed any change in visual acuity during the dynamic phase of the test.

Using the DIE test, Longridge and Mallinson (1984) reported the ability of the DVA test to screen for aminoglycoside vestibulotoxicity. A group of eight subjects with documented aminoglycoside toxicity were selected to perform the DIE test. Six of these subjects were unable to identify any of the optotypes from the DIE test with head movement. One patient had normal caloric responses and was able to perform the DIE test with abnormal results, and one patient was unable to be tested due to osteomyelitis. Interestingly, when blood serum was monitored during therapy none of this group had toxic levels. According to the authors, these results provided evidence that the DIE test was an appropriate screening tool for aminoglycoside vestibulotoxicity.

Longridge and Mallinson (1987a, 1987b) provided further support for use of the clinical DVA test in the prediction of vestibular dysfunction. This investigation evaluated the relationship between DIE test performance and the magnitude of caloric reduction. The authors recruited 244 patients with abnormal caloric tests to undergo DIE testing. Multiple regression testing revealed a significant correlation between visual acuity during head movement and degree of caloric reduction. Specifically, the greater the degree of caloric reduction the poorer the DIE test score.

Demer et al. (1994) used a computerized paradigm to measure DVA performance. The authors compared a group of 13 normal subjects with two patients presenting with complete bilateral vestibular system weakness. The two subjects with vestibular dysfunction demonstrated reduced DVA performance compared to the normal group. The authors suggested that DVA testing during imposed head motion is a quantitative and clinically feasible measure of oscillopsia that reflects functionally significant abnormalities in the VOR.

Herdman et al. (1998) presented data describing DVA performance in patients with bilateral and unilateral vestibular deficits using a computerized system. DVA test performance was found to be significantly different when scores obtained from patients with unilateral and bilateral vestibular loss were compared to their normal counterparts. Furthermore, in the UVH group, there was a significant difference in DVA performance for head movements toward the affected side, compared to the unaffected side. When the authors examined the sensitivity and specificity of the test for age-matched normals compared to the treatment groups, the DVA test was shown to have a sensitivity of 94.5% and specificity of 95.2%.

However, evidence from other studies fails to support the reported relationship between DVA test performance and vestibular dysfunction. Burgio, Blakely, and Myers (1992) found a poor relationship between vestibular dysfunction and DVA performance. This study evaluated 115 patients referred to a clinic for dizziness and compared them to 17 control subjects. The experimental group consisted of 25 patients with unilateral caloric weakness (25% to 100%), 10 with a bilateral weakness (total SPV of 0 to 21 deg/s), and 80 with normal ENGs who had complaints of dizziness. The investigators found that the DVA test was highly specific (100%) but had poor sensitivity. Their results suggested that the DVA test did not detect vestibular loss or subjective dizziness in more than 50% of the cases with significant unilateral impairment.

The inconsistency in findings among the various studies above is due to several factors. First, differences in methodology when performing the DVA test exist between the aforementioned studies. With recent advances in the technology used for the assessment of dizzy patients, computerized systems are now available for DVA testing (O'Leary & Davis, 1990). These systems require that the head be moving at or above a critical oscillation frequency prior to exposure to visual stimuli. This prevents the subject from reading the optotypes when the head is slowed to change direction. Herdman et al. (1998) employed such a system and reported the highest sensitivity to date for DVA testing.

A second source of variability is the frequency of subject head movement during the test. The pursuit system has been shown to contribute to gaze stabilization at lower frequencies. Lee, Dumford, and Crowley (1997) assessed DVA performance from 27 normal patients using voluntary head rotation at frequencies ranging from 0.7 to 4 Hz. The authors found that there was a natural decrement in visual acuity with increasing frequency of horizontal head movement. The authors suggested that the ocular motor system becomes an ineffective system for ocular stabilization at frequencies above 2 Hz, and that the VOR functions as the primary control system for visual stabilization during lower frequencies associated with ambulation. According to their results, to obtain an accurate measure of how well the VOR is compensating for head movement, the head should be oscillated no slower than 2 Hz. Many of the studies described previously were performed with head oscillations at frequencies below 2 Hz (Barber, 1984; Longridge & Mallinson, 1984, 1987a, 1987b).

In patients with UVH, the ability to read the optotype is improved when oscillating the head toward the intact or better end organ. In paradigms where performance is not measured for each half-cycle this may result in spuriously good DVA performance. This variable can be controlled by computerized DVA systems, where left and right head movement performance can be separated, thereby increasing the sensitivity of the test to unilateral end-organ dysfunction.

A fourth source of interstudy variability is the method used to calculate the DVA score. The two common methods are the traditional Snellen distance 20/XX system (e.g., 20/20, 20/100, etc.), and the LogMAR scale. Computerized DVA systems typically use the measurement parameter "logarithm of the minimum angle of resolution" or LogMAR. The LogMAR scale is a conversion method that transforms the geometric sequence of a traditional Snellen chart to a linear scale. The LogMar scale describes performance as visual acuity loss. Specifically, vision loss is represented by a positive score, whereas better visual acuity is represented by a negative score. Many of the earlier studies discussed above have described DVA performance by indicating how many lines of the Snellen chart visual acuity dropped with head movement. This interpretation of lines lost is only accurate when all steps between lines are equal, which is not the case in the Snellen chart.

A fifth variable to consider in assessing the sensitivity of DVA is the degree of vestibular system compensation patients with UVH have attained. Herdman, Schubert, Das, and Tusa (2003) reported the effect of vestibular exercises on the recovery of DVA during head movement in patients with UVH. The sample consisted of 21 patients with UVH who were culled from an ambulatory referral center. Of this total, 13 of the patients performed vestibular exercises designed to increase VOR gain, whereas eight of the patients performed placebo exercises. Subjects in the treatment group receiving vestibular exercises showed a significant improvement in DVA performance, whereas those performing the placebo exercises did not. In contrast, Longridge and Mallinson (1987a, 1987b) used the conventional DVA test to explore the relationship between DVA performance and central nervous system compensation. The factors age, degree of caloric impairment, and time from onset of disease process were compared with scores from the DIE test. The investigators found no correlation between DIE test performance and central vestibular system compensation.

The clinical utility of the DVA test appears to be influenced somewhat by technique and experience of the examiner. The original DVA test using a standard Snellen chart or DIE chart can be extremely

useful in predicting severe vestibular dysfunction. Specifically, the clinical utility has been proven when the examiner suspects bilateral vestibular dysfunction from aminoglycoside vestibulotoxicity or a severe unilateral lesion (Burgio et al., 1992; Demer et al., 1994; Longridge & Mallinson, 1984). However, today's computerized DVA systems although superior, are relatively rare in balance clinics. They allow the examiner to document central nervous system compensation after rehabilitation, predict the side of the lesion in unilateral involvement, and grossly quantify the severity of bilateral vestibular hypofunction. Regardless of the system used, it is important that whenever the results from the DVA test are abnormal, a full balance function workup should be recommended. When results are determined to be normal, the referral should be made based on a thorough case history.

HYPERVENTILATION-INDUCED NYSTAGMUS

Introduction

Hyperventilation may produce a variety of apparent vestibular symptoms in patients, including faintness, light-headedness, unsteadiness, giddiness, and true vertigo. Early reports suggested that hyperventilation was often caused by anxiety-related disorders (Drachman & Hart, 1972). Hyperventilation-induced nystagmus has since been demonstrated in patients with vestibular-related disorders. Subsequent authors agreed that it is important to note that hyperventilation elicits responses of dizziness in many patients with normal vestibular systems as well as patients with peripheral or central vestibular lesions, perilymphatic fistula, or epidermoid tumor (Bance, O'Driscoll, Patel, & Ramsden, 1998; Choi, Cho, Koo, Park, & Kim, 2005; Drachman & Hart, 1972; Kroenke et al., 1992; Sama, Meikle, & Jones, 1995; Singer, 1958). In most patients, elicited sensations are not described as true vertigo. It is important to be cognizant of the possibility of unmasking previously undetected vestibular anomalies with hyperventilation (Bance et al., 1998). Careful observation of patient responses to hyperventilation, when combined with the results of other tests, may help to distinguish patients with vestibular or central nervous system anomalies from normals and those affected by psychosomatic or anxiety-related dizziness. A wide range of disorders may cause hyperventilation-induced dizziness or nystagmus. When elicited, hyperventilation-induced nystagmus is significantly more common in retrocochlear pathologies than in end-organ disease (Robichaud, DesRoches, & Bance, 2002), and almost ubiquitous in cases of vestibular schwannoma (Bance et al., 1998). An increase in down-beating nystagmus can be observed in patients with cerebellar lesions (Walker & Zee, 1999). Leigh and Zee (1999) described a patient who exhibited hyperventilation-induced nystagmus due to a lesion of the petrous apex. In most cases, nystagmus beats toward the lesioned ear, whereas in others, such as complete unilateral lesions, it will beat away from the lesioned side. Some authors suggest that emergent nystagmus should beat ipsilaterally due to short-term improvement in axonal conduction caused by changes in the concentration of free calcium ions in the blood (Bance et al., 1998; Minor, Haslwanter, Straumann, & Zee, 1999; Walker & Zee, 1999). Hain (2006) has observed that this tendency also explains the presence of hyperventilation-induced nystagmus in patients with complete lesions of the vestibular apparatus on one side, or of patients who have undergone vestibular nerve section. In these situations the enhancement in conduction can only be produced by the intact side. Other authors argue that dizziness resulting from hyperventilation is caused by a decrease in the partial pressure of carbon dioxide in the blood (Bance et al., 1998). This results in reduced neural activity in the VOR due to the concurrent drop in oxygen delivered to the cells as a result of vasoconstriction. It is thought that the reduction in activity may reveal an underlying paretic nystagmus. It is generally agreed, however, that the test for hyperventilation-induced nystagmus is not diagnostic of vestibular or central abnormalities by itself. Combined with other tests described herein, it can be a valuable tool in the quest to identify compensated peripheral losses and explain the origin of dizziness complaints.

Technique

All testing should be conducted while the patient is wearing Frenzel lenses or light-occluding VNG goggles to prevent VOR cancellation. In a standing position, the patient should be instructed to take deep, rapid breaths for 30 to 60 s, averaging approximately one breath per second (Minor et al., 1999). The examiner should observe the movements of the eyes before hyperventilation commences to note any existing nystagmus. Once hyperventilation commences, the examiner should carefully observe the movements of the eyes for the appearance of, or reversal of, nystagmus. The examiner also should be watchful for changes in body sway during and after hyperventilation. It is useful to stabilize the patient with a hand on the shoulder to help prevent a fall and to increase examiner awareness of any light-headedness, dizziness, or vertigo.

Results

Normal Results

Normal subjects should exhibit no nystagmus. The sensation of light-headedness or dizziness should not be taken as a positive test result. An increase in sway in the sagittal plane may also appear in normal subjects (Sakellari et al., 1997).

Abnormal Results

Patients with incomplete unilateral peripheral lesions may exhibit nystagmus in the horizontal plane which appears, or is enhanced, for up to 60 s or more following hyperventilation (Sakellari et al., 1997). The direction of the fast phase of the nystagmus is ipsilesional (Chee & Tong, 2002; Walker & Zee, 1999). Patients with a complete unilateral peripheral lesion due to surgery exhibit a contralesional beating nystagmus (Bance et al., 1998). Hyperventilation may result in nystagmus in cases of bilateral incomplete lesions. Alterations in neural conduction due to blood gas and blood chemistry changes disrupt central vestibular compensation for unbalanced peripheral vestibular input. Central lesions such as demyelination due to multiple sclerosis, or cerebellar ischemia due to infarct may also result in hyperventilation-induced nystagmus. The direction of nystagmus cannot be predicted in such cases. Walker and Zee (1999) reported that hyperventilation enhanced the slow phase velocity of down-beating nystagmus in patients with cerebellar lesions.

Mechanism

Nystagmus of both peripheral and central origin can be affected by hyperventilation (Bance et al., 1998; Minor et al., 1999; Sakellari et al., 1997). Two theories exist to explain the seemingly contradictory test results seen in patients with similar histories and symptoms:

1. Increased metabolic activity induces changes in nerve conduction, and is most applicable to patients with peripheral lesions such as vestibular schwannoma. Tumors of the VIIIth cranial nerve cause focal demyelination by compressing the nerve bundle. It is argued that hyperventilation increases metabolic activity in the nerve, allowing the nerve to overcome the blockage to conduction caused by demyelination. This serves to produce stronger signals from the side of the lesion, due to decreased neural firing thresholds, than are typically received by the central vestibular system thereby disrupting central compensation (Walker & Zee, 1999). Hyperventilation causes an increase in blood pH as carbon dioxide is expelled from the body. As blood gas levels and blood chemistry largely govern metabolic rate, neural firing patterns are subject to change during and immediately following hyperventilation. When the alkalinity of the blood is increased, the theoretical carrying capacity of the blood serum for calcium ions decreases, thereby lowering the threshold of nerve activation (Bance et al., 1998). Central compensation is thereby disrupted, with greater activity from the lesioned side than is normally encountered by the central system, resulting in an ipsilesional beating nystagmus.
2. Hyperventilation reduces blood flow to the central nervous system, thereby starving the cells of oxygen. As discussed above, decreased blood carbon dioxide concentration causes an increase in pH, which elicits a vasoconstriction response in the body. This theory is further supported by the physiologic principle of the Bohr effect (Monday & Tetreault, 1980). This effect causes hemoglobin to increase its binding affinity for oxygen with increasing blood pH (Giardina, Mosca, & De Rosa, 2004). Although the concentration of oxygen in the blood is increased relative to the

resting state, the increase in binding affinity renders oxygen in the blood less available to tissues, hindering the action of the electron transport chain in mitochondria and inhibiting continued firing of the nerves. Central compensation for unilateral vestibular impairment thus would be disrupted, revealing the underlying contralesional beating nystagmus. This explanation of hyperventilation-induced nystagmus is more appropriate for cases of complete unilateral vestibular loss, as in patients who have undergone vestibular nerve section.

Test Performance

Authors' reports of the sensitivity and specificity of the hyperventilation test vary widely (Table 7–4). Monday and Tetreault (1980) failed to record nystagmus in 19 normal subjects who reported dizziness during hyperventilation. Subjects underwent ENG testing before and after 90-s periods of hyperventilation. Hyperventilation was not shown to affect the slow phase velocity of nystagmus elicited by caloric stimulation but was shown to increase the number of positions in which nystagmus could be elicited during positional testing (see Table 7–4). The authors speculated that this effect was due to induced hypoxia. Development of physiologic explanations for the observed phenomena led to investigation of the relationship between retrocochlear pathologies and hyperventilation-induced dizziness. Wilson and Kim (1981) measured eye movements in subjects under conditions of increased (breathing oxygen) and decreased (hyperventilation) available oxygen blood gas levels in 18 patients with acoustic neuroma. The authors noted that hyperventilation was more likely to induce nystagmus (8% of subjects) than was oxygen (2.5%), and that in cases where both conditions elicited nystagmus, the eye movements were in opposite directions. It was further suggested that hyperventilation had little localizing value. Bance et al. (1998) reported 100% (i.e., 32 of 32 subjects) sensitivity in patients with complete unilateral loss of vestibular function due to surgical intervention for acoustic neuroma. Additionally, 23 of 28 patients with acoustic neuroma who did not undergo surgery exhibited hyperventilation-induced

Table 7-4. Comparison of Studies Evaluating the Hyperventilation Test

Study	*n*	Controls	Disorder	Condition	Sensitivity	Specificity
Monday & Tetreault (1980)	19	0	Vestibular normal, reported dizziness during hyperventilation		Could not calculate	100.00%
Wilson & Kim (1981)	18	0	Acoustic neuroma	Breathing O$_2$	3%	Could not calculate
				Hyperventilation	8%	Could not calculate
Bance, O'Driscoll, Patel, & Ramsden (1998)	32	29	Complete unilateral vestibular loss	Surgery for acoustic neuroma	100%	96.50%
	28	29	Acoustic neuroma	No surgery	82%	96.50%
Minor, Haslwanter, Staumann, & Zee (1999)	6	0	Unilateral vestibular schwannoma		100%	Could not calculate
Robichaud, DesRoches, & Bance (2002)	24	0	Acoustic neuroma		58%	Could not calculate
	38	0	Vestibular end organ lesion		18%	Could not calculate
Totals	165	28			53%	97.67%

nystagmus (i.e., 82% sensitivity). Normal volunteers exhibited hyperventilation-induced nystagmus in only 1 of 29 cases (i.e., 96.5% specificity). The authors further reported that the hyperventilation test was more sensitive and specific than the head-shaking test in this sample of subjects. Similar results were reported by Minor et al. (1999), where 6 of 6 patients with confirmed unilateral vestibular schwannoma exhibited hyperventilation-induced nystagmus (i.e., 100% sensitivity). In each case, hyperventilation replicated the subjective sensations of dizziness, vertigo, or unsteadiness reported by the patients. Following resection of the tumor, the authors reported elimination of the hyperventilation-induced nystagmus in 4 of 6 subjects. In a follow-up study to Bance et al. (1998), Robichaud et al. (2002) reported hyperventilation-induced nystagmus in 14 of 24 patients (i.e., 58% sensitivity) with confirmed acoustic neuroma, versus 7 of 38 patients (i.e., 18% sensitivity) with end-organ lesions.

The wide range of sensitivity and specificity reported in the literature suggests that the results of the hyperventilation test should not be considered to have localizing value, and that the results should be interpreted with caution.

VALSALVA-INDUCED NYSTAGMUS

Introduction

The self-induced change of middle ear and intracranial pressure commonly known as the Valsalva maneuver (VM) is capable of inducing eye movements in patients with craniocervical junction abnormalities and disorders affecting the inner ear. These anomalies may include Arnold-Chiari malformation, perilymphatic fistula, superior canal dehiscence, and other anomalies that involve the oval window, round window, saccule, or ossicles. The VM is named in honor of one of its early proponents, Antonio Mario Valsalva (1666–1723), although documentation of the technique exists from the 16th century and earlier as a treatment for deafness and method for removing foreign bodies from the ear canal (Lustig & Jackler, 1999). Hennebert first described eye movements induced by changes in middle ear pressure in the early 20th century. This phenomenon is now known as Hennebert's sign and describes a conjugate eye movement away from the affected ear with positive pressure applied to the external auditory meatus. A movement toward the affected ear is expected with applied negative pressure. The presence of such a movement allows the examiner to deduce the presence of an anomalous connection between the inner ear and the external environment (Goebel, 2001).

Technique

Two variants of the VM should be performed by the patient: one designed to increase air pressure in the sinuses and middle ear, the other designed to increase venous pressure in the cranium. In both cases, the subject should wear Frenzel or VNG goggles to prevent VOR suppression, and to permit the observation and documentation of eye movements (Zee & Fletcher, 1996). The patient also should be instructed to report any sensations of dizziness or vertigo induced by the test procedure, including blurred vision, oscillopsia, or diplopia (Brandt & Strupp, 2005). Eye movements should be observed during and immediately following pressurization and relaxation for both tests. The positive air pressure variant is performed by increasing barometric pressure in the sinuses, middle ear, and pharynx. Patients should be instructed to take a deep breath, pinch the nose, and close the mouth tightly, then blow as if equalizing the pressure of the ears when descending from altitude on an airplane. The patient should maintain the pressure for 10 to 15 s. The result is an increase in middle ear pressure (Walker & Zee, 2000). Following recovery from any elicited responses, the patient should strain against a closed glottis and lips for a similar duration, as if pressurizing the lungs to help stabilize the trunk while lifting a heavy weight. This variant serves to raise the intracranial pressure by inducing increases in central venous pressure (Walker & Zee, 2000). Either or both techniques may induce nystagmus in patients with the anomalies described above, and both therefore should be included in the bedside test battery.

Results

Normal Results

Although Hennebert's sign has been reported in normal subjects, the VM should not elicit sensations of dizziness or vertigo in the great majority of patients. The examiner, therefore, should be careful to distinguish between a shift of the eyes (positive Hennebert's sign) and nystagmus. No elicited conjugate eye movements should be observed under Frenzel or VNG goggles.

Abnormal Results

Increased middle ear or intracranial pressure as a result of either variant of the Valsalva maneuver will elicit a conjugate movement of the eyes toward the contralesional ear in the cases of lateral and anterior canal involvement. If the patient maintains increased intracranial pressure, a corrective saccade toward the ipsilateral ear will be observed. Thus, nystagmus will "beat" toward the affected ear. The direction of the fast phase of nystagmus thereby may provide information regarding the site of lesion. Horizontal nystagmus indicates involvement of the lateral semicircular canal and will beat toward the affected ear. Torsional and down-beating vertical nystagmus indicates a site of lesion in the anterior canal, whereas vertical up-beating nystagmus with a torsional component suggests the involvement of the posterior canal (Davies, 2004). The direction of torsion provides information regarding the laterality of the lesion. The fast phase of the torsional nystagmus will beat in a clockwise direction for lesions of the left ear, and counterclockwise for lesions of the right ear.

Mechanism

Increased pressure in the middle ear acts on abnormal connections between the labyrinth and the external environment to induce a pressure gradient within the cochlea. These abnormalities may exist as a hypermobility of the oval and round window membranes, defects of the bony structures surrounding the lateral aspect of the membranous labyrinth such as erosion due to cholesteatoma or chronic otitis media leading to dehiscence or fistula of the posterior or lateral canal, or defects of the floor of the middle cranial fossa leading to superior canal dehiscence (Brandt & Strupp, 2005; Goebel, 2001). The increased pressure within the affected labyrinth simulates movement of the head as it stimulates neural firing by displacing the cupula of the semicircular canal. The increased neural discharge rate drives the VOR such that a compensatory eye movement away from the affected ear is generated (Hennebert's sign).

In the case of straining against a closed glottis, increased pressure within the middle fossa is generated through changes in central venous pressure. Increasing and maintaining pressure within the thoracic cavity decreases venous return through the jugular vein, thereby raising intracranial pressure (Minor et al., 2001). An abnormal connection between the middle fossa and the vestibular labyrinth such as occurs in the case of superior canal dehiscence will induce a pressure change in the affected canal and elicit down-beating, torsional nystagmus beating toward the affected ear. Conversely, a dehiscence of the posterior canal will elicit up-beating and torsional nystagmus with the fast phase oriented toward the affected ear (Brantberg, Bagger-Sjoback, Mathiesen, Witt, & Pansell, 2006).

Test Performance

A review of the literature (Table 7–5) suggests that the Valsalva test is useful in screening dizzy patients for the presence of canal dehiscence and perilymphatic fistula. The phenomenon, however, has also been reported in the presence of several other disorders, including cholesteatoma. Brantberg, Greitz, and Pansell (2004) reported a case of superior canal dehiscence where abnormal bone development in the middle cranial fossa was not the cause of the dehiscence. The patient exhibited pressure-induced vertigo despite the location of the dehiscence close to the common crus. Similarly, Tilikete, Krolak-Salmon, Tuy, and Vighetto (2004) reported the case of a subject with bilateral superior canal dehiscence. In this case, both Valsalva-induced vertigo and Tullio's sign could be elicited, with upward and counterclockwise torsional beating nystagmus. Halmagyi et al. (2003) described a patient who underwent three stapedectomy surgeries despite the audiometric finding of conductive hearing loss with preserved ipsilat-

eral and contralateral acoustic reflexes, symptoms of superior canal dehiscence. The patient reported hypersensitivity to bone-conducted sounds (Tullio's phenomenon), and exhibited a VEMP at abnormally soft sound intensities and Valsalva-induced vertigo. Rambold, Heide, Sprenger, Haendler, and Helmchen (2001) reported the case of a patient who experienced Valsalva-elicited contralateral horizontal nystagmus with the diagnosis of perilymphatic fistula. The patient also exhibited pulse synchronous oscillations of the eyes.

Several studies have been conducted investigating the sensitivity of the Valsalva test. Reported sensitivity has varied. Hillman, Kertesz, Hadley, and Shelton (2006) reported vertigo evoked by VM in only 12 of 27 (44%) subjects with superior canal dehiscence. Of the 12 subjects, 8 could elicit nystagmus during the Valsalva or simulated heavy lifting, corresponding to a sensitivity of 29%. Minor (2000) reported Valsalva-induced nystagmus in 10 of 17 subjects (i.e., a sensitivity of 58%) subsequently identified with SCD. In a later study the VM showed 82% sensitivity in a cohort of 28 patients previously diagnosed with SCD (Minor et al., 2001). Symptoms could be evoked in some of these patients by pressing on the tragus of the ear. The authors noted that nystagmus could continue for several beats after the release of pressure. Cremer, Minor, Carey, and Della Santina (2000) reported that 8 of 11 subjects with SCD exhibited nystagmus following VM (i.e., 73% sensitivity). Brantberg, Bergenius, Mendel, Witt, Tribukait, and Ygge (2001) reported that 8 of 8 (100%) subjects with superior canal dehiscence experienced pressure-induced vertigo. The subjects reported that the vertigo worsened during periods of upper respiratory infection.

The presence of a positive Valsalva test therefore should be considered evidence of an abnormal connection between the middle ear and inner ear, or the intracranial space and the middle ear.

FUKUDA STEPPING

Introduction and History

The Fukuda stepping task is designed to identify the presence of a peripheral vestibular system

Table 7–5. Comparison of Studies Evaluating Valsalva-Induced Nystagmus

Study	n	Controls	Disorder	Condition	Sensitivity	Specify
Brantberg, Greitz, & Pansell (2004)	1		Dehiscence of the common crus		100%	Could not calculate
Tilikete, Krolak-Salmon, Truy, & Vighetto (2004)	1		Bilateral SCD		100%	Could not calculate
Halmagyi et al. (2003)	1		SCD		100%	Could not calculate
Rambold, Heide, Sprenger, Haendler, & Helmchen (2001)	1		Perilymphatic fistula		100%	Could not calculate
Hillman, Kertesz, Hadley, & Shelton (2006)	27		SCD		29%	Could not calculate
Minor (2000)	17		SCD		58%	Could not calculate
Minor, Cremer, Carey, Della Santina, Streubel, & Weg (2001)	28		SCD		82%	Could not calculate
Cremer, Minor, Carey, & Della Santina (2000)	11		SCD		73%	Could not calculate
Brantberg, Bergenius, Mendel, Witt, Tribukait, & Ygge (2001)	8		SCD		100%	Could not calculate
Totals	95				82%	Could not calculate

impairment manifested as an asymmetry in lower extremity vestibulospinal reflex "tone." It represents a simplification of Unterberger 's "Treversuch" test (Unterberger, 1938) and Hirsch's "Waltzing" test (Hirsch, 1940) intended for the clinical environment and patients who are easily able to stand, unsupported. Whereas Unterberger's and Hirsch's tests included caloric stimulation followed by a stepping task, Fukuda (1959a) indicated that the performance of the stepping task without caloric stimulation was of more clinical value in the identification of peripheral vestibular weakness. This recommendation arose from the observation that middle ear patholo-gies can influence the results of caloric stimulation due to alteration of thermal conductivity across the middle ear space (Fukuda, 1959a). Similar tests of the vestibulospinal reflex have been described including Fukuda's vertical writing test (1959b). However, differential connections between the vestibular labyrinth and the upper and lower limbs, ease of implementation, and test-retest reliability have resulted in superior sensitivity and specificity for the Fukuda stepping test and its variants. Unterberger observed that stepping tests were of limited use in cases of spontaneous nystagmus due to the tendency of the patient to stagger or fall when walking with the eyes closed (Peitersen, 1964). As such, good judgment must be used in selecting patients appropriately for the test.

Technique

With the arms extended at a 90° angle in front of the body and the eyes closed, the patient marches in place for 50 steps. Fukuda (1959a) recommended a stepping rate of approximately 110 steps per minute. The angle, direction, and distance of deviation from the origin should be recorded. It is helpful to make use of a reference mark system such as a band of tape on the floor oriented along the sagittal plane at the start of the test (Figure 7–2), or a thin, dense rubber mat with a polar pattern marked on it. These features improve the ability of the examiner to assess the angle of deviation from the starting position.

Results

Normal Results

The original work by Fukuda (1959a) on 500 normal subjects (Video 7–7) suggested that normal subjects could complete 50 steps without significant angular deviation from the starting position (i.e., normal

rotation ≤30°). It is common for normal subjects to drift as much as 50 cm (~18 inches) in the forward direction, but it is uncommon to observe backward deviation from the origin. Moffat, Harries, Baguley, and Hardy (1989) suggest that this result may, in fact, be a sign of nonorganic dysequilibrium. Fukuda (1959) suggested that it was not uncommon for normal subjects to rotate slightly in the direction of their dominant hand; however, subsequent research by Nyabenda, Briart, Deggouj, and Gersdorff (2004) indicated that handedness did not affect the outcome of the test.

Abnormal Results

A rotation of greater than 45 degrees (Video 7–8) in either direction is considered to be abnormal (Fukuda, 1959; Furman & Cass, 2003). Other authors have considered the presence of marked sway, staggering, or a fall as an abnormal result (Moffat et al., 1989). Results typically coincide with the results of the past-pointing test.

Mechanism

Unilateral lesions of the peripheral vestibular system result in a rotation of the body, which coincides

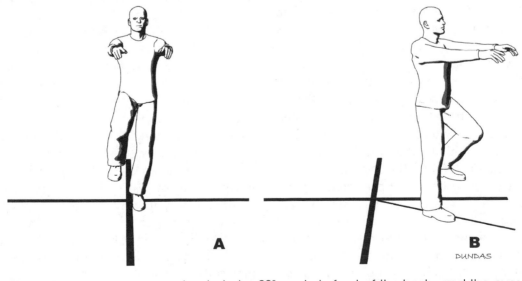

Figure 7–2. With the arms extended at a 90° angle in front of the body, and the eyes closed, the patient marches in place for 50 steps. **A.** Normal Fukuda stepping test result. **B.** Abnormal Fukuda stepping test result with rotation greater than 45°. Courtesy of J. A. Dundas.

with the direction of the slow component of the nystagmus, that is, in the direction of the lesioned peripheral vestibular system labyrinth. The body rotation results from the unbalanced static activity of the two end organs. The imbalance is interpreted centrally as rotation in the yaw plane toward the contralesioned ear. This results in a reflexive deviation of the body toward the ipsilesioned ear. The positive stepping test appears to persist after central VOR compensation is complete. It is present in disorders that affect peripheral vestibular system function, including Ménière's disease (Peitersen, 1964), labyrinthectomized patients (Peitersen, 1964), and acoustic neuroma/vestibular schwannoma (Moffat et al., 1989). In most pathologies, the patient rotates toward the side of lesion. However, in the case of acoustic neuroma/vestibular schwannoma, numerous authors have reported that the patient may rotate either toward or away from the side of lesion (Peitersen, 1964, 1967; Moffat et al., 1989), thus, test results should not necessarily be considered as constituting lateralizing information.

Test Performance

A study by the present authors found that the Fukuda stepping test exhibited 70% sensitivity (95% confidence interval 50% to 90%) and 59% specificity (44% to 74%) in identifying peripheral vestibular impairment. These findings were in agreement with the available literature. Moffat et al. (1989) reported 71% sensitivity for the Fukuda test in a sample of 100 subjects with unilateral acoustic neuroma. As all subjects in this study must be considered abnormal, it was impossible to assess the specificity of the test on this sample. Peiterson (1964) conducted stepping tests in patients with a variety of pathologies. Of 18 subjects with unilateral Ménière's disease, 12 consistently rotated toward the lesioned ear, and 5 away. The 18th patient did not consistently rotate to one side. Five of seven patients with bilateral Ménière's disease rotated away from the ear with more impaired function. The author speculates that this apparent anomaly may be due to the comparatively recent damage to the less impaired ear and the relative lack of compensation accomplished since lesion. All eight patients who had undergone surgical fenestration of the labyrinth rotated toward

the side of surgery. A similar result was found in patients with labyrinthine fistula due to complications from otitis media. The average rotation across all conditions was over 90°.

Norré, Forrez, and Beckers (1989) investigated the sensitivity of various vestibulospinal tests among patients diagnosed with either Ménière's disease or vestibular neuritis. Utilizing a 30-second stepping test, the authors reported 27% sensitivity among 75 subjects with Ménière's disease and 26% sensitivity among 39 subjects diagnosed with unilateral vestibular neuritis. The authors noted that the stepping test could reveal deficits in vestibulospinal reflex compensation when vestibulo-ocular reflex compensation was complete.

The Fukuda stepping test therefore can be considered a useful test of peripheral vestibular "tone" as expressed by the lower extremities. It is appropriate for the clinician to implement the test in the screening of subjects for vestibular disorders. It is not appropriate, however, to make use of the result of the test in isolation to attempt to lateralize or localize lesions of the vestibular system as several pathologies may induce test results contrary to the "rule of thumb" that patients should rotate toward the site of lesion.

SUMMARY

The results of informal tests of vestibular function such as those described in this chapter are commonly considered to be well-established criteria for the appropriate referral of patients for diagnostic testing. However, a review of published literature regarding the tests in question does not support such a conclusion. Rather, the tests may be most appropriately used to alert the examiner that special care should be taken during a particular subtest when laboratory testing is being performed, or that additional testing is warranted. Although the tests reviewed in this chapter tend to exhibit high specificity, their attendant low sensitivity renders them relatively unsuitable for clinical use. As such, informal assessment tools should not be considered to be substitutes for electrophysiologic testing, imaging studies, or other diagnostic testing. If bedside tests are to be included in the screening and referral process, new or improved versions and combinations of the tests must be developed, investigated, and proven by clinician scientists. Without such developments, it is likely that reliance on bedside tests of vestibular function may lead to missed diagnoses or inappropriate referrals for testing and follow-up care.

VIDEOS ASSOCIATED WITH THIS CHAPTER

Video 7–1. Video of spontaneous vestibular nystagmus.

Video 7–2. Normal head thrust animation.

Video 7–3. Abnormal head thrust animation.

Video 7–4. Normal head-shake animation.

Video 7–5. Abnormal head-shake animation.

Video 7–6. Abnormal head-shake real-patient video.

Video 7–7. Normal Fukuda animation.

Video 7–8. Abnormal Fukuda animation.

REFERENCES

Alexander, G. (1912). Die Ohrenkrankheiten im Kindesalter. In M. Pfaundler & A. Schossmann (Eds.), *Handbuch der Kinderheilkunde* (pp. 84–96). Leipzig, Germany: Vogel.

Angelaki, D. E., & Perachio, A. A. (1993). Contribution of irregular semicircular canal afferents to the horizontal vestibule-ocular response during constant velocity rotation. *Journal of Neurophysiology, 69,* 996–999.

Bance, M. L., O'Driscoll, M., Patel, N., & Ramsden, R. T. (1998). Vestibular disease unmasked by hyperventilation. *Laryngoscope, 108*(4), 610–614.

Bárány, R. (1907). Untersuchungen uber Verhalten des Vestibularapparates bei Kopftraumen und ihre practische Bedeuntung. *Verhandugen der Deutxchen Otol Gessellschaft,* pp. 252–266.

Barber, H. O. (1984). Vestibular neurophysiology. *Otolaryngology-Head and Neck Surgery, 92,* 151–157.

Beynon, G. J., Jani, P., & Baguley, D. M. (1998) A clinical evaluation of head impulse testing. *Clinical Otolaryngology, 106,* 6–9.

Borries, G. V. (1923). Klinische Untersuchungen uber diedurch Kopfbewegungen und Kopfstellungen ausgelosten Nystagmussantalle. *Monatschr Ohrenheilk, 57,* 644–683.

Brandt, T., & Strupp, M. (2005). General vestibular testing. *Clinical Neurophysiology, 116,* 406–426.

Brantberg, K., Bagger-Sjoback, D., Mathiesen, T., Witt, H., & Pansell, T. (2006). Posterior canal dehiscence syndrome caused by an apex cholesteatoma, *Otology and Neuro-Otology, 27*(4), 531–534.

Brantberg, K., Bergenius, J., Mendel, L., Witt, H., Tribukait, A., & Ygge, J. (2001). Symptoms, findings and treatment in patients with dehiscence of the superior semicircular canal. *Acta Otolaryngolica, 121*(1), 68–75.

Brantberg, K., Greitz, D., & Pansell, T. (2004). Subarcuate venous malformation causing audio-vestibular symptoms similar to those in superior canal dehiscence syndrome. *Otology and Neuro-Otology, 25*(6), 993–997.

Brickner, R. M. (1936). Oscillopsia: A new symptom commonly occurring in multiple sclerosis. *Archives of Neurological Psychiatry, 36,* 586–589.

Burgio, D. L., Blakley, B. W., & Myers, S. F. (1991). An evaluation of the head-shaking nystagmus test. *Acta Oto-Laryngologica Supplement, 540,* 27–33.

Burgio, D. L., Blakely, B. W., & Myers, S. F. (1992). The high-frequency oscillopsia test. *Journal of Vestibular Rehabilitation, 2,* 221–226.

Cass, S. P., Kartush, J. M., & Graham, M. D. (1992). Patterns of vestibular function following vestibular nerve section. *Laryngoscope, 102,* 388–394.

Chee, N. W., & Tong, H. M. (2002). Acoustic neuroma presenting as exercise-induced vertigo. *Journal of Laryngology and Otology, 116*(8), 630–632.

Choi, K. D., Cho, H. J., Koo, J. W., Park, S. H., & Kim, J. S. (2005). Hyperventilation-induced nystagmus in vestibular schwannoma. *Neurology, 64*(12), 2062.

Cohen, B., Henn, V., Raphan, T., & Dennett, D. (1981). Velocity storage, nystagmus, and visual vestibular interactions in humans. *Annals of the New York Academy of Sciences, 374,* 421–433.

Cohen, B., Matsuo, V., & Raphan, T. (1977). Quantitative analysis of the velocity characteristics of optokinetic nystagmus and optokinetic afternystagmus. *Journal of Physiology, 270,* 321–344.

Cremer, P. D., Halmagyi, G. M., Aw, S. T., Curthoys, I. S., McGarvie, L. A., Todd, M. J., . . . Hannigan, I. P. (1998). Semicircular canal plane head impulses detect absent function of individual semicircular canals. *Brain, 121,* 699–716.

Cremer, P. D., Minor, L. B., Carey, J. P., & Della Santina, C. C. (2000). Eye movements in patients with superior canal dehiscence syndrome align with the abnormal canal. *Neurology, 55*(12), 1833–1841.

Davies, R. (2004). Bedside neuro-otological examination and interpretation of commonly used investigations. *Journal of Neurology, Neurosurgery, and Psychiatry, 75*(Suppl. 4), 32–44.

Dayal, V. S., Tarantino, L. Farkashidy, J., & Paradisgarten, A. (1974). Spontaneous and positional nystagmus: A reassessment of clinical significance. *Laryngoscope, 84*(11), 2033–2044.

Demer, J. L., Honrubia, V., & Baloh, R. W. (1994). Dynamic visual acuity: A test of oscillopsia and vestibulo-ocular reflex function. *American Journal of Otology, 16,* 97–103.

Drachman, D. A., & Hart, C. W. (1972). An approach to the dizzy patient. *Neurology, 22*(4), 323–334.

Fetter, M., & Dichgans, J. (1990). Adaptive mechanisms of VOR compensation after unilateral peripheral vestibular lesions in humans. *Journal of Vestibular Research, 1,* 9–22.

Fisher, C. M. (1969). The neurological examination of the comatose patient. *Acta Neurologica Scandinavica, 45*(Suppl. 36), 1–56.

Foster, C. A., Foster, B. D., Spindler, J., & Harris, J. P. (1994). Functional loss of the horizontal doll's eye reflex following unilateral vestibular lesions. *Laryngoscope, 104*(4), 473–478.

Fujimoto, M., Rutka, J., & Mai, M. (1993). A study into the phenomenon of head-shaking nystagmus: Its presence in a dizzy population. *Journal of Otolaryngology, 22*(5), 376–379.

Fukuda, T. (1959a). The stepping test: Two phases of the labyrinthine reflex. *Acta Oto-Laryngologica, 50*(2), 95–108.

Fukuda, T. (1959b). Vertical writing with eyes covered: A new test of vestibulo-spinal reaction. *Acta Oto-Laryngologica, 50,* 26–36.

Furman, J. M., Balaban, C. D., & Pollack, I. F. (1997). Vestibular compensation in a patient with a cerebellar infarction. *Neurology, 48,* 916–920.

Furman, J. M., & Cass, S. P. (2003). *Vestibular disorders* (2nd ed.). New York, NY: Oxford University Press.

Giardina, B., Mosca, D., & De Rosa, M. C., (2004). The Bohr effect of haemoglobin in vertebrates: An example of molecular adaptation to different physiological requirements. *Acta Physiologica Scandia, 182*(3), 229–244.

Goebel, J. A. (2001). The ten-minute examination of the dizzy patient. *Seminars in Neurology, 21*(4), 391–398.

Goebel, J. A., & Garcia, P. (1992) Prevalence of post-head shake nystagmus in patients with caloric deficits and vertigo. *Otolaryngology-Head and Neck Surgery, 106,* 121–127.

Goldberg, J. M., & Fernandez, C. (1971). Physiology of peripheral neurons innervating semicircular canals of the squirrel monkey. I. Resting discharge and response to constant angular acceleration. *Journal of Neurophysiology, 34,* 634–660.

Guidetti, G., Monzani, D., & Civiero, N. (2002) Head shaking nystagmus in the follow-up of patients with vestibular diseases. *Clinical Otolaryngology, 27,* 124–128.

Guidetti, G., Monzani, D., & Rovatti, V. (2006). Clinical examination of labyrinthine-defective patients out of the vertigo attack: Sensitivity and specificity of three low-cost methods. *Acta Otorhinolaryngol Italia, 26,* 96–101.

Hain, T. C. (2006). *Hyperventilation in dizzy persons.* Retrieved November 16, 2006, from http://www.dizziness-and-balance.com/practice/hyperventilation.htm

Hain, T. C., Fetter, M., & Zee, D. S. (1987). Head-shaking nystagmus in patients with unilateral peripheral vestibular lesions. *American Journal of Otolaryngology, 8,* 36–47.

Hain, T. C., & Spindler, J. S. (1993). *Head-shaking nystagmus. The vestibulo-ocular reflex and vertigo.* New York, NY: Raven Press.

Hall, S. F., & Laird, M. E. (1992). Is head-shaking nystagmus a sign of vestibular dysfunction? *Journal of Otolaryngology, 21,* 209–212.

Halmagyi, G. M., Aw, S. T., McGarvie, L. A., Todd, M. J., Bradshaw, A., Yavor, R., & Fagan, P. A. (2003). Superior semicircular canal dehiscence simulating otosclerosis. *Journal of Laryngology and Otology, 117,* 553–557.

Halmagyi, G. M., Black, R. A., Thurtell, M. J., & Curthoys, I. S. (2003). The human horizontal vestibulo-ocular reflex in response to active and passive head impulses after unilateral vestibular deafferentation. *Annals of the New York Academy of Sciences, 1004,* 325–336.

Halmagyi, G. M., & Curthoys, I. S. (1988). A clinical sign of canal paresis. *Archives of Neurology, 45,* 737–739.

Halmaygi, G. M., Curthoys, I. S., & Cremer, P. D., (1990). The human horizontal vestibule-ocular reflex in response to high-acceleration stimulation before and after unilateral vestibular neurectomy. *Experimental Brain Research, 81,* 479–490.

Harvey, S. A., & Wood, D. J. (1996). The oculocephalic response in the evaluation of the dizzy patient. *Laryngoscope, 104,* 473–478.

Harvey, S. A., Wood, D. J., & Feroah, T. R. (1997). Relationship of the head impulse tests and head-shake nystagmus in reference to caloric testing. *American Journal of Otology, 18,* 207–213.

Herdman, S. J., Schubert, M. C., Das, V. E., & Tusa, R. J. (2003). Recovery of dynamic visual acuity in unilateral vestibular hypofunction. *Archives of Otolaryngology-Head and Neck Surgery, 129,* 819–824.

Herdman, S. J., Tusa, R. J., Blatt, P., Suzuki, A., Venuto, P. J., & Roberts, D. (1998). Computerized dynamic visual acuity test in the assessment of vestibular deficits. *American Journal of Otology, 19,* 790–796.

Hillman, T. A., Kertesz, T. R., Hadley, K., & Shelton, C. (2006). Reversible peripheral vestibulopathy: The treatment of superior canal dehiscence. *Otolaryngology-Head and Neck Surgery, 134*(3), 431–436.

Hirsch, C. (1940). A new labyrinthine reaction: The waltzing test. *Annals of Otolaryngology, 49,* 232–238.

Igarashi, M., & Ishikawa, K. (1985). Post-labyrinthectomy balance compensation with preplacement of cerebellar vermis lesion. *Acta Otolaryngolica, 99*(3–4), 452–458.

Iwasaki, S., Ito, K., Abbey, K., & Murofushi, T. (2004). Prediction of canal paresis using head shaking nystagmus test. *Acta Oto-Laryngologica, 124,* 803–806.

Jacobson, G. P., Newman, C. W., & Safadi, I. (1990) Sensitivity and specificity of the head-shaking test for detecting vestibular system abnormalities. *Annals of Oto-Rhino-Laryngology, 99,* 539–542.

Jacobson, G. P., Pearlstein, R., Henderson, J., Calder, J. H., & Rock, J. (1998). Recovery nystagmus revisited. *Journal of the American Academy of Audiology, 9,* 263–271.

Kamei, T., & Kornhuber, H. H. (1964). Spontaneous and head-shaking nystagmus in normals and in patients with central lesions. *Canadian Journal of Otolaryngology, 3,* 372–380.

Kaufman, G. D., Anderson, J. H., & Beitz, A. J. (1992). Brainstem Fos expression following acute unilateral labyrinthectomy in the rat. *NeuroReport, 3*(10), 829–832.

Kelly, D. H. (1985). Visual processing of moving stimuli. *Journal of the Optometry Society of America, 2*(2), 216–225.

Kroenke, K., Lukas, C. A., Rosenberg, M. L., Scherokman, B., Herbers, J. E. Jr., Wehrle, P. A., & Boggi, J. O. (1992). Causes of persistent dizziness. A prospective study of 100 patients in ambulatory care. *Annals of Internal Medicine, 117*(11), 898–904.

Lee, M. H., Durnford, S. J., & Crowley, J. S. (1997). Visual vestibular interaction in the dynamic visual acuity test during voluntary head rotation. *Aviation Space Environmental Medicine. 68,* 111–117.

Lehnen, N., Aw, S. T., Todd, M. J., & Halmagyi, G. M. (1994). Head impulse test reveals residual semicircular canal function after vestibular neurectomy. *Neurology, 62,* 2294–2296.

Leigh, R. J., & Zee, D. S. (1999). *The neurology of eye movements* (3rd ed.). New York, NY: Oxford University Press.

Longridge, N. S., & Mallinson, A. I. (1984). A discussion of the dynamic eligible E test: A new method of screening for aminogylcoside vestibulotoxicity. *Otolaryngology-Head and Neck Surgery, 92,* 671–676.

Longridge, N. S., & Mallinson, A. I. (1987a). The dynamic illegible E (DIE) tests. A simple technique for assessing the ability of the vestibulo-ocular reflex to overcome vestibular pathology. *Journal of Otolaryngology, 16,* 97 103.

Longridge, N. S., & Mallinson, A. I. (1987b). The dynamic illegible E-test. *Acta Otolarynigologica (Stockholm), 103,* 273–279.

Lustig, L. R., & Jackler, R. K. (1999). The history of otology through eponyms II: The clinical examination. *American Journal of Otology, 20*(4), 535–550

McClure, J. A., & Lycett, P. (1978). Recovery nystagmus. *Journal of Otolaryngology, 7*(2), 141–148.

Miller, J. W., & Ludvigh, E. J. (1962). The effect of relative motion on visual acuity. *Surveys in Ophthalmology, 7,* 83–116.

Minor, L. B. (2000). Superior canal dehiscence syndrome. *American Journal of Otology, 21*(1), 9–19.

Minor, L. B., Cremer, P. D., Carey, J. P., Della Santina, C. C., Streubel, S. O., & Weg, N. (2001). Symptoms and signs in superior canal dehiscence syndrome. *Annals of the New York Academy of Sciences, 942,* 259–273.

Minor, L. B., Haslwanter, T., Straumann, D., & Zee, D. S. (1999). Hyperventilation-induced nystagmus in patients with vestibular schwannoma. *Neurology, 53*(9), 2158–2168.

Moffat, D. A., Harries, M. L. L., Baguley, D. M., & Hardy, D. G. (1989). Unterberger's stepping test in acoustic neuroma. *Journal of Laryngology and Otology, 103,* 839–841.

Monday, L. A., & Tetreault, L. (1980). Hyperventilation and vertigo. *Laryngoscope, 90,* 1003–1010.

Moritz, W. Z. (1951). An analysis of nystagmus due to movement of the head. *Laryngology, Rhinology, and Otology, 30*(6), 269–275.

Norré, M. E., Forrez, G., & Beckers, A. (1989). Vestibulo-spinal findings in two syndromes with spontaneous vertigo attacks. *Annals of Otology Rhinology and Laryngology, 98,* 191–195.

Nyabenda, A., Briart, C., Deggouj, N., & Gersdorff, M. (2004). A normative study of the vestibulospinal and rotational tests. *Advances in Physiotherapy, 6*(3), 122–129.

O'Leary, D. P., & Davis, L. L. (1990). High frequency auto-rotational testing of the vestibulo-ocular reflex. *Neurology Clinics, 8*(2), 297–312.

Peitersen, E. (1964). Vestibulospinal reflexes VII: Alterations in the stepping test in various disorders of the inner ear and vestibular nerve. *Archives of Otolaryngology, 79,* 481–486.

Peitersen, E. (1967). Vestibulospinal reflexes X: Theoretical and clinical aspects of the stepping test. *Archives of Otolaryngology, 85,* 192–198.

Perez, N., & Rama-Lopez, J. (2003). Head impulse and caloric tests in patients with dizziness. *Otology and Neuro-Otology, 24,* 913–917.

Rambold, H., Heide, W., Sprenger, A., Haendler, G., & Helmchen, C. (2001). Perilymph fistula associate with pulse-synchronous eye oscillations. *Neurology, 56*(12), 1769–1771.

Raphan, T., Matsuo, V., & Cohen, B. (1979). Velocity storage in the vestibule-ocular reflex arc (VOR). *Experimental Brain Research, 35,* 229–248.

Robichaud, J., DesRoches, H., & Bance, M. (2002). Is hyperventilation-induced nystagmus more common in retrocochlear vestibular disease than in end-organ vestibular disease? *Journal of Otolaryngology, 31*(3), 140–143.

Sakellari, V., Bronstein, A. M., Corna, S., Hammon, C. A., Jones, S., & Wolsley, C. J. (1997). The effects of hyperventilation on postural control mechanisms. *Brain, 120*(9), 1659–1673.

Sama, A., Meikle, J. C., & Jones, N. S. (1995). Hyperventilation and dizziness: Case reports and management. *British Journal of Clinical Practice, 49*(2), 79–82.

Schubert, M. C., Tusa, R. J., Grine, L. E., & Herdman, S. J. (2004). Optimizing the sensitivity of the head thrust test for identifying vestibular hypofunction. *Physical Therapy, 84,* 151–158.

Serra, A., & Leigh, R. J. (2002). Diagnostic value of nystagmus: Spontaneous and induced ocular oscillations. *Journal of Neurology, Neurosurgery, and Psychiatry, 73,* 615–618.

Shepard, N. T. (1998). *Caloric weakness needed to achieve a positive head thrust test.* XXth Regular Meeting of the Bárány Society, Equilibrium in research and equilibriometry in modern treatment. Wurzberg, Germany: Elsevier.

Singer, E. P. (1958). The vestibulospinal test in unilateral neurolabrinthitis. *New York State Journal of Medicine, 58*(9), 1494–1500.

Takahashi, S., Fetter, M., Koenig, E., & Dichgans, J. (1990). The clinical significance of head-shaking nystagmus in the dizzy patient. *Acta Otolaryngolgica (Stockholm), 109,* 8–14.

Tseng, H. Z., & Chao, W. Y. (1997). Head-shaking nystagmus: A sensitive indicator of vestibular dysfunction. *Clinical Otolaryngology and Allied Sciences, 22*(6), 549–552.

Tilikete, C., Krolak-Salmon, P., Truy, E., & Vighetto, A. (2004). Pulse-synchronous eye oscillations revealing bone superior canal dehiscence. *Annals of Neurology, 56*(4), 556–560.

Unterberger, S. (1938). Neue objective registrierbare vestibularis-Drehrealktion erhalten durch Treten auf der Stelle. Der Tretversuch! *Archiv fur Ohren Nasen un Kehlopfheilkunde, 145,* 478–492.

Vicini, C., Casani, A., & Ghilardi, P. (1989). Assessment of head shaking in neuro-otological practice. *ORL Journal of Otorhinolaryngol and Related Specialties, 51,* 8–13.

Vogel, K. (1929) Differential diagnostische Anhaltspunkte fur die Erkennung von Schadigungen des Gleichgewichsapparates nach Schadelverletzungen. *Deutsche Med Wochenschr, 7,* 268–270.

Walker, M. F., & Zee, D. S. (1999). The effect of hyperventilation on downbeat nystagmus in cerebellar disorders. *Neurology, 53*(7), 1576–1579.

Walker, M. F., & Zee, D. S. (2000). Bedside vestibular examination. *Otolaryngology Clinics of North America, 33*(3), 495–506.

Wei, D., Hain, T. C., & Proctor, L. R. (1989). Head-shaking nystagmus: Associations with canal paresis and hearing loss. *Acta Oto-Laryngologica (Stockholm), 108,* 362–367.

Westheimer, G., & McKee, S. P. (1975). Visual acuity in the presence of retinal image motion. *Journal of Optometry Society of America, 65,* 847–850.

Wilson, W. R., & Kim, J. W. (1981). Study of ventilation testing with electronystagmography. *Annals of Otology Rhinology and Laryngology, 90*(1 Pt. 1), 56–59.

Zee, D. S., & Fletcher, W. A. (1996). Bedside examination. In R. W. Baloh & C. M. Halmagyi (Eds.), *Disorders of the vestibular system* (pp. 178–190). New York, NY: Oxford University Press.

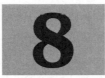

8

Assessing Dizziness-Related Quality of Life

Gary P. Jacobson, Craig W. Newman, and Erin G. Piker

INTRODUCTION

This chapter presents a description of the tools that are available to measure dizziness-related quality of life (DRQoL). The reasons to measure DRQoL in the context of the balance function assessment are discussed. How these measures are created is presented. Some of the more commonly used measures are described. Last, we illustrate how DRQoL measures have been used in clinic-based research.

Why is it important to measure a patient's DRQoL? There are at least three answers to that question. First, based on past research it has been shown repeatedly that measures of impairment (e.g., caloric test results) do not correlate significantly with measures of DRQoL unless the loss of peripheral vestibular system function is profound and bilateral (Jacobson & Calder, 2000). So, with few notable exceptions, we know that DRQoL measures represent unique information that cannot be predicted based on measures of impairment. For example, the magnitude of caloric asymmetry does not correlate with measures of DRQoL. No phase, gain, or vestibulo-ocular reflex (VOR) asymmetry measures correlate with DRQoL measures. Cervical or ocular vestibular evoked myogenic potential (i.e., cVEMP, oVEMP) latency or amplitude measures do not predict DRQoL measures (McCaslin, Jacobson, Grantham, Piker, & Verghese,

2011; Pelosi et al., 2013; Piker, Jacobson, McCaslin, & Grantham, 2008).

A second reason to administer DRQoL measures is to demonstrate to payers that the services we offer are efficacious. These can be diagnostic services that lead to accurate diagnosis and treatment. These services can be medical or surgical as well (i.e., administered in a pre- versus posttreatment paradigm).

A final reason to administer DRQoL measures is to obtain information that can lead to the correct diagnosis. An excellent example is a disease called *chronic subjective dizziness* (CSD) (Staab, 2012) (also see Chapter 30). CSD often occurs secondary due to a significant anxiety disorder that may or may not coexist with a vestibular impairment. These patients often do not complain of true vertigo but instead complain of continuous dizziness. For this group of patients the administration of a self-report measure of anxiety, and the information derived from that measure, may lead to targeted and accurate treatment (e.g., the administration of an anxiolytic medication) of the patient.

In this chapter we describe the evolution of the World Health Organization's (WHO) definitions of disability and handicap and the importance of this classification scheme in quantifying DRQoL. The psychometric characteristics of an acceptable measurement device are described. A comprehensive list of dizziness-specific questionnaires currently available to clinicians and researchers is provided, as well as a list of commonly used generic questionnaires. The scoring/interpretation and application of the most commonly used instruments to assess DRQoL are presented. Finally, representative data obtained from studies employing dizziness questionnaires in pre- and posttreatment paradigms are described. The latter application for documenting treatment efficacy is especially important in light of today's health care environment.

WORLD HEALTH ORGANIZATION (1980) ICIDH

The International Classification of Impairments, Disabilities, and Handicaps (ICIDH) is a classification system developed by the WHO in 1980 used for describing the consequences of health conditions (WHO, 1980). In this schema, the WHO defines "health" as a multidimensional concept that encompasses three domains of function, namely, "physical," "social," and "mental" states. According to the WHO, "health" is a "state of complete physical, mental and social well-being and not mere absence of disease or infirmity." In the past, the assessment of patients complaining of dizziness focused on the evaluation of dizziness *impairment*, effectively representing only one dimension of "health." The WHO (1980) defined *impairment* as "Any temporary or permanent loss or abnormality of a body structure or function, whether physiological or psychological." Using this definition, an example of dizziness impairment would be the functional absence of a vestibular end organ. The identification of the impairment could be accomplished through bithermal caloric testing (i.e., quantifying a significant unilateral weakness), or rotary chair step testing (i.e., quantifying a significantly reduced slow-phase nystagmus velocity time constant).

Under the 1980 WHO model, *disability* is defined as "A restriction or inability to perform an activity in a manner or within the range that is considered normal." Using this definition, an example of dizziness disability would be a fear of falling that may result in a patient's inability to engage in a vocation that depends on intact vestibular system function (e.g., a house painter). In contrast, the WHO defines *handicap* as "A social, economic or environmental disadvantage resulting from an impairment or disability." Using the WHO definition, an example of a dizziness handicap would be the self-imposed social isolation that occurs when a patient fears having an incapacitating spell of vertigo in public.

We suggest that a *balance system impairment* describes an abnormality in any of the three interdependent sensory systems required for individuals to maintain postural stability including vision, proprioception, and the vestibular system. A *balance system disability/handicap* occurs when a balance impairment is severe enough to affect an individual's physical and/or psychosocial function.

In addition to the physical manifestations, it is known that vertigo imparts significant psychological comorbidities that impact dizziness disability/handicap. The reasons for this are manifold. First, vertigo is difficult to see. Vertigo does not leave a mark on the skin; it is not something that can be measured with a thermometer. Thus, during vertiginous episodes patients appear only to be extremely ill and disoriented. Second, and with few exceptions, vertigo attacks occur without warning and the symptoms are profound. It is this unpredictability that produces the anxiety, depression, and panic observed in this patient sample (Monzani, Casolari, Guidetti, & Rigatelli, 2001). Third, there are known links between balance control and anxiety that are largely based on shared neural circuits that mediate autonomic function (e.g., pallor, sweating, nausea) (Yates & Miller, 1998). Finally, there appears to be overlapping psychopharmacology including sensitivity to different classes of antidepressants (Blakley, 1999; Ramos, 2006; Simon et al., 2005; Staab , Ruckenstein, & Amsterdam, 2004). This close association suggests the possibility of a common neurologic mechanism linking balance and anxiety, and these connections may be the basis for the association between dizziness and the somatic effects of psychological disorders.

For these reasons, it is accepted that the assessment of the dizzy patient should be multifactorial and should include metrics designed to inform the examiner not only whether vestibular system function is normal, but also to what extent any existing impairment is affecting the patient's psychosocial function. It is important to assess multiple dimensions of function because disability and handicap resulting from a given vestibular system impairment will vary unpredictably from individual to individual in the same way that a given hearing impairment may impart differing levels of handicap from individual to individual.

WORLD HEALTH ORGANIZATION (2001) ICF

In acknowledgment of the complexities associated with the definition of disability and handicap, in 2001 the 191 member states of the WHO approved a revision to the WHO 1980 system that is called the International Classification of Functioning Disability and Health (ICF) (WHO, 2002). The 2001 classification system differs radically from the 1980 ICIDH system. Instead of customizing the terms *impairment*, *disability*, and *handicap* for the effects of diseases and disorders, the new system includes a taxonomy that permits the description of the *magnitude* of disability and handicap for diseases and disorders that are identified in the ICD-10 coding system.

Definition of Terms

Areas of assessment in the ICF are classified as *domains*. The presence and severity of a problem in functioning (body, person, or societal levels) are "qualifiers." For example, a qualifier for the *body function* and *structure* domains indicates the presence of an impairment of function or structure that can be graded on a five-point scale (e.g., no impairment, mild, moderate, severe, complete impairment). For the *activity limitation* and *participation restriction* domains (i.e., formerly referred to as *disability* and *handicap*, respectively) there are two important qualifiers: *performance* (i.e., how the individual performs in their current environment using assistive devices or personal assistance) and *capacity* (i.e., the individual's ability to execute a task or action in a "standardized" environment) that assumes a "naked person" assessment. That is, capacity without personal assistance or use of assistive devices. Having access to performance and capacity data enables the ICF user to determine the gap between capacity and performance.

The new ICF classification system acknowledges contextual factors that include both exogenous, *environmental factors* (e.g., social norms, political factors,

institutions), and endogenous *personal factors* (e.g., coping skills, education, past experience). Collectively, these factors can influence the magnitude of both activity limitations and participation restrictions. In this way the ICF represents an attempt to describe how activity limitation and functioning represent complex interactions between health conditions and contextual factors. It is not surprising, therefore, that the ICF has been described as a *biopsychosocial model*. In the ICF neither the terms *disability* nor *handicap* are used. Instead, these data are captured as activity limitations and participation restrictions that occur as a result of changes in body function and structure that result from a disease or disorder.

In the ICF model, disability involves dysfunction at one or more levels of impairment, activity limitation, and/or participation restriction. Formal definitions of these components of ICF are shown in Table 8–1. For each construct of body function and body structure (i.e., numerically coded) the rater/clinician assigns a number representing the magnitude of the impairment (e.g., for body structure the 0–9 scale includes such choices as 0 = no change in structure, 1 = total absence, 2 = partial absence, etc.). The coding extends further (i.e., given the magnitude of impairment in the specific body function

Table 8-1. Definitions from the ICF

Body functions: physiologic functions of body systems
Body structures: anatomic parts of the body such as organs, limbs, and their components
Impairments: problems in body function or structures such as significant deviation or loss
Activity: execution of a task or action by an individual
Participation: involvement in a life situation
Activity limitations: difficulties an individual may have in executing activities (i.e., formerly referred to as disability)
Participation restrictions: problems an individual may experience in involvement in life situations (i.e., formerly referred to as handicap)
Environmental factors: make up the physical, social, and attitudinal environment in which people live and conduct their lives.

Source: World Health Organization (2002), p. 10.

and structure) to include an assessment of how both performance and capacity aspects of activity limitation and participation restriction are affected. Further coding includes the assignment of a number to represent how environmental factors affect activity and participation. For purposes of dizziness and unsteadiness, under the classification of "body function" the vestibular system falls under the heading "Sensory functions and pain." Under the classification "body structure" the vestibular system falls under the heading "The eye, ear, and related structures." "Sensations associated with hearing and vestibular function" is one of the body functions in the classification schema. The area falls under the general heading "hearing and vestibular functions." The area is further subclassified into sensations of "dizziness," "falling," and "nausea associated with vertigo." There is another subheading under "hearing and vestibular functions" called "vestibular functions." Under that subheading are the subclassifications "vestibular function of position," "vestibular function of balance," and, "vestibular function of determination of movement." That is, any one or more of these functions could be affected by a disease or disorder. Using this classification scheme, practitioners can evaluate the impact that a disease or disorder has on function and structure.

Not only does the ICF (WHO, 2002) allow the practitioner to code the magnitude of activity limitation and participation restriction caused by a vestibular impairment (i.e., a change in vestibular system function and structure occurring as a result of disease) but also how contextual factors, both personal and environmental, augment the activity limitation and participation restrictions. The formal quantitative assessment of dizziness-induced activity limitation and participation restriction provides us with a method for determining the extent that the contextual factors influence these spheres. The measures provide semiobjective evidence of change in physical, social, mental, and functional health that can be used to evaluate the human benefits and the financial value of selected programs and interventions. In this way, these devices serve as standardized outcome measures. Over and above this, the quantification of dizziness activity limitation and participation restriction provides third-party payers with evidence that the rehabilitative services we provide are both beneficial and cost effective.

TOOLS FOR MEASURING DRQOL

Factors to Consider When Selecting a Tool for Clinical or Research Application

When choosing a questionnaire to assess DRQoL, careful consideration should be given to the content of the tool (e.g., domains of assessment) as well as to its ultimate application (e.g., to assess treatment-related change). An appropriate measure to include in an evaluation should be supported by evidence demonstrating that it is acceptable to the patient, reliable, valid, and responsive (i.e., sensitive to change). The adequacy of each of these latter criteria should be based on evidence discerned from the psychometric characteristics of the selected measurement tool. Furthermore, a number of practical issues need to be considered prior to using a specific measure in clinical practice or when incorporating a dizziness questionnaire as part of a research methodology. These include such factors as ease of administration (i.e., burden on the patient, clinician, or researcher), scoring, and interpretation.

The purpose of this section is to assist the reader in becoming a more informed consumer of the literature when evaluating and selecting a "candidate" dizziness assessment tool. Such insight will help clinicians and researchers evaluate the quality of available instruments in order to choose a tool that is most appropriate for the intended application. A few key areas of questionnaire attributes and psychometric standards are reviewed below. Further, a brief overview of the importance of econometric evaluation will be presented. For a more in-depth discussion, the interested reader is referred to Fitzpatrick, Davey, Buxton, and Jones (1998), Hyde (2000), Shum, O'Gorman, and Myors (2006), and Siegel, Weinstein, Russell, and Gold (1996).

Appropriateness

Are the items comprising the inventory appropriate to the concerns of the patient and clinician, or, to the researcher addressing specific questions in a study or clinical trial?

A fundamental factor when selecting a quality of life measure is to identify an instrument which contains items that clearly matter to patients and are relevant to the intended clinical or research application, as well (Gill & Feinstein, 1994; Guyatt & Cook, 1994). This is accomplished by evaluating the theoretic constructs (domains) underlying the development of the tool. For example, is DRQoL represented by the items comprising the questionnaire? Is the tool assessing activity limitation or participation restriction described by the WHO model? Or is it assessing other constructs such as global health, maladaptive thinking and behaviors, or self-efficacy (i.e., confidence in one's ability to complete a task such as walk, reaching, bending)? Accordingly, when selecting a measurement tool, it needs to be focused on the patient's concern so that the obtained data provide insight about the patient and is ultimately of value to the respondent (Noble, 2013).

Reliability

Does the tool produce results that are reproducible and internally consistent?

Reliability is an important psychometric property of a questionnaire because it is critical to establish that treatment-related changes in scores are due to intervention per se and not related to measurement error. There are two major types of reliability that are of interest to clinicians—*internal consistency reliability* and *reproducibility*.

Internal consistency reliability reflects the interitem consistency of responses or relationships among scale or subscale items. For example, if a dizziness questionnaire contains items addressing the emotional consequences of dizziness (e.g., Does your dizziness make you frustrated? Does your dizziness make you angry? Does your dizziness make you depressed?), it is reasonable to assume that scores on each item would be correlated with scores on all other items within an "emotional subscale" of a larger questionnaire. Accordingly, individual items within a single domain should be highly correlated with each other and with the summed score of items within the same scale or subscale (i.e., item-total correlation). In this connection, there must be a balance between items within a measure that are too homogeneous or too diverse (Hyde, 2000). That is, if the items within a questionnaire tap into constructs that are too diverse, they may not warrant a total score. In contrast, it is undesirable to develop a scale that is composed of several items with only minor wording changes. Cronbach's alpha is the statistical method

for computing internal consistency reliability (values range from 0 to 1). A low alpha (e.g., below 0.5) suggests that the items do not come from the same conceptual domain (Bowling, 1997).

The two major components of reproducibility are *test-retest reliability* and *stability*. The degree of reliability is based on assessments between baseline measurement and subsequent administrations of the questionnaire. The time interval between administrations needs to be of sufficient length so that respondents do not recall their answers, yet not so long that the underlying health condition has changed. In general, test-retest refers to short-term, day-to-day fluctuations in test scores. In contrast, test stability measures changes that may occur in test scores when longer periods of time have elapsed (Demorest & DeHaven, 1993). When test stability is evaluated, it is incumbent upon the clinician to determine whether the patient has experienced changes in the underlying health condition that would reduce the apparent reproducibility of the questionnaire. An approach is to ask a transition question at the follow-up assessment (e.g., Is your dizziness better, the same, or worse than when you answered this questionnaire last time?). Pearson product moment correlation coefficients are often used to assess reliability (i.e., commonly cited minimal standards for reliability coefficients are 0.7 for group data).

Application of Bland Altman graphical plots (Bland & Altman, 1986) have been advocated to address the extent of agreement (i.e., in contrast to the strength of association estimated by correlations) between two administrations of an instrument. Using this graphic technique, difference values between test and retest are plotted as a function of the mean test and retest scores for each subject. The underlying assumption is that the difference score should be zero because the same measurement tool was used for both administrations without any intervening intervention. Accordingly, the mean of the test and retest scores provide the best estimate of the patient's true score.

Validity

Does the tool measure what it claims to measure?

The validity of a questionnaire is its ability to yield relevant, appropriate, meaningful, and useful information. This is reflected by the extent to which the measurement tool assesses what it was intended to measure for a specific purpose or set of purposes. A variety of strategies exist to evaluate the psychometric properties of validity including content validity (Does the questionnaire includes items necessary to represent the concept being measured?), construct validity (Does the questionnaire measure the underlying concept of interest to the clinician or researcher?), face validity (Do the items sufficiently represent different hypothesized domains? Do the items "look reasonable"?), criterion validity (Does the questionnaire correlate with a "gold standard" or an already well-established measure of the same characteristic/criterion?) (Fitzpatrick et al., 1998). In essence, the validity of a measurement tool is its ability to yield "truthful," "correct," and "real" information about the patient or subject. For a complete discussion of the various facets of validity the interested reader is referred to Bannigan and Watson (2009) and Hyde (2000).

Responsiveness

Is the tool sensitive enough to detect changes over time that matter to the patient?

A goal of evidence-based practice is to assess the effectiveness of medical, surgical, or rehabilitative treatment. Accordingly, the psychometric characteristic of responsiveness is of utmost importance when selecting a dizziness instrument that will be used to detect treatment-related changes in behavior and performance that are important to patients. An assessment tool's ability to detect clinically significant changes related to treatment effects (i.e., outcome studies) is especially critical in clinical trials (Norman, Stratford, & Regehr, 1997). Guyatt, Feeny, and Patrick (1993) distinguished between two different types of responsive questionnaires: *discriminative tools* are used to evaluate quality of life differences between patients at a point in time in order to establish their clinical status and intervention needs; *evaluative tools* are used to evaluate quality of life differences within a patient during a period of time in order to assess treatment-related changes. Accordingly, questionnaires selected to detect changes in DRQoL must have high sensitivity to change, or responsiveness. It is noteworthy that it is possible to have reliable questionnaires that are not responsive and responsive questionnaires that are not reliable.

For example, a repeated administration of a DRQoL tool may give the same results with each administration (e.g., test-retest reliability), yet it is unresponsive if it does not detect improvement in function that has been known to occur.

A variety a statistical techniques have been developed to assess responsiveness including effect size (Kazis, Anderson, & Meenan, 1989), standardized response mean (Liang, Fossel, & Larson, 1990), relative efficiency (Liang, Larson, Cullen, & Schwartz, 1985), sensitivity and specificity (Deyo & Inui, 1984), and receiver operating characteristics (Deyo & Centor, 1986). Of these latter approaches, the most common standardized expression of responsiveness is effect size.

Effect Size. This statistical technique yields a value reflecting observed treatment effects in terms of standard deviation units of the questionnaire (Lipsey, 1990; Stewart & Archbold, 1992). Below are effect size calculations for (a) treatment studies involving pre- and posttreatment measures; and for (b) studies in which a treatment group is compared to a control group. It is noteworthy that effect size calculations are useful only for evaluating group data and are not appropriate for estimation of differences for individual patient data.

a.
$$Effect\ size = \frac{Mean\ difference\ size\ for\ group}{Standard\ deviation\ of\ difference\ scores}$$

b.
$$Effect\ size = \frac{Intervention\ group\ mean - Control\ group\ mean}{Average\ standard\ deviation}$$

Guidelines have been developed (Cohen, 1988) for interpreting effect size values (Cohen's *d*) for outcome studies, with larger *d* scores representing outcome measures reflecting greater responsiveness or larger treatment effects: $d < 0.20$ are inconsequential or nonsignificant; $d = 0.20$ to 0.50, small; $d = 0.5$ to 0.8, moderate; and $d > 0.80$, large. Unfortunately, developers of dizziness-related outcome measures have not routinely included calculations of effect size in their norming and standardization studies. This is a call for future reevaluation of currently available questionnaires or the development of new tools designed specifically to evaluate responsiveness to treatment-related changes by applying effect size statistical techniques.

Precision

How precise are the scores, or numerical properties, of the tool?

Response format influences the precision of an instrument. At one end of the continuum is a simple "yes"/"no" format, having the advantage of simplicity. Yet, this type of response format does not allow the respondent to report degrees of difficulty or severity as it relates to the construct being evaluated. The Dizziness Handicap Inventory (DHI) employs a three-item response format of "yes," "sometimes," or "no" (Jacobson & Newman, 1990). In contrast, the Vestibular Disorders of Daily Living Scale (Cohen, Kimball, & Adams, 2000) uses a 10-item Likert rating scale in response to the effects of vertigo and balance disorders on independence in routine activities of daily living (1 = independent; 10 = too difficult, no longer perform). Intrinsic variables associated with the respondent such as cognitive function, motivation, recall effects (memory), honesty, willingness to disclose sensitive information, and response bias (responding "positively" or "negatively" to items) may all play a role in response precision.

Acceptability

Is the tool acceptable to the patient?

It is critical that the questionnaire used in clinical practice is acceptable to the patient and does not present undue burden on the individual to complete. In this connection, it is important to avoid or minimize distress to patients already coping with the consequences of balance disorders and potentially other health issues. There are at least four steps involved in answering questionnaires, each making a cognitive demand on the patient. These include:

- comprehension of the question;
- recall of the requested information from memory;
- evaluation of the connection between the retrieved information and the item posed on the questionnaire; and
- communication of the response (Bowling, 2005).

Furthermore, the mode of questionnaire administration (e.g., face-to-face, paper/pencil, e-mail, telephone, computer assisted) may affect the cognitive burden placed on the respondent. Similarly, the literacy level of the respondent needs to be appreciated especially when a self-report written format is used to obtain responses. Clinicians should not assume that patient's reading skills are at a level to handle a questionnaire in written form versus a face-to-face interview format (Noble, 2013). Variables such as visual layout of the items and response format, appearance, and length of the questionnaire could potentially impact response compliance.

Cultural and language bias are additional factors related to acceptability. For example, cultural and linguistic variations within the same language may present barriers and misunderstandings of item content. That is, questionnaires developed in one culture do not necessarily evaluate the same factor, even within national boundaries (Langguth, Searchfield, Biesinger, & Greimel, 2011). Translation of a questionnaire into another language can introduce changes in meaning and must be accomplished using specific procedures including use of several independent translations that are compared, backward translations, and testing acceptability of the translation by respondents (Hambleton & Patsula, 1998; Leplege & Verdieer, 1995). Clinicians and researchers must be aware of potential cultural and language differences when selecting a particular tool for a given patient population.

Feasibility

Is the tool easy to administer, score, and interpret?

In addition to considerations of how burdensome the tool is to the patient, it is also important to consider the impact on the clinician and researcher in collecting and processing the information (Aaronson, 1992; Erickson, Taeuber, & Scott, 1995). During the collection phase, staff effort and costs are associated with questionnaire administration. The time and resources required to collect, process, and analyze data from a questionnaire are typically not reported so evidence regarding feasibility is often unavailable (Fitzpatrick et al., 1998); however, in a busy clinical practice, dizziness questionnaires that are brief, easy to administer, and simple to score and interpret are considered most feasible.

Usefulness

The usefulness of the selected tool should be evaluated in relation to its standardization and norming. For example, normative referenced scores compare an individual's score to a distribution of scores obtained by an appropriate reference group. Accordingly, normative data in the form of estimated population means of the distribution, standard deviations, standard error of measurement (S_e), and percentiles provide the clinician with information about what is considered typical or atypical for the target population or for a given individual (Demorest & DeHaven, 1993). For example, Kinney, Sandridge, and Newman (1997) reported four severity categories (described later in this chapter) for the DHI based on quartile ranges for a sample of patients being treated for Ménière's disease.

From an outcomes perspective, determining significant treatment-related change in perceived DRQoL for a given individual patient is clinically useful in order to quantify the impact of a specific intervention. Assessing the difference between two scores on two occasions can be derived from the application of 95% confidence intervals (CI) based on S_e. The S_e is interpreted as the standard deviation of independently obtained scores around an individual's true score (Demorest & Walden, 1984). Using this approach, Jacobson and Newman (1990) determined that the S_e for the DHI was 6.23. Based on 95% CI estimates, pretreatment and posttreatment DHI scores would have to differ by more than 18 points for clinical efforts to be considered statistically and clinically effective.

Scoring Methods

Scaling Item Responses

The term *scaling* refers to how numbers are assigned to each of the items comprising the assessment tool. The *response set* is the choice of items that the respondent has for answering a given question. The use of rating scales permits the patient a method for quantifying the magnitude estimation of the attribute being measured, using such tools as numeric rating scales (i.e., Likert scale) or the visual analog scale (VAS).

Numeric Rating Scales (NRSs). NRSs are useful in providing numerical estimates of dizziness severity or dimensions of DRQoL. The majority of tools use somewhat arbitrary but commonsense methods. For example, the Vertigo Handicap Questionnaire uses a 5-point scale (0 = never; 1 = occasionally; 2 = sometimes; 3 = often; 4 = always) to quantify dimensions of activity limitation (e.g., "I can move around quickly and freely") and participation restriction (e.g., "My vertigo means that my family life is restricted").

Visual Analog Scale (VAS). The VAS is an alternative scaling technique that uses a line of fixed length (typically 100 mm), with anchors at each end of the line appropriate for the attribute being measured. Using this technique, the patient is required to place an "X" or vertical line on the horizontal line corresponding to their perceived judgment. In this way, the clinician or researcher is able to quantify accurately the respondent's judgment by simply measuring the distance (in millimeters) along the horizontal line between the two anchors. For example, Figure 8–1 illustrates the use of VAS to evaluate the domains of activity limitation (e.g., feeling anxious) and participation restriction (e.g., interference with everyday activities).

In addition to being used as a static (i.e., one-time) measure, the VAS could be employed as a useful tool for measuring change (Scott & Huskisson, 1979). For example, the VAS could be used to evaluate the degree of treatment-related change following 3 months of physical therapy. When used to measure change, the patient could be given the baseline VAS and then asked to indicate his or her present state by marking a second "X" on the same VAS. The difference between the two marks would provide the estimate of change (e.g., improvement or worsening of perceived DRQoL). The clinician needs to be aware of caveats when using a VAS. That is, there are no guarantees that the response reflects accurately and precisely the underlying perceptual attribute being measured (Streiner & Norman, 1995) and that factors such as memory, physical, or visual problems may affect responses (Gagliese, 2001), thereby limiting their applicability.

Patient Global Impression of Change (PGIC) Scale. Especially useful as an outcome measure, a PGIC scale may help to quantify in a single summary

OVER THE PAST WEEK, ON AVERAGE:

How **anxious** has your dizziness made you feel? Mark an **X** on the line.

Not Anxious ——————————— *Extremely Anxious*
At All

How much did your dizziness **interfere** with your ability to enjoy everyday social and leisure activities? Mark an **X** on the line.

Did Not Interfere ——————————— *Completely Interfered*
At All

Figure 8–1. Examples of visual analog scales.

global score a patient's impression of change following treatment. In this connection, a single question is directed to the patient asking him or her to indicate the amount of change following intervention. For example, a patient may be asked, "Since you have completed vestibular rehabilitation, how would you describe the changes with your balance problems?" and may be given the following 7-item PGIC scale (Hurst & Bolton, 2004):

- No change (or worse)
- Almost the same, hardly any change at all
- A little better, but no noticeable change
- Somewhat better, but the change has not made any real difference
- Moderately better, and a slight but noticeable change
- Better, and definite improvement that has made a real and worthwhile difference

- A great deal better, and a considerable improvement that has made all the difference

The most obvious advantage of this type of self-report scaling is its brevity, requiring little time to complete. On the other hand, PGIC scales may be difficult for some patients because they require a "mental subtraction" by asking the patients to quantify both their present state (e.g., posttreatment) and initial state (e.g., pretreatment) (Norman et al., 1997).

Econometric Evaluation

Econometric techniques are becoming increasingly popular given today's health care environment. In this connection, an econometric technique such as cost-utility analysis (CUA) captures the cost per quality of life units gained expressed as quality-adjusted life years (QALYs). Therefore, QALY is a measure of both the quality and quantity of life lived in relation to a particular disease/condition burden (Detsky & Laupacis, 2007). QALYs are calculated using cost of treatment, obtained benefit (based on pre/post quality of life measures), and life expectancy (based on actuarial tables) (Chisolm & Abrams, 2008). Recently, Yardley and colleagues (2012) applied a QALY analysis to compare the cost effectiveness of routine medical care, booklet-based vestibular rehabilitation (i.e., provision of booklets providing advice on undertaking home exercises and cognitive behavioral techniques) only, or booklet-based vestibular rehabilitation with telephone support. The cost per QALY was calculated using EuroQol (EQ-5D) scores obtained at 0, 12 weeks, and one year following treatment; dizziness-related costs; and clinician costs. Results indicated that booklet self-management with telephone support was the most cost-effective approach while the "routine care group" was least cost effective. Application of QALY and other forms of health econometric techniques (e.g., incremental cost-effectiveness analyses) will continue to expand as clinicians will need to justify the value of recommending different forms of intervention to patients, providers, third-party payers, and policy makers.

General and Disease-Specific Measurement Tools

Self-report measures can be classified as "general" or "disease/disorder specific." General scales assess constructs that are relevant to a broad range of health conditions (e.g., anxiety, personality traits). The advantage of using a general measurement tool is that the results can be compared across patient groups of various disorders (i.e., results are generalizable). For example, one could measure levels of anxiety in patients with dizziness and compare that to levels of anxiety in patients with rheumatoid arthritis. However, there are several disadvantages to using general scales. First, the instrument has to cover a wide range of disorders; thus it may be lengthy, time consuming, and include questions irrelevant to the patient. Second, general questionnaires may be unresponsive to small changes in your specific patient. Last, results from general questionnaires may be confounded by other health problems.

Table 8–2 lists the general/generic questionnaires that have either been shown to have good reliability and/or validity in populations of dizzy patients or have been used to assess convergent validity in the development of dizziness-specific questionnaires. These scales assess constructs including quality of life, general health/disability, anxiety, depression, and coping.

In contrast to general scales, disease-specific measurement tools are designed to assess constructs particular to a condition or illness of interest. The advantages of using a disease-specific scale include the following: (1) all items are, by definition, relevant to the patient; (2) the measures tend to be brief to administer; (3) the content validity is often high as items are specific to the needs and concerns of patient; and (4) disease-specific scales are considered more appropriate for measuring treatment outcome. The greatest disadvantage to using a disease-specific tool is the loss of generalizability since scores cannot be compared across disease conditions. The DHI is one of the first, the most heavily studied, and most often utilized dizziness self-report scale in the clinical setting. Since the DHI's creation in 1990, 17 additional questionnaires have been developed specifically for patients with dizziness, vertigo, and/or unsteadiness.

Tables 8–3 through 8–6 show each of the dizziness-specific questionnaires available to clinicians and researchers. The factors to consider when choosing a self-report instrument for clinical or research purposes are discussed above. One additional factor is simply considering what you want to measure. We have categorized the 18 dizziness-specific questionnaires based on the construct(s) each aims to quantify. Categories include those tools aimed to measure dizziness symptoms, dizziness handicap and quality of life, a mix of symptoms and handicap, or tools designed to measure the effects of specific diseases within a dizzy population (such as Ménière's disease).

It is beyond the scope of this chapter to present an in-depth discussion regarding the psychometric characteristics of each dizziness-specific questionnaire available to the clinician or researcher. The historical framework for measuring self-report dizziness and several of the most heavily researched and used questionnaires are discussed in greater detail in the following sections of this chapter.

Table 8–2. General/Generic Scales Often Used in Dizzy Populations for Both Clinical Research, Clinical Assessment, and Outcomes

Name	Purpose
Basic Symptom Inventory-53 (BSI-53) (Derogatis & Melisaratos, 1983; Ruckenstein & Staab, 2001)	To reflect the psychological systems of psychiatric, medical, and normal individuals
Beck Anxiety Index (BAI) (Beck, Epstein, Brown, & Steer, 1988)	To measure the severity of anxiety in psychiatric populations
Beck Depression Inventory (BDI) (Beck, Ward, Mendelson, Mock, & Erbaugh, 1961)	Measures characteristic attitudes and symptoms of depression
European Quality of Life Scale (EQ-5D) (1990)	To describe and measure health states and health outcome
General Health Questionnaire (GHQ-12) (Goldberg & Hillier, 1979)	Focuses on the inability to carry out normal functions and the appearance of new and distressing experiences
Hospital Anxiety and Depression Scale (HADS) (Zigmond & Snaith, 1983)	To determine levels of anxiety and depression in an outpatient setting
Medical Outcomes Study Short form (SF-36) (Stewart, Hays, & Ware, 1988)	Yields an eight-scale profile of functional health and well-being
Patient Intentions Questionnaire (PIQ) (Salmon & Quine, 1989)	To measure patients' expectations and what they want from the clinician during a given visit
PRIME-MD Patient Health Questionnaire (PHQ) (Spitzer, Kroenke, & Williams, 1999)	Diagnostic tool for mental health disorders used by health care professionals
Sense of Coherence Scale (SOC) (Antonovsky, 1993)	To assess how people view life and to identify general coping resources used to maintain health in stressful situations
Sickness Impact Profile (SIP) (Gilson et al., 1975)	To measure quality of life and level of dysfunction that result from disability or illness
State-Trait Anxiety Inventory (STAI) (Spielberger, 1984)	To measure trait and state anxiety and to distinguish anxiety from depressive syndromes
Ways of Coping (Folkman & Lazarus, 1980)	To measure the thoughts and actions people use to handle stressful situations
World Health Organization Disability Assessment Schedule II (WHO-DAS II) (Ustun et al., 2010)	To assess health and disability across all diseases, including mental, neurological, and addictive disorders
World Health Organization Quality of life—Brief (WHOQoL-Bref) (1995)	To assess individual perceptions of quality of life in the context of their culture and value system, personal goals, standards, and concerns

Table 8–3. Tools Designed to Measure Dizziness Symptoms

Name (Reference)	Validation	Items, Subscales	Scoring	Purpose, Examples
European Evaluation of Vertigo (EEV) (Megnigbeto, Sauvage, & Launois, 2001)	Validated in adults with episode of vertigo occurring during the previous week (*n* = 123)	Five items (illusion of movement, duration of the illusion, motion intolerance, neurovegetative signs, instability)	0 to 4-point scale	To assess vertigo symptoms and associated vestibular symptoms independent of handicap e.g., rate your "motion intolerance"
Modified Falls Efficacy Scale (MFES) (Hill, Schwarz, Kalogeropoulos, & Gibson, 1996)	Validated in healthy community dwelling elderly adults (*n* = 111) and in older adults referred to a Falls and Balance Clinic (*n* = 68)	14 activities	Rated on a 10-point visual analogue scale from "not at all confident" to "completely confident"	To measure self-perceived fear of falling during the performance of 14 common activities e.g., "How confident are you that you can use public transport without falling?"
Motion Sensitivity Quotient (MSQ) (Smith-Wheelock, Shepard, & Telian, 1991)	Validated in 15 dizzy patients	16 questions regarding dizziness with movement	Yields two scores: intensity (1- to 5-point scale) and duration (1- to 3-point scale) Total score is the sum of the intensity and duration scores	To quantify the severity of symptoms evoked by movements e.g., supine to sitting (rate intensity and duration of dizziness or vertigo)
Visual Vertigo Analog Scale (VVAS) (Dannenbaum, Chilingaryan, & Fung, 2011)	Validated in adults with vestibular diseases (*n* = 102)	Nine items that typically induce visual vertigo	Patients rate the intensity of their dizziness on each item by drawing a vertical line on a 10-cm anchored line	To provide a quantitative evaluation of visual vertigo e.g., "Rate the dizziness you experience when under fluorescent lights"
Vertigo Symptom Scale (VSS) (Yardley, Masson, Verschuur, Haacke, & Luxon, 1992)	Validated in adults with dizziness and/or vertigo (*n* = 127)	36 Items total Two subscales: (1) vertigo severity, and (2) autonomic and anxiety symptoms	Six-point scale: 0 (never) to 5 (very often)	To assess and differentiate symptoms of vertigo from autonomic/anxiety symptoms e.g., "How often in the past month have you had the following symptoms: nausea, vomiting?"

Table 8-4. Tools Designed to Measure Dizziness Handicap and Quality of Life

Name (Reference)	Validation	Items, Subscales	Scoring	Purpose, Examples
Activities-Specific Balance Confidence Scale (ABC) (Powell & Myers, 1995)	Validated in community-dwelling adults 65 years and older (n = 60)	16 Items	Scores range from 0 (no confidence) to 100 (complete confidence)	To assess loss of balance confidence in senior citizens and to discriminate between "fallers" and "nonfallers" e.g., "How confident are you that you will *not* lose your balance or become unsteady when you walk up or down stairs?"
Dizziness Handicap Inventory (DHI) (Jacobson & Newman, 1990)	Validated in adults referred for vestibular testing (n = 106)	25 items, three subscales (emotional, functional, physical)	Items rated and scored as "yes" (4 points), "sometimes" (2 points), and "no" (0 points)	To evaluate the self-perceived handicapping effects imposed by vestibular system disease e.g., "Does looking up increase your problem?"
Vestibular Disorders Activities of Daily Living (VADL) (Cohen & Kimball, 2000)	Validated in adults seen for vestibular rehabilitation (n = 94)	28 items, three subscales (functional, ambulation, instrumental)	10-point scale: 1 (independent) to 10 (too difficult, no longer perform)	To assess self-perceived disablement in patients with vestibular impairments by assessing independence in routine activities of daily living e.g., "Indicate the level that most accurately describes how you perform the task: Carrying things while walking"
Vertigo Handicap Questionnaire (VHQ) (Yardley & Putman, 1992)	Validated in adults with chronic dizziness and/or vertigo complaints from 6 months to 5 years (n = 84)	25 items, four subscales (restriction of activity, social anxiety, fears about vertigo, severity of vertigo attacks)	5-point scale: 0 (no handicap) to 4 (maximum handicap)	To assess patient-perceived common beliefs, behavior, and difficulties (i.e., handicap) associated with vertigo

Table 8–5. Tools Designed to Measure a Blend of Symptoms, Disability, Handicap, and/or Quality of Life

Name (Reference)	Validation	Items, Subscales	Scoring	Purpose, Examples
Dizziness Belief Scale (DBS) (Yardley, Beech, & Weinman, 2001)	Validated in adults with complaints of dizziness and disequilibrium (*n* = 159)	Eleven beliefs about negative consequences of dizziness	Five-point scale: strongly agree to strongly disagree	To evaluate the negative anticipated consequences of dizziness e.g., "When I am dizzy I will let people down"
Dizzy Factor Inventory (DFI) (Hazlett, Tusa, & Waranch, 1996)	Validated in adults referred to neurologist for complaints of dizziness (*n* = 184)	44 items, three subscales (symptom factors, responses of significant others to dizzy patient, activity level)	Five-point scale: word anchors change according to content of item	To be used as preliminary screening device and to aid in the selection of further diagnostic testing or treatment strategies
Dizziness Needs Assessment (DiNA) (Kruschinski, Klaassen, Breull, Broll, & Hummers-Pradier, 2010)	Validated in German-speaking adults 65 years and older seen by general practitioners and reporting dizziness (*n* = 123)	18 items, four subscales (handicap and mobility, empathy and help, causes, doctor realizes suffering)	Seven-point Likert scale	To assess priorities of elderly patients with dizziness
UCLA Dizziness Questionnaire (UCLA-DQ) (Honrubia, Bell, Harris, Baloh, & Fisher, 1996)	Validated in adults seen in neurotology clinic with complaints of dizziness (*n* = 362)	Five items: frequency, severity, limitation of daily activities, general quality of life, fear of dizziness	Five-point ranking scale with anchors specific to item	To obtain an overview of patient's subjective analysis of their condition and provide the clinician with information not usually available at the time of the visit e.g., "When I am dizzy, my symptoms are most often: (1) very mild, (2) mild, (3) moderate, (4) moderate to severe, (5) severe"
Vestibular Activities and Participation (VAP) (Alghwiri et al., 2012)	Validated in adults (*n* = 58) with balance or vestibular disorders	34 items	Five-point Likert scale indicating level of difficulty with an item from "none" to "unable to do"	To examine activities and participation according to the *International Classification of Functioning Disability and Health* e.g., "Because of your dizziness/imbalance, how much difficulty did you have recently in carrying out your daily routine?"

Table 8-5. *continued*

Name (Reference)	Validation	Items, Subscales	Scoring	Purpose, Examples
Vestibular Disability Index (VDI) (Prieto, Santed, Cobo, & Alonso, 1999)	Validated in Spanish-speaking adults (*n* = 130) referred to ENT and neurology clinics for vertigo, dizziness, and/or imbalance	36 items, two subscales (Symptom Subscale, Health-Related Quality of Life Subscale)	Six-point Likert scale: 1 (all the time) to 6 (none of the time)	To assess symptoms and quality of life in dizzy patients
Vestibular Rehabilitation Benefit Questionnaire (VRBQ) (Morris, Lutman, & Yardley, 2009)	Validated in adults (*n* = 124) referred for vestibular rehabilitation therapy	22 items, three subscales (Dizziness and Anxiety, Motion-Provoked Dizziness, Quality of Life)	Seven-point bipolar scale: −6 (not at all dizzy) to 6 (extremely dizzy)	To assess outcome of vestibular rehabilitation therapy, especially for longitudinal application e.g., "Moving my head *slowly* from side to side makes me feel . . . "

Table 8-6. Tools Designed to Measure the Effects of Specific Diseases on Quality of Life

Name (Reference)	Validation	Items, Subscales	Scoring	Purpose, Examples
Ménière's Disease Patient-Oriented Severity Index (MD-POSI) (Gates, 2000)	Validated in adults with Ménière's disease enrolled in a Meniett device clinical trial (*n* = 61)	20 items	Six-point scale: 0 (none) to 5 (worse ever)	To quantify the morbidity (balance, hearing, memory) of Ménière's disease and effects of the disease on the personal, social, and occupational aspects of a patient's life e.g., "During my most recent typical Ménière's attacks I had trouble with hearing"
Penn Acoustic Neuroma Quality of Life Scale (PANQOL) (Shaffer, Cohen, Bigelow, & Ruckenstein, 2010)	Validated in adults with acoustic neuromas (*n* = 143)	26 items, seven domain scores (anxiety, facial dysfunction, general health, balance, hearing loss, energy, and pain)	Five-point Likert scale: 1 (strongly disagree) to 5 (strongly agree)	To assess quality of life in patients with acoustic neuromas e.g., "I act differently around people because of problems moving my face"

Historical Framework for the Measurement of Change in Dizziness/Vertigo Severity

In 1985, the Committee on Hearing and Equilibrium Subcommittee of the American Academy of Ophthalmology and Otolaryngology (AAOO) described a method for quantifying the effects of treatment for the control of definitive spells of vertigo. The metric was calculated as the average number of definitive spells of vertigo per month in the 6-month period *prior* to treatment, divided by the average number of spells per month occurring in the 24-month period *after* treatment. If the observation period prior to treatment is less than 6 months, then the numerator is the average number of spells occurring per month in the pretreatment interval. The result of the calculation is multiplied by 100. The result was categorized into one of five categories: "0" (i.e., Classification group *A*) representing complete control of definitive spells; 1 to 40 (i.e., Classification group *B*) representing substantial control of definitive spells; 41 to 80 (i.e., Classification group *C*) representing limited control of definitive spells; 81 to 120 (i.e., Classification group *D*) representing insignificant control over definitive spells; and >120 (i.e., Classification group *E*) representing poorer control (over baseline) of definitive spells. There was also included a Classification group *F* representing the situation where "secondary treatment was initiated due to disability from vertigo" (Committee on Hearing and Equilibrium guidelines for the evaluation of hearing preservation in acoustic neuroma (vestibular schwannoma). American Academy of Otolaryngology-Head and Neck Surgery Foundation, 1995).

Although the latter classification schema was simple to employ, the interpretation was difficult. For example, the definition of a *definitive* spell of vertigo may vary from one clinician to another. The measurement technique is critically dependent on the patient being a reliable historian in his or her recollections of numbers of definitive vertiginous spells. Finally, this measurement technique does not capture the impact that spells of vertigo have on a patient's ability to carry out activities that are considered normal for the individual nor does the technique quantify the effects of dizziness on psychosocial function. For example, and based on what we understand about headache handicap, it is

possible for one patient who has 20 definitive but shorter-lasting and less severe vertiginous spells to demonstrate less activity limitation and/or participation restriction than another patient who has two, severe and incapacitating definitive spells, of 4-hour duration (or longer) who has become ill in a public place.

In 1995, a second metric was developed by the American Academy of Otolaryngology (AAO) to augment the original classification metrics. This *Functional Level Scale* was developed to address the disabling accompaniments of vertigo. For this measure, a patient makes a single decision of which statement best reflects his or her current status. The statements are shown in Table 8–7. According to the AAO, "The raw data of the functional level scale should be reported for each patient at each time interval recorded (baseline, 2 years, etc.). The treatment outcome regarding disability should be expressed as improved, changed, or worse for each patient" (Committee on Hearing and Equilibrium guidelines for the evaluation of hearing preservation in acoustic neuroma (vestibular schwannoma). American Academy of Otolaryngology-Head and Neck Surgery Foundation, 1995).

Commonly Used Self-Report Tools for Assessing DRQoL

Motion Sensitivity Quotient (MSQ)

Smith-Wheelock, Shepard, and Telian (1991) described a device referred to as the Motion Sensitivity Quotient (MSQ). The MSQ represents a method of quantifying the severity of symptoms evoked by Norre and Becker 's (1989) stereotyped movements of the head and head/body that were designed for vestibular habituation therapy. The authors have taken 16 of these movements and devised a quantitative rather than qualitative method for documenting dizziness (Figure 8–2).

That is, for each of Norre and Becker 's 16 positioning movements, the patient is asked to respond whether the symptoms of dizziness occurred, and if so, at what intensity using a scale from 1 to 5 (i.e., 1 = mild and 5 = severe). Finally, patients are asked for each position to report the duration of their symp-

Table 8–7. The Functional Level Scale Developed by the American Academy of Otolaryngology (AAO)

Regarding my current state of overall function, not just during attacks (check the one that best applies):

1. My dizziness has no effect on my activities at all.

2. When I am dizzy I have to stop what I am doing for a while, but it soon passes and I can resume activities. I continue to work, drive, and engage in any activity I choose without restriction. I have not changed any plans or activities to accommodate my dizziness.

3. When I am dizzy, I have to stop what I am doing for a while, but it does pass and I can resume activities. I continue to work, drive, and engage in most activities I choose, but I have had to change some plans to make some allowance for my dizziness.

4. I am able to work, drive, travel, take care of my family, or engage in most essential activities, but I must exert a great deal of effort to do so. I must constantly make adjustments in my activities and budget my energies. I am barely making it.

5. I am unable to work, drive, or take care of my family. I am unable to do most of the active things that I used to. Even essential activities must be limited. I am disabled.

6. I have been disabled for 1 year or longer and/or I receive compensation (money) because of my dizziness or balance problem.

Source: Committee on Hearing and Equilibrium Guidelines for the Diagnosis and Evaluation of Therapy in Ménière's Disease. American Academy of Otolaryngology-Head and Neck Foundation, Inc. 1995. *Otolaryngology-Head and Neck Surgery,113,* 181–185.

toms on a scale from 0 to 3 (i.e., 0 = 0–4 seconds; 1 = 5–10 seconds, 2 = 11–29 seconds, and 3 = >30 seconds). The total score is obtained by summing the intensity (i.e., maximum of 3 × 16 = 48) and duration scores (i.e., maximum 5 × 16 = 80) for each of the 16 positions where symptoms were evoked and multiplying that number by the number of positionings (i.e., maximum of 16) where symptoms were elicited. The resulting product is divided by the maximum score of 2048 and then multiplied by 100 to convert the number to a percentage. Higher percentage scores reflect greater symptom severity.

The psychometric characteristics of the MSQ have been reported by Akin and Davenport (2003). The subject sample consisted of 15 patients (mean age 65 years) and 10 control subjects (mean age 66 years). If the patient reported dizziness prior to testing the magnitude of the dizziness was estimated by the patient (on the 5-point scale) and that value was subtracted from the estimated magnitude during testing.

The authors reported 100% sensitivity for the MSQ. That is, all patients reported dizziness on the MSQ. The range of values in the patient group was 0.2 to 91.4. The mean value was 21.6. The positions yielding the greatest number of positive responses were 4 (supine to sitting), 5 (Hallpike left), 6 (up from left Hallpike), 7 (Hallpike right), 8 (up from right Hallpike), 10 (head up from left knee), 13 (sitting, head turns [5′] 180 degrees), 14 (sitting, head tilts [5′] pitch), 15 (180-degree turn to right, standing), and 16 (180-degree turn to left, standing). The range of values in the control group was 0 to 0.5 with an average value of 0.06. Accordingly, the test specificity was 80%. The MSQ was administered at baseline, and then 24 h later. For a smaller subgroup of eight patients, the MSQ was administered on one additional occasion, 90 min after the baseline measure. The intraclass correlation coefficients (ICC) for the 90-min and 24-hr intervals were 0.98 and 0.96, respectively. Additionally, the ICC scores from the

	Intensity (maximum 5 points)	Duration (maximum 3 points)	Score
1. Baseline symptoms			
2. Sitting to supine			
3. Supine to left side			
4. Supine to right side			
5. Supine to sitting			
6. Left Hallpike			
7. Left Hallpike to sitting			
8. Right Hallpike			
9. Right Hallpike to sitting			
10. Sitting to nose to left knee			
11. Sitting to erect left			
12. Sitting to nose to right knee			
13. Sitting to erect right			
14. Sitting with head rotation			
15. Sitting with head flexion and extension			
16. Standing and turning to the right 180 degrees			
17. Standing and turning to the left 180 degrees			

Intensity: Scale from 0–5 (0 = no symptoms, 5 = severe symptoms)
Duration: Scale from 0–3 (5–10 sec = 1 point, 11–30 sec = 2 points, >30 sec = 3 points)
Motion sensitivity quotient: [(sum (duration + intensity) × number of dizziness-provoking positions)/2,048] × 100

Figure 8–2. The Motion Sensitivity Quotient (MSQ). From Smith-Wheelock, M., Shepard, N. T,. and Telian, S. A. (1991). Physical therapy program for vestibular rehabilitation. *American Journal of Otology, 12,* 218–225. Reprinted with permission from Wolters Kluwer Health.

two examiners was assessed and found to be 0.99, reflecting strong interrater reliability.

Although the MSQ would appear to be a very good outcome measure reflecting the magnitude of decrease in motion-provoked symptoms, the measure provides little detail as to the origin of the total score. That is, as noted by Akin and Davenport (2003), a score of 25 (for example) does not tell the clinician whether the score was generated by low-intensity, short-duration dizziness occurring for multiple positions, or by longer-duration, higher-intensity vertigo occurring on fewer positions. Thus, the total score on the metric provides limited information about specific motion-provoked dizziness.

Vertigo Symptom Scale (VSS)

The VSS was developed by Yardley, Todd, Lacoudraye-Harter, and Ingham (1992) and Yardley, Masson,

Verschuur, Haacke, and Luxon (1992) in an effort to address the known relationship between vertigo, anxiety, and emotional disturbance. For example, it is known that increased somatic awareness toward tinnitus can result in decreases in tinnitus-related quality of life. In the same manner, increased vigilance directed toward sensations of disequilibrium and vertigo can result in increases in anxiety and depression, in turn resulting in panic and agoraphobia. This can further escalate into hyperventilation syndrome that may have the effect of creating chronic vertigo and so on. In fact, as noted by Yardley, Masson, et al. (1992) and Yardley, Todd, et al. (1992), patients with spells of vertigo may experience the same symptoms during a spell (e.g., dizziness/unsteadiness, nausea, trembling, and sweating) that patients with panic disorder experience during a panic attack. The authors stated that their goal in creating the VSS was to develop a self-report measure of vertigo severity that was not contaminated "by symptomatology caused by anxiety, and which could therefore be used, in preference to vestibular test results, to examine the relative influence of vertigo and anxiety on reported handicap and distress."

The scale consists of 36 items describing common symptoms that are reported by, or observed from, patients with vertigo. These items were derived from an interview study reported above (Yardley, Todd, et al., 1992). The scale is shown in Figure 8–3.

The patient is asked, "How often in the past 12 months have you had the following symptoms?" (i.e., the symptoms include pains in the heart or chest region, tension/soreness in muscles, feeling of pressure in the ear). The patient is asked to circle the, "appropriate number to indicate about how many times you have experienced each of the symptoms listed . . . during the past 12 months or since the vertigo started, if (the patient has had the) vertigo for less than one year." The responses and point values associated with them are, "Never" (zero points), "A few times" (1–3 times a year [1 point]), "Several times" (4–12 times a year [2 points]), "Quite often" (on average, more than once a month [3 points]), and "Very often" (on average, more than once a week [4 points]).

Responses obtained from 138 patients were analyzed using a factor analysis to determine what factor (i.e., subscale) structure existed in this device. The result of the factor analysis showed that 44% of the variance could be explained by three factors. The first factor, explaining 24% of the variance, described complaints suggesting somatization and anxiety (i.e., Anxiety/Autonomic symptom subscale—AA). Representative symptoms included tension/soreness in muscles, heart pounding or fluttering, and/or heavy feeling in the arms or legs. The second factor explaining approximately 12% of the variance, consisted of symptoms lasting longer than an hour that are characteristic of those observed in patients with acute vertigo (i.e., Acute attack of vertigo subscale—VACU). These items included "feeling that things are spinning or moving lasting more than one hour," "unsteadiness so severe that you fall over," and "nausea (feeling sick), stomach churning." The third factor (i.e., Vertigo of short duration subscale—VSH) explaining 8% of the variance, consisted of items describing dizziness and unsteadiness symptoms of short duration. These items included, "feeling that things are spinning or moving lasting up to one hour," and "feeling unsteady, about to lose balance lasting up to one hour."

The investigators employed the data from the factor analysis to create two primary subscales: the vertigo subscale and the anxiety and autonomic symptom subscale, each containing two further subscales. The vertigo subscale contained items comprising the VSH and VACU subscales. The anxiety and autonomic symptom subscale contained items that comprised the somatization (SOM, e.g., heavy feeling in the arms and legs) and autonomic symptoms (AU, e.g., feeling faint, about to black out) subscales.

The concurrent and construct validity of this scale were reported to be robust. For example, patients with spontaneous episodic vertigo had higher acute vertigo and total vertigo scores. Patients with positional vertigo demonstrated intermediate acute vertigo and total vertigo scores. Magnitude of scores on the AA subscale was significantly correlated with measures of state and trait anxiety (i.e., $r = .55$ and $.44$, respectively). Both the AA and VER subscales were significantly correlated (i.e., $r = .33$ and $.37$, respectively) with self-reported handicap. There was no predictable relationship between quantitative measures of vestibular system function (e.g., caloric test asymmetry) and subscale or total scores on the VSS.

VERTIGO SYMPTOM SCALE

Please circle the appropriate number to indicate about how many times you have experienced each of the symptoms listed below during the past 12 months (or since the vertigo started, if you have had vertigo for less than one year).

The range of responses are:

0	1	2	3	4
Never	A few times (1–3 times a year)	Several times (4–12 times a year)	Quite often (on average, more than once a month)	Very often (on average, more than once a week)

How often **in the past 12 months** have you had the following symptoms:

1. A feeling that things are spinning or moving around, lasting:
   (PLEASE ANSWER ALL THE CATEGORIES)

a) less than 2 minutes	0	1	2	3	4
b) up to 20 minutes	0	1	2	3	4
c) 20 minutes to 1 hour	0	1	2	3	4
d) several hours	0	1	2	3	4
e) more than 12 hours	0	1	2	3	4

2. Pains in the heart or chest region   0   1   2   3   4

3. Hot or cold spells   0   1   2   3   4

4. Unsteadiness so severe that you actually fall   0   1   2   3   4

5. Nausea (feeling sick), stomach churning   0   1   2   3   4

6. Tension/soreness in your muscles   0   1   2   3   4

7. A feeling of being lightheaded, "swimmy" or giddy, lasting:
   (PLEASE ANSWER ALL THE CATEGORIES)

a) less than 2 minutes	0	1	2	3	4
b) up to 20 minutes	0	1	2	3	4
c) 20 minutes to 1 hour	0	1	2	3	4
d) several hours	0	1	2	3	4
e) more than 12 hours	0	1	2	3	4

8. Trembling, shivering   0   1   2   3   4

9. Feeling of pressure in the ear(s)   0   1   2   3   4

10. Heart pounding or fluttering   0   1   2   3   4

Figure 8–3. The Vertigo Symptoms Scale (VSS). From Yardley, L., and Hallam, R. S. (1996). Psychosocial aspects of balance and gait disorders. *continues*

11. Vomiting	0	1	2	3	4
12. Heavy feeling in arms or legs	0	1	2	3	4
13. Visual disturbances (e.g., blurring, flickering, spots before the eyes)	0	1	2	3	4
14. Headache or feeling of pressure in the head	0	1	2	3	4
15. Unable to stand or walk properly without support	0	1	2	3	4
16. Difficulty breathing, short of breath	0	1	2	3	4
17. Loss of concentration or memory	0	1	2	3	4
18. Feeling unsteady, about to lose balance, lasting: (PLEASE ANSWER ALL THE CATEGORIES)					
a) less than 2 minutes	0	1	2	3	4
b) up to 20 minutes	0	1	2	3	4
c) 20 minutes to 1 hours	0	1	2	3	4
d) several hours	0	1	2	3	4
e) more than 12 hours	0	1	2	3	4
19. Tingling, prickling, or numbness in parts of the body	0	1	2	3	4
20. Pains in the lower part of your back	0	1	2	3	4
21. Excessive sweating	0	1	2	3	4
22. Feeling faint, about to black out	0	1	2	3	4

Scoring, administration, validation, and statistical properties. To obtain a measure of vertigo severity, simply sum the patient's responses to the following items on the long version of the VSS: 1a to 1e, 4, 5, 7a to 7e, 11, 15, 18a to 18e. A measure of somatic anxiety can be obtained by summing items 2, 3, 6, 8 to 10, 12 to 14, 16, 17, 19 to 22.

The VSS scales and subscales have very good statistical reliability (Cronbach's alpha typically .80 or better) and the two subscales of the long form of the VSS are only modestly correlated (.33). Test-retest reliability of both the VSS scales has been shown to be good.

The discriminant, concurrent, and predictive validity of the VSS have been well established in U.K. patient samples, and have been confirmed cross-culturally in a Spanish speaking Mexican sample. Both scales distinguish between patients complaining of disorientation and healthy controls. The Vertigo scale is unrelated to standard measures of anxiety and depression, but is correlated with handicap and with objective measures of perceptual disorientation following vestibular surgery. The Autonomic/Anxiety scale is correlated with measures of anxiety and depression and with objective measures of psychophysiological arousal, and is a longitudinal predictor of change in symptoms, handicap, and emotional distress over a seven-month period.

Figure 8-3. *continued* In A. M. Bronstein, T. Brandt, and M. Woollacott (Eds.), *Clinical disorders of balance, posture and gait.* London, UK: Arnold. See text for details. Courtesy of Dr. Lucy Yardley.

Dizziness Handicap Inventory (DHI)

In response to a perceived need to have a standardized measure of self-report activity limitation and participation restriction resulting from dizziness and unsteadiness, Jacobson and Newman (1990) developed a measure called the DHI. The DHI seemed a natural progression from the work of one of the authors (CWN) on the development of a Hearing Handicap Inventory for Adults (HHIA) (Newman, Weinstein, Jacobson, & Hug, 1990). As such, the intent of the authors was to create the DHI using the HHIA as a template. The initial (alpha) version of the DHI consisted of 37 statements that were generated based on the authors' experience evaluating patients who were dizzy, light-headed, or unsteady. The items did not contain the word "dizzy" or "dizziness" but instead contained the phrase "your problem" (e.g., Because of your problem, are you depressed?). The items were grouped a priori into "subscales" based on their content alone. The subscales were labeled "functional" (i.e., the item was designed to probe how "the problem" affected the patient's ability to execute normal everyday activities), "emotional" (i.e., the item was designed to probe how "the problem" affected their emotional well-being), and "physical" (i.e., the item was designed to probe how "the problem" was affected by movement of the head or head and body together). The patient was asked to respond to each item by choosing either a "yes," "sometimes," or "no" response. In scoring the DHI, a "yes" response is awarded four points, a "sometimes" response is awarded two points, and a "no" response is awarded 0 points. The alpha version of the DHI (i.e., αDHI) was administered to 63 consecutive patients (mean age 49 years).

The initial administration of the αDHI was used to reduce the 37-item version to a more manageable, smaller version. Cronbach's alpha coefficient analysis showed that 12 items could be discarded because they were not predictive of the individual subscale scores where they were placed. Thus, the analysis of the data from the αDHI yielded a 25-item beta version of the DHI (i.e., the βDHI). This was administered to 106 consecutive patients (mean age 48 years) seen in our balance disorders clinic. The construct validity of the DHI was established in this investigation. Subjects were asked to state whether their dizziness occurred occasionally (<12 times/

year), frequently (≥12 times/year but not continuously) or continuously. For the total DHI score and functional and emotional subscales, an increase in event frequency did result in an increase in subscale scores. This did not occur for the physical subscale.

An unexpected finding was no significant relationship between subject age and total and subscale scores. Jacobson and Newman (1990) did not evaluate gender effects; however, this was later evaluated by Robertson and Ireland (1995) who reported increased self-report handicap for females for the physical subscale ($p = .02$) and total DHI score ($p = .02$).

In a third investigation, Jacobson and Newman (1990) assessed the short-term (i.e., within a single day) test-retest reliability of the DHI for 14 patients (mean age 45 years). Pearson product-moment correlation coefficients were high for total ($r = .97$) and subscale scores (i.e., functional subscale $r = .94$, emotional subscale $r = .97$ and physical subscale $r = .92$). From this data set it was possible to establish the 95% confidence interval for change. The standard error of measurement was 6.23 points suggesting that pretreatment and post-treatment scores would have to differ by at least 18 points (i.e., 95% confidence interval for a true change) for the change to have occurred not due to chance alone. The final version of the DHI is shown in Figure 8–4.

In an attempt to develop severity categories on the DHI, Jacobson and McCaslin (unpublished data) calculated interquartile ranges for the total DHI score for a clinical sample of 200 consecutive dizzy patients. This assessment suggested that a DHI total score of 0 to 14 points could be classified as no activity limitation and participation restriction, a score of 16 to 26 could be classified as mild activity limitation and participation restriction, a score of 28 to 44 points could be classified as moderate activity limitation and participation restriction and a total score of 46 points or greater could be classified as a severe activity limitation and participation restriction. These values are reasonably close to those reported by Kinney, Sandridge, and Newman (1997) who using a smaller patient sample ($N = 51$) suggested that total DHI scores were: 0 to 14 points, 16 to 34 points, 36 to 52 points, and >54 points for the no handicap, mild, moderate, and severe handicap groups, respectively.

Shortened versions of the DHI have been developed. A 10-item screening version of the DHI

Dizziness Handicap Inventory

Instructions: The purpose of this questionnaire is to identify difficulties that you may be experiencing because of your dizziness or unsteadiness. Please answer "yes," "no," or "sometimes" to each question. <u>Answer each question as it pertains to your dizziness problem only.</u>

	Yes (4)	Some-times (2)	No (0)
P1. Does looking up increase your problem?			
E2. Because of your problem do you feel frustrated?			
F3. Because of your problem do you restrict your travel for business or recreation?			
P4. Does walking down the aisle of a supermarket increase your problem?			
F5. Because of your problem do you have difficulty getting into or out of bed.			
F6. Does your problem significantly restrict your participation in social activities such as going out to dinner, the movies, dancing, or to parties?			
F7. Because of your problem do you have difficulty reading?			
P8. Does performing more ambitious activities like sports, dancing, household chores, such as sweeping or putting dishes away, increase your problem?			
E9. Because of your problem are you afraid to leave your home without having someone accompany you?			
E10. Because of your problem have you been embarrassed in front of others?			
P11. Do quick movements of your head increase your problem?			
F12. Because of your problem do you avoid heights?			
P13. Does turning over in bed increase your problem?			
F14. Because of your problem is it difficult for you to do strenuous housework or yardwork?			
E15. Because of your problem are you afraid people may think that you are intoxicated?			
P16. Because of your problem is it difficult for you to go for a walk by yourself?			
P17. Does walking down a sidewalk increase your problem?			
E18. Because of your problem is it difficult for you to concentrate?			
F19. Because of your problem is it difficult for you to walk around your house in the dark?			
E20. Because of your problem are you afraid to stay home alone?			
E21. Because of your problem do you feel handicapped?			
E22. Has your problem placed stress on your relationships with members of your family and friends?			
E23. Because of your problem are you depressed?			
F24. Does your problem interfere with your job or household responsibilities?			
P25. Does bending over increase your problem?			

F = FUNCTIONAL	E = EMOTIONAL	P = PHYSICAL	TOTAL SCORE

Figure 8–4. The Dizziness Handicap Inventory (DHI). Maximum self-report handicap is 100 points. From Jacobson, G. P., and Newman, C. W. (1990). The development of the Dizziness Handicap Inventory. *Archives of Otolaryngology-Head and Neck Surgery, 116,* 424–427. Copyright © 1990 American Medical Association. All rights reserved. See text for details. Reprinted with the permission of the publisher.

(DHI-S) was initially developed by Jacobson and Calder (1998). The response format was identical to the DHI. Thus, with a 10-item scale, the maximum score was 40 points (i.e., representing maximum self-report dizziness-related activity limitation and participation restriction) and the minimum score was 0 points. Items comprising the DHI-S represented those items having the highest item-total correlation coefficients from the Jacobson and Newman (1990) investigation. The DHI-S consisted of four items from the functional subscale, four items from the emotional subscale, and two items from the physical subscale. Scores on the DHI-S were highly correlated with the longer, 25-item DHI (i.e., $r = .86$). The 95% confidence interval for change was four points. The DHI-S is shown in Figure 8–5.

Subsequently, Tesio, Alpini, Cesarani, and Perucca (1999) employed a Rasch analysis (i.e., a probabilistic measurement model) to the full DHI and created a 13-item version of the instrument (i.e., a "Short Form" DHI). It was the investigators' objective to create a "simpler, yet more valid, instrument from the *older* DHI." Although the methods for reducing the number of items differed, it is striking that five of the items comprising the DHI-S (Jacobson & Calder, 1998) were included in the Shortened Form of the DHI (Tesio et al., 1999) and these items have been designated in boldface type on the DHI-S shown in Figure 8–5.

Several investigators have attempted to establish the criterion validity of the DHI. Jacobson, Newman, Hunter, and Balzer (1991) conducted Pearson

Dizziness Handicap Inventory—Screening Version

Instructions: The purpose of this questionnaire is to identify difficulties that you may be experiencing because of your dizziness or unsteadiness. Please answer "yes," "no," or "sometimes" to each question. <u>Answer each question as it pertains to your dizziness problem only.</u>

		Yes (4)	Some-times (2)	No (0)
F1.	**Because of your problem do you restrict your travel for business or recreation?**			
F2.	Does your problem significantly restrict your participation in social activities such as going out to dinner, going to the movies, dancing, or to parties?			
E3.	Because of your problem are you afraid to leave your home without having someone accompany you?			
E4.	Because of your problem have you been embarrassed in front of others?			
P5.	**Does walking down a sidewalk increase your problem?**			
E6.	Because of your problem is it difficult for you to concentrate?			
F7.	**Because of your problem is it difficult for you to walk around your house in the dark?**			
E8.	**Because of your problem are you depressed?**			
F9.	Does your problem interfere with your job or household responsibilities?			
P10.	**Does bending over increase your problem?**			
F = FUNCTIONAL	**E = EMOTIONAL**	**P = PHYSICAL**	**TOTAL SCORE**	

Figure 8-5. Dizziness Handicap Inventory-Screening version (DHI-S). Maximum self-report handicap is 40 points. From Jacobson, G. P., and Calder, J. H. (1998). A screening version of the Dizziness Handicap Inventory (DHI-S). *American Journal of Otology, 19,* 804–808. The boldface items also appear in the "Short Form of the Dizziness Handicap Inventory" (Tesio et al., 1999). See text for details. The DHI-S is reprinted with the permission of Wolters Kluwer Health.

product-moment correlations between DHI total and subscale scores and balance function test results. The authors reported that, in general, there were no significant relationships observed between DHI total and subscale scores and electronystagmographic (ENG) or rotational test variables. There was a significant weak-to-moderate correlation, however, observed between sensory organization test (SOT) condition 5 (i.e., eyes closed, platform sway-referenced) on computerized dynamic posturography and DHI total ($r = -.40$) and functional ($r = -.44$) and emotional ($r = -.42$) subscales. That is, as self-report activity limitation and participation restriction increased, postural stability scores decreased.

The latter findings are reasonably consistent with those of Perez, Martin, and Garcia-Tapia (2003) who found a weak-moderate correlation between the SOT composite score and the DHI total score ($r = -.35$, $p < .01$). It was suggested by Jacobson et al. (1991) that 77% of self-report dizziness handicap was unaccounted for by physiologic measures of vestibular or balance function. Interestingly, these findings were not supported by a later investigation by Robertson and Ireland (1995) who reported no correlation coefficient greater than 0.25 for comparisons between the DHI and the SOT of the Equitest computerized dynamic posturography. More recently Loughran, Gatehouse, Kishore, and Swan (2006) evaluated, in a group of 159 patients, the relationship between the DHI and the results of the Clinical Test for the Sensory Interaction on Balance (CTSIB) (a measure similar to the SOT). The investigators reported weak positive correlations between the CTSIB "Firm surface, eyes open" condition (equivalent to Condition 1 of the SOT), and the total and subscale scores on the DHI (strongest correlation was 0.27). The investigators also reported weak positive correlations between the "Firm surface, eyes closed" condition (equivalent to Condition 2 of the SOT) and the total and subscale scores on the DHI (strongest correlation was 0.37). Finally, there was a weak positive correlation observed between the composite score on the CTSIB and the total score and emotional and functional subscale scores (i.e., strongest correlation was 0.21). The investigators surmised that there was a generally poor relationship between self-report measures of dizziness handicap, and functional, quantitative measures of postural stability. They further stated that the reason for the lack of

concordance may have occurred due to the fact that the two devices were measuring different aspects of "health status."

Finally, Whitney, Wrisley, Brown, and Furman (2004) evaluated the relationship between the DHI and five functional measures of balance including performance on the Dynamic Gait Index (DGI), Five Times Sit to Stand Test (FTSST), the Activities Specific Balance Confidence (ABC) scale, gait speed, and the Timed "Up and Go" test. Patients were then stratified into "mild (0–30 points)," "moderate (31–60 points)," and "severe (61–100)" self-report handicap groups based on their total DHI scores. The investigators also asked the patients to keep a record of the numbers of falls that occurred during the 4 weeks prior to the visit when the evaluation was conducted. The results are shown in Table 8–8 from Whitney et al. (2004). There were significant group differences observed on the DGI, FTSST, ABC, and number of falls. That is, the patients with the greatest total DHI scores were also the patients with the greatest functional impairments. The authors concluded that patients with total DHI scores exceeding 60 points are most likely significantly functionally impaired and at increased risk for falling.

It bears mentioning that the factor structure of the DHI has been evaluated by both Asmundson, Stein, and Ireland (1999) and Perez, Garmendia, Garcia-Granero, Martin, and Garcia-Tapia (2001). Remember that the subscales of the DHI were developed empirically. This means that we grouped items into subscales based on their content without determining whether our subjective judgments could withstand a statistical challenge. Asmundson et al. (1999) formally evaluated the factor structure of the DHI. The investigators administered the DHI to 95 patients in their balance disorders clinic. They conducted a principal components analysis on the data set with an oblique rotation in an attempt to find subsets of items that measured a common factor (e.g., functional, emotional, physical characteristics of dizziness and unsteadiness). The authors reported both two-factor (i.e., they referred to as "General Functional Limitations" and "Postural Difficulties") and three-factor solutions (i.e., "Disability in Activities of Daily Living," "Phobic Avoidance," "Postural Difficulties") which did not support the initial, a priori assignment of individual items to subscales. It was suggested that both the subscale structure

Table 8-8. Medians or Means and Standard Deviations of the DGI, TUG, FTSST, ABC, Number of Reported Falls in the Past 4 Weeks, and Gait Speed for Each of the Three DHI Groups

	Mild DHI (0–30) (n = 23)	Moderate DHI (31–60) (n = 44)	Severe DHI (61–100) (n = 18)	Significance Level
Median DGI	19 (n = 23)	17 (n = 41)	12 (n = 18)	p < 0.05
Mean TUG (s)	12 ± 3 (n = 22)	11 ± 4 (n = 43)	14 ± 5 (n = 17)	p = 0.79
Mean FISST (s)	15 ± 5 (n = 19)	15 ± 5 (n = 39)	20 ± 9 (n = 15)	p < 0.05
Mean ABC	74 ± 14 (n = 23)	55 ± 22 (n = 44)	28 ± 16 (n = 18)	p < 0.001
Fallers	1 (n = 23)	1 (n = 43)	6 (n = 18)	p < 0.001
Gait speed (m/s)	1.02 ± 0.2 (n = 17)	1.04 ± 0.2 (n = 37)	0.9 ± 0.2 (n = 16)	p = 0.15

Source: Adapted from Whitney, S. L., Wrisley, D. M., Brown, K. E., & Furman, J. M. (2004). Is perception of handicap related to functional performance in persons with vestibular dysfunction? *Otology and Neurotology, 25,* 139–143. Reproduced with permission of the publisher.

might be altered, and/or the total score be used as a single global measure of self-report dizziness activity limitation and participation restriction.

Similarly, Perez et al. (2001) conducted a factor analysis of the DHI. The investigators observed a three-factor solution for the DHI. The authors referred to factor 1 as "Vestibular Handicap" because the items comprising this factor dealt with levels of independence, limited use of transportation, ability to carry out job or house responsibilities, and social integration. The second factor was referred to as "Vestibular Disability" and consisted of items describing precipitating factors for positional vertigo. The third factor was referred to as "Visuovestibular Disability" because the items comprising this factor are those where "visual-vestibular interaction must be dealt with correctly in order to maintain stability." Since these two reports were published we have abandoned the calculation of subscale scores and use only the DHI total score in our clinical practice.

To date (i.e. September 2014), the original paper (Jacobson & Newman, 1990) has been referenced 857 times in the world literature. Also, of the date of this writing there have been 15 translations of the DHI (i.e., see http://www.proqolid.org). The translations include Arabic, Chinese, Croatian, Dutch, French, German, Hebrew, Hungarian, Italian, Norwegian, Polish, Portuguese, Russian, Spanish, and Swedish. The process of translation is not for the faint of heart. An excellent template for the translation of

measures can be found in the study by Kurre et al. (2009). In this study the investigators described the process by which they created a German-language version of the DHI (Kurre et al., 2009). First the primary investigator contacted an author of the original English language version of the DHI to clarify the intent/meaning of several items. They then began by performing a translation into German of the original English-language DHI. After this, a different set of translators accomplished a translation of the German-language DHI back into English. By doing this it was possible to assess whether the first translation preserved the meaning present in the original English-language version of the scale. Once judged worthy, the scale was discussed with patients to determine whether the items were clearly stated, and, if the items covered the breadth of disabilities/handicaps that are associated with dizziness, vertigo, and unsteadiness disorders and diseases. Once the items for the scale were created the investigators proceeded through the steps required to establish the validity and reliability of the scale a process that was described earlier.

Vertigo Handicap Questionnaire (VHQ)

The VHQ was developed in 1992 by Yardley and Putman. The device emanated from an investigation by Yardley et al. (1992) that consisted of a structured interview designed to generate statements specific to the psychological and social consequences of vertigo. The subjects in the interview study were 16 females and 7 males (mean age 50 years, range = 19–72 years). Major "themes" represented in the 176 statements of the subjects included, "Practical restrictions on lifestyle resulting from vertigo," "Effects of recurrent vertigo on social relations," "Self-generated rules," and "Emotional responses to vertigo." The resulting VHQ was designed to "permit reliable, quantitative comparisons to be made between groups over time."

The questionnaire interview investigation yielded 46 statements that related to dizziness, handicap, and psychological consequences of vertigo. The statements were used to create a series of items to which patients responded using a 5-point Likert scale with the anchors being zero or "no handicap" and 4 points or "maximum handicap."

The sample consisted of 84 patients. Analysis of data showed that the initial iteration of the scale contained items that were redundant, irrelevant, nondiscriminating, or ambiguous. The investigators reduced the 46-item device to a 25-item device that demonstrated high internal consistency reliability (Cronbach's alpha coefficient = 0.93) and test-retest reliability. This scale is shown in Figure 8–6.

The final device consisted of 25 statements that are answered using a 5-point Likert scale with the anchors being "Never" (scored as zero) and "Always" (scored as 4 points). Representative items are, "I find that the vertigo does restrict me socially," and "I feel less confident than I used to." The maximum score for the VHQ is 100 points representing maximum vertigo handicap. The instructions to the patients were, "The statements below describe ways in which vertigo can affect people's lives. (Throughout the questionnaire the word 'vertigo' is used to describe the feeling which you may call dizziness, giddiness, or unsteadiness.). We would like you to indicate whether vertigo has affected your life in any of these ways by circling a number between 0 and 4. The response categories are, 0 = never, 1 = occasionally, 2 = sometimes, 3 = often, and 4 = always."

In addition to the 25 probe items there is a final item (#26) designed to inquire about vertigo-related activity limitation. The item asks, "Are you currently employed?" (Answer "yes" or "no"). If the answer is "yes," then the patient is asked to answer the following questions using a "yes/no" format: "Have you changed the kind of work you do because of your vertigo?" and "Does vertigo cause you any difficulties at work?" If the answer to #26 is "no" the patient is asked to answer the question, "Did you give up work because of vertigo?"

The 25-item scale was developed into subscales consisting of "Anxiety and Depression" (e.g., "I get anxious in case I have an unexpected attack of vertigo."), "Restriction of Activity" (e.g., "I avoid making plans in advance in case I can't get there on the day."), "Social Anxieties" (e.g., "People are understanding about the problems that the vertigo causes."), "Fears about Vertigo" (e.g., "I sometimes think that there may be something seriously wrong."), and "Severity of Vertigo Attacks" (e.g., "I can usually go on with whatever I am doing during attacks)." Interestingly, the investigators reported that items comprising the "Social Anxieties," "Restriction of Activity," and "Fears about Vertigo" subscales were associated with dizziness-related anxiety and depression; however, the items comprising the "Severity of Vertigo Attacks" subscale were not.

Yardley, Todd, et al. (1992) reported that VHQ scores are correlated significantly with measures of trait and state anxiety and depression. The same investigators reported that 42% of the variance in the VHQ score could be explained by measures of vertigo severity (VSS), autonomic symptom scores (AU), and depression. Of course, this means that fully 82% of the variability in the VHQ is unaccounted for in these measures. To our knowledge (http://www.proqolid.org) the VHQ has been translated into at least Dutch, French, German, Spanish, Swedish, and Turkish.

Subjective Disability Scale (SDS) and Posttherapy Symptom Score (PSS)

The Subjective Disability Scale (SDS) was first described by Shepard, Smith-Wheelock, Telian, and Raj (1993). The measure was developed for providing a means of assessing the clinical outcomes of vestibular rehabilitative therapy. The SDS is simple to conduct because it requires only the assignment of a patient to one of six categories before and then after treatment. The disability categories as reported by the authors are shown in Table 8–9.

Vertigo Handicap Questionnaire (VHQ)

The statements below describe ways in which vertigo can affect people's lives. (Throughout the questionnaire the word "vertigo" is used to describe the feelings which you may call dizziness, giddiness, or unsteadiness.)
We would like you to indicate whether vertigo has affected your life in any of these ways by circling a number between 0 and 4. The response categories are:

0	1	2	3	4
never	occasionally	sometimes	often	always

Please read each statement and then circle a number to indicate how much of the time (if at all) vertigo affects your life in this way at present.

1. I find that the vertigo does restrict me socially.	Never	0	1	2	3	4	Always
2.* I can still take part in active leisure pursuits (e.g., swimming, dancing, sports).	Never	0	1	2	3	4	Always
3. Some of my friends or relations get impatient because of the vertigo.	Never	0	1	2	3	4	Always
4.* I can move around quickly and freely.	Never	0	1	2	3	4	Always
5. I feel less confident than I used to.	Never	0	1	2	3	4	Always
6.* I am happy to go out alone.	Never	0	1	2	3	4	Always
7. My vertigo means that my family life is restricted.	Never	0	1	2	3	4	Always
8. I find some of my less active hobbies difficult (e.g., sewing, reading).	Never	0	1	2	3	4	Always
9.* I am still able to travel despite the vertigo.	Never	0	1	2	3	4	Always
10. I try to avoid bending over.	Never	0	1	2	3	4	Always
11.* My family takes the vertigo in its stride.	Never	0	1	2	3	4	Always
12. My friends are unsure how to react and do not really understand.	Never	0	1	2	3	4	Always
13. I think that there may be something seriously wrong with me.	Never	0	1	2	3	4	Always
14.* People are understanding about the problems that the vertigo causes.	Never	0	1	2	3	4	Always
15. I get anxious in case I have an unexpected attack of vertigo.	Never	0	1	2	3	4	Always
16.* During an attack of vertigo I can carry on with whatever I am doing.	Never	0	1	2	3	4	Always

Figure 8-6. The Vertigo Handicap Questionnaire (VHQ). In A. M. Bronstein, T. Brandt, and M. Woollacott (Eds.), *Clinical disorders of balance, posture and gait.* New York, NY: Oxford University Press. See text for details. Reprinted with the permission of the author. *continues*

17. I find the attacks frightening.	Never	0	1	2	3	4	Always
18.* I am able to walk long distances.	Never	0	1	2	3	4	Always
19. The vertigo worries me.	Never	0	1	2	3	4	Always
20. I avoid making plans in advance in case I cannot get there on the day.	Never	0	1	2	3	4	Always
21.* I find I can carry out everyday activities without difficulty (e.g., shopping, gardening, jobs around the house.)	Never	0	1	2	3	4	Always
22. I am afraid of spoiling things for others.	Never	0	1	2	3	4	Always
23. I get rather depressed because of the vertigo.	Never	0	1	2	3	4	Always
24.* During an attack of vertigo, if I just sit down I am fine.	Never	0	1	2	3	4	Always
25. If I have an attack of vertigo in public I get embarrassed.	Never	0	1	2	3	4	Always

26. Are you currently employed? (Please tick)   Yes _____ No _____
If you answered "Yes" to question 26 please answer question b) and c) only.
If you answered "No" to question 26 please answer question a) only.

a) Did you give up work because of vertigo?   Yes _____ No _____

b) Have you changed the kind of work you do?   Yes _____ No _____

c) Does vertigo cause you any difficulties at work?   Yes _____ No _____

<u>Scoring and administration.</u> To obtain the total handicap score (out of 80) simply sum responses to items 1 to 25 of the VHQ, after first reversing the scores on the asterisked* items (so that 0 = 4, 4 = 0, etc.).

Statistical properties and normative values (based on a sample of 120 outpatients referred for investigation of balance disorder). The VHQ has very good reliability (alpha = 0.86); the mean handicap scorer was 43.6 with a standard deviation of 17.24. Test-retest reliability of the VHQ has been shown to be good.

Figure 8-6. *continued*

In addition to the SDS, the authors reported another measure that addressed the magnitude of symptoms following vestibular rehabilitative therapy. In order to conduct the Post-Therapy Symptom Score (PSS) patients were assigned to one of five groups based on symptom severity. The groups are shown in Table 8–10.

The investigators reported on 152 patients who completed therapy and had been enrolled in a vestibular rehabilitation "maintenance" program. The age range of the patients was 20 to 89 years (mean age = 52 years, SD 16 years). Reported in the investigation were the group pre- and posttherapy disability scores and their posttherapy symptoms scores. The

Table 8–9. The Subjective Disability Scale

0	No disability; negligible symptoms
1	No disability; bothersome symptoms
2	Mild disability; performs usual work duties, but symptoms interfere with outside activities
3	Moderate disability; symptoms disrupt performance of both usual work duties and outside activities
4	Recent severe disability; on medical leave or had to change job because of symptoms
5	Long-term severe disability; unable to work for over 1 year or established permanent disability with compensation payments

Source: From Shepard, N. T., Telian, S. A., Smith-Wheelock, M., and Raj, A. (1993). Vestibular and balance rehabilitation therapy. *Annals of Otology, Rhinology, and Laryngology, 102,* 198–205. See text for details. Reprinted with permission of the publisher.

Table 8–10. Posttherapy Symptom Score (PSS)

0	No symptoms remaining at the end of therapy
1	Marked improvements in symptoms, mild symptoms remaining
2	Mild improvement, definite persistent symptoms remaining
3	No change in symptoms relative to pretherapy period
4	Symptoms worsened with therapy activities on a persistent basis relative to the pretherapy period

Source: From Shepard, N. T., Telian, S. A., Smith-Wheelock, M., and Raj, A. (1993). Vestibular and balance rehabilitation therapy. *Annals of Otology, Rhinology, and Laryngology, 102,* 198–205. See text for details. Reprinted with permission of the publisher.

authors reported that 85% of their sample showed a reduction of symptoms and 80% showed a reduction of their SDS by one point. Those with the greatest pretreatment disability scores (i.e., a score of 5) demonstrated the least amount of change. Additionally, 9% of the patients demonstrated no change and 6% demonstrated a worsening of their symptoms as a result of therapy. Specifically, the average pretreatment disability score was 3.0 and the average posttreatment disability score was 1.4 ($p < .001$). None of the subjects showed a worsening of their SDS following therapy.

Activities-Specific Balance Confidence (ABC) Scale

In 1995, Powell and Myers reported the development of a device that was designed to serve as a measure of "situation-specific" balance confidence in community-dwelling elderly who are functioning at a moderate to high level of mobility and independence. The device, called "The Activities Specific Balance Confidence Scale" (i.e., ABC Scale), shown in Figure 8–7, consists of a standardized question, "How confident are you that you will not lose your balance or become unsteady when you . . . " that is followed by 16 conditions (e.g., "walk around the house?" or "walk up or down stairs?").

This measure is a departure from other instruments in that it evaluates self-efficacy. Assessment of self-efficacy beliefs is important to estimate the confidence an individual has for performing a set of skills required to succeed at a specific task or goal (Bandura, 1986). Self-efficacy also influences choices of activities and motivational levels that contribute to a patient's acquisition and refinement of new abilities as well as effort, resilience, and perseverance in the face of difficulties (Smith & West, 2006).

On the ABC Scale, patients are asked to rate on a scale of 0 to 100% how confident they are performing the activities. In addition to the individual item scores, an average score is calculated across all items. Items comprising the ABC Scale were derived from interviews with both clinicians and patients. Clinicians were asked to "name the 10 most important activities essential to independent living that while requiring some position change or walking, would be safe and nonhazardous to most elderly persons." Patients were asked, "Are you afraid of falling during any normal daily activities, and if so, which ones?" Based on their responses, 12 unique items were generated. Additionally, four items from the Falls Efficacy Scale (i.e., "light housekeeping," "reaching," "simple shopping," and "walking around the house") were included in the ABC Scale. The investigators pointed out that the words in the instruction set, "will not lose your balance or become unsteady" were chosen as losses of balance may, but do not have to, progress to a fall.

The Activities-Specific Balance Confidence (ABC) Scale*

Administration:

The ABC can be self-administered or administered via personal or telephone interview. Larger typeset should be used for self-administration, whereas an enlarged version of the rating scale on an index card will facilitate in-person interviews. Regardless of method of administration, each respondent should be queried concerning their understanding of instructions, and probed regarding difficulty answering specific items.

Instructions to Participants:

For each of the following, please indicate your level of confidence in doing the activity without losing your balance or becoming unsteady from choosing one of the percentage points on the scale from 0% to 100%. If you do not currently do the activity in question, try and imagine how confident you would be if you had to do the activity. If you normally use a walking aid to do the activity or hold onto someone, rate your confidence as if you were using these supports. If you have any questions about answering any of these items, please ask the administrator.

Instructions for Scoring:

The ABC is an 11-point scale and ratings should consist of whole numbers (0-100) for each item. Total the ratings (possible range = 0–1600) and divide by 16 to get each subject's ABC score. If a subject qualifies his or her response to items #2, #9, #11, #14, or #15 (different ratings for "up" vs. "down" or "onto" vs. "off"), solicit separate ratings and use the lowest confidence of the two (as this will limit the entire activity, for instance the likelihood of using the stairs.)

For *each* of the following activities, please indicate your level of self-confidence by choosing a corresponding number from the following rating scale:

```
        0%    10    20    30    40    50    60    70    80    90    100%
  no confidence                                              completely confident
```

"How confident are you that you will not lose your balance or become unsteady when you . . .

. . . walk around the house? ____%

. . . walk up or down stairs? ____%

. . . bend over and pick up a slipper from the front of a closet floor? ____%

. . . reach for a small can off a shelf at eye level? ____%

. . . stand on your tiptoes and reach for something above your head? ____%

. . . stand on a chair and reach for something? ____%

. . . sweep the floor? ____%

. . . walk outside the house to a car parked in the driveway? ____%

. . . get into or out of a car? ____%

. . . walk across a parking lot to the mall? ____%

. . . walk up or down a ramp? ____%

. . . walk in a crowded mall where people rapidly walk past you? ____%

. . . are bumped into by people as you walk through the mall? ____%

. . . step onto or off an escalator while you are holding onto a railing? ____%

. . . step onto or off an escalator while holding onto parcels such that you cannot hold onto the railing? ____%

. . . walk outside on icy sidewalks? ____%

Figure 8-7. The Activities-Specific Balance Confidence (ABC) scale. From Powell, L. E., and Myers, A. M. (1995). The Activities Specific Balance Confidence (ABC) Scale. *Journals of Gerontology: Medical Science*, 50A, M28-M34. See text for details. Reprinted with the permission of Oxford University Press.

Internal consistency reliability was high for items comprising the ABC Scale (coefficient alpha = 0.96). A step-wise deletion of items did not improve the coefficient alpha. The test-retest reliability of the ABC Scale has been found to be excellent using a 2-week interval (r = .92) (Powell & Myers, 1995) or a 4-week interval (r = .91) (Miller, Deathe, & Speechley, 2003). Powell and Myers (1995) reported moderate correlations (r = .49) between scores from the ABC Scale and the Physical Self-Efficacy Scale (Ryckman, Robbins, Thornton, & Cantrell, 1982), and the Falls Efficacy Scale (Tinetti, Richman, & Powell, 1990). Additionally, Miller et al. (2003) reported a strong positive correlation (r = .72) between scores on the ABC Scale and scores on the Two-Minute Walking test and a strong negative correlation between scores on the ABC Scale and those on the Timed Up and Go test. That is, as the elapsed time to complete the TUG test decreased, balance confidence increased.

When the ABC Scale was administered to subgroups of patients who had fallen in the past year, or who had sustained an injury due to a fall, these subgroups scored lower on the ABC, but not significantly so, compared to a group that had not fallen in the past year or who had fallen and not been injured. ABC Scale scores were significantly different when scores from high-mobility subjects and low-mobility subjects were compared.

However, only a small subset of patients presenting to a vestibular disorders clinic have a history of falls. The question becomes, to what extent is a scale such as the ABC Scale appropriate and valid for use in a vestibular disorders clinic. Whitney, Hudak, and Marchetti (1999) attempted to address this question. Support for such an investigation could be found in the results of a previous study where functional reach and scores on the DHI were compared (Mann, Whitney, Redfern, Borello-France, & Furman, 1996). The authors reported that, as functional reach increased, DHI scores decreased. In their study, Whitney et al. (1999) evaluated the relationship between the ABC Scale and the DHI. Both the ABC and DHI scales were administered to 71 patients almost equally split between those younger than and those older than 65 years of age. The investigators reported a moderately strong correlation coefficient of −0.63 between the average ABC score and the total DHI score. That is, lower scores on the DHI (representing low self-perceived dizziness handicap) were associated with increased balance confidence when performing everyday tasks. Although no age-related effects had been reported for dizziness handicap, the investigators evaluated independently the correlations of the DHI and ABC scales for those younger than versus those older than 65 years of age. The investigators did not find a significant difference between groups. The authors concluded that their data suggested that dizziness handicap was not a result of age-related changes in the balance system, but that the ABC and DHI scales might supply complementary information. That is, the ABC Scale is a measure of self-efficacy providing information about how confident a patient is to perform activities of daily living (ADLs), whereas the DHI is a self-report measure of dizziness handicap providing information about how the participation restriction impacts psychosocial function and reduced independence.

UCLA Dizziness Questionnaire (UCLA-DQ)

Honrubia, Bell, Harris, Baloh, and Fisher (1996) developed a device called the UCLA Dizziness Quotient (UCLA-DQ) and it is shown in Figure 8–8. The UCLA-DQ was designed to quantify the frequency, severity, and impact of dizziness-related quality of life.

The device consists of five items. There are five possible responses for each of the five items ranging from lowest severity/impact to greatest severity/impact. The first two items are designed to quantify self-reports of dizziness frequency and severity. The product of the scores from these two items has been referred to by Bamiou, Davies, McKee, and Luxon (1999) as the Dizziness Index (DI). Because the minimum score for each item is 1 point and the maximum is 5 points, the minimum and maximum DI scores are 1 point and 25 points, respectively. The final three items of the UCLA-DQ measure the effect of dizziness on activities of daily living (e.g., working, driving, shopping, taking care of a family, and taking care of self), the effect of dizziness on overall quality of life (e.g., social activities, intimate relationships, work, leisure activities), and the magnitude of the patient's fear they will become dizzy.

In the original report the device was administered to 362 dizzy patients. The patients also

---

UCLA Dizziness Questionnaire (UCLA-DQ)

1. I have this problem

   ____ Rarely   ____ Sometimes   ____ About half of the time   ____ Usually   ____ Always

2. When I have this problem, my symptoms are most often:

   ____ Very mild   ____ Mild   ____ About half of the time   ____ Usually   ____ Always

3. When I experience this problem, it has the following effect on my daily activities such as walking, driving, shopping, taking care of family, and taking care of myself:

   ____ I continue all of my daily activities without restriction, although I make allowances for the problem

   ____ I continue most of my activities, although I make allowances for my problem

   ____ I continue some of my activities, but I find that my problem causes me to be unable to continue most functions

   ____ I am unable to continue any of my daily activities

4. What impact does my problem have on the overall quality of my life? Examples: participating in social activities, sharing intimate relationships, making plans for the future, obtaining or maintaining work, and participating in leisure activities:

   ____ My problems has no impact on the overall quality of my life

   ____ My problem has some impact on the overall quality of my life

   ____ My problem has moderate impact on the overall quality of my life

   ____ My problem has a great deal of impact on the overall quality of my life

   ____ My problem has a severe impact on the overall quality of my life

5. Regarding my fear of becoming dizzy or unsteady:

   ____ I never worry about becoming dizzy or unsteady

   ____ I seldom worry about becoming dizzy or unsteady

   ____ I sometimes worry about becoming dizzy or unsteady

   ____ I frequently worry about becoming dizzy or unsteady

   ____ I always worry about becoming dizzy or unsteady

Figure 8–8. The UCLA Dizziness Questionnaire (UCLA-DQ). From Honrubia, V., Bell, T. S., Harris, M. R., Baloh, R. W., and Fisher, L. M. (1996). Quantitative evaluation of dizziness characteristics and impact on quality of life. *American Journal of Otology, 17,* 595–602. See text for details. Reprinted with permission from Wolters Kluwer Health.

completed standardized measures of anxiety and depression. Additionally, the first four items were reworded in such a way that they could be completed by the patient's physician so that the level of agreement between the beliefs of the patient and physician could be compared.

The investigators reported that higher frequencies and severities of dizziness were associated with greater negative impacts on daily activities, qual-

ity of life, and fears of becoming vertiginous. The authors reported that patients in the BPPV, general peripheral vertigo, and migraine diagnostic categories demonstrated the greatest self-report dizziness severity. The group whose dizziness affected the greatest negative impact on quality of life was patients with psychogenic dizziness and the least impact was observed for patients with BPPV. The assessment of agreement between patients and their physicians showed that the physicians underestimated the impact that dizziness had on the patient's quality of life.

Monzani, Casolari, Guidetti, and Rigatelli (2001) conducted an investigation to determine whether anxiety and depression occurred more frequently in a group of dizzy patients in comparison to a group of control subjects. Additionally, the investigators sought to determine whether anxiety and depression associated with vertigo occurred more frequently in subgroups of vestibular disease. Finally, they attempted to determine whether patients with increased anxiety and depression showed increases in vertigo related activity limitation and participation restriction. The investigators utilized the UCLA-DQ to answer the latter question. The investigators reported that vertiginous patients demonstrated greater levels of anxiety and depression compared to controls. Additionally, fear of becoming dizzy and total UCLA-DQ score also were significantly different between the two groups. The investigators reported that patient age, illness duration, fear of dizziness, and total UCLA-DQ were positively correlated with measures of anxiety and depression.

Last, Perez et al. (2003) conducted an investigation designed to determine the relationships between vestibular handicap (i.e., as measured with the total DHI score) and vertigo severity (i.e., as measured by the DI of the UCLA-DQ) for five subgroups of patients defined by their patterns of performance on caloric testing, rotational testing, and posturographic testing (i.e., composite score on the SOT subtest of the Equitest protocol). The authors reported agreement between dizziness severity and handicap measures (i.e., $r = .42$ between DHI total score and the DI measure from the UCLA-DQ). The authors reported a -0.21 correlation between the SOT composite score and the DI, and a correlation coefficient of -0.35 between the DHI total score and the DI.

Vestibular Disorders Activities of Daily Living (VADL) Scale

In 2000, Cohen and Kimball reported their experiences developing a device designed to assess what impact (if any) vertigo and disequilibrium had on a patient's ability to carry out activities of daily living. Their device called the Vestibular Disorders Activities of Daily Living Scale (VADL) actually represented the evolution of an earlier device reported by Cohen (1992). The VADL is shown in Figure 8–9.

Item generation was facilitated through systematic consultation with 31 occupational and physical therapists. The 30 items were empirically subgrouped into functional (i.e., items dealing with self-care and "intimate activities"), ambulation (i.e., items addressing walking and climbing stairs), and instrumental (i.e., items addressing "home management," productivity, and leisure activities) subscales.

An initial iteration of the VADL underwent psychometric testing. In response to each of the 30 probe items, patients were requested to respond along a 10-point continuum (or not applicable, NA). A "1" response represents the ability of the patient to carry out the activity completely independently (i.e., "I am not disabled, perceive no change in performance from before developing an inner ear impairment."), whereas a "10" response represents the patient's inability to perform the activity at all (i.e., "I no longer perform the activity due to vertigo or a balance problem."). Scores ranged from 1 to 8 on the total scale, 1 to 5 for the functional subscale, 1 to 8 on the ambulation subscale, and 1 to 10 on the instrumental subscale. According to the investigators most subjects scored between 1 and 4 points. The result of this administration showed that items were either answered with the NA response or showed poor internal consistency/reliability. The final 28-item scale demonstrated strong internal consistency/reliability (alpha = 0.97 for total score, 0.92 for functional subscale, 0.96 for ambulation subscale, and 0.91 for the instrumental subscale). The test-retest reliability (i.e., 2-hr intertest interval) of the VADL was found to be excellent for the total score ($r_c = 1.00$, 95% CI = 0.99–1.00), functional subscale ($r_c = 0.87$, 95% CI = 0.67–0.95), ambulation subscale ($r_c = 0.95$, 95% CI = 0.87–0.98), and instrumental subscale ($r_c = 0.97$, CI = 0.92–0.99).

A subsequent investigation by Cohen and colleagues (Cohen et al., 2000) compared a sample of normal individuals to two patient groups (i.e., BPPV and chronic vestibulopathy) to determine how the patient groups differed in their total and subscale scores. The investigators compared results of the VADL to those obtained on measures of vestibular impairment. Finally, the authors compared the responses obtained from patients to those obtained

Vestibular Disorders of Daily Living Scale

This scale evaluates the effects of vertigo and balance disorders on independence in routine activities of daily living. Please rate your performance on each item. If your performance varies due to intermittent dizziness or balance problems please use the greatest level of disability. For each task indicate the level which most accurately describes how you perform the task. If you never do a particular task, please check the box in the column NA. The rating scales are explained on the bottom of the page.

Independence Rating

1 = Independent	6 = Must Use an Object for Help
2 = Uncomfortable, No Change in Ability	7 = Must Use Special Equipment
3 = Decreased Ability, No Change in Manner of Performance	8 = Need Physical Assistance
	9 = Dependent
4 = Slower, Cautious, More Careful	10 = Too Difficult, No Longer Perform
5 = Prefer Using an Object for Help	NA

Task	1	2	3	4	5	6	7	8	9	10	NA
F-1 Standing up from lying down											
F-2 Standing up from sitting on the bed or chair											
F-3 Dressing the upper body (e.g., shirt, brassiere, undershirt)											
F-4 Dressing the lower body (e.g., pants, skirt, underpants)											
F-5 Putting on socks or stockings											
F-6 Putting on shoes											
F-7 Moving in or out of the bathtub or shower											
F-8 Bathing yourself in the bathtub or shower											
F-9 Reaching overhead (e.g., to a cupboard or shelf)											
F-10 Reaching down (e.g., to the floor or a shelf)											
F-11 Meal preparation											
F-12 Intimate activity (e.g., foreplay, sexual activity)											
A-13 Walking on level surfaces											
A-14 Walking on uneven surfaces											
A-15 Going up steps											
A-16 Going down steps											
A-17 Walking in narrow spaces (e.g., corridor, grocery store aisle)											
A-18 Walking in open spaces											
A-19 Walking in crowds											
A-20 Using an elevator											
A-21 Using an escalator											
I-22 Driving a car											
I-23 Carrying things while walking (e.g., package, garbage bag)											
I-24 Light household chores (e.g., dusting, putting items away)											
I-25 Heavy household chores (e.g., vacuuming, moving furniture)											
I-26 Active recreation (e.g., sports, gardening)											
I-27 Occupational role (e.g., job, child care, homemaking, student)											
I-28 Traveling around the community (car, bus)											

Figure 8–9. The Vestibular Disorders of Daily Living Scale (VADL). From Cohen, H. S., and Kimball, K. T. (2000). Development of the Vestibular Disorders Activities of Daily Living Scale. *Archives of Otolaryngology-Head and Neck Surgery, 126,* 881–887. Copyright © (2000) American Medical Association. All rights reserved. Reprinted with the permission of the American Medical Association. Note that *F* = Functional, *A* = Ambulation, and *I* = Instrumental. *continues*

Explanation of Independence Rating Scale

This scale will help us to determine how inner ear problems affect your ability to perform each task. Please indicate your current performance on each task, as compared to your performance before developing an inner ear problem, by checking one of the columns in the center of the page. Pick the answer that most accurately describes how you perform the task.

1. I am **not disabled**, perceive no change in performance from before developing an inner ear impairment.

2. I am **uncomfortable** performing the activity but **perceive no difference** in the quality of my performance.

3. **I perceive a decrement** in the quality of my performance, **but have not changed** the manner of my performance.

4. **I have changed** the manner of my performance (e.g., I do things more slowly or carefully than before, or I do things without bending).

5. **I prefer using an ordinary object** in the environment for assistance (e.g., stair railing) but I am not dependent on the object or device to do the activity.

6. **I must use** an ordinary object in the environment for assistance, but I have not acquired a device specifically designed for the specific activity.

7. I must use **adaptive equipment** designed for the particular activity (e.g., grab bars, cane, reachers, bus with lift, wedge pillow).

8. I require another person for **physical assistance** or, for an activity involving two people, I need unusual physical assistance.

9. I am **dependent** on another person to perform the activity.

10. **I no longer perform** the activity due to vertigo or a balance problem.

NA. **I do not usually perform this task** or **I prefer not to answer** this question.

Figure 8–9. *continued*

from their caregivers/significant others to assess levels of concordance. The investigators found that VADL and DHI scores were moderately correlated. That is, greater levels of self-report functional independence were associated with lesser levels of self-report activity limitation and participation restriction. Not surprisingly, the normal subjects appeared less impaired than the patients on the total and subscale scores. Patients felt they were more independent than perceived by their caregivers/ significant others.

No significant relationships were observed between VADL total or subscale scores and vertigo intensity. The latter observations are similar to the finding reported earlier by Jacobson and Newman (1990). Vertigo frequency was weakly correlated with total VADL score and instrumental subscale score, another finding similar to that reported by Jacobson and Newman (1990). Additionally, weak but significant relationships were observed among SOT conditions 5 and 6 and composite score (Equitest protocol) and VADL total and functional and instrumental subscale scores. This relationship was similar to that observed by Jacobson et al. (1991) for the DHI.

In light of high test-retest reliability, the authors contend that the VADL may be of use in the pre- and posttreatment assessments of patients who have undergone vestibular rehabilitative therapy. In this connection, Cohen and Kimball (2003) used the VADL as an outcome measure in an investigation to determine whether vestibular rehabilitative therapy could have a positive impact on activities of daily living. Specifically, the investigators evaluated whether a home program of head movement exercises could decrease vertigo, and improve functional independence and psychosocial functioning in a subgroup of patients with a diagnosis of chronic, uncompensated, peripheral vestibular system impairment. Finally, the authors sought to determine whether chronologic age or length of time since onset of symptoms would have an effect on the efficacy of therapy. Subjects were asked to rate both the frequency and intensity of their vertigo on a 10-point scale (i.e., 10 being the maximum worse situation in each case). Subjects also completed the VHQ, the VSS, the DHI, and the VADL. Subjects were then assigned to one of three treatment groups each requiring subjects to perform stereotyped repetitive head movements five times per day. Subjects assigned to Group 1 were asked to perform slow head movements while they were seated. Subjects in Group 2 were asked to perform rapid head movements while both seated and standing. Subjects in Group 3 were asked to do the same exercises as those in Group 2 but had their progress monitored and their efforts reinforced by a weekly telephone call. These home exercises were performed for 4 weeks and then the dependent variables were remeasured. The investigators reported that improvements in vertigo intensity occurred for all treatment groups over a 6-month period with the greatest improvements occurring in the first 30 to 45 days. These changes were highly associated with changes in VADL total scores ($p = .004$). Vertigo frequency also decreased significantly over a 6-month period with the greatest changes occurring in the first 30 to 45 days across all groups. These improvements in vertigo frequency were associated with significant improvements in VADL total score ($p = 0.03$) and ambulation subscale score ($p = 0.03$). These significant changes in VADL total score and ambulation subscale score were associated with like changes in the DHI total score. The strong relationship between scores on the VADL and the DHI was proof of convergent validity of the VADL. Finally, from a practical perspective the findings of this investigation suggested that even a minimal home exercise program could affect positive changes in patient symptoms.

EXAMPLES OF HOW THE DHI HAS BEEN USED AS A TOOL TO ASSESS OUTCOMES

Tables 8–11 and 8–12 summarize representative published reports of how the DHI has been used to assess changes in DRQoL following nonmedical, medical, or surgical treatment. For these investigations a statistically significant reduction in self-perceived dizziness activity limitation and participation was used as evidence of subjective benefit (the treatment was effective). Alternatively, no change or an increase in reported activity limitation and participation restriction suggested no improvement (i.e., the treatment was ineffective).

SUMMARY

The assessment of the vertiginous, "dizzy," and unsteady patient has evolved from a quantification of impairment only, to an assessment of impairment coupled with the measurement of the impact that impairment has on psychosocial function. The addition of this information is valuable because there is generally a weak predictive relationship between the two forms of measurement. In this regard, Table 8–13 shows several examples of investigations illustrating a generally poor relationship between impairment of the peripheral vestibular system and self-reported dizziness disability/handicap. Thus, self-report measures provide unique data that can become important, for example, in the assessment of severity of a disease and in the quantification of improvement following treatment. This chapter aimed to (1) introduce the reader to contemporary concepts in classification of impairment, disability, and handicap (i.e., dizziness-related activity limitation and participation restriction); (2) describe characteristics that define an appropriate measure of dizziness DRQoL; (3) list the validated tools available to measure DRQoL; (4) discuss, in detail, several of the more commonly used devices for assessing these spheres; and finally, (5) summarize how one such measure has been used as a dependent variable in clinic-based research.

Table 8–11. Examples of How the DHI Has Been Used in the Area of BPPV

Authors	Year	Subjects	Purpose	Results	Conclusions
Huebner, Lytle, Doettl, Plyler, & Thelin	2013	63 patients with BPPV	To determine the effectiveness of PRMs for patients with subjective BPPV compared with objective BPPV	Significant reductions in the total DHI score were observed for both patients with subjective and objective BPPV. Baseline total DHI scores were not significantly different. Significant improvements were observed for both objective and subjective BPPV groups. There was no significant group difference in the magnitude of the improvements	PRMs are equally effective for patients with subjective and those with objective BPPV
Jung, Koo, Kim, Kim, & Song	2012	73 patients with BPPV randomly assigned to PRM group or the PRM + medication group	To determine changes in self-report dizziness handicap for patients who are treated with anxiolytics for residual dizziness/vertigo after PRM compared to a group who did not receive anxiolytics	Both groups demonstrated significant improvements in DHI scores with significantly greater improvements for the group that received the added medication	The adjuvant therapy of anxiolytics may be helpful for patients with BPPV even when PRMs are successful
Gamiz and Lopez-Escamez	2004	28 adults over the age of 60 years	To assess the magnitude of dizziness-related quality of life in a sample of elders with BPPV and then 30 days after a PRM has been performed	The DHI-S (maximum 40 points) on average decreased from 17.19 points prior to treatment to 9.70 points at posttreatment + 30 days	BPPV has a significant negative effect on DRQoL and those effects can be reduced by performing the PRM
Whitney, Marchetti, & Morris	2005	383 patients with a number of types of vestibular diagnoses	To determine whether patient performance on a custom adaptation of the DHI would be predictive of whether a patient had BPPV	Scores on a five-item and even a two-item adaptation of the DHI (containing many of the items from the physical subscale) were predictive of those patients with BPPV	This adaptation of the DHI that is sensitive to motion-provoked vertigo can assist clinicians in identifying those individuals most likely to have BPPV before the formal assessment has been performed

Table 8–12. Investigations of Treatments for SCD and Vestibular Schwannoma Where the DHI Was Used as a Dependent Variable

Authors	Year	Subjects	Purpose	Results	Conclusions
Bogle, Lundy, Zapala, & Copenhaver	2013	20 patients	To evaluate the change in self-report dizziness handicap before and following cartilage cap occlusion in superior semicircular canal dehiscence	Group pre- and postoperative total DHI scores were not significantly different. Patients with total scores in the moderate-severe range showed a statistically significant change (those will mild starting scores did not)	The cartilage cap occlusion represents an alternative to the middle cranial fossa approach to SCD
Crane, Minor, & Carey	2008	19 adult patients	To determine whether canal plugging to eliminate SCD is associated with greater handicap than that observed preoperatively	Preoperative handicap (mean = 44 points) was significantly reduced postoperatively (mean postop total score of 18 points) with the exception of two patients	Self-report handicap is significantly improved after plugging the superior canal. The greatest improvements occurred for those individuals with the highest preop values. Those patients with primarily auditory symptoms showed the least net change in total DHI score
Shaia et al.	2006	28 patients	To examine the long-term efficacy of posterior canal plugging for SCD	Mean follow-up time was 40 months. Mean preop score was 70 points. Mean postop score was 13 points. These differences were statistically significant	Canal occlusion is successful and associated with improvement in self-report dizziness disability handicap
Park et al.	2011	59 patients	To assess DRQoL in patients with vestibular schwannoma who are treated with gamma knife surgery	Baseline function was measured and then measures were conducted at follow-up intervals of 1, 3, 6, 12, and 18 months postop. There were no significant differences in DHI postoperatively	Authors suggested that these findings should be shared with patients considering surgical versus nonsurgical approaches to the removal of VS
Wockym, Hannley, Runge-Samuelson, Jensen, & Zhu	2008	55 patients	To measure changes in balance function that might occur with gamma knife surgery	Follow-up was between 6 months and +60 months. Significant change in the total DHI score (pre versus post treatment) was observed only for the elderly group where balance improved	The improvement in DHI score postoperatively should be considered for the elderly who often are unsteady
Pollock et al.	2006	82 patients	To determine whether surgical removal or radiosurgery was the best technique to treat small to medium size schwannoma	Normal facial function and better hearing occurred in the radiosurgery group. DHI scores were statistically better for the radiosurgery group	Investigators suggested that radiosurgery for vestibular schwannoma was "the best management strategy for the majority of VS patients"

Table 8–13. Examples of Investigations Illustrating the Poor Relationship Between Vestibular System Impairment and Measures of Dizziness Disability/Handicap

Authors	Year	Subjects	Results	Conclusions
Jacobson & Calder	2000	N = 72, groups = normal exam, unilateral and bilateral impairments	Significant differences in DHI total scores for comparisons between normal and bilateral loss, and between normal and unilateral loss	As occurs with studies of self-reported hearing disability/handicap and hearing impairment, the differences in total score were significant only between normal and bilateral loss groups
Jacobson & McCaslin	2003	N = 122, groups = normal results, unilateral compensated, unilateral partially compensated, unilateral uncompensated	Significant differences in the total DHI score were observed only between those with normal examinations and the three impaired groups. There were no significant differences in the total DHI score between impaired groups.	The DHI is providing information that cannot be predicted on the basis of impairment alone
McCaslin et al.	2011	N = 92, (62 patients, and 30 controls). Experimental groups were: Group 1, abnormal cVEMP, normal caloric; Group 2, abnormal caloric, normal cVEMP; Group 3, abnormal cVEMP and abnormal caloric; Group 4, normal caloric and normal cVEMP. All patients underwent VNG, rotary chair and posturography testing	Patients with abnormal cVEMP showed significantly impaired postural stability when compared to normals. The group with abnormal cVEMP had better postural stability than the group with abnormal caloric responses alone and the group with both abnormal caloric testing and abnormal cVEMP. Patients with an abnormal cVEMP did not differ significantly on the DHI compared to the other impaired groups	The DHI is providing information that cannot be predicted on the basis of impairment alone
Pelosi et al.	2013	N = 61 (31 with isolated unilateral oVEMP impairment), and 30 with normal vestibular function test results	There were no significant group differences for DHI total scores. Also there were no significant group differences on the HADS.	Although the patients with isolated unilateral utricle impairments had greater postural instability and rocking sensation (not apparent to others) there were no significant group differences in self-report dizziness disability handicap

REFERENCES

Aaronson, N. K. (1992). Assessing the quality of life of patients in cancer clinical trials: Common problems and common sense solutions. *European Journal of Cancer, 28A*(8–9), 1304–1307.

Akin, F. W., & Davenport, M. J. (2003). Validity and reliability of the Motion Sensitivity Test. *Journal of Rehabilitation Research and Development, 40*(5), 415–421.

Alghwiri, A. A., Whitney, S. L., Baker, C. E., Sparto, P. J., Marchetti, G. F., Rogers, J. C., & Furman, J. M. (2012). The development and validation of the vestibular activities and participation measure. *Archives of Physical Medicine and Rehabilitation, 93*(10), 1822–1831.

Antonovsky, A. (1993). The structure and properties of the sense of coherence scale. *Social Science and Medicine, 36*(6), 725–733.

Asmundson, G. J., Stein, M. B., & Ireland, D. (1999). A factor analytic study of the dizziness handicap inventory: Does it assess phobic avoidance in vestibular referrals? *Journal of Vestibular Research, 9*(1), 63–68.

Bamiou, D. E., Davies, R. A., McKee, M., & Luxon, L. M. (1999). The effect of severity of unilateral vestibular dysfunction on symptoms, disabilities and handicap in vertiginous patients. *Clinical Otolaryngology and Allied Sciences, 24*(1), 31–38.

Bandura, A. (1986). *Social foundations of thought and action: A social cognitive theory.* Englewood Cliffs, NJ: Prentice Hall.

Bannigan, K., & Watson, R. (2009). Reliability and validity in a nutshell. *Journal of Clinical Nursing, 18*(23), 3237–3243.

Beck, A. T., Epstein, N., Brown, G., & Steer, R. A. (1988). An inventory for measuring clinical anxiety: Psychometric properties. *Journal of Consulting and Clinical Psychology, 56*(6), 893–897.

Beck, A. T., Ward, C. H., Mendelson, M., Mock, J., & Erbaugh, J. (1961). An inventory for measuring depression. *Archives of General Psychiatry, 4*, 561–571.

Blakley, B. W. (1999). Antidepressants and dizziness. *Journal of Otolaryngology, 28*(6), 313–317.

Bland, J. M., & Altman, D. G. (1986). Statistical methods for assessing agreement between two methods of clinical measurement. *Lancet, 1*(8476), 307–310.

Bogle, J. M., Lundy, L. B., Zapala, D. A., & Copenhaver, A. (2013). Dizziness handicap after cartilage cap occlusion for superior semicircular canal dehiscence. *Otology and Neurotology, 34*(1), 135–140.

Bowling, A. (1997). *Measuring health: A review of quality of life measurement scales* (2nd ed.). Berkshire, England: Open University Press, McGraw-Hill.

Bowling, A. (2005). Mode of questionnaire administration can have serious effects on data quality. *Journal of Public Health (Oxford), 27*(3), 281–291.

Chisolm, T. H., & Abrams, H. B. (2008). Outcome measures and evidence-based practice. In H. Hosford-Dunn, R. J. Roeser, & M. Valente (Eds.), *Audiology: Practice management* (2nd ed., pp. 171–194). New York, NY: Thieme.

Cohen, H. (1992). Vestibular rehabilitation reduces functional disability. *Otolaryngology-Head and Neck Surgery, 107*(5), 638–643.

Cohen, H., & Kimball, K. T. (2000). Development of the vestibular disorders activities of daily living scale. *Archives of Otolaryngology-Head and Neck Surgery, 126*(7), 881–887.

Cohen, H. S., & Kimball, K. T. (2003). Increased independence and decreased vertigo after vestibular rehabilitation. *Otolaryngology-Head and Neck Surgery, 128*(1), 60–70.

Cohen, H. S., Kimball, K. T., & Adams, A. S. (2000). Application of the vestibular disorders activities of daily living scale. *Laryngoscope, 110*(7), 1204–1209.

Cohen, J. (1988). *Statistical power analysis for the behavioral sciences* (2nd ed.). Hillsdale, NJ: Lawrence Erlbaum.

Committee on Hearing and Equilibrium guidelines for the evaluation of hearing preservation in acoustic neuroma (vestibular schwannoma). American Academy of Otolaryngology-Head and Neck Surgery Foundation (1995). *Otolaryngology-Head and Neck Surgery, 113*(3), 179–180.

Crane, B. T., Minor, L. B., & Carey, J. P. (2008). Superior canal dehiscence plugging reduces dizziness handicap. *Laryngoscope, 118*(10), 1809–1813.

Dannenbaum, E., Chilingaryan, G., & Fung, J. (2011). Visual vertigo analogue scale: An assessment questionnaire for visual vertigo. *Journal of Vestibular Research, 21*(3), 153–159.

Demorest, M. E., & DeHaven, G. P. (1993). Psychometric adequacy of self-assessment scales. *Seminars in Hearing, 14*(4), 314–325.

Demorest, M. E., & Walden, B. E. (1984). Psychometric principles in the selection, interpretation, and evaluation of communication self-assessment inventories. *Journal of Speech and Hearing Disorders, 49*(3), 226–240.

Derogatis, L. R., & Melisaratos, N. (1983). The Brief Symptom Inventory: An introductory report. *Psychological Medicine, 13*(3), 595–605.

Detsky, A. S., & Laupacis, A. (2007). Relevance of cost-effectiveness analysis to clinicians and policy makers. *JAMA, 298*(2), 221–224.

Deyo, R. A., & Centor, R. M. (1986). Assessing the responsiveness of functional scales to clinical change: An analogy to diagnostic test performance. *Journal of Chronic Diseases, 39*(11), 897–906.

Deyo, R. A., & Inui, T. S. (1984). Toward clinical applications of health status measures: sensitivity of scales to clinically important changes. *Health Services Research, 19*(3), 275–289.

Erickson, P., Taeuber, R. C., & Scott, J. (1995). Operational aspects of Quality-of-Life Assessment. Choosing the right instrument. *Pharmacoeconomics, 7*(1), 39–48.

EuroQol—a new facility for the measurement of health-related quality of life. (1990). *Health Policy, 16*(3), 199–208.

Fitzpatrick, R., Davey, C., Buxton, M. J., & Jones, D. R. (1998). Evaluating patient-based outcome measures for use in clinical trials. *Health Technology Assessment, 2*(14), i–iv, 1–74.

Folkman, S., & Lazarus, R. S. (1980). An analysis of coping in a middle-aged community sample. *Journal of Health and Social Behavior, 21*(3), 219–239.

Gagliese, L. (2001). Assessment of pain in elderly people. In D. C. Turk & R. Melzack (Eds.), *Handbook of pain assessment* (2nd ed., pp. 119–133). New York, NY: Guilford.

Gamiz, M. J., & Lopez-Escamez, J. A. (2004). Health-related quality of life in patients over sixty years old with benign paroxysmal positional vertigo. *Gerontology, 50*(2), 82–86.

Gates, G. A. (2000). Clinimetrics of Meniere's disease. *Laryngoscope, 110*(3 Pt 3), 8–11.

Gill, T. M., & Feinstein, A. R. (1994). A critical appraisal of the quality of quality-of-life measurements. *JAMA, 272*(8), 619–626.

Gilson, B. S., Gilson, J. S., Bergner, M., Bobbit, R. A., Kressel, S., Pollard, W. E., & Vesselago, M. (1975). The sickness impact profile. Development of an outcome measure of health care. *American Journal of Public Health, 65*(12), 1304–1310.

Goldberg, D. P., & Hillier, V. F. (1979). A scaled version of the General Health Questionnaire. *Psychological Medicine, 9*(1), 139–145.

Guyatt, G. H., & Cook, D. J. (1994). Health status, quality of life, and the individual. *JAMA, 272*(8), 630–631.

Guyatt, G. H., Feeny, D. H., & Patrick, D. L. (1993). Measuring health-related quality of life. *Annals of Internal Medicine, 118*(8), 622–629.

Hambleton, R. K., & Patsula, L. (1998). Adapting tests for use in multiple languages and cultures. *Social Indicators Research, 45*(1–3), 153–171.

Hazlett, R. L., Tusa, R. J., & Waranch, H. R. (1996). Development of an inventory for dizziness and related factors. *Journal of Behavioral Medicine, 19*(1), 73–85.

Hill, K. D., Schwarz, J. A., Kalogeropoulos, A. J., & Gibson, S. J. (1996). Fear of falling revisited. *Archives of Physical Medicine and Rehabilitation, 77*(10), 1025–1029.

Honrubia, V., Bell, T. S., Harris, M. R., Baloh, R. W., & Fisher, L. M. (1996). Quantitative evaluation of dizziness characteristics and impact on quality of life. *American Journal of Otology, 17*(4), 595–602.

Huebner, A. C., Lytle, S. R., Doettl, S. M., Plyler, P. N., & Thelin, J. T. (2013). Treatment of objective and subjective benign paroxysmal positional vertigo. *Journal of the American Academy of Audiology, 24*(7), 600–606.

Hurst, H., & Bolton, J. (2004). Assessing the clinical significance of change scores recorded on subjective outcome measures. *Journal of Manipulative and Physiological Therapeutics, 27*(1), 26–35.

Hyde, M. L. (2000). Reasonable psychometric standards for self-report outcome measures in audiological rehabilitation. *Ear and Hearing, 21*(Suppl. 4), 24S–36S.

Jacobson, G. P., & Calder, J. H. (1998). A screening version of the Dizziness Handicap Inventory (DHI-S). *American Journal of Otology, 19*(6), 804–808.

Jacobson, G. P., & Calder, J. H. (2000). Self-perceived balance disability/handicap in the presence of bilateral peripheral vestibular system impairment. *Journal of the American Academy of Audiology, 11*(2), 76–83.

Jacobson, G. P., & McCaslin, D. L. (2003). Agreement between functional and electrophysiologic measures in patients with unilateral peripheral vestibular system impairment. *Journal of the American Academy of Audiology, 14*(5), 231–238.

Jacobson, G. P., & Newman, C. W. (1990). The development of the Dizziness Handicap Inventory. *Archives of Otolaryngology-Head and Neck Surgery, 116*(4), 424–427.

Jacobson, G. P., Newman, C. W., Hunter, L., & Balzer, G. K. (1991). Balance function test correlates of the Dizziness Handicap Inventory. *Journal of the American Academy of Audiology, 2*(4), 253–260.

Jung, H. J., Koo, J. W., Kim, C. S., Kim, J. S., & Song, J. J. (2012). Anxiolytics reduce residual dizziness after successful canalith repositioning maneuvers in benign paroxysmal positional vertigo. *Acta Oto-Laryngologica, 132*(3), 277–284.

Kazis, L. E., Anderson, J. J., & Meenan, R. F. (1989). Effect sizes for interpreting changes in health status. *Medical Care, 27*(Suppl. 3), S178–S189.

Kinney, S. E., Sandridge, S. A., & Newman, C. W. (1997). Long-term effects of Meniere's disease on hearing and quality of life. *American Journal of Otology, 18*(1), 67–73.

Kruschinski, C., Klaassen, A., Breull, A., Broll, A., & Hummers-Pradier, E. (2010). Priorities of elderly dizzy patients in general practice. Findings and psychometric properties of the "Dizziness Needs Assessment" (DiNA). *Zeitschrift Fur Gerontologie Und Geriatrie, 43*(5), 317–323.

Kurre, A., van Gool, C. J., Bastiaenen, C. H., Gloor-Juzi, T., Straumann, D., & de Bruin, E. D. (2009). Translation, cross-cultural adaptation and reliability of the german version of the dizziness handicap inventory. *Otology and Neurotology, 30*(3), 359–367.

Langguth, B., Searchfield, G. D., Biesinger, E., & Greimel, K. V. (2011). History and questionnaires. In A. R. Møller, L. B., D. DeRidder, & T. Kleinjung (Eds.), *Textbook of tinnitus* (pp. 387–404). New York, NY: Springer.

Leplege, A., & Verdieer, A. (1995). The adaptation of health status measures: Methodological aspects of translation procedures. In S. Shumaker & R. Berson (Eds.), *The international assessment of health-related quality of life: Theory, translation, measurement and analysis* (pp. 93–101). Oxford, England: Rapid Communications of Oxford.

Liang, M. H., Fossel, A. H., & Larson, M. G. (1990). Comparisons of five health status instruments for orthopedic evaluation. *Medical Care, 28*(7), 632–642.

Liang, M. H., Larson, M. G., Cullen, K. E., & Schwartz, J. A. (1985). Comparative measurement efficiency and sensitivity of five health status instruments for arthritis research. *Arthritis and Rheumatology, 28*(5), 542–547.

Lipsey, M. W. (1990). *Design sensitivity: Statistical power for experimental research.* Newbury Park, CA: Sage.

Loughran, S., Gatehouse, S., Kishore, A., & Swan, I. R. (2006). Does patient-perceived handicap correspond to the modified clinical test for the sensory interaction on balance? *Otology and Neurotology, 27*(1), 86–91.

Mann, G. C., Whitney, S. L., Redfern, M. S., Borello-France, D. F., & Furman, J. M. (1996). Functional reach and single leg stance in patients with peripheral vestibular disorders. *Journal of Vestibular Research, 6*(5), 343–353.

McCaslin, D. L., Jacobson, G. P., Grantham, S. L., Piker, E. G., & Verghese, S. (2011). The influence of unilateral saccular impairment on functional balance performance and self-report dizziness. *Journal of the American Academy of Audiology, 22*(8), 542–549.

Megnigbeto, C. A., Sauvage, J. P., & Launois, R. (2001). [The European Evaluation of Vertigo (EEV) scale: A clinical validation study]. *Revue de Laryngologie-Otologie-Rhinologie, 122*(2), 95–102.

Miller, W. C., Deathe, A. B., & Speechley, M. (2003). Psychometric properties of the Activities-specific Balance Confidence Scale among individuals with a lower-limb amputation. *Archives of Physical Medicine and Rehabilitation, 84*(5), 656–661.

Monzani, D., Casolari, L., Guidetti, G., & Rigatelli, M. (2001). Psychological distress and disability in patients with vertigo. *Journal of Psychosomatic Research, 50*(6), 319–323.

Morris, A. E., Lutman, M. E., & Yardley, L. (2009). Measuring outcome from vestibular rehabilitation, part II: Refinement and validation of a new self-report measure. *International Journal of Audiology, 48*(1), 24–37.

Newman, C. W., Weinstein, B. E., Jacobson, G. P., & Hug, G. A. (1990). The Hearing Handicap Inventory for Adults: Psychometric adequacy and audiometric correlates. *Ear and Hearing, 11*(6), 430–433.

Noble, W. (2013). Self-assessment in adult audiologic rehabilitation: Research applications. In J. J. Montano & J. B. Spitzer (Eds.), *Adult audiologic rehabilitation* (2nd ed., pp. 75–88). San Diego, CA: Plural.

Norman, G. R., Stratford, P., & Regehr, G. (1997). Methodological problems in the retrospective computation of responsiveness to change: The lesson of Cronbach. *Journal of Clinical Epidemiology, 50*(8), 869–879.

Norre, M. E., & Beckers, A. (1989). Vestibular habituation training for positional vertigo in elderly patients. *Archives of Gerontology and Geriatrics, 8*(2), 117–122.

Park, S. S., Grills, I. S., Bojrab, D., Pieper, D., Kartush, J., Maitz, A., . . . Chen, P. (2011). Longitudinal assessment of quality of life and audiometric test outcomes in vestibular schwannoma patients treated with gamma knife surgery. *Otology and Neurotology, 32*(4), 676–679.

Pelosi, S., Schuster, D., Jacobson, G. P., Carlson, M. L., Haynes, D. S., Bennett, M. L., . . . Wanna, G. B. (2013). Clinical characteristics associated with isolated unilateral utricular dysfunction. *American Journal of Otolaryngology, 34*(5), 490–495.

Perez, N., Garmendia, I., Garcia-Granero, M., Martin, E., & Garcia-Tapia, R. (2001). Factor analysis and correlation between Dizziness Handicap Inventory and Dizziness Characteristics and Impact on Quality of Life scales. *Acta Oto-Laryngologica Supplementum, 545*, 145–154.

Perez, N., Martin, E., & Garcia-Tapia, R. (2003). Dizziness: Relating the severity of vertigo to the degree of handicap by measuring vestibular impairment. *Otolaryngology-Head and Neck Surgery, 128*(3), 372–381.

Piker, E. G., Jacobson, G. P., McCaslin, D. L., & Grantham, S. L. (2008). Psychological comorbidities and their relationship to self-reported handicap in samples of dizzy patients. *Journal of the American Academy of Audiology, 19*(4), 337–347.

Pollock, B. E., Driscoll, C. L., Foote, R. L., Link, M. J., Gorman, D. A., Bauch, C. D., . . . Johnson, C. H. (2006). Patient outcomes after vestibular schwannoma management: A prospective comparison of microsurgical resection and stereotactic radiosurgery. *Neurosurgery, 59*(1), 77–85; discussion 77–85.

Powell, L. E., & Myers, A. M. (1995). The Activities-specific Balance Confidence (ABC) Scale. *Journals of Gerontology. Series A, Biological Sciences and Medical Sciences, 50A*(1), M28–34.

Prieto, L., Santed, R., Cobo, E., & Alonso, J. (1999). A new measure for assessing the health-related quality of life of patients with vertigo, dizziness or imbalance:

The VDI questionnaire. *Quality of Life Research, 8*(1–2), 131–139.

Ramos, R. T. (2006). Antidepressants and dizziness. *Journal of Psychopharmacology, 20*(5), 708–713.

Robertson, D. D., & Ireland, D. J. (1995). Dizziness Handicap Inventory correlates of computerized dynamic posturography. *Journal of Otolaryngology, 24*(2), 118–124.

Ruckenstein, M. J., & Staab, J. P. (2001). The Basic Symptom Inventory-53 and its use in the management of patients with psychogenic dizziness. *Otolaryngology-Head and Neck Surgery, 125*(5), 533–536.

Ryckman, R. M., Robbins, M. A., Thornton, B., & Cantrell, P. (1982). Development and validation of a physical self-efficacy scale. *Journal of Personality and Social Psychology, 42*(5), 891–900.

Salmon, P., & Quine, J. (1989). Patients' intentions in primary care: Measurement and preliminary investigation. *Psychology and Health, 3*(2), 103–110.

Scott, J., & Huskisson, E. C. (1979). Accuracy of subjective measurements made with or without previous scores—an important source of error in serial measurement of subjective states. *Annals of the Rheumatic Diseases, 38*(6), 558–559.

Shaffer, B. T., Cohen, M. S., Bigelow, D. C., & Ruckenstein, M. J. (2010). Validation of a disease-specific quality-of-life instrument for acoustic neuroma: The Penn Acoustic Neuroma Quality-of-Life Scale. *Laryngoscope, 120*(8), 1646–1654.

Shaia, W. T., Zappia, J. J., Bojrab, D. I., LaRouere, M. L., Sargent, E. W., & Diaz, R. C. (2006). Success of posterior semicircular canal occlusion and application of the Dizziness Handicap Inventory. *Otolaryngology-Head and Neck Surgery, 134*(3), 424–430.

Shepard, N. T., Smith-Wheelock, M., Telian, S. A., & Raj, A. (1993). Vestibular and balance rehabilitation therapy. *Annals of Otology Rhinology and Laryngology, 102*(3), 198–205.

Shum, D., O'Gorman, J., & Myors, B. (2006). *Psychological testing and assessment.* New York, NY: Oxford University Press.

Siegel, J. E., Weinstein, M. C., Russell, L. B., & Gold, M. R. (1996). Recommendations for reporting cost-effectiveness analyses. Panel on Cost-Effectiveness in Health and Medicine. *Journal of the American Medical Association, 276*(16), 1339–1341.

Simon, N. M., Parker, S. W., Wernick-Robinson, M., Oppenheimer, J. E., Hoge, E. A., Worthington, J. J., . . . Pollack, M. H. (2005). Fluoxetine for vestibular dysfunction and anxiety: A prospective pilot study. *Psychosomatics, 46*(4), 334–339.

Smith, S. L., & West, R. L. (2006). The application of self-efficacy principles to audiologic rehabilitation: A tutorial. *American Journal of Audiology, 15*(1), 46–56.

Smith-Wheelock, M., Shepard, N. T., & Telian, S. A. (1991). Physical therapy program for vestibular rehabilitation. *American Journal of Otology, 12*(3), 218–225.

Spielberger, C. D. (1984). *State-trait anxiety inventory: A comprehensive bibliography.* Palo Alto, CA: Consulting Psychologists Press.

Spitzer, R. L., Kroenke, K., & Williams, J. B. (1999). Validation and utility of a self-report version of PRIME-MD: The PHQ primary care study. Primary Care Evaluation of Mental Disorders. Patient Health Questionnaire. *JAMA, 282*(18), 1737–1744.

Staab. (2012). Chronic subjective dizziness. *Continuum (Minneapolis, Minnesota), 18*(5 Neuro-otology), 1118–1141.

Staab, J. P., Ruckenstein, M. J., & Amsterdam, J. D. (2004). A prospective trial of sertraline for chronic subjective dizziness. *Laryngoscope, 114*(9), 1637–1641.

Stewart, A. L., Hays, R. D., & Ware, J. E., Jr. (1988). The MOS short-form general health survey. Reliability and validity in a patient population. *Medical Care, 26*(7), 724–735.

Stewart, B. J., & Archbold, P. G. (1992). Focus on psychometrics—nursing intervention studies require outcome measures that are sensitive to change .1. *Research in Nursing & Health, 15*(6), 477–481.

Streiner, D. L., & Norman, G. R. (1995). *Health measurement scales: A practical guide to their development and use* (2nd ed.). New York, NY: Oxford University Press.

Tesio, L., Alpini, D., Cesarani, A., & Perucca, L. (1999). Short form of the Dizziness Handicap Inventory: Construction and validation through Rasch analysis. *American Journal of Physical Medicine and Rehabilitation, 78*(3), 233–241.

Tinetti, M. E., Richman, D., & Powell, L. (1990). Falls efficacy as a measure of fear of falling. *Journals of Gerontology, 45*(6), P239–P243.

Ustun, T. B., Chatterji, S., Kostanjsek, N., Rehm, J., Kennedy, C., Epping-Jordan, J., . . . Pull, C. (2010). Developing the World Health Organization Disability Assessment Schedule 2.0. *Bulletin of the World Health Organization, 88*(11), 815–823.

Wackym, P. A., Hannley, M. T., Runge-Samuelson, C. L., Jensen, J., & Zhu, Y. R. (2008). Gamma knife surgery of vestibular schwannomas: Longitudinal changes in vestibular function and measurement of the Dizziness Handicap Inventory. *Journal of Neurosurgery,* (Suppl. 109), 137–143.

Whitney, S. L., Hudak, M. T., & Marchetti, G. F. (1999). The activities-specific balance confidence scale and the dizziness handicap inventory: A comparison. *Journal of Vestibular Research, 9*(4), 253–259.

Whitney, S. L., Marchetti, G. F., & Morris, L. O. (2005). Usefulness of the dizziness handicap inventory in the screening for benign paroxysmal positional vertigo. *Otology and Neurotology, 26*(5), 1027–1033.

Whitney, S. L., Wrisley, D. M., Brown, K. E., & Furman, J. M. (2004). Is perception of handicap related to functional performance in persons with vestibular dysfunction? *Otology and Neurotology, 25*(2), 139–143.

WHO. (1980). *International Classification of Impairments, Disabilities and Handicaps: A manual of classification relating to the consequences of disease* (pp. 1–205). Published in accordance with resolution WHA 29.35 of the Twenty-ninth World Health Assembly, Geneva. Geneva, Switzerland: Author.

WHO. (2002). http://www.cdc.gov/nchs/icd.htm

The World Health Organization Quality of Life assessment (WHOQOL): Position paper from the World Health Organization. (1995). *Social Science and Medicine, 41*(10), 1403–1409.

Yardley, L., Barker, F., Muller, I., Turner, D., Kirby, S., Mullee, M., . . . Little, P. (2012). Clinical and cost effectiveness of booklet based vestibular rehabilitation for chronic dizziness in primary care: Single blind, parallel group, pragmatic, randomised controlled trial. *British Medical Journal, 344*, e2237.

Yardley, L., Beech, S., & Weinman, J. (2001). Influence of beliefs about the consequences of dizziness on handicap in people with dizziness, and the effect of therapy on beliefs. *Journal of Psychosomatic Research, 50*(1), 1–6.

Yardley, L., & Hallam, R. S. (1996). Psychosocial aspects of balance and gait disorders. In A. M. Bronstein, T. Brandt, & M. H. Woolacott (Eds.), *Clinical disorders of balance, posture and gait* (pp. 251–267). London, UK: Arnold.

Yardley, L., Masson, E., Verschuur, C., Haacke, N., & Luxon, L. (1992). Symptoms, anxiety and handicap in dizzy patients: Development of the vertigo symptom scale. *Journal of Psychosomatic Research, 36*(8), 731–741.

Yardley, L., & Putman, J. (1992). Quantitative analysis of factors contributing to handicap and distress in vertiginous patients: A questionnaire study. *Clinical Otolaryngology and Allied Sciences, 17*(3), 231–236.

Yardley, L., Todd, A. M., Lacoudraye-Harter, M. M., & Ingham, R. (1992). Psychosocial consequences of recurrent vertigo. *Psychology and Health, 6*(1–2), 85–96.

Yates, B. J., & Miller, A. D. (1998). Physiological evidence that the vestibular system participates in autonomic and respiratory control. *Journal of Vestibular Research, 8*(1), 17–25.

Zigmond, A. S., & Snaith, R. P. (1983). The Hospital Anxiety and Depression Scale. *Acta Psychiatrica Scandinavica, 67*(6), 361–370.

Background and Technique of Ocular Motility Testing

Neil T. Shepard and Michael C. Schubert

INTRODUCTION

In the evaluation of the dizzy patient, the eyes provide the most direct access to the evaluation of the peripheral vestibular system anatomy and physiology. However, the pathways from the labyrinthine structures involve significant neurologic substrate in the brainstem and cerebellum with controlling influence from higher centers in the midbrain and cerebral cortex. Therefore, correct interpretation of eye movements relative to the periphery rely on normal function of the central pathways. Also, symptoms of dizziness can result from lesions in the central neural pathways or at the central nuclei. Secondary to these issues, it becomes important to use the eyes as our window into the central nervous system controlling structures for eye movements that function independently of the peripheral vestibular system. The anatomy and physiology of the ocular motor system is presented in detail in Chapter 2. The purpose of this chapter is to describe the routine procedures available for assessing these central ocular motor structures with interpretation of those results provided in Chapter 10. The discussion is limited to test protocols that can be routinely performed in the vast majority of hospital and private office facilities. The reader interested in more depth of discussion of both the routine and esoteric protocols and their interpretation is referred to other dedicated publications (Leigh & Zee, 2006).

As one approaches the assessment of the ocular motor system functioning independently of the peripheral vestibular system (during head still examinations), four principal ocular control events are evaluated. These include the following:

1. Saccade testing—This is the ability to move the eyes in a rapid single movement to refixate a target of interest onto the fovea (the most sensitive part of the retina) for clear viewing.
2. Smooth pursuit tracking—This is the ability to track the movement of a target of interest maintaining the image on the fovea with smooth continuous eye movements as opposed to tracking with the use of repeated saccades.
3. Gaze stability—This refers to the ability to maintain gaze stable without the generation of other eye movements (principally jerk nystagmus) while looking straight ahead (primary), left, right, up, and down.
4. Optokinetic nystagmus—This is the development of reflexive eye movements in the form of jerk nystagmus during the visualization of moving objects that fill 80% to 90% or greater of the visual field of view. Ostensibly, the purpose for the generation of the nystagmus is to assist clear visual viewing when the head is in constant velocity motion, or the head is still and objects of interest are moving in a regular manner, or both are moving at constant velocities that are

not equal, thus rendering the vestibulo-ocular reflex unable to maintain clear visual world viewing.

ELECTRODE VERSUS VIDEO TECHNIQUES

Chapter 5 provides a complete discussion of the eye movement recording techniques; however, it is useful to briefly review issues specific to the ocular motor assessment when using different recording methods. The primary advantage of using a computerized system for ENG or VNG is the ability to perform ocular motor testing in a manner that uses a repeatable and controllable stimulus with the ability to compare the analysis of the patient's performance to a quantitative normative database that can be both age and gender specific as required. Secondary to the importance of accurate stimulus presentation and comparison against age and gender-sensitive normative performance, this chapter does not discuss the testing with noncomputerized systems.

As the affordability and availability of video nystagmography systems has increased, a significant percentage of facilities providing for the evaluation and management of the dizzy patient have changed to video-recording techniques. It is important to realize that the use of electrode recording is still needed in virtually all facilities for those eyes that cannot be adequately recorded and quantified with a video system and especially when performing tests of this nature on children under the age of five (see Chapter 25 for detailed discussion). Specific to the ocular motor testing is the representation of the velocity of the eye. Accurate representation of peak speeds that can achieve 400 to 500 degrees/second requires sampling rates of greater than 100 Hz (Leigh & Zee, 2006). Although the electrode systems can provide for 100-Hz rate of sampling, the majority of video systems are only between 30 and 60 Hz. The consequence of this low rate of sample is that you do not get accurate peak velocity but an averaged velocity for the fast eye movements like those encountered in performing saccades. It is important to recognize this issue as we talk about peak velocity in the interpretation of the saccade. This does not render the test unreliable as the normative data against which individual performance is compared

are also taken from sampling at less than 100 Hz. This situation would also reduce the sensitivity of the use of eye velocity to differentiate the effects of certain disorders or medications on the status of patients. New ANSI standards released in 2009 contain recommendations for equipment parameters that address this issue and recognize the changes in video camera equipment that will improve affordability of high-speed camera systems (American National Standard ANSI S3.45-2009).

The other concern in ocular motor testing is the level of background noise in the recording trace. This is of particular interest in identifying square wave jerks, a form of saccade intrusions, which can be a small as 0.5 to 1 degrees of subtended arc movement of the eye (Leigh & Zee, 2006). In this regard, the video systems are superior to the use of the electrodes techniques because of the reduction in background noise. Second, the use of individual eye recordings during an electronystagmography (ENG)/videonystagmography (VNG) is primarily only needed during certain ocular motor tasks (saccades and occasionally smooth pursuit). When this is attempted with the use of the electrode system, even in systems where the use of medial canthus electrodes are not needed, the signal-to-noise ratio is effectively reduced by a factor of two. This makes recognizing a small eye movement more difficult in the presence of that level of background noise. Using a video system, the signal-to-noise level does not change in going from monocular to binocular recordings; however, to do binocular recordings will require two cameras in some, but not all, of the commercial systems available.

SACCADE TESTING

Technical Considerations

To assess saccadic eye movement, targets need to be presented that require sudden rapid movements of the eyes. In the past this has been accomplished with the use of fixed targets placed on a wall or screen such that when the patient was seated at a particular distance from the target plane eye movements to each target from the center would require a 10- to 15-degree subtended arc movement of the eyes. This task was used for calibration of the system and for a cursory evaluation of volitional saccades. With the use of computerized systems, targets can now be presented via light bars or through video projection systems. More importantly, the task can be either that of presenting fixed position targets or targets that appear randomly in different positions in the horizontal or vertical planes. Also, it is possible to present the targets at random time intervals together with the random location. Although fixed target location and timing are used for certain paradigms, producing volitional saccades (predictable targets), the use of random saccade testing is preferable in the overall evaluation to elicit reflexive saccades (ability to react when a target of interest suddenly appears at a new location). A more complete discussion of the protocols for clinical use follows below. Targets fixed or random are usually presented within a ±30-degree range of subtended arc movement of the eye. As mentioned above it is with saccade tasks specifically that the use of a broad band-pass filter of 10 to 100 Hz and a sampling rate of a minimum of 60 Hz with 100 Hz or higher are advised by the new ANSI standards for ENG/VNG (American National Standard ANSI S3.45-2009).

It is also with this task that individual eye evaluation is the preferred technique. This is secondary to the need to recognize disorders involved with dysconjugate eye movements such as intranuclear ophthalmoplegia (see Chapter 10 for details). Although individual eye recording with smooth pursuit can elucidate nonyoked eye movements, the effect is more easily detected during saccade testing. If using EOG for this task, additional electrodes may need to be placed near the medial canthus of each eye paired with those at the lateral canthus to obtain individual horizontal eye movements. A second pair of vertical electrodes would then allow for complete individual eye monitoring in the vertical plane. By adding the additional electrodes and using full individual eye recordings the signal to noise ratio is reduced by a factor of two. Recording torsional eye rotation is not possible with electrodes due to the absence of a change in the relative polarity for rotations about the roll plane.

Parameters for Analysis

The features of saccadic eye movements used for the clinical analysis are measures of the delay of the eye movement after the target has moved (latency), the speed at which the eye moves (eye velocity), and the accuracy of the movement. Each of these parameters is considered as a function of the excursion of the eye movement, not the distance the target has moved. Therefore, if you have a 15-degree target movement to the left but the eye only moves 12 degrees, the latency, velocity, and accuracy are calculated and presented as a function of a 12-degree movement (Figure 9–1).

Refer to the bottom two panels of Figure 9–1 as we define each of the analysis parameters:

- Velocity—the plot on the left presents the main sequence plot. This is a plot of the peak velocity of the eye movement during the trajectory from the initial point of regard to the new eye location. Note that if the sampling rate is less than 100 Hz the plot is more representative of the average velocity not truly peak velocity. The eye velocities are plotted as a function of the excursion distance of the eye in degrees of subtended arc movement.
- Accuracy—the center plot gives the percentage of the distance the eye moved in its first single movement relative to that of the target as a function of eye movement excursion. One hundred percent indicates that the eye moved the same distance as the target in a single major excursion. Values over 100% indicate an overshoot, whereas those under 100% show an undershoot.
- Latency—the final plot to the right reflects the lapsed time in milliseconds from the initiation of the target movement to the initiation of the eye movement, again as a function of eye movement excursion.

In each of the plots, the abnormal region defined as two standard deviations below the mean in the main sequence plot, two standard deviations above and below the mean in the accuracy plot, and two standard deviations above the mean in the latency plot are shown by the stippled region. Age-related normative data are not indicated for routine clinical analysis of saccade testing by either fixed, random, or remembered paradigms (Hain, 1993; Leigh & Zee, 2006; Shepard & Telian, 1996). A sample of normative data for individual eye recordings

Saccade-Random

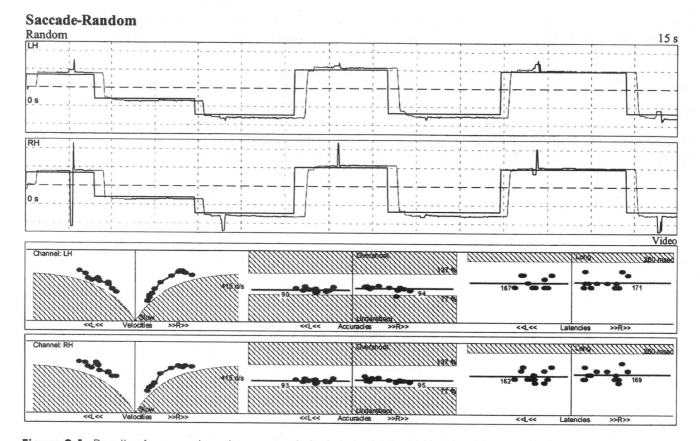

Figure 9–1. Results of a normal random saccade test via individual eye video recordings on a 49-year-old female diagnosed with unilateral vestibular hypofunction secondary to vestibular neuronitis. The top two panels provide a sample of the traces showing the target in the dark line and the left and right recorded eye movements in the lighter line. The left eye is in the top panel with the right eye in the second panel. The third and fourth panels give the quantitative analysis for the saccade test. Each dot represents the analysis of a single saccade out of the total of 30 presented for the test. From the left to the right in both the third and fourth panels the plots are for velocity (main sequence plot), accuracy, and latency all as a function of the excursions of the eyes. The left eye analysis is in panel three with the right eye analysis in the fourth panel.

(electro-oculography techniques) from 46 subjects of age 19 to 49, 15 of age 50 to 69, 8 from 70 to 79, and 7 from 80 to 88 is shown in Figure 9–2. In the figure the population responses with means and two standard deviation ranges are given for all three parameters discussed above. In the main sequence plot in Figure 9–2, abduction velocities are lower than adduction velocities. This is a finding that has been reported previously (Boghen, Troost, Daroff, Dell'Osso, & Birkett, 1974) again by the use of electro-oculography (EOG) recording techniques. In this work it was determined that a consistent relationship between the peak velocity and the size of the excursion of the saccade was present—the larger the excursion of

the saccade the higher the peak velocity up to about 500 degrees/second. It was also demonstrated that the duration of the saccade also lengthened with the increase in excursion up to about 100 ms. This duration is shorter than that needed to obtain visual feedback implying that adjustments in the speed of the saccade and the final destination of the eye movement cannot be adjusted while the saccadic eye movement is in progress. Comparisons with other eye movement recording techniques suggest that this may be unique to the use of EOG techniques as use of scleral search coils and infrared reflections show the opposite (Leigh & Zee, 2006). In a direct comparison between video-oculography (VOG) and

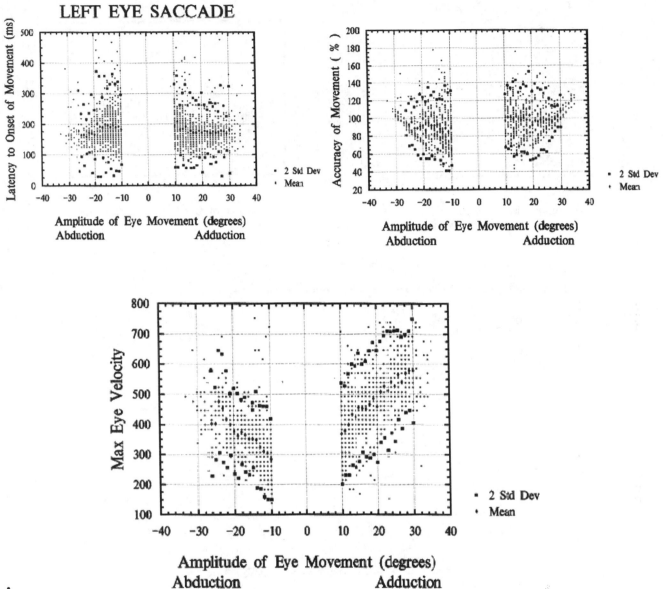

A

Figure 9–2. A. Shown are the individual eye data for a random saccade paradigm for the left eye of the 76 subjects with age distributions as given in the text. The graph on the top left gives latency to onset of saccade eye movements, the top right plots percent accuracy, and the bottom graph shows the peak velocity all as a function of the excursion of the eye. *continues*

search coils for saccade, smooth pursuit and optokinetic nystagmus in both an artificial and human eye during roll plane rotation, the mean difference between the VOG and the search coil was 0.56, 0.78, and 0.18 degrees of rotation for the roll, pitch, and yaw (horizontal) planes, respectively (Imai et al., 2005). The implication from this is that normative data for saccade testing need to be those developed from the video recordings but if EOG techniques are used then the normative ranges for comparison should be those developed with the EOG technique. It has not been demonstrated, irrespective of the recording technique, that age-related normative ranges are needed for the clinical study of saccades.

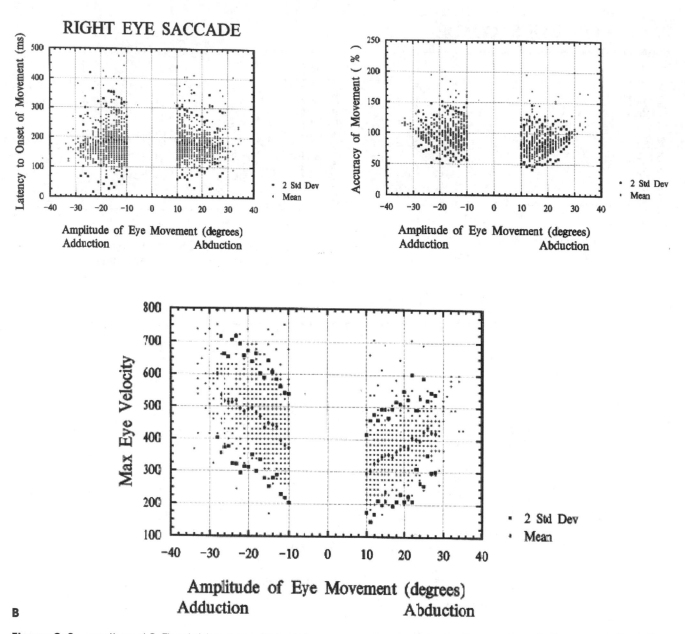

Figure 9-2. *continued* **B.** The right eye results for latency, accuracy, and velocity are given in the same orientation as in part A. From Shepard, N. T., and Telian, S. A., 1996, pp. 100–103. Used with permission.

Protocols

Fixed Time and Location

The simplest of the protocols used with a computerized system presents the target in a fixed location with a fixed time interval between the target presentations. In this format the same analysis parameters would be used to characterize performance; however, the abscissa for each plot should have only minimal variation in eye excursion. This situation has the target positions known to the patient after the first two presentations and tasks a somewhat different neurologic substrate than when the location and time between target presentations are random (Leigh & Zee, 2006).

Random Saccades

The protocol presents a target randomly within the horizontal or vertical plane then disappears and immediately reappears in a new location (Video 9–1). The task stimulates a reactionary saccadic eye movement to a new target of interest (see Figure 9–2). This protocol has become a frequently used paradigm associated with the use of computerized systems, either ENG or VNG. In this protocol both the position of the target and the time interval between target presentations can be randomized. As discussed in Chapter 10 the neurologic substrate assessed with this test emphasizes posterior cerebellum and various areas of the brainstem (Leigh & Zee, 2006). The random saccade test is more challenging than the fixed position and timing task. As a result it is suspected to bring forth more subtle abnormalities in the central ocular motor pathways involved in saccade production than the fixed position/time paradigm.

Antisaccade Test

This protocol allows for testing of the ability to suppress a reflexive saccade. It is used to suggest possible abnormalities dominantly in the frontal eye fields (Machado & Rafal, 2004). Unlike the other routine paradigms, analysis of this test is simply the ability to make the eyes move opposite the target movement. The test is performed by the presentation of a fixed position and timing stimulus in the horizontal plane. The patient is instructed and coached to move the eyes in the direction opposite of the target movement. This may require a short practice, but once the patient begins with the correct execution of the task they can typically continue with multiple saccades in succession. Once a demonstration of correct performance over 5 to 10 saccades is noted, the test is terminated. Analysis is qualitative as the computerized systems currently on the market do not usually provide for a means to analyze automatically. Children can perform this task by adolescence (Fukaushima, Hatta, & Fukushima, 2000) and the latency to execution of the task increases with increasing age (Butler, Zacks, & Henderson, 1999).

Although other protocols can and have been used with saccade testing the ones given above represent the principal tests used in the routine evaluation of the dizzy patient. The interested reader is referred to other sources for additional evaluation protocols (Leigh & Zee, 2006).

SMOOTH PURSUIT TRACKING

Technical Considerations

General filter setting would be the same as for saccade testing with a low-pass filter at 100 Hz and a high-pass filter, if used, at 3 to 10 Hz. Like saccade testing a 60-Hz notch filter can be used as required. For pursuit tracking the issue of the sampling rate of the video or electrode system is not as critical as in saccade testing given the much slower eye velocity being captured. Whereas many systems will provide for binocular individual eye recording, the simultaneous individual eye recording is not as clinically revealing as with saccade evaluation. However, if this feature is available in the video systems, it can be of use as usually a selection of either the right or the left eye can be used for analysis, thus allowing for optimization of the analysis if a poor recording was obtained for technical reasons for only one eye.

What is critical with this evaluation is the use of age-sensitive normative data. Changes in performance of pursuit tracking can be seen starting in the third or fourth decades of life (Paige, 1994). Figure 9–3 shows the effects of age and the frequency of target presentation on the outcome parameter of pursuit velocity gain (discussed below). A full set of normative data for individual eye electrode recordings for all outcome parameters as a function of age are reprinted in Table 9–1 for reference (Shepard & Telian, 1996). The data given in Table 9–1 are from subjects ranging in age from 20 to 80 years with 8 to 10 normal subjects in each decade. These data are for horizontal smooth pursuit testing. Statistical analysis showed significant differences at the $p = 0.05$ level criteria for age grouping shown in the table. For all the smooth pursuit frequencies the excursion of the target was a 17.5-degree peak (movement to either side of center). These data were developed using EOG technique. The authors are not aware of published normative data as a function

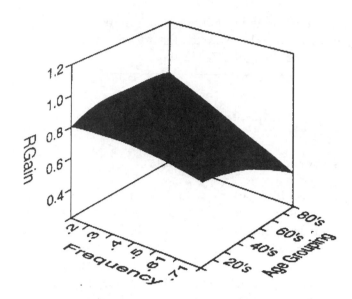

Figure 9–3. A modeling of smooth pursuit data acquired from normal volunteers as a function of age groupings (on the x-axis) and frequency of target movement (on the y-axis). The pursuit outcome parameter of velocity gain (see text for explanation) for the left eye is shown on the z-axis. The modeled data were developed using a negative exponential weighting function. From Shepard, N. T., and Telian, S. A., 1996, p. 26. Used with permission.

of age developed using video recordings. It is the use of age-sensitive normative data that improves the overall performance of smooth pursuit testing, not by increasing sensitivity but by increasing the specificity of the test.

Attention to the stimulus for smooth pursuit tracking by fixed velocity (ramp) or varying acceleration/velocity (sinusoidal) target protocols (see below) can maximize performance. The brighter the target and the larger the target are both features that improve performance (Hutton & Tegally, 2005). Even if the visual field is filled with the stimulus it is the central portion of the fovea that dominates the response (van den Berg & Collewijin, 1986; Van Die & Collewijin, 1986).

For smooth pursuit tracking as well as for saccade testing, these are novel tasks for the patient. Even though the ocular motor tasks are used throughout an individual's daily routines they are not used in a focused and isolated manner as when testing. Therefore, to achieve maximum performance the

tasks may have to be repeated with coaching multiple times. It is important not to accept the first trial for saccades or pursuit tracking as adequate performance unless the first trial is either normal or explainable by age-related normative data.

Parameters for Analysis

Here as with saccades the specifics of the analysis are dependent on the manufacture of the equipment being used, unless the facility has the capability to develop their own computer sampling and analysis techniques. That said there are three parameters more commonly seen with routine ENG/VNG analysis of smooth pursuit. These usually assume the use of a sinusoidal protocol (see discussion below). For this discussion refer to Table 9–1 and Figure 9–4.

Velocity gain is indirectly a measure of how sinusoidal the eye movement was in comparison to the target. The gain value is calculated by a ratio of peak eye velocity divided by peak target velocity. Figure 9–4 presents a plot of the overall combined velocity gain without regard to movement of the eye leftward or rightward. Other examples of velocity gain displays showing the individual gain for eye movements in each direction are provided with the discussion of analysis in Chapter 10. If the eye tracked the target in a perfect manner, the gain would be expected to be one. As saccadic disruptions in the eye movement occur, this introduces discontinuities that reduce the sinusoidal behavior of the eye movement and result in gain values less than unity. The mathematical process to determine the actual gain is manufacturer specific. As noted in the left-most plots in the second and third panels of Figure 9–4, the stippled region represents the age-related low range of normal (two standard deviations below the mean) for persons 49 years old.

Asymmetry, shown in the middle plot of panels 2 and 3 in Figure 9–4, is simply the percentage difference for velocity gain for the right or left eye moving rightward and leftward. This provides a means to indicate asymmetric performance in smooth pursuit tracking for rightward versus leftward eye movements.

Phase angle, the third parameter, provides a measure of how much the eye is lagging or leading

Table 9-1. Normative Data

Age 20–49 Years						
	0.2	**0.3**	**0.4**	**0.5**	**0.61**	**0.71**
Gain L	0.82 0.42–1.22	0.84 0.64–1.04	0.82 0.62–1.02	0.83 0.63–1.03	0.72 0.32–1.12	0.71 0.37–0.95
Gain R	0.85 0.45–1.25	0.84 0.58–1.1	0.87 0.67–1.07	0.82 0.62–1.02	0.78 0.52–1.04	0.73 0.39–0.97
Phase	−0.36 6.36–5.64	−0.13 4.13–3.87	−0.25 4.25–3.75	−1.85 7.85–4.15	−2.36 8.36–3.64	−4.72 12.72–3.2

Age 50–69 Years						
	0.2	**0.3**	**0.4**	**0.5**	**0.61**	**0.71**
Gain L	0.86 0.56–1.16	0.82 0.60–1.04	0.82 0.58–1.06	0.78 0.50–1.06	0.69 0.39–0.99	0.61 0.27–0.95
Gain R	0.83 0.53–1.13	0.84 0.56–1.12	0.80 0.56–1.04	0.76 0.40–1.12	0.73 0.43–1.03	0.66 0.32–1.00
Phase	−0.4 6.40	−0.79 4.79–3.21	−0.89 4.89–3.11	−2.38 8.38–3.62	−5.06 13.06–2.9	−7.89 17.89–2.1

Age 70–79 Years						
	0.2	**0.3**	**0.4**	**0.5**	**0.61**	**0.71**
Gain L	0.90 0.68–1.12	0.82 0.60–1.04	0.75 0.45–1.05	0.7 0.34–1.06	0.63 0.27–0.99	0.48 0.08–0.88
Gain R	0.87 0.59–1.15	0.85 0.65–1.05	0.8 0.6–1.00	0.7 0.4–1.00	0.68 0.46–0.9	0.5 0.24–0.76
Phase	0.13 3.87–4.13	−0.01 3.81–3.79	−1.4 −6.8–4.0	−2.32 −10.3–5.7	−4.2 −11.4–3.0	−3.7 −12.7–5.3

Age 80–89 Years						
	0.2	**0.3**	**0.4**	**0.5**	**0.61**	**0.71**
Gain L	0.77 0.49–1.05	0.81 0.61–1.01	0.76 0.54–0.97	0.7 0.54–0.96	0.61 0.27–0.95	0.6 0.38–0.82
Gain R	0.83 0.57–1.09	0.8 0.5–1.1	0.71 0.39–1.03	0.61 0.31–0.91	0.63 0.29–0.97	0.6 0.23–0.87
Phase	−0.49 4.29–3.32	−2.64 −12–6.8	−2.3 −6.3–1.7	−4.07 −14.1–5.9	−7.8 −15.8–0.2	−8.9 −20.9–3.1

the target. In general, given the instructions to follow or track the target it is expected that the eyes will be in phase with the target or be minimally lagging behind. Patients who consistently lead the target do so with saccadic movements and usually do not understand the task requested of them.

Pursuit repeat 1

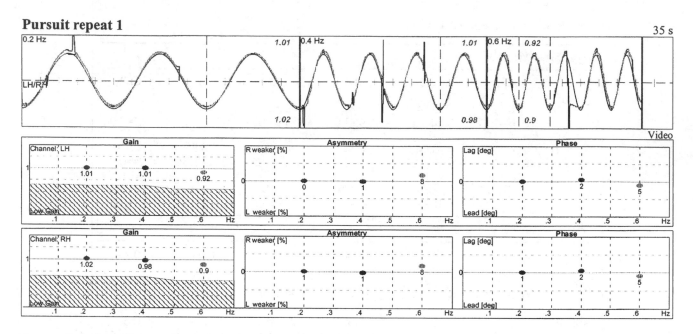

Figure 9-4. Smooth pursuit analysis shown is from a 49-year-old female being evaluated for possible vestibular neuritis event. The top panel shows the left eye raw movement and the right raw eye trace, superimposed for each of the three frequencies tested; 0.2, 0.4, and 0.6 Hz. The testing was done using a video-recording system with the peak excursion of the target at 15° subtended arc. The second and third panels provide the analysis for velocity gain, asymmetry in velocity gain in percentage, and phase angle between the target movement and the eye movement in degrees each as a function of frequency of the target, as seen from left to right (refer to the text for an explanation of the parameters). The second panel is for the left eye whereas the third is for the right.

Protocols

Sinusoidal Target

This represents the most commonly used method for testing smooth pursuit tracking abilities. The target is presented via a light bar or projection system moving with a sinusoidal trajectory (see Video 9–1). The peak excursion of the target would be fixed between 15 and 20 degrees of subtended arc movement to either side of center. The excursion is maintained the same and the frequency of the target is varied between 0.2 and 0.8 Hz, thereby increasing the difficulty of the task. It is suggested that subtle abnormalities may be detected by increasing the task difficulty to evaluate the smooth pursuit system across its full physiologic range. However, in doing such and given the age effect on smooth pursuit, it is critical to have age-sensitive normative data to prevent false-positive identifications of pathology that actually represent degraded performance secondary to age alone. It is

this paradigm that typically uses some version of the three major analysis parameters in interpretation.

Fixed Velocity Pursuit

For some patients the sinusoidal movements of a target produces nausea, this results in poor performance or inability to complete the task. An alternative is the fixed-velocity smooth pursuit task. In this paradigm the target can be presented moving left to right (or the reverse) at a speed of 20 to 40 deg/s. Each target traverses the light bar or within the video projection field and a new target is presented at the same speed and in the same direction. After several samples, the direction is reversed now moving right to left at the same speed. The alternative to constant direction is to use a triangular waveform to produce the stimulus target movement. In this case the target moves left to right and then reverses back right to left. Be aware that, as the target makes a sudden stop and sudden change in direction, smooth pursuit performance will be less than perfect as the smooth pursuit system does not handle abrupt changes without introducing a saccadic eye movement to track the target.

To increase the sensitivity of the test to more subtle abnormalities, the speed is increased up to 40 deg/s. Speeds up to 70 deg/s are possible but the smooth pursuit tracking system's performance is significantly poorer at these high speeds (Meyer, Lasker, & Robinson, 1985). As in the sinusoidal task age-sensitive normative data for each of the speeds tested should be available for testing. The analysis in this situation is significantly simpler as it is just the eye velocity divided by the target velocity to produce the gain value.

Both the fixed velocity and sinusoidal protocols are in a category of predictable target smooth pursuit tracking. There are other paradigms that are not of a predictable target nature. These are used more for research purposes instead of routine clinical investigations and are not discussed in this context. The interest reader is referred to other literature (Hain, 1993; Leigh & Zee, 2006). Interestingly since children do not develop the ability to track small objects until around 4 months of age, large repeated targets can be used (optokinetic protocol) to provide an estimate of smooth pursuit tracking in the very young. This is possible since optokinetic eye movements are highly dominated by smooth pursuit, not the optokinetic generator (see below for further discussion of optokinetic testing and Chapter 25 for further discussion of testing in children).

GAZE STABILITY

This evaluates a patient's ability to maintain gaze on a target in primary position or eccentric positions (right, left, up, or down) in a steady manner without the production of eye movements, principally jerk nystagmus, or presence of saccadic intrusions (see Chapter 10 for description). The sole purpose of saccade and pursuit testing is the identification of central brainstem/cerebellar lesions, whereas abnormalities in gaze stability can occur from either a central or peripheral vestibular system lesion. Criteria for differentiating between central and peripheral lesions are discussed in Chapter 10.

Technical Considerations

Filter settings and sampling rates would be the same as that for smooth pursuit tracking and usually individual eye recordings would not be necessary. However, if one eye is observed with a visual occluding camera while the other has vision, a form of nystagmus known as latent nystagmus (jerk nystagmus that has its fast component away from the occluded eye) can result from an ocular misalignment (Dell'Osso, Ellenberger, Abel, & Flynn, 1983) and may not be representative of either a peripheral or central lesion. Because of this when using a video system with a single visual occluding camera it is always best to check gaze stability with both eyes viewing the target prior to the formal recording of gaze stability.

Parameters for Analysis

In the majority of abnormal gaze stability, the type of eye movement is that of jerk nystagmus. If the nystagmus is persistent in primary gaze, it is referred to as fixation present, spontaneous designating the direction of the beat, and one can give the average slow component velocity. When jerk nystagmus is noted in any of the eccentric positions, it is referred to as fixation present gaze-evoked nystagmus, again designating the direction of the fast component. A specific nomenclature is used when nystagmus is horizontal and direction fixed. Designation as to fixation present or fixation removed is made along with an indication as to the direction of the nystagmus beat. Next, it is indicated whether the nystagmus was present when gazing only in the direction of the fast component (first degree), in the direction of the fast component and in primary second degree), or in the direction of the beat, primary, and while gazing away from the beat of the nystagmus (third degree). Last, it is indicated whether the nystagmus followed Alexander's law (see Chapter 2 for a full explanation —if it follows Alexander's law the nystagmus will increase in its briskness (slow component velocity) as the gaze is directed further in the direction of the fast component of the nystagmus). For example, the phrase "third degree, left-beating gaze evoked nystagmus with fixation present following Alexander's law" implies a left-beating nystagmus that is present with fixation when the individual is looking at a target to the right, primary, and left, and the nystagmus increases in intensity as the gaze is shifted toward the direction of the fast component, to the left. In all other situations, when nystagmus changes direction or another nonjerk nystagmus eye movement is noted, a verbal description of those movements is required.

Although these are descriptive techniques instead of quantitative analysis as used for saccades and smooth pursuit, they are adequate for the analysis of gaze-stability testing as the primary focus is the presence or absence of abnormal eye movements. This is especially true when one encounters saccadic intrusions, although some minor analysis of the eye movement recording may be needed to distinguish between certain forms of saccadic intrusions (see Chapter 10).

Protocol

Gaze stability testing is usually performed first with fixation present using a target in the primary position. The target is then moved 30 degrees (this would be considered the minimum subtended arc movement to elicit gaze-evoked nystagmus) to the right, left, up, or down. If the subtended arc movement exceeds 30 degrees laterally or up, the possibility of physiologic endpoint nystagmus is increased. However, physiologic endpoint nystagmus is not persistent when fixation is present decaying to stable eye movement typically within seconds (Leigh & Zee, 2006). Between each of the eccentric gaze positions, it is important to return to the primary position to observe for rebound nystagmus (a jerk nystagmus that beats in the direction of the last movement of the eyes). Each of the positions (primary, eccentric, and primary for rebound) should be held for at least 10 s to observe for nystagmus. Avoid prolonged eccentric gaze (greater than 1 min) as that can produce a rebound nystagmus in normal subjects (Leigh & Zee, 2006). In all positions, other than testing for rebound, the nystagmus, if seen, should be persistent; rebound nystagmus will decay. Following gaze stability with fixation present it is repeated with fixation removed asking the patient to gaze straight ahead, then to the right, left, up, and

down each time returning to center between each of the eccentric positions. It is not necessary to try and control the position of the eccentric eye locations laterally or up or down. Some patients will move the eyes to the extreme in the lateral directions and this may produce physiologic endpoint nystagmus that without a visual target can be persistent. This is recognized by the following features: (1) the nystagmus is symmetric looking to the right or left; (2) it is of typically low slow component velocity (<5 deg/s); and, (3) there was no persistent nystagmus in the visual fixation present condition. If these characteristics are noted then the nystagmus may be written off as physiologic endpoint and ignored in the interpretation.

OPTOKINETIC NYSTAGMUS (OKN)

Technical Considerations

The production of true optokinetic nystagmus (OKN) involves a combination of the neurologic substrate involved with smooth pursuit tracking together with areas that respond to moving visual stimuli in a full field format but do not respond to head movement, the optokinetic areas (Leigh & Zee, 2006). Furthermore, when viewing a full field (90% or more of the visual field filled with the repeated moving targets) stimulus, the initiation of the nystagmus is dominantly a result of smooth pursuit tracking with the OKN component added as the stimulus is continued requiring seconds to fully develop. The response then continues as a combination of both smooth pursuit tracking and optokinetics with smooth pursuit dominant. Therefore, to evaluate OKN function in isolation from smooth pursuit one must take advantage of a perseveration of nystagmus caused by stimulation of the optokinetic system when the person is suddenly put into the dark after a minimum of 30 s worth of stimulation (called optokinetic after nystagmus [OKAN]). As soon as the target has been extinguished for 1 s the smooth pursuit system no longer has any influence and the OKAN is a direct result of the activity of the optokinetic system reflected through the area of the brainstem referred to as the velocity storage system (Tijssen, Straathof, Hain, & Zee, 1989). To produce the OKN stimulation through retinal stimulation and signals transmitted via the accessory optic track, the stimulus needs to fill a minimum of 90% of the visual field and be capable of producing a circularvection effect (the illusion of circular motion when not moving) (Leigh & Zee, 2006).

Based on the above discussion, the size of the target used in testing for OKN must basically fill the visual field with its movements. Therefore, light bars are not tapping into the optokinetic system even though they can produce a nystagmus that looks like that of OKN but is created primarily by the smooth pursuit system. Light bar stimuli do not produce OKAN which would be the indicator of optokinetic system stimulation and the means by which it can be directly evaluated. The projection systems have a better opportunity to produce true optokinetic system stimulation even though for a standard ENG/VNG system this is projected onto a flat surface. The most efficient manner to provide for optokinetic system stimulation is having the subject seated within a full-field stimulus configuration. An example of such is provided in a rotary chair environment with a projection light system in the ceiling is shown in Figure 9–5. Other arrangements may consist of a patterned cloth enclosure that surrounds the patient and the entire cloth system is placed into motion. Even with all of the appropriate arrangements of a full field stimulus and the production of the sensation of circularvection, the OKN response is still dominated by the smooth pursuit system and hence the same normative data is used for analysis of sinusoidal OKN as is used for smooth pursuit (seen discussion on protocols below).

Filter settings and sampling rates would be as set for gaze stability testing. The nystagmus would have parametric features of slow component and fast component velocity similar to that of other jerk nystagmus.

When testing for OKN the instructions given the patient are critical as the form of the nystagmus can be easily altered. If the patient is to capture and follow a single target out of the optokinetic visual presentation (e.g., stripes, checkerboard, random dots) the nystagmus will have a large excursion for the slow component giving a course appearance to the jerk nystagmus; this is referred to as "look" nystagmus. If the instructions are to have the patient stare or gaze in the center of the target display and

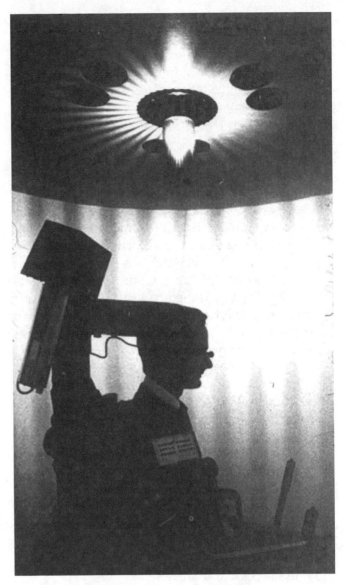

Figure 9-5. An immersive optokinetic stimulation system as a component of a rotational chair system. From Shepard, N. T., and Telian, S. A., 1996. Used with permission.

try to count the targets as they go by this results in a low-amplitude slow component nystagmus called "stare" nystagmus. "Look" nystagmus emphasizes the smooth pursuit component, whereas "stare" nystagmus increases the optokinetic component in a full-field presentation but the OKN component is still less than the smooth pursuit portion. Patients can inadvertently eliminate the OKN response by "staring through" the target to an imagined stationary target on the other side of the display. If this type of full-field stimulus in daily routine causes the patient symptoms, they may have adopted this "looking through" strategy as a means for controlling the unwanted sensations. Therefore, shaping the character of the nystagmus is important along with an appropriately sized visual presentation if stimulation of the optokinetic system is to be achieved.

Parameters for Analysis

The analysis for OKN is performed by calculating the velocity gain of the eye movement response. This is defined as the peak eye velocity divided by the target velocity. The velocity gain is used for either the fixed velocity or sinusoidal protocols (see protocol section below). The gain is calculated for target movement to the right and to the left. These gains are expected to be symmetric (within a 25% difference range) with a minimum 0.5 for the fixed velocity target protocol with speeds up to 60 deg/s.

For the sinusoidal target profile, velocity gain is the dominant outcome parameter. In this protocol the velocity gain is expected to fall within the ranges given for smooth pursuit tracking at the same frequency (see Table 9–1). This results from the domination of the neurologic substrate responsible for smooth pursuit in the production of OKN. Additionally, phase angle can be calculated for the sinusoidal protocol with results expected to be within the range given for smooth pursuit. Again, in this protocol the outcome parameters are given for both target movement to the right and the left.

When testing for OKAN (this response can only be generated using a fixed velocity target), three outcome parameters are used to quantify the response. Velocity gain is calculated from the slow component eye velocity determined at 2 s after extinguishing the lights of the target and test area divided by the target speed. The second is the time constant of decay of the slow component eye velocity. The time constant is defined as the length of time from the extinguishing of the lights to when the slow component eye velocity decays to 37% of its amplitude at 2 s after the lights were turned off. The final outcome parameter is called the slow cumulative eye position (SCEP). The SCEP is the sum of the amplitudes of the slow component eye movements for 45 s from the time the lights are extinguished (Hain et al., 1994). Even

though the analysis of OKAN reflects the optokinetic system separately from smooth pursuit the acquisition of the response is technically very difficult to obtain and shows significant variability. Therefore, it is not used in a routine manner and the interested reader is referred to other sources for more detailed information (Leigh & Zee, 2006).

Protocols

Fixed Velocity Target With and Without Optokinetic After Nystagmus

For an OKN-only protocol the full-field stimulus is rotated at a constant speed ranging from 20 to 60 deg/s for a minimum of 30 s to a maximum of 60 s. The direction of the target is reversed and the stimulus repeated. This paradigm may be repeated at a second speed. The gain is expected to decrease as the speed of the target is increased for target velocities greater than 60 deg/s (Baloh, Yee, & Honrubia, 1982).

In a protocol for both OKN and OKAN the same fixed velocity target is used but the presentation is typically for 60 s. The lights are extinguished and recording of eye movements is continued for another 60 s. Secondary to the significant variability in the OKAN response, other more complex paradigms have been developed to minimize the variance (Leigh & Zee, 2006).

Sinusoidal Target Movement

In this paradigm, the stimulus is presented at a frequency similar to that used during smooth pursuit tracking. The stimulus is typically presented for 30 to 60 s with peak target speed between 20 and 40 deg/s. The sinusoidal nature of the stimulus does not allow for the production of OKAN and therefore only OKN analysis can be produced representing primarily a smooth pursuit following eye movement.

VIDEO ASSOCIATED WITH THIS CHAPTER

Video 9–1. Shown is a random saccade paradigm using random position in the horizontal plane with fixed timing. This is followed by a sinusoidal smooth pursuit tracking protocol performed at three discrete frequencies of 0.2, 0.4, and 0.6 Hz.

REFERENCES

American National Standards Institute. (2009). *ANSI S3.45-200X American National Standards procedures for testing basic vestibular function.* New York: Acoustical Society of America.

Baloh, R. W., Yee, R. D., & Honrubia, V. (1982). Clinical abnormalities of optokinetic nystagmus. In G. Lennerstrand, D. S. Zee, & E. L. Keller (Eds.), *Functional basis of ocular motility disorders.* Oxford, UK: Pergamon Press.

Boghen, D., Troost, B. T., Daroff, R. B., Dell'Osso, L. F., & Birkett, J. E. (1974). Velocity characteristics of normal human saccades. *Investigative Ophthalmology and Visual Science, 13,* 619–623.

Butler, K. M., Zacks, R. T., & Henderson, J. M. (1999). Suppression of reflexive saccades in younger and older adults: Age comparisons on an antisaccade task. *Memory and Cognition, 27,* 584–591.

Dell'Osso, L. F., Ellenberger, C., Abel, L. A., & Flynn, J. T. (1983). The nystagmus blockage syndrome: Congenital nystagmus, manifest latent nystagmus or both? *Investigations in Ophthalmology and Visual Science, 24,* 1580–1587.

Fukushima, J., Hatta, T., & Fukushima, K. (2000). Development of voluntary control of saccadic eye movements. I. Age-related changes in normal children. *Brain and Development, 22,*173–180.

Hain, T. (1993). Background and technique of ocular motility testing. In G. P. Jacobson, C. W. Newman, & J.M. Kartush (Eds.), *Handbook of balance function testing* (pp. 83–100). St. Louis, MO: Mosby.

Hain, T. C., Herdman, S. J., Holliday, M., Mattox, D., Zee, D. S., & Byskosh, A. T. (1994). Localizing value of opto-kinetic afternystagmus. *Annals of Otology, Rhinology, und Laryngology, 103,* 806–811.

Hutton, S. B., & Tegally, D. (2005). The effects of dividing attention on smooth pursuit eye tracking. *Experimental Brain Research, 163,* 306–313.

Imai, T., Sekine, K., Hattori, K., Takeda, N., Koizuka, I., Nakamae, K., . . . Kubo, T. (2005). Comparing the accuracy of video-oculography and the scleral search coil system in human eye movement analysis. *Auris Nasus Larynx, 32,* 3–9.

Leigh, J. R., & Zee, D. S. (2006). *The neurology of eye movements* (4th ed.). New York, NY: Oxford University Press.

Machado, L., & Rafal, R. D. (2004). Control of fixation and saccades during an anti-saccade task: An investigation in humans with chronic lesions of oculomotor cortex. *Experimental Brain Research, 156,* 55–63.

Meyer, C. H., Lasker, A. G., & Robinson, D. A. (1985). The upper limit of human smooth pursuit velocity. *Vision Research, 25*(4), 561–563.

Paige, G. D. (1994). Senescence of human visual-vestibular interactions: Smooth pursuit, optokinetic, and vestibular control of eye movements with aging. *Experimental Brain Research, 98,* 355–372.

Shepard, N. T., & Telian, S. A. (1996). *Practical management of the balance disorder patient.* San Diego, CA: Singular.

Tijssen, M. A. J., Straathof, C. S. M., Hain, T. C., & Zee, D. S. (1989). Optokinetic afternystagmus in humans: Normal values of amplitude, time constant and asymmetry. *Annals of Otology, Rhinology, and Laryngology, 98,* 741–746.

Van Die, G. C., & Collewijin, H. (1986). Control of human optokinetic nystagmus by the central and peripheral retina: Effects of partial visual field masking, scotopic vision and central retinal scatomata. *Brain Research, 383,* 185–194.

Van den Berg, A.V., & Collewijin, H. (1986). Human smooth pursuit: Effects of stimulus extent and of spatial temporal constraints of the pursuit trajectory. *Vision Research, 29,*1209–1222.

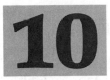

Interpretation and Usefulness of Ocular Motility Testing

Neil T. Shepard, Michael C. Schubert, and Scott D. Z. Eggers

INTRODUCTION

Chapter 9 provided a discussion of the technical aspects of the routine clinical evaluation of the ocular motor systems involved with gaze stability, saccade production, smooth pursuit tracking, and the optokinetic system. The purpose of the present chapter is to present the interpretation parameters for each of these tests and how they can be used in routine clinical investigations of the dizzy patient, principally for the purpose of site-of-lesion determination.

To better understand the interpretation of these tests and how they can be used to localize lesions to the central nervous system (CNS), the reader is referred to Chapter 2 and other sources (Leigh & Zee, 2006) for a review of the neurologic pathways involved in each of the ocular motor tasks listed above. In a review of that nature, you find overlaps in the neural pathways especially between gaze stability to an eccentric target and saccade production, gaze stability to a primary target and smooth pursuit, smooth pursuit and optokinetic activity. Therefore, although the tests for ocular motor functioning can be used to indicate CNS involvement, and, in some cases, suggest differential lesions within the CNS, specific site-of-lesion determination clearly is not always possible. In many cases, both brainstem and cerebellar structures may be implicated, and further differentiation with physiologic test-

ing alone is not possible with routine clinical techniques. There are, however, other combinations of results that are highly suggestive of specific regions of the brainstem or cerebellum involved in abnormal ocular motor control. Through the use of specific patient examples of abnormal eye movements, the following discussion attempts to delineate the global CNS indicators from those with more specific site-of-lesion implications.

GAZE STABILITY TESTING

Of the four routine ocular motor tests, this is the only one in which lesions of either the peripheral or central vestibular and ocular motor systems can produce abnormalities. Therefore, it is best to lay out distinguishing and contrasting features that will allow for this peripheral versus CNS differentiation. Therefore we start with spontaneous nystagmus that is typically seen in primary (straight-ahead gaze) that is direction fixed. In other than during acute onset (within the first 72 hr) of symptoms this nystagmus is seen only with fixation removed. This nystagmus then continues with the fast component in the same direction with gaze in eccentric directions. Because this nystagmus is seen without provocation of eccentric gaze it is referred to as spontaneous nystagmus. The principal abnormality noted in gaze stability testing would be the development of nystagmus or other repetitive eye movement in place of steady fixation. When it is jerk nystagmus and seen only on eccentric gaze, the abnormality is referred to as gaze-evoked nystagmus. The general characterizations of spontaneous and gaze-evoked nystagmus of peripheral origin are given in Table 10–1; characterizations associated with gaze-evoked nystagmus of central origin are given in Table 10–2 (Leigh & Zee, 2006). Although all of the characteristics listed can be observed, the dominant ones for determining that the gaze-evoked nystagmus is of peripheral origin are the enhancement in the nystagmus in the same direction with fixation removed, direction-fixed nature obeying Alexander's law, and post-head-shake testing (although this can be seen in cerebellar lesions it is rare and sensitivity/specificity for identification of peripheral lesion is 30% to 35%/90% to 95%—see Chapter 7 text for a complete discussion). For gaze-evoked nystagmus of central origin, the dominant characteristic is that of direction-changing nystagmus, pure vertical or pure torsional nystagmus.

Video 10–1 demonstrates these features for a peripheral lesion. The patient is a 77-year-old female with the diagnosis of vestibular neuronitis. She has a documented severe right peripheral hypofunction via head thrust direct examination and caloric irrigation testing during her laboratory evaluation. Her smooth pursuit tracking and saccade testing are all within normal limits. In the video, she is seen with just a hint of first degree (seen only when gazing in the direction of the fast component), left-beating, gaze-evoked, nystagmus with fixation present. When fixation is removed, she develops second degree (seen when gazing in the direction of the fast component and in center gaze), left-beating gaze-evoked nystagmus. Both with and without fixation her nystagmus follows Alexander's law. Alexander's law, simply stated, indicates that nystagmus will increase in its slow component velocity as gaze is directed farther in the direction of the fast component of nystagmus, a result of an uncompensated peripheral asymmetry (Kasai & Zee, 1978). Finally, the head-shake test is given and her post-head-shake nystagmus is a third degree (seen when gazing in

Table 10–1. Characteristics of Gaze-Evoked Nystagmus of Peripheral Origin

- *Acute lesion*—in a peripheral lesion nystagmus is usually only visible with fixation present when the lesion is acute in nature.

- *Direction-fixed*—nystagmus with fixation present or absent should be direction fixed in nature with the patient sitting, head in primary position. (Nystagmus direction may vary when testing positional and be of peripheral origin.) May have both horizontal and vertical components but must have a horizontal component to be considered of peripheral origin—that is, pure vertical nystagmus is taken as central until proven otherwise (see text for explanation).

- *Alexander's law*—the horizontal nystagmus should follow Alexander's law; that is, the nystagmus increases in its intensity as the patient gazes further in the direction of the fast component of the nystagmus (this applies to horizontal nystagmus component only).

- *Enhanced with fixation removed*—this is the primary determiner of the periphery being the source of the nystagmus. When fixation is removed nystagmus is brought forth when absent with fixation or nystagmus intensity increases if it was seen with fixation present.

- *Nystagmus enhanced with head-shake test*—if ongoing direction fixed nystagmus of peripheral origin is present, it can usually be enhanced with head-shake testing

- *Linear slow component*—on the tracing of the nystagmus the slow component is a linear trace (*straight line*).

Table 10–2. Characteristics of Gaze-Evoked Nystagmus of Central Origin

- *Acute or chronic*—when nystagmus is seen with fixation it can be from an acute or chronic (beyond 12 weeks) lesion. The nystagmus persists following the lesion onset without any significant diminution in intensity with time.

- *Direction-fixed or changing*—although the nystagmus could be direction fixed in nature such as pure up or down beat it is likely to be direction changing based on the direction of gaze; that is, right beat with right gaze, left beat with left gaze, and so on. This also applies to a form of nystagmus called "rebound" nystagmus. With rebound nystagmus the direction of the beat is always in the last direction that the eye moved. Also, pure vertical or pure torsional nystagmus even though direction fixed is taken as indicative of central involvement until proven otherwise.

- *Rarely in primary*—it is rare to have horizontal nystagmus persist in the primary (straight ahead) gaze position (can be there for a brief interval when rebound is present and returning from eccentric gaze). Pure vertical or pure torsional nystagmus can persist in the primary gaze position with central involvement.

- *Enhanced with fixation present*—typically, nystagmus is increased in its intensity with fixation present and no change or a reduction in the nystagmus is seen when fixation is removed.

- *Vertical nystagmus post-head-shake test*—it would be unusual to see horizontal nystagmus enhanced with horizontal head shake when the nystagmus is of central origin only. It is possible that following either a horizontal or vertical head-shake test the nystagmus produced is that of pure vertical when a central lesion is the source of the nystagmus.

- *Decreasing speed of slow component*—the horizontal nystagmus trace many times will show a slow component that is nonlinear implying a slowing in the speed of the eye as it moves from an eccentric horizontal position toward the primary gaze position.

the direction of the fast component, center gaze, and when gaze is directed away from the fast component), left-beating, gaze-evoked, nystagmus again following Alexander's law.

In contrast, Videos 10–2A and 10–2B show right-beating nystagmus on gaze right (see Video 10–2A) and left-beating on gaze left (see Video 10–2B). These are eye movements recorded during the patient's videonystagmography (VNG) testing. She was a 46-year-old female with diffuse cerebellar and brainstem involvement secondary to prior long-term alcohol abuse. In this case, when fixation is removed (not shown in the video), gaze-holding abnormalities continue, but there is no enhancement of the nystagmus.

Gaze-evoked nystagmus can be produced for gaze right and left as shown in Videos 10–1 and 10 2, but also up and down. Video 10–3 demonstrates abnormal gaze holding on up gaze for the

same patient in Videos 10–2A and 10–2B. Figure 10–1 shows tracings from a VNG of a 54-year-old male with multiple sclerosis. In the figure, no nystagmus is noted in primary (center) gaze; however, on up gaze a persistent up-beating nystagmus is seen and no nystagmus on down gaze. This patient also has gaze-holding deficits when gazing to the right and left as shown in Figure 10–2.

Prior to discussions of special forms of primary or eccentric gaze stability abnormalities, consider the situation of pure vertical nystagmus noted in primary gaze which is persistent with fixation present and removed. Video 10–4 illustrates this type of nystagmus in the form of pure down-beating nystagmus in primary gaze that is exacerbated on lateral gaze but is persistent in nature. The case from Video 10–4 is a female in her seventies with a diagnosed cervical-cranial junction abnormality (discussed further in the site-of-lesion section). Video 10–5 also shows this

Vertical Gaze - 0 degrees   Vertical Gaze - 30 deg Up   Vertical Gaze - 30 deg Dow

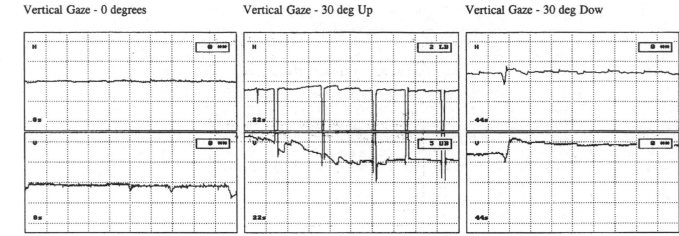

Figure 10–1. Gaze recordings of a male 54-year-old patient with multiple sclerosis. Each of the panels present the horizontal (*upper half*) and the vertical (*lower half*) video eye movement recordings. The panel on the left is gaze in primary position. The panel in the center shows results from gaze up with the panel on the right representative of results for gaze down. In the center panel the horizontal trace (*upper half*) shows several eye blinks indicated by the large asymmetric sharp downward excursions of the trace. No persistent horizontal nystagmus is noted. In the lower half of the center panel a vertical up-beat nystagmus is noted. No horizontal or vertical nystagmus is seen for primary or down gaze tracings.

type of nystagmus superimposed on a patient's gaze-evoked nystagmus on gaze left and right. The patient in Video 10–5 also illustrates disrupted pursuit tracking (discussed below). As fixation is removed in the patient in Video 10–5, it is noted that no change in gaze-evoked nystagmus intensity is seen, another characteristic of gaze-evoked nystagmus of central origin (see Table 10–2). However, an exacerbation in his vertical nystagmus with the head-shake test is seen (see Tables 10–1 and 10–2).

Is pure vertical down- or up-beating nystagmus to be considered of peripheral or central origin? In answering this question, it is useful to consider the specific eye movements that are provoked in a normal subject when each of the semicircular canals is stimulated individually. The movements considered below are the compensatory eye movement (slow component of nystagmus), the vestibulo-ocular reflex (VOR), when the canal in question is stimulated, not the beat or fast component. The direction of the nystagmus is referenced to the left/right of the subject's (or patient's) head frame of reference for all forms of eye movement, horizontal, vertical and torsional. For torsional the superior pole of the eye is used as the point of reference to describe the movement of the eye (see further description in Chapter 2):

- Horizontal (lateral) canals right and left—VOR response would be to the left and right, respectively.
- Anterior (superior) canals right and left—VOR response would be up for both with a torsional movement to the left for the right canal, and to the right for the left canal.
- Inferior (posterior) canals right and left—VOR response would be down for both with a torsional movement to the left for the right canal, and to the right for the left canal.

Using the above descriptions of the VOR responses for each of the canals, the only way to produce a down-beating nystagmus from the periphery would be with simultaneous stimulation of both anterior canals. The VOR response would be pure up with the torsional components canceling and the beat would be down. To have this happen via a pathological insult would require that both anterior canals have simultaneous irritative lesions or have simultaneous paretic lesions of both posterior and horizontal canals. Currently, there is only one condition that has been reported that is a peripheral disorder known to produce at least transient pure down-beating nystagmus: bilateral superior canal dehiscence (Deutchlander, Strupp, Jahn, Quiring, &

Horiz. Gaze Right - Eyes Open

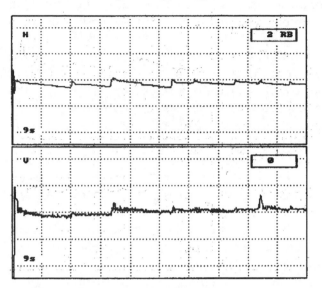

Horiz. Gaze Right - Rebound

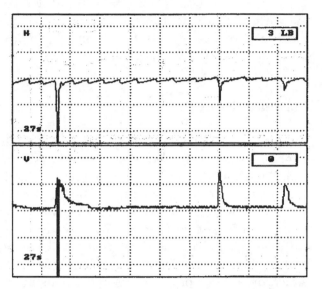

Horiz. Gaze Left - Eyes Open

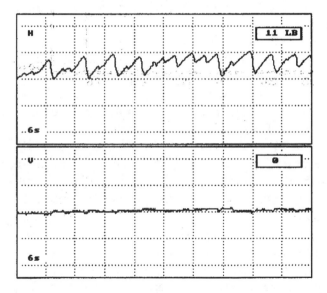

Horiz. Gaze Left - Rebound

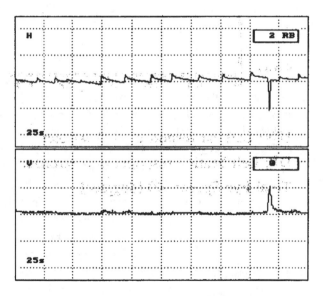

Figure 10–2. Gaze recordings of a 54-year-old male patient with multiple sclerosis. The top two panels give the horizontal and vertical eye movement traces during gaze right, right-beating nystagmus (*panel on top left*), and the resulting nystagmus on return to center gaze, left-beating nystagmus (*panel on top right*). In each panel the top trace is the horizontal eye movement and the bottom trace is the vertical movement. The two bottom panels give the same information for gaze left, left-beating nystagmus (*bottom left*), and the nystagmus on returning to center gaze from gaze left, right-beating nystagmus (*bottom right*).

Brandt, 2004). Otherwise, the likelihood of a peripheral disorder capable of causing pure vertical up- or down-beating nystagmus is so remote that pure vertical nystagmus should be considered of central

origin until proven otherwise. This same rationale may be applied with the use of the specific individual canal eye signatures to pure torsional (note that occasionally posterior canal BPPV can appear with primary gaze as pure torsional to the observer when visual fixation is not removed but will have the vertical component introduced with change in the direction of gaze away from primary) and pure up-beating nystagmus (Leigh & Zee, 2006).

Rebound Nystagmus

Another aspect of gaze-evoked nystagmus of central origin is a feature referred to as rebound nystagmus (Gordon, Hain, Zee, & Fetter, 1986). In this situation nystagmus is produced beating in the last direction the eye moved as the eye is returned to primary position from eccentric gaze. The Bárány Society has developed a proposed International Classification for Vestibular Disorders (ICVD) document in which definitions of disorders and nystagmus are proposed. For rebound nystagmus the proposed definition is, "Nystagmus appearing transiently upon return to the straight-ahead gaze position after sustained eccentric gaze, with the fast phases beating away from the original direction of eccentric gaze" (personal communication from Scott Eggers, Chapter 2). Even for a normal individual if the eccentric gaze is held for an extended period of time one to two beats of nystagmus may be visualized. What is being tested for is a burst of nystagmus lasting several seconds with the fast component in the last direction of movement of the eye (Hood, 1981). For example, if persistent gaze-evoked right-beating nystagmus is noted on right gaze then on return to center, a leftward eye movement, a brief event of left-beating nystagmus is seen that does not persist. Figure 10–2 illustrates this for the patient diagnosed with multiple sclerosis. The rebound nystagmus can be seen on return from both right and left gaze.

Sites of Lesion

When gaze-evoked nystagmus is direction fixed in character, follows Alexander's law, and is enhanced with fixation removed, it is considered of peripheral origin most likely beating away from the involved side. However, this is not always the case. The nystagmus will certainly beat toward the more active neural side, but that could be an irritative labyrin-

thine lesion as seen in Ménière's disease (Bance, Mai, Tomlinson, & Rutka, 1991; McClure & Lycett, 1983). Therefore, the presence of gaze-evoked nystagmus of peripheral origin has two possible lesion sites, labyrinthine hypofunction on the side away from the beat or an irritative lesion on the side ipsilateral to the beat. It will require further information from the patient's history and presenting symptoms together with other tests and presenting signs to resolve the periphery involved.

When the gaze-evoked nystagmus is of central origin by its characteristics the possible lesion sites will depend on whether the gaze-evoked nystagmus is in a horizontal or vertical direction. The primary neurologic substrate responsible for maintaining binocular horizontal gaze to the left or right involves the nucleus prepositus hypoglossi (NPH) and the medial vestibular nucleus (MVN) (Leigh & Zee, 2006; McConville, Tomlinson, King, Paige, & Na, 1994; Sylvestre, Choi, & Cullen, 2003). These structures would be ipsilateral to the direction of gaze and therefore one can have gaze-evoked nystagmus during only left or right gaze suggesting a unilateral lesion in this region of the brainstem. While these are the primary central structures in horizontal, eccentric gaze, realize that areas of the vestibulocerebellum (flocculus and paraflocculus) participate to enhance the neural integration process in the brainstem needed for maintaining horizontal eccentric gaze (Zee, Yamazaki, Butler, & Gücer, 1981). The ability to move the eye in a saccade movement from primary to a left or right position requires a different region of the brainstem (burst neurons of the parapontine reticular formation [PPRF]) (Van Gisbergen, Robinson, & Geilen, 1981) and is discussed in the saccade section of this chapter.

Vertical gaze-evoked nystagmus during up or down gaze suggests a different site of lesion. The primary region for neural integration during gaze holding up or down is engendered by the interstitial nucleus of Cajal of the midbrain (Fukushima, Kaneko, & Fuchs, 1992). However, this is not the only structure in the midbrain that contributes to gaze holding, and lesions in the cerebellum and brainstem can affect vertical gaze holding (Leigh & Zee, 2006). The vertical gaze-evoked nystagmus is most often seen in association with horizontal gaze-evoked nystagmus with cerebellar flocculus/paraflocculus lesions secondary to the loss of influence of the cerebellum on the horizontal and vertical neural integrators (see full discussion of these pathways in Chapter 2).

As discussed above pure vertical or torsional nystagmus in primary position is to be considered of central origin until proven otherwise. For up and down beats the most likely lesion sites are in the midline from the low posterior fossa at the level of the pontomedullary junction to the pontomesencephalic junction (Brandt & Dieterich, 2000). For down-beat nystagmus one of the common causes would be craniocervical junction pathology. This can be of a mechanical compression form as in Arnold-Chiari malformation or from other pathologies affecting the low posterior fossa, but most commonly the vestibulocerebellum (Walker & Zee, 2005; Zee et al., 1981). In contrast, up-beating nystagmus is more likely to originate from the lower brainstem and medullary regions (Pierrot-Deseilligny & Milea, 2005). The patient illustrated in Video 10–4 had a mechanical compression of the midline pontomedullary region by the dens process secondary to a congenitally foreshortened C1 and severe progressive kyphotic condition. It is important to realize that lesions in the low posterior fossa that may produce pure downbeat nystagmus may not disrupt other ocular motor functions such as horizontal saccades or pursuit yet may cause disruption in vertical especially downward pursuit from the down-beat nystagmus in paraflocculus lesions. Therefore, on an ENG/VNG when pure vertical nystagmus is noted with or without fixation in a persistent manner, such as during positional testing, lesions of the low posterior fossa need to be ruled out.

In contrast to the pure vertical nystagmus of central origin, which is more likely from a midline lesion, pure torsional in primary gaze and torsional with a horizontal component as a form of gaze-evoked nystagmus of central origin is more likely to result from a lesion that lateralizes to the right or left in the pontomedullary/medullary area ipsilesional or above the pons contralesional (Brandt & Dieterich, 2000). With two-dimensional ENG/VNG, pure torsional nystagmus will not be recognized and a combined torsion and horizontal nystagmus (Video 10–6) will appear as a diagonal nystagmus. On VNG the same printout traces will result as with

ENG yet during testing the examiner will be able to observe the actual eye movements and comment on such in the report. An example of the pure torsion in primary gaze (right torsional nystagmus) changing to a mixed right torsional nystagmus with right horizontal nystagmus on gaze right is seen in Video 10–6. This female, in her forties, suffered a posterior inferior cerebellar artery (PICA) ischemic stroke on the right resulting in a dorsolateral medullary infarct producing the nystagmus noted in the video. In this situation the nystagmus, both the torsion and the horizontal components, beat toward the lesion side; however, this is not an irritative-style lesion as referred to with a peripheral labyrinthine insult but a possible complex combination of increased inhibition in the vestibular nucleus ipsilateral and decreased excitation of the contralateral brainstem reticular formation (Solomon, Galetta, & Liu 1995). The final point illustrated in the video is that of ocular-lateral pulsion (Waespe & Wichmann, 1990). As shown when the fixation point in primary gaze is eliminated by having the patient close his or her eyes, the eyes deviate consistently toward the lesion side, to the right. This can be seen on an ENG/VNG if recording is ongoing when fixation is removed. This is shown in Figure 10–3 for a 65-year-old male also suffering from a PICA distribution stroke event on the left.

It is also possible to have combinations of gaze-evoked nystagmus of both peripheral and central origin. Videos 10–7A and 10–7B demonstrate a patient with Bruns' nystagmus (Bruns, 1908) in addition to a persistent down beat during direct video examination. Bruns' nystagmus is commonly a manifestation of a cerebellar-pontine angle mass lesion or may be seen even after resection of a mass in this region from damage by the tumor to the labyrinth and the brainstem/cerebellum ipsilateral to the tumor. On gaze contralateral to the tumor a gaze-evoked nystagmus is seen that is usually smaller in amplitude and higher in frequency than the gaze-evoked nystagmus on ipsilateral gaze. The gaze-evoked nystagmus to the contralateral side is likely a result of an uncompensated peripheral vestibular hypofunction from the compressive effects of the mass lesion. The gaze-evoked nystagmus on ipsilateral gaze results from gaze-holding abnormalities from the CNS damage (Leigh & Zee, 2006).

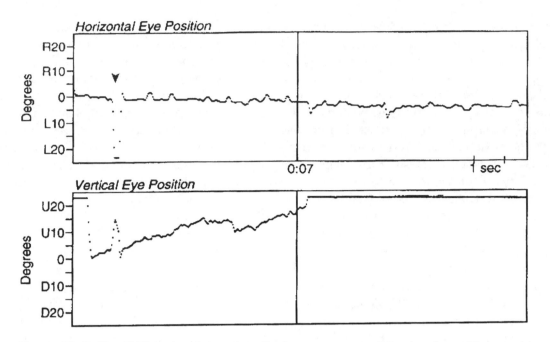

Figure 10-3. The ENG horizontal and vertical eye movement tracing for a 65-year-old male with a left-sided dorsolateral medullary distribution stroke. The top panel shows the horizontal eye movements with the bottom panel demonstrating the vertical eye movement. As indicated by the arrow, the patient went from a lighted condition to a dark condition and had an immediate deviation of the eyes to the left returning to the center when fixation was restored. His ocular lateral pulsion was noted during routine ocular motor testing when changing from fixation present during gaze testing to fixation removed by eye closure. Reprinted with permission from Shepard and Telian, 1996.

When fixation is removed, one can see the contralateral gaze nystagmus enhance, whereas the ipsilateral gaze-evoked nystagmus remains unchanged; features expected for gaze nystagmus of peripheral and central origin (see Tables 10–1 and 10–2). The patient in Videos 10–7A and 10–7B had a Chiari malformation with surgical repair at age 15 resulting in the persistent down-beating nystagmus. At age 47, she was diagnosed with a vestibular schwannoma on the left side. She underwent a tumor resection procedure via a retrosigmoid approach with preservation of VIIIth nerve function as evidenced by preserved hearing. In Video 10–7A, fixation is present and she demonstrates a persistent down beat with a large amplitude left-beating, gaze-evoked nystagmus on gaze left and small amplitude, weak right-beating nystagmus on gaze right. In Video 10–7B, fixation has been removed and no change is seen in the down-beating or left-beating nystagmus but the right-beating nystagmus is significantly enhanced.

Saccade Intrusions and Oscillations

During the execution of gaze testing, especially with primary gaze evaluation, another group of abnormal eye movements may be observed that are collectively referred to as saccadic intrusions and oscillations (Leigh & Zee, 2006). These are seen with fixation present and when seen are suggestive of cerebellar and/or brainstem involvement. Characteristics of each of these eye movements are described below. Associated video examples are provided for some of the eye movements described. It is important to realize that during the execution of an ENG/VNG the larger amplitude movements in this grouping may well obscure other spontaneous or positional nystagmus. However, the recognition of these movements as something other than "random eye noise" is critical in the evaluation of the patient's condition. None of the saccadic intrusions or oscillations is a result of peripheral system involvement although square-wave jerks and voluntary ("party") flutter are both seen in normal subjects. Therefore, when identified the implication is involvement in the brainstem and/or cerebellar region. The reader desiring a more in-depth discussion of each of these including pathogenesis and treatments for the conditions is referred to Leigh and Zee (2006).

Square-Wave Jerks

These are the 0.5- to 5-degree subtended arc movements in a direction away from point of fixation, with intersaccade intervals up to 200 ms. These movements occur in normal individuals at frequencies less than 20 to 30 per minute becoming more frequent with age (Herishanu & Sharpe, 1981). They represent likely cerebellar or upper motor neuron pathology when the frequency exceeds this range (Leigh & Zee, 2006). Video 10–8 shows the eye movements of a 68-year-old male diagnosed with a form of spinocerebellar atrophy. He had a 12-year history of slow progressive imbalance and upper limb coordination difficulties. The eye movements are repeated

saccades first taking his gaze away from the target and then returning to the target. No gaze-evoked nystagmus is seen on lateral gaze right or left. He demonstrates saccadic disrupted smooth pursuit. Fixation is then removed and the square-wave jerks continue. He shows no nystagmus following head-shake test but continues with his square-wave jerks. Figure 10–4 shows horizontal and vertical eye movement tracings for a male in his thirties (unusually young for this disorder) with multiple system atrophy, another form of spino-cerebellar atrophy. The figure illustrates his frequent square-wave jerks.

Macro Square-Wave Jerks

These are the 5- to 15-degree subtended arc movements in a direction away from the point of fixation, with intersaccade intervals of up to 150 ms that are typically shorter than that of square-wave jerks. They represent pathology of brainstem and/or cerebellum (Leigh & Zee, 2006). Figure 10–5 illustrates macro square-wave jerks recorded during a VNG while testing smooth pursuit. This was from a 20-year-old

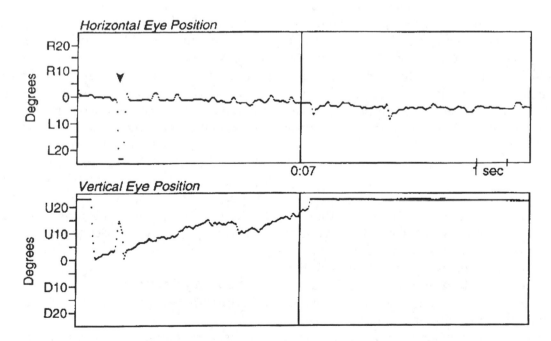

Figure 10–4. Recording of square-wave jerks from a male in his thirties with multiple system atrophy. The top panel is a sample of his horizontal eye trace recorded using electro-oculography techniques. Note the presence of repeated square-wave jerks. The bottom panel shows the tracing of his vertical eye movements. These recordings were made during gaze stability testing. Each trace represents 14 s of recording.

SMOOTH PURSUIT: WAVEFORM

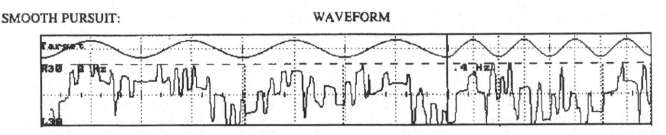

Figure 10–5. An attempt at smooth pursuit testing during a VNG on a 20-year-old female with significant cerebellar damage from a head injury. The horizontal eye tracing illustrates macro square-wave jerks. The top trace in the figure shows the trajectory of the sinusoidal target. The bottom trace is the horizontal eye movement recorded from the right eye.

female with significant cerebellar damage from a closed head injury and traumatic brain injury. Even though her eyes were in constant motion from the macro square-wave jerks a complete VNG was performed being able to detect right-beating positional nystagmus and a full set of caloric irrigations showing no peripheral asymmetry.

Macro Saccadic Oscillations

These are eyes moving in both directions laterally around a fixation point with intersaccade intervals of 150 to 200 ms. The finding is suggestive of cerebellar involvement (Selhorst, Stark, Ochs, & Hoyt, 1976). [The proposed Bárány Society ICVD definition is, "Oscillations around a fixation point due to saccadic hypermetria, typically consisting of runs of (usually horizontal) saccades that build up and then decrease in amplitude, with intersaccadic intervals of about 200 msec."]

Ocular Flutter

These are bursts (typically 2 to 5 s in length) of eye movement in horizontal or horizontal and vertical dimensions. The eyes are taken away from the point of fixation without intersaccade intervals. When the flutter occurs in both horizontal and vertical directions simultaneously it is referred to as opsoclonus. Although ocular flutter and opsoclonus can originate from either brainstem or cerebellar lesions, one must consider the possibility of paraneoplastic cerebellar degeneration when opsoclonus is noted (Bataller et al., 2003). Video 10–9 was obtained during a direct bedside examination from a 71-year-old

female subsequently diagnosed with paraneoplastic cerebellar degeneration secondary to breast cancer. The video illustrates ocular flutter with opsoclonus (also see the discussion of ocular flutter in Chapter 2 of this text).

Voluntary (Party) Flutter

This is a form of flutter behavior in which the eyes are disconjugate in their movement by converging and diverging. The movements are unable to be sustained longer than 20 to 30 s. The movements can be provoked by voluntarily performing a near target convergence or with no target fixation converge the eyes. A person can gain control over the movement and use it for "entertaining" others, hence the name "party nystagmus." It is not representative of a pathological process (Hotson, 1984). It occurs as a combination of convergence, likely for initiation, with small repeated saccades (Yee, Spiegel, Yamada, Abel, & Zee, 1994). It is distinguished from pathologic ocular flutter in that as the eyes are converging the pupils will contract where as in pathologic flutter the eyes move in the same direction together and there is no pupillary contraction.

Infantile Nystagmus (Congenital Nystagmus)

Another form of nystagmus noted during gaze testing as well as during casual observation of a patient is that of infantile nystagmus syndrome. The older term of congenital nystagmus, while in the literature is being dropped since the nystagmus usually develops within the first 8 to 12 weeks and is not present at birth. Appearance is that of a horizontal beating nystagmus in an eye reference frame as opposed to head reference, typically mixed with pendular nystagmus. Infantile nystagmus may be accentuated by visual attention or arousal and suppressed by convergence, inattention, eye closure, or sleep. The amplitude, frequency, and waveform can vary with eye position, typically increasing on lateral gaze (right-beating in right gaze, left-beating in left gaze) but diminishing in intensity in a null zone, leading individuals to adopt a head position that minimizes the oscillations. Infantile nystagmus may occur in the setting of other visual sensory disorders or with a normal visual system. Therefore, this nystagmus can appear as a direction-changing, gazed-evoked nystagmus with nystagmus present in primary eye position (mild forms may have primary position nystagmus absent). Although it may not change significantly, with fixation removed the usual presentation would be to note that the nystagmus reduces in frequency of the beat, regularity, and slow component velocity (SCV). If not recognized as infantile nystagmus this finding could easily be confused as an indication of CNS pathology. In the majority of patients the infantile nystagmus has little or nothing to do with the reason why the patient has sought evaluation for dizziness. In that sense it becomes a "noise" interference that must be dealt with during the ENG/VNG evaluation. There are specific characteristics that distinguish ongoing, fixation present nystagmus as infantile:

1. A history of the ongoing eye movements since as early as the patient can remember. The patient may be able to relate incidences of being teased by other children because of the ongoing eye movement activity (Hertle, Maldanado, Maybodi, & Yang, 2002). However, forms of this type of nystagmus may develop later in life (Gresty, Bronstein, Page, & Rudge, 1991).
2. Nystagmus is usually horizontal even during up or down gaze in an eye reference plane.
3. The nystagmus can be slowed with convergence and during gaze just lateral to primary called the null point. By handing the patient something to read and watching how they position the material, they will likely move the material in closer

than expected and to the right or left from primary gaze by a turn of their head. In this position they take advantage of both the quieting of the nystagmus with convergence and the null point.
4. Trace recordings will many times show the slow component of the nystagmus to be one of increasing velocity. This presentation is just the opposite of the decreasing velocity noted in gaze-evoked nystagmus of central origin (see Table 10–2). Figure 10–6 illustrates in a schematized form the nystagmus seen in gaze-evoked nystagmus of central and peripheral origin. Compare that to the nystagmus tracings from ENG testing from a patient with infantile nystagmus shown in Figure 10–7. The trace in Figure 10–7 illustrates the increasing velocity of the slow component drift of the eyes to the left.

The above description is the more common presentation of infantile nystagmus. It can, however, take other forms and be associated with other ocular system abnormalities. One example of a variation is shown in Video 10–10 recorded during VNG evaluation of a 16-year-old female with migraine-related dizziness. The nystagmus seen in the video is effectively direction changing, gaze-evoked nystagmus on lateral gaze. On investigation by neurology and magnetic resonance imaging (MRI), it was determined that this was a mild form of congenital nystagmus secondary to ocular misalignment for which she had been treated years prior. For a complete description of the variants, associated abnormalities, and discussion of the pathogenesis of congenital nystagmus the reader is referred to Leigh and Zee (2006).

SACCADE TESTING

Discussed in Chapter 9 were several protocols for testing saccadic activity. These are all well documented in the literature for ENG or VNG applications (Jacobson, Newman, & Kartush, 1993; Leigh & Zee, 2006; Shepard & Telian, 1996). Therefore, we concentrate our interpretation discussion on what has become the most common protocol used for routine clinical evaluation of saccadic eye movements, the random saccade paradigm, with a brief

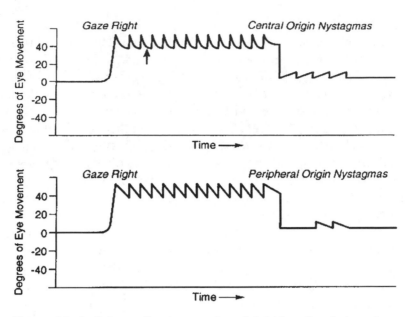

Figure 10-6. Schematized examples of right-beating jerk nystagmus of central origin in the top trace and of peripheral origin in the bottom trace. Note that in the top trace the slow component of the nystagmus shows a decreasing velocity. In the bottom trace the slow component has a constant (linear) velocity. Reprinted with permission from Shepard and Telian, 1996.

Congenital Nystagmus

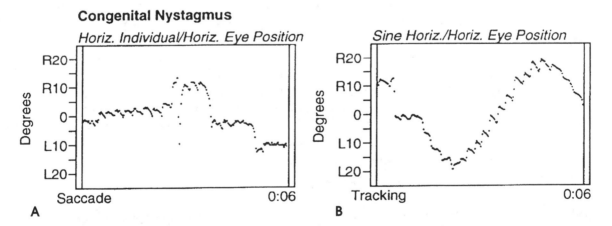

Figure 10-7. A. Recording from a patient with infantile nystagmus. Note that the slow component of the nystagmus demonstrates an increasing velocity curve for the right-beating nystagmus. This sample was taken during ENG saccade testing. **B.** Trace recorded during smooth pursuit testing in the same patient. The right-beating nystagmus is superimposed on the pursuit tracking but also shows the increasing velocity behavior for the slow component of the superimposed right beat. Reprinted with permission from Shepard and Telian, 1996.

discussion on antisaccades. Recognize that, in general, the interpretation of a fixed saccade paradigm will be similar to that detailed below for the random saccade paradigm.

As indicated in Chapter 9, the parameters used for analysis of a saccadic eye movement are the latency to onset after the presentation of a target at a new location, the accuracy with which that movement is made, and the peak velocity of the eye during the movement. The combined use of these three allows for possible suggestions of localization of involvement within the CNS based on the neurologic substrate responsible for the performance aspects of each of the three outcome parameters. Unlike gaze stability testing where abnormal findings can be of either central or peripheral vestibular system origin, saccade testing abnormalities do not occur as a result of peripheral vestibular system lesions, but can be of origin that is no CNS lesions (Tables 10–3 to 10–5). A detailed discussion of the current state of knowledge of the neural pathways responsible for saccade production is provided in Leigh and Zee (2006); only a brief summary of the salient aspects of that information is presented below. The neural substrate information is then used to develop the interpretation suggestions given for abnormalities related to saccade velocity, accuracy, and latencies or combinations of these parameters in Tables 10–3, 10–4, and 10–5, respectively.

For a horizontal or vertical reflexive saccade via the random saccade paradigm, the initiation of the movement results from the presentation of a target of interest in a new location. The horizontal reflexive eye movement bringing gaze to the new target is primarily engendered by excitatory burst

Table 10-3. Abnormalities of Saccade Velocity

- Slowing both eyes, all directions with full ocular range-of-motion
  - Fatigue, medications, drowsiness
  - PPRF for horizontal movements and RIMLF for vertical
  - Cerebral hemispheres, superior colliculus, cerebellum
  - Early in myasthenia gravis especially with repeated activity—glissades, initial fast movement and slowing as the target is approached (Leigh & Zee, 2006)
- Slowing either eye, restricted directions
  - For horizontal PPRF
  - For vertical RIMLF
  - For horizontal on adduction only (monocular or binocular)—MLF lesion on the side of the slowing (INO)
  - Cranial nerves III, IV, VI, or muscle palsy
- Abnormally fast
  - Later in myasthenia gravis of ocular type (Leigh & Zee, 2006)
  - Calibration errors
  - Restriction syndromes (see text for explanation)

Table 10-4. Abnormalities of Accuracy

- Hypometria (undershoot)
  - Fatigue, medications, drowsiness
  - Bilateral—cerebellar dorsal vermis (Leigh & Zee, 2006)
  - Unilateral—ipsilateral cerebellar/brainstem
  - Visual acuity or visual field cuts
  - Myasthenia gravis for large saccades
  - Brainstem burst neuron providing too short of a burst
  - Cerebral hemispheric—contralateral to the lesion more likely if the patient demonstrates neglect (Meienberg, Harrer, & Wehren, 1986)
- Hypermetria (overshoot)
  - Cerebellar
  - Bilateral—cerebellar fastigial nucleus (Leigh & Zee, 2006)

Table 10-5. Abnormalities of Latency

- Both eyes in all directions
  - Fatigue, medication, drowsiness
  - Frontal eye fields, but likely for remembered or antisaccade tasks as opposed to reflexive random saccade paradigm
  - Visual deficits—severe reductions in acuity, amblyobia (Ciuffreda, Kenyon, & Stark, 1978)
- Both eyes for fixed saccade paradigms—learned or commanded tasks
  - Basal ganglia as in Parkinson's and other disorders of motor initiation where target location and timing of movement is regular (Lasker & Zee, 1997; Lasker, Zee, & Hain, 1987)
- Abnormally short latency
  - Highly unusual—most likely patient anticipating target movement, needs reinstruction
- Superior colliculus and pathways to reticular formation in the brainstem (Leigh & Zee, 2006)

neurons (EBNs) in the paramedian pontine reticular formation (PPRF) in the caudal pons (van Gisbergen, Robinson, & Gielen, 1981). For vertical and torsional saccades the excitatory burst neurons are part of the rostral interstitial nucleus of the medial longitudinal fasciculus (riMLF) in the rostral mesencephalon (King & Fuchs, 1979; Vilis, Hepp, Schwarz, & Henn, 1989). These premotor neurons initiate bursts of activity approximately 12 ms prior to the actual initiation of the eye movement. However, while the premotor neurons connect with cranial nerve nuclei III and VI, the neural circuit also involves activity from inhibitory and omnipause neurons in the brainstem and midbrain areas in a complex network allowing for the activity of the EBN to initiate eye movements (see Chapter 2 in this text for a more detailed discussion) with velocities proportional to the neural firing rate (Leigh & Zee, 2006). There is a growing body of evidence that for both horizontal and vertical voluntary saccades areas other than simply frontal eye fields of the frontal lobe, brainstem and midbrain circuits are involved. These include the superior colliculus, cerebellum, various regions of the frontal lobe, the posterior parietal cortex, basal ganglia, and thalamus. A synthesis of this literature is provided by Leigh and Zee (2006).

Primary control over the velocity of the saccadic movement is engendered by the PPRF in the pons. Yet not all saccadic slowing disorders are from the pons region of the brainstem. A useful generality is that global slowing (both eyes in both directions with full ocular range of motion) could involve either the PPRF or the riMLF (see Chapter 2 for complete discussion), yet higher centers such as the superior colliculus or cerebral hemispheres need to be considered. If the slowing is restricted to involve only one eye or a single direction, then slowing of abduction is most likely a sixth nerve palsy with monocular slowing of adduction would be most likely INO with ipsilateral MLF lesion (see Chapter 2 for a full discussion of the effects of lesions in these areas). See Table 10–3 for other considerations.

In the performance of saccade testing, more so than during other portions of the ENG/VNG, individual eye recordings should be made if at all possible. It is during saccade testing that disconjugate eye movements are accentuated. The hallmark eye movement disorder causing disconjugate movement is that of internuclear ophthalmoplegia (INO). In this disorder the adducting (moving toward the midline) eye is abnormally slow. Recognition of the condition immediately implies a lesion in the medial longitudinal fasciculus (MLF) on the side of the eye with the adduction slowing (Leigh & Zee, 2006). Additionally, when INO is bilateral, there is a presumptive diagnosis of multiple sclerosis until proven otherwise. Video 10–11 shows the eye movements of a 44-year-old male with multiple sclerosis. The eye movements were captured during VNG saccade testing and illustrate bilateral INO. Figure 10–8 shows the recorded analysis for the eye movement in Video 10–11. Video 10–12 shows the eye movements of a 30-year-old male during random saccade testing with Figure 10–9 illustrating the recorded analysis for Videos 10–8 through 10–12. In this example, the eye movements and analysis are consistent with left-side unilateral INO. The patient was shown to have had an ischemic stroke on the left involving the left MLF pathway.

Abnormally fast saccades typically occur as a result of the saccade being prematurely halted before reaching the target (restriction syndrome) (Leigh & Zee, 2006). This can occur as a result of disease process that reduces the range of motion of an eye (such as myasthenia gravis) or a mechanical restriction in range of motion (such as trauma or a mass lesion), making the saccade too fast for its actual recorded amplitude, though likely normal velocity for its larger intended amplitude (Leigh & Zee, 2006). During ENG or VNG testing inaccurate calibration needs to be ruled out as a cause for apparent abnormally fast saccade performance.

The cerebellum, specifically the dorsal vermis and fastigial nucleus regions, are major contributors to the accuracy with which saccades are performed (Leigh & Zee, 2006). Yet although overshoot dysmetria (hypermetria) is considered a strong indication of cerebellar involvement, the possibilities for involvement in the presences of hypometric (undershoot dysmetria) saccades are considerably broader (Leigh & Zee, 2006). Patients with severe visual acuity deficits, especially macular degeneration, may perform the saccades to targets by using multiple smaller saccades, because during a random saccade task the target direction is clear but placing the target on the fovea becomes difficult. Patients with visual field cuts that involve a full or partial hemisphere (hemianopia) will produce hypometric saccades. Here also combinations of brainstem and cerebellar lesion may

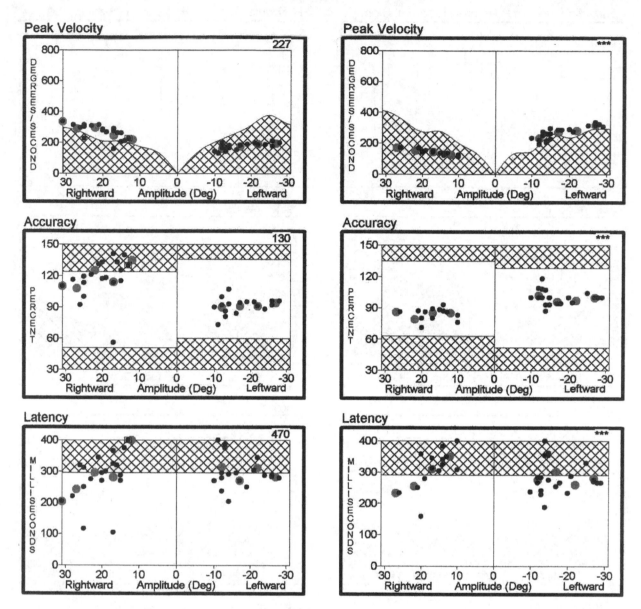

Figure 10–8. The recorded eye movement from individual eye recordings for the 44-year-old male in Video 10–11 who was subsequently diagnosed with multiple sclerosis. The column of results on the left is for the right eye with the right column representing the left eye. The top two panels indicate peak velocity; the middle two show accuracy, and the bottom two are for latency all as a function of the excursion of the eyes. The larger light color dots represent average performance for the parameter at the specific excursion with the small black dots the performance for individual saccades. The velocity panels clearly show, as seen in the video, slowing of each eye on adduction indicating bilateral INO. Additionally, abnormal slowing is noted for both eyes dominantly on movements to the right. Note that analysis is done based on needing 50% of the individual saccades to be outside the normal range for a particular aspect of the study to be considered abnormal.

result in mild to severe undershooting of the target (Leigh & Zee, 2006).

Another aspect of saccade accuracy is related to the mentioned ocular lateralpulsion introduced in the section on gaze testing (a full discussion of the anatomy and examination findings is given in Chapter 2). This directional bias of saccades is most commonly ipsipulsion, with hypermetric saccades (overshoot) to the lesion side, and hypometric saccades to the contralateral side (undershoot).

Saccade - Individual Eyes

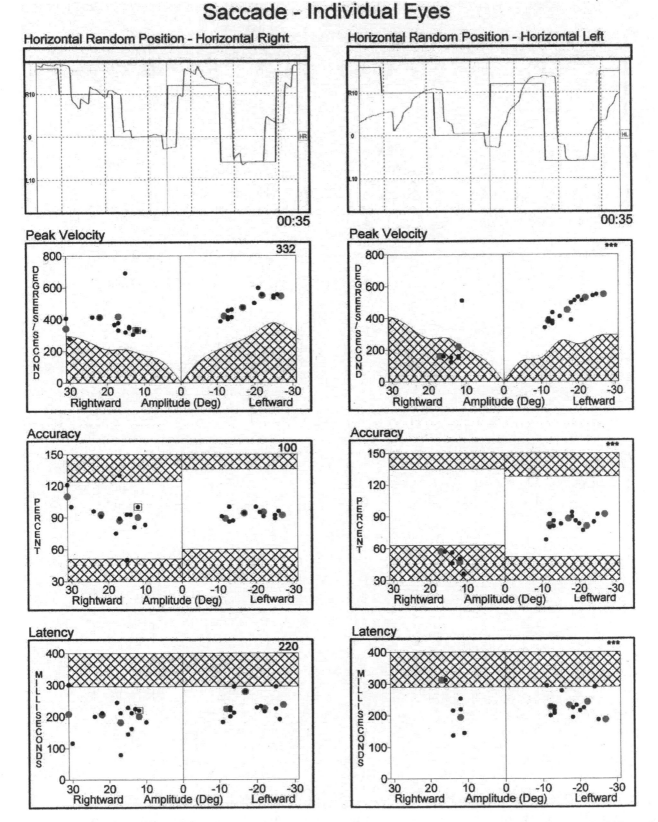

Figure 10-9. Saccade performance from the 30-year-old male in Video 10–12 demonstrating left-side INO and subsequently diagnosed with a left-side brainstem stroke. See legend for Figure 10–8 for details of the figure layout. Additionally, the top two panels show samples of the raw eye movement for five saccades. The lighter trace is the actual eye movements with the black trace the target movement. Right eye represented on the left and left eye on the right. In the velocity plot for the left eye significant slowing is noted for adduction.

The bias in eye movement to the lesion side is seen in conditions like the examples in Video 10–6. This is also seen in a more involved form of dorsolateral medullary infarction (with specific signs beyond that in the patient in Video 10–6) called Wallenberg's syndrome (Leigh & Zee, 2006). The general bias for active saccade movement toward the lesion side is due to disruption of fibers from the inferior olivary nucleus in the medulla through the inferior cerebellar peduncle that modulate the neural firing pattern of the dorsal vermis Purkinje cells ipsilateral to the lesion. Through a combination of disruptions in complex excitatory and inhibitory pathways this results in the clinical picture of overshoot in horizontal saccades in one direction and undershoot in the contralateral direction (Leigh & Zee, 2006). Realize that the example presented in Video 10–6 shows ipsipulsion (ocular lateral pulsion is the older term), but the reverse can occur with the hypermetric saccade being contralesional (for a full discussion of the literature in this area and possible models see Leigh & Zee, 2006, pp. 149, 163).

The last attribute of a saccade is the length of time to initiation of the eye movement (latency) once a target of interest appears or a command is given to gaze at an already existing target within the visual field. Lesions in the PPRF or riMLF involving the burst neurons could cause delays in the initiation of the eye movement horizontally or vertically but this would represent an unusual situation. The process to initiate the burst neuron activity involves multiple other central areas that could result in delayed onset of burst neuron activity and ultimately in an increase in latency for the desired saccade. The involvement may be from visual acuity problems, and amblyopia (Ciuffreda, Kenyon, & Stark, 1978) to visual eye fields in the frontal cortex (Leigh & Zee, 2006). Likely more with latency than either velocity or accuracy the state of the patient regarding medication, drowsiness, and attention highly influences the results. It is with latency more so than with velocity or accuracy that the paradigm differences between fixed (volitional or commanded) saccades and the random paradigm reflexive saccades are seen. Basal ganglia involvement can cause increased latencies to fixed saccades yet show normal initiation timing with random saccades (Leigh & Zee, 2006).

Once drugs, inattention, drowsiness, fatigue, and impaired visual acuity are ruled out then any abnormality with saccade performance must be considered as a potential indicator of CNS or peripheral ocular motor involvement. It would not be reasonable to consider peripheral vestibular system involvement as a possible source for disruptions in any of the saccade parameters discussed above.

When performing an antisaccade paradigm the primary means for analysis during an ENG or VNG is percent error. This would be a ratio of the number of saccadic eye movements that were made in the direction of the target movement to the number made in the opposite direction (the desired response). With practice you should expect patients to be able to perform the antisaccade task with a percent of error near zero for an interval of 5 to 10 s. When overall performance from the start to the end of the task was investigated in a large number of young healthy male subjects the percent error has been noted to be 23% with a large variance of 17% (Evdokimidis et al., 2002). If performance is such that correct sustained saccades cannot be obtained for 5 to 10 s then involvement in the eye fields of the frontal cortex must be considered (Leigh & Zee, 2006).

SMOOTH PURSUIT TRACKING

The principal parameters for interpreting smooth pursuit tracking are paradigm specific. Tasks for evaluation of pursuit abilities can use initiation-focused, nonpredictable target movement, apparent or actual movement of the background together with the target, the most widely used protocol is that described in Chapter 9, predictable sinusoidal or fixed-velocity target movement. For this type of paradigm the velocity gain and phase of the eye movement with regard to the target are used (see Chapter 9 for further explanations) for the sinusoidal target with velocity gain as the main factor when using fixed-velocity stimuli. As with other ocular motor tasks these parameters are highly susceptible to the state of the subject, but unlike gaze stability and saccades, smooth pursuit tracking is the task most sensitive to age. A sample of age-sensitive normative data is provided in Chapter 9 giving both velocity gain and phase values. Other such data demonstrating the effects of age on various aspects of smooth pursuit are available in the literature (Paige, 1994;

Spooner, Sakala, & Baloh, 1980; Zackon & Sharpe, 1987). For a discussion of other paradigms to investigate features of smooth pursuit tracking other than sustained pursuit (predicable steady state targets like sinusoids), the reader is referred to Leigh and Zee (2006).

The neurologic substrate (for a complete description see the discussion in Chapter 2 of this text) for the generation and sustaining of accurate smooth pursuit tracking starts with retinal stimulation and involves multiple areas of the cortex with projections through the pontine area of the brainstem to the cerebellum and onto the nuclei of the extraocular muscles. These pathways are suggested from both primate and human studies (Berman et al., 1999; Leigh & Zee, 2006). The complexity of the multiple pathways and the various contributions of the individual components make specific site-of-lesion identification within the pathways difficult at best even when multiple protocols are used to investigate patient performance. For a thorough discussion of the hypotheses based on a synthesis of a large body of literature the reader is referred to Leigh and Zee (2006). In the routine clinical evaluation by ENG/VNG, only target stimuli that investigate the sustainable nature of smooth pursuit are used, thus limiting the ability to identify abnormalities (more likely cerebral cortex) that may impact on only the initiation phase of the pursuit performance (Leigh & Zee, 2006).

No specific differentiation in lesion site has been determined when comparing reduced velocity gain for sustained target presentation at fixed-velocity versus changing velocity stimuli of the sinusoidal target. Lesions could involve large cerebral infarcts, basal ganglia regions, pontine projection pathways to the cerebellum, and various areas of the cerebellum (Leigh & Zee, 2006). The principal region of the cerebellum involved in the production of smooth pursuit eye movements is that of the paraflocculus of the vestibulocerebellum (Rambold, Churchland, Selig, Jasmin, & Lisberger, 2002). The dorsal vermis of the cerebellum is involved in the initial movement of pursuit during the onset of the task (open-loop period) but does not seem to participate in the steady-state aspects of the performance seen with fixed velocity or sinusoidal (increasing acceleration) protocols (Takagi, Zee, & Tamargo, 2000).

Therefore, although there are numerous other neurologic substrate contributions to various aspects of the performance of pursuit contingent on the specific task, the vestibulocerebellum is a common final pathway that is always involved in the production of the eye movements. Even though it is a significant oversimplification, an interpretive suggestion is that persistent abnormalities of pursuit using sustained target tasks may relate to lesions in the vestibulocerebellum (especially with coexisting gaze-evoked nystagmus) or the immediate projection pathways from the pontine nuclei of the brainstem. One must always be cognizant of the other pathway possibilities that could be involved in pursuit disruptions.

The use of the phase parameter for sinusoidal target tasking is a measure of the temporal arrangement between target and eye movements. In general, at younger ages the phase angle should be close to zero for properly performed smooth pursuit. As we age or as the task becomes more difficult, by increasing the frequency of target movement the phase lag becomes more apparent. A leading phase is not usually taken as an indication of pathologic activity but rather as anticipatory behavior on the part of the patient. The leading could be anxiety regarding the testing situation or simply a lack of understanding the task. Most often this is corrected with reinstruction of the patient and repeating of the task. It is typical that reduction in gain will be seen with abnormal phase lag. However, when the phase lag is outside the normal range with velocity gain normal and reinstruction and repeated testing does not remove the abnormality, possible central system involvement should be considered but it would be less likely to involve the dorsolateral pontine nuclei or the vestibulocerebellum (Leigh & Zee, 2006).

Pursuit disruptions can be bidirectional or unidirectional. When asymmetric gain is encountered, lesion sites can again range from the cortex to the pontine nuclei and vestibulocerebellum. In most cases, the pursuit abnormality is toward the lesion side due to a double deccusation between the cortex and ocular motor nuclei. The magnitude of the gain disruption is usually greater for lesions in the lower system pathways versus lesion in the cortex (Leigh & Zee, 2006). Video 10–13 and Figure 10–10 demonstrate asymmetrical pursuit in a 20-year-old male with indications of cortex and subcortical

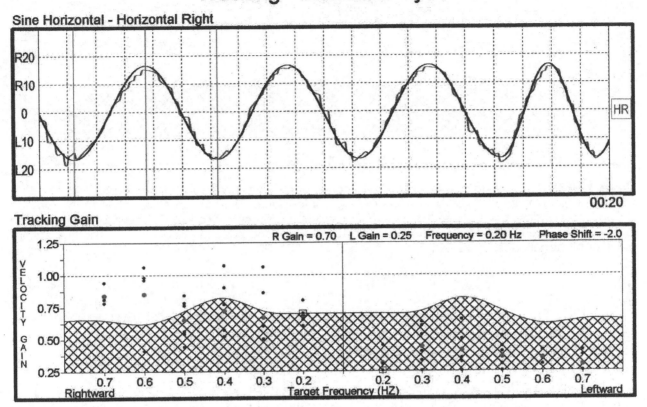

Figure 10–10. The top panel shows the target and the recorded eye movements for the right eye from a 20-year-old male following a severe closed head injury accident. The bottom panel gives the quantitative analysis for the eye movements shown in the top panel and Video 10–13. In the analysis the larger gray dots are the average performance over several cycles of the target movement with the small black dots the velocity gain for an individual cycle. All are shown as a function of frequency of target movement for a fixed target excursion of 20 degrees to each side of center. Note the significant asymmetry in performance for left versus right. See the text for discussion of the asymmetry.

involvement resulting from a closed head injury accident. The eye movements demonstrate classic saccadic disruptions to the attempt to move the eyes in a smooth manner when tracking the light bar target. This is referred to as "cog wheeling" pursuit. Note that the performance of the pursuit worsens for leftward movements yet improves for rightward movements as the frequency of the target increases. The analysis of his eye movement shown in Figure 10–10 brings up the question as to whether pursuit is interpreted as abnormal when performance at the lower frequencies is abnormal, yet as the difficulty of the task increases the performance returns to the normal region as shown for eye movement to the right in this figure. Could it be possible to have

lesions in areas other than the cerebellum that may cause abnormalities at the lower frequencies yet normal performance at the more rapid movements? It would take comparisons of fixed-velocity paradigms and the accelerating target paradigm (as used in this example) to suggest that situation (Leigh & Zee, 2006). However, in most situations if the sinusoidal pursuit returns to a normal range as the frequency of the target for a fixed excursion is increased, the study is taken as normal especially when the performance is symmetrical. Video 10–14 demonstrates pursuit abnormality that is strictly unidirectional with no abnormal performance to the right as a contrast with the example in Video 10–13. The quantitative analysis for this video is shown in Figure 10–11.

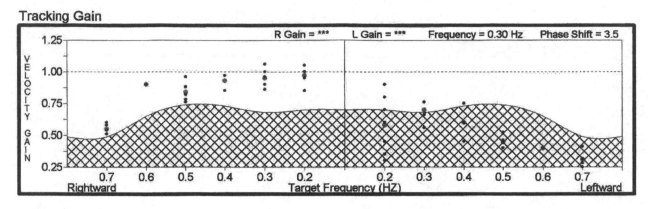

Figure 10–11. Quantitative analysis for the eye movements shown in Video 10–14 from a 33-year-old male with diagnosed traumatic brain injury. See the legend for Figure 10–10 for an explanation of the symbols shown in the analysis panel. Note that this analysis shows strictly unidirectional pursuit disruption compared to the asymmetric pursuit performance in Figure 10–10 suggesting possible abnormalities in both directions of different magnitudes.

The patient is a 33-year-old male also with a closed head injury and diagnosed traumatic brain injury. Video 10–15 demonstrates abnormal pursuit that is bidirectional and symmetric. This is from the 46-year-old female with diffuse brainstem and cerebellar involvement secondary to alcohol abuse. The quantitative analysis for her eye movements is given in Figure 10–12.

There can be interactions between saccade performance and that of smooth pursuit that can give the appearance of unidirectional pursuit abnormalities that is a false positive. This is illustrated in Videos 10–16 and 10–17. These videos show random saccade performance (see Video 10–16) followed by smooth pursuit performance (see Video 10–17) in a 52-year-old female with multiple sclerosis. As can be seen in Video 10–16 the patient is displaying bilateral INO with significant slowing of each eye on adduction. Therefore, when viewing her performance for smooth pursuit, it would appear that as each eye adducts with the pursuit task the eye is moving smoothly while the abducting eye has a saccadic appearance. The smooth movements of each eye on the pursuit task for adduction are a result of the effects of the INO causing saccades to not be produced as is seen when abducting movement is made. It is the combination of the INO and the central system lesion to the pursuit neuro-substrate that gives the appearance of unidirectional pursuit abnormality.

OPTOKINETIC EVALUATION

As discussed in Chapter 9, the technical aspects to evaluate the optokinetic system are significant. They require filling at least 90% of the visual field with the target, then quantitatively analyzing the optokinetic nystagmus (OKN) with velocity gain (eye velocity divided by target velocity) for target movement to the left and right, and lastly obtaining and analyzing optokinetic after nystagmus (OKAN) to get an isolated review of the optokinetic system without the influence of smooth pursuit (Leigh & Zee, 2006). Even if all of the technical points are achieved, abnormalities of OKN regarding asymmetric velocity gain in the absence of abnormalities of smooth pursuit tracking are likely related to unilateral peripheral hypofunction resulting in a bias of the nystagmus beating away from the hypofunction or as a result of abnormalities in the visual pathways including the eye (Baloh, Yee, & Honrubia, 1982; Valmaggia, Proudlock, & Gottlob, 2003). In general, if asymmetrical performance for OKN gains is to be reflective of central vestibular system lesions of the cerebellum/brainstem regions, it would be expected that abnormalities would be noted for the more specific tests for these regions: smooth pursuit tracking and saccade testing. The principal reason for the lack of sensitivity to CNS lesions with OKN is that the production of OKN is dependent on two overlapping

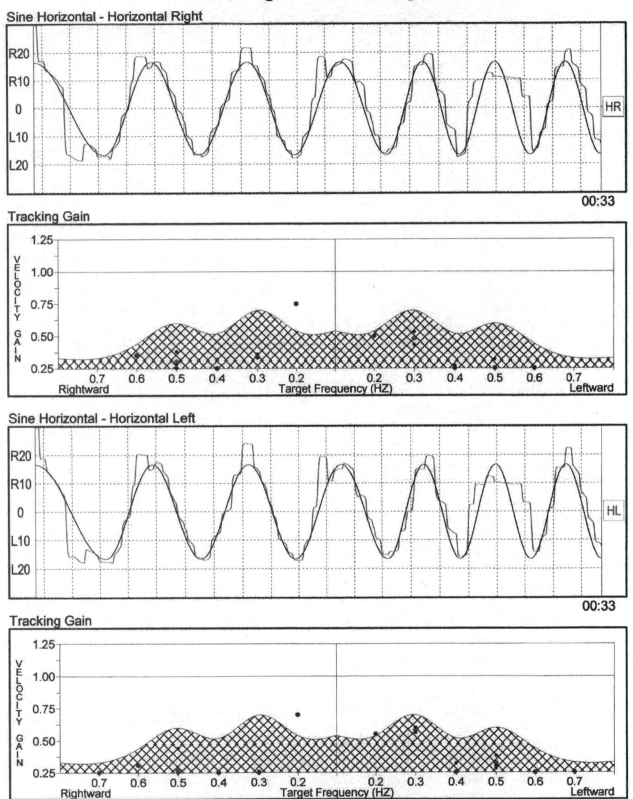

Tracking - Individual Eyes

Figure 10–12. Quantitative analysis for the eye movements from the 46-year-old female shown in Video 10–15. Shown are the sample recordings for both the right eye in the upper panel and the left eye in the lower panel. The quantitative analysis for each eye is shown below the eye tracings. See text for further information and Figure 10–10 legend for explanation of the symbols on the figure.

systems sharing neurologic substrate: the optokinetic system and the smooth pursuit system. This has been shown in a variety of primate and human studies summarized in Leigh and Zee (2006) and in recent work with functional MRI studies in human subjects (Bense et al., 2006; Konen, Kleiser, Seitz, & Bremmer, 2005). As would therefore be expected, the gain for OKN does decline with age in a manner parallel to that of smooth pursuit at least up to ages under 75 years with some suggested stabilization after age 75 (Kerber, Ishiyama, & Baloh, 2006; Valmaggia et al., 2004).

Because of this overlap between pursuit and OKN, a common manner for analysis is the comparison of the velocity gains from OKN to smooth pursuit for a given patient in order to suggest whether OKN performance is abnormal yet possibly explainable based on abnormalities in pursuit if present.

To investigate lesions affecting the optokinetic system activity of the velocity storage system in the vestibular nuclei in the pons, OKAN must be used together with OKN. Hypothetically, abnormalities of gain asymmetry may not be seen with OKN, yet asymmetries in initial slow component velocity (initial gain), the time constant of decay, or the slow cumulative eye velocity of the OKAN may be noted implicating the region of the velocity storage integrator (Leigh & Zee, 2006). The reader is, however, reminded as to the significant variability and difficulty in reliably acquiring the OKAN response. Because of the technical issues and the lack of sensitivity and specificity in lesion detection, this combination is not considered currently to be part of a routine ocular motor investigation and beyond the scope of this chapter. For a full discussion of these issues the interested reader is referred to the literature (Hain & Zee, 1991; Hain et al., 1994; Leigh & Zee, 2006).

In routine clinical ocular motor testing, the evaluation of OKN is the least useful of the tests we have discussed. Yet it can be brought into play in specific situations precisely because of its relationship to smooth pursuit. The first is in the evaluation of smooth pursuit testing in children. Smooth pursuit gains are lower and phase lag larger in children (8 to 19 years of age) than adults or children reaching adult values for horizontal movement of the eyes between 12 and 15 years of age (Salman, Sharpe, Lilakas, Dennis, & Steinbach, 2006). Yet to test smooth pursuit in an infant, although obtainable, is not an easy task. Studies concentrating on children in the first year of life have shown, as in the adults, that pursuit and optokinetic systems work together to produce OKN and that the evaluation of pursuit may be approximated with evaluation of OKN velocity gains (Rosander & von Hofsten, 2002; Valmaggia et al., 2004; Von Hofsten & Rosander, 1996, 1997) (see Chapter 25 for further discussion). The second use of OKN can be in the adult with severely disrupted pursuit performance. In situations of this type OKN would also be expected to be significantly abnormal. Thus, OKN testing may serve as a cross-check for the pursuit findings. In patients who cannot complete a smooth pursuit task secondary to complaints of symptom generation with sinusoidal movements, OKN velocity gain with fixed velocity movement and a small target (like that of a light bar) may serve to approximate pursuit performance.

The foregoing discussion provides general guidelines for interpretation of the routine ocular motor studies used in the evaluation of the dizzy and balance disorder patient population. Although the principal utility of these studies is to investigate the possible involvement of the central vestibular and ocular motor control regions of the CNS, other uses for investigation of eye movement disorders not related to dizziness are well documented and are discussed in Leigh and Zee (2006) for the interested reader. Additionally, the area of eye movement abnormalities using the above investigational tools for characterization of psychiatric disease not related to dizziness has recently been described in the literature. A summary article is available that synthesizes this area of work (Trillenberg, Lencer, & Heide, 2004).

VIDEOS ASSOCIATED WITH THIS CHAPTER

Video 10–1. Shown is the direct eye movement examination in the following order; fixation present, fixation removed, and finally head-shake testing. The patient is a 77-year-old female with diagnosis of right vestibular hypofunction secondary to vestibular-neuronitis.

See text discussion for details of what is occurring in the video.

Video 10–2. A. Right-beating, gaze-evoked nystagmus on right gaze for a 46-year-old female with diffuse brainstem and cerebellar involvement. **B.** The same patient on left gaze producing left-beating, gaze-evoked nystagmus.

Video 10–3. Demonstrated is vertical up-beating nystagmus on gaze up in a 46-year-old female with central involvement secondary to alcohol abuse. This video was taken during the execution of the ocular motor testing of her VNG.

Video 10–4. A female in her mid-seventies with a persistent down-beating nystagmus. The video direct office examination is with fixation present with gaze in primary position, to the left, up, and finally to the right. Note that the down beat is pure with no horizontal or torsional components. This was the result of a cranio-cervical junction abnormality other than an Arnold-Chiari malformation; see text for further discussion.

Video 10–5. Direct video examination of a male in his mid-forties with a significant traumatic brain injury from a closed head injury. For details of what is being shown in the video, see the text discussion.

Video 10–6. Pure right torsional nystagmus in center (primary) gaze with a combined right torsional and right horizontal beating nystagmus on right gaze in this female in her mid-forties. On returning to primary gaze from the right she is asked to close her eyes and on opening the eyes can be seen to be deviated to the right. For further details about her case see the text discussion.

Video 10–7. A. Bruns' nystagmus in the 49-year-old female who is status post a Chiari surgical repair at age 15 and a vestibular schwannoma resection on the left at age 47. **B.** Video eye examination now with fixation removed. See the text discussion for further details.

Video 10–8. A 68-year-old male diagnosed with a form of spinocerebellar atrophy. The

video illustrates square-wave jerks. See text for details.

Video 10–9. Ocular flutter with opsoclonus in a 71-year-old female. For case details refer to the text.

Video 10–10. Gaze-evoked nystagmus on right and left gaze in a 16-year-old female. This was determined to be a mild form of congenital nystagmus and not representative of active CNS pathology. See the text for details.

Video 10–11. Bilateral INO in a 44-year-old male who was subsequently diagnosed with multiple sclerosis. The patient is performing random saccade testing during his VNG.

Video 10–12. A 30-year-old male performing random saccade testing during his VNG. Seen is unilateral, left-side INO subsequently shown to be a result of an ischemic stroke on the left involving the left MLF pathways.

Video 10–13. The eye movements seen are from a 20-year-old male during the smooth pursuit testing from his VNG. Demonstrated is his asymmetric pursuit with saccadic disruptions significantly greater for eye movements to the left. Yet minor difficulties are noted for movement to the right. The quantitative analysis of these eye movements as a function of frequency is given in Figure 10–10.

Video 10–14. The smooth pursuit performance is from a 33-year-old male with traumatic brain injury. The analysis of the pursuit tracking is given in Figure 8–11. See text for details.

Video 10–15. In this recording the pursuit abnormality is symmetrical for both right- and leftward movements. As with Videos 10–13 and 10–14, the performance is shown over a variety of frequencies. The patient is a 46-year-old female with cerebellar and brainstem involvement from alcohol abuse. Figure 10–12 shows her quantitative analysis.

Video 10–16. This is a recording of random saccade performance in a 52-year-old female with multiple sclerosis. Individual eyes are shown. For details of the case see the text.

Video 10–17. Individual eye recordings during smooth pursuit tracking task in the same 52-year-old female shown in Video 10–16. See the text for further explanations of the case.

REFERENCES

Baloh, R. W., Yee, R. D., & Honrubia, V. (1982). Clinical abnormalities of optokinetic nystagmus. In G. Lennerstrand, D. S. Zee, & E. L. Keller (Eds.), *Functional basis of ocular motility disorders* (pp. 311–320). Oxford, UK: Pergamon.

Bance, M., Mai, M., Tomlinson, D., & Rutka, J. (1991). The changing direction of nystagmus in acute Meniere's disease: Pathophysiological implications. *Laryngoscope, 101,* 197–201.

Bataller, L., Rosenfeld, M. R., Graus, F., Vilchez, J. J., Cheung, N.-K., & Dalmau, J. (2003). Autoantigen diversity in the opsoclonus-myoclonus syndrome. *Annals of Neurology, 53,* 347–353.

Bense, S., Janusch, B., Vucurevic, G., Bauermann, T., Schlindwein, P., Brandt, T., . . . Dieterich, M. (2006). Brainstem and cerebellar fMRI-activation during horizontal and vertical optokinetic stimulation. *Experimental Brain Research, 174,* 312–323.

Berman, R. A., Colby, C. L., Genovese, C. R., Voyvodic, J. T., Luna, B., Thulborn, K. R., & Sweeney, J. A. (1999). Cortical networks subserving pursuit and saccadic eye movements in humans: An FMRI study. *Human Brain Mapping, 8,* 209–225.

Brandt, T., & Dieterich, M. (2000). Assessment and management of central vestibular disorders. In S. Herdman (Ed.), *Vestibular rehabilitation* (2nd ed., pp. 264–297). Philadelphia, PA: F. A. Davis.

Bruns, L. (1908). *Die geschwulste des nervensystems.* Berlin, Germany: S. Karger.

Ciuffreda, K. J., Kenyon, R. V., & Stark, L. (1978). Increased saccadic latencies in amblyopic eyes. *Investigative Ophthalmology and Visual Science, 17,* 697–702.

Deutschlander, A., Strupp, M., Jahn, K., Quiring, F., & Brandt, T. (2004). Vertical oscillopsia in bilateral superior canal dehiscence syndrome. *Neurology, 62*(5), 784–787.

Evdokimidis, I., Smyrnis, N., Constantinidis, T. N., Stefanis, N. C., Avramopoulos, D., Paximadis, C., . . . Stefanis, C. N. (2002). The antisaccade task in a sample of 2006 young men. I. Normal population characteristics. *Experimental Brain Research, 147,* 45–52.

Fukushima, K., Kaneko, C. R., & Fuchs, A. F. (1992). The neuronal substrate of integration in the oculomotor system. *Progress in Neurobiology, 39,* 609–639.

Gordon, S., Hain, T., Zee, D., & Fetter, D. (1986). Rebound nystagmus. *Society of Neuroscience Abstracts, 12,* 1091.

Gresty, M. A., Bronstein, A. M., Page, N. G., & Rudge, P. (1991). Congenital-type nystagmus emerging in later life. *Neurology, 41,* 653–656.

Hain, T. C., Heroman, S. J., Holliday, M., Mattox, D., Zee, D. S., & Byskosh, A. I. (1994). Localizing value of optokinetic afternystagmus. *Annals of Otology, Rhinology and Laryngology, 103,* 806–811.

Hain, T. C., & Zee, D. S. (1991). Abolition of optokinetic afternystagmus by aminoglycoside ototoxicity. *Annals of Otology, Rhinology and Laryngology, 100,* 580–583.

Herishanu, Y. O., & Sharpe, J. A. (1981). Normal square wave jerks. *Investigative Ophthalmology and Visual Science, 20,* 268–272.

Hertle, R. W., Maldanado, V. K., Maybodi, M., & Yang, D. (2002). Clinical and ocular motor analysis of the infantile nystagmus syndrome in the first 6 months of life. *British Journal of Ophthalmology, 86,* 670–675.

Hood, J. D. (1981). Further observations on the phenomenon of rebound nystagmus. *Annals of the New York Academy of Sciences, 374,* 532–539.

Hotson, J. R. (1984). Convergence-initiated voluntary flutter: A normal intrinsic capability in man. *Brain Research, 294,* 299–304.

Jacobson, G. P., Newman, C. W., & Kartush, J. M. (Eds.). (1993). *Handbook of balance function testing.* St. Louis MO: Mosby.

Kasai, T., & Zee, D. S. (1978). Eye-head coordination in labyrinthine-defective human beings. *Brain Research, 144,* 123–141.

Kerber, K. A., Ishiyama, G. P., & Baloh, R. W. (2006). A longitudinal study of oculomotor function in normal older people. *Neurobiology and Aging, 27,* 1346–1353.

King, W. M., & Fuchs, A. F. (1979). Reticular control of vertical saccadic eye movements by mesencephalic burst neurons. *Journal of Neurophysiology, 42,* 861–867.

Konen, C. S., Kleiser, R., Seitz, R. J., & Bremmer, F. (2005). An fMRI study of optokinetic nystagmus and smooth-pursuit eye movement in humans. *Exponential Brain Research, 165,* 203–216.

Lasker, A. G., & Zee, D. S. (1997). Ocular motor abnormalities in Huntington's disease. *Vision Research, 37,* 3639–3645.

Lasker, A. G., Zee, D. S., & Hain, T. C. (1987). Saccades in Huntington's disease: Initiation defects and distractibility. *Neurology, 37,* 364–370.

Leigh, J. R., & Zee, D. S. (2006). *The neurology of eye movements* (4th ed). New York, NY: Oxford University Press.

McClure, J. A., & Lycett, P. (1983). Vestibular asymmetry. Some theoretical and practical considerations. *Archives of Otolaryngology, 109,* 682.

McConville, K., Tomlinson, R. D., King, W. M., Paige, G., & Na, E. Q. (1994). Eye position signals in the vestibular nuclei: Consequences for models of integrator function. *Journal of Vestibular Research, 4,* 391–400.

Meienberg, O., Harrer, M., & Wehren, C. (1986). Oculographic diagnosis of hemineglect in patients with homonymous hemianopia. *Journal of Neurology, 233,* 97–101.

Paige, G. D. (1994). Senescence of human visual-vestibular interactions: Smooth pursuit, optokinetic, and vestibular control of eye movements with aging. *Experimental Brain Research, 98,* 355–372.

Pierrot-Deseilligny, C., & Milea, D. (2005). Vertical nystagmus: Clinical facts and hypotheses. *Brain, 128,* 1237–1246.

Rambold, H., Churchland, A., Selig, Y., Jasmin, L., & Lisberger, S. G. (2002). Partial ablations of the flocculus and ventral paraflocculus in monkeys cause linked deficits in smooth pursuit eye movements and adaptive modification of the VOR. *Journal of Neurophysiology, 87,* 912–924.

Rosander, K., & von Hofsten, C. (2002). Development of gaze tracking of small and large objects. *Experimental Brain Research, 146,* 257–264.

Salman, M. S., Sharpe, J. A., Lillakas, L., Dennis, M., & Steinbach, M.J. (2006). Smooth pursuit eye movements in children. *Experimental Brain Research, 169,* 139–143.

Selhorst, J. B., Stark, L., Ochs, A. L., & Hoyt, W. F. (1976). Disorders in cerebellar ocular motor control. II Macrosaccadic oscillation. An oculographic control system and clinico-anatomic analysis. *Brain, 99,* 509–522.

Shepard, N. T., & Telian, S. A. (1996). *Practical management of the balance disorder patient.* San Diego, CA: Singular.

Solomon, D., Galetta, S. L., & Liu, G. T. (1995). Possible mechanisms for horizontal gaze deviation and lateropulsion in the lateral medullary syndrome. *Journal of Neuro-Ophthalmology, 15,* 26–30.

Spooner, J. W., Sakala, S. M., & Baloh, R. W. (1980). Effect of aging on eye tracking. *Archives of Neurology, 37,* 575–576.

Sylvestre, P. A., Choi, J. T., & Cullen, K. E. (2003). Discharge dynamics of oculomotor neural integrator neurons during conjugate and disjunctive saccades and fixation. *Journal of Neurophysiology, 90,* 739–754.

Takagi, M., Zee, D. S., & Tamargo, R. J. (2000). Effects of lesions of oculomotor cerebellar vermis on eye movements in primate: Smooth pursuit. *Journal of Neurophysiology, 83,* 2047–2062.

Trillenberg, P., Lencer, R., & Heide, W. (2004). Eye movements and psychiatric disease. *Current Opinion in Neurology, 17,* 43–47.

Valmaggia, C., Proudlock, F., & Gottlob, I. (2003). Optokinetic nystagmus in strabismus: Are asymmetries related binocularity? *Investigative Ophthalmology and Visual Science, 44,* 5142–5150.

Valmaggia, C., Rutsche, A., Baumann, A., Pieh, C., Bellaiche Shavit, Y., Proudlock, F., & Gottlob, I. (2004). Age related change of optokinetic nystagmus in healthy subjects: A study from infancy to senescence. *British Journal of Ophthalmology, 88,* 1577–1581.

Van Gisbergen, J. A. M., Robinson, D. A., & Gielen, S. (1981). A quantitative analysis of the generation of saccadic eye movements by burst neurons. *Journal of Neurophysiology, 45,* 417–442.

Vilis, T., Hepp, K., Schwarz, U., & Henn, V. (1989). On the generation of vertical and torsional rapid eye movements in the monkey. *Experimental Brain Research, 77,* 1–11.

Von Hofsten, C., & Rosander, K. (1996). The development of gaze control and predictive tracking in young infants. *Vision Research, 36,* 81–96.

Von Hofsten, C., & Rosander, K. (1997). Development of smooth pursuit tracking in young infants. *Vision Research, 37,* 1799–1810.

Waespe, W., & Wichmann, W. (1990). Oculomotor disturbances during visual-vestibular interaction in Wallenberg's lateral medullary syndrome. *Brain, 113,* 821–846.

Walker, M. F., & Zee, D. S. (2005). Asymmetry of the pitch vestibulo-ocular reflex in patients with cerebellar disease. *Annals of the New York Academy of Sciences, 1039,* 349–358.

Yee, R. D., Spiegel, P. H., Yamada, T., Abel, L. A., & Zee, D. S. (1994). Voluntary saccadic oscillations resembling ocular flutter and opsoclonus. *Journal of Neuro-ophthalmology, 14,* 95–101.

Zackon, D. H., & Sharpe, J. A. (1987). Smooth pursuit in senescence. *Acta Oto-Laryngologica (Stockh.), 104,* 290–297.

Zee, D. S., Yamazaki, A., Butler, P. H., & Gücer, G. (1981). Effects of ablation of flocculus and paraflocculus on eye movements in primate. *Journal of Neurophysiology, 46,* 878–899.

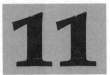

Technique and Interpretation of Positional Testing

Richard A. Roberts

INTRODUCTION

The purpose of this chapter is to review the techniques and interpretation of results obtained when patients undergoing vestibular assessment are moved into specific positions (positioning) and when they are maintained in static positions (positionals). There is somewhat of a paradox regarding the information provided to the clinician by these techniques. On one hand, positioning allows the clinician to identify the most common cause of vertigo, benign paroxysmal positional vertigo (BPPV). The results typically provide information regarding not only the involved ear but also the involved semicircular canal, results that are essential for successful management. The results of positioning are most often unequivocal.

On the other hand, positional testing may yield results that could be consistent with central or peripheral involvement while consideration must be given to effects of drugs and alcohol on results. Determination of the involved ear can be difficult using results of positional testing alone. Clinicians may become frustrated trying to determine if observed nystagmus is "clinically significant." If the nystagmus is termed clinically significant, the results may be interpreted as "nonspecific" or "nonlocalizing" which are terms that are not helpful. This is discussed, but also our view that any nystagmus

should be considered along with history, symptoms, and other remarkable findings for appropriate interpretation.

VESTIBULO-OCULAR REFLEX

Optimal visual perception of a target image is accomplished when that image is directed to the most sensitive areas of the retina in the area of the foveola. Poletti, Listorti, and Rucci (2013) have shown that the foveola is not uniform in its sensitivity and microsaccades help move target images onto the most sensitive areas for visual tasks with no head movement. Maintaining the target image grows more challenging during natural head movements. The purpose of the vestibulo-ocular reflex (VOR) is to maintain the location of a viewed image on the foveola of the retina during active head motion (Demer, Oas, & Baloh, 1993; Longridge & Mallinson, 1987). The vestibular system provides information regarding head movement so that compensatory eye movements may be produced to avoid slippage of the image from this area of the retina (Dannenbaum, Paquet, Hakim-Zadek, & Feldman, 2005; Roberts & Gans, 2007). VOR activity is elicited during head or head and body movement from one position to another in the normal system by an imbalance in neural activity from the end organs to the vestibular nuclei. The medial longitudinal fasciculus connects the output of the vestibular nuclei to appropriate cranial nerve nuclei to cause changes in the extraocular muscles so that the eyes move in a manner corresponding to the end organ activity (McCaslin, 2013). The VOR activity can be observed as nystagmus corresponding to the plane of head movement using video-oculography (VOG) and no fixation target (vision-denied condition). Nystagmus is no longer present in a normal system after an individual has stopped moving from one position to another because there is no imbalance in neural activity from the end organs. Continuing with this logic, when nystagmus is present in an individual who is maintaining a static position, there should not be an asymmetry in neural input from the end organs and there should not be any nystagmus. If nystagmus is observed when the patient is in a particular position, there must be an imbalance in neural activity either within the vestibular periphery or the central vestibular pathways. This is referred to as *positional nystagmus*. A positioning nystagmus results when the act of moving the individual from one position to another causes an abnormal interaction between displaced otoconial debris and semicircular canal cupula. This interaction ultimately leads to an asymmetry in the tonic resting discharge rate of the two end organs. The nystagmus resulting from positioning is essential for identification of BPPV. After a discussion of spontaneous nystagmus, we consider positioning techniques followed by static positional testing.

SPONTANEOUS NYSTAGMUS

Prior to determining if placement of a patient into various positions causes a nystagmus response, it is important to identify the presence of nystagmus in a "neutral" position (Figure 11–1). This is essentially the gaze center position with the patient seated. We prefer to test in a vision-denied condition using VOG as opposed to Frenzel's lenses which, in many cases, can still allow fixation with a patient's focus on variances in light or even the inside of the goggle. If no nystagmus is observed in this neutral position, nystagmus observed in other positions should be attributable to the specific test position(s) as the orientation of the head relative to the ground has

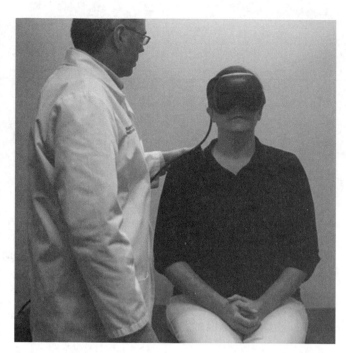

Figure 11–1. The patient is in the neutral seated position used to test for spontaneous nystagmus. The patient is in a vision-denied condition with video-oculography goggles used to observe and record all eye movements. If nystagmus is present with vision denied, the test is repeated with a fixation stimulus. Reprinted with permission from Alabama Hearing & Balance Associates, Inc.

been altered from the neutral, sitting position. This would be termed *positional nystagmus* (Table 11–1). If no nystagmus is present in the gaze center position with the patient seated, but nystagmus is present with eccentric placement of the eyes only (i.e., gaze right, left, up, etc.) or in gaze center with a fixation stimulus, then this is a gaze-evoked nystagmus. It is given that name because it is the act of gazing that provokes the nystagmus.

If a spontaneous nystagmus is present, the examiner should determine if it is modulated or if the direction is changed during eccentric gaze. Also, it is important to determine if the spontaneous nystagmus can be decreased with visual fixation. These measures are among the many that can assist the clinician in making a determination regarding differentiation of central and peripheral involvement. In some cases, the nystagmus may not alter with change in position. This has been interpreted as a purely spontaneous nystagmus. In other cases, the nystagmus observed during the neutral posi-

Table 11-1. Differentiation of Spontaneous and Positional Nystagmus

Type of Nystagmus	Position
Spontaneous	Present in neutral position (sitting with vision denied)
Positional	Present in positional tests (supine, head right or right lateral, head left or left lateral) only
Spontaneous and positional	Present in neutral position and changes in direction or intensity during positional tests
Gaze	Present with eccentric gaze with vision or vision denied
	Present in gaze center with visual fixation stimulus

tion may change in direction and/or intensity with change in position. This would represent a spontaneous and positional nystagmus.

Interpretation of Spontaneous Nystagmus

Central Nervous System Involvement

Vertical nystagmus (up-beating or down-beating) is most often interpreted as an indicator of central nervous system (CNS) involvement. Down-beating nystagmus has been most commonly reported with degeneration of the cerebellum, lesions at the craniocervical junction (Arnold-Chiari malformations), multiple sclerosis, vertebrobasilar insufficiency (VBI), and drug intoxication (Baloh & Honrubia, 2001; Brandt, 1990; Leigh & Zee, 2001). There is sufficient evidence that down-beating nystagmus can also be an indicator of peripheral vestibular involvement with anterior canal BPPV (Bertholon, Bronstein, Davies, Rudge, & Thilo, 2002; Ogawa et al., 2009; Zapala, 2008), but that is provoked with change in position (positioning techniques) as opposed to spontaneous nystagmus and is discussed in the section on BPPV. We have observed down-beating nystagmus in older patients with CNS changes reported on imaging studies. It is not uncommon for these changes to be interpreted as normal for

the patient's age. Baloh and Honrubia (2001) suggest that the presence of down-beating nystagmus is common with degeneration of the cerebellar flocculus and paraflocculus given a release of inhibitory pathways on the inherent upward eye movement bias from the six semicircular canals.

Up-beating nystagmus is commonly associated with brainstem and/or cerebellar infarct or tumor, multiple sclerosis, and drug intoxication effects (Baloh & Honrubia, 2001; Brandt, 1990; Leigh & Zee, 2001). This type of vertical nystagmus tends to be less prevalent than down-beating nystagmus. Whereas down-beating nystagmus is not uncommon in the older population with CNS involvement, the presence of an up-beating nystagmus may be a stronger clinical indicator. Imaging studies may need to be considered if they have not already been obtained.

Some common factors that should be considered regarding interpretation of spontaneous nystagmus are provided in Table 11–2. Vertical nystagmus is considered indicative of CNS involvement if the presence of a visual fixation stimulus causes no suppression of the nystagmus. This is often considered a classic rule when differentiating peripheral and central causes of nystagmus, but there is evidence beyond anecdotal observation that nystagmus resulting from CNS involvement can be suppressed with visual fixation (Choi, Oh, Park, et al., 2007). Additionally, the examiner must keep in mind that multiple medications, alcohol, and even nicotine have all been implicated as causes of vertical spontaneous nystagmus (Brandt, 1991; Sibony, Evinger, & Manning, 1987). Fetter, Haslwanter, Bork, and Dichgans (1999) used magnetic search coil technology to measure an up-beating nystagmus in all 10 of their subjects following consumption of 0.8 g of alcohol per kilogram of body weight. They concluded that the up-beating nystagmus represented the effect of alcohol on the central vestibular pathways underlying the vertical VOR. This nystagmus was independent of head position relative to gravity which is a finding that differs from the established positional alcohol nystagmus (PAN I and PAN II). It is important for the clinician to be aware of and consider the potential of nystagmus effects from these substances even in cases where patients are resolute in their assertions about 48-hr restriction. The reality is that some patients forget or may intentionally provide misleading statements. It may be difficult in certain

Table 11-2. Interpretation of Spontaneous Nystagmus

Peripheral	Central
Direction-fixed horizontal or torsional nystagmus	Vertical nystagmus (up-beating or down-beating)
Suppression of nystagmus with fixation	No suppression of nystagmus with fixation
Follows Alexander's law	Direction-changing nystagmus in neutral position including the following: • Congenital nystagmus • Periodic alternating nystagmus
Expect fast phase toward intact ear except for the following: • Irritative nystagmus • Recovery nystagmus	May be present as a result of the following: • Pharmacy • Alcohol • Tobacco

cases to differentiate between CNS involvement and the effect of medications.

Spontaneous nystagmus that changes direction is also typical of CNS involvement. Congenital nystagmus usually presents with a horizontal fast and slow phase. This nystagmus may change direction with alteration in eccentric gaze. Congenital nystagmus is a result of abnormalities in the chiasm neural pathways (Tusa, Zee, Hain, & Simonsz, 1992). Periodic alternating nystagmus is another type of spontaneous nystagmus that changes direction within the neutral sitting position. These changes can occur independent of eye and body position. There are many reported etiologies for periodic alternating nystagmus including cerebellar and brainstem impairments (e.g., brainstem infarcts, demyelinating diseases) (Leigh & Zee, 2001).

Peripheral Vestibular Involvement

Spontaneous nystagmus related to an acute unilateral labyrinthine involvement will present as a direction-fixed horizontal nystagmus and may have a torsional component. The magnitude of the vertical component may be diminished somewhat by the canceling effect of the two opposing vertical semicircular canals from the intact ear. The fast phase of the nystagmus beats toward the intact ear consistent

with Ewald's second law. The asymmetry in neural firing between the labyrinths favors the intact ear, which is similar to the pattern of neural firing present at the vestibular nuclei in response to acceleration of the head. It would also be expected that this spontaneous nystagmus would follow Alexander's law. That is, with eccentric gaze toward the fast phase of the nystagmus, there is an increase in nystagmus velocity. Eccentric gaze toward the slow phase of the nystagmus will decrease the nystagmus velocity.

As opposed to a spontaneous nystagmus with a central origin, the spontaneous nystagmus resulting from peripheral insult will usually disappear within days or weeks with static compensation (Baloh, 1998; Zee, 2000; also, see Chapter 4 in this text). This occurs as the resting neural activity is restored to balance at the level of the vestibular nuclei. It is noted that this will happen in the absence of any change in information from the involved end organ. It is further noted that the reduction or absence of spontaneous nystagmus does not mean the patient has fully "compensated" to the peripheral vestibulopathy. Rather, this is an indicator that static compensation has occurred, but not necessarily complete dynamic compensation.

Whereas spontaneous nystagmus with a CNS origin does not typically suppress with fixation, spontaneous nystagmus with a peripheral vestibular origin will suppress with fixation except within approximately 24 hr of the onset of the dysfunction (Zee, 2000). After that, the spontaneous nystagmus will be present only in a vision-denied condition. A direction-fixed horizontal nystagmus that follows Alexander's law and suppresses with fixation supports a peripheral vestibular problem affecting the ear opposite the fast phase of the nystagmus. As there is still the possibility that this could represent CNS involvement, the clinician must correlate all findings with results from other tests, and most importantly, with the history and symptoms of the patient.

Rarely, a spontaneous nystagmus may beat toward the involved ear if an "irritative" peripheral lesion is present (Jacobson, Pearlstein, Henderson, Calder, & Rock, 1998). This has been reported particularly for patients with Ménière's disease (Leigh & Zee, 2001; Marques & Perez-Fernandez, 2012; Matsuzaki & Kamei, 1995). Marques and Perez-Fernandez (2012) reported that 13.3% of their patients with definite, unilateral Meniere's disease exhibited an irritative nystagmus. Consideration should also be given to the possibility that irritative nystagmus may sometimes represent a form of recovery nystagmus.

Recovery Nystagmus

Another interesting finding that might be observed during testing for spontaneous nystagmus is recovery nystagmus. This is nystagmus with fast phase that beats toward the involved ear (Jacobson et al., 1998; Zee, 2000). This may seem confusing at first given the previous section. The clinician must recall that with an acute unilateral peripheral vestibulopathy, the initial asymmetry in neural activity at the vestibular nuclei is eliminated by restoring the tonic balance at this level. In cases where the activity may not achieve perfect balance, the neural activity could be greater at the ipsilesional vestibular nuclei, causing a secondary nystagmus beating toward the involved ear. Jacobson et al. (1998) discuss this possibility. Some support may also be found in a report by Parnes and Riddell (1993). These authors described three patients who developed an irritative nystagmus (beating toward the involved ear) following treatment with transtympanic gentamicin for Ménière's disease. The authors speculated that a temporary ototoxic effect may have occurred in

the nontreatment ear that might explain this nystagmus. Another explanation could be that a temporary asymmetry favoring the ipsilesional vestibular nuclei may have occurred during the time that the mechanisms underlying static compensation were attempting to restore the balance at this level of the central vestibular pathway.

The term *recovery nystagmus* may be more aptly named for a situation in which the peripheral vestibulopathy may not be permanent (i.e., some cases of vestibular neuritis). The initial phase of spontaneous nystagmus would be expected to beat toward the unaffected ear. This should disappear as the neural tone is restored at the vestibular nuclei. However, if the tone is balanced between the vestibular nuclei and then the involved ear begins to recover function, an asymmetry would exist again with greater neural firing at the ipsilesional vestibular nuclei. This would cause the spontaneous nystagmus to beat toward the involved, but recovering, ear. Jacobson et al. (1998) provide a comprehensive rationale for the possible underpinnings of recovery nystagmus. The finding of recovery nystagmus may also be observed following a dynamic head-shaking stimulus (Choi, Oh, Kim, et al., 2007; Hain & Spindler, 1993).

PATHOPHYSIOLOGY OF BENIGN PAROXYSMAL POSITIONAL VERTIGO (BPPV)

Cupulolithiasis and Canalithiasis

BPPV is the most common cause of vertigo in patients with vestibular disorders (Bath et al., 2000; Gans, 2000; Hornibrook, 2011). Strupp, Dieterich, and Brandt (2013) reported that among 17,718 patients evaluated at their respective centers, the most common diagnosis was of BPPV at 17.7% (3,036). In another investigation, data collected from 4,294 patients with vertigo from 13 countries over 28 months indicated that 26.9% had BPPV (Agus, Benecke, Thum, & Strupp, 2013). It should be of great interest that pretreatment health-related quality of life measures in patients with BPPV were comparable to measures of patients with HIV/AIDS, age-related macular degeneration, and hepatitis B (Roberts et al., 2009). Clearly, this treatable vestibular disorder has a negative impact on the lives of many people.

The symptoms of BPPV, primarily intense vertigo with rotary nystagmus, are caused by an abnormal interaction of the semicircular canal cupula and displaced otoconia from the utricle. Schucknecht's (1969) description of cupulolithiasis was based on his observation of basophilic deposits on the posterior semicircular canal (PSCC) cupula within the temporal bones of patients with a history of positional vertigo (Figure 11–2). The normal cupula has a specific gravity similar to the surrounding endolymph and is sensitive to angular acceleration. The

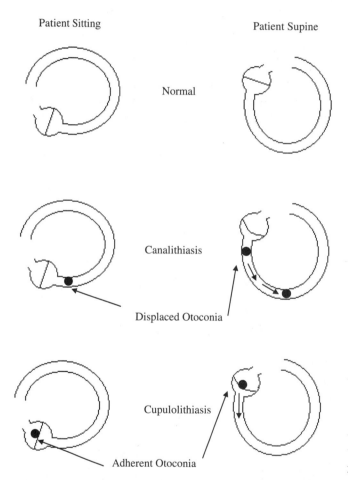

Patient Sitting   Patient Supine

Normal

Canalithiasis

Displaced Otoconia

Cupulolithiasis

Adherent Otoconia

Figure 11-2. *Top panel:* Posterior semicircular canal in normal patient sitting upright and then in supine position. *Middle panel:* Canalithiasis of the posterior semicircular canal is shown. Note the debris moving with change in position from sitting to supine and its effect on the cupula. *Lower panel:* Cupulolithiasis of the posterior semicircular canal is shown. Note the otoconial debris adherent to the cupula and its effect from sitting to supine.

presence of otoconia causes an increase in mass of the cupula, making the semicircular canal sensitive to linear acceleration. According to this theory, moving the patient into a provoking position deflects the heavy cupula. This causes the nystagmus and vertigo. The expectation would be that the nystagmus and vertigo would be persistent, remaining to a large extent (aside from some influence of central adaptation) as long as the patient remains in the provoking position. Such a persistent response is rarely observed in the clinic which makes it difficult to support a purely cupulolithiasis explanation.

Alternatively, Hall, Ruby, and McClure (1979) suggested that the displaced otoconia were not necessarily adherent to the cupula but were present as mobile densities within the canal. The presence of otoconial debris was directly observed as an operative finding and reported by Parnes and McClure (1992). These authors adapted the term *canalithiasis* to describe their findings. With canalithiasis, it is believed the mass of otoconia moves within the semicircular canal after change in head position. This movement displaces the endolymphatic fluid, deflecting the cupula of the involved canal and eliciting the nystagmus and vertigo (see Figure 11–2).

The presence of mobile debris within the semicircular canal (canalithiasis) is consistent with typical clinical findings for BPPV. These findings include latency from movement into provoking position until onset of symptoms, rotary nystagmus, vertigo, transient duration, and reversal of nystagmus direction with movement opposite the provoking position. These signs and symptoms are also consistent with a model of how otoconial debris would move through canals of this size and be able to generate the force needed to deflect the cupula (Squires, Weidman, Hain, & Stone, 2004). The model of Squires et al. also provides explanations of why there are variations in latency and intensity that do not require changes in the size of the particulate matter. For example, their model suggests that for a given otoconium, the greatest transcupular pressure (which would lead to the largest magnitude response) occurs with movement through the center of the semicircular canal duct. Less pressure is exerted with movement down the walls of the duct. The model even offers an explanation for the commonly observed onset latency of the response. The authors suggest that as the otoconia move through the ampulla toward the duct, there is little exertion of transcupular pressure until the debris begin to move through the canal duct. This can also explain variations in onset latency which would be related to position of the mass of otoconial debris within the semicircular canal (ampulla, canal duct) when the patient moves into a provoking position.

Jackson, Morgan, Fletcher, and Krueger (2007) found that among 260 patients identified with BPPV, 39 (17.6%) exhibited symptoms consistent with cupulolithiasis. Considering the three canals, the authors reported cupulolithiasis was most common in HC-BPPV (41.9%), followed by AC-BPPV with 27.3%. Furthermore, the authors reported that 6.3% of their patients with posterior canal involvement were diagnosed with cupulolithiasis. Our own clinical experience is in agreement that if cupulolithiasis exists, it is more common with HC-BPPV and AC-BPPV. However, not many patients present with symptoms of BPPV consistent with expectations with cupulolithiasis (i.e., symptom duration greater than 60 s, no onset latency, etc.). We are rather in agreement with Radtke and Lempert (2005) who wrote that "cupulolithiasis is an outdated concept." If there is adherent debris attached to the cupula or possibly within some aspect of the canal, it is more likely a rare occurrence.

The type of nystagmus observed most often with BPPV is a rotary up-beating nystagmus with an oblique movement toward the involved ear. This type of nystagmus is observed because the posterior canal is the most often affected by BPPV and this canal is connected through the VOR pathway to the ipsilateral superior oblique and the contralateral inferior rectus extraocular muscles (Baloh & Honrubia, 2001; Hornibrook, 2011). This is shown in Figure 11–3A. When the horizontal canal is affected, a linear horizontal nystagmus is observed which may be either geotropic or ageotropic. The horizontal canal is connected through the VOR pathway to the ipsilateral medial rectus and contralateral lateral rectus extraocular muscles (Baloh & Honrubia, 2001; Hornibrook, 2011) (see Figure 11–3B). Figure 11–3C shows that a rotary down-beating nystagmus is observed with anterior canal involvement given its VOR pathway connections with the ipsilateral superior rectus and contralateral inferior oblique extraoc-

ular muscles (Baloh & Honrubia, 2001; Hornibrook, 2011). This information is shown in Table 11–3.

Clinicians can modify, to an extent, the nystagmus response with vertical canal involvement by having the patient move their eyes. For example, the response with posterior canal BPPV can be made to have a more vertical aspect by having the patient gaze away from the involved ear. Gazing toward the involved ear should create a more torsional eye movement. At times this can be rather striking as patients may cause this type of response by moving their eyes without clinician prompting. This must be kept in mind because, although down-beating nystagmus has historically been interpreted as an indicator of a CNS issue, there are reports in the literature that suggest purely down-beating nystagmus may also be indicative of anterior canal BPPV (Bertholon et al., 2002; Ogawa et al., 2009; Zapala, 2008).

In a series of 50 consecutive patients with down-beating nystagmus, Bertholon et al. (2002) reported that 24% (12) had no other indicators of CNS involvement, but actually had symptoms and other findings consistent with BPPV. They note an upward bias in vertical slow phase eye velocity based on calculations of angular eye velocity vectors derived from known canal geometry which is in agreement with Baloh and Honrubia (2001). Using these calculations, they suggest that anterior canal BPPV would favor a more vertical nystagmus as opposed to the more torsional nystagmus expected with posterior canal BPPV. Zapala (2008) stated that in the absence of other central symptoms and findings, patients with down-beating nystagmus should be treated for anterior canal BPPV even when the nystagmus response is persistent. Recall that adherent otoconial debris (i.e., cupulolithiasis) would be expected to cause nystagmus with a more persistent duration. Ogawa et al. (2009) shared findings from four patients similar to Bertholon et al. (2002) and Zapala (2008) but are more conservative in their exclusion of CNS involvement. We are in agreement with Zapala (2008) for appropriate cases but caution that even in Bertholon et al.'s series, 76% of their patients did have CNS involvement.

Careful consideration of history and symptoms, along with a sufficient knowledge with repositioning maneuvers for BPPV treatment, should allow the experienced clinician to differentiate questionable BPPV responses from more serious CNS issues.

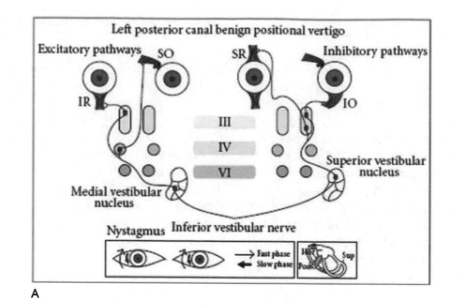

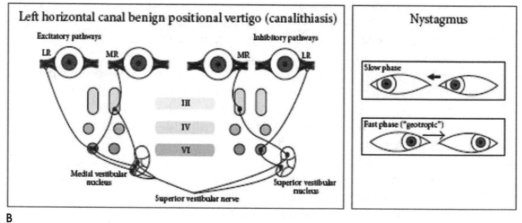

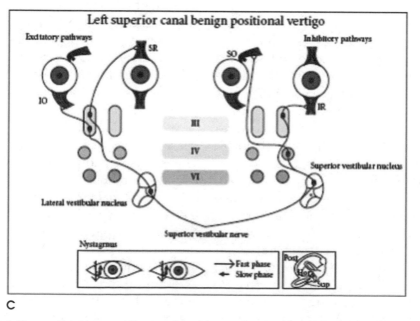

Figure 11–3. A. The path of innervation and nystagmus in a patient with left posterior canal benign paroxysmal positional vertigo (BPPV). **B.** The path of innervation and nystagmus in a patient with left horizontal canal BPPV. **C.** The path of innervation and nystagmus in a patient with left anterior canal BPPV. Created by Jeremy Hornibrook. Courtesy of the Hindawi Publishing Corporation.

Table 11-3. Semicircular Canal Involvement and Associated Nystagmus

Canal	Nystagmus Fast Phase	Paired Extraocular Muscles
Posterior	Rotary up-beating	Ipsilateral superior oblique Contralateral inferior rectus
Horizontal (lateral)	Horizontal	Ipsilateral medial rectus Contralateral lateral rectus
Anterior (superior)	Rotary down-beating	Ipsilateral superior rectus Contralateral inferior oblique

Simply put, repositioning maneuvers are highly effective for BPPV and there should be no change in patient status with a CNS origin. We have advocated this for differentiation of migrainous positional vertigo from horizontal canal BPPV (Roberts, Gans, & Kastner, 2006). Zapala (2008) has advocated this for differentiation of CNS issues from anterior canal BPPV (when there is no obvious sign of central involvement).

Semicircular Canal Involvement

Although BPPV has been reported to affect all three semicircular canals, the posterior canal is reported to be the involved canal in 61% to 97% of BPPV cases (de la Meilleure et al., 1996; Honrubia, Baloh, Harris, & Jacobson, 1999; Moon et al., 2006; Ruckenstein, 2001). There is no debate about that. This is believed to be related to the inferior orientation of the PSCC relative to the utricle. The majority of investigations indicate that horizontal canal BPPV is the second most common involvement, accounting for 1% to 32% of cases (Cakir et al., 2006; de la Meilleure et al., 1996; Fife, 1998; Macias, Lambert, Massingale, Ellensohn, & Fritz, 2000). Though always theoretically possible, the increased use of VOG has confirmed that the anterior canal can also be the involved canal. Most reports place this as the least common form of BPPV ranging from 1% to 21% of cases. Herdman, Tusa, and Clendaniel (1994) and Jackson et al. (2007) are in the minority of investigations reporting a higher incidence of anterior canal compared to horizontal canal involvement with 12% and 21.2% reported, respectively. At this point, the evidence tends to favor anterior canal involvement

being less common than horizontal canal BPPV. Table 11–4 presents a list of selected studies in this area. It remains possible that there are more cases of anterior canal than previously thought. Clinicians may not have been looking for this so they did not see it. Any torsional nystagmus may have been attributed to posterior canal involvement. Use of VOG with recording can be helpful in differentiation of vertical canal involvement.

Another interesting finding with BPPV is that it is most commonly unilateral. Bilateral BPPV has been reported to range from a low of 4% to upward of 15% of cases (Gans & Harrington-Gans, 2002; Longridge & Barber, 1978). There is evidence that bilateral involvement is more common following head trauma compared to other causes of BPPV (Katsarkas, 1999; Liu, 2012). Liu (2012) reported significantly more bilateral BPPV (25%) in patients with posttraumatic BPPV compared to only 2% of patients with other causes of BPPV. Patients with posttraumatic BPPV were also significantly more likely (55%) to have BPPV affecting more than one canal compared to only 6.5% of other patients with BPPV. Soto-Varela, Rossi-Izquierdo, and Santos-Pérez (2013) report similar results to Liu. They also noted that in their series, patients with multicanal, but unilateral BPPV, were more likely to have a history of recurrent BPPV.

The right ear is more often affected by BPPV than the left ear (Epley, 1992; Korres et al., 2002; Roberts, Gans, DeBoodt, & Lister, 2005; Roberts, Gans, & Montaudo, 2006). In a review of 18 studies, von Brevern, Seelig, Neuhauser, and Lempert (2004) found only two that reported more left ear than right ear involvement. From all the data, the authors estimated that the right ear was the involved ear 1.41 times more often than the left (95% CI 1.37 to 1.45).

Table 11–4. Incidence of Benign Paroxysmal Positional Vertigo (BPPV) Among Semicircular Canals

Study	*n*	PC	HC	AC
Herdman, Tusa, & Clendaniel (1994)	59	63.6	1.3	11.7
Fife (1998)	424	91	6	3
Wolf, Boyev, Manokey, & Mattox (1999)	107	95.3	1.9	2.8
Honrubia, Baloh, Harris, & Jacobson (1999)	292	93.5	5.1	1.4
Ruckenstein (2001)	86	96.5	2.3	1.2
Korres & Balatsouras, (2004)	122	90.2	8.2	1.6
Cakir et al. (2006)	169	85.2	11.8	1.2
Moon et al. (2006)	1,692	60.9	31.9	2.2
Jackson, Morgan, Fletcher, & Krueger (2007)	260	66.9	11.9	21.2
Celebisoy, Polat, & Akyurekli (2008)	157	87.9	9	1.3
De Stefano et al. (2011)	412	70.9	27	2.4
Soto-Varela, Rossi-Izquierdo, & Santos-Pérez (2013)	614	88.4	6.4	5.2

They suggested this may be related to patient sleeping position (i.e., patients are more likely to sleep on their right sides than their left sides). Lopez-Escamez, Gamiz, Finana, Perez, and Canet (2002) also reported a significant association between affected ear and side during bed rest.

POSITIONING TECHNIQUES FOR ELICITING BENIGN PAROXYSMAL POSITIONAL VERTIGO (BPPV)

It is important for the clinician to realize that the BPPV response can fatigue with repeated changes in position due to dispersal of the displaced otoconia within the affected semicircular canal. For this reason, clinicians are instructed to perform appropriate positioning testing to identify the presence of BPPV prior to positional testing. It is also emphasized that testing for BPPV is an essential component of the vestibular and equilibrium evaluation given that this problem is the most common vestibular cause of vertigo.

For over 60 years, the gold standard for diagnosis of BPPV has been the Dix-Hallpike maneuver (Dix & Hallpike; 1952; Hornibrook, 2011; Lanska & Remler, 1997). This maneuver has been described for many years in virtually every article and book that discusses dizziness and vertigo, although some authorities have questioned whether there are better ways to obtain the same information (Gans, 2000; Sakata, Ohtsu, & Sakata, 2004). Safer, more comfortable adaptations have been suggested with no loss of sensitivity (Cohen, 2004; Gans, 2000; Humphriss, Baguley, Sparkes, Peerman, & Moffat, 2003).

Among the major issues of concern when assessing patients for BPPV is the risk of ischemia of the posterior circulation in patients with vertebrobasilar insufficiency (Choi et al., 2005; Humprhiss et al., 2003; Nagashima, Iwama, Sakata, & Miki, 1970; Sakata et al., 2004) which is sometimes termed "Bow Hunter's Syndrome" (Ikeda, Villelli, Shaw, & Powers, 2013; Yamaguchi, Nagasawa, Yamakawa, & Kato, 2012), The possibility of vertebrobasilar dissection is also of concern (Albuquerque et al., 2011; de Bray, Penisson-Benier, Dubas, & Emile, 1997; Young & Chen, 2003). Apart from dissection, position-induced vascular insufficiency may be caused by cervical spondylotic-induced compression of the vertebrobasilar area (Cornelius et al., 2012; Olszewski, Majak, Pietkiewicz, Luszcz, & Repetowski, 2006).

It is apparent in the literature that positioning of the patient so that hyperextension of the neck may occur should be avoided in such patients because of the risk (Cohen, 2004; Humphriss et al., 2003; Sakata et al., 2004). One method that has been reported by Humphriss et al. (2003) and which we have used for many years to determine which

patients may be at risk for possible vertebrobasilar ischemia is termed the Vertebral Artery Screening Test (VAST). Although some question the validity of VAST and place its sensitivity in the range from 0 to 57% (Hutting et al., 2013), we are in agreement with Asavasopon, Jankoski, and Godges (2005) that these tools can be helpful in certain cases. Figure 11–4 depicts this screening test. In a seated position, the patient is asked to rotate the head to the right and then hyperextend the neck (i.e., look up). The

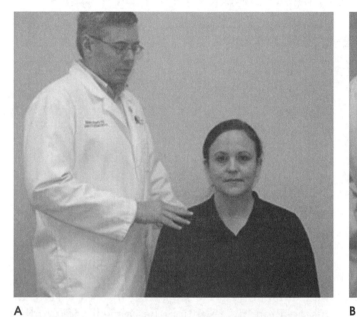

A

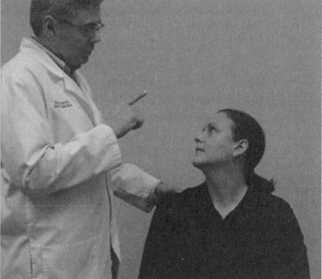

B

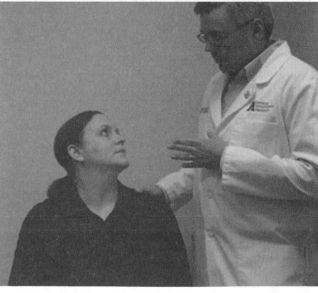

C

Figure 11-4. The examiner is performing a vertebral artery screening test (VAST). **A.** The patient is seated with the examiner in position to observe any provoked nystagmus. **B.** The head is rotated to the right and the neck hyperextended within the cervical range of comfort of the patient and held for 20 to 30 s. **C.** After returning to the neutral position, the head is rotated to the left and the neck hyperextended again for 20 to 30 s. Reprinted with permission from Alabama Hearing & Balance Associates, Inc.

patient is instructed to move only within their range of comfort which gives the clinician some idea of cervical range of motion. The position is maintained for 20 to 30 s and the patient is questioned about symptoms of dizziness, lightheadedness, nausea, blurred vision, double vision, and so forth, while the clinician watches for nystagmus and listens to the patient's speech for dysarthria (Magarey et al., 2004). This is repeated with rotation and hyperextension to the opposite side. If a positive result is noted or if cervical range of motion is limited, the clinician should consider an alternative assessment technique (side-lying or fully supported Hallpike) in place of the methods that require hyperextension (traditional Dix-Hallpike or modified Dix-Hallpike).

For quite some time, it was thought that the Hallpike maneuver had to be performed in what might be described as an aggressive manner. As this was uncomfortable and potentially problematic in many patients experiencing lower back or cervical spine problems and especially elderly patients, the test was sometimes eliminated from the clinical protocol. In fact, some have suggested that the maneuver never be performed with elderly patients (Sakata et al., 2004). This is unfortunate as BPPV is the leading peripheral cause of vertigo (Bath et al., 2000; Strupp et al., 2013), and it is well established that its presence can adversely affect postural stability in a population already at risk for falling (Blatt, Georgakakis, Herdman, Clendaniel, & Tusa, 2000; Oghalai, Manolidis, Barth, Stewart, & Jenkins, 2000). Furthermore, it is unlikely that patients who are provoking themselves with everyday activities, such as lying back and rolling over, are rapidly forcing themselves into an uncomfortable body position while merely lying back in bed. The provocation of BPPV symptoms is based on a change in the orientation of the semicircular canal relative to the earth-gravitational vector. The provocation of symptoms has less to do with rapid positioning of the patient except that it is possible more debris could move at one time, causing a greater effect on the cupula. If the involved semicircular canal is moved so that displaced otoconial debris is no longer at a low point in the canal, gravity will cause the debris to move to the lowest point which, again, is why patients provoke symptoms in everyday situations.

There are a variety of modifications to the standard Dix-Hallpike maneuver that appear to remain sensitive in provoking the symptoms of the patient without requiring excessive stress or strain on the cervical spine or lower back. These modifications should also avoid the potential for triggering VBI. Tests for BPPV of the posterior or anterior semicircular canal are presented first, followed by testing for BPPV of the horizontal semicircular canal.

Posterior/Anterior Semicircular Canal

Modified Hallpike Test

For the modified Hallpike, the examiner begins in a position standing behind the patient (Gans & Harrington-Gans, 2002; Gans & Yellin, 2007; Roberts et al., 2005) as in the Epley maneuver for BPPV treatment (Epley, 1992), rather than to the side as is done in the traditional Dix-Hallpike (Dix & Hallpike, 1952). The examiner instructs the patient to turn his or her head slightly toward the test ear (45 degrees away from midline) while providing support to the patient's neck and back. This allows the examiner to sit as the patient is eased into the provoking supine position. The neck of the patient is slightly hyperextended but always supported while the head is off the examination table as shown in Figure 11–5. In this position, the examiner has a clear view of the eyes of the patient while maintaining excellent body mechanics.

We again note that this modification is consistent with the first position of most versions of canalith repositioning maneuver (CRM) (Epley, 1992; Gans & Harrington-Gans, 2002; Herdman, Tusa, Zee, Proctor, & Mattox, 1993). This simple modification to the traditional Dix-Hallpike test results in enhanced ease of performance for both the patient and the examiner. The examiner is also in a much better position to provide support to the patient if there is a strong subjective component along with provocation of BPPV (Gans, 2000; Gans & Yellin, 2007). The modified Hallpike should not be used for patients in whom hyperextension of the neck is contraindicated (Gans & Yellin, 2007).

Bertholon et al. (2002) have suggested that a supine, head-hanging position may be helpful

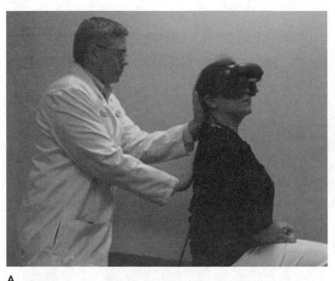

A

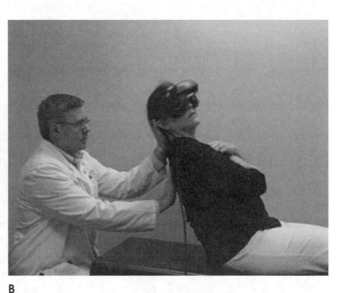

B

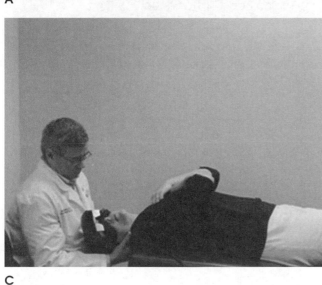

C

Figure 11–5. The examiner is performing a modified Hallpike to check the right posterior semicircular canal for benign paroxysmal positional vertigo (BPPV). **A.** The patient is seated on the examination table with back to the examiner. The head of the patient is turned toward the ear to be tested (right ear in this example). The examiner is positioned behind the patient and provides support to the back and neck of the patient. **B.** The patient is lowered to the examination table as the examiner sits. **C.** The neck of the patient is hyperextended and the head is maintained 45 degrees toward the test ear. The examiner supports the neck and head of the patient and has a clear view of the eyes of the patient. The maneuver is repeated for the left ear. Reprinted with permission from Alabama Hearing & Balance Associates, Inc.

in identification of anterior canal BPPV in some patients (Figure 11–6). In their report, two of 12 patients diagnosed with AC-BPPV only experienced provocation of symptoms using this position. The authors explained that the additional downward positioning of the head (hyperextension of the neck) may be crucial for provoking anterior canal BPPV as only then the ampullary segment will approach a vertical down-pointing position. Ogawa et al. (2009) report on four cases with possible AC-BPPV who also only provoked using similar positioning. Given that nine of Bertholon et al.'s 12 patients could be identified with Dix-Hallpike positioning alone, it would seem that supine, head-hanging should be

reserved only for special cases. For example, if history and symptoms are consistent with BPPV but typical positioning is not effective, supine position with head hanging may be considered. We would caution clinicians to consider this only for patients in whom hyperextension of the neck is not contraindicated. Recall that Zapala (2008) was able to provoke AC-BPPV using side-lying positioning which is discussed next.

Side-Lying Maneuver

For patients with conditions that contraindicate neck hyperextension (i.e., VBI, cervical spondylosis, limited

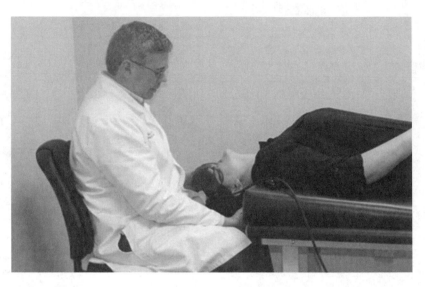

Figure 11-6. The examiner is performing supine head-hanging technique for anterior canal benign paroxysmal positional vertigo (BPPV). Note the level of neck hyperextension. This positioning maneuver may be useful for patients who do not provoke with other techniques and in whom the hyperextension is not contraindicated. Reprinted with permission from Alabama Hearing & Balance Associates, Inc.

range of motion, etc.), Humphriss et al. (2003) suggest that the traditional Dix-Hallpike maneuver should not be performed. They advocated that the side-lying maneuver is an appropriate substitute. Cohen (2004) is in agreement and found no significant difference in sensitivity when she compared side-lying to traditional Dix-Hallpike testing. This maneuver is identical to the first position of the Semont liberatory maneuver (SLM) (Gans & Harrington-Gans, 2002; Herdman et al., 1993; Semont, Freyss, & Vitte, 1988) and the Gans repositioning maneuver (GRM) (Roberts, Gans, & Montaudo, 2006). As shown in Figure 11–7, the maneuver is typical of a patient's normal movement as he or she prepares to lie in bed on his or her side. The head of the patient is turned 45 degrees away from the ear to be tested. This head position is important, as after the patient is positioned on the side, the posterior semicircular canal of the test ear will be in a plane that will cause any displaced otoconia to move to the lowest point in the canal. The patient is then placed on the test side using a lateral positioning. A major advantage of the side-lying maneuver is that the head and neck of the patient are fully supported on the exam table. This was an important reason Zapala (2008) reported for

using side-lying to identify anterior canal BPPV. The side-lying maneuver is particularly advantageous for those patients whose lower back discomfort or other restrictions, such as obesity, do not allow them to comfortably sit or bend at the waist. The side-lying maneuver, however, may be contraindicated for any patient who has significant hip issues or has undergone a recent hip replacement.

Fully Supported Hallpike

In the case of patients who may have contraindications to neck hyperextension but also cannot lie comfortably on their side given issues such as recent hip replacement, rotator cuff surgery, and so forth, another option exists, the fully supported Hallpike. The fully supported Hallpike is performed in the same way as the modified Hallpike with the exception that the patient is positioned so that the head and neck are fully supported on the table in the supine position rather than with hyperextension of the neck which occurs with the head off the table. Figure 11–8 depicts this maneuver. For the majority of patients with PC-BPPV, this maneuver should be capable of provoking their symptoms as it mimics

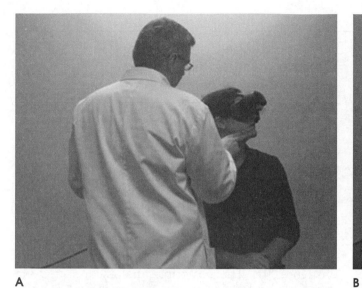

A

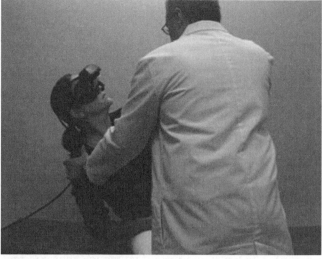

B

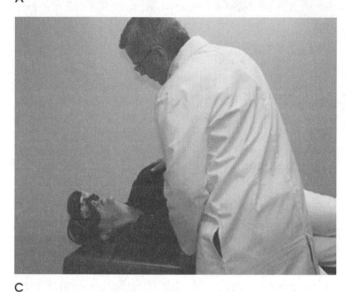

C

Figure 11-7. The examiner is performing a side-lying maneuver to check the right posterior semicircular canal for benign paroxysmal positional vertigo (BPPV). **A.** The patient is seated near the center of the examination table in the side-lying position. The head of the patient is turned away from the ear to be tested. **B.** The patient is positioned on the right side. **C.** The legs of the patient are brought up onto the examination table. Note that the head of the patient is supported by the examination table, avoiding hyperextension of the neck. The examiner has a clear view of the eyes of the patient. The maneuver is repeated to check the left ear. Reprinted with permission from Alabama Hearing & Balance Associates, Inc.

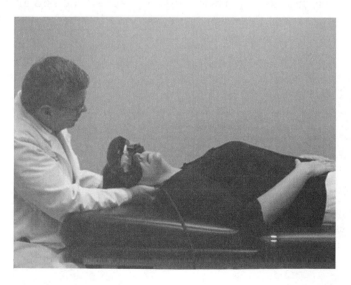

Figure 11-8. The patient is in the fully supported Hallpike position to check for right posterior semicircular canal benign paroxysmal positional vertigo (BPPV). The head of the patient is fully supported on the examination table with the head turned 45 degrees toward the test ear (right ear in this example). The examiner is seated behind the patient. Note that the examiner has clear view of the eyes of the patient. Maneuver is repeated to test left ear. Reprinted with permission from Alabama Hearing & Balance Associates, Inc.

lying flat in bed with the head turned slightly. This maneuver is probably best suited for the more frail patients who have comorbidities that contraindicate assessment for BPPV with either modified Hallpike or side-lying (Gans & Yellin, 2007).

Horizontal Canal Benign Paroxysmal Positional Vertigo

Horizontal semicircular canal BPPV (HC-BPPV) presents with a nystagmus fast phase that changes direction with head positioning in the plane of the horizontal semicircular canal. This nystagmus is horizontal as opposed to the rotary nystagmus observed with vertical semicircular canal BPPV. HC-BPPV is sometimes provoked with the Hallpike maneuver, but that is not always the case so other techniques must be available. The Roll test, as described in the section on Positional Testing, will always provoke HC-BPPV, and the nystagmus will usually be geotropic (beating toward the ground regardless of position on the right or left side) or ageotropic (beating away from the ground regardless of position on the right or left side). Many clinicians have observed a change in the direction of nystagmus on repeat testing, and there is at least one report that describes direction-fixed nystagmus with HC-BPPV that ultimately transforms to the geotropic type (Califano, Vassallo, Melillo, Mazzone, & Salafia, 2013). The changing nystagmus patterns can make it difficult to determine the involved ear in some cases. We cover this and some suggestions for making that determination in the next section.

Interpretation and Usefulness of Positioning Results

The most common finding observed during positioning testing is a paroxysmal and transient rotary nystagmus. The patient should experience a subjective sensation coincident with the nystagmus. The nystagmus is typically up-beating and toward the affected ear. This is not surprising as these findings are expected with BPPV of the posterior semicircular canal which is by far the most common variant (de la Meilleure et al., 1996; Honrubia et al., 1999; Ruckenstein, 2001). The posterior canal is connected via the VOR pathway to the ipsilateral superior oblique and the contralateral inferior rectus muscles which, when activated, produce a slow downward deviation of the eyes followed by a torsional up-beating movement (i.e., a rotary up-beating nystagmus) (Baloh & Honrubia, 2001).

If a down-beating rotary nystagmus is provoked, also transient and paroxysmal, BPPV is affecting the anterior semicircular canal. This variant is less common and may not be recognized unless the clinician incorporates VOG recordings (Gans, 2000). A down-beating rotary nystagmus is observed because the anterior semicircular canal is connected to the ipsilateral superior rectus and contralateral inferior oblique (Baloh & Honrubia, 2001). A purely vertical down-beating nystagmus can also be observed with AC-BPPV (Bertholon et al., 2002; Zapala, 2008). As shown in Table 11–5, with both posterior and anterior semicircular canal BPPV, it is common for the nystagmus to reverse if the patient is returned to an upright position following provocation of symptoms.

Table 11–5. Interpretation of Positioning Results

Characteristics	Peripheral	Central
Nystagmus	Rotary (BPPV)	Rotary, vertical, or horizontal
Duration	Transient (<1 min)	Persistent
Onset latency	Short onset latency often observed	Not expected
Reversal of nystagmus	Change in direction on sitting	Not expected
Subjective dizziness	Vertigo always	May or may not be present

Even though BPPV presents in the typical manner almost exclusively, there are accounts of what can be termed subjective BPPV (Huebner, Lytle, Doettl, Plyler, & Thelin, 2013). The only difference is that no nystagmus is present during vertigo provocation. Haynes et al. (2002) reported on 35 patients with a presenting history and symptoms consistent with BPPV. The patients reported transient vertigo during Hallpike testing, but no nystagmus was observed by the clinician. The authors used the SLM to treat these patients and success was achieved in 86% (i.e., 30) after 1.59 treatments, on average. Huebner et al. (2013) reported no difference in treatment outcome for patients with typical (objective) BPPV compared to patients with subjective BPPV. Both studies confirm that BPPV may be present in the absence of characteristic nystagmus for some patients. We would caution clinicians not to overgeneralize this finding to mean that numerous BPPV treatments should be imposed on all patients presenting with atypical symptoms. Whenever identification of an "atypical variant" or a "nonclassic form" of BPPV is considered, the possibility increases substantially that the patient may not have BPPV.

Common characteristics observed with HC-BPPV are found in Table 11–6. Geotropic nystagmus (beating toward the ground) is thought to reflect a canalithiasis variant and is reported to occur 60% to 83% of the time with involvement of the horizontal canal (Cakir et al., 2006; Honrubia et al., 1999; Steenerson, Cronin, & Marbach, 2005; White, Coale, Catalano, & Oas, 2005). This means that when the patient is positioned so that the ear is toward the ground, the fast phase of the nystagmus will also move toward the ground (e.g., left-beating with the patient in the left lateral position and right-beating with the patient in the right lateral position). The nystagmus will be present when the patient is on either the right side or the left side, but the side with the more intense symptoms should be treated (Appiani, Catania, & Gagliardi, 2001; Fife, 1998; White et al., 2005). Figure 11–9 depicts what is believed to occur with the canalithiasis variant of HC-BPPV. Positioning of the affected ear downward toward the ground should move the displaced otoconia from the long arm of the lateral canal toward the ampulla. This should cause a flow of endolymphatic fluid so that a utriculopetal displacement of the cupula (i.e., toward the utricle) occurs and increases neural firing on that side. As the neural firing is greater on this side, the nystagmus beats toward the dependent ear and the ground.

If the patient is positioned on the opposite side with the affected ear upward and the unaffected ear toward the ground, the otoconial debris is believed to move farther away from the ampulla, causing movement of endolymph also away from the ampulla. This creates an utriculofugal displacement of the cupula (away from the utricle) to occur which results in an inhibitory effect on neural firing for the affected ear. As the relative difference in neural firing is greater from the dependent ear, a nystagmus with fast phase toward the unaffected ear will be present. This nystagmus would be expected to be of lower intensity compared to positioning the affected ear downward which should be helpful in determining the involved canal.

An ageotropic nystagmus (beating away from the ground) is less common with HC-BPPV, occurring from 17% to 40% of the time (Honrubia et al., 1999; Steenerson et al., 2005). As with HC-BPPV with geotropic nystagmus, positioning on either side is expected to elicit a nystagmus response. Most literature suggests this represents a cupulolithiasis variant and the side with the less intense response is the one that must be treated (Casani, Vannucci, Fattori, & Berrettini, 2002; White et al., 2005).

Table 11–6. Characteristics of Horizontal Canal Benign Paroxysmal Positional Nystagmus

Horizontal Canal Benign Paroxysmal Positional Nystagmus (HC-BPPV)
Paroxysmal
Transient duration (except for cupulolithiasis type which may last longer)
Horizontal nystagmus: <ul><li>Geotropic—Side with more intense response has displaced otoconia</li><li>Ageotropic—Side with less intense response has displaced otoconia</li></ul>
Strong subjective impression of vertigo

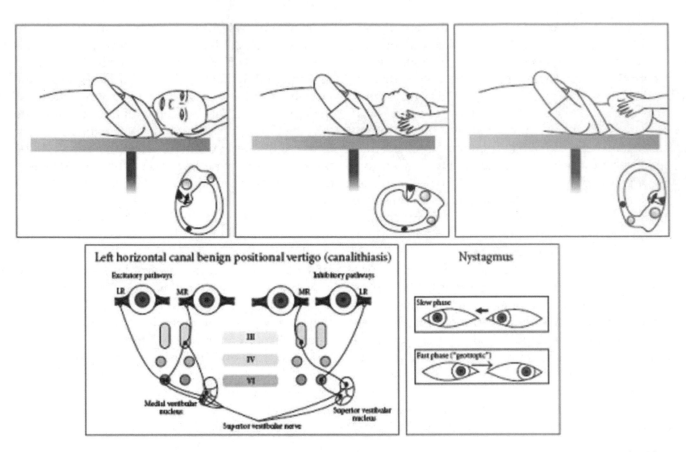

Figure 11–9. Representation of canalithiasis variant of horizontal canal benign paroxysmal positional vertigo (HC-BPPV) with geotropic nystagmus. Upper panel shows patient during roll testing with mobile otoconial debris in the left horizontal semicircular canal. Lower panel shows the innervation and nystagmus resulting with otoconial debris moving toward the cupula with positioning on the left side. This causes an increase in neural firing. The fast phase of the nystagmus will beat toward the ground which is toward the left. Positioning on the right side will cause the otoconial debris in the left horizontal semicircular canal to move away from the cupula, causing decreased neural firing and a nystagmus beating toward the ground which is toward the right. Created by Jeremy Hornibrook. Courtesy of the Hindawi Publishing Corporation.

Figure 11–10 depicts what is believed to occur with the cupulolithiasis variant of HC-BPPV. The debris may be adherent to the utricle or canal side of the cupula (Chiou, Lee, Tsai, Yu, & Lee, 2005). Positioning of the affected ear downward toward the ground is believed to cause a utriculofugal displacement of the otoconia-weighted cupula, which results in an inhibitory effect on neural firing from the horizontal canal. An ageotropic nystagmus with fast phase toward the unaffected ear results because the neural firing from the unaffected ear is relatively greater. When the affected ear is positioned upward, away from the ground, a utriculopetal displacement of the otoconia-weighted cupula is believed to occur. This is excitatory and creates a stronger ageotropic

nystagmus toward the uppermost ear. Some have suggested that ageotropic nystagmus may also be present when the otoconial debris is not adherent to the cupula but is located in the anterior portion of the lateral canal (Casani et al., 2002). This makes a great deal of sense and probably explains why the nystagmus can switch direction at times with repeating the positions. In fact, given the observed effects with PC- BPPV that are most often consistent with mobile debris (canalithiasis), one could also reason mobile debris would be more likely to be present with HC-BPPV.

The switching of nystagmus and responses to either side with similar magnitude have made the process of identifying involved ear difficult

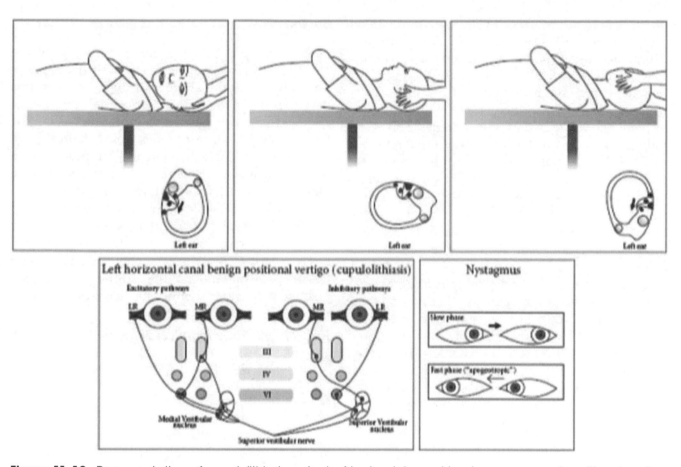

Figure 11–10. Representation of cupulolithiasis variant of horizontal canal benign paroxysmal positional vertigo (HC-BPPV) with ageotropic nystagmus. Upper panel shows patient with otoconial debris attached to the left horizontal semicircular canal cupula. When patient is positioned onto the left side, otoconial debris pulls cupula away from the utricle, causing decreased neural firing. The fast phase of the nystagmus will beat away from the ground which is toward the right. When the patient is positioned on the right side, the otoconial debris pushes the cupula toward the utricle, causing increased neural firing and a nystagmus beating away from the ground which is toward the left. Created by Jeremy Hornibrook. Courtesy of the Hindawi Publishing Corporation.

in some cases. Koo, Moon, Shim, Moon, and Kim (2006) investigated nystagmus patterns provoked in patients moved from sitting to supine in an effort to help lateralize involved horizontal canal. They found a tendency for nystagmus to beat toward the involved ear for HC-BPPV with geotropic nystagmus and away from the involved ear for ageotropic HC-BPPV. Choung, Shin, Kahng, Park, and Choi (2006) found that neck flexion "bow" and hyperextension "lean" place the head in positions that can also be helpful in identification of involved ear with HC-BPPV. After HC-BPPV was identified, the investigators had patients bow the head forward 90 degrees while in a seated position. Nystagmus was recorded and then patients leaned the head back-

wards 45 degrees and nystagmus response was also recorded. They recorded nystagmus beating toward the involved ear during bowing with HC-BPPV with geotropic nystagmus (canalithiasis) and toward the involved ear with leaning with HC-BPPV with ageotropic nystagmus (cupulolithiasis). We agree that these methods of identifying with certainty the involved ear in HC-BPPV are important from a scientific standpoint. From a practical standpoint, the clinician may prefer to simply treat both ears when there is lack of certainty and no resolution of symptoms after initial treatment.

Nystagmus due to CNS involvement may also be present during positioning testing. Purely vertical nystagmus can be observed with involvement of the cerebellum, Arnold-Chiari malformations, multiple sclerosis, vertebrobasilar insufficiency, and drug intoxication (Baloh & Honrubia, 2001; Brandt, 1990; Leigh & Zee, 2001). As previously noted, if a patient with nystagmus due to BPPV gazes away from the involved ear, the verticality of the nystagmus enhances due to the rectus muscles. This is still rather easy to distinguish because nystagmus due to CNS disease will most often persist while the patient is kept in the provoking position, whereas the duration is usually transient with BPPV. This is shown in Table 11–5. Nystagmus without vertigo may also be present. In the absence of a subjective impression of dizziness, a CNS origin or possibly pharmacologic influence may be supported. Still, there are reports of purely down-beating nystagmus with anterior canal BPPV (Bertholon et al., 2002; Zapala, 2008). In the absence of other CNS indicators, BPPV treatment may be considered given its high efficacy (Roberts, Gans, & Kastner, 2006; Zapala, 2008). As stated previously, repeated BPPV treatment without successful resolution of symptoms is not encouraged. In these cases CNS disease may be the origin of the nystagmus.

POSITIONAL TESTING AND NYSTAGMUS

Positional Testing

Movement of the head or the head and body into various static positions can cause nystagmus with or without subjective dizziness. The positional nystagmus is thought to occur as a result of reduction in suppression of asymmetric semicircular canal function, impaired otolith function, or central vestibular pathway involvement. The typical test positions we include are supine, head right or body right, and head left or body left.

All testing is initially performed in a vision-denied condition with VOG. If nystagmus is observed in any static position, we test for suppression of the positional nystagmus with fixation. The rationale behind this order of testing is that both central and peripheral causes of positional nystagmus are present in the absence of visual fixation, and only central causes may be present with fixation. If no positional nystagmus is observed with vision denied, it is unlikely to be present with fixation. Use of this rationale makes positional testing more efficient over time.

Supine

During this position, the patient is lying on the examination table but the head and neck are supported by the examiner. Neck flexion of 30 degrees is used to position the head in appropriate orientation relative to the body. This is opposed to having the head of the patient rest on the table (Figure 11–11). This is a comfortable position and our practice is to return patients to this neutral position between the other static positions. Nystagmus may be present in this position as discussed for spontaneous nystagmus, but Koo et al. (2006) find this position useful for identification of involved ear with horizontal canal BPPV. Nearly 60% of their patients had a horizontal nystagmus when moved from sitting to the supine position that helped identify the ear to be treated.

Head Right/Body Right and Head Left/Body Left

The point of these positions is to change the orientation of the labyrinth to the earth gravitational vector (Figure 11–12). This is thought to provoke abnormal VOR activity in cases where the otolith system of the lesioned ear is closest to the ground. There may be a lack of suppression of asymmetric semicircular canal afferent activity which leads to positional nystagmus. There are also CNS issues and other effects (i.e., alcohol) that may produce positional nystagmus.

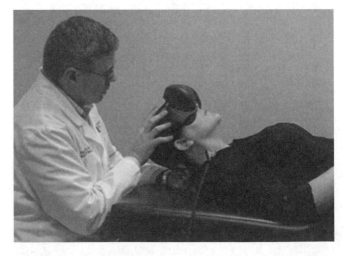

Figure 11–11. The patient is in the supine position. Note slight neck flexion to place the neck in appropriate orientation. Testing is completed in vision-denied condition and repeated with visual fixation stimulus if nystagmus is observed. Reprinted with permission from Alabama Hearing & Balance Associates, Inc.

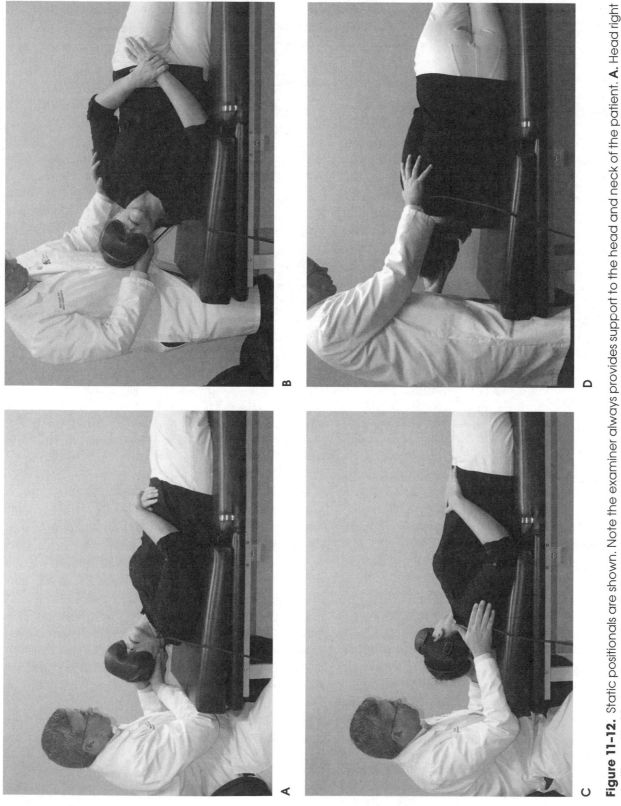

Figure 11–12. Static positionals are shown. Note the examiner always provides support to the head and neck of the patient. **A.** Head right position with 90-degree rotation. **B.** Right lateral position. **C.** Head left position with 90-degree rotation. **D.** Left lateral position. Note that all positions are performed in vision-denied condition and repeated with visual fixation stimulus if nystagmus is observed. Reprinted with permission from Alabama Hearing & Balance Associates, Inc.

271

Although it is possible to elicit HC-BPPV during vertical semicircular canal assessment with Hallpike maneuver variations, it is important to realize that HC-BPPV will not always be elicited by this positioning. The head positioning discussed here does place the horizontal semicircular canals in a position to cause movement of otoconial debris (Cakir et al., 2006; Gans & Yellin, 2007). When it is not possible or advisable to turn the head into eccentric positions because of limited cervical range of motion, placement into a lateral position (sometimes referred to as the Roll test) offers a viable alternative.

Appropriate assessment for positional nystagmus and HC-BPPV requires the head to be rotated 90 degrees with the ear toward the ground. For many individuals, including older adults who may have cervical spondylosis or osteoarthritis and other patients with restricted cervical range of motion, 90 degree rotation of the head is impossible. That patient must be moved into a lateral positioning to achieve this orientation of the ear to the earth. Some believe the decision to move from head right to body right, for example, is to eliminate neck torsion issues which could trigger symptoms having a cervicogenic origin (see Cervical Vertigo Screening Test). In fact, it is very important to consider the orientation between the labyrinth and the earth gravitational vector to decide when to institute the positions.

Interpretation and Usefulness of Positional Nystagmus

Notwithstanding the often cited study conducted by Barber and Wright (1973), we do not share the view that it is normal to observe positional nystagmus in a large percentage of the population. Rather, there must be an asymmetry in the vestibular afferent tone of either the periphery or the CNS. We do agree that this may also be present as a result of alcohol consumption or other pharmacologic influences. A careful case history should help differentiate such causes. We feel that in the majority of cases, it is possible to avoid the terminology "nonlocalizing finding" to describe the presence of positional nystagmus. This is possible when positional nystagmus is correlated with a thorough clinical history and identification of symptoms, as well as careful integration of other

diagnostic measures. We discuss this method of interpretation of positional nystagmus and also the older methods.

Central Nervous System Involvement

Most of the nystagmus characteristics discussed under the section "Interpretation of Spontaneous Nystagmus" are also valid for positionally provoked nystagmus with some exceptions. As for spontaneous nystagmus, vertical (i.e., up- or down-beating) nystagmus present during positional testing is an indicator of CNS involvement or pharmacologic influence. Damage to the cerebellum, Arnold-Chiari malformations, multiple sclerosis, VBI, and pharmacological effects may all cause vertical positional nystagmus (Brandt, 1991). This nystagmus may or may not be accompanied by vertigo. If there is nystagmus, but there is no subjective impression of vertigo or dizziness by the patient, CNS involvement is supported (Table 11–7).

We have observed ageotropic positional nystagmus in older patients and no vertigo or other dizziness is reported. In these cases, there may be age-related ischemic changes reported on imaging studies. We have also observed patients with migrainous positional vertigo (MPV) (Roberts, Gans, & Kastner, 2006) who also present with ageotropic nystagmus. von Brevern, Radtke, Clarke, and Lempert (2004) presented results of 10 patients with "pseudo-BPPV" who actually had migrainous vertigo. Four of the patients had positionally provoked nystagmus with concomitant vertigo during their episodes. All manner of nystagmus was reported in various static positions: geotropic, ageotropic, torsional, and downbeat. In two patients the episodes of positional nystagmus were transient, whereas in others the duration of the episodes ranged from hours to weeks. In other patients, the nystagmus was persistent in a given position, which is what we have observed for MPV and also in our older patients who have no vertigo. Both age-related CNS changes and migraine may be the cause of positional nystagmus. Lack of fixation suppression of positional nystagmus supports CNS involvement, but it is also not uncommon for some suppression to occur. As with spontaneous nystagmus, medication effects could also cause positional nystagmus.

Table 11–7. Interpretation of Positional Nystagmus

Peripheral	Central
Direction fixed horizontal or torsional nystagmus	Vertical nystagmus (up-beating or down-beating)
Suppression of nystagmus with fixation except HC-BPPV	No suppression of nystagmus with fixation
Expect fast phase toward intact ear except for the following: • Irritative nystagmus • Recovery nystagmus • HC-BPPV	Ageotropic nystagmus with or without subjective dizziness • Must exclude HC-BPPV
Enhances dynamically post head shake	May be present as a result of the following: • Pharmacy • Alcohol • Tobacco
May not be persistent within position	Does not enhance dynamically Usually persists while in position

Peripheral Vestibular Involvement

Placing a patient with spontaneous nystagmus resulting from an acute unilateral labyrinthine involvement into various positions may alter the nystagmus. Likewise, when restoration of vestibular tone occurs with static compensation, placing the patient into different positions with different levels of neural firing from the periphery may provoke a positional nystagmus. This positional nystagmus of peripheral origin would be expected to be direction-fixed and horizontal with the fast phase of the nystagmus beating toward the intact ear consistent with Ewald's second law. As described above, there remains the possibility of an irritative or recovery nystagmus, which may deviate from this expectation.

Any time the examiner observes positional nystagmus, an attempt should be made to measure fixation suppression. As with spontaneous nystagmus, suppression of positional nystagmus would be expected with a peripheral origin, but lack of suppression would be expected with CNS involvement (except in cases of HC-BPPV). As there is certainly the possibility that a direction-fixed horizontal nys-

tagmus that suppresses with visual fixation could represent CNS involvement, the clinician must correlate findings with the history and symptoms of the patient.

For example, a patient who reports an episode of vertigo with nausea and emesis for two days following an upper respiratory infection may present with a direction-fixed right-beating nystagmus in left lateral position that suppresses with vision. In this case there is support for a clinical impression of positional nystagmus of peripheral origin. If we now correlate this finding with other videonystagmography results such as a right-beating nystagmus post-head-shake and a left unilateral weakness on caloric testing, there is greater support for the existence of an uncompensated peripheral vestibulopathy. Now, if we add in other results such as degraded dynamic visual acuity and/or abnormal postural stability with a vestibular pattern, then we can report with some degree of certainty that this positional nystagmus supports the presence of the uncompensated left peripheral vestibulopathy, as opposed to its presence as a "nonlocalizing finding."

On the other hand, another patient who denies true vertigo and has a history of cerebrovascular disease, may present with the same type of positional nystagmus, direction fixed and beating to the right. We may observe no enhancement of the nystagmus with head shake and there may be no caloric weakness. There may be degraded oculomotor function though and a CNS pattern on postural stability testing. By combining these bits of information, and if the nystagmus does not suppress with visual fixation, it may be possible to ascribe the nystagmus to a CNS origin.

Positional Alcohol Nystagmus

Another type of positional nystagmus pattern that may be encountered in the clinic is either a geotropic or ageotropic nystagmus related to excessive alcohol consumption. Positional alcohol nystagmus (PAN) actually has two phases (i.e., referred to as PAN I and PAN II), and the nystagmus direction varies for each phase (Table 11–8). In PAN I, a difference in specific gravity occurs between the semicircular canal cupulae and the surrounding endolymph. These normally have the same specific gravity so that the canals are mainly sensitive to angular acceleration in the plane of the canal. However, there is a temporal difference in which alcohol diffuses into the cupula faster compared to the endolymph. The alcohol, which is lighter than the endolymph, causes the cupulae to become lighter than normal, making them sensitive to changes in head position relative to the gravity. Approximately 30 min after ingestion of alcohol, these changes in specific gravity may be manifested as a positionally provoked geotropic nystagmus (i.e., beating toward the lower ear) (Fetter et al., 1999; Money, Myles, & Hoffert, 1974). As the alcohol diffuses into the endolymph, the difference in specific gravity becomes negligible again and the PAN I is no longer observable.

The second phase of PAN (PAN II) begins between 5 to 10 hr after alcohol is no longer being ingested. Now, the opposite occurs. Alcohol diffuses from the cupulae before the endolymph, making the cupulae denser than the surrounding fluid. Again, a positionally provoked nystagmus can be recorded, but with the nystagmus beating toward the upper ear (ageotropic nystagmus). PAN was originally described as occurring due to changes in the buoyancy of the cupulae due to changes in the specific gravity of the cupulae and endolymph. Much of this work was done by Aschan and colleagues (e.g., Aschan, 1958; Aschan, Bergstedt, Goldberg, & Laurell, 1956).

Classic Interpretation of Positional Nystagmus

For some time, it has been clinical practice to interpret the presence of some positional nystagmus as normal (Barber & Stockwell, 1980). The evidence often cited for this is found in Barber and Wright (1973). The authors tested a random sample of 112 participants with reportedly normal health status and no history of dizziness. The participants were tested using electro-oculography recording techniques with patients placed in eight different positions: upright, supine, right lateral, left lateral, head hanging, head-hanging right, head-hanging left, and caloric test position (i.e., supine with head elevated 30 degrees). The authors reported that 82% (i.e., 92) of their participants had measurable positional nystagmus. Based on these data, the authors developed suggested criteria for clinically significant abnormal positional nystagmus. Within their eight positions, the authors felt that positional nystagmus was pathologic in the following cases: a single beat with intensity 14 deg/s or greater; spontaneous nystagmus; burst of nystagmus with average intensity of

Table 11–8. Characteristics of Positional Alcohol Nystagmus (PAN)

PAN Phase	Specific Gravity Difference	Nystagmus
Initial (PAN I)	30 min after ingestion of alcohol • Cupula lighter than endolymph	Geotropic
Intermediate	No difference in specific gravity between cupula and endolymph	No nystagmus
Second (PAN II)	5 to 10 hr after discontinuing alcohol ingestion • Cupula is heavier than endolymph	Ageotropic

9 deg/s or greater; persistent or intermittent nystagmus in six or more positions; or a combination of persistent and intermittent positional nystagmus in eight positions (Table 11–9). These criteria are still used by many clinicians for determination of abnormal positional nystagmus.

Aschan (1961) proposed a classification system for positional and positioning nystagmus based on the duration of the nystagmus and whether it is direction fixed or direction changing. Type I is persistent and direction changing. If this type of nystagmus occurs in a single head position, it is typically of central origin. On the other hand, HC-BPPV may also present in this manner, but with the difference that a change in position will change the direction of the nystagmus. Type II is direction fixed regardless of position and can be present with peripheral or CNS involvement. Most often this represents the direction-fixed spontaneous nystagmus that occurs in a unilateral, uncompensated peripheral impairment. Type III nystagmus is transient in duration while the patient remains in the provoking position. Of course, this type is observed most often with cases of BPPV.

More recently, Shepard and Telian (1996) suggested the following criteria for clinically significant positional nystagmus: nystagmus intensity more than 5 deg/s; less than 6 deg/s, but persistent in four or more of 8 to 11 positions; less than 6 deg/s and sporadic, but present in all positions tested; and direction changing within a given head position. This is shown in Table 11–9 and suggests that even a low-intensity positional nystagmus is of clinical significance.

The fact that 82% of normal participants had positional nystagmus seems like a remarkably large percentage. However, others report similar results.

Coats (1993) reported that 82.3% (42 of 51 healthy participants) had positional nystagmus under closed lids in at least one of five positions. Data from several studies that reported on positional nystagmus are shown in Table 11–10. McAuley, Dickman, Mustain, and Anand (1996) reported that 88% (43 of 49 participants) with no vestibular symptoms, normal audiometric hearing, and normal performance on dynamic posturography had positional nystagmus recorded using ENG techniques. Nystagmus presence was determined by the identification of at least three beats of nystagmus within a 20 s time period using electronystagmography techniques. Sunami et al. (2004) has reported similar results for positional nystagmus in normal participants using modern videonystagmography techniques. Using this technique, Sunami et al. (2004) reported that 73% (65 of 89) healthy participants had nystagmus in at least one position.

Interestingly, Barber and Wright (1973) observed that positional nystagmus was more common if testing was performed after calorics compared to positional testing prior to caloric stimulation. If the data of their participants who received caloric stimulation first is excluded, then the prevalence of positional nystagmus from their report decreases from 82% to 73%. Then 40% of their instances of positional nystagmus were classified as either "doubtful, possible nystagmus" or "doubtful, probable nystagmus." Within these two categories, the nystagmus was considered intermittent 75% of the time when classified as "doubtful, possible nystagmus" and 77% of the time when classified as "doubtful, probable nystagmus." Investigators and clinicians should give consideration to these facts, as well as the criterion of three nystagmus beats within a relatively large 20-s window used by McAuley et al. (1996).

Table 11-9. Classic Parameters to Interpret Positional Nystagmus

Barber & Wright (1973)	Shepard & Telian (1996)
Single nystagmus beat 14°/s or greater	Nystagmus intensity greater than 5°/s
Burst of nystagmus 9°/s or greater	Less than 6°/s, but persistent in four or more of 8 to 11 positions
Persistent or intermittent nystagmus in six or more positions	Less than 6°/s and sporadic, present in all positions tested
Persistent and intermittent nystagmus in eight positions	Direction-changing nystagmus in a single head position

Table 11–10. Studies Reporting on Positional Nystagmus

Study	ENG/VNG	Sample	Percent (%)	n
Barber & Wright (1973)	ENG	Normal	82	112
Coats (1993)	ENG	Normal	82.3	51
McAuley, Dickman, Mustain, & Anand (1996)	ENG	Normal	88	49
Van der Stappen, Wuyts, & Van de Heyning (2000)	ENG	Normal	7.5	40
Hajioff, Barr-Hamilton, Colledge, Lewis, & Wilson (2000)	ENG	Older normal	27	96
Sunami et al. (2004)	VNG	Normal	73	89
Johkura, Momoo, & Kuroiwa (2008)	VNG	Normal controls	19	155
		Chronic dizziness	61	200

It is possible that "normal" positional nystagmus is not that common.

Van der Stappen, Wuyts, and Van de Heyning (2000) only observed positional nystagmus in 7.5% (3 of 40) of their healthy participants. Testing was completed using ENG with eyes closed in nearly total darkness. Hajioff et al. (2000) report data using an ENG technique similar to Van der Stappen et al. (2000) but with an older group of healthy participants. The average age of the participants in their investigation was 51 years. The age range of the participants in Hajioff et al. was 66 to 89 years with a median of 76 years. As in other studies completed using ENG, data were obtained in both eyes open and eyes closed conditions. They report that 27% (26 of 96) participants had positional nystagmus.

In an interesting study of positional nystagmus in patients with chronic dizziness, Johkura, Momoo, and Kuroiwa (2008) only observed positional nystagmus in 19% (30 of 155) of their healthy control group using VNG techniques. The mean age of these participants was 71.8 years. These participants were matched for age and gender to their experimental group with chronic dizziness. The prevalence data for this experimental group with chronic dizziness was 61% (122 of 200).

We are more in agreement with the view of Shepard and Telian (1996) and would urge clinicians to interpret the presence of positional nystagmus in the context of the patient's history and symptoms and the results of other quantitative tests. The value of validating a patient's complaint of vertigo when in a static position by recording their eye movements cannot be overstated.

CERVICAL VERTIGO SCREENING TEST

It is established that connections exist between the cervical dorsal roots and the vestibular nuclei with the neck proprioceptors and joint receptors serving a role in eye-hand coordination, perception of balance, and postural adjustments (Brown, 1992; Wrisley, Sparto, Whitney, & Furman, 2000). Zuo et al. (2013) report evidence for bidirectional nerve fiber connections between cervical spinal and sympathetic ganglia, providing a possible neuroanatomical basis for the pathogenesis of cervical vertigo. Others suggest the basis may sometimes relate to the influence of cervical changes on vertebrobasilar circulation (Piñol, Ramirez, Saló, Ros, & Blanch, 2013; Yacovino, 2012).

Clendaniel and Landel (2007) and Wrisley et al. (2000) provide excellent reviews of both examination and treatment of cervical vertigo. They note that patients with a possible cervicogenic origin typically present with dysequilibrium, light-headedness, ataxia, unsteadiness, and so forth, along with cervical pain and limited cervical motion. There is often a history of neck injury. It should be noted by the clinician that true vertigo is not a common symptom of cervical vertigo. Vertebrobasilar insufficiency

(Olszewski et al., 2006; Piñol et al., 2013; Yacovino, 2012) and altered cervical proprioceptive signals are both potential etiologies and should be investigated when tests for cervical vertigo evoke true vertigo (Magarey et al., 2004).

Wrisley et al. (2000) have created a decision tree to guide the clinician through the process of evaluating and managing (and referring when appropri-

ate) patients with possible cervicogenic dizziness. Clendaniel and Landel (2007) suggest that tests for cervical vertigo should include an evaluation of cervical range of motion, palpation of cervical spine musculature, and mobility testing of the cervical spine. We perform a simple screening in cases where a cervicogenic origin is suspected (Figure 11–13). The patient is seated on a swivel chair and

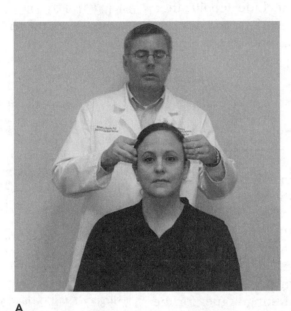

A

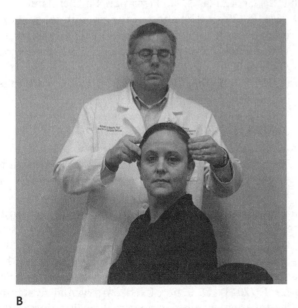

B

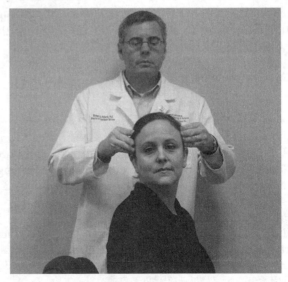

C

Figure 11–13. Cervical vertigo screening test is shown. The patient is asked to fixate on a visual target. **A.** The examiner is positioned behind the patient and attempts to assist in stabilizing the head. **B.** The patient moves the body to the right with the head maintained center. This position is held for 20 to 30 s. **C.** Following a brief return to the neutral center position, the patient moves the body to the left with the head maintained center. This position is held for 20 to 30 s. Reprinted with permission from Alabama Hearing & Balance Associates, Inc.

the head is immobilized. The patient then "walks" his or her body to one side while keeping the head immobile (to limit changes in vestibular information). After holding this position for 30 to 40 s, the patient is returned to the neutral position and then the screening is repeated for the opposite side. If a cervicogenic origin is confirmed via cervical spine imaging and/or other clinical evaluation, referral to physical therapy for appropriate treatment is indicated and may include mobilization and manipulation, active range of motion, restricted mobility, increased muscle tone, trigger points, and so forth (Clendaniel & Landel, 2007; Wrisley et al., 2000).

SUMMARY

Positioning and positional subtests provide important information in the evaluation and management of the patient with dizziness and imbalance. Several practical options to evaluate patients for all forms of BPPV, VBI, and cervical origins of symptoms have been presented. The fact that peripheral vestibular involvement or CNS involvement may provide similar findings during testing argues for the imperative need for correlation with patient history and symptoms, in addition to results of other diagnostic evaluation, to arrive at the true origin of the nystagmus.

REFERENCES

Agus, S., Benecke, H., Thum, C., & Strupp, M. (2013). Clinical and demographic features of vertigo: Findings from the REVERT registry. *Frontiers in Neurology, 10*, 4–48.

Albuquerque, F., Hu, Y., Dashti, S., Abla, A., Clark, J., Alkire, B., . . . McDougall, C. (2011). Craniocervical arterial dissections as sequelae of chiropractic manipulation: Patterns of injury and management. *Journal of Neurosurgery, 115*(6), 1197–1205.

Appiani, G., Catania, G., & Gagliardi, M. (2001). A liberatory maneuver for the treatment of horizontal canal paroxysmal positional vertigo. *Otology and Neurotology, 22*, 66–69.

Asavasopon, S., Jankoski, J., & Godges, J. (2005). Clinical diagnosis of vertebrobasilar insufficiency: Resident's case problem. *Journal of Orthopaedic and Sports Physical Therapy, 35*(10), 645–650.

Aschan, G. (1958). Different types of alcohol nystagmus. *Acta Oto-Laryngologica, 140*, 69–78.

Aschan, G. (1961). The pathogenesis of positional nystagmus. *Acta Oto-Laryngologica Supplement, 159*, 90–93.

Aschan, G., Bergstedt, M., Goldberg, L., & Laurell, L. (1956). Positional nystagmus in man during and after alcohol intoxication. *Quarterly Journal of Studies of Alcohol, 17*, 381–405.

Baloh, R. (1998). Differentiating between peripheral and central causes of vertigo. *Otolaryngology-Head and Neck Surgery, 119*, 55–59.

Baloh, R., & Honrubia, V. (2001). *Clinical neurophysiology of the vestibular system* (3rd ed.). New York, NY: Oxford University Press.

Barber, H., & Stockwell, C. (1980). *Manual of electronystagmography* (2nd ed.). St. Louis, MO: Mosby.

Barber, H., & Wright, G. (1973). Positional nystagmus in normals. *Advances in Oto-Rhino-Laryngology, 19*, 276–285.

Bath, A., Walsh, R., Ranalli, P., Tyndel, F., Bance, M., Mai, R., & Rutka, J. A. (2000). Experience from a multidisciplinary "dizzy" clinic. *American Journal of Otology, 21*, 92–97.

Bertholon, P., Bronstein, A., Davies, R., Rudge, P., & Thilo, K. (2002). Positional down beating nystagmus in 50 patients: Cerebellar disorders and possible anterior semicircular canalithiasis. *Journal of Neurology, Neurosurgery, and Psychiatry, 72*, 366–372.

Blatt, P., Georgakakis, G., Herdman, S., Clendaniel, R., & Tusa, R. (2000). The effect of the canalith repositioning maneuver on resolving postural instability in patients with benign paroxysmal positional vertigo. *American Journal of Otology, 21*, 356–363.

Brandt, T. (1990). Positional and positioning vertigo and nystagmus. *Journal of Neurological Science, 95*, 3–28.

Brandt, T. (1991). *Vertigo, its multisensory syndromes.* London, UK: Springer-Verlag.

Brown, J. (1992). Cervical contributions to balance: Cervical vertigo. In A. Berthoz, P. P. Vidal, & W. Graf (Eds.), *The head neck sensory motor system* (pp. 644–647). New York, NY: Oxford University Press.

Cakir, B., Ercan, I., Cakir, Z., Civelek, S., Sayin, I., & Turgut, S. (2006). What is the true incidence of horizontal semicircular canal benign paroxysmal positional vertigo? *Otolaryngology-Head and Neck Surgery, 134*, 451–454.

Califano, L., Vassallo, A., Melillo, M., Mazzone, S., & Salafia, F. (2013). Direction-fixed paroxysmal nystagmus lateral canal benign paroxysmal positioning vertigo (BPPV): Another form of lateral canalolithiasis. *Acta Otorhinolaryngologica Italica, 33*(4), 254–260.

Casani, A., Vannucci, G., Fattori, B., & Berrettini, S. (2002). The treatment of horizontal canal positional vertigo: Our experience in 66 cases. *Laryngoscope, 112*, 172–178.

Celebisoy, N., Polat, F., & Akyurekli, O. (2008). Clinical features of benign paroxysmal positional vertigo in Western Turkey. *European Neurology, 59*(6), 315–319.

Chiou, W., Lee, H., Tsai, S., Yu, T., & Lee, X. (2005). A single therapy for all subtypes of horizontal canal positional vertigo. *Laryngoscope, 115,* 1432–1435.

Choi, K., Oh, S., Kim, H., Koo, J., Cho, B., & Kim, J. (2007). Recovery of vestibular imbalances after vestibular neuritis. *Laryngoscope, 117,* 1307–1312.

Choi, K., Oh, S., Park, S., Kim, J., Koo, J., & Kim, S. (2007). Head-shaking nystagmus in lateral medullary syndrome. *Neurology, 68,* 1337–1344.

Choi, K., Shin, H., Kim, J., Kim, S., Kwon, O., Koo, J., . . . Roh, J. -K. (2005). Rotational vertebral artery syndrome: Oculo-graphic analysis of nystagmus. *Neurology, 65,* 1287–1290.

Choung, Y., Shin, Y., Kahng, H., Park, K., & Choi S. (2006). "Bow and lean test" to determine the affected ear of horizontal canal benign paroxysmal positional vertigo. *Laryngoscope, 116*(10), 1776–1781.

Clendaniel, R., & Landel, R. (2007). Cervicogenic dizziness. In S. Herdman (Ed.), *Vestibular rehabilitation* (3rd ed.). Philadelphia, PA: F. A. Davis.

Coats, A. (1993). Computer-quantified positional nystagmus in normals. *American Journal of Otolaryngology, 14,* 314–326.

Cohen, H. (2004). Side-lying as an alternative to the Dix-Hallpike test of the posterior canal. *Otology and Neurotology, 25,* 130–134.

Cornelius, J., George, B., N'dri Oka, D., Spiriev, T., Steiger, H., & Hänggi D. (2012). Bow-hunter's syndrome caused by dynamic vertebral artery stenosis at the cranio-cervical junction—a management algorithm based on a systematic review and a clinical series. *Neurosurgical Review, 35*(1), 127–135.

Dannenbaum, E., Paquet, N., Hakim-Zadek, R., & Feldman, A. (2005). Optimal parameters for the clinical test of dynamic visual acuity in patients with a unilateral vestibular deficit. *Journal of Otolaryngology, 34,* 13–19.

de Bray, J., Penisson-Benier, I., Dubas, F., & Emile, J. (1997). Extracranial and intracranial vertebrobasilar dissections: Diagnosis and prognosis. *Journal of Neurology Neurosurgery and Psychiatry, 63,* 46–51.

de la Meilleure, G., Dehaene, I., Depondt, M., Damman, W., Crevits, L., & Vanhooren, G. (1996). Benign paroxysmal positional vertigo of the horizontal canal. *Journal of Neurology Neurosurgery and Psychiatry, 60,* 68–71.

Demer, J., Oas, J., & Baloh, R. (1993). Visual-vestibular interaction in humans during and passive vertical head movement. *Journal of Vestibular Research, 3,* 101–114.

De Stefano, A., Kulamarva, G., Citraro, L., Neri, G., & Croce, A. (2011). Spontaneous nystagmus in benign paroxysmal positional vertigo. *American Journal of Otolaryngology, 32*(3), 185–189.

Dix, R., & Hallpike, C. (1952). The pathology, symptomatology and diagnosis of certain common disorders of the vestibular system. *Annals of Otology, Rhinology and Laryngology, 6,* 987–1016.

Epley, J. (1992). The canalith repositioning procedure: For treatment of benign paroxysmal positional vertigo. *Otolaryngology-Head and Neck Surgery, 119,* 399–404.

Fetter, M., Haslwanter, T., Bork, M., & Dichgans, J. (1999). New insights into positional alcohol nystagmus using three-dimensional eye-movement analysis. *Annals of Neurology, 45,* 216–223.

Fife, T. (1998). Recognition and management of horizontal canal benign positional vertigo. *American Journal of Otology, 19,* 345–351.

Gans, R. (2000). Overview of BPPV: Pathophysiology and diagnosis. *The Hearing Review, 7,* 38–43.

Gans, R., & Harrington-Gans, P. (2002). Treatment efficacy of benign paroxysmal positional vertigo (BPPV) with canalith repositioning maneuver and Semont liberatory maneuver in 376 patients. *Seminars in Hearing, 23,* 129–142.

Gans, R., & Yellin, W. (2007). Assessment of vestibular function. In R. Roeser, M. Valente, & H. Hosford-Dunn (Eds.), *Audiology: Diagnosis* (pp. 540–566). New York, NY: Thieme.

Hain, T., & Spindler, J. (1993). Head-shaking nystagmus. In J. Sharpe & H. Barber (Eds.), *The vestibulo-ocular reflex and vertigo* (pp. 217–228). New York, NY: Raven Press.

Hajioff, D., Barr-Hamilton, R., Colledge, N., Lewis, S., & Wilson, J. (2000) Re-evaluation of normative electronystagmography data in healthy ageing. *Clinical Otolaryngology and Allied Sciences, 25,* 249–252.

Hall, S., Ruby, R., & McClure, J. (1979). The mechanics of benign paroxysmal vertigo. *Journal of Otolaryngology, 8,* 151–158.

Haynes, D., Resser, J., Labadie, R., Girasole, C., Kovach, B., Scheker, L., & Walker, D. C. (2002). Treatment of benign positional vertigo using the Semont maneuver: Efficacy in patients presenting without nystagmus. *Laryngoscope, 112,* 796–801.

Herdman, S., Tusa, R., & Clendanial, R. (1994). Eye movement signs in vertical canal benign paroxysmal positional vertigo. In A. Fuchs, T. Brandt, U. Buttner, & D. Zee (Eds.), *Contemporary ocular motor and vestibular research: A tribute to David A. Robinson* (pp. 385–387). Stuttgart, Germany: Georg Thieme-Verlag.

Herdman, S., Tusa, R., Zee, D., Proctor, L., & Mattox, D. (1993). Single treatment approaches to benign paroxysmal positional vertigo. *Archives of Otolaryngology-Head and Neck Surgery, 119,* 450–454.

Honrubia, V., Baloh, R., Harris, M., & Jacobson, K. (1999). Paroxysmal positional vertigo syndrome. *American Journal of Otology, 20,* 465–470.

Hornibrook, J. (2011). Benign paroxysmal positional vertigo (BPPV): History, pathophysiology, office treatment and future directions. *International Journal of Otolaryngology, 2011,* 1–13.

Huebner, A., Lytle, S., Doettl, S., Plyler, P., & Thelin J. (2013). Treatment of objective and subjective benign paroxysmal positional vertigo. *Journal of the American Academy of Audiology, 24*(7), 600–606.

Humphriss, R., Baguley, D., Sparkes, V., Peerman, S., & Moffat, D. (2003). Contraindications to the Dix-Hallpike manoeuvre: A multidisciplinary review. *International Journal of Audiology, 42,* 166–173.

Hutting, N., Verhagen, A., Vijverman, V., Keesenberg, M., Dixon, G., & Scholten-Peeters, G. (2013). Diagnostic accuracy of premanipulative vertebrobasilar insufficiency tests: A systematic review. *Manual Therapy, 18*(3), 177–182.

Ikeda, D., Villelli, N., Shaw, A., & Powers C. (2014). Bow hunter's syndrome unmasked after contralateral vertebral artery sacrifice for aneurysmal subarachnoid hemorrhage. *Journal of Clinical Neuroscience, 21*(6), 1044–1046.

Jackson, L., Morgan, B., Fletcher, J., & Krueger, W. (2007). Anterior canal benign paroxysmal positional vertigo: An underappreciated entity. *Otology and Neurotology, 28,* 218–222.

Jacobson, G., Pearlstein, R., Henderson, J., Calder, J., & Rock, J. (1998). Recovery nystagmus revisited. *Journal of the American Academy of Audiology, 9,* 263–271.

Johkura, K., Momoo, T., & Kuroiwa, Y. (2008) Positional nystagmus in patients with chronic dizziness. *Journal of Neurology Neurosurgery and Psychiatry, 79,* 1324–1326.

Katsarkas, A. (1999). Benign paroxysmal positional vertigo (BPPV): Idiopathic versus post-traumatic. *Acta Oto-Laryngologica, 119,* 745–749.

Koo, J., Moon, I., Shim, W., Moon, S., & Kim, J. (2006). Value of lying down nystagmus in the lateralization of horizontal semicircular canal benign paroxysmal positional vertigo. *Otology and Neurotology, 27,* 367–371.

Korres, S., & Balatsouras, D. (2004). Diagnostic, pathophysiologic, and therapeutic aspects of benign paroxysmal positional vertigo. *Otolaryngology-Head and Neck Surgery, 131,* 438–444.

Korres, S., Balatsouras, D., Kaberos, A., Economou, C., Kandiloros, D., & Ferekidis E. (2002). Occurrence of semicircular canal involvement in benign paroxysmal positional vertigo. *Otology and Neurotology, 23,* 926–932.

Lanska, D., & Remler, B. (1997). Benign paroxysmal positioning vertigo: Classic descriptions, origins of provocative positioning technique, and conceptual developments. *Neurology, 48,* 1167–1177.

Leigh, R., & Zee, D. (2001). *The neurology of eye movements* (3rd ed.). New York, NY: Oxford University Press.

Liu, H. (2012). Presentation and outcome of post-traumatic benign paroxysmal positional vertigo. *Acta Oto-Laryngologica, 132*(8), 803–806.

Longridge, N., & Barber, H. (1978). Bilateral paroxysmal positioning nystagmus. *Journal of Otolaryngology, 7,* 395–400.

Longridge, N., & Mallinson, A. (1987). The dynamic illegible E (DIE) test: A simple technique for assessing the ability of the vestibulo-ocular reflex to overcome vestibular pathology. *Journal of Otolaryngology, 16,* 97–103.

Lopez-Escamez, J. A., Gamiz, M. J., Finana, M., Perez, A., & Canet, I. (2002). Position in bed is associated with left or right location in benign paroxysmal positional vertigo of the posterior semicircular canal. *American Journal of Otolaryngology, 23,* 263–266.

Macias, J., Lambert, K., Massingale, S., Ellensohn, A., & Fritz J. (2000). Variables affecting treatment in benign paroxysmal positional vertigo. *Laryngoscope, 110,* 1921–1924.

Magarey, M., Rebbeck, T., Coughlan, B., Grimmer, K., Rivett, D., & Refshauge, K. (2004). Pre-manipulative testing of the cervical spine review, revision and new clinical guidelines. *Manual Therapy, 9,* 95–108.

Marques, P., & Perez-Fernandez, N. (2012). Bedside vestibular examination in patients with unilateral definite Ménière's disease. *Acta Oto-Laryngologica, 132*(5), 498–504.

Matsuzaki, M., & Kamei, T. (1995). Stage-assessment of the progress of continuous vertigo of peripheral origin by means of spontaneous and head-shaking nystagmus findings. *Acta Otolayrngologica Supplement, 519,* 188–190.

McAuley, J., Dickman, J., Mustain, W., & Anand, V. (1996). Positional nystagmus in asymptomatic human subjects. *Otolaryngology-Head and Neck Surgery, 114,* 545–553.

McCaslin, D. (2013). Anatomy and physiology of the vestibular system. In *Electronystagmography and videonystagmography ENG/VNG* (pp. 15–37). San Diego, CA: Plural.

Money, K., Myles, W., & Hoffert, D. (1974). The mechanism of positional alcohol nystagmus. *Canadian Journal of Otolaryngology, 3,* 302–313.

Moon, S., Kim, J., Kim, B., Kim, J., Lee, H., Son, S., . . . Lee, W. (2006). Clinical characteristics of benign paroxysmal positional vertigo in Korea: A multicenter study. *Journal of Korean Medical Science, 21*(3), 539–543.

Nagashima, C., Iwama, K., Sakata, E., & Miki, Y. (1970). Effect of temporary occlusion of a vertebral artery on human vestibular system. *Journal of Neurosurgery, 33,* 338–394.

Ogawa, Y., Suzuki, M., Otsuka, K., Shimizu, H., Inagaki, T., Hayashi, M., . . . Kitajima, N. (2009). Positional and positioning down-beating nystagmus without central nervous system findings. *Auris Nasus Larynx, 36*(6), 698–701.

Oghalai, J., Manolidis, S., Barth, J., Stewart, M., & Jenkins, H. (2000). Unrecognized benign paroxysmal positional vertigo in elderly patients. *Otolaryngology-Head and Neck Surgery, 122,* 630–634.

Olszewski, J., Majak, J., Pietkiewicz, P., Luszcz, C., & Repetowski, M. (2006). The association between positional vertebral and basilar artery flow lesion and prevalence of vertigo in patients with cervical spondylosis. *Otolaryngology-Head and Neck Surgery, 134,* 680–692.

Parnes, L., & McClure, J. (1992). Free-floating endolymph particles: A new operative finding during posterior semicircular canal occlusion. *Laryngoscope, 102,* 988–992.

Parnes, L., & Riddell, D. (1993). Irritative spontaneous nystagmus following intratympanic gentamicin for Ménière's disease. *Laryngoscope, 103,* 745–749.

Piñol, I., Ramirez, M., Saló, G., Ros, A., & Blanch, A. (2013). Symptomatic vertebral artery stenosis secondary to cervical spondylolisthesis. *Spine, 38*(23), E1503–E1505.

Poletti, M., Listorti, C., & Rucci M. (2013). Microscopic eye movements compensate for nonhomogeneous vision within the fovea. *Current Biology, 23*(17), 1691–1695.

Radtke, A., & Lempert, T. (2005). Self treatment of benign paroxysmal positional vertigo: Semont maneuver vs. Epley procedure. *Neurology, 64,* 583.

Roberts, R., Abrams, H., Sembach, M., Lister, J., Gans, R., & Chisolm, T. (2009). Utility measures of health-related quality of life in patients treated for benign paroxysmal positional vertigo. *Ear and Hearing, 30,* 369–376.

Roberts, R., & Gans, R. (2007). Comparison of horizontal and vertical dynamic visual acuity in patients with vestibular dysfunction and nonvestibular dizziness. *Journal of the American Academy of Audiology, 18,* 236–244.

Roberts, R., Gans, R., DeBoodt, J., & Lister, J. (2005). Treatment of benign paroxysmal positional vertigo: Necessity of postmaneuver patient restrictions. *Journal of the American Academy of Audiology, 16,* 357–366.

Roberts, R., Gans, R., & Kastner, A. (2006). Differentiation of migrainous positional vertigo (MPV) from horizontal canal benign paroxysmal positional vertigo (HC-BPPV). *International Journal of Audiology, 45,* 224–226.

Roberts, R., Gans, R., & Montaudo, R. (2006). Efficacy of a new treatment maneuver for posterior canal benign paroxysmal positional vertigo. *Journal of the American Academy of Audiology, 17,* 598–604.

Ruckenstein, M. (2001). Therapeutic efficacy of the Epley canalith repositioning maneuver. *Laryngoscope, 111,* 940–945.

Sakata, E., Ohtsu, K., & Sakata, H. (2004). Pitfalls in which otolaryngologists often are caught in the diagnosis and treatment of vertigo. *International Tinnitus Journal, 10,* 31–34.

Schuknecht, H. (1969). Cupulolithiasis. *Archives of Otolaryngology, 90,* 765–778.

Semont, A., Freyss, G., & Vitte, E. (1988). Curing the BPPV with a liberatory maneuver. *Advances in Otorhinolaryngology, 42,* 290–293.

Shephard, N., & Telian, S. (1996). Electronystagmography evaluation. In *Practical management of the balance disorder patient* (pp. 51–84). San Diego, CA: Singular.

Sibony, P., Evinger, C., & Manning, K. (1987). Tobacco induced primary-position upbeat nystagmus. *Annals of Neurology, 21,* 53–58.

Soto-Varela, A., Rossi-Izquierdo, M., & Santos-Pérez, S. (2013). Benign paroxysmal positional vertigo simultaneously affecting several canals: A 46-patient series. *European Archives of Otorhinolaryngology, 270*(3), 817–822.

Squires, T., Weidman, M., Hain, T., & Stone, H. (2004). A mathematical model for top-shelf vertigo: The role of sedimenting otoconia in BPPV. *Journal of Biomechanics, 37,* 1137–1146.

Steenerson, R., Cronin, G., & Marbach, P. (2005). Effectiveness of treatment techniques in 923 cases of benign paroxysmal positional vertigo. *Laryngoscope, 115,* 226–231.

Strupp, M., Dieterich, M., & Brandt, T. (2013). The treatment and natural course of peripheral and central vertigo. *Deutsches Ärzteblatt International, 110*(29–30), 505–516.

Sunami, K., Tochino, R., Zushi, T., Yamamoto, H., Tokuhara, Y., Iguchi, H., . . . Yamane, H. (2004). Positional and positioning nystagmus in healthy subjects under videonystagmoscopy. *Acta Oto-Laryngologica Supplement, 554,* 35–37.

Tusa, R., Zee, D., Hain, T., & Simonsz, H. (1992). Voluntary control of congenital nystagmus. *Clinics in Visual Science, 7,* 195–210.

Van der Stappen, A., Wuyts, F., & Van de Heyning P. (2000) Computerized electronystagmography: Normative data revisited. *Acta Oto-Laryngologica, 120,* 724–730.

von Brevern, M., Radtke, A., Clarke, A., & Lempert, T. (2004). Migrainous vertigo presenting as episodic positional vertigo. *Neurology, 62,* 469–472.

von Brevern, M., Seelig, T., Neuhauser, H., & Lempert, T. (2004). Benign paroxysmal positional vertigo predominantly affects the right labyrinth. *Journal of Neurology Neurosurgery Psychiatry, 75,* 1487–1488.

White, J., Coale, K., Catalano, P., & Oas, J. (2005). Diagnosis and management of lateral semicircular canal benign paroxysmal positional vertigo. *Otolaryngology-Head and Neck Surgery, 133,* 278–284.

Wolf, J. S., Boyev, K. P., Manokey, B. J., & Mattox, D. E. (1999). Success of the modified epley maneuver in treating benign paroxysmal positional vertigo. *Laryngoscope, 109*(6), 900–903.

Wrisley, D., Sparto, P., Whitney, S., & Furman, J. (2000). Cervicogenic dizziness: A review of diagnosis and treatment. *Journal of Orthopaedic & Sports Physical Therapy, 30*(12), 755–766.

Yacovino, D. (2012). Cervical vertigo: Myths, facts, and scientific evidence. *Neurologia*, S0213-4853(12)00211-3.

Yamaguchi, Y., Nagasawa, H., Yamakawa, T., & Kato, T. (2012). Bow hunter's syndrome after contralateral vertebral artery dissection. *Journal of Stroke and Cerebrovascular Diseases, 21*(8), 916.

Young, Y., & Chen, C. (2003). Acute vertigo following cervical manipulation. *Laryngoscope, 113*, 659–662.

Zapala, D. (2008). Down-beating nystagmus in anterior canal benign paroxysmal positional vertigo. *Journal of the American Academy of Audiology, 19*(3), 257–266.

Zee, D. (2000). Vestibular adaptation. In S. Herdman (Ed.), *Vestibular rehabilitation* (2nd ed., pp. 77–87). Philadelphia, PA: F. A. Davis.

Zuo, J., Han, J., Qiu, S., Luan, F., Zhu, X., Gao, H., & Chen, A. (2013). Neural reflex pathway between cervical spinal and sympathetic ganglia in rabbit: Implication for pathogenesis of cervical vertigo. *The Spine Journal*, S1529-9430(13), 01871–01878.

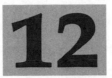

Background and Technique of Caloric Testing

Kamran Barin

OVERVIEW

The function of the vestibulo-ocular reflex (VOR) can be evaluated by stimulating the vestibular system and measuring the eye movement responses. Head movements provide the natural and physiologic stimulation for the vestibular system, but under most conditions, it is not possible to restrict such stimuli to one labyrinth at a time. As a result, caloric irrigations have been used historically as a more practical method for testing vestibular function in clinical settings. In the caloric test, the external auditory canal is irrigated by a medium that has a significantly different temperature compared to the body temperature. The temperature gradient eventually reaches the labyrinth and under the appropriate conditions can result in cupular deflections that produce vestibular responses.

Despite a number of limitations, caloric irrigations offer a major advantage over other types of vestibular stimulation. Unlike head movements, which always stimulate both labyrinths simultaneously, caloric irrigations allow each labyrinth to be evaluated independently (Baloh & Honrubia, 2001). Also, caloric stimulation can be generated by relatively small-sized and inexpensive equipment.

This chapter describes the procedures for administering the caloric test and analyzing the responses. The underlying principles of the caloric test are also discussed so that the examiner can recognize the limitations and artifacts when they occur.

BACKGROUND

Mechanism of Caloric Stimulation

The first detailed description of the caloric test and its underlying mechanism are attributed to Robert Bárány (Baloh, 2002). It is interesting to note that the publication year of this book coincides with the 100th anniversary of Bárány receiving the Nobel Prize in medicine in 1914 for "his work on the physiology and pathology of the vestibular apparatus" (excerpt from nobelprize.org).

In his now well-known book published almost a century ago, Bárány (1907) described caloric irrigations administered in the supine position with the head placed at an angle of 30 degrees with respect to the horizontal plane (Figure 12–1A). In this head position, known as the caloric test position, the lateral (horizontal) semicircular canals become aligned with the plane of gravity. In the absence of caloric stimulation, no responses are evoked from the lateral canals because the cupula and the surrounding endolymph have the same densities and are not affected by gravity. When the external auditory canal is irrigated with a medium that is considerably cooler or warmer than the body temperature, a temperature gradient is generated across the lateral canal of the irrigated ear. According to Bárány, the temperature gradient changes the density of the endolymph on the side of the canal closest to the site of irrigation.

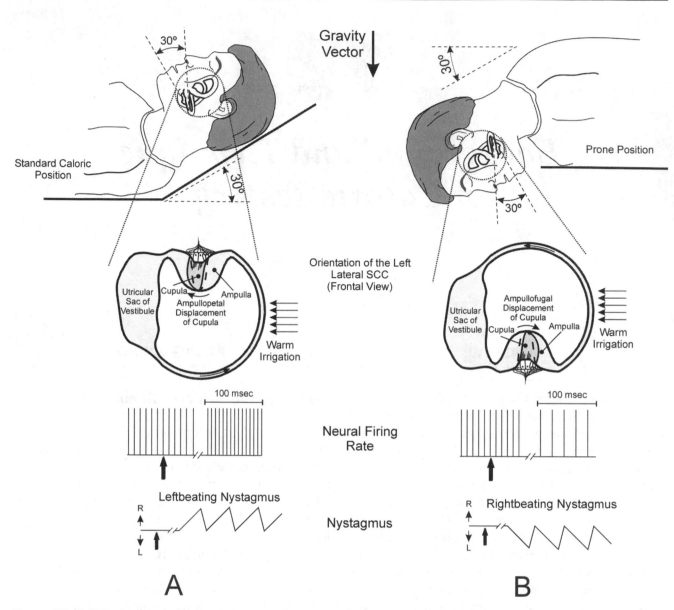

Figure 12-1. Effects of caloric stimulation on the neural firing and the eye movement responses with the patient. **A.** Supine with the head tilted up 30°. **B.** Prone with the head tilted down 30°. Solid arrows indicate the onset of irrigation. Based on Barin, K. (2009). Clinical neurophysiology of the vestibular system. In J. Katz, L. Medwetsky, R. Burkhart, and L. Hood, (Eds.), *Handbook of Clinical Audiology* (6th ed.). Philadelphia, PA: Lippincott Williams & Wilkins.

If that explanation is correct, warm irrigations in the standard caloric test position should cause the endolymph to become lighter and rise, thus generating an ampullopetal deflection of the cupula. Such a deflection should cause an excitatory response from the lateral canal and generate nystagmus with its fast phases beating toward the irrigated ear (see Figure 12–1A). Conversely, cool irrigations should cause the endolymph to become heavier and sink, thus generating an inhibitory response from the irrigated ear. The nystagmus fast phases should beat away from

the side of irrigation. The relationship between the temperature in the irrigated ear and the direction of the evoked nystagmus fast phases is summarized by the acronym COWS—cold opposite, warm same.

For many years, experimental findings were consistent with the above explanation and supported Bárány's predictions regarding the mechanism of caloric irrigations. The first serious challenge to this hypothesis came from one of the Spacelab-I experiments in which caloric responses were observed in the absence of gravity (Scherer, Brandt, Clarke,

Merbold, & Parker, 1986). This finding could not be explained based on Bárány's hypothesis because the change of the endolymph density depends on the presence of gravity. Alternative hypotheses have since emerged, including the direct effect of temperature on the vestibular nerve (Hood, 1989) and gravity-independent changes in the volume or pressure of the endolymph (Gentine, Eichhorn, Kopp, & Conraux, 1991). However, there are a number of compelling experimental findings that cannot be explained by any mechanism other than the one proposed by Bárány. For example, Figure 12–1B shows what happens when caloric irrigations are administered with the patient in the prone position with the head tilted 30 degrees downward. The lateral canals are still in the vertical plane but their orientation with respect to gravity is the reverse of that in the standard caloric position. If the caloric stimulations are mediated entirely by gravity-independent mechanisms, the nystagmus direction should be the same in the supine and prone positions. However, the exact opposite is expected under the Bárány's hypothesis. That is, warm irrigations in the prone position should generate nystagmus with the fast phases beating away from the irrigated ear. The reason is that the rise of lighter endolymph should now cause an ampullofugal flow of the endolymph, which should result in the inhibition of the irrigated lateral canal. Similarly, cool irrigations in the prone position should generate nystagmus with the fast phases beating toward the irrigated ear, indicating excitation of the irrigated lateral canal.

Coats and Smith (1967) demonstrated that the direction of nystagmus was indeed different in the supine and prone positions. Furthermore, the intensity of the nystagmus was slightly higher for the supine position. They concluded that the primary component of caloric stimulation was the change in the endolymph density. Additionally, they proposed that there was a secondary component involving direct stimulation of the vestibular nerve. The first component is gravity dependent as postulated by Bárány whereas the second component is gravity independent. Coats and Smith (1967) attributed the difference in the nystagmus intensity in different head positions to the fact that in the supine position, the two components are added but in the prone position, the two components are subtracted. This explains why caloric responses in the supine position are slightly larger than those in the prone

position. Today, the general consensus on the mechanism of caloric stimulation is similar to the views expressed by Coats and Smith (1967). That is, caloric stimulation consists of two components, one gravity dependent, and the other gravity independent. Hood (1989) suggested that the contribution of the gravity-independent component was very small (~10%) and the change in the endolymph density was the dominant mechanism underlying caloric responses.

Another topic of interest in caloric testing concerns the method by which the heat is transferred from the external auditory canal to the labyrinth. Initially, conduction via the bony connection between the external meatus and the lateral canal was assumed to be the primary pathway for heat transfer (Schmaltz, 1932). Subsequent studies, however, have highlighted the importance of the middle-ear space in caloric stimulation (see O'Neill, 1995, for a review). Two different modes of heat transfer have been proposed: convection through the air within the middle ear cleft (O'Neill, 1987) or radiation (Feldmann, Huttenbrink, & Delank, 1991). The study by Pau, Sievert, Just, and Wild (2001) supports the notion that at the onset, radiation is the main mode of heat transfer. However, conduction through the bone and convection through the middle ear air may play a role later on during the caloric irrigation.

The debate about the nature and mechanism of caloric stimulation is not just a matter of academic interest but has profound clinical implications. It is now clear that caloric stimuli are highly variable and depend on characteristics that are different from one individual to another. The effect of some of these differences, such as a perforated tympanic membrane, is obvious. Other differences, such as the dimensions of the internal meatus, have a less obvious and more puzzling effect on the caloric stimulus (O'Neill, 1995). New methods for measuring the heat transfer through the middle ear are becoming available (Nishizawa, 2002). These methods can enhance our understanding of the precise mechanisms of caloric stimulation and could someday lead to improvements in the test procedures.

Limitations of Caloric Test

The caloric test suffers from a number of shortcomings. First, caloric stimuli are not calibrated (Stockwell, 1997). Even though the external stimulus is the same, the effect on the labyrinth differs from one patient to another and sometimes from one ear to another in the same patient. Therefore, one cannot compare the sensitivity of the labyrinths in different patients by comparing the absolute responses to caloric stimuli. The variability in the caloric stimulus can be reduced to a manageable level by comparing the responses of the right and left ears of the same patient. In such a case, one has to make a key assumption that both labyrinths receive *equal* stimulation. Therefore, caloric responses from the right and left ears are expected to be equal in an individual with normal vestibular function. In practice, the difference between right and left responses of a normal person can be relatively large due to the variability of the caloric stimulus. Furthermore, the assumption of both labyrinths receiving equal stimulation is not valid when perforations or other anatomical anomalies are present.

The second limitation of the caloric test is that it is primarily a test of the lateral semicircular canals and their afferent neural pathways. Although caloric responses from the anterior and posterior semicircular canals are possible (Fetter, Aw, Haslwanter, Heimberger, & Dichgans, 1998), the distance from the external auditory canal makes it impractical for the temperature gradient to effectively reach the vertical canals. In some individuals, caloric irrigations do provoke small vertical and torsional nystagmus from the anterior and posterior canals but horizontal nystagmus from the lateral canal dominates the overall response (Aw, Haslwanter, Fetter, Heimberger, & Todd, 1998).

The third limitation of the caloric test is that it generates extremely low-frequency stimulation of the vestibular system. The vestibular receptors respond best to brief head movements within the frequency range of about 0.1 to 3 Hz. The caloric stimulus is estimated to be equivalent to head movements with the frequency of approximately 0.003 Hz (Hamid, Hughes, & Kinney, 1987). The estimates for the frequency response of the caloric test should be interpreted cautiously because it is based on eye movement responses without the knowledge of the precise input to the labyrinth. Nonetheless, it is clear that the frequency of caloric stimulation is well below the optimal operational range of the vestibular receptors. As a result, some compare testing the vestibular system with the caloric stimulus to testing the auditory system at frequencies that are not commonly included in the clinical testing.

Finally, caloric irrigations are distressing and poorly tolerated by some patients. If the patient experiences severe vertigo and nausea before completing the caloric test, the results are rarely useful. It is the responsibility of the examiner to try to the best of his or her ability to predict when the patient is likely to become ill and discontinue the irrigation before the onset of severe symptoms.

Given the limitations of the caloric test and the introduction of newer vestibular tests such as the vestibular-evoked myogenic potentials (VEMP) and video head impulse testing (vHIT), some have advocated abandoning the caloric test as a routine part of evaluation for dizzy patients. However, it is important to recognize that despite these limitations, the caloric test has withstood the test of time and has been the single most useful test of the labyrinth and its afferent pathways. This is especially true for identifying unilateral vestibular abnormalities. Therefore, it seems premature to assume that newer tests of vestibular function can replace the caloric test especially based on theoretical evidence and case reports. More time and more large-scale studies of vHIT and VEMP are needed to compare their efficacy and usefulness with the caloric test in typical clinical settings.

CALORIC IRRIGATORS

There are three types of caloric irrigators in clinical use today: open-loop water, air, and closed-loop water. The open-loop water irrigators were developed first and are still used in some clinics. The air caloric devices became available in the 1960s and are currently the most widely used irrigators (personal communication with MicroMedical and GN Otometrics). The closed-loop water irrigators, also called the Brookler-Grams system, were developed in the 1980s. Very few clinics use the closed-loop water irrigators now because they are no longer manufactured commercially.

All three irrigator types are capable of delivering caloric stimulation at precise temperatures. Almost all commercially available caloric irrigators today have a built-in timer and a flow meter to regulate the duration and the volume of irrigation. Furthermore, for computerized electronystagmography (ENG) and videonystagmography (VNG) systems, the irrigation temperature can be controlled by the computer to minimize the need for operator intervention. Nonetheless, there are a number of differences among the different systems that are noteworthy. More detailed descriptions of each irrigator type and the differences among them are discussed in this section.

Open-Loop Water Irrigators

A typical open-loop water irrigator contains one or two reservoirs that are filled with water. Most laboratories use tap water. Others use distilled water to reduce mineral deposits. It is best to follow the manufacturer's recommendations on the use of tap water versus distilled water. Some irrigators connect directly to the water line, thus eliminating the need to manually fill the water reservoirs.

Most modern open-loop water irrigators consist of two separate reservoirs for cool and warm water. As both cool and warm water are kept at or near the irrigation temperatures, very little time (typically less than a minute) is required for the water to reach the desired temperature when switching between cool and warm irrigations. Older irrigator models contain only one reservoir where the water is cooled or heated depending on the temperature setting. As a result, much longer time (typically several minutes) is needed for the temperature to stabilize when switching temperatures.

The water is transferred from the reservoir to the delivery point through an insulated hose. Some models of open-loop water irrigators regulate the temperature at the reservoirs and not at the delivery point. Therefore, before irrigation, the system has to be purged of the water that has stayed in the hose and replaced with the water from the reservoir that is at the appropriate temperature. Modern open-loop water systems eliminate the need for purging by constantly circulating the water between the reservoirs and the irrigator tip. Therefore, the water at the tip is always at the desired temperature and ready for irrigation.

The design of the irrigator tip that delivers the water to the ear varies depending on the manufacturer and the model. Some irrigators use a simple piece of tube. Others are more elaborate and resemble hand-held otoscopes, which illuminate the ear canal during the irrigation. In open-loop water irrigators, it is necessary to recover the water from the ear during the irrigation and dispose of it later. A simple container that fits conveniently under the ear and is large enough to hold the irrigated water is adequate for this purpose. Regardless of the design, the examiner must use universal precautions to disinfect the irrigator tip for different patients.

As noted, most open-loop water irrigators have a switch to start the irrigation and to trigger a timer. The switch is either built into the irrigator tip or housed within a foot pedal. Some nystagmographs can also be triggered by a switch so that the irrigation, the timer, and the eye movement recordings can all start simultaneously. In some irrigators that are packaged as a part of computerized ENG/VNG systems, the warm or cool irrigation setting can be selected by the computer.

The standard temperatures for warm and cool water irrigations are 44°C and 30°C, respectively (Table 12–1). These temperatures represent 7°C above and below the normal body temperature of 37°C. The temperature variation at the irrigator tip should be less than ±0.5°C according to the American National Standards Institute (ANSI, 2009) and less than ±0.4°C according to the British Society of Audiology (BSA, 2010). In many irrigators, the irrigation temperature can be adjusted over a wide range (e.g., 25°C to 50°C). However, the standard temperatures are usually preset so that they can be selected quickly.

Traditionally, the standard flow rate and duration of irrigation for open-loop water systems have been set at 250 mL for 30 seconds (BSA, 2010). Most normative limits for the caloric test are derived using those values (Barber & Stockwell, 1980). However, there is no universal agreement on the flow rate and duration of caloric irrigations. Flow rates of 200 to 500 mL/min and durations of 30 to 40 s have been used in different studies and recommended by different organizations (American Academy of Neurology, 1996; ANSI, 2009; Henry, 1999). For example, ANSI (2009) recommends 200 mL/min of water delivered for 40 s. Because of the differences in the total amount of water delivered to the ear, the values recommended by different standards

Table 12–1. Irrigation Parameters Reported in the Literature and Recommended by Different Organizations

	Most Commonly Cited in the Literature			Recommended by ANSI (2009)			Recommended by BSA (2010)		
	Open-Loop Water	Air	Closed-Loop Water	Open-Loop Water	Air	Closed-Loop Water	Open-Loop Water	Air	Closed-Loop Water
Volume	250 mL	8 L	—	200 ± 20 mL/min	X	350 ± 35 mL/min	250 ± 10 mL	8 ± 0.4 L	X
Duration	30 s	60 s	45 s	40 ± 1 s	X	40 ± 1 s	30 s	60 s	X
Temperature (warm/cool)	44°C/ 30°C	50°C/ 24°C	46°C/ 28°C	44°C/ 30°C ± 0.5°C	X	44°C/ 27°C ± 0.4°C	44°C/ 30°C ± 0.4°C	50°C/ 24°C ± 0.4°C	X

are not expected to generate the same level of caloric stimulation. Therefore, regardless of which flow rate or duration is used, each laboratory either must develop its own normative values or use values derived from studies that use similar irrigation parameters.

The use of open-loop water irrigators requires a few precautions. First, irrigating an ear with water is contraindicated when the tympanic membrane is perforated. See the section on Specialized Caloric Tests for a detailed discussion of testing a perforated ear. Second, the electrical safety of the irrigator must be reviewed regularly to ensure that it is properly grounded and electrically isolated. Although all of the devices in a vestibular laboratory must meet stringent patient safety requirements, open-loop irrigators require special attention because of the direct contact of the patient with water. Third, the water in the reservoirs must be replaced frequently to prevent growth of algae and bacteria (Baguley, Whipp, & Farrington, 1991). This is a good precautionary measure even though there has not been a reported case of infection from water caloric irrigations. Finally, open-loop water irrigators must undergo regular maintenance at least once a year, to clean the mineral deposits. Also as with all irrigator types, the temperatures in the water caloric systems must be checked and calibrated annually. For the details of the calibration procedure see Jacobson and Newman (1993).

Air Irrigators

A typical air irrigator consists of an air pump to push the air through the system. The air pump can be either external or built into the irrigator unit. A flow controller measures and controls the amount of air that is delivered to the ear. A thermoelectric unit regulates the temperature of the air. Some irrigators can heat the air but do not cool it. Therefore, these irrigators cannot achieve cool temperatures that are below the ambient temperature. Other irrigators can cool as well as heat the air. Cool air is usually produced by forcing the air through a coil surrounded by a water-filled radiator. The air temperature is controlled by cooling the water. The air in most modern air caloric systems is delivered to the ear by an otoscopic head with a tube routed through the tip. A small thermistor located at the end of the air delivery tube measures the temperature just before it enters the ear canal and provides the feedback necessary for precise control of the temperature. This is the major difference between modern and older air caloric systems. Because the heat capacity of air is far less than that of water (Fleming, Proctor, Dix, & Metz, 1978), the temperature at the irrigator tip can be significantly different compared to the temperature at the heating or cooling site within the irrigator. Regulating the temperature at the irrigator tip ensures that the desired temperature is delivered to the ear canal.

Air irrigators also have a timer and a switch similar to those in the open-loop water systems. However, as the airflow is continuous, the switch starts only the timer and does not affect the flow of air.

The standard temperatures for warm and cool air irrigations are 50°C and 24°C, respectively (see Table 12–1). These temperatures represent 13°C above and below the normal body temperature. The maximum recommended temperature variation at the irrigator tip is ±0.4°C according to BSA (2010). As discussed later, there are no equivalent irrigation parameters for air calorics in ANSI. Irrigators that do not cool the air may not achieve the standard temperature for cool irrigation if the ambient temperature is not below 22°C. Therefore, they are not recommended for routine clinical testing at the standard temperatures.

In air irrigators, the actual temperature in the ear canal depends on the design of the delivery tip. The recommended temperatures of 50°C and 24°C are for irrigator tips where the air flows freely in and out of the ear canal. Some air irrigators seal the ear canal during the irrigation and cause the temperature at the tympanic membrane to be significantly different compared to the temperature at the irrigator tip. Using the standard temperatures, especially for warm irrigations, can pose a patient safety issue because the excess temperature can cause a burning sensation in the ear canal. Therefore, any facility that uses this type of irrigator must follow the manufacturer's temperature settings and establish its own normative values.

The standard flow rate and duration for air irrigators are 8 L/min and 60 s, respectively. Again, the standard temperatures, flow rate, and duration are usually preset, but many irrigators allow adjustments, if needed.

Caloric testing with air is technically more challenging than testing with water (Proctor, 1977). The examiner must visualize and direct the irrigator tip toward the tympanic membrane throughout the irrigation. The effectiveness of this task can be improved by otoscopic inspection of the ear canal before *each* irrigation. This will remind the examiner about the shape of the canal and assist with directing the irrigator tip.

Caloric testing with air in patients with small and tortuous ear canals can be difficult. Using a narrow (pediatric) tip in place of a standard irrigator tip often produces more robust caloric responses in these patients. It has been assumed that the use of narrower irrigator tip causes the ear canal to open further and the temperature gradient to be presented closer to the tympanic membrane. However, the use of a narrow tip can also increase the speed of airflow, which has been shown to increase caloric response intensities (Lightfoot & Milner, 2010). The increase in intensity should not affect the caloric asymmetry as long as all four irrigations are delivered using the same tip.

Air irrigators must also undergo regular maintenance and temperature calibration. The user should periodically check the water level in the cooling air irrigators and the air filter should be replaced in all air irrigators. However, temperature calibration in air irrigators is far more complicated and it should be performed by the manufacturer. Proper temperature calibration requires making measurements within a simulated ear canal. It is not clear if manufacturers take that level of precaution in their recommended maintenance procedures.

Closed-Loop Water Irrigators

A closed-loop water irrigator is essentially an open-loop water irrigator with a balloon-like elastic barrier fitted to the end of the irrigator tip. Instead of flowing directly into the ear canal, the water fills the balloon, which expands in the ear. The heat transfer occurs through the wall of the balloon without any direct contact between the water and the ear. The desired temperature at the tip is maintained by circulating the water between the water reservoir and the balloon. In the commercial version of the closed-loop irrigator, the balloon consists of a disposable silicone sheath.

Although the idea was not a new one (Ono & Kanzaki, 1976), the first commercially viable closed-loop irrigator was described by Brookler, Baker, and Grams (1979). The system has a timer and switches, which control the duration of the irrigation by inflating and deflating the balloon at precise intervals. Another feature of the commercial system is the ability to simultaneously irrigate both ears by having two separate hoses and delivery tips.

There is controversy about the standard irrigation parameters for the closed-loop systems. Brookler et al. (1979) used 46°C and 28°C for warm and cool irrigation temperatures for the duration of 45 s. These temperatures represent 9°C above and below the normal body temperature. Subsequently, the manufacturer's recommended parameters lowered the warm temperature to 44°C and the duration to 40 s, presumably to reduce patient discomfort. The recommended temperature for cool irrigation was further lowered to 27°C by ANSI (2009). There are no equivalent irrigation parameters for the closed-loop system in BSA standards. It is unclear whether the closed-loop water irrigation parameters recommended by the manufacturer or ANSI can generate caloric stimulation equivalent to that generated by open-loop water or air systems. Again, each laboratory must choose normative values that are developed based on using corresponding irrigation parameters.

The examiner should be aware there is a slight chance of the balloon bursting in the ear canal during the irrigation. The chances can be further reduced by using a new balloon for each patient. Apparently, the high cost of disposable balloons has led some laboratories to disinfect and reuse them. This is not recommended as it increases the possibility of the balloons bursting during the irrigation.

Like all caloric irrigators, closed-loop systems require regular maintenance and calibration. However, this is becoming increasingly more difficult because as noted, closed-loop irrigators are no longer manufactured at this time.

Comparison of Different Caloric Irrigation Methods

Several studies have compared the reliability of different types of caloric irrigators (Jacobson & Newman, 1993). The majority of these studies have concluded that all three irrigator types provide adequate caloric stimulation with comparable test-retest reliability (see Anderson, 1995, for a review). However, this has not been a unanimous conclusion. In particular, the results from early studies that compared air and open-loop irrigation methods were mixed. For example, studies by Tole (1979), Zangemeister and Bock (1980), and Greven, Oosterveld, Rademakers, and Voorhoeve (1979) found air irrigations to be less effective than water irrigations.

However, these studies were based on irrigation parameters that were significantly different from those listed in Table 12–1. Furthermore, as discussed before, air calorics are technically more challenging and require a longer learning period (Suter, Blanchard, & Cook-Manokey, 1977). Other studies that have directly compared the two methods have found no significant differences between air and open-loop water irrigations (e.g., Benitez, Bouchard, & Choe, 1978; Ford & Stockwell, 1978; Munro & Higson, 1996).

Although there is strong evidence that air irrigators provide acceptable caloric stimulation, the ANSI recommendation does not include them as a standard method for caloric testing (ANSI, 2009). It is stated that the decision to exclude air calorics in the ANSI standard is based on the lack of published data "to establish response variability equivalent to water calorics" (ANSI 2009). In addition to the previously cited articles, there are two recent publications that seem to contradict the above statement. Zapala, Olsholt, and Lundy (2008) in a large-scale retrospective study showed that the sensitivity and specificity of both air and water calorics were similar for differentiating between normal and abnormal patients. In addition, they showed that the differences between warm and cool irrigation responses were higher for water calorics and that the air calorics produced more uniform responses. Zapala et al. (2008) used slightly different temperatures for air calorics than those listed in Table 12–1 and they have advocated a similar procedure to calibrate caloric parameters as they did for the study.

Similarly, Marques Perrella de Barros and Caovilla (2012) showed that there were no significant differences in unilateral weakness and directional preponderance for air versus water calorics in 40 healthy individuals. They did report higher nystagmus intensities for individual irrigations for water calorics compared to those for air calorics. This may explain the anecdotal reports that patients generally experience more discomfort during water calorics.

The exclusion of air in the ANSI standard has been largely ignored by the clinical community. Today, the sale of air irrigators continues to outpace the sale of open-loop water irrigators by a large margin (personal communication with GN Otometrics and MicroMedical).

Similar discrepancies have been reported in studies that have examined the reliability of closed-loop irrigators. Initially, Brookler et al. (1979) tested 296 patients with both open-loop and closed-loop irrigation systems and adjusted the irrigation parameters of the closed-loop system until the responses were equivalent to those of the open-loop irrigators. The parameters that produced equivalent responses were reported to be 45 s of irrigation at 28°C for cool irrigations and 46°C for warm irrigations. In some of the subsequent studies however, caloric responses from the closed-loop irrigators were reported to either be weaker (Karlsen, Mikhail, Norris, & Hassanein, 1992) or have lower test-retest reliability compared to the responses from the open-loop irrigators (Henry, 1999; Henry & DiBartolomeo, 1993). It should be noted that the irrigation parameters in these studies were not the same as those proposed by Brookler et al. (1979). Currently, the BSA recommended procedure does not include the use of closed-loop irrigators either because they are no longer manufactured, or because there are conflicting reports about their test-retest reliability (BSA, 2010).

In a thorough review of the previous literature, Anderson (1995) concluded that all three irrigation methods produce acceptable caloric responses with similar test-retest reliability. He attributed the discrepancy among the different studies to variables that are difficult to control, such as the psychological state of the patient. More recent studies support his conclusions. As such, the choice of the irrigation method is a matter of personal preference with some consideration to the advantages and disadvantages of each method.

The main advantage of the open-loop system is that the irrigations are relatively simple and do not require a great deal of technical skill. The main disadvantage is the inconvenience. The returned water from the ear must be collected, the irrigator must be cleaned often, and in the older systems, the irrigator must be purged before irrigation. Also, some patients find the open-loop systems unpleasant because they produce strong caloric responses. Finally, the open-loop irrigators cannot be used in patients with tympanic membrane perforations. The main advantage of air and closed-loop systems is their convenience. There is no water to collect and they can be used in patients with tympanic membrane perforations.

The main disadvantage of the air irrigators is that they require more technical skill and a longer learning process. Some patients also find the irrigations to be too warm or too cold as the temperatures are more extreme compared to the open-loop irrigators. The main disadvantage of the closed-loop irrigators is the cost because the silicone sheaths must be replaced for each patient. Also, there is uncertainty as to what irrigation parameters should be used in closed-loop irrigators to generate caloric stimulation equal to that of the air and open-loop systems.

In summary, all three irrigation methods provide acceptable caloric stimulation. However, the examiner must acquire the necessary skill to perform appropriate irrigations using whichever method he or she chooses. Furthermore, it should be noted that design differences for different irrigator models, especially for air irrigators, can influence the strength of the caloric stimulation. As a result, each clinic must either establish its own normative values or calibrate the caloric stimuli using methods similar to those described by Zapala et al. (2008).

PERFORMING THE CALORIC TEST

The most common form of caloric testing is the bithermal caloric test, which was first described by Fitzgerald and Hallpike (1942). In this test, each ear is irrigated twice—once with warm temperature and once with cool temperature. This generates both excitatory and inhibitory responses from both ears. The validity of the caloric test is based on the assumption that both ears receive adequate and approximately equal stimulation. Some of the factors that affect the strength of caloric stimulation can be controlled by the examiner, such as the temperature and the duration of irrigations. It is the responsibility of the examiner to ensure that the controllable test parameters remain constant from one irrigation to another. Other factors are not controllable, such as the ear anatomy. The examiner must make a note of those uncontrolled factors that may affect the validity of the caloric test.

In this section, the proper method for administering the standard bithermal caloric test is described in detail. Practical considerations for performing a valid test are explored.

Preliminary Procedures

Many of the preliminary procedures for the caloric test are the same as those necessary for all of the subtests in ENG. For example, the patients must be advised about stopping certain medications at least 48 hr before the test and a note must be made of medications that cannot be stopped.[1] Authorization for testing should be reconfirmed with the referring physician when the patient has a history of seizures, cardiovascular disease, or severe neck or back problems. The patients' eye movements must be inspected before the test and the recording technique should be modified accordingly if disconjugate eye movements are observed.

A few preliminary procedures are unique to the caloric test. The ears should be inspected carefully before the test. If there is cerumen blocking the ear canal, it should be removed before the irrigations. Even when the cerumen is not completely blocking the tympanic membrane, the examiner may want to remove it because the irrigation medium can push the cerumen deeper into the ear canal and impede the heat transfer. When removing the cerumen, it is best to *spoon* it out instead of washing the ear canal with water. This is especially important for the users of air caloric systems because the remaining moisture in the ear canal may produce a cooling effect during warm irrigations and result in the nystagmus initially beating in the opposite direction of what is expected for warm irrigations.

During the ear inspection, the examiner must make a note of any anatomic anomalies, such as those caused by surgery or trauma. Even when the ears look normal, anatomic changes may affect the heat transfer and interfere with caloric testing. Therefore, differences in the caloric responses from different ears should be interpreted cautiously when there is a history of ear surgery. Similarly, the ear inspection should note any evidence of tympanic membrane perforation, middle ear fluid, or otitis externa.

Before the test, the examiner should explain the procedure to the patient in an honest but nonthreat-ening manner. Developing good rapport is important because many patients are apprehensive about the caloric test. It is best to reassure the patient that the sensation of motion during caloric irrigations is expected and will not last long. The patient should then be placed in the supine position with the head raised up about 30 degrees. The irrigation system should be switched on and prepared for testing according to the guidelines of the previous section. To reduce changes in the corneoretinal potential (CRP) in ENG and light leaks in VNG, the entire test should be conducted in a dimly lit room. At this point, the examiner can proceed with administering the caloric test.

Standard Bithermal Caloric Test Procedure

The eye movements must be calibrated at the beginning of the caloric test (see the next section about calibrations between irrigations). Next, visual fixation should be eliminated. In ENG, this can be accomplished by recording the eye movements with eyes closed. In VNG, the fixation is eliminated by covering the goggles and recording the eye movements in complete darkness with eyes open. At this time, the examiner should start the eye movement recording system and begin alerting the patient. The presence of any preexisting nystagmus should be noted. The irrigation should begin promptly and should last anywhere from 30 to 60 s depending on the irrigation system (see Table 12–1). Once the irrigation ends, the examiner should continue alerting the patient by asking a series of questions at a steady pace. Most patients do not require vigorous alerting but some patients are difficult to keep alert. In those patients, the examiner must be more vigilant and change the type and pace of questions to maintain patient alertness. The caloric response continues to get stronger and usually reaches its peak around 30 s after the end of the irrigation (about 60–90 s from the onset of the irrigation). About 10 to 15 s after the response reaches its peak and begins to decline, the

---

[1]Many laboratories, as well as both ANSI and British standards, require the patient to stop medications that are not life-supporting for at least 48 hr before the test. However, there is no general agreement about the necessity and effectiveness of this approach, especially for long-term users of certain medications such as antidepressants. If the results are ambiguous for a patient who is tested while on medications, the examiner should consider repeating the test at a later date after the patient stops taking them.

examiner should ask the patient to fixate on a stationary target. In ENG, this can be done by simply asking the patient to open his or her eyes and to look straight ahead at a target. Some VNG systems have a built-in light within the goggles that can be turned on for fixation. Otherwise, the goggle cover should be removed so that the patient can fixate on a target. The examiner must make sure that the patient is actually fixating. Some patients, who are experiencing dizziness during the irrigation, are reluctant to fixate. The fixation period is usually 10 to 15 s, after which the fixation should be eliminated again. The tracings should be marked to identify the beginning and the end of fixation. Eye movement recordings should continue until the caloric response subsides (usually 2 to 3 min from the onset of irrigation). After a waiting period, the remaining irrigations should be performed in the same manner.

Practical Considerations in Performing the Caloric Test

Although the above procedure is straightforward, there are many controversies and practical considerations that must be addressed.

Recalibration Before Each Irrigation

The ANSI (2009) standard as well as an earlier report by the Committee on Hearing, Bioacoustics, and Biomechanics (CHABA, 1992) recommend recalibration of eye movements before each irrigation. However, the most recent BSA recommendation has reversed the earlier standard and no longer requires it (BSA, 2010). The concept of recalibration before each irrigation was a reasonable one for the users of older noncomputerized ENG equipment. However, for more modern computerized ENG and VNG systems, recalibration before each irrigation is an outdated recommendation that should be reconsidered. In ENG, eye movements are estimated indirectly by measuring the CRP. Because the CRP changes over time, the calibration process must be repeated several times during ENG (Proctor, Hansen, & Rentea, 1980). In VNG, eye movements are estimated directly by measuring the movements of the pupils. Therefore, recalibrations are unnecessary as long as the orientation of the cameras does not

change with respect to the patient's eyes. Even routine removal and replacement of the goggles have been shown to have minimal effect on the calibration (Andrew & Meredith, 2009).

In noncomputerized ENGs, the standard calibration is performed initially and subsequent recalibrations usually involve *verifying* the previous calibration and making minor adjustments when necessary. In computerized ENGs and VNGs, recalibration means discarding the previous calibration and performing an entirely new calibration. Norman and Brown (1999) have demonstrated that in computerized ENGs, there is an average difference of about 17% between two calibrations without any change in the CRP. Such a difference means that recalibration between irrigations can significantly increase the variability of the caloric test. To avoid this problem in computerized ENG and VNG, either one should avoid recalibration between irrigations or should use the same procedure used in noncomputerized ENGs. That is, verify the existing calibration and make changes only when necessary. Most of the commercially available computerized ENG and VNG systems do not currently have an explicit option for verifying the previous calibration. Until such an option becomes available, one can use workaround procedures to overcome this limitation. For example, the examiner can use a mock saccade or tracking test to verify the calibration. Recalibration is not warranted when the amplitudes of target and eye movements are equal.

Testing with Eyes Open in Total Darkness

Both the ANSI and British standards recommend performing the caloric test with eyes open in total darkness (ANSI, 2009; BSA, 2010). This recommendation is based primarily on a study by Baloh, Solingen, Sills, and Honrubia (1977) in which caloric responses were measured via ENG under different fixation conditions. They reported better morphology for the caloric nystagmus and lower variability for the response parameters when the test was conducted with eyes open in total darkness as compared to when the test was conducted with eyes closed. This finding may be related to the upward deviation of the eyes, known as the Bell's phenomenon, that occurs with eye closure (Jacobson & Newman, 1993).

The above recommendation is aimed at the ENG users because in VNG, the test is always conducted with eyes open in total darkness under the goggles. However, the original authors themselves, as well as other authors, have acknowledged the difficulty of maintaining a completely dark environment in a clinical ENG laboratory (Baloh et al., 1977; BSA, 2010). Even a small light leak may enable the patient to fixate, thus negating any benefits derived from testing without eye closure. In addition, a number of studies have demonstrated adequacy of recording caloric responses with ENG where the fixation was eliminated by eye closure (Barber & Stockwell, 1980; Jacobson & Newman, 1993; Karlsen, Goetzinger, & Hassanein, 1980). Therefore, if the ENG laboratory is capable of providing a completely dark environment, the caloric test can be conducted with eyes open in total darkness. Otherwise, eye closure is an acceptable and much simpler method for eliminating fixation.

Alerting Tasks

In any vestibular test that is performed in the absence of fixation, including the caloric test, it is necessary to keep the patient alert during the test (Barber & Stockwell, 1980; Jacobson & Newman, 1993). The purpose of alerting tasks is to maintain a steady stimulation of the higher cortical level brain activity that is most likely needed to generate the fast phases of nystagmus (Barin, 2009). As a result, the requirement for alerting tasks is independent of the eye movement measurement method.

A number of studies have examined the effect of different alerting tasks on the caloric response parameters (e.g., Davis & Mann, 1987; Formby et al., 1992). The most effective alerting tasks are those requiring interaction of the patient with the examiner in which the patient is required to recall items from the memory, such as names of states, cities, and so forth. The alerting tasks should be moderately challenging and on topics that are of interest to the patient. It is the responsibility of the examiner to monitor the caloric responses and modify the pace and the difficulty of the alerting task if suddenly the nystagmus disappears or becomes intermittent. It is best to have an accessible list of potential questions with different difficulty levels to refer to, when needed.

Order of Irrigations

The ANSI and British standards recommend performing the irrigations in the bithermal caloric test in a specific order (ANSI, 2009; BSA, 2010). Warm irrigations are to be performed first followed by cool irrigations in both standards. The ANSI standard requires the right ear to be irrigated first for both warm and cool temperatures. The BSA standard allows either the right or left ear to be irrigated first as long as the same order is used for both temperatures.

The main reason for the recommended sequence is in the ANSI standard is the systematic decline in the intensity of caloric responses from the first to the last irrigation. Furman and Jacob (1993) first described this phenomenon and attributed it to central adaptation mechanisms. To reduce this bias, they suggested modifying the formulas used for quantifying the caloric responses or changing the order of irrigations. However, it is now clear that the underlying premise of the order effect in bithermal caloric testing may have been inaccurate. Lightfoot (2004) demonstrated that the order effect was specific to ENG and was not present in VNG. That is, the order effect is unrelated to the adaptation mechanisms and it reflects the systematic change in the CRP over time. As a result, careful verification of the calibration (but not necessarily recalibration) before each irrigation can minimize or eliminate the order effect in both ENG and VNG regardless of in what order the irrigations are performed.

The main advantage of performing warm irrigations first is that under certain conditions, the examiner can interpret the caloric results without performing the cool irrigations (BSA, 2010). See the discussion on monothermal caloric testing below. However, there may be a disadvantage to starting with warm irrigations. Noaksson, Schulin, Kovacsovics, and Ledin (1998) have shown that starting with warm irrigations results in significantly stronger responses for warm irrigations. On the other hand, starting with cool irrigations can reduce the typical difference between warm and cool responses.

Based on the above discussion, it is clear that the order of irrigations recommended by ANSI (2009) and BSA (2010) is appropriate, but it is not the only acceptable sequence. For example, there is no evidence that starting the irrigations with cool temperature will have a significant effect on the outcome of the caloric test. In fact, when the bithermal caloric testing is planned from the outset, performing cool irrigations first may have the advantage of reducing the difference between the intensity of responses for warm and cool temperatures (Noaksson et al., 1998). Therefore, the examiner is free to start with either warm or cool irrigations as long as the ears are irrigated in the same order for each temperature.

Waiting Period Between Irrigations

The ANSI standard recommends waiting 5 min from the end of the recording for one irrigation to the beginning of the next irrigation (ANSI, 2009). The purpose of the wait period is to reduce residual effects of the previous irrigation. However, the ANSI standard does not specify what constitutes the end of recording after each irrigation. That is, it is not clear whether the recording should be stopped after a fixed period of time from the onset of the irrigation or should continue until the caloric nystagmus dissipates completely.

In most patients, the caloric-induced nystagmus dissipates within 3 min after the onset of the irrigation. However, there is strong evidence that the temperature gradient across the labyrinth persists much longer and depending on the strength of the caloric response, may require over 10 min to return to its preirrigation state (Barnes, 1995). The effect of this residual temperature gradient varies from one patient to another and from one irrigation to another. Therefore, maintaining a fixed time interval between successive irrigations may actually increase the variability of the caloric test. The most recent version of the BSA standard has tried to address this issue by recommending a minimum of 7-min interval between the start of two consecutive irrigations with consideration for extending the interval for patients who continue to exhibit caloric-induced nystagmus after the wait period (BSA, 2010).

A study by Beattie and Koester (1992) provides a direct method for determining the appropriate waiting period between irrigations. They measured the peak slow-phase velocity (SPV) of the caloric nystagmus for two successive irrigations where the end of one irrigation was separated from the beginning of the next irrigation by 1, 2, 3, 5, or 15 min. They did not find statistically significant differences for the peak SPVs when the time interval was 3, 5, or 15 min. These results suggest that as long as the nystagmus from one irrigation has subsided, the residual temperature gradient will not have a significant effect on the caloric responses of the following irrigation. In fact, Beattie and Koester (1992) recommend starting the irrigation immediately after the cessation of nystagmus from the previous irrigation. This will reduce the required time for caloric testing but it may also lead to patient discomfort. Therefore, a better method is to wait a fixed period of time (3 to 5 min) after the caloric nystagmus has returned to its baseline before starting the next irrigation. The baseline represents either the return to the level of spontaneous nystagmus SPV or complete disappearance of nystagmus when there is no spontaneous nystagmus.

The examiner can make use the waiting period productively by analyzing the caloric responses of the preceding irrigation. That way, at the end of the caloric test, the examiner can quickly determine whether the test is valid or if any irrigation requires repeating.

Monothermal Caloric Testing

A number of studies have considered the use of monothermal caloric tests either as a replacement or as a screening test for bithermal caloric testing (for a review, see Enticott, Dowell, & O'Leary, 2003; Jacobson, Calder, Shepherd, Rupp, & Newman, 1995; Murnane, Akin, Lynn, & Cyr, 2009). Torok's monothermal caloric test, which is intended as an adjunct test to the bithermal caloric test, is discussed later in this chapter. The advantages of monothermal caloric testing include shorter test time and possibly reduced patient discomfort. However, previous studies that have compared monothermal and bithermal caloric tests have resulted in contradictory findings. The inconsistencies are most likely due to differences in the irrigation parameters and test procedures.

Some studies have entirely dismissed the use of monothermal caloric testing in clinical settings due to its presumed low sensitivity and specificity (e.g., Keith, Pensak, & Katbamna, 1991; Shupak, Kaminer,

Gilbey, & Tal, 2010). However, several other studies have demonstrated that under certain conditions, monothermal caloric testing can be used as a screening test for the bithermal caloric test (e.g., Bush et al., 2013; Lightfoot et al., 2009; Murnane et al., 2009). Yet significant disagreements remain about the other aspects of the monothermal caloric test.

A few studies recommend using the cool temperature for monothermal testing. However, the majority of the studies have demonstrated that warm monothermal calorics offer a better sensitivity and specificity over cool monothermal calorics. Also, different studies have adopted different rules for precluding the use of monothermal caloric test in some patients. For example, Barber, Wright, and Demanuele (1971) recommend against using monothermal caloric tests when the nystagmus intensity from each ear is less than 11 deg/s. Jacobson and Means (1985) and Jacobson et al. (1995) have added abnormalities in oculomotor tests or presence of any type of nystagmus in the static or dynamic position tests as criteria for not using the monothermal caloric test.

Some studies have used the same normative values for both monothermal and bithermal testing (e.g., Enticott et al., 2003; Keith, et al, 1991). These studies have produced relatively low false-negative rates for monothermal testing (Enticott et al., 2003). That is, there are very few instances where the monothermal test indicates a normal finding and the bithermal test does not. On the other hand, false-positive rates for the monothermal test can be very high if the same normative values are used for both tests (Enticott et al., 2003). That is, there are many instances where the monothermal test indicates an abnormal finding but the bithermal test does not. To address this shortcoming, other studies have established distinct normative values for the monothermal test (e.g., Jacobson & Means, 1985; Jacobson et al., 1995, Murnane et al., 2009). Using this approach, Jacobson et al. (1995) have demonstrated high sensitivity and specificity for predicting bithermal test abnormalities from monothermal test results, especially when additional restrictions were imposed on the caloric response parameters.

Although methodological differences make it difficult to directly compare the results from different studies, it is possible to develop a rational approach to monothermal caloric testing if the outcomes of these studies are considered collectively. The most

effective application of monothermal caloric test seems to be in predicting when the completion of bithermal caloric test is likely to result in a normal finding. That way, the test can be terminated after the first two irrigations if the examiner can predict with a high probability a normal outcome for the bithermal caloric test.

The BSA (2010) has adopted a standard for predicting the normality of the bithermal caloric test based on the results of the first two irrigations. The standard, which is based on a study by Lightfoot et al. (2009), recommends terminating the caloric test after the first two warm irrigations if the asymmetry between the right and left responses is less than 15%. Furthermore, the patient should not have spontaneous nystagmus greater than 4 deg/s, and the responses should be greater than 8 deg/s for both irrigations (to exclude patients with bilateral caloric weakness). For patients who meet the above criteria, the outcome of normal bithermal caloric testing can be predicted accurately in 95% of them, whereas 29% of the patients who do not meet the criteria end up with normal results after completing the bithermal caloric test (Lightfoot et al., 2009).

Murnane et al. (2009), using a larger sample size and a robust statistical approach, have developed criteria for monothermal caloric testing that are similar to the BSA (2010) standard. They recommend an upper limit of 10% for the asymmetry between the right and left responses, which is a stricter criterion than the BSA standard. Therefore, the outcome of normal bithermal caloric testing can be predicted in a higher percentage of the patients but at the same time, a higher percentage of patients who undergo all four irrigations end up with normal bithermal caloric results.

In summary, warm monothermal caloric testing can be a useful screening test as long as certain exclusionary rules are applied and appropriate normal limits are used. The recommended standard by BSA (2010) is appropriate for most laboratories. However, alternative criteria such as those proposed by Jacobson et al. (1995) or Murnane et al. (2009) are also acceptable for monothermal caloric testing. As described by BSA (2010), there are compromises associated with the use of monothermal calorics of which the examiner should be aware. Therefore, it is best to reserve the monothermal test for patients who are unable to complete the bithermal test.

Number of Fixation Suppression Tests

Only two tests of fixation suppression, one for each direction of nystagmus, are needed (Alpert, 1974). As a result, most examiners perform the fixation suppression test only during two caloric irrigations of the same temperature (usually warm irrigations). However, to compare the suppression results for different nystagmus direction, nystagmus intensities just before fixation should be approximately equal. This will not be possible when the fixation suppression test is performed only for the same-temperature irrigations and when there is a significant difference between the responses from the two ears. This problem can be avoided by following the recommended procedure in the previous section and testing the fixation suppression in all four irrigations. The examiner can then choose two irrigations where the nystagmus intensities just before fixation are close for different nystagmus directions.

Minimum Age of Patients in Caloric Testing

Caloric testing requires considerable cooperation even from adult patients. Very young children may not tolerate having an irrigator tip in their ears or being kept in a dark room for an extended period of time (Cyr, 1980). In the literature, the youngest children who have undergone caloric testing are reported to be 4 or 5 years old (Melagrana, D'Agostino, Pasquale, & Taborelli, 1996; Melagrana, D'Agostino, Tarantino, Taborelli, & Calevo, 2002). Generally, caloric testing is not recommended in children under the age of 6 and in developmentally delayed adults with a mental equivalent age of 6 or under. The age limit can be modified in rare cases where the child is very cooperative.

ANALYSIS OF CALORIC RESPONSES

A number of nystagmus parameters, including duration, frequency, or amplitude, have been used in the past to quantify caloric responses (Jacobson & Newman, 1993). Currently, there is general agreement that the nystagmus slow-phase velocity (SPV) is the most practical measure of its intensity (ANSI, 2009; BSA, 2010). In computerized ENG and VNG systems, the task of calculating SPV is, for the most part, automated. However, in noncomputerized ENG systems, calculations have to be performed manually.

To measure the nystagmus SPV, the examiner must first know the scales for the time and eye movement axes. The scale for the time axis is determined by the settings on the equipment, and the scale for the eye movement axis is determined by the calibration. For the example in Figure 12–2, 10 mm on the time axis represents 1 s and 10 mm on the eye movement

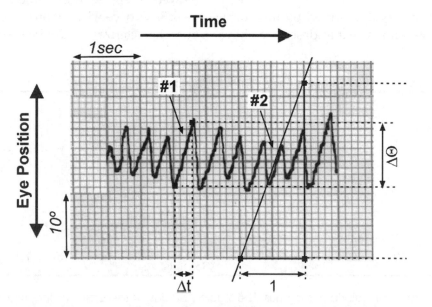

Figure 12–2. Calculating nystagmus slow-phase velocity (SPV).

axis represents 10 degrees. Nystagmus SPV is calculated by determining the distance that the eyes travel during the slow phase and dividing that by the amount of time it takes for the eyes to travel that distance (see Figure 12–2). For example, for the nystagmus beat identified as #1:

$$SPV = \Delta\Theta/\Delta t = 10 \text{ degrees}/0.3 \text{ s } 33 \approx \text{deg/s}$$

An easier, and perhaps more accurate method, is to draw a best-fitting line through the slow phase of nystagmus and measure the slope of this line. The time base can be set to any value that simplifies the calculations. It is usually set to 1 s. For the nystagmus beat identified as #2:

$$SPV = \Delta\Theta'/1 = 27 \text{ degrees}/1 \text{ s} = 27 \text{ degrees/s}$$

In noncomputerized ENG, the SPV is always expressed as a positive (unsigned) number except for caloric irrigations where the nystagmus is in the opposite direction of what is expected. In computerized ENG and VNG, the SPV is expressed as a signed number, with positive numbers representing rightward slow phases and negative numbers representing leftward slow phases. The equations in this chapter are derived based on the assumption that the SPVs will be represented by signed numbers.

SPV Profile of Caloric Responses

Caloric responses can be quantified by measuring the SPV of each nystagmus beat as described above.

Although the strength and direction of caloric nystagmus can vary, the profile of its SPV remains essentially the same from one irrigation to another (Figure 12–3). Caloric responses do not start immediately at the onset of the irrigation. It takes about 15 to 20 s from the onset of the irrigation before nystagmus appears. The nystagmus intensity rises to its peak approximately 60 to 90 s after the onset of the irrigation and begins to decline thereafter. The caloric nystagmus dissipates altogether after 2 to 3 min.

In computerized ENG and VNG systems, the SPV profiles for all four irrigations are usually displayed side by side to simplify the task of comparing the responses (Figure 12–4A). In this type of display, the combination of SPV profiles for warm and cool irrigations of each ear is called a *caloric pod* because of its distinct shape.

An alternative method for displaying the caloric responses is the *butterfly chart*. In its original form, nystagmus frequencies were used to quantify caloric responses (Claussen & von Schlachta, 1972), but a more recent variation of the butterfly chart uses peak SPVs (Figure 12–4B). A butterfly chart consists of a rectangular grid with the vertical axis on one side representing responses of the right ear and the vertical axis on the opposite side representing responses of the left ear. The horizontal axis is scaled to represent the difference between the responses of the right and left ears. The peak SPVs for warm irrigations of the right and left ears are marked on the appropriate axes and a line is drawn between them. A similar line is drawn between the peak SPVs of cool irrigations. The intersection of these lines characterizes the difference between the two ears.

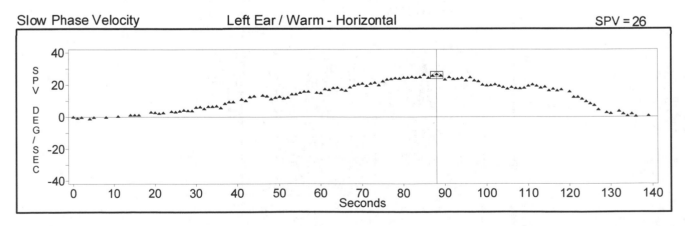

Figure 12–3. SPV profile of caloric nystagmus. The tracing begins at the onset of the irrigation. The peak of the caloric response is identified by a box.

Caloric - Both Eyes

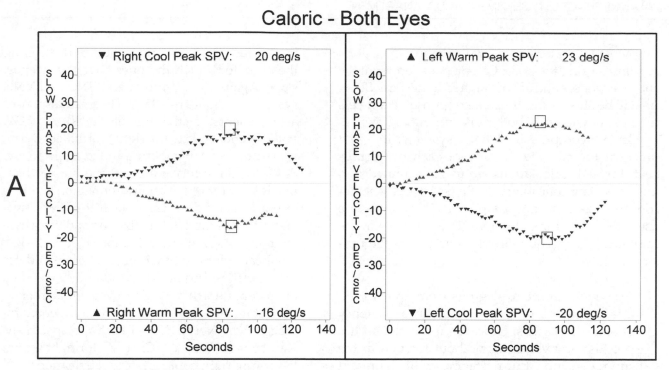

Caloric Weakness: 9% in the right ear
Directional Preponderance: 9% to the left

Caloric - Both Eyes

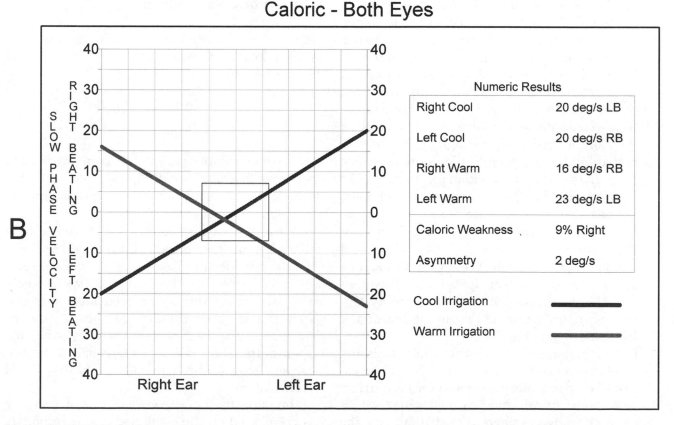

Figure 12-4. Display of the caloric test results: **A.** Pods. The peak caloric response for each irrigation is identified by a box. **B.** Butterfly chart. The horizontal axis represents caloric weakness in percent. The vertical axes represent the peak caloric responses and also asymmetry in degrees per second. The center box represents the normal limits for caloric weakness and asymmetry.

Most laboratories prefer displaying the caloric responses using the pods. Caloric pods represent the entire responses and are not limited to the peak SPVs. As will be shown shortly, some response parameters require knowledge of both peak and initial SPVs.

In noncomputerized ENG systems, it is not practical to calculate the SPV of each nystagmus beat. Instead, calculations are usually limited to a few important time intervals. Regardless of whether computerized or noncomputerized systems are used, there are three different time intervals in the caloric test that require careful analysis of the nystagmus SPV:

1. As noted, caloric nystagmus from an ear with intact tympanic membrane usually has a latency of about 15 to 20 s. However, if the patient has preexisting nystagmus without fixation in the supine position, this nystagmus will be present during the first 10 to 15 s after the onset of irrigation (Figure 12–5A). In that case, the baseline of the caloric response will shift by the SPV of the preexisting nystagmus and will no longer be zero. In addition, the response will return to this baseline once the caloric nystagmus subsides. When present, the intensity of the preexisting nystagmus should be calculated by averaging the SPV of three to five representative beats. In the computerized systems, the baseline shift (SPV of the preexisting nystagmus) can be estimated by drawing a best-fitting horizontal line through the SPV points within the first 10 to 15 s after the onset of the response. In this chapter, the baseline shifts are represented by the symbols *BaseRW*, *BaseLW*, *BaseRC*, and *BaseLC* for right warm, left warm, right cool, and left cool irrigations, respectively. These values should be approximately the same for all four irrigations and should also match the SPV of the nystagmus without fixation in the supine position of the static position testing.

2. Caloric responses usually reach their maximum level around 60 to 90 s after the onset of irrigation. The peak caloric response for each irrigation should be calculated by averaging the SPV of three to five nystagmus beats that have the highest velocities (Figure 12–5B). In noncomputerized ENG, these beats can be identified by drawing a line for each nystagmus beat (or at

least a few representative ones) and selecting the beats for which the lines have the steepest slope. Again, the computerized ENG and VNG systems automate this task. The peak responses are represented by the symbols *PeakRW*, *PeakLW*, *PeakRC*, and *PeakLC* for right warm, left warm, right cool, and left cool irrigations, respectively.

3. A 10- to 15-s interval around the time of fixation is used for the fixation suppression test. The examiner should average the SPV of three nystagmus beats right before fixation and three nystagmus beats right after fixation (Figure 12–5C). The beats that occur within 1 s before and 1 s after fixation, should be avoided because they often contain artifacts. The nystagmus intensities before and after fixation are represented by the symbols *NoFixXX* and *FixXX*, respectively. *XX* denotes *RW*, *LW*, *RC*, or *LC*, for right warm, left warm, right cool, or left cool irrigations.

Total Caloric Responses

The first step in analyzing the caloric responses is to calculate total responses from the right (*TotRE*) and the left ear (*TotLE*):

$$TotRE = PeakRC - PeakRW$$
$$TotLE = PeakLW - PeakRC$$

The total response from each ear represents the opening of the caloric pod (Figure 12–6). Note that the peak SPVs are signed numbers and the formulas are algebraic operations.

When the total responses from both the right and the left ears are very small, the caloric test indicates the presence of bilateral caloric weakness. As seen in the next few sections, when a bilateral weakness exists, the equations for the remaining response parameters do not produce valid results because the denominator approaches zero. Therefore, when the responses from both ears are very small, the examiner *must* stop and not proceed with the rest of the calculations.

Traditionally, the criterion for bilateral weakness has been based on the combined caloric responses from both ears. For example, Barber and Stockwell (1980) use *TotRE* + *TotLE* < 30 deg/s and Jacobson and Newman (1993) use *TotRE* + *TotLE* < 22 deg/s.

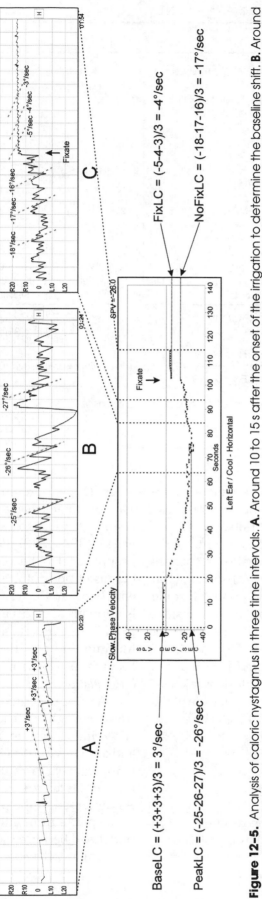

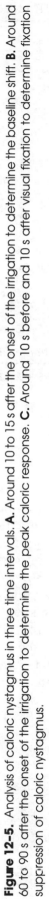

BaseLC = (+3+3+3)/3 = 3°/sec

PeakLC = (-25-26-27)/3 = -26°/sec

FixLC = (-5-4-3)/3 = -4°/sec

NoFixLC = (-18-17-16)/3 = -17°/sec

Figure 12–5. Analysis of caloric nystagmus in three time intervals. **A.** Around 10 to 15 s after the onset of the irrigation to determine the baseline shift. **B.** Around 60 to 90 s after the onset of the irrigation to determine the peak caloric response. **C.** Around 10 s before and 10 s after visual fixation to determine fixation suppression of caloric nystagmus.

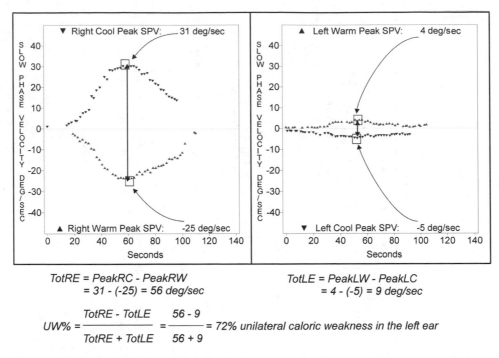

$$TotRE = PeakRC - PeakRW$$
$$= 31 - (-25) = 56 \ deg/sec$$

$$TotLE = PeakLW - PeakLC$$
$$= 4 - (-5) = 9 \ deg/sec$$

$$UW\% = \frac{TotRE - TotLE}{TotRE + TotLE} = \frac{56 - 9}{56 + 9} = 72\% \ unilateral \ caloric \ weakness \ in \ the \ left \ ear$$

Figure 12–6. Calculation of total caloric responses from each ear and unilateral caloric weakness.

Under that criterion, some cases where there is adequate response from one ear and minimal response from the other ear will be misidentified as bilateral weakness. Another criterion, proposed by the British standard, requires all four irrigation responses to be very small (less than 8 deg/s) for bilateral weakness (BSA, 2010). Under that criterion, some cases where there is a strong spontaneous nystagmus but no caloric responses from either ear will not be identified as bilateral weakness. To avoid these issues, one can use the criteria of $TotRE < 12$ deg/s and $TotLE < 12$ deg/s for bilateral caloric weakness. The threshold value of 12 deg/s is a composite of the thresholds used by Barber and Stockwell (1980) and Jacobson and Newman (1993).

Unilateral Caloric Weakness

The difference between the caloric responses from the right and left ears is quantified by

$$UW\% = (TotRE - TotLE / TotRE + TotLE) \times 100$$

where $UW\%$ represents *unilateral weakness in percent*. This parameter has also been called *percent reduced vestibular response* (ANSI, 2009) and *percent canal paresis* (BSA, 2010). Because unilateral weakness is proportional to the intensity of caloric responses and because caloric stimuli are uncalibrated, the difference between the responses of the right and left ears is normalized by dividing it by the sum of responses from both ears. This equation is equivalent to the formula that was first proposed by Jongkees and Philipszoon (1964) and is now referred to as the *Jongkees equation*.

A value of zero for $UW\%$ indicates the responses from the right and left ears are equal. A positive $UW\%$ indicates a unilateral weakness in the left ear, and a negative $UW\%$ indicates a unilateral weakness in the right ear. A value of +100% or −100% for $UW\%$ indicates total lack of caloric response from one ear. As discussed in the previous section, when there is no response from either ear, the equation becomes undefined because the denominator is zero.

Unilateral weakness is commonly expressed relative to the weaker ear, such as, "$UW\%$ unilateral weakness in the *weaker* ear." When there is minimal response from one ear and UW% is approaching either +100% or −100%, instead of using the percentage, it is best to express the lack of response as "no response to the standard caloric stimulus from the *nonresponsive* ear."

It is important to understand what UW% tells us about vestibular function. One may assume that UW% represents the loss of horizontal VOR function in the weaker ear relative to the other ear. However, as Wexler (1994) has pointed out, this assumption is incorrect because of the nonlinearity of Jongkees equation. That is, a change in the horizontal VOR function does not produce a proportional change in UW%. For example, as shown in Figure 12–7, a 50% loss of hair cells in the lateral canal or their afferent nerve fibers results in only 33% unilateral weakness using Jongkees equation. Wexler (1994) proposed an alternative formula to characterize the difference between the caloric responses of the right and left sides:

$$LP\% = \left[1 - \frac{\text{Total Caloric Response of the Weaker Ear}}{\text{Total Caloric Response of the Stronger Ear}} \right] \times 100$$

Linear paresis (LP%) is a direct one-to-one representation of the relative loss of horizontal vestibular function between the ears. Despite its advantages, most laboratories have not adopted this approach.

Directional Preponderance

In the standard bithermal caloric test, two irrigations are expected to generate right-beating nystagmus (right warm and left cool), and two irrigations are expected to generate left-beating nystagmus (right cool and left warm). In a normal individual, caloric responses in one direction are approximately equal to those in the other direction. However, some patients have a directional preponderance where the responses in one direction are stronger than the

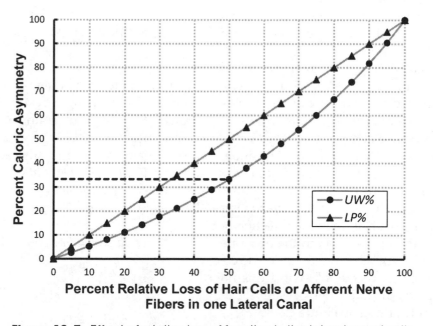

Figure 12–7. Effect of relative loss of function in the lateral canal or its afferent nerve fibers on the resulting caloric asymmetry. Circles represent caloric asymmetry calculated using the Jongkee's formula (*UW%*) and triangles represent caloric asymmetry calculated using Wexler's linear paresis formula (*LP%*). Based on Wexler, D. B. (1994). Nonlinearity of the Jongkees difference equation for vestibular hypofunction. *Otolaryngology-Head and Neck Surgery, 111*(4), 485–487.

responses in the other direction (Fitzgerald & Hall-pike, 1942).

The difference between right-beating and left-beating caloric responses is commonly quantified by

$$DP\% = (TotRB - TotLB / TotRB + TotLB) \times 100$$

where $DP\%$ represents directional preponderance in percent. $TotRB$ represents total responses from the irrigations that are expected to generate right-beating nystagmus, and $TotLB$ represents total responses from the irrigations that are expected to generate left-beating nystagmus:

$$TotRB = -PeakRW - PeakLC$$

$$TotLB = PeakRC + PeakLW$$

A value of zero for $DP\%$ indicates right-beating and left-beating responses are equal. A positive $DP\%$ indicates right-beating responses are stronger than left-beating responses, and a negative $DP\%$ indicates left-beating responses are stronger than right-beating responses. Directional preponderance is commonly expressed relative to the stronger nystagmus direction, such as, "$DP\%$ directional preponderance to the *stronger nystagmus direction*."

There are several issues with the concept of directional preponderance that limit its usefulness. For example, it is now clear that there are two types of directional preponderance. The most common type is due to the presence of preexisting nystagmus without fixation in the standard caloric test position. For this type, caloric responses are approximately equal in both directions but the baseline is shifted by an amount equal to the SPV of the preexisting nystagmus. Therefore, peak SPVs in the direction of the shift are higher than peak SPVs in the opposite direction (Figure 12–8A). A second type of directional preponderance can occur when there is no preexisting nystagmus but the caloric responses in one direction are truly stronger (Figure 12–8B). This type of directional preponderance, which is called *gain asymmetry*, was first identified by Halmagyi, Cremer, Anderson, Murofushi, and Curthoys (2000). Gain asymmetry is extremely rare and was reported in just 1% of the patients. On the other hand, directional preponderance due to baseline shift is quite common.

The above equation does not differentiate between two types of directional preponderance. The criterion for interpreting nystagmus in the position test is based on its intensity in different head positions. Therefore, when directional preponderance is due to preexisting nystagmus, it does not seem appropriate to normalize the baseline shift as it is done in the equation for $DP\%$ (Stockwell, 1987). The consequence of normalizing the baseline shift is illustrated in Figure 12–9. The same level of baseline shift can generate significantly different values for directional preponderance depending on the strength of the overall caloric responses. On the other hand, gain asymmetry is proportional to the strength of caloric responses. Therefore, in case of gain asymmetry, normalizing the difference between right-beating and left-beating responses is appropriate as long as the baseline shift is subtracted from all caloric responses.

The following procedure is recommended for calculating both the baseline shift and the gain asymmetry. An overall baseline shift can be determined by averaging the baseline shift of all four irrigations:

$$BaseAvg = \frac{BaseRW + BaseLW + BaseRC + BaseLC}{4}$$

In computerized systems, this parameter can be estimated by drawing a best-fitting horizontal line through the SPV points within the first 10 to 15 s of all four irrigations (see Figure 12–8A).

For gain asymmetry, the caloric portion of the response ($CalRW$, $CalLW$, $CalRC$, or $CalLC$) should be determined by subtracting the baseline shift from the peak SPV for each irrigation:

$$CalRW = PeakRW - BaseAvg,$$

$$CalLW = PeakLW - BaseAvg,$$

$$CalRC = PeakRC - BaseAvg,$$

$$CalLC = PeakLC - BaseAvg.$$

Total responses without the effect of baseline shift can be derived from

$$CalRB = -CalRW - CalLC,$$

$$CalLB = CalRC + CalLW.$$

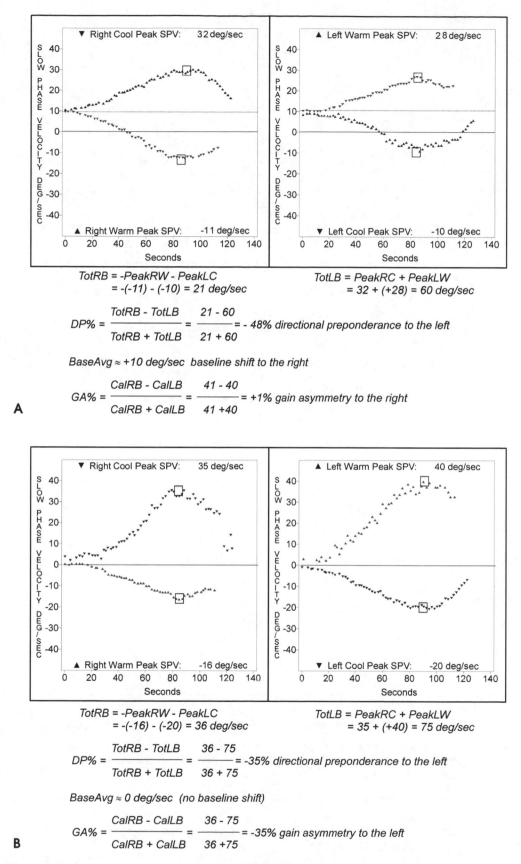

$$TotRB = -PeakRW - PeakLC$$
$$= -(-11) - (-10) = 21 \text{ deg/sec}$$

$$TotLB = PeakRC + PeakLW$$
$$= 32 + (+28) = 60 \text{ deg/sec}$$

$$DP\% = \frac{TotRB - TotLB}{TotRB + TotLB} = \frac{21 - 60}{21 + 60} = -48\% \text{ directional preponderance to the left}$$

$BaseAvg \approx +10$ deg/sec baseline shift to the right

$$GA\% = \frac{CalRB - CalLB}{CalRB + CalLB} = \frac{41 - 40}{41 + 40} = +1\% \text{ gain asymmetry to the right}$$

A

$$TotRB = -PeakRW - PeakLC$$
$$= -(-16) - (-20) = 36 \text{ deg/sec}$$

$$TotLB = PeakRC + PeakLW$$
$$= 35 + (+40) = 75 \text{ deg/sec}$$

$$DP\% = \frac{TotRB - TotLB}{TotRB + TotLB} = \frac{36 - 75}{36 + 75} = -35\% \text{ directional preponderance to the left}$$

$BaseAvg \approx 0$ deg/sec (no baseline shift)

$$GA\% = \frac{CalRB - CalLB}{CalRB + CalLB} = \frac{36 - 75}{36 + 75} = -35\% \text{ gain asymmetry to the left}$$

B

Figure 12-8. Different types of directional preponderance. **A.** Baseline shift. **B.** Gain asymmetry. Note that directional preponderance and gain asymmetry are expressed with respect to the direction of nystagmus fast phases and baseline shift is expressed with respect to the direction of nystagmus slow phases.

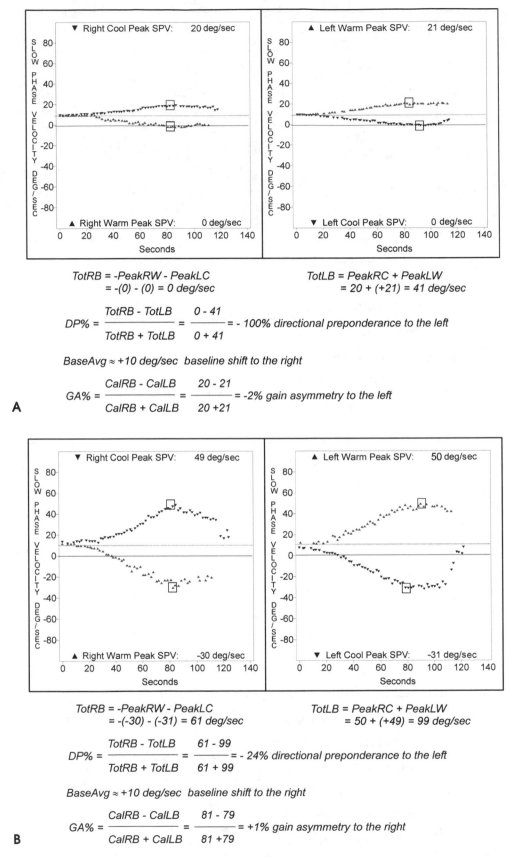

Figure 12-9. The effect of the strength of caloric responses on the directional preponderance. **A.** Weak overall response. **B.** Strong overall response. Note that the directional preponderance is significantly different for about the same amount of baseline shift and gain asymmetry.

Gain asymmetry is then calculated from (Barin & Stockwell, 2002)

$$GA\% = \frac{CalRB - CalLB}{CalRB + CalLB} \times 100$$

where $GA\%$ represents gain asymmetry in percent.

Fixation Index

Fixation suppression for each direction of nystagmus is quantified by the ratio of nystagmus intensity before and after fixation:

$$FI_{rb}\% = \frac{FixRW}{NoFixRW} \times 100 \quad \text{or} \quad \frac{FixLC}{NoFixLC} \times 100$$

$$FI_{lb}\% = \frac{FixRW}{NoFixRW} \times 100 \quad \text{or} \quad \frac{FixLW}{NoFixLW} \times 100$$

where $FI_{rb}\%$ and $FI_{lb}\%$ represent the fixation index in percent for each direction of nystagmus. As noted, the fixation index should be calculated from the irrigations where the nystagmus intensities just before fixation are close for different nystagmus directions. When nystagmus is fully suppressed, the fixation index will be 0%. When nystagmus is partially suppressed, the fixation index will be between 0% and 100%. When nystagmus is enhanced, the fixation index will be greater than 100%.

Analysis of Monothermal Caloric Responses

Sometimes caloric responses are available only for one temperature. This can be either by design, as in the case of monothermal screening test, or by necessity, as in the case of a patient who is unable to complete the test after two irrigations. The equation of $UW\%$ can be modified for monothermal testing. First, if there is baseline shift due to preexisting nystagmus, its effect must be subtracted from the peak SPV. An average baseline shift can be calculated from the baseline shift for two irrigations:

$$BaseWAvg = (BaseRW + BaseLW)/2,$$
(for warm monothermal caloric tests)

or

$$BaseCAvg = (BaseRC + BaseLC)/2,$$
(for cool monothermal caloric tests).

Responses without the effect of baseline shift can be derived from

$$CalRW = PeakRW - BaseWAvg,$$
$$CalLW = PeakLW - BaseWAvg,$$
(for warm monothermal caloric tests)

or

$$CalRC = PeakRC - BaseCAvg,$$
$$CalLC = PeakLC - BaseCAvg$$
(for cool monothermal caloric tests)

$UW\%$ for monothermal caloric testing can be calculated from one the following equations:

$$UW\% =$$
$$(-CalRW - CalLW)/(-CalRW + CalLW) \times 100,$$
(for warm monothermal caloric tests)

or

$$UW\% = (CalRC + CalLC)/(CalRC - CalLC) \times 100,$$
(for cool monothermal caloric tests)

ARTIFACTS AND TECHNICAL ERRORS IN CALORIC TESTS

Physiologic artifacts and technical errors can contaminate the caloric responses and affect the validity of the test results (Becker, 1978). Some of the sources of artifacts and errors for caloric tests are the same as those that affect all of the subtests in ENG. For example, eye blinks in ENG, noisy tracings, and crosstalk between the horizontal and vertical channels can contaminate the entire ENG test. Other sources are more specific, and perhaps more critical to the caloric test (Kileny and Kemink, 1986). They include faulty or poor irrigations, incorrect identification of peak caloric responses, failure to maintain a constant level of alertness throughout the test, and faulty calibrations. It is the responsibility of the examiner to reduce the possibility of these errors. However, because of the complexity of the procedures and the inherent variability of the stimulus, the caloric test can sometimes produce invalid results despite the examiner's best efforts. It is important to recognize invalid test results and take corrective action, when possible.

An invalid caloric test should be suspected when the results cannot be explained by any known physiology or pathology of the VOR (Barin, 2006). There are at least four types of valid caloric responses. In the first type, all four caloric irrigations generate approximately equal responses (see Figure 12–4A). This type of response is seen in patients with normal VOR and in patients with bilateral hypo- or hyperactive VOR function. In the second type, responses of each ear to warm and cool irrigations are approximately equal, but the total responses from one ear are significantly different from the total responses of the other ear (see Figure 12–6). This type of response is seen in patients with unilaterally reduced VOR function. In the third type, total responses from both ears are approximately equal but the baseline of the caloric responses are shifted in one direction causing the nystagmus intensity in one direction to be stronger than the nystagmus intensity in the opposite direction (see Figure 12–8A). This type of response is seen in patients who have nystagmus without fixation in the supine position. In the fourth type, the

nystagmus intensity in one direction is truly stronger than the nystagmus intensity in the opposite direction without any baseline shift (see Figure 12–8B). This type of response is seen in patients with the rare abnormality of gain asymmetry (Halmagyi et al., 2000). Any combination of these four types also represents a valid caloric test. When the test results do not match one of the valid caloric response types, the examiner must not proceed with interpreting the test until all possible sources of technical error have been ruled out.

There is no definitive method for identifying invalid caloric tests, but there is a simple observation that can alert the examiner to that possibility. In almost all of the valid caloric test types, the baseline shifts for the right and left ears are approximately equal. The only exception can occur in a patient who has both gain asymmetry and unilateral weakness. Although theoretically possible, there has not been a report of such a case so far. Therefore, invalid test results should be suspected when the baseline shifts from the right and left ears differ significantly (Stockwell, 1994). The baseline shift for each ear can be approximated by finding the midpoint between the peak caloric responses. Figure 12–10 shows an example where there is a significant difference

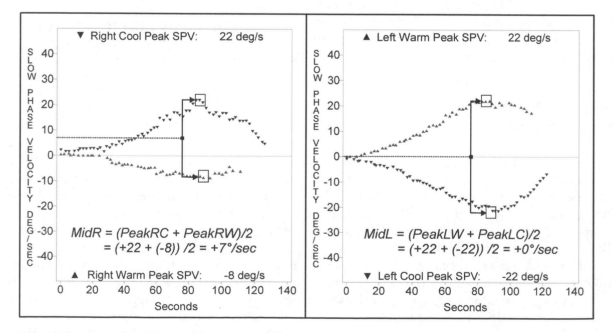

Figure 12–10. Verifying the validity of the caloric test results by comparing the response midpoints from the right and left ears. In this caloric test, one irrigation generates much weaker response compared to the other three irrigations.

between the response midpoints of the right and left ears. The exact amount of difference between midpoints that indicates an invalid test is not known. Some commercially available ENG systems have used a threshold of less than 5 deg/s for valid results. The threshold most likely depends on the overall strength of the response with lower values for the weaker overall response strengths and higher values for the stronger overall response strengths.

When invalid caloric test results are suspected, the first step is to verify that the SPV profiles are estimated accurately. Computerized ENG and VNG systems derive the SPV profiles using an algorithm that distinguishes between the fast and slow phases of nystagmus. Even the most sophisticated algorithms are not perfect in this task and occasionally miscalculate nystagmus SPVs. This can lead to misidentification of the response peak (Figure 12–11). Therefore, if the system allows it, the examiner should inspect the tracings for all irrigations and correct the SPV of outliers. Two key guidelines must be kept in mind when identifying the outliers and cleaning the SPV profile. First, the shape of caloric responses remains essentially the same even though the strength and direction can vary. Second, because the frequency of caloric responses is very low, the intensities of adjacent nystagmus beats cannot differ significantly. Figure 12–11 shows how cleaning the tracings using these two guidelines can affect the estimate of the peak caloric response. Figure 12–3 represents the SPV profile after cleaning the tracing in Figure 12–11.

One of the most common examples of an invalid caloric test is when the response from one irriga-

tion is significantly less intense than the responses from the other three irrigations (see Figure 12–10). The most likely cause of this error is poor irrigation, but faulty calibrations and lack of patient alertness are also possible. Regardless of the cause, the examiner should repeat one or more of the irrigations. It is very likely that these results are generated by a patient who has normal VOR function and all four caloric irrigations should have generated approximately equal responses. Therefore, the examiner should first repeat the irrigation that has produced the weak response (right warm for Figure 12–11). If this does not resolve the error, the examiner should then repeat the irrigation of the same ear that was performed with the other temperature (right cool for Figure 12–11). This allows for the less likely event that the patient has a unilateral weakness. If the error is still present after repeating two irrigations, the entire caloric test should be repeated at a later date. Performing more than six irrigations in the same setting is not recommended because of the central adaptation issues, as well as patient comfort.

Sometimes, one irrigation, usually the first one, generates much stronger responses compared to the other three irrigations (Figure 12–12). The most likely cause of this finding is hyperalertness during the first irrigation but faulty calibrations and poor irrigation of the same ear with the other temperature are also possible. The examiner should first repeat the irrigation that has produced the strong response, which is significantly different from the responses of the other three irrigations. If this does not resolve the error, the examiner should then repeat the irrigation

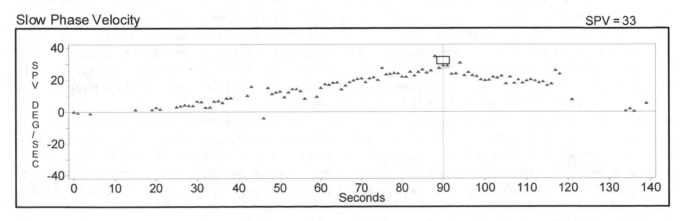

Figure 12–11. SPV profile of caloric nystagmus in Figure 12–3 before cleaning the tracings. The estimated peak response changes from 26 deg/s to 33 deg/s, a difference of 27%.

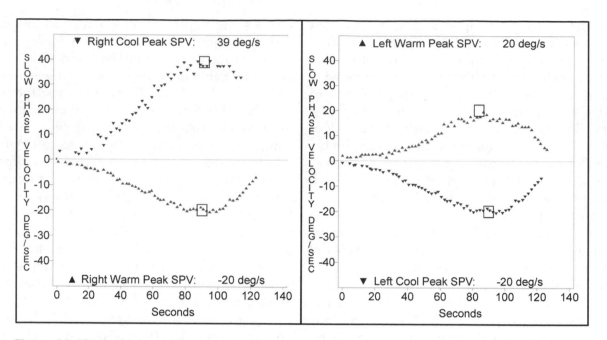

Figure 12–12. Caloric results with one irrigation generating a much stronger response compared to the other three irrigations.

of the same ear that was performed with the other temperature. This allows for the less likely event that the patient has a unilateral weakness in the other ear.

A special case of a single irrigation producing unusually strong responses occurs when the strong response is produced by one of the warm irrigations and repeating the irrigations as described before does not resolve the issue. There have been several anecdotal reports that some patients, most commonly those with the diagnosis of migraine, produce responses for one of the warm irrigations that are significantly stronger than the responses for the other three irrigations (personal communication with several clinicians). A few studies have reported rare cases of unilateral hyperactive caloric responses (e.g., Huygen, Nicolasen, Verhagen, & Theunissen, 1989). However, it is not clear if the hyperactivity was present for both irrigation temperatures or limited to the warm irrigations. Also, a few studies have reported unilateral caloric weakness in a subset of patients with migraine (e.g., Celebisoy, Gökçay, Sirin, & Biçak, 2008). Again, it is not clear if the caloric weakness could be attributed to a strong response from the warm irrigation of the contralateral ear. As the evidence is lacking in these cases, it is

best to view the presence of strong caloric responses for a single warm irrigation as a technical error until more studies become available.

Figure 12–13 shows another type of error where the responses for one temperature are significantly different than the responses for the other temperature in both ears. This is called the *temperature effect* and can be caused by a faulty irrigator, faulty calibrations, or a patient who has significantly higher or lower than normal body temperature. Fortunately, calculations of the response parameters such as *UW%* and *DP%*, are not compromised by temperature effect. However, identification of other types of error becomes more difficult in the presence of the temperature effect. Therefore, if temperature effect occurs frequently, the examiner should have the irrigator checked and the irrigation temperatures calibrated.

Repeating an erroneous irrigation is not always necessary unless it can change the outcome of the overall test. For example, assume the peak caloric response for the right warm irrigation in Figure 12–12 is 30 deg/s instead of 39 deg/s. Regardless of what repeating the right cool or right warm irrigation produces, the result of the overall test is not likely to change.

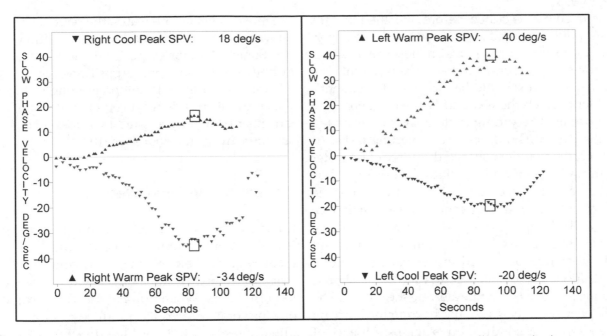

Figure 12–13. Caloric results showing irrigations for one temperature generating much stronger responses compared to the other temperature.

There are less common types of error that can affect the caloric test. A careful review of the test as well as a comprehensive knowledge of the equipment and the VOR physiology can help the examiner to recognize and avoid technical errors.

SPECIALIZED CALORIC TESTS

Two types of specialized caloric tests are discussed in this section. These tests are not part of the standard ENG/VNG test battery. They are reserved for specific patient populations.

Ice Water Caloric Test

When the standard caloric stimulus fails to provoke a response from an ear, ice water caloric testing should be performed in that ear (Proctor, 1992). The purpose of the ice water caloric test is to verify the results of the bithermal caloric test and to determine if there is any residual function remaining in the test ear. Bilateral ice water tests are indicated if neither ear responds to the standard caloric stimulus. How-

ever, in those cases, some form of rotation testing (see Chapters 14 and 15 is more effective and more informative than the bilateral ice water test.

Determining the absence of a caloric response is not always easy, especially in the presence of spontaneous or positional nystagmus. When the total response from either ear is very small, for example, less than 6 deg/s (*TotRE* or *TotLE* <6 deg/s), one can consider the ear to be a candidate for ice water testing. This value is derived empirically based on the inherent variability in identifying peak caloric responses of each irrigation.

Before irrigating an ear with ice water, the patient's ear should be examined to make sure there is no tympanic membrane perforation. Ice water testing must not be performed in an ear with perforated eardrum. Then the examiner should mix some water with ice cubes and let it stand for a few minutes. It is best to keep sterile ice cubes and sterile water in the refrigerator and use them for the ice water caloric test. Alternatively, regular ice cubes and cold water from a water fountain can be used. A small syringe should be placed in the ice water mix until the time of the irrigation. The patient should be placed in the standard caloric position and the eye movements should be calibrated. Visual fixation should be removed as described before and the patient's head should be turned so that the test ear is uppermost. The examiner can place an otoscope tip in the ear and use it as a funnel to inject the water into the ear canal. A towel should be placed on the patient's shoulder to catch the water after the irrigation. The eye movement recording system should be started and the patient should be given alerting tasks. At this time, the examiner should draw 2 cc of ice water into the syringe and inject it into the ear canal. It is best not to deliver more than 2 cc because that is the average volume of the ear canal. Any additional ice water is likely to run out of the ear. After 20 s, the ice water should be emptied out into the towel and the head should be placed in the standard caloric test position. The eye movement recording should continue for 30 to 60 s while alerting the patient. The eye movement tracings should be examined for any evidence of caloric-induced nystagmus. Absence of such nystagmus indicates total loss of function in the lateral semicircular canal or its afferent pathways. Sometimes a small response is present indicating a severe but not a complete loss of function.

BSA (2010) has recommended a procedure for the basic ice water caloric testing that for the most part matches the procedure described above. However, sometimes a more comprehensive type of ice of water testing is needed. For example, interpretation of the ice water caloric test becomes complicated if there is any spontaneous or positional nystagmus. The intensity of this nystagmus can change depending on the level of alertness. Ice water caloric testing in the prone position can distinguish between caloric-induced responses and changes in the intensity of spontaneous/positional nystagmus due to different levels of alertness (Proctor, 1987). After administering the ice water in the supine position and recording the eye movements for 30 to 40 s, the examiner should ask the patient to turn into the prone position with the head hanging downward by 30 degrees (see Figure 12–1B). Alternatively, the patient can sit up and bend forward to place the head at an angle of 30 degrees with respect to the horizontal plane. Caloric-induced nystagmus will either disappear or reverse directions in the prone position. That will indicate presence of residual vestibular function in the test ear. If nystagmus does not change direction, it indicates total loss of function in the lateral semicircular canal and its afferent pathways. After recording the

eye movements for 30 to 40 s, the patient should be returned to the standard caloric test position.

Some laboratories perform the ice water test in both supine and prone positions regardless of whether or not there is any preexisting nystagmus. This prevents misidentifying a latent form of spontaneous nystagmus, referred to as *pseudonystagmus*, as caloric nystagmus (Greisen, 1972).

Caloric Test in Perforated Ear

Caloric testing of a patient with a perforated ear is possible but a number of issues must be considered. First, as the use of water is contraindicated, irrigations must be done either with air or closed-loop irrigators. When air is used, warm irrigations of a perforated ear often produce nystagmus that initially beats in the opposite direction of what is expected for warm irrigations (Barber, Harmand, & Money, 1978). This is most likely due to the cooling effect that dry air has on the moist mucous membrane within the middle ear cavity. Once the mucous membrane heats up after the initial cooling, the nystagmus will reverse direction. Second, the heat transfer from the external auditory canal to the labyrinth is faster and more intense in a perforated ear because the tympanic membrane no longer acts as a barrier. As a result, the onset of caloric responses is usually much earlier and the intensity is much stronger in a perforated ear compared to those in an intact ear. Finally, caloric responses from two ears cannot be compared quantitatively because the main assumption of the caloric test—that both ears are receiving equal stimulation—is no longer valid in case of a perforated ear. Therefore, the purpose of caloric testing in a patient with a perforated ear is to simply determine whether or not there is any response from that ear.

Based on the above discussion, full caloric testing in a patient with a perforated ear is not recommended. A modified procedure can provide the necessary information and minimize patient discomfort. The examiner should first perform a cool irrigation of the nonperforated ear as in the standard caloric test. Then, the perforated ear should be irrigated with cool temperature. If caloric nystagmus appears (usually within the first 10 to 15 s), the examiner should immediately stop the irrigation and report that caloric responses are present. If no nystagmus appears, the examiner should report that there is no response from the perforated ear to the standard air or closed-loop water stimuli.

ALTERNATE CALORIC TESTS

Alternate methods of performing the caloric test have been proposed to improve the sensitivity and the comfort of the test (Wetmore, 1986). Two of these methods, simultaneous caloric testing and Torok's monothermal caloric testing, have received more clinical attention compared to other alternate caloric tests. Both tests are offered as an adjunct to the standard bithermal caloric test. In this section, the proper methods for administering these tests are described. The usefulness and interpretation of the tests are discussed in Chapter 13.

Simultaneous Caloric Test

Simultaneous caloric testing has been popularized by Brookler and his colleagues (Brookler, 1976, 2002; Hoffman, Brookler, & Baker, 1979). In this test, both ears are simultaneously irrigated, first with the cool medium and then with the warm medium. For practical reasons, simultaneous caloric testing with air is not possible. Only open-loop or closed-loop water irrigators can be used. Both types of irrigators have to be modified to allow the water from the reservoir to be carried to two separate irrigator tips. The irrigation temperatures and volumes are the same for both the standard and simultaneous caloric tests. However, the duration of irrigation is increased to 1 min in the simultaneous caloric test for both irrigator types.

The analysis of simultaneous caloric testing requires inspecting the eye movement tracings and determining if nystagmus is present or absent. If present, the nystagmus direction must also be identified. The criterion for the presence of nystagmus is identifying three nystagmus beats within a 10-s period (Hoffman et al., 1979). No other quantification is needed. For each irrigation, there are three possible outcomes—no nystagmus, right-beating nystagmus, or left-beating nystagmus. As there are

two irrigations, there are a total of nine different response patterns in the simultaneous caloric test. Brookler (1976) has categorized these patterns into four different types. Type I represents absence of nystagmus for both warm and cool irrigations. Type II represents nystagmus that beats in different directions for warm and cool irrigations. Type III represents nystagmus that beats in the same direction for both warm and cool irrigations. All of the remaining patterns are categorized as Type IV.

The premise of simultaneous caloric testing is that in a patient who has normal VOR pathways, simultaneous excitation or inhibition of the labyrinth will produce no nystagmus. The test is advocated as a more sensitive adjunct to the standard bithermal caloric test because both ears are stimulated with the exact same irrigation. However, small differences in the heat transfer from the right and left ears will generate nystagmus in the simultaneous caloric test, which can be mistakenly classified as abnormal. In the standard caloric testing, those differences are averaged and normalized. Furthermore, their effect is taken into account by choosing a relatively wide range for normal responses. As there are no such safeguards in the simultaneous caloric test, the false-positive rates are expected to be high (Furman, Wall, & Kamerer, 1988). More details on the interpretation of the test are provided in Chapter 13.

Torok Differential Monothermal Caloric

Torok (1970) proposed a different type of caloric test, in which each ear is irrigated by two stimuli of different strengths. The weak stimulus consists of 10 mL of water at 20°C irrigated over 5 s. During the irrigation, the patient is seated upright with the head tilted 30 degrees downward. In this position, the lateral canal is in the horizontal plane and caloric stimulation is not expected to generate a significant response. The patient remains in this position for 60 s after the irrigation. Then the patient is rapidly tilted back into the standard caloric test position. This generates a sudden caloric stimulus as the lateral canal becomes aligned with the plane of gravity. After a wait period, the other ear is irrigated using the exact same procedure. The strong stimulus consists of 100 mL of water, also at 20°C, irrigated over 20 s. For these irrigations, the entire test is conducted with the patient in the standard caloric test position. Again, the same procedure is repeated for the other ear.

In the original version of the test described by Torok (1970), the eye movements are recorded by an infrared photoelectric device with the patient's eyes open and fixating. Caloric responses are quantified by the nystagmus frequency. Nystagmus beats are counted in two 5-s periods that contain the most intense response, then averaged to get the culmination frequency. Finally, the ratio of culmination frequencies for the strong versus the weak stimulus is used to quantify *recruitment* and *decruitment* of caloric responses (Kumar, 1981; Torok, 1976). Recruitment exists when the response to the strong stimulus is unusually larger than the response to the weak stimulus. Decruitment exists when the response to the strong stimulus is less than or equal to the response to the weak stimulus.

Some investigators have modified the test procedures for Torok's monothermal caloric test. For example, some have recorded the nystagmus by ENG and have quantified the responses by the peak SPV (Wexler, Harker, Voots, & McCabe, 1991). Others have used either air or different water temperatures for irrigation (Ghosh & Kacker, 1979; Parker & Hamid, 1985). These modifications have been criticized by the originator of the technique and others, who believe the modified procedures are not optimal and contribute to the variability of the test (Kumar, 1995; Torok, 1979).

Torok (1970) suggested that identifying recruitment and decruitment of caloric responses provided a method for distinguishing labyrinthine from retrolabyrinthine lesions, which is not possible with the standard bithermal caloric test (Bhansali, Stockwell, Bojrab, & Schwan, 1989; Linstrom & Stockwell, 1993). However, that viewpoint has not been universally accepted (e.g., Proctor, Frazer, Glackin, & Smith, 1983). Currently, Torok's differential monothermal caloric test has not found widespread use in the United States.

SUMMARY

Caloric testing is time consuming and technically challenging. The examiner must be careful to avoid the pitfalls and artifacts. However, caloric testing remains the most important part of vestibular function tests as it provides information not available from other tests.

REFERENCES

Alpert, J. N. (1974). Failure of fixation suppression: A pathologic effect of vision on caloric nystagmus. *Neurology, 24*, 891–896.

American Academy of Neurology. (1996). Electronystagmography: Report of the Therapeutics and Technology Assessment Subcommittee. *Neurology, 46*(6), 1763–1766.

Anderson, S. (1995). Caloric irrigators: Air, open-loop water and closed-loop water. *British Journal of Audiology, 29*(2), 117–128.

Andrew, S., & Meredith, R. (2009). Verification of chart videonystagmography calibration. *BSA News 58* (December), 11–14.

ANSI. (2009). Procedures for testing basic vestibular function. *American National Standards Institute*, ANSI/ASA S3.45-2009 (Revision of ANSI S3.45-1999).

Aw, S. T., Haslwanter, T., Fetter, M., Heimberger, J., & Todd, M. J. (1998). Contribution of the vertical semicircular canals to the caloric nystagmus. *Acta Oto-Laryngologica, 118*(5), 618–627.

Baguley, D. M., Whipp, J., & Farrington, M. (1991). A microbiological hazard in caloric testing. *British Journal of Audiology, 25*(6), 427–428.

Baloh, R. W. (2002). Robert Bárány and the controversy surrounding his discovery of the caloric reaction. *Neurology, 58*(7), 1094–1099.

Baloh, R. W., & Honrubia, V. (2001). *Clinical neurophysiology of the vestibular system*. New York, NY: Oxford University Press.

Baloh, R. W., Solingen, L., Sills, A. W., & Honrubia, V. (1977). Caloric testing. 1. Effect of different conditions of ocular fixation. *Annals of Otology, Rhinology and Laryngology, 86*(5 Pt. 3, Suppl. 43), 1–6.

Bárány, R. (1907). *Physiologie und pathologie des bogengangapparates beim menschen*. Vienna, Austria: Deuticke.

Barber, H. O., Harmand, W. M., & Money, K. E. (1978). Air caloric stimulation with tympanic membrane perforation. *Laryngoscope, 88*(7 Pt. 1), 1117–1126.

Barber, H. O., & Stockwell, C. W. (1980). *Manual of electronystagmography* (pp. 159–187). St Louis, MO: Mosby.

Barber, H. O., Wright, G., & Demanuele, F. (1971). The hot caloric test as a clinical screening device. *Archives of Otolaryngology, 94*(4), 335–337.

Barin, K. (2006). *Common errors in ENG/VNG*. In Audiology Online.com posted 7/17/2006. Retrieved December 1,

2013, from http://www.audiologyonline.com/articles/common-errors-in-eng-vng-978

Barin, K. (2009). Clinical neurophysiology of the vestibular system. In J. Katz, L. Medwetsky, R. Burkhart, & L. Hood (Eds.), *Handbook of clinical audiology* (6th ed., pp. 431–466). Philadelphia, PA: Lippincott Williams & Wilkins.

Barin, K., & Stockwell, C. W. (2002). Directional preponderance revisited. *Insights in Practice*, ICS Medical, 1–6.

Barnes, G. (1995). Adaptation in the oculomotor response to caloric irrigation and the merits of bithermal stimulation. *British Journal of Audiology, 29*(2), 95–106.

Beattie, R. C., & Koester, C. K. (1992). Effects of interstimulus interval on slow phase velocity to ipsilateral warm air caloric stimulation in normal subjects. *Journal of the American Academy of Audiology, 3*(5), 297–302.

Becker, G. D. (1978). Sources of error in interpretation of caloric tests. *Otolaryngology, 86*(5), 830–833.

Benitez, J. T., Bouchard, K. R., & Choe, Y. K. (1978). Air calorics: A technique and results. *Annals of Otology, Rhinology, and Laryngology, 87*(2 Pt. 1), 216–223.

Bhansali, S. A., Stockwell, C. W., Bojrab, D. I., & Schwan, S. A. (1989). Evaluation of the monothermal caloric test. *Laryngoscope, 99*(5), 500–504.

British Society of Audiology (BSA). (2010). *Recommended procedure: The caloric test.* Berkshire, UK: Author.

Brookler, K. H. (1976). The simultaneous binaural bithermal: A caloric test utilizing electronystagmography. *Laryngoscope, 86*(8), 1241–1250.

Brookler, K. H. (2002). Importance of simultaneous binaural bithermal caloric testing. *Ear, Nose, and Throat Journal, 81*(4), 199.

Brookler, K. H., Baker, A. H., & Grams, G. (1979). Closed loop water irrigator system. *Otolaryngology-Head and Neck Surgery, 87*(3), 364–365.

Bush, M. L., Bingcang, C. M., Chang, E. T., Fornwalt, B., Rayle, C., Gal, T. J., . . . Shinn, J. B. (2013). Hot or cold? Is monothermal caloric testing useful and cost-effective? *Annals of Otology, Rhinology, and Laryngology, 122*(6), 412–416.

Celebisoy, N., Gökçay, F., Sirin, H., & Biçak, N. (2008). Migrainous vertigo: Clinical, oculographic and posturographic findings. *Cephalalgia: An International Journal of Headache, 28*(1), 72–77.

Claussen, C. F., & von Schlachta, I. (1972). Butterfly chart for caloric nystagmus evaluation. *Archives of Otolaryngology, 96*(4), 371–375.

Coats, A. C., & Smith, S. Y. (1967). Body position and the intensity of caloric nystagmus. *Acta Oto-Laryngologica, 63*(6), 515–532.

Committee on Hearing, Bioacoustics, and Biomechanics (CHABA). (1992). Evaluation of tests for vestibular function. *Aviation, Space, and Environmental Medicine, 63*(2 Suppl.), A1–A34.

Cyr, D. G. (1980). Vestibular testing in children. *Annals of Otology, Rhinology and Laryngology Supplement, 89*(5, Pt. 2), 63–69.

Davis, R. I., & Mann, R. C. (1987). The effects of alerting tasks on caloric induced vestibular nystagmus. *Ear and Hearing, 8*(1), 58–60.

Enticott, J. C., Dowell, R. C., & O'Leary, S. J. (2003). A comparison of the monothermal and bithermal caloric tests. *Journal of Vestibular Research: Equilibrium and Orientation, 13*(2–3), 113–119.

Feldmann, H., Huttenbrink, K. B., & Delank, K. W. (1991). Transport of heat in caloric vestibular stimulation. Conduction, convection or radiation? *Acta Oto-Laryngologica, 111*(2), 169–175.

Fetter, M., Aw, S., Haslwanter, T., Heimberger, J., & Dichgans, J. (1998). Three-dimensional eye movement analysis during caloric stimulation used to test vertical semicircular canal function. *American Journal of Otology, 19*(2), 180–187.

Fitzgerald, G., & Hallpike, C. S. (1942). Studies in human vestibular function. I. Observations of the directional preponderance of caloric nystagmus resulting from cerebral lesions. *Brain, 65*, 115–137.

Fleming, P. M., Proctor, L. R., Dix, R. C., & Metz, W. A. (1978). Results of new air caloric testing method among normal subjects. I. Biphasic testing. *Annals of Otology, Rhinology, and Laryngology, 87*(2 Pt. 1), 248–256.

Ford, C. R., & Stockwell, C. W. (1978). Reliabilities of air and water caloric responses. *Archives of Otolaryngology, 104*(7), 380–382.

Formby, C., Kuntz, L. A., Rivera-Taylor, I. M., Rivera-Mraz, N., Weesner, D. R., Butler-Young, N. E., & Ahlers, A. E. (1992). Measurement, analysis, and modelling of the caloric response. 2. Evaluation of mental alerting tasks for measurement of caloric-induced nystagmus. *Acta Oto-Laryngologica Supplement, 498*, 19–29.

Furman, J. M., & Jacob, R. G. (1993). Jongkees' formula re-evaluated: Order effects in the response to alternate binaural bithermal caloric stimulation using closed-loop irrigation. *Acta Oto-Laryngologica, 113*(1), 3–10.

Furman, J. M., Wall, C., III, & Kamerer, D. B. (1988). Alternate and simultaneous binaural bithermal caloric testing: A comparison. *Annals of Otology, Rhinology, and Laryngology, 97*(4 Pt. 1), 359–364.

Gentine, A., Eichhorn, J. L., Kopp, C., & Conraux, C. (1991). Modelling the action of caloric stimulation of the vestibule. II. The mechanical model of the semicircular canal considered as an inflatable structure. *Acta Oto-Laryngologica, 111*(1), 10–15.

Ghosh, P., & Kacker, S. K. (1979). Vestibular recruitment and decruitment. *Acta Oto-Laryngologica, 88*(3–4), 227–234.

Greisen, O. (1972). Pseudocaloricnystagmus. *Acta Oto-Laryngologica, 73*, 341–343.

Greven, A. J., Oosterveld, W. J., Rademakers, W. J., & Voorhoeve, R. (1979). Caloric vestibular test with the use of air. *Annals of Otology, Rhinology, and Laryngology, 88*(1 Pt. 1), 31–35.

Halmagyi, G. M., Cremer, P. D., Anderson, J., Murofushi, T., & Curthoys, I. S. (2000). Isolated directional preponderance of caloric nystagmus: I. Clinical significance. *American Journal of Otology, 21*(4), 559–567.

Hamid, M. A., Hughes, G. B., & Kinney, S. E. (1987). Criteria for diagnosing bilateral vestibular dysfunction. In M. D. Graham, & J. L. Kemink, (Eds.), *The vestibular system: Neurophysiologic and clinical research* (pp. 115–118). New York, NY: Raven Press.

Henry, D. F. (1999). Test-retest reliability of open-loop bithermal caloric irrigation responses from healthy young adults. *American Journal of Otology, 20*(2), 220–222.

Henry, D. F., & DiBartolomeo, J. D. (1993). Closed-loop caloric, harmonic acceleration and active head rotation tests: Norms and reliability. *Otolaryngology-Head and Neck Surgery, 109*(6), 975–987.

Hoffman, R. A., Brookler, K. H., & Baker, A. H. (1979). The accuracy of the simultaneous binaural bithermal test in the diagnosis of acoustic neuroma. *Laryngoscope, 89*(7 Pt. 1), 1046–1052.

Hood, J. D. (1989). Evidence of direct thermal action upon the vestibular receptors in the caloric test. A reinterpretation of the data of Coats and Smith. *Acta Oto-Laryngologica, 107*(3–4), 161–165.

Huygen, P. L., Nicolasen, M. G., Verhagen, W. I., & Theunissen, E. J. (1989). Contralateral hyperactive caloric response in unilateral labyrinthine weakness. *Acta Oto-Laryngologica, 107*(1–2), 1–4.

Jacobson, G. P., Calder, J. A., Shepherd, V. A., Rupp, K. A., & Newman, C. W. (1995). Reappraisal of the monothermal warm caloric screening test. *Annals of Otology, Rhinology, and Laryngology, 104*(12), 942–945.

Jacobson, G. P., & Means, E. D. (1985). Efficacy of a monothermal warm water caloric screening test. *Annals of Otology, Rhinology, and Laryngology, 94*(4 Pt. 1), 377–381.

Jacobson, G. P., & Newman, C. W. (1993). Background and technique of caloric testing. In G. P. Jacobson, C. W. Newman, & J. M. Kartush (Eds.), *Handbook of balance testing function* (pp. 156–192). St. Louis, MO: Mosby.

Jongkees, L. B. W., & Philipszoon, A. J. (1964). Electronystagmography. *Acta Oto-Laryngologica Supplement 189*, 1–111.

Karlsen, E. A., Goetzinger, C. P., & Hassanein, R. (1980). Effects of six conditions of ocular fixation on caloric nystagmus. *Archives of Otolaryngology, 106*(8), 474–476.

Karlsen, E. A., Mikhail, H. H., Norris, C. W., & Hassanein, R. S. (1992). Comparison of responses to air, water, and closed-loop caloric irrigators. *Journal of Speech and Hearing Research, 35*(1), 186–191.

Keith, R. W., Pensak, M. L., & Katbamna, B. (1991). Prediction of bithermal caloric response from monothermal stimulation. *Otolaryngology-Head and Neck Surgery, 104*(4), 499–502.

Kileny, P., & Kemink, J. L. (1986). Artifacts and errors in the electronystagmographic (ENG) evaluation of the vestibular system. *Ear and Hearing, 7*(3), 151–156.

Kumar, A. (1981). Diagnostic advantages of the Torok monothermal differential caloric test. *Laryngoscope, 91*(10), 1678–1694.

Kumar, A. (1995). Post caloric nystagmus: An analysis of culmination frequency and maximum slow phase velocity. *Acta Oto-Laryngologica Supplement, 520*(Pt. 1), 220–224.

Lightfoot, G. R. (2004). The origin of order effects in the results of the bi-thermal caloric test. *International Journal of Audiology, 43*(5), 276–282.

Lightfoot, G., Barker, F., Belcher, K., Kennedy, V., Nassar, G., & Tweedy, F. (2009). The derivation of optimum criteria for use in the monothermal caloric screening test. *Ear and Hearing, 30*(1), 54–62.

Lightfoot, G., & Milner, L. (2010). The dependency of air caloric stimulus effectiveness on delivery tip characteristics. *International Journal of Audiology, 49*(10), 772–774.

Linstrom, C. J., & Stockwell, C. W. (1993). Clinical evaluation of the monothermal caloric test. *Otolaryngology-Head and Neck Surgery, 108*(1), 27–35.

Marques Perrella de Barros, A. C., & Caovilla, H. H. (2012). From nystagmus to the air and water caloric tests. *Brazilian Journal of Otorhinolaryngology, 78*(4), 120–125.

Melagrana, A., D'Agostino, R., Pasquale, G., & Taborelli, G. (1996). Study of labyrinthine function in children using the caloric test: Our results. *International Journal of Pediatric Otorhinolaryngology, 37*(1), 1–8.

Melagrana, A., D'Agostino, R., Tarantino, V., Taborelli, G., & Calevo, M. G. (2002). Monothermal air caloric test in children. *International Journal of Pediatric Otorhinolaryngology, 62*(1), 11–15.

Munro, K. J., & Higson, J. M. (1996). The test-retest variability of the caloric test: A comparison of a modified air irrigation with the conventional water technique. *British Journal of Audiology, 30*(5), 303–306.

Murnane, O. D., Akin, F. W., Lynn, S. G., & Cyr, D. G. (2009). Monothermal caloric screening test performance: A relative operating characteristic curve analysis. *Ear and Hearing, 30*(3), 313–319.

Nishizawa, S. (2002). Observations on conduction of caloric stimulation to the middle ear cavity by thermoscanning. *Laryngoscope, 112*(3), 504–508.

Noaksson, L., Schulin, M., Kovacsovics, B., & Ledin, T. (1998). Temperature order effects in the caloric reaction. *International Tinnitus Journal, 4*(1), 71–73.

Norman, M., & Brown, E. (1999). Variations in calibration for computerized electronystagmography. *British Journal of Audiology, 33*(1), 1–7.

O'Neill, G. (1987). The caloric stimulus. Temperature generation within the temporal bone. *Acta Oto-Laryngologica, 103*(3–4), 266–272.

O'Neill, G. (1995). The caloric stimulus: Mechanisms of heat transfer. *British Journal of Audiology, 29*(2), 87–94.

Ono, H., & Kanzaki, J. (1976). A new caloric tester using ear canal balloon. *Revue De Laryngologie-Otologie-Rhinologie, 97*(5–6), 223–230.

Parker, W., & Hamid, M. (1985). Vestibular responses to different caloric stimulus intensities. *American Journal of Otology, 6*(5), 378–386.

Pau, H. W., Sievert, U., Just, T., & Wild, W. (2001). Heat radiation during caloric vestibular test: Thermographic demonstration in temporal bone experiments. *Annals of Otology, Rhinology, and Laryngology, 110*(11), 1041–1044.

Proctor, L. R. (1977). Air caloric test: Irrigation technique. *Laryngoscope, 87*(8), 1383–1390.

Proctor, L. R. (1987). Caloric stimulation in face-down position. In M. D. Graham & J. L. Kemink, (Eds.), *The vestibular system: Neurophysiologic and clinical research.* New York, NY: Raven Press.

Proctor, L. R. (1992). The ice water caloric test. *ENG Report,* ICS Medical, 69–72.

Proctor, L. R., Frazer, R. K., Glackin, R. N., & Smith, C. R. (1983). "Recruitment/decruitment" of caloric responses: Effect of anatomical variables. *Advances in Oto-Rhino-Laryngology, 30,* 150–155.

Proctor, L., Hansen, D., & Rentea, R. (1980). Corneoretinal potential variations: Significance in electronystagmography. *Archives of Otolaryngology, 106*(5), 262–265.

Scherer, H., Brandt, U., Clarke, A. H., Merbold, U., & Parker, R. (1986). European vestibular experiments on the Spacelab-1 mission: 3. Caloric nystagmus in microgravity. *Experimental Brain Research, 64*(2), 255–263.

Schmaltz, G. (1932). The physical phenomena occurring in the semicircular canals during rotatory and thermic stimulation. *Journal of Laryngology Otology, 47,* 35–62.

Shupak, A., Kaminer, M., Gilbey, P., & Tal, D. (2010). Monothermal caloric testing in the screening of vestibular function. *Aviation, Space, and Environmental Medicine, 81*(4), 369–374.

Stockwell, C. W. (1987). Directional preponderance. *ENG Report,* ICS Medical, 37–40.

Stockwell, C. W. (1994). Three common errors in ENG testing. *ENG Report,* ICS Medical, 85–88.

Stockwell, C. W. (1997). Vestibular testing: Past, present, future. *British Journal of Audiology, 31*(6), 387–398.

Suter, C. M., Blanchard, C. L., & Cook-Manokey, B. E. (1977). Nystagmus responses to water and air caloric stimulation in clinical populations. *Laryngoscope, 87*(7), 1074–1078.

Tole, J. R. (1979). A protocol for the air caloric test and a comparison with a standard water caloric test. *Archives of Otolaryngology, 105*(6), 314–319.

Torok, N. (1970). A new parameter of vestibular sensitivity. *Annals of Otology, Rhinology, and Laryngology, 79*(4), 808–817.

Torok, N. (1976). Vestibular decruitment in central nervous system disease. *Annals of Otology, Rhinology, and Laryngology, 85*(1 Pt. 1), 131–135.

Torok, N. (1979). Pitfalls in detecting vestibular decruitment with air calorics. *Journal of Oto-Rhino-Laryngology, 41*(3), 143–146.

Wetmore, S. J. (1986). Extended caloric tests. *Ear and Hearing, 7*(3), 186–190.

Wexler, D. B. (1994). Nonlinearity of the Jongkees difference equation for vestibular hypofunction. *Otolaryngology-Head and Neck Surgery, 111*(4), 485–487.

Wexler, D. B., Harker, L. A., Voots, R. J., & McCabe, B. F. (1991). Monothermal differential caloric testing in patients with Meniere's disease. *Laryngoscope, 101*(1 Pt. 1), 50–55.

Zangemeister, W. H., & Bock, O. (1980). Air versus water caloric test. *Clinical Otolaryngology and Allied Sciences, 5*(6), 379–387.

Zapala, D. A., Olsholt, K. F., & Lundy, L. B. (2008). A comparison of water and air caloric responses and their ability to distinguish between patients with normal and impaired ears. *Ear and Hearing, 29*(4), 585–600.

Interpretation and Usefulness of Caloric Testing

Kamran Barin

OVERVIEW

The caloric test has been the most important test of vestibular function for over half a century. It is the most challenging and time-consuming part of the electronystagmography (ENG) test battery. Yet despite its limitations, the caloric test is still one of the most sensitive tests for detecting common vestibular abnormalities. The proper method for administering the test and quantifying the response parameters were described in Chapter 12. The interpretation of abnormalities in the caloric test and their clinical significance are discussed in this chapter. For accurate interpretation of the caloric test, the validity of the results must be established first. Therefore, as described in the previous chapter, the examiner must eliminate artifacts and technical errors before interpreting the test.

BITHERMAL CALORIC TEST FINDINGS IN NORMAL SUBJECTS

Several studies have examined caloric responses of healthy individuals and have established normal limits for many of the response parameters (see Barber & Stockwell, 1980, and CHABA, 1992, for a review of early studies). The key studies that have contributed to the more common normal limits include those by Barber and Wright (unpublished data as referenced by Barber & Stockwell, 1980), Sills, Baloh, and Honrubia (1977), and Jacobson, Newman, and Peterson (1993). Table 13–1 shows the most commonly used values as well as alternative values used by some laboratories. Some of the values have been adjusted from the original studies to reflect the recommended procedures in Chapter 12. Also, some of the parameters such as *UW%* and *DP%* are represented by signed numbers. The signs should be disregarded by taking the absolute value of these parameters when comparing them to the normative values.

Normal Limits for Unilateral Weakness

The work of Barber and Wright (unpublished data) is by far the largest ($n > 100$) among the early studies to establish normal limits of caloric responses. Based on using both open-loop water and air irrigators, they reported normal limits of 25% for unilateral weakness. The study by Sills et al. (1977) was smaller ($n = 43$) but included several response parameters such as nystagmus amplitude, nystagmus frequency, as well as nystagmus slow-phase velocity. Based on these data, Baloh and Honrubia (2001) recommended normal limits of 25% for unilateral weakness. Jacobson

Table 13–1. Normal Limits for Caloric Response Parameters (Common Values and Alternative Values Used by Some Laboratories)

	Common	Alternative
Unilateral weakness	$\lvert UW\% \rvert$ <25%	20%–30%
Directional preponderance	$\lvert DP\% \rvert$ <30%	25%–50%
Baseline shift	$\lvert BaseAvg \rvert$ <6°/s	—
Gain asymmetry	$\lvert GA\% \rvert$ <25%?	30%
Bilateral weakness	TotRE >12°/s **or** TotLE >12°/s	TotRE + TotLE > 22–30 deg/s
Hyperactivity	TotRE <140°/s **and** TotLE <140°/s	Alternative 1 (Jacobson et al., 1993): TotRE <110°/s **and** TotLE <110°/s
		Alternative 2 (Barber & Stockwell, 1980): PeakRC **and** PeakLC <50–60 deg/s **and** PeakRW **and** PeakLW <80 deg/s
Fixation suppression	FI% <0.6	0.5–0.7

Note. See Chapter 12 for the formulas to calculate *UW%* (unilateral weakness); *DP%* (directional preponderance); *BaseAvg* (baseline shift); *GA%* (gain asymmetry); *TotRE & TotLE* (total responses from the right and left ear, respectively); *PeakRC, PeakRW, PeakLC, PeakLW* (peak caloric responses for right cool, right warm, left cool, and left warm irrigations); *FI%* (fixation index).

et al. (1993) used both parametric and nonparametric statistics on a sample of 100 healthy individuals to establish their normal limits. The approximate normal limits based on combining the results from both statistical methods yielded values of 20% for unilateral weakness. In another study, Henry (1999) compared the caloric responses in a sample of 20 individuals using open- versus closed-loop water irrigators. For unilateral weakness, the upper limit of 25% was recommended for open-loop irrigators and 30% for closed-loop irrigators. Van der Stappen, Wuyts, and Van de Heyning (2000) used a computerized ENG system to measure caloric responses of 40 normal subjects. Their normal limit for unilateral weakness was 22%.

In summary, almost all of the relevant studies agree that the upper normal limit for unilateral weakness is within the range of 20% to 25%. Each laboratory is free to choose the value within this range that produces the best combination of sensitivity and specificity for their specific clinical settings.

As discussed in Chapter 12, it is important to recognize that even the lower normative value of 20% for unilateral weakness represents a substantial loss of 33% in the lateral canal or its afferent neural pathway.

Normal Limits for Directional Preponderance

There are more discrepancies among different studies regarding the normative values for directional preponderance. Barber and Wright (unpublished data) reported the normal limit of 23% for directional preponderance. This is lower than the normal limit of 30% and 27% reported by Baloh and Honrubia (2001) and Jacobson et al. (1993), respectively. However, Van der Stappen et al. (2000) have determined a surprisingly low value of 19% for the normative limit of directional preponderance.

The discrepancies may be related to the fact that, as noted in Chapter 12, directional preponderance consists of two components: baseline shift and gain asymmetry. As the baseline shift is caused by preexisting nystagmus in the supine position, its normal limit is derived from the criterion for nystagmus in the static position test. Most laboratories consider horizontal nystagmus without fixation to be clinically insignificant if the intensity is less than 4 to 6 deg/s (Isaacson & Rubin, 2001; Shepard & Telian, 1996). Currently, there are no studies of gain asymmetry in normal individuals. Halmagyi, Cremer, Anderson, Murofushi, and Curthoys (2000) used the normal limit of 30% for gain asymmetry. However, this limit is derived from the normal limit for directional preponderance, which does not directly correspond to gain asymmetry. It seems logical for gain asymmetry to have a lower normal limit than directional preponderance because the latter includes baseline shift. Until a formal study is conducted, one can use 25% as the normal limit for gain asymmetry, which is lower than the common limit for directional preponderance.

In recent years, it has become clear that directional preponderance is of limited clinical value (Hain, 2012), and as a result, some laboratories no longer use it. Those who wish to continue using directional preponderance should consider separating the contribution of the baseline shift and gain asymmetry because they represent two distinct abnormalities.

Normal Limits for Total Caloric Responses

The sum of peak caloric responses from four irrigations represents the total caloric response and is used to determine hypoactivity (bilateral weakness) and hyperactivity of the vestibular pathways. It should be stated at the outset that the caloric test is not a particularly useful test to detect bilateral vestibular hypoactivity. Therefore, it should not be surprising that there are considerable differences among different studies about the normal limits for total caloric responses. These differences are related to the high variability of caloric stimulus and individual differences in heat transfer from the external auditory canal to the labyrinth.

Barber and Stockwell (1980) estimated the lower normal limit to be 30 deg/s for total caloric responses. That is, when the sum of peak caloric responses from four irrigations is less than 30 deg/s, caloric responses are considered bilaterally weak. Jacobson et al. (1993) considered the lower normal limit for total caloric responses to be 22 deg/s. Similarly, Van der Stappen et al. (2000) determined the 95% confidence limit for the sum of all four irrigation responses to be 27 deg/s in the computerized ENG.

Most of the above studies that have established a threshold for bilateral weakness stipulate that the limit should apply only when caloric responses from the right and left ears are symmetric. Unfortunately, the formula for unilateral weakness is of little use in determining symmetry when the total response is very small. To address this issue, some have recommended imposing a lower normal limit on the peak caloric responses of individual irrigations (e.g., BSA, 2010). However, that approach is also not ideal because some patients who have strong spontaneous nystagmus but minimal caloric responses from either ear will not be correctly classified as cases of bilateral caloric weakness. As a result, it is more appropriate to define the threshold for bilateral weakness based on total responses from each ear. Stockwell (1993) defines the caloric test to be bilaterally weak when total responses from each ear are less than 12 deg/s. Using this approach eliminates the possibility of misidentifying the test as bilateral weakness when the responses of only one ear are very small.

Since the caloric test is of limited value in identifying patients with bilateral vestibular hypoactivity, one can simplify the process. If a patient is suspected of having bilateral caloric weakness using any of the above criteria, another test, such as the rotation test or the head impulse test, should be included in the evaluation protocol.

The normative limits for hyperactive caloric responses have also been defined differently in different studies. Barber and Stockwell (1980) consider caloric responses as hyperactive when peak slow-phase velocities exceed 50 deg/s for each of the cool irrigations or 80 deg/s for each of the warm irrigations. Jacobson et al. (1993) use the criteria of total cool and warm responses of greater than 99 deg/s and 146 deg/s, respectively, and total caloric response of greater than 221 deg/s from both ears. Again, to account for asymmetric caloric responses and presence of spontaneous nystagmus, one can use total responses from either ear as the criterion for hyperactivity (see Table 13–1).

Normal Limits for Fixation Suppression

The fixation index (FI%) represents the patient's ability to suppress vestibular nystagmus. As with most caloric response parameters, there is no general agreement as to the normal limit for the fixation index. Some studies have suggested any suppression of nystagmus (FI% < 100%) indicates normal fixation suppression (Coats, 1970). In other studies, the normal range includes any value less than 50% (Demanez & Ledoux, 1970). Alpert (1974) recommends a normal limit of less than 60% or 70%. Today, most laboratories use FI% of 60% as the upper limit of normal fixation (Jacobson et al., 1993).

There are a number of problems with the way the fixation index is quantified and its normal limit is established (Schuchman & Uri, 1986). The ability to suppress vestibular nystagmus is age and most likely, gender dependent, but these factors are not considered in the fixation index (Jacobson et al., 1993). Furthermore, to generate a valid fixation suppression test, the optimal nystagmus intensities just before fixation should be approximately 20 to 40 deg/s. If the nystagmus intensities are much higher than the optimal values, even normal subjects may not be able to fully suppress the nystagmus. Conversely, if the nystagmus intensities are much lower than the optimal values, the fixation task may not be challenging enough to reveal abnormalities even in patients with defective fixation suppression. Finally, suppression of vestibular nystagmus is a voluntary task. Therefore, an abnormal fixation index may simply reflect the patient's unwillingness to fixate. Because of these limitations, failure of fixation suppression should be interpreted cautiously.

Age-Related Changes of Caloric Response Parameters

Age-related changes in both peripheral and central vestibular pathways are well documented (e.g., Bergstrom, 1973; Park, Tang, Lopez, & Ishiyama, 2001; Rosenhall, 1973; Tang, Lopez, & Baloh, 2001-2002). However, the effect of aging on many of the caloric response parameters is far less conclusive (Bruner & Norris, 1971). Van der Laan and Oosterveld (1974) reported that total caloric responses increased up to the age of 40 years and then declined with increas-

ing age. Similar findings were reported by Mulch and Petermann (1979) who studied 102 normal subjects between the ages of 11 and 70. Peterka, Black, and Schoenhoff (1990–1991) measured total caloric responses, unilateral weakness, and directional preponderance in 216 healthy individuals between the ages of 7 and 81. They found small age-related changes in these parameters but the differences were not statistically significant. Finally, Mallinson and Longridge (2004) measured the slow-phase velocity of caloric-induced nystagmus and concluded that caloric responses do not decline with age.

Based on the above studies, it is reasonable to assume that the normal limits for unilateral weakness, directional preponderance, and total caloric responses are the same for different age groups. The lack of age-related changes in the caloric response parameters in view of changes in the vestibular structures is most likely due to the fact that age-related changes affect both labyrinths approximately the same way.

One response parameter that does seem to be age dependent is the fixation index (Jacobson & Henry, 1989). It is well known that the ability to suppress vestibular nystagmus declines with age. However, establishing age-adjusted normal limits for the fixation index has proved to be difficult due to the limitations of the fixation suppression test. As a result, the normal limit for the fixation index is applied to all age groups, which as stated earlier, further limits the usefulness of the fixation suppression test.

Establishing Normal Limits for Each Laboratory

Although reasonable agreement has emerged on the normal limits for some of the caloric response parameters, there are significant differences in the estimated values from different studies. These differences are not just because of the inherent variability of caloric responses, but also because of the differences in the equipment, irrigation parameters, statistical analysis methods, and other factors. As a result, there are no universally accepted normal values for the caloric response parameters. Even some organizations such as ANSI that recommend standardized test procedures have avoided addressing the issue of normal limits (ANSI, 2009). Instead, the general recommendation is for each laboratory to establish its own normal limits.

Those who wish to establish their own normal limits must consider a number of key issues. First, to avoid contamination of data, clear criteria must be established as to who can be considered a normal individual and eligible to participate in the study.

Second, most laboratory normal limits are derived based on a small sample of normal individuals, whereas commonly used values are usually based on a much larger sample. Confidence limits that are based on small sample sizes tend to be more variable and may not accurately reflect the true normal limits of the population. An alternative to using locally derived laboratory norms is to compare them with the values listed in Table 13–1. If the differences are not statistically significant, it is more logical to continue using the commonly accepted values to maintain consistency with other laboratories and to avoid errors due to a small sample size.

Finally, the statistical procedures used for analyzing the response parameters must be appropriate for the underlying distribution of the data (see Jacobson et al., 1993, for a review of statistical methods). In particular, most studies use two standard deviations from the mean as the 95% confidence limit for the normal population. This approach is acceptable if the sample size is at least 100 and becomes more accurate once the sample size exceeds 200. Most laboratory norms are established based on a far fewer number of normal individuals (e.g., Van Der Stappen et al., 2000). In those cases, using two standard deviations from the mean underestimates the normal limit even when the requirements for the underlying distribution are met (Glantz, 1997). For example, when the number of study subjects is 40, it is more accurate to use 2.346 times the standard deviation from the mean to establish the normal limit (Lewis, 1966). The reason for this discrepancy is that using two standard deviations assumes that the population standard deviation is known, whereas, in fact, it is estimated from the measured data.

Clinical Significance of Normal Caloric Responses

It is important to recognize that normal caloric test results do not necessarily indicate intact VOR path-

ways. The caloric test is primarily a test of the lateral semicircular canals and their afferent pathways, and it does not adequately evaluate other vestibular structures. Therefore, the caloric test may indicate normal responses, even when there are abnormalities in the vertical semicircular canals, the otolith organs, or their neural pathways.

Furthermore, the range of normal limits for caloric response parameters is large. As a result, subtle abnormalities may not be detected. For example, a unilateral weakness must be greater than 20% to 25% before the caloric test can be classified as abnormal. However, it is not clear what the threshold of asymmetry in the VOR pathways is before the patient begins to experience symptoms. It is likely that the threshold is far less than 20%. In short, a normal caloric test result does not mean normal vestibular function and the patient diagnosis should still be established in the context of history, physical exam, and other diagnostic test findings.

BITHERMAL CALORIC TEST FINDINGS IN PATIENTS

Caloric test findings have been studied in patients with various diseases originating from different parts of the VOR pathways, including the labyrinth, the vestibular nerve, or the central nervous system. Jacobson et al. (1993) have summarized the results of these studies in a comprehensive list of different caloric findings for each disease. It is obvious from these studies that caloric abnormalities cannot identify a specific disease. Instead, they provide information about the function of different structures within the VOR pathways that can be damaged by a number of different pathologies.

In this section, the interpretation and clinical significance of abnormal findings for each of the response parameters are discussed.

Interpretation and Clinical Significance of Unilateral Weakness

An abnormal unilateral caloric weakness exists when the total responses from one ear are significantly weaker than the total responses from the opposite ear (see Figure 12–6). It indicates a lesion involving the lateral (horizontal) semicircular canal or its afferent neural pathways in the weaker ear. This finding is usually considered as the single most clinically useful finding in the ENG test battery. Aside from the benign paroxysmal positional-type nystagmus in the Dix-Hallpike maneuver, an abnormal unilateral weakness is the only finding that localizes the lesion to the peripheral vestibular system (labyrinth or vestibular nerve) and identifies the damaged side.

Several important factors should be considered about the peripheral vestibular lesions and their effect on the unilateral caloric weakness:

1. The finding of unilateral caloric weakness can occur as a result of damage to the hair cells, damage to vestibular nerve fibers, or blockage of the vestibular nerve at the root entry zone to the brainstem (Baloh & Honrubia, 2001). However, unilateral caloric weakness cannot differentiate between damage to the hair cells and damage to the vestibular nerve fibers.

2. Damage to the central vestibular pathways does not seem to produce a unilateral weakness. For example, Uemura and Cohen (1973) found that a focal lesion in the vestibular nuclei of monkeys does not result in a unilateral caloric weakness unless it involves the root entry zone of the eighth nerve.

3. The damage to the hair cells or the nerve fibers has to be confined to one side or at least should affect one side more significantly to produce a unilateral caloric weakness. Conditions that affect both sides approximately equally, such as vestibulotoxicity or aging, do not result in a significant unilateral weakness.

4. The damage must involve the hair cells in the lateral canal or the superior portion of the vestibular nerve to generate a unilateral weakness in the caloric test. Furthermore, the loss of function must be substantial. As noted earlier, at least 30% to 40% of the hair cells in the lateral canal or their nerve fibers have to be damaged for the unilateral caloric weakness to exceed the normative limits.

5. The finding of abnormal unilateral caloric weakness is most common in otological diseases. However, any other type of disease that can damage the hair cells or affect the function of

vestibular nerve can also result in a unilateral weakness in the caloric test.

The underlying cause of hair cell damage can be due to (1) infection, (2) trauma, (3) ischemia affecting the labyrinthine blood supply, and (4) toxic agents. Other causes, such as metabolic disorders are possible but not well understood.

An example of an otological disease that causes hair cell damage and usually results in a unilateral caloric weakness is labyrinthitis. The disease can be due to the primary infection of the labyrinth or secondary to a middle ear disease. The cochlea is also involved as hearing loss is a common feature of labyrinthitis.

An example of trauma-induced unilateral weakness is labyrinthine concussion. The underlying mechanism is usually shock damage to the hair cells but head trauma may also affect the vestibular nerve.

Another example of an otological disease that affects the hair cell function is Ménière's disease and its variations. An abnormal unilateral caloric weakness is a common finding in patients with Ménière's disease, but it is not a required criterion for the diagnosis. The presence and the extent of caloric weakness usually depend on the stage of the disease and the elapsed time since the last attack (Mateijsen et al., 2001). In the early stages of the disease, a unilateral caloric weakness is often present shortly after the onset of the attack but dissipates after a few days or weeks. In the later stages of the disease, the weakness becomes persistent and is often progressive. More information about the caloric test findings at various stages of compensation following a Ménière's attack is provided later in this chapter and also in Chapter 4.

Pathologies that affect the blood supply to the peripheral vestibular structures can also produce a unilateral weakness in the caloric test. The labyrinth receives blood supply through one vessel only and therefore is susceptible to ischemic events. Brief interruptions of the blood supply to the labyrinth can cause reversible damage to the hair cells and result in fluctuating vestibular symptoms. These symptoms can be attributed to etiologies such as migraine, if one accepts the vascular origin of such diseases. If the ischemia persists beyond a few minutes, damage to the hair cells in the affected vestibular structures will become permanent (Baloh & Honrubia, 2001). For example, an infarct of the internal auditory artery will damage both the cochlea and the hair cells in the entire labyrinth and produces test findings that are similar to those of labyrinthitis. Likewise, anterior vestibular artery infarctions damage the hair cells in the lateral and anterior canals and produce caloric test findings that are similar to those produced by the superior nerve vestibular neuritis. When the blood supply disruptions are caused by infarcts and strokes of different kinds, usually the imaging studies can identify the underlying pathology. However, in case of transient ischemic attacks, the imaging studies are often not helpful. In those cases, the only distinguishing factors between vascular and nonvascular origins of vertigo and unilateral caloric weakness are the patient history and the presence or absence of risk factors for cerebrovascular disease.

One of the most common pathologies that produce unilateral caloric weakness is vestibular neuritis. Baloh and Honrubia (2001) have suggested that a complete or near complete loss of unilateral caloric response is more common with vestibular nerve lesions than those affecting the hair cell function. The underlying mechanism is infection of the vestibular nerve. It is now known that there are different types of vestibular neuritis that result in different findings in the caloric test. One type of vestibular neuritis is believed to cause degeneration of vestibular nerve and result in permanent loss of vestibular function (Manzari, Burgess, MacDougall, & Curthoys, 2013). This type of vestibular neuritis results in a unilateral caloric weakness that persists indefinitely. Another type of vestibular neuritis presumably causes inflammation of the vestibular nerve but does not permanently damage it. Once the inflammation subsides, the vestibular function is restored and the unilateral weakness disappears. Finally, recent reports have identified an uncommon form of vestibular neuritis that involves only the inferior branch of the vestibular nerve (Kim & Kim, 2012). This type of neuritis does not produce a caloric weakness and will be missed without another test such as vestibular-evoked myogenic potential (VEMP) testing.

Another example of vestibular nerve pathology that produces unilateral weakness is vestibular schwannoma (acoustic neuroma). The mechanism is the compression of the vestibular nerve by the tumor arising from the schwann cells. Although the diagnosis of vestibular schwannoma is usually made through imaging studies, the caloric test can provide useful information about the proximity of the tumor to the vestibular nerve. Absence or severe reduction of caloric responses along with mild to moderate hearing loss suggests the tumor is impinging the vestibular portion of the eighth nerve more than the auditory portion. The opposite suggests more involvement of the auditory portion of the eighth nerve. This information can help with evaluating the chance of hearing preservation and the prognosis for the severity of postsurgery vertigo symptoms.

Occasionally, central nervous system (CNS) lesions can cause unilateral weakness in the caloric test if they involve the root entry zone of the eighth nerve. For example, approximately 50% of patients with multiple sclerosis experience vestibular symptoms some time during the course of the disease. This is likely due to the demyelization process, which may cause blockage of neural transmission from the vestibular nerve to the central vestibular structures. When the blockage is unilateral, the caloric test will reveal unilateral weakness. One may be able to differentiate between peripheral vestibular and CNS lesions that cause unilateral caloric weakness because the latter usually produce other central findings in the ENG test.

Theoretically, a unilateral caloric weakness can occur as a result of hyperactive responses from the contralateral ear. However, this is extremely rare and on the basis of caloric test results, is virtually indistinguishable from unilateral lesions that damage the ipsilateral ear. Huygen, Nicolasen, Verhagen, and Theunissen (1989) reported 10 such cases in a group of 600 patients. In nine of those patients, there was a hearing loss on the side of weaker caloric responses. They attributed this finding to the loss of commissural inhibition following temporary vestibular decompensation. When observed, the examiner must rule out technical issues such as undetected tympanic membrane perforation, faulty irrigations, or faulty calibrations.

In summary, unilateral caloric weakness is a highly significant finding that can localize the lesion to the labyrinth or the vestibular nerve and further lateralize it to one ear. In the acute stage of the lesion, this finding is usually accompanied by a baseline shift (directional preponderance), which is discussed in the next section.

Interpretation and Clinical Significance of Directional Preponderance

An abnormal directional preponderance exists when nystagmus responses in one direction are significantly stronger than nystagmus responses in the opposite direction. It indicates presence of an asymmetry in the horizontal VOR pathways but provides no localizing information. That is, abnormal directional preponderance can originate from the labyrinths, vestibular nerves, vestibular nuclei, or the CNS.

Early studies attributed directional preponderance to CNS lesions (Fitzgerald & Hallpike, 1942). However, in these studies, what was called directional preponderance was in fact asymmetric fixation suppression because caloric responses were observed with eyes open and in the presence of vision. In later studies, directional preponderance was found in patients with labyrinthine or vestibular nerve lesions as well as in patients with CNS lesions (Baloh, Sills, & Honrubia, 1977; Coats, 1966; Stahle, 1958). Furthermore, directional preponderance has also been reported in normal subjects (Coats, 1965).

As discussed in Chapter 12, directional preponderance consists of two different components: baseline shift and gain asymmetry. Historically, these two components have been interpreted together but clinical implications of directional preponderance can be better explained if they are considered separately.

A baseline shift exists when the patient has preexisting nystagmus in the absence of fixation in the standard caloric test position. The caloric responses are added to the preexisting nystagmus when they are in the same direction and subtracted from it when they are in opposite directions. As a result, even when the caloric-induced responses are equally strong in both directions, the overall nystagmus intensities become greater for the irrigations where the caloric responses are in the direction of the preexisting nystagmus (see Figure 12–8A). This type of directional preponderance is caused by a shift in the baseline of the caloric responses. The amount of baseline shift is equal to the slow-phase velocity of the preexisting nystagmus. This is the more common form of directional preponderance and accounts for approximately 99% of abnormal directional preponderance findings in the caloric test (Halmagyi et al., 2000).

The interpretation of baseline shift is the same as the interpretation of spontaneous or positional nystagmus in the absence of fixation. The nystagmus intensity, as well as the amount of baseline shift, has to be large enough (typically, greater than 4 to 6 deg/s) before it can be considered abnormal. Abnormal baseline shift is a nonlocalizing finding, which indicates an imbalance in the resting neural activity of either the primary vestibular neurons in the peripheral vestibular system or the secondary vestibular neurons in the central vestibular pathways.

Although baseline shift is nonlocalizing, it is frequently present in patients with abnormal unilateral caloric weakness. This is not surprising because unilateral peripheral vestibular lesions result in spontaneous nystagmus with its slow phase typically toward the damaged ear. The nystagmus is most intense initially during the acute phase of the lesion and gradually subsides as the patient undergoes vestibular compensation (see below for more details). Therefore, a finding of abnormal unilateral caloric weakness and baseline shift in the direction of the weaker ear is consistent with an uncompensated peripheral vestibular lesion on the side of the weaker ear (Figure 13–1).

On rare occasions, nystagmus following a unilateral peripheral vestibular lesion beats toward the damaged side, and as a result, the baseline shift is in the opposite direction of the weaker ear. In patients with Ménière's disease, this finding is due to *recovery nystagmus* (Jacobson, Pearlstein, Henderson, Calder, & Rock, 1998). A few non-Ménière's patients also exhibit this phenomenon. In that case, the risk factors for cerebrovascular diseases should be considered. It is plausible that the disruption of blood supply in these patients can affect multiple sites within the VOR pathways thus causing unilateral caloric weakness due to the loss of peripheral vestibular function and nystagmus due to the damage to central structures. However, other explanations are possible (see Chapter 4).

A gain asymmetry exists when caloric responses are truly stronger in one direction without any preexisting nystagmus (see Figure 12–8B). Baloh and Honrubia (2001) have suggested that such an abnormality is likely to be caused by a central lesion. However, Halmagyi et al. (2000) found evidence of CNS lesions in only 5% of patients with abnormal gain asymmetry. Instead, about half of the patients

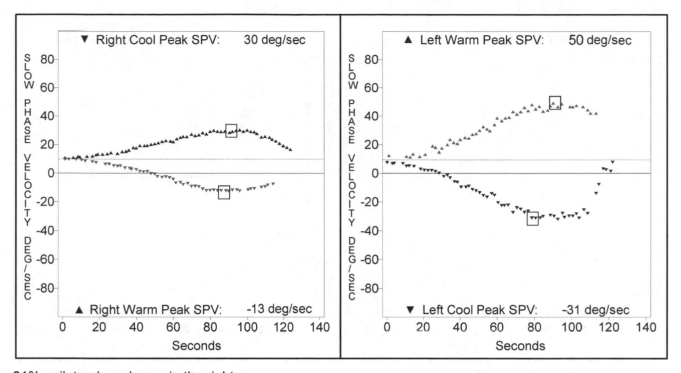

31% unilateral weakness in the right ear
29% directional preponderance to the left (10 deg/sec baseline to the right +3% gain asymmetry to the right)

Figure 13-1. Caloric responses of a patient with a significant unilateral weakness and a significant baseline shift toward the weaker ear. Note that the directional preponderance and gain asymmetry are expressed with respect to the direction of nystagmus fast phases and the baseline shift is expressed with respect to the direction of nystagmus slow phases.

had either benign paroxysmal positioning vertigo or Ménière's disease. For the rest of these patients, no definitive diagnosis could be established. Halmagyi and his associates stated that gain asymmetry is a benign and transient abnormality. In a companion paper, they attributed gain asymmetry to an increase in the dynamic response of the medial vestibular nucleus brought on by intermittent hyperactivity of primary vestibular neurons (Cartwright, Cremer, Halmagyi, & Curthoys, 2000).

Gain asymmetry is an extremely rare finding. Therefore, one must be cautious to rule out technical errors. When confirmed, gain asymmetry still does not provide definitive localizing information (Halmagyi et al., 2000).

Overall, the clinical value of directional preponderance is marginal. It can originate from the labyrinths, vestibular nerves, central vestibular structures, or the CNS. As noted, because of its limited usefulness, some laboratories do not include direc-

tional preponderance in the interpretation of the caloric test. When the baseline shift is the underlying cause of abnormal directional preponderance and accompanied by a unilateral caloric weakness, it can help the examiner to determine the level of compensation after a unilateral peripheral vestibular lesion.

Interpretation and Clinical Significance of Bilateral Weakness

An abnormal bilateral weakness exists when total caloric responses from both ears are absent or markedly weak (Figure 13–2). This finding is far less common than an abnormal unilateral caloric weakness and does not always indicate bilateral loss of vestibular function. Because of the possibility of inadequate heat transfer to the labyrinth, inadequate patient alertness, or suppression of caloric responses by medications, an additional test is needed to confirm

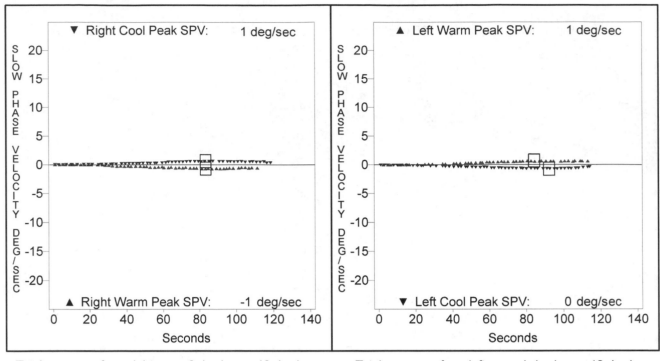

Total response from right ear = 2 deg/sec < 12 deg/sec   Total response from left ear = 1 deg/sec < 12 deg/sec

Figure 13–2. Caloric responses of a patient with a significant bilateral caloric weakness.

the presence of bilateral vestibular hypoactivity (Furman & Kamerer, 1989; Stockwell, 1993).

The most effective procedure for confirming bilateral vestibular hypoactivity is either by using the rotation chair test or by using the head impulse test (Jacobson & Newman, 1991; Petersen, Straumann, & Weber, 2013). There are three possible outcomes in rotation testing for patients who have bilateral weakness in the caloric testing (Baloh, Sills, & Honrubia, 1979). The finding of below normal gains for all rotation frequencies confirms total bilateral loss of horizontal vestibular function. The finding of abnormal gains in low frequencies only (0.01 to 0.05 Hz) suggests a partial loss of horizontal VOR. The gain in very low frequencies (0.01 and 0.02 Hz) is better correlated with the presence of bilateral caloric weakness compared to the gain at higher frequencies (Myers, 1992). Finally, the finding of normal gain in all frequencies indicates normal horizontal VOR and most likely, faulty caloric irrigations or lack of patient alertness.

Another alternative to rotation testing for confirming bilateral vestibular hypoactivity is the head impulse test (Halmagyi, 2005). Patients with bilateral vestibular hypoactivity are expected to have corrective refixation saccades to both right and left head impulses.

When rotation or head impulse testing is not available, bilateral ice water testing can be used as a last resort to confirm presence of bilateral vestibular hypoactivity (Stockwell, 1993). If ice water, which is a stronger stimulus than standard caloric stimuli, generates a strong response from one or both ears, the vestibular function is not likely to be bilaterally hypoactive. On the other hand, absent or weak responses to ice water indicate total or partial loss of bilateral vestibular function, respectively.

The most common symptom in patients with bilateral vestibular hypoactivity, also called Dandy's syndrome, is unsteadiness. Some patients also complain of oscillopsia and even episodic vertigo. Hearing loss is present in some but not all patients (Vibert, Liard, & Hausler, 1995). Compensation after a bilateral vestibular lesion is limited, and the patients are more likely to have impaired balance indefinitely (Telian, Shepard, Smith-Wheelock, & Hoberg, 1991; Vibert et al., 1995).

Bilateral loss of vestibular function has been associated with several etiologies originating from both peripheral and central vestibular pathways (Simmons, 1973). However, in many cases the cause is unknown (Baloh, Jacobson, & Honrubia, 1989; Sargent, Goebel, Hanson, & Beck, 1997). The most common pathology of a peripheral origin is vestibulotoxicity (Brandt, 1996). Infections that affect the labyrinths or vestibular nerves, such as bilateral vestibular neuritis, meningitis, or chronic otitis media, can also cause bilateral vestibular hypoactivity (Telian et al., 1991). Other causes include bilateral Ménière's disease and congenital malformations (Honrubia et al., 1985). Bilateral loss of vestibular responses can also be due to central pathologies such as cerebellar degeneration and tumors (Rinne, Bronstein, Rudge, Gresty, & Luxon, 1995). Head trauma, vascular diseases, and autoimmune diseases have also been reported as possible causes for bilateral loss of vestibular function (Syms, & House, 1997).

Occasionally, bilateral caloric weakness is accompanied by a baseline shift (Figure 13–3), indicating presence of spontaneous nystagmus (Stockwell, 1993). This could mean that although responses from both ears are weak, one ear is less responsive than the other. Thus, the baseline shift in such cases is similar to that seen in unilateral lesions. However, the baseline shift can be an unrelated lesion affecting other parts of the VOR pathways.

Some patients with a defective saccadic system have an unusual caloric test result that mimics bilateral caloric weakness. Caloric irrigations in these patients generate nystagmus slow phases in the appropriate direction (Yokota et al., 1991). However, because of the saccadic impairment, nystagmus fast phases are not activated and the eyes remain deviated to one side. This type of abnormality can be detected during the saccade test. In that case, the absence of caloric nystagmus should not be misinterpreted as bilateral caloric weakness. If these patients are asked to fixate, nystagmus responses may appear because fixation redirects the eyes to the center gaze. Again, this should not be misinterpreted as failure of fixation suppression discussed below (Jacobson et al., 1993).

Overall, the finding of bilateral caloric weakness is of moderate clinical value. It is important to first determine if the finding is in fact due to bilateral

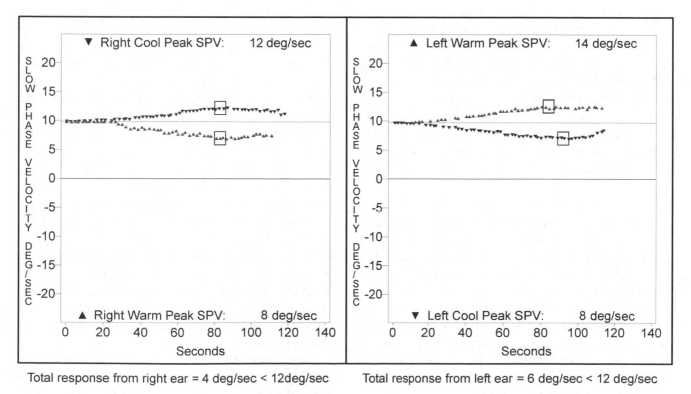

Total response from right ear = 4 deg/sec < 12deg/sec   Total response from left ear = 6 deg/sec < 12 deg/sec

10 deg/sec baseline shift to the right

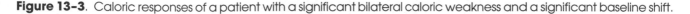

Figure 13–3. Caloric responses of a patient with a significant bilateral caloric weakness and a significant baseline shift.

loss of vestibular function. If so, it indicates bilateral lesion of the lateral semicircular canals, their afferent pathways, or the CNS.

Interpretation and Clinical Significance of Hyperactive Responses

Caloric hyperactivity exists when total responses from one or both ears exceed the normal limit. It is a rare finding and the examiner must make sure that it is not due to technical errors or artifacts. For example, heat transfer from the external auditory canal to the labyrinth can be enhanced in patients with a tympanic membrane perforation or with an open or altered mastoid (Barber & Stockwell, 1980).

Occasionally, one caloric irrigation can produce very strong responses due to overalertness of the patient or presence of strong preexisting nystagmus. Using total caloric responses from each ear as the criterion for abnormality eliminates the possibility of falsely identifying such responses as hyperactive. Faulty calibrations can also produce responses that may appear hyperactive. As noted in Chapter 12, there have been anecdotal reports about some patients generating unusually strong responses for one of the warm irrigations, which are reproducible and do not resolve after repeating the appropriate irrigations. This finding has been associated with the diagnosis of migraine-associated vertigo but currently there are no studies to confirm this association. Until such studies become available, it is best to treat these cases as technical errors but make a note when the recommended procedures fail to resolve the error.

Once technical errors are ruled out, hyperactive caloric responses indicate a central lesion most likely caused by the loss of VOR inhibitory function at the vestibular nuclei. Baloh, Konrad, and Honrubia (1975) have demonstrated high incidence of hyperresponsive calorics in patients with cerebellar atrophy. Animal studies are consistent with the notion that lesions of the cerebellar nodulus produce hyperactive caloric responses (Fredrickson & Fernandez, 1964). However, the results should be interpreted cautiously because the responses were recorded without eliminating vision.

Caloric hyperactivity is usually bilateral but there are reports of patients with hyperactive responses from one ear only (Ikeda & Watanabe, 1997). Such a finding could be due to technical errors noted above. It is also possible that the patient may have two different lesions: a central lesion involving the vestibular nuclei that produces hyperactive responses and a peripheral vestibular lesion involving the weaker ear. Finally, it is possible, but unlikely, that unilateral caloric hyperactivity can be caused by a peripheral vestibular lesion on the hyperactive side (Huygen et al., 1989; Kimm & Donaldson, 1980).

Overall, clinical value of caloric hyperactivity is moderate because the results can be contaminated by technical errors. The finding indicates a central lesion most likely involving the cerebellum.

Interpretation and Clinical Significance of Failure of Fixation Suppression

Failure of fixation suppression exists when the intensity of caloric nystagmus is not sufficiently reduced by fixation (Figure 13–4). It indicates a central lesion involving the parietal-occipital cortex, the pons, or the cerebellum. However, failure of fixation suppression is most common with lesions of the midline cerebellum (Baloh & Honrubia, 2001).

The fixation suppression test examines the interaction of visual and vestibular pathways. There is strong evidence that *the smooth pursuit system* is involved in suppressing vestibular nystagmus (Chambers & Gresty, 1982; Halmagyi, & Gresty, 1979). The pursuit system makes it possible to track a small moving target by keeping its image on the fovea (the most sensitive part of retina). When a target moves across the retina, it causes *retinal slip*, which triggers the pursuit system to move the eyes in a way that minimizes the retinal slip and keeps the target image on the fovea. When a patient is asked to fixate on a stationary target during the caloric test, the slow phase of nystagmus causes the target image to move across the retina and generate retinal slip. The pursuit system will move the eyes in the opposite direction of nystagmus slow phases and suppress the nystagmus.

If the role of the smooth pursuit system in suppressing caloric nystagmus is accepted, one would expect the findings in the fixation suppression test to mimic those of the tracking test, essentially making the fixation test redundant (Barnes, Benson, & Prior,

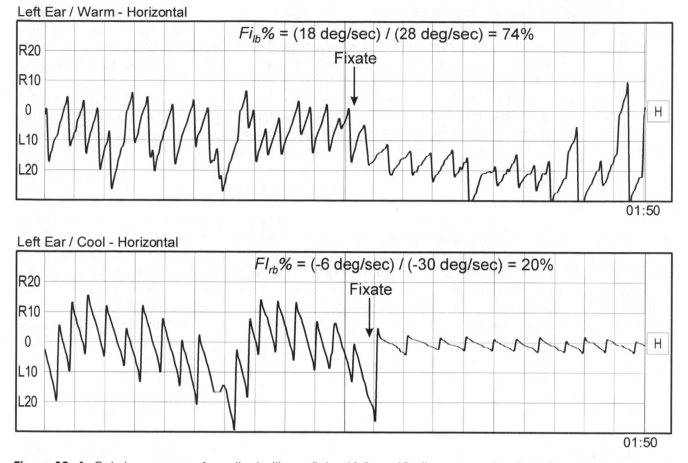

Figure 13–4. Caloric responses of a patient with a unilateral failure of fixation suppression (for left-beating nystagmus).

1978). For example, patients with defective pursuit for rightward target movements often have failure of fixation suppression for caloric irrigations that generate left-beating nystagmus. Other investigators have argued that a distinct mechanism—*vestibular cancellation*—is primarily responsible for fixation suppression (e.g., Tomlinson & Robinson, 1981). In their view, the vestibular cancellation system reduces nystagmus intensity and then the pursuit system eliminates the residual nystagmus once the target image is placed near the fovea. If this view is accepted, the fixation suppression test is not redundant and its findings may not always match those of the tracking test.

A number of studies have demonstrated close association between impaired fixation suppression and abnormal smooth pursuit (e.g., Halmagyi, & Gresty, 1979). Other studies have shown the findings in the fixation suppression test and the tracking test do not always match (e.g., Barin & Davis, 2003). However, these studies do not prove involvement

of another mechanism besides the smooth pursuit system in suppressing caloric nystagmus. They may simply reflect the differences in the test procedures for the tracking and fixation suppression tests. Although fixation suppression and smooth pursuit mechanisms appear to be closely associated, based on the above discussion, the fixation suppression test does not seem to be redundant. In rare cases, there are patients with normal smooth pursuit systems who fail to adequately suppress vestibular nystagmus, and vice versa.

The pathways that mediate fixation suppression of vestibular nystagmus reside in different sites within the CNS. As a result, many different etiologies of central origin can cause failure of fixation suppression. Bilateral cases are usually associated with diffuse lesions such as cerebellar degeneration, whereas unilateral cases are usually associated with more focal lesions such as cerebellopontine angle tumors (Jacobson et al., 1993).

Overall, failure of fixation suppression is a moderately significant finding that indicates a central lesion, often involving the cerebellar flocculus or the surrounding structures. The fixation test is a simple test to administer and can sometimes detect oculomotor abnormalities that are not identified in other parts of ENG. There are some limitations associated with the fixation test that affect its usefulness and require more careful interpretation of the results.

Rare Abnormalities in Caloric Testing

This section describes a number of highly unusual and rare findings that have been reported in the caloric test. Most of these reports date back to the time before sophisticated test equipment became available and before our understanding of the underlying physiology had evolved. There have been no convincing cases of such abnormalities in recent years. This raises the possibility of technical issues with at least some of these findings. Because these findings are extremely rare, the examiner must assume a technical error unless proven otherwise.

Caloric Inversion

Caloric inversion exists when *all four* irrigations produce responses that beat opposite of the expected direction (Barber & Stockwell, 1980). This type of finding has been associated with posterior fossa lesions but there are other more plausible explanations.

If the direction of nystagmus is reversed for only one or two irrigations, the caloric test should not be considered inverted. Such cases usually occur when there is a strong preexisting nystagmus and caloric responses from one or both ears are weak. For example, in Figure 13–3, all four irrigations produce left-beating nystagmus, which means right warm and left cool nystagmus responses are beating opposite of the expected direction. This is clearly not a case of caloric inversion, and it is caused by the presence of strong preexisting left-beating nystagmus and bilaterally weak caloric responses.

If the nystagmus direction is reversed only when using warm air as caloric stimulus, the examiner should consider the possibility of residual moisture or tympanic membrane perforation in the irrigated ear. The cause of this finding was described in Chapter 12.

Finally, there are other technical errors that can produce an apparent caloric inversion. Some of these errors are difficult to detect. For example, if the right and left electrodes are reversed or if the polarity of the eye movement amplifier is switched, all four irrigations will appear to beat opposite of the expected direction. The examiner must consider this possibility and make sure that the direction of eye movements are recorded correctly.

Caloric Perversion

Caloric perversion exists when irrigations produce *purely* vertical nystagmus (Barber & Stockwell, 1980). Some authors also consider the caloric responses to be perverted if the nystagmus intensity for the vertical component is stronger than the nystagmus intensity for the horizontal component (Elidan, Gay, & Lev, 1985; Jacobson et al., 1993). It should be noted that the finding of vertical nystagmus in caloric testing does not always indicate an abnormality unless one of the above conditions is met (Barber & Stoyanoff, 1986).

Animal studies have demonstrated that focal lesions of vestibular nuclei can produce caloric perversion (Uemura & Cohen, 1973). This finding has been attributed to the disruption of the interconnecting fibers in the vestibular commissure. In humans, caloric-induced vertical nystagmus has been reported in diseases of both peripheral and central vestibular pathways as well as in normal individuals (Aw, Haslwanter, Fetter, Heimberger, & Todd, 1998; Norre, 1987; Toupet, & Pialoux, 1981).

Early studies of caloric perversion were based on ENG recordings. Vertical eye movements are difficult to measure in ENG because of noisy tracings and eye blink artifacts. On the other hand, in VNG, the accuracy and signal-to-noise ratio for vertical eye movements are nearly as good as those for horizontal eye movements. With more widespread use of VNG, it has become clear that caloric-induced responses from the vertical semicircular canals are common in both normal and patient populations (Fetter, Aw, Haslwanter, Heimberger, & Dichgans, 1998). As a result, in some patients, the concept of caloric perversion as a separate and distinct abnormality must be reevaluated. For example, a patient with a focal damage to the lateral semicircular canal but intact anterior and posterior semicircular canals may generate purely vertical nystagmus in caloric testing (Norre, 1987). Identifying this abnormality as caloric perversion is questionable because it misses the more plausible finding of caloric weakness and the possible need for rotation or ice water testing to confirm the extent of loss.

Premature Caloric Reversal

Caloric responses usually dissipate about 3 min after the onset of irrigation. At the end of this period, occasionally, a weak nystagmus reappears but this time, beating in the opposite direction. This finding, called *caloric reversal*, is more common when irrigations produce strong responses. Caloric reversal has been attributed to the central compensation mechanisms although it is more likely due to the cupula overshooting the resting position and bending in the opposite direction.

Barber and Stockwell (1980) have described an abnormality in which the caloric reversal occurs much earlier than anticipated. They attribute this abnormality, called *premature caloric reversal*, to lesions of the cerebellar system. Jacobson et al. (1993) suggest overadaptation in the vestibular nuclei from one side following a vestibular lesion can cause this abnormality. So far, premature caloric reversal has been reported in a handful of patients (Monday, Lemieux, St Vincent, & Barbeau, 1978; Monday, Lesperance, Lemieux, & Saint-Vincent, 1984). Most of these patients suffered from Friedreich's ataxia.

For a true premature caloric reversal, Barber and Stockwell (1980) require the nystagmus direction to change no later than 140 s from the onset of the irrigation, the intensity of the secondary nystagmus to be greater than 6 to 7 deg/s, and the tympanic membrane to be intact. The last requirement is to prevent misinterpretation of warm air caloric responses in an ear with tympanic membrane perforation as premature caloric reversal. As discussed in Chapter 12, warm air irrigations in the presence of tympanic membrane perforation or moisture can cause nystagmus to beat opposite of the expected direction initially and then reverse direction shortly after. Perhaps, complete dissipation of the nystagmus after the reversal should be added to the criteria proposed by Barber and Stockwell (1980) for premature caloric reversal. The reason is that an apparent premature caloric reversal can occur for some irrigations if there is preexisting nystagmus in the caloric test position (Figure 13–5). Sometimes the presence of this nystagmus is missed due to lack of adequate alertness and other technical issues.

After careful review of the reported cases of premature caloric reversal and its underlying mechanism, there is reasonable doubt about the existence of such a finding as a distinct clinical abnormality. In almost all cases, there is a simpler and more logical explanation for the finding. For example, Kim, Lee, Yi, and Baloh (2012) have recently presented the case of a patient with a tumor of the fourth ventricular who demonstrated an apparent premature caloric reversal. However, there are a number of methodological issues that cast serious doubt on the validity of this finding. First, the recording and analysis

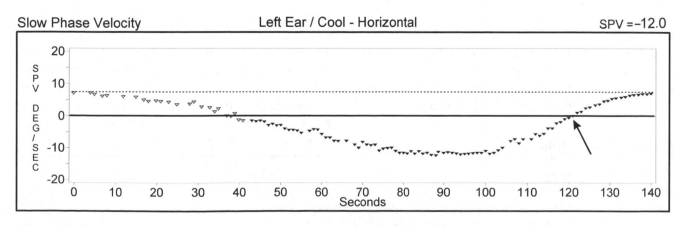

Figure 13–5. Responses of a patient with a caloric reversal (*identified by arrow*) caused by the presence of spontaneous nystagmus. This should not be confused with premature caloric reversal. As alerting usually starts at the end of irrigation, the initial part of the response (*gray triangles*) may be missed.

of caloric responses start 20 s after the end of the irrigation (Figure 13–6). As a result, the opportunity to verify presence or absence of preexisting nystagmus at the onset of the irrigation is lost. Second, only monothermal cool caloric testing is performed despite the fact that the patient has gaze-evoked nystagmus. In addition, when there is an unusual finding such as this one, it is mandatory to perform a full caloric test to verify if the premature reversal occurs for both temperatures. Although it is reported that the patient has no spontaneous nystagmus and despite the methodological issues, the caloric responses in Figure 13–6 are consistent with the presence of right-beating spontaneous nystagmus with the approximate intensity of 10 to 15 deg/s. This nystagmus is seen at the end of both right and left caloric responses and it persists until the recordings stop. If this was a true case of premature caloric reversal, the nystagmus should have dissipated or at least started to decline, which is not the case here. As noted, this nystagmus may be missed for various reasons during the spontaneous nystagmus or the static position test.

The patient is also reported to have perverted caloric nystagmus during the cool irrigation of the left ear. This conclusion is also doubtful because the vertical nystagmus during the right cool irrigation does not seem to be strong. Overall, the caloric test in this patient can be interpreted based on the common findings of mild left unilateral weakness and baseline shift (based the monothermal caloric results in the presence of right-beating spontaneous nystagmus). The weakness in the left ear should be confirmed by performing the bithermal caloric test. Based on the available data, the caloric test in this patient does not necessarily indicate a central lesion, and the results seem to be unrelated to the fourth ventricular tumor. However, the presence of gaze-evoked nystagmus should have provided ample evidence for considering a central pathology.

Caloric Dysrhythmia

Caloric dysrhythmia refers to a condition where there is considerable beat-to-beat variability in the amplitude, frequency, or the velocity of nystagmus (Proctor & Lam, 2002). In some cases, caloric-induced nystagmus may cease entirely for short periods of time before reappearing. The cerebellum is involved

in regulating the characteristic of nystagmus and, therefore, has been implicated in caloric dysrhythmia (Baloh & Honrubia, 2001). However, a number of studies have demonstrated presence of this condition in normal individuals (e.g., Mehra, 1964). As a result, the diagnostic value of caloric dysrhythmia is minimal.

Caloric dysrhythmia has been linked to fatigue and inattention (Baloh & Honrubia, 2001). A recent study by Proctor and Lam (2002) suggests that dysrhythmia is specific to certain individuals and does not improve by more vigorous alerting. They also report that it is a prevalent condition affecting 40% of the patients undergoing caloric testing.

When it is severe, dysrhythmia can interfere with accurate analysis of caloric responses. Specifically, automated computer algorithms are often incapable of differentiating between regular and irregular beats. That is the main reason for manually inspecting the nystagmus slow-phase velocity profile and making changes when necessary (see Chapter 12).

Direction of gaze may be an important factor in caloric dysrhythmia. For example, Alexander's law states that the intensity of vestibular nystagmus increases when gaze is directed toward the fast phases. More widespread use of VNG should allow for monitoring and controlling the gaze direction during the caloric test.

Caloric Test Findings During Vestibular Compensation

Vestibular pathways undergo compensatory changes following a unilateral lesion in the peripheral vestibular system (Curthoys, 2000; Zee 2000). Although the test-retest variability of the caloric test does not make it an ideal tool for serial testing, important information can be gained by recognizing how the caloric test findings change at different stages of vestibular compensation (Proctor & Glackin, 1985). A brief discussion of vestibular compensation and its effect on the caloric test findings will be presented here. More information on this topic can be found in Chapter 4.

Immediately after a lesion that involves the lateral canal or the superior portion of the vestibular nerve, the resting neural activity from the damaged

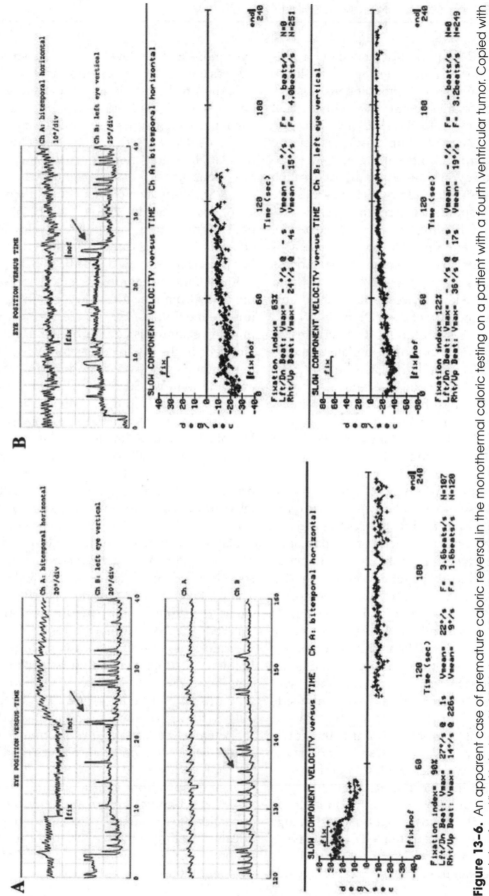

Figure 13–6. An apparent case of premature caloric reversal in the monothermal caloric testing on a patient with a fourth ventricular tumor. Copied with permission from Kim, H. A., Lee, H., Yi, H. A., and Baloh, R. W. (2012). Unusual caloric responses in a patient with a fourth ventricular ependymoma. *Neurological Sciences: Official Journal of the Italian Neurological Society and of the Italian Society of Clinical Neurophysiology, 33*(2), 383–385.

side declines and the caloric test will show a unilateral weakness on the side of lesion. In addition, the patient will have strong spontaneous nystagmus without fixation most commonly with the fast phases beating away from the side of lesion. The nystagmus at this stage of compensation is usually so strong that it cannot be fully suppressed with fixation. The caloric test will show a significant baseline shift toward the side of lesion, which signifies the presence of strong spontaneous nystagmus.

Within hours following the onset of the lesion, vestibular compensation mechanisms become activated. The first step in the compensation process involves *clamping* of the resting neural activity from the intact side at the level of vestibular nuclei. This will reduce the asymmetry of the VOR pathway and improve the patient's symptoms. The caloric test at this stage will continue to show a unilateral weakness on the side of lesion and a baseline shift. The baseline shift should be less intense compared to the earlier stage. Sometimes the clamping of the intact side is so severe that the caloric responses will be weak bilaterally (Stockwell & Graham, 1988). For these cases, bilateral vestibular loss is confined to low frequencies and should quickly convert to a unilateral caloric weakness within few days.

Over the course of several days, the clamping of the intact side is reduced as the resting activity is restored to the vestibular nuclei of the damaged side. As a result, the intensity of the spontaneous nystagmus, as well as the level of baseline shift in the caloric test, will decline accordingly. This process continues until *static compensation* is achieved. At this stage, there will be minimal spontaneous nystagmus and baseline shift. The patient's symptoms will be reduced also as long as the head remains stationary. Throughout this process, the caloric test will continue to show unilateral weakness on the side of lesion.

The process of compensation and the corresponding findings in the caloric test are mostly the same regardless of whether the lesion occurs suddenly, as in labyrinthitis or trauma, or gradually, as in vestibular schwannoma. The only difference is that when the vestibular loss is gradual, the change in the level of asymmetry in the VOR pathways is incremental. As a result, the severity of the patient's symptoms as well as the intensity of spontaneous nystagmus and the level of baseline shift are not as large as those at the onset of a sudden vestibular loss.

The process of static compensation described above is for stable lesions. For fluctuating lesions, such as Ménière's disease, the compensation process is usually altered, which affects the caloric test results. There are a few reports of vestibular testing at various stages of Ménière's disease (e.g., Meissner, 1981; Nishikawa & Nishikawa, 1986; Watanabe, 1996). For example, Watanabe (1996) recorded a patient's nystagmus immediately following an acute attack of Ménière's disease. Initially, the nystagmus fast phases were toward the affected side but within a minute, the nystagmus reversed and began beating away from the side of lesion. Bance, Mai, Tomlinson, and Rutka (1991) have postulated that the initial nystagmus is caused by the excitation of the hair cells in the involved ear following the rupture of membranous labyrinth and mixing of perilymph and endolymph. Subsequently, the neural firing from the hair cells in the involved ear declines and the nystagmus direction becomes consistent with the loss of labyrinthine function in that ear. At this time, the compensation process proceeds to the clamping stage as described before. If the rupture of the membrane heals and function is restored to the damage labyrinth during the clamping stage, the asymmetry in the VOR pathways will be reversed and the nystagmus will now beat toward the side of lesion. This nystagmus is called *recovery nystagmus* (Jacobson et al., 1998; McClure, Copp, & Lycett, 1981). The nystagmus will disappear or change direction again depending on how the compensation process proceeds. Based on this discussion, it is clear that the caloric test findings can vary in patients with Ménière's disease depending on the stage and the long-term course of the disease. A caloric weakness may or may not be present and the baseline shift may be toward or away from the affected side.

Finally, the last stage of vestibular compensation, *dynamic compensation*, involves reprogramming the VOR pathways to deal with the long-term effect of losing input from one labyrinth. Unfortunately, caloric test findings before and after dynamic compensation are the same. This is one of the limitations of caloric testing, which can identify and lateralize a lesion but cannot determine the level of functional compensation.

INTERPRETATION OF
ICE WATER CALORIC TEST

As described in Chapter 12, the ice water caloric test is performed when there is no clearly identifiable response to standard caloric irrigations. If there is spontaneous nystagmus, the test should be performed in both supine and prone positions (Proctor, 1992). This will allow the examiner to differentiate between caloric-induced responses and changes in the intensity of spontaneous nystagmus. Some lab-

oratories perform the ice water test in both supine and prone positions regardless of whether or not there is any preexisting nystagmus. This prevents misidentifying a latent form of spontaneous nystagmus, referred to as *pseudonystagmus*, as caloric nystagmus (Greisen, 1972).

Ice water caloric responses are typically analyzed qualitatively and classified as absent, weak, or strong (normal). Figure 13–7 shows these three types of responses for ice water caloric testing in the supine position. In Figure 13–7A, no nystagmus is generated in response to ice water. This result represents total

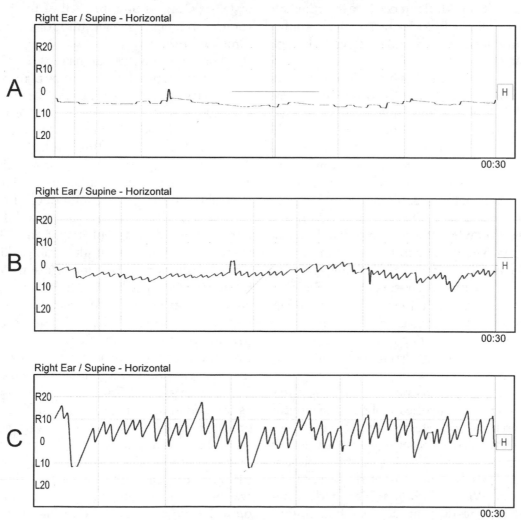

Figure 13–7. Three types of responses to ice water caloric testing in the supine position from different patients. **A.** Absent response. **B.** Weak response. **C.** Strong response. All three patients failed to generate a response to standard caloric stimuli.

loss of lateral semicircular canal or its afferent neural pathways. The patient in Figure 13–7B generates a weak response (~5 deg/s) to ice water. As there is no preexisting nystagmus, the results indicate residual function in the irrigated ear. If there is any question about the presence or absence of preexisting nystagmus, the test should be performed in the prone position also (see below). Finally, on rare occasions, strong nystagmus is generated in response to ice water (Figure 13–7C). This indicates that the standard caloric test has been faulty and the patient has adequate caloric responses from the irrigated ear.

Currently, there are no guidelines about the intensity of ice water-induced nystagmus for classifying the response as weak or strong. However, the decision is usually not difficult because intermediate responses are unlikely. That is, the response is either very strong (typically >20 deg/s) or very weak (typically <10 deg/s).

Figure 13–8 shows three types of responses for ice water caloric testing in both supine and prone positions. All three patients have preexisting nystagmus. In Figure 13–8A, the nystagmus direction for supine and prone positions is the same. This indicates absent response to ice water and is consistent with total loss of lateral semicircular canal or its afferent neural pathways. In Figure 13–8B, weak nystagmus is present in the supine position and changes direction when the patient is placed in the prone position. The change in the direction of nystagmus indicates that there is an ice water–induced caloric response, which is consistent with the presence of residual function in the irrigated ear. In Figure 13–8C, strong nystagmus is present in the supine position and changes direction in the prone position. Again, this indicates faulty irrigations in the standard caloric test.

As indicated before, absence of caloric responses, even to ice water, does not mean total loss of labyrinthine function because the test is limited to the lateral semicircular canal. Also, because caloric irrigations are low-frequency stimuli, it is possible, although unlikely, that a patient with absent responses to ice water may have VOR function at high frequencies. Finally, ice water testing can be done bilaterally if responses to standard caloric testing are absent from both ears. However, as discussed earlier, bilateral ice water caloric testing should be used only when rotational or head impulse testing is not available.

INTERPRETATION OF SIMULTANEOUS CALORIC TEST

The simultaneous caloric test has been proposed as an adjunct to the standard caloric test (Brookler, 1971). Brookler (1976) has suggested that the two tests together are more sensitive in identifying vestibular abnormalities.

In the simultaneous caloric test, both ears are irrigated simultaneously with either cool or warm temperatures. The responses are evaluated qualitatively based on the presence and direction of nystagmus. There are three possible outcomes for each irrigation—no nystagmus, right-beating nystagmus, or left-beating nystagmus. All of the possible outcomes can be categorized into four different types (Brookler, 1976).

For Type I, no nystagmus is generated for either warm or cool irrigations. This type of response occurs in normal subjects as well as patients with bilaterally hypoactive or hyperactive caloric responses. The results from the standard caloric test must be used to differentiate among the three different possibilities. According to Brookler (1976), most patients with a Type I response in the simultaneous caloric test have normal responses in the standard caloric test.

For Type II, nystagmus beats in different directions for warm and cool irrigations. This type of response is similar to unilateral weakness in the standard caloric test. The side of lesion is determined by the nystagmus direction following the cool irrigation (or opposite of the nystagmus direction following the warm irrigation). The reason is that cool irrigations generate inhibitory responses from both ears. If one ear is hypoactive, the neural activity in that ear will not be inhibited as much as it will be from the intact ear. This will cause an asymmetry as the neural activity from the affected ear will be greater than the neural activity from the intact ear. As a result, nystagmus will be generated with its fast phases beating toward the ear with stronger neural firing, in this case, the hypoactive side. Similarly, warm irrigations will generate an asymmetry in the opposite direction and the nystagmus fast phases will beat away from the hypoactive side. In a study by Brookler (1976), 60% of the patients with a Type II response in the simultaneous caloric test had normal responses in the standard caloric test. However,

Ice Water Caloric Test

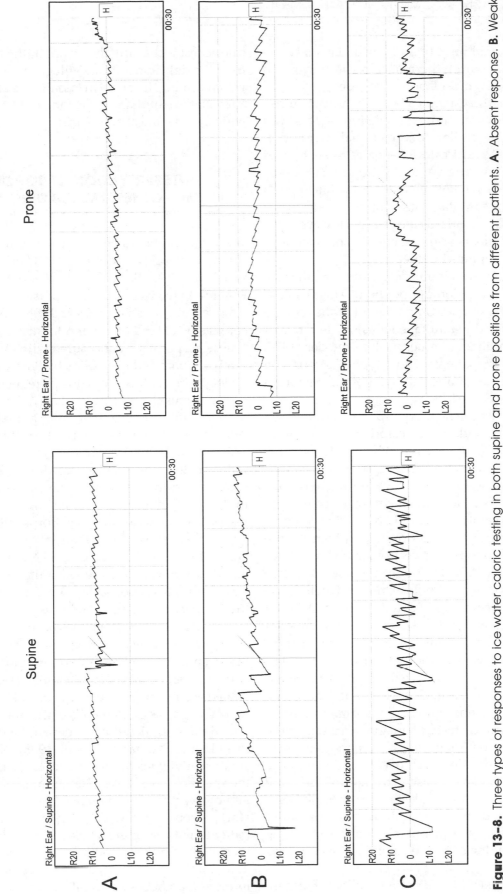

Figure 13–8. Three types of responses to ice water caloric testing in both supine and prone positions from different patients. **A.** Absent response. **B.** Weak response. **C.** Strong response. All three patients had left-beating spontaneous nystagmus (right baseline shift) and all failed to generate a response to standard caloric stimuli.

he used a normal limit of 30% for unilateral weakness in the standard bithermal caloric test, which is higher than what most laboratories use.

For Type III, nystagmus beats in the same direction for both warm and cool irrigations. This type of response is similar to directional preponderance in the standard caloric test and as such, does not have a localizing value. In the same study by Brookler (1976), 80% of the patients with a Type III response in the simultaneous caloric test had normal responses in the standard caloric test. However, 58% of the same patients also had either spontaneous or positional nystagmus in ENG.

For Type IV, nystagmus is present for either the warm or cool irrigation but not both. This is a nonspecific finding that encompasses all of the remaining outcomes in the simultaneous caloric test. It does not have a localizing value. In the Brookler (1976) study, 77% of the patients with a Type IV response in the simultaneous caloric test had normal responses in the standard caloric test.

There have been no randomized case-controlled studies of the simultaneous caloric test. One study by Brookler (1976) that was cited here included 1,180 patients who underwent both standard and simultaneous caloric testing. Based on the above results, Brookler and his colleagues have suggested that the simultaneous caloric test should be used in conjunction with the standard caloric test to increase the sensitivity of identifying vestibular abnormalities (Brookler, 1976, 2002; Hoffman, Brookler, & Baker, 1979). However, one should consider whether the two tests were compared fairly (Wetmore, 1986). In the simultaneous caloric test, any nystagmus, even weak nystagmus, is considered abnormal. This is equivalent to lowering the normal limit of unilateral weakness and directional preponderance for the standard caloric test. If we do so, patients in the Brookler (1976) study who had a normal finding in the standard caloric test but an abnormal one in the simultaneous one, may now have abnormal findings in both tests. However, one should expect the false-positive rate to increase as the normal limits are lowered. Furman, Wall, and Kamerer (1988) systematically changed the normal limits and compared the simultaneous and standard caloric tests. They concluded that the standard caloric test was indeed superior in distinguishing between normal individuals and patients with VOR abnormalities (Furman, 1989). The main disadvantage of the simultaneous caloric test is that any difference in the heat transfer from the right and left ears will generate nystagmus, which can be mistakenly classified as abnormal. As a result, the simultaneous caloric test has not gained widespread clinical acceptance.

INTERPRETATION OF TOROK'S MONOTHERMAL CALORIC TEST

Torok's monothermal caloric test is unique in that it compares caloric responses to weak and strong stimuli (Torok, 1970). Both stimuli use room temperature water with the weak stimulus consisting of 10 mL of water administered over 5 s and the strong stimulus consists of 100 mL of water administered over 20 s. Caloric responses are measured with eyes open in a dimly lit room and quantified by the nystagmus frequency. The ratio of nystagmus frequencies for the strong versus the weak stimulus is compared to the normal limits and classified as either *recruitment* or *decruitment* when it falls outside those limits (Kumar, 1981; Torok, 1976). Kumar (1981) has indicated that ratios greater than 3.5 (4.6 according to Torok, 1970) signify recruitment, which suggests the response to the strong stimulus is unusually larger than the response to the weak stimulus. Torok (1976) has suggested that ratios of less than 1.1 (1.3 according to Torok, 1970, and 1.2 according to Kumar, 1981) signify decruitment, which suggests the response to the strong stimulus is not sufficiently large compared to the response to the weak stimulus.

Vestibular recruitment has been associated with labyrinthine lesions, whereas vestibular decruitment has been associated with retrolabyrinthine lesions (Kumar, 1981; Torok, 1976). Kumar (1981) demonstrated vestibular recruitment in 39 out of 47 patients with a diagnosis of Ménière's disease and vestibular decruitment in 51 out of 54 patients with posterior fossa lesions. Kumar and Patni (1998) demonstrated 90% sensitivity for the Torok's monothermal test but the specificity was 25%. The findings of other studies however, have been mixed. For example, Wexler, Harker, Voots, and McCabe (1991) found far fewer patients with Ménière's disease who had recruitment in the Torok's monothermal caloric test (10% to 20%). Similarly, decruitment has been demonstrated in more than 50% of normal subjects tested in two different studies (de la Fuente-Arjona, & Marco-

Algarra, 1993; Mangabeira-Albernaz, Gananca, Martinelli, Novo, & Rodrigues de Paiva, 1979). Proctor, Frazer, Glackin, and Smith (1983) have attributed these findings in normal subjects to the variations in the temporal bone structure.

Some of the above studies that have failed to confirm Torok's findings have been criticized because they did not exactly replicate the recommended test procedure (Kumar, 1995; Torok, 1979). For example, some studies used nystagmus slow-phase velocities to quantify the responses instead of nystagmus frequency and some studies conducted the test in the absence of vision (e.g., Parker & Hamid, 1985). However, even the studies that have used the exact procedure as described by Torok, have resulted in less conclusive findings. For example, Bhansali, Stockwell, Bojrab, and Schwan (1989) demonstrated decruitment in six out of eight patients with vestibular nerve or central vestibular lesions and recruitment in two patients with active Ménière's disease. Nine out of 10 normal individuals in their study had normal responses to the Torok's monothermal caloric test. On the other hand, Linstrom and Stockwell (1993) tested nine patients with labyrinthine lesions and 25 patients with retrolabyrinthine lesions. In patients with retrolabyrinthine lesions, 56% had decruitment but only 42% correctly identified the side of lesion. Decruitment was also observed in 63% of patients with unilateral

Ménière's disease without any retrolabyrinthine lesions. Recruitment was never observed on the side of the Ménière's disease.

Overall, Torok's monothermal caloric test does offer a unique way of examining the VOR pathways. As the patient is tested with eyes open, it combines the caloric responses with the effects of fixation suppression. The test seems to be moderately sensitive to retrolabyrinthine lesions but the findings are not highly specific. More randomized case-controlled studies are needed to establish the utility of the Torok's monothermal caloric test. Until then, routine use of the test is not warranted.

SUMMARY

Table 13–2 provides a summary of common abnormalities in the caloric test. The caloric test is routinely used in patients with dizziness. Although it does not identify a specific etiology, so far, it has proved to be one of the single most useful tests for detecting unilateral peripheral vestibular lesions. In many cases, the caloric test can determine the side of lesion. The information from the caloric test must be used along with history, physical examination, and other tests to make a diagnosis and devise management plans.

Table 13–2. Common Abnormalities in the Caloric Test and Their Localization and Clinical Value

Abnormality	Clinical Value	Localization
Unilateral caloric weakness	High	Indicates a lesion involving the lateral semicircular canal or its afferent neural pathways in the weaker ear
Directional preponderance	Low	None—Indicates a peripheral vestibular lesion in either ear or a central vestibular lesion
Baseline shift	Moderate	None—Indicates a peripheral vestibular lesion in either ear or a central vestibular lesion
Gain asymmetry	Unknown	None—Indicates a peripheral vestibular lesion in either ear or a central vestibular lesion
Bilateral weakness	Moderate	Indicates a peripheral vestibular lesion in *both* ears or a central vestibular lesion
Hyperactivity	Moderate	Indicates a central lesion most likely involving the cerebellum
Failure of fixation suppression	Moderate	Indicates a central lesion

REFERENCES

Alpert, J. N. (1974). Failure of fixation suppression: A pathologic effect of vision on caloric nystagmus. *Neurology, 24*, 891–896.

ANSI. (2009). Procedures for testing basic vestibular function. *American National Standards Institute*, BSR S3.45-2009(Revision of ANSI S3.45+1999).

Aw, S. T., Haslwanter, T., Fetter, M., Heimberger, J., & Todd, M. J. (1998). Contribution of the vertical semicircular canals to the caloric nystagmus. *Acta Oto-Laryngologica, 118*(5), 618–627.

Baloh, R. W., & Honrubia, V. (2001). *Clinical neurophysiology of the vestibular system*. New York, NY: Oxford University Press.

Baloh, R. W., Jacobson, K., & Honrubia, V. (1989). Idiopathic bilateral vestibulopathy. *Neurology, 39*(2 Pt. 1), 272–275.

Baloh, R. W., Konrad, H. R., & Honrubia, V. (1975). Vestibulo-ocular function in patients with cerebellar atrophy. *Neurology, 25*(2), 160–168.

Baloh, R. W., Sills, A. W., & Honrubia, V. (1977). Caloric testing. 3. Patients with peripheral and central vestibular lesions. *Annals of Otology, Rhinology and Laryngology Supplement, 86*(5 Pt. 3 Suppl. 43), 24–30.

Baloh, R. W., Sills, A. W., & Honrubia, V. (1979). Impulsive and sinusoidal rotatory testing: A comparison with results of caloric testing. *Laryngoscope, 89*(4), 646–654.

Bance, M., Mai, M., Tomlinson, D., & Rutka, J. (1991). The changing direction of nystagmus in acute Meniere's disease: Pathophysiological implications. *Laryngoscope, 101*(2), 197–201.

Barber, H. O., & Stockwell, C. W. (1980). *Manual of electronystagmography*, St. Louis, MO: Mosby, 159–187.

Barber, H. O., & Stoyanoff, S. (1986). Vertical nystagmus in routine caloric testing. *Otolaryngology-Head and Neck Surgery, 95*(5), 574–580.

Barin, K., & Davis, L. R. (2003). The fixation suppression test. *Insights in Practice*, ICS Medical, 1–5.

Barnes, G. R., Benson, A. J., & Prior, A. R. (1978). Visual-vestibular interaction in the control of eye movement. *Aviation, Space, and Environmental Medicine, 49*(4), 557–564.

Bergstrom, B. (1973). Morphology of the vestibular nerve. II. The number of myelinated vestibular nerve fibers in man at various ages. *Acta Oto-Laryngologica, 76*(2), 173–179.

Bhansali, S. A., Stockwell, C. W., Bojrab, D. I., & Schwan, S. A. (1989). Evaluation of the monothermal caloric test. *Laryngoscope, 99*(5), 500–504.

Brandt, T. (1996). Bilateral vestibulopathy revisited. *European Journal of Medical Research, 1*(8), 361–368.

British Society of Audiology (BSA). (2010). Recommended procedure: The caloric test. Author.

Brookler, K. H. (1971). Simultaneous bilateral bithermal caloric stimulation in electronystagmography. *Laryngoscope, 81*(7), 1014–1019.

Brookler, K. H. (1976). The simultaneous binaural bithermal: A caloric test utilizing electronystagmography. *Laryngoscope, 86*(8), 1241–1250.

Brookler, K. H. (2002). Importance of simultaneous binaural bithermal caloric testing. *Ear, Nose, and Throat Journal, 81*(4), 199.

Bruner, A., & Norris, T. W. (1971). Age-related changes in caloric nystagmus. *Acta Oto-Laryngologica. Supplementum, 282*, 1–24.

Cartwright, A. D., Cremer, P. D., Halmagyi, G. M., & Curthoys, I. S. (2000). Isolated directional preponderance of caloric nystagmus: II. A neural network model. *American Journal of Otology, 21*(4), 568–572.

Chambers, B. R., & Gresty, M. A. (1982). Effects of fixation and optokinetic stimulation on vestibulo-ocular reflex suppression. *Journal of Neurology, Neurosurgery, and Psychiatry, 45*(11), 998–1004.

Coats, A. C. (1965). Directional preponderance and unilateral weakness as observed in the electronystagmographic examination. *Annals of Otology, Rhinology, and Laryngology, 74*(3), 655–668.

Coats, A. C. (1966). Directional preponderance and spontaneous nystagmus as observed in the electronystagmographic examination. *Annals of Otology, Rhinology, and Laryngology, 75*(4), 1135–1159.

Coats, A. C. (1970). Central electronystagmographic abnormalities. *Archives of Otolaryngology, 92*(1), 43–53.

Committee on Hearing, Bioacoustics, and Biomechanics (CHABA). (1992). Evaluation of tests for vestibular function. *Aviation, Space, and Environmental Medicine, 63*(2, Suppl.), A1–A34.

Curthoys, I. S. (2000). Vestibular compensation and substitution. *Current Opinion in Neurology, 13*(1), 27–30.

de la Fuente-Arjona, L., & Marco-Algarra, J. (1993). Vestibular decruitment: An indicator of central pathology? *Laryngoscope, 103*(7), 793–797.

Demanez, J. P., & Ledoux, A. (1970). Automatic fixation mechanisms and vestibular stimulation. Their study in central pathology with ocular fixation index during caloric tests. *Advances in Oto-Rhino-Laryngology, 17*, 90–98.

Elidan, J., Gay, I., & Lev, S. (1985). On the vertical caloric nystagmus. *Journal of Otolaryngology, 14*(5), 287–292.

Fetter, M., Aw, S., Haslwanter, T., Heimberger, J., & Dichgans, J. (1998). Three-dimensional eye movement analysis during caloric stimulation used to test vertical semicircular canal function. *American Journal of Otology, 19*(2), 180–187.

Fitzgerald, G., & Hallpike, C. S. (1942). Studies in human vestibular function. I. Observations of the directional preponderance of caloric nystagmus resulting from cerebral lesions. *Brain, 65,* 115–137.

Fredrickson, J. M., & Fernandez, C. (1964). Vestibular disorders in fourth ventricle lesions. Experimental studies in the cat. *Archives of Otolaryngology, 80,* 521–540.

Furman, J. M. (1989). Simultaneous caloric testing. *ENG Report,* ICS Medical.

Furman, J. M., & Kamerer, D. B. (1989). Rotational responses in patients with bilateral caloric reduction. *Acta Oto-Laryngologica, 108*(5–6), 355–361.

Furman, J. M., Wall, C., III, & Kamerer, D. B. (1988). Alternate and simultaneous binaural bithermal caloric testing: A comparison. *Annals of Otology, Rhinology, and Laryngology, 97*(4 Pt. 1), 359–364.

Glantz, S. A. (1997). *Primer of biostatistics* (4th ed., pp. 207–211). New York, NY: McGraw-Hill.

Greisen, O. (1972). Pseudocaloric nystagmus. *Acta Oto-Laryngologica, 73*(4), 341–343.

Hain, T. C. (2012). *Caloric test.* In Dizziness-and-Balance. com, posted 5/30/2012. Retrieved December 7, 2013, from http://www.dizziness-and-balance.com/testing/ENG/caloric_test.htm

Halmagyi, G. M. (2005). Diagnosis and management of vertigo. *Clinical Medicine, 5*(2), 159–165.

Halmagyi, G. M., Cremer, P. D., Anderson, J., Murofushi, T., & Curthoys, I. S. (2000). Isolated directional preponderance of caloric nystagmus: I. Clinical significance. *American Journal of Otology, 21*(4), 559–567.

Halmagyi, G. M., & Gresty, M. A. (1979). Clinical signs of visual-vestibular interaction. *Journal of Neurology, Neurosurgery, and Psychiatry, 42*(10), 934–939.

Henry, D. F. (1999). Test-retest reliability of open-loop bithermal caloric irrigation responses from healthy young adults. *American Journal of Otology, 20*(2), 220–222.

Hoffman, R. A., Brookler, K. H., & Baker, A. H. (1979). The accuracy of the simultaneous binaural bithermal test in the diagnosis of acoustic neuroma. *Laryngoscope, 89*(7 Pt. 1), 1046–1052.

Honrubia, V., Marco, J., Andrews, J., Minser, K., Yee, R. D., & Baloh, R. W. (1985) Vestibulo-ocular reflexes in peripheral labyrinthine lesions: III. Bilateral dysfunction. *American Journal of Otolaryngology, 6*(5), 342–352.

Huygen, P. L., Nicolasen, M. G., Verhagen, W. I., & Theunissen, E. J. (1989). Contralateral hyperactive caloric response in unilateral labyrinthine weakness. *Acta Oto-Laryngologica, 107*(1–2), 1–4.

Ikeda, M., & Watanabe, I. (1997). Evaluation of hyperactive caloric responses in patients with inner ear diseases. *ORL, Journal for Oto-Rhino-Laryngology, 59*(6), 326–331.

Isaacson, J. E., & Rubin, A. M. (2001). Performing the physical exam: Detecting spontaneous and gaze-evoked nystagmus. In J. A. Goebel (Ed.), *Practical management of the dizzy patient* (pp. 61–71). Philadelphia, PA: Lippincott Williams & Wilkins.

Jacobson, G. P., & Henry, K. G. (1989). Effect of temperature on fixation suppression ability in normal subjects: the need for temperature- and age-dependent normal values. *Annals of Otology, Rhinology, and Laryngology, 98*(5 Pt. 1), 369–372.

Jacobson, G. P., & Newman, C. W. (1991). Rotational testing. *Seminars in Hearing, 12*(3), 199–225.

Jacobson, G. P., Newman, C. W., & Peterson, E. L. (1993). Interpretation and usefulness of caloric testing. In G. P. Jacobson, C. W. Newman, & J. M. Kartush, (Eds.), *Handbook of balance testing function* (pp. 193–233). St. Louis, MO: Mosby Yearbook.

Jacobson, G. P., Pearlstein, R., Henderson, J., Calder, J. H., & Rock, J. (1998). Recovery nystagmus revisited. *Journal of the American Academy of Audiology, 9*(4), 263–271.

Kim, H. A., Lee, H., Yi, H. A., & Baloh, R. W. (2012). Unusual caloric responses in a patient with a fourth ventricular ependymoma. *Neurological Sciences: Official Journal of the Italian Neurological Society and of the Italian Society of Clinical Neurophysiology, 33*(2), 383–385.

Kim, J. S, & Kim, H. J. (2012). Inferior vestibular neuritis. *Journal of Neurology, 259*(8), 1553–1560.

Kimm, J., & Donaldson, J. A. (1980). Hyperactive vestibular response of peripheral origin. *American Journal of Otology, 1*(4), 238–239.

Kumar, A. (1981). Diagnostic advantages of the Torok monothermal differential caloric test. *Laryngoscope, 91*(10), 1678–1694.

Kumar, A. (1995). Post caloric nystagmus: An analysis of culmination frequency and maximum slow phase velocity. *Acta Oto-laryngologica Supplement, 520*(Pt. 1), 220–224.

Kumar, A., & Patni, A. (1998). Vestibular decruitment, hyperactivity, and rebound caloric nystagmus. *American Journal of Otology, 19*(2), 188–195.

Lewis, A. E. (1966). *Biostatistics (Chap. 12).* New York, NY: Reinhold.

Linstrom, C. J., & Stockwell, C. W. (1993). Clinical evaluation of the monothermal caloric test. *Otolaryngology-Head and Neck Surgery, 108*(1), 27–35.

Mallinson, A. I., & Longridge, N. S. (2004). Caloric response does not decline with age. *Journal of Vestibular Research, 14*(5), 393–396.

Mangabeira-Albernaz, P. L., Gananca, M. M., Martinelli, M. C., Novo, N. F., & Rodrigues de Paiva, E. (1979). Vestibular decruitment. A study of the phenomenon in a normal population. *ORL Journal for Oto-Rhino-Laryngology, 41*(3), 135–142.

Manzari, L., Burgess, A. M., MacDougall, H. G., & Curthoys, I. S. (2013). Vestibular function after vestibular neuritis. *International Journal of Audiology, 52*(10), 713–718.

Mateijsen, D. J., Hengel, P. W., Kingma, H., Oreel, M. A., Wit, H. P., & Albers, F. W. (2001). Vertigo and electronystagmography in uni- and bilateral Meniere's disease. *ORL Journal for Oto-Rhino-Laryngology, 63*(6), 341–348.

McClure, J. A., Copp, J. C., & Lycett, P. (1981). Recovery nystagmus in Meniere's disease. *Laryngoscope, 91*(10), 1727–1737.

Mehra, Y. N. (1964). Electronystagmography. A study of caloric tests in normal subjects. *Journal of Laryngology and Otology, 78*, 520–529.

Meissner, R. (1981). Behavior of the nystagmus in Meniere's attack. *Archives of Oto-Rhino-Laryngology, 233*(2), 173–177.

Monday, L. A., Lemieux, B., St. Vincent, H., & Barbeau, A. (1978). Clinical and electronystagmographic findings in Friedreich's ataxia. *Canadian Journal of Neurological Sciences, 5*(1), 71–73.

Monday, L., Lesperance, J., Lemieux, B., & Saint-Vincent, H. (1984). Follow-up study of electronystagmographic findings in Friedreich's ataxia patients and evaluation of their relatives. *Canadian Journal of Neurological Sciences, 11*(4 Suppl.), 570–573.

Mulch, G., & Petermann, W. (1979). Influence of age on results of vestibular function tests. Review of literature and presentation of caloric test results. *Annals of Otology, Rhinology and Laryngology. Supplement, 88*(2 Pt. 2 Suppl. 56), 1–17.

Myers, S. F. (1992). Patterns of low-frequency rotational responses in bilateral caloric weakness patients. *Journal of Vestibular Research, 2*(2), 123–131.

Nishikawa, K., & Nishikawa, M. (1986). Nystagmus during attack in Meniere's disease. *Auris, Nasus, Larynx, 13*(Suppl. 2), S147–S151.

Norre, M. E. (1987). Caloric vertical nystagmus: The vertical semicircular canal in caloric testing. *Journal of Otolaryngology, 16*(1), 36–39.

Park, J. J., Tang, Y., Lopez, I., & Ishiyama, A. (2001). Age-related change in the number of neurons in the human vestibular ganglion. *Journal of Comparative Neurology, 431*(4), 437–443.

Parker, W., & Hamid, M. (1985). Vestibular responses to different caloric stimulus intensities. *American Journal of Otology, 6*(5), 378–386.

Peterka, R. J., Black, F. O., & Schoenhoff, M. B. (1990–1991). Age-related changes in human vestibulo-ocular reflexes: Sinusoidal rotation and caloric tests. *Journal of Vestibular Research, 1*(1), 49–59.

Petersen, J. A., Straumann, D., & Weber, K. P. (2013). Clinical diagnosis of bilateral vestibular loss: Three simple bedside tests. *Therapeutic Advances in Neurological Disorders, 6*(1), 41–45.

Proctor, L. R. (1992). The ice water caloric test. *ENG Report*, ICS Medical, 69–72.

Proctor, L. R., Frazer, R. K., Glackin, R. N., & Smith, C. R. (1983). "Recruitment/decruitment" of caloric responses: Effect of anatomical variables. *Advances in Oto-Rhino-Laryngology, 30*, 150–155.

Proctor, L., & Glackin, R. (1985). Factors contributing to variability of caloric test scores. *Acta Oto-Laryngologica, 100*(3–4), 161–171.

Proctor, L. R., & Lam, A. P. (2002). Dysrhythmia of caloric nystagmus. *Laryngoscope, 112*(10), 1730–1736.

Rinne, T., Bronstein, A. M., Rudge, P., Gresty, M. A., & Luxon, L. M. (1995) Bilateral loss of vestibular function. *Acta Oto-Laryngologica Supplement, 520*(Pt. 2), 247–250.

Rosenhall, U. (1973). Degenerative patterns in the aging human vestibular neuro-epithelia. *Acta Oto-Laryngologica, 76*(2), 208–220.

Sargent, E. W., Goebel, J. A., Hanson, J. M., & Beck, D. L. (1997). Idiopathic bilateral vestibular loss. *Otolaryngology-Head and Neck Surgery, 116*(2), 157–162.

Schuchman, G., & Uri, N. (1986). The variability of fixation suppression of caloric-induced nystagmus. *Journal of Laryngology and Otology, 100*(7), 765–768.

Shepard, N. T., & Telian, S. A. (1996). *Practical management of the balance disorder patient.* San Diego, CA: Singular.

Sills, A. W., Baloh, R. W., & Honrubia, V. (1977). Caloric testing 2. Results in normal subjects. *Annals of Otology, Rhinology and Laryngology, 86*(5 Pt. 3, Suppl. 43), 7–23.

Simmons, F. B. (1973). Patients with bilateral loss of caloric response. *Annals of Otology, Rhinology, and Laryngology, 82*(2), 175–178.

Stahle, J. (1958). Electro-nystagmography in the caloric and rotatory tests: A clinical study. *Acta Oto-Laryngologica Supplement, 137*, 1–83.

Stockwell, C. W. (1993). Bilateral weakness. *ENG Report*, ICS Medical, 73–75.

Stockwell, C. W., & Graham, M. D. (1988). Vestibular compensation following labyrinthectomy and vestibular neurectomy. In J. Nadol (Ed.), *Second international symposium on Meniere's disease* (pp. 489). Amsterdam, the Netherlands: Kugler & Ghedini.

Syms, C. A. 3rd, & House, J. W. (1997). Idiopathic Dandy's syndrome. *Otolaryngology-Head and Neck Surgery, 116*(1), 75–78.

Tang, Y., Lopez, I., & Baloh, R. W. (2001–2002). Age-related change of the neuronal number in the human medial vestibular nucleus: A stereological investigation. *Journal of Vestibular Research, 11*(6), 357–363.

Telian, S. A., Shepard, N. T., Smith-Wheelock, M., & Hoberg, M. (1991). Bilateral vestibular paresis: Diagnosis and treatment. *Otolaryngology-Head and Neck Surgery, 104*(1), 67–71.

Tomlinson, R. D., & Robinson, D. A. (1981). Is the vestibulo-ocular reflex cancelled by smooth pursuit? In A. Fuchs & W. Becker (Eds.), *Progress in oculomotor research* (pp. 533–539). New York, NY: Elsevier/North-Holland.

Torok, N. (1970). A new parameter of vestibular sensitivity. *Annals of Otology, Rhinology, and Laryngology, 79*(4), 808–817.

Torok, N. (1976). Vestibular decruitment in central nervous system disease. *Annals of Otology, Rhinology, and Laryngology, 85*(1 Pt. 1), 131–135.

Torok, N. (1979). Pitfalls in detecting vestibular decruitment with air calorics. *Journal of Oto-Rhino-Laryngology, 41*(3), 143–146.

Toupet, M., & Pialoux, P. (1981). [The perverted nystagmus (author's transl)]. *Annales D'oto-laryngologie et de Chirurgie Cervico Faciale, 98*(7–8), 319–338.

Uemura, T., & Cohen, B. (1973). Effects of vestibular nuclei lesions on vestibulo-ocular reflexes and posture in monkeys. *Acta Oto-Laryngologica. Supplement, 315,* 1–71.

Van der Laan, F. L., & Oosterveld, W. J. (1974). Age and vestibular function. *Aerospace Medicine, 45*(5), 540–547.

Van der Stappen, A., Wuyts, F. L., & Van de Heyning, P. H. (2000). Computerized electronystagmography: Normative data revisited. *Acta Oto-Laryngologica, 120*(6), 724–730.

Vibert, D., Liard, P., & Hausler, R. (1995). Bilateral idiopathic loss of peripheral vestibular function with normal hearing. *Acta Oto-Laryngologica, 115*(5), 611–615.

Watanabe, T. K. (1996). Nystagmus during an acute attack of Meniere's disease. *ENG Report*, ICS Medical.

Wetmore, S. J. (1986). Extended caloric tests. *Ear and Hearing, 7*(3), 186–190.

Wexler, D. B., Harker, L. A., Voots, R. J., & McCabe, B. F. (1991). Monothermal differential caloric testing in patients with Meniere's disease. *Laryngoscope, 101*(1 Pt. 1), 50–55.

Yokota, T., Tsuchiya, K., Yamane, M., Hayashi, M., Tanabe, H., & Tsukagoshi, H. (1991). Geotropic ocular deviation with skew and absence of saccade in Creutzfelt-Jakob disease. *Journal of the Neurological Sciences, 106*(2), 175–178.

Zee, D. S. (2000). Vestibular adaptation. In S. J. Herdman, (Ed.), *Vestibular rehabilitation* (pp. 77–90), Philadelphia, PA: F. A. Davis.

Background and Introduction to Whole-Body Rotational Testing

Adam M. Goulson, James H. McPherson, and Neil T. Shepard

INTRODUCTION

The ability to evaluate the peripheral vestibular system in greater detail has been a topic of focus by many researchers over centuries. The development and use of electronystagmography (ENG) and more commonly videonystagmography (VNG) testing, specifically caloric irrigation, has been considered the gold standard in the evaluation of a patient with vestibular and balance complaints. However, caloric testing evaluates the function of the horizontal semicircular canals only and stimulates the peripheral system in a frequency range equivalent to 0.004 to 0.008 Hz (by modeling the temporal course of the caloric response as equivalent sinusoidal rotation). In order to evaluate the peripheral vestibular system beyond the low frequencies, the use of whole-body rotational testing should be considered.

Whole-body rotational testing involves the patient being seated in a darkened enclosed room in a chair mounted atop a computer-controlled torque motor with the head coupled securely to the chair. This allows a precise and repeatable stimulus to be presented to the head by rotating the whole body with the vertical axis of rotation through the center of the head. The eye movements (jerk nystagmus provoked by the rotations) of the patients are measured with the slow phase velocity (vestibular component) being extracted and used to evaluate the

function of the vestibular system. Currently, this is primarily completed using two different paradigms: sinusoidal harmonic acceleration and velocity step test. Additionally, evaluation of otolith function, specifically utricular function, can be evaluated by using off-vertical axis rotation (OVAR) and unilateral centrifugation (UC) paradigms. The technique and interpretation of these tests are described in detail in this and the following chapter.

HISTORICAL BASIS OF ROTATIONAL TESTING

In the latter part of the 19th century it was recognized that the vestibular labyrinth of the ear performed a function separate from hearing. Robert Bárány was among the first to attempt assessment of vestibular function in a systematic manner developing a caloric test and rotational tests.

By the time Bárány (1907) described his rotating chair test, the use of "spinning" or "swinging" devices had been documented in the literature from about the early 1800s. Hayner (1818) (as cited by Grusser, 1984, in Cohen & Raphan, 2004), reported that "swinging" was a popular "treatment" for mental illness in the 1800s. The patient was rotated while seated and/or supine at a constant velocity, primarily in normal room light. If seated, the axis of rotation was vertical and the patient would experience a sensation of angular acceleration and deceleration at the start of "swinging" and when the device slowed to a stop. In light, during constant velocity rotation, the response of the semicircular canals would adapt away and the resulting nystagmus and the sensation of rotation would be the result of optokinetic stimulation. If the patient was treated while supine, centrifugation was involved as the patient would be rotated in a bed, with the head pointed outward, at the end of a long beam. The sensation of motion would, again, occur at the onset of acceleration and deceleration in keeping with the descriptions of Mach (1875) (as cited by Grusser, 1984, in Cohen & Raphan, 2004), the semicircular canals were "transducers of angular acceleration, not angular velocity." While the therapeutic value of these "treatments" may be in question today, they no doubt provided investigators of the day with evidence of independent receptors for sensing rotation.

Likewise, Purkinje (1820) who was one of the first researchers credited with establishing research on the vestibular system, replicated research completed by Erasmus Darwin (as cited by Grusser, 1984, in Cohen & Raphan, 2004) in an attempt to demonstrate that specific and separate motion receptors are responsible for sensing movement. This was done by rotating a subject in a chair and describing both the per-rotary and postrotary eye movements. He concluded that the movement of the brain, specifically the cerebellum, was the source of the receptors for sensing movement.

Flourens (1830), another researcher credited with establishing research on the vestibular system, established the relationship between compensatory eye movement and semicircular canal stimulation. Early work describing the corneoretinal potential had been published by DuBois-Reymond (1849) and Dodge (1903), and they presented a systematic categorization of eye movements. Among the five types of eye movements described was the reactive compensatory eye movement provoked by rotating a subject in light with eyes closed or with eyes open in the dark. In this instance, a compensatory nystagmus was evoked with the fast phase in the direction of rotation.

Bárány described a manually operated rotating chair that produced observable, postrotatory nystagmus. For his test, as shown in Figure 14–1, Bárány seated the subject in a chair with the subject's head

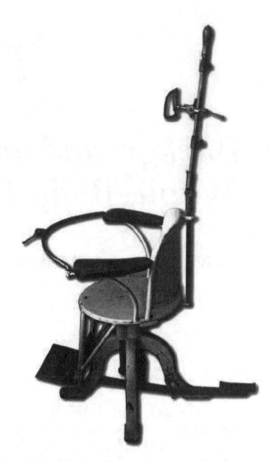

Figure 14–1. Bárány-like chair. This chair has a handle on top to rotate patient manually and a foot brake on the side to stop rotation to observe nystagmus. The chair was produced by V. Mueller & Company, Chicago, IL.

tipped forward 30 degrees bringing the horizontal semicircular canals into the plane of rotation with the axis of rotation being through the center of the head. The chair was rotated 10 times over 20 s and then stopped abruptly. The duration of the postrotatory nystagmus was measured in seconds by visual observation, and inferences were made regarding horizontal semicircular canal function.

The test was conducted in both clockwise and counterclockwise directions. There were numerous difficulties reported during the development of this test, including poor control of the manually applied stimulus and the highly inconsistent effects of visual suppression causing variability both between and within subjects. These difficulties obviously affected the clinical utility of rotational testing but interest in rotary stimulation of the vestibular mechanism continued.

Historically, three types of angular acceleration have been attempted clinically to evaluate the horizontal semicircular canal system. The Bárány chair is an example of impulsive stimulation where the chair was stopped quickly following rotation. Later studies of constant and sinusoidal stimuli were carried out. Van Egmond, Groen, and Jongkees (1949) reported a method of impulsive rotation that was intended to improve the reliability of the stimulus. In their test the subject was slowly accelerated to several velocities and then stopped suddenly. They coined the term *cupulometry*, referring to the plot of postrotatory turning sensations and nystagmus versus the logrithmic value of the stimulus magnitude. Though an improvement, these tests proved to be quite unreliable and insensitive to vestibular lesions due to continued problems with producing repeatable stimuli and accurate recording of evoked nystagmus.

Raphan, Matsuo, and Cohen (1979) reported on the discovery of a central storage mechanism that they called *velocity storage* and modeled this concept with the use of a "leaky" integrator. The velocity storage integrator stores information regarding head velocity to produce compensatory eye movements especially at lower frequencies and beyond the time that cupula deflection is occurring. When the cupula is deflected the velocity storage integrator, which is regulated by the nodulus of the cerebellum, begins to charge up. This mechanism extends the measured response and sensation of motion beyond that of the stimulation of cupula or peripheral labyrinth alone. It known that the cupula time constant is approximately 6 to 8 s (the time it would take for the cupula deflection to return to 37% of its maximum deflected value at the start of deceleration), and the canal ocular time constant is 14 to 18 s (the time it takes for the slow component eye velocity to decay to 37% of the maximum velocity at the start of the deceleration). During acceleration the cupular and canal ocular time constants have the same values but are defined at the time taken to achieve 63% of the maximum cupular deflection and maximum slow component velocity of the nystagmus, respectively. The ability to measure the canal ocular time constant during rotational chair testing allows for a determination of possible site-of-lesion within the peripheral (shortened time constant) or central (lengthened time constant) vestibular system.

SINUSOIDAL HARMONIC ACCELERATION

As pointed out by Cyr (1991), patients tolerate rotational testing better than caloric testing, the potential mechanical artifacts related to delivery of the caloric stimulus are obviated, the rotational stimulus is more a natural physiologic stimulus than caloric stimulation, multiple test frequencies may be presented, and the vestibulo-ocular reflex (VOR) may be monitored more accurately because of better stimulus/response control. Cyr also noted the primary disadvantage of rotary chair testing is that both vestibular labyrinths are involved simultaneously, one being stimulated (side to which the chair is rotated) and one being inhibited (the one on the side away from direction of rotation).

During the 1960s and 1970s, as electrooculography (EOG) became a more prevalent clinical tool, the issue of response measurement during rotational testing became better understood and less problematic. The damped torsion swing test developed by Van de Calseyde and Dupondt (1974) is an example of the application of a single-frequency sinusoidal stimulus with EOG recording of evoked nystagmus. In this test the intensity and duration of the stimulus were determined by a combination of the characteristics of the spring driving the chair and the subject's weight. The intensities of the right-beating and left-beating responses were calculated and plotted as a function of the maximal amplitude of chair swing looking at the variable of age. Ultimately, the torsion swing test proved to be unreliable and was frequently insensitive to peripheral vestibular disorders.

It was also during this time period that Cramer (1963), examining the dynamic characteristics of the VOR, described the phase and gain of rotation-induced eye movements in the cat. He reported that above 0.1 Hz the vestibular-oculomotor system operates as an integrating accelerometer with eye movement being 180 degrees out of phase with head rotation. His measurements were not clinically practical as they required complex calculations done by hand, but they did bring systems engineering techniques to vestibular research. The work of Jones and Milsum (1965) and that of Niven, Hixom, and Correia (1965) pushed ahead an understanding of the physiologic systems allowing stabilization of visual images on the retina and phase relationships evoked by rotational stimuli in the frequency range 0.02 to 0.2 Hz in human subjects.

In the early 1970s there were two advances in technology that had a major impact on rotational testing. The precision torque motor became available solving most of the stimulus control problems and small computers were becoming available and more common in clinical settings. The early DC torque motors would typically generate 30 to 100 footpounds of torque; however, with modern AC torque motors higher values can be achieved (Figure 14–2). The AC torque motor used in the contemporary chair generates 340 foot-pounds of torque. The concept of torque in rotational testing is critical for rapid acceleration of patients, without regard to their weight, during velocity step testing. The use of more powerful torque motors allows the examiner to avoid spuriously reduced gain values in heavier patients, (i.e., as pointed out by Shepard and Telian, 1996) by ensuring that the chair is appropriately calibrated to achieve the desired acceleration and peak velocities, particularly for higher-frequency rotation.

Mathog (1972) reported gain and symmetry data for 22 normal and 53 abnormal subjects using multifrequency, sinusoidal stimulation in darkness with eyes open. He was among the first to present such data using a motor directly driving the chair that provided no cues to the subject from vibration or noise.

Also in the early 1970s reports were appearing in the literature describing both off- and online digital analysis of voluntary and involuntary eye movements (Allum, Tole, & Weiss, 1975; Baloh, Kumley, Sills, & Honrubia, 1975; Baloh, Langhofer, Honrubia, & Yee, 1980; Engelken & Wolfe, 1977; Honrubia, Katz, Strelioff, & Ward, 1971; Ranacher, 1977; Schilder, Pasik, & Pasik, 1973). These efforts allowed for experiments in both animal and human models designed to investigate questions regarding the type of stimulus best suited for rotational testing.

The evolution of the techniques described herein has allowed the documentation and quantification of human responses to rotational stimuli by measuring eye movement during head motion. Figure 14–3 summarizes the analysis of harmonic acceleration for a normal patient. The frequency tested is 0.16 Hz and the chair peak velocity is 50 deg/s. The upper curve shows the chair velocity in degrees per second. The lower curve shows the average composite eye displacement velocity in degrees per second for the slow phases of the eye motion (the vestibular portion or the VOR) for these four cycles. The data at the bottom of the figure show the normative data as well as the subject's responses for phase, gain, asymmetry, spectral purity, and saccade factor. The clinical use of sinusoidal harmonic acceleration testing requires the understanding of the parameters used. A description of each parameter is provided with reference back to Figure 14–3.

Measurement Parameters

It has become accepted that in the evaluation of the peripheral vestibular system using rotational stimuli, three primary parameters are measured. The parameters represent phase, gain, and symmetry of the VOR (Shepard & Telian, 1996). The parameter characterizing the spectral purity of the evoked nystagmus is also useful in determining the quality of the data. One last parameter, saccade factor, is a value that is selected to represent the data (slow-phase velocity) which are collected. As discussed by Shepard and Telian, the concept of phase is "the least intuitive of the three but has the greatest clinical significance in its ability to document peripheral system dysfunction." Phase measurements characterize the timing relationship between motion of the head and the VOR and allow for the quantification of phase lead or lag.

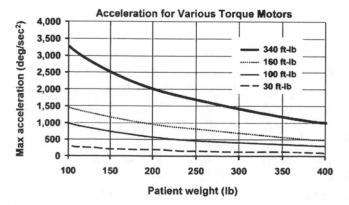

Figure 14-2. Maximum acceleration verses patient weight for motors generating 30, 100,160, and 340 ft-lb of torque.

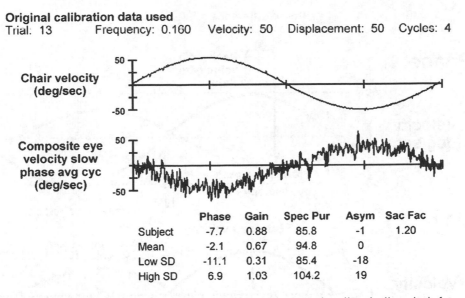

Original calibration data used
Trial: 13   Frequency: 0.160   Velocity: 50   Displacement: 50   Cycles: 4

	Phase	Gain	Spec Pur	Asym	Sac Fac
Subject	-7.7	0.88	85.8	-1	1.20
Mean	-2.1	0.67	94.8	0	
Low SD	-11.1	0.31	85.4	-18	
High SD	6.9	1.03	104.2	19	

Figure 14-3. Summary of analysis for harmonic acceleration in the dark for a patient at 0.16 Hz for four cycles of rotation. The smooth upper line represents the velocity of the chair and the lower noisy line represents the average composite slow-phase eye velocity. At the bottom of the figure, Mayo Clinic normative mean values for 0.16 Hz are –2.1 degrees for phase, 0.67 for gain, 94.8% for spectral purity, and the asymmetry is 0.0%. Also shown are the limits of ±2 standard deviations.

Figure 14–4 displays the three primary parameters phase, gain, and symmetry used to analyze harmonic accelerations (Brey, 2002). Each of these parameters is calculated as a function of the frequency at which the chair is oscillated. *Phase* lead is the value, in degrees, to which compensatory eye movements lead or lag movement of the head. At the lower frequencies of rotation (0.01 to 0.08 Hz) the phase value of the average slow component eye velocity leads the average head velocity (chair velocity). As the frequency of rotation increased the average slow component eye velocity changes to lagging behind the head velocity. In other words, the eye can accomplish its compensatory movement prior to the head completing its movement in the opposite direction (see the example in Figure 14–4A). This is only the case if the head is moving in a pure sinusoidal manner. In daily routine head movements the head always leads the eye movements since our head movements are transient in nature and not sinusoidal. Therefore, this relationship between eye movement and head movement where the eye movement can lead the head movement is unique to this testing situation. It has been demonstrated that disorders in the peripheral vestibular labyrinth or vestibular nerve will result in phase leads that are greater than that observed in normal subjects. An exception to this common interpretation of test data (Shepard & Telian, 1996) occurs when damage affects the vestibular nuclei (i.e., part of the central vestibular system) which may result in an abnormally increased phase lead. This will be discussed further in Chapter 15. Another concept relating to measurement of phase is abnormally decreased phase lead for the lower frequencies. Decreased phase lead is felt to be related to lesions in the cerebellum (Waespe, Cohen, & Raphan, 1985) and, anecdotally, in our laboratory this appears to be a common test finding in patients with other indications of central vestibular system involvement.

A second measurement parameter in rotary chair testing is *gain* (refer to Figure 14–4B). If the function of the VOR is to produce an eye movement that compensates for head movement, then under perfect conditions the vestibular portion (i.e., slow-phase eye velocity) of the response to rotation should be a mirror image of head velocity producing a gain value (output divided by input, i.e., average

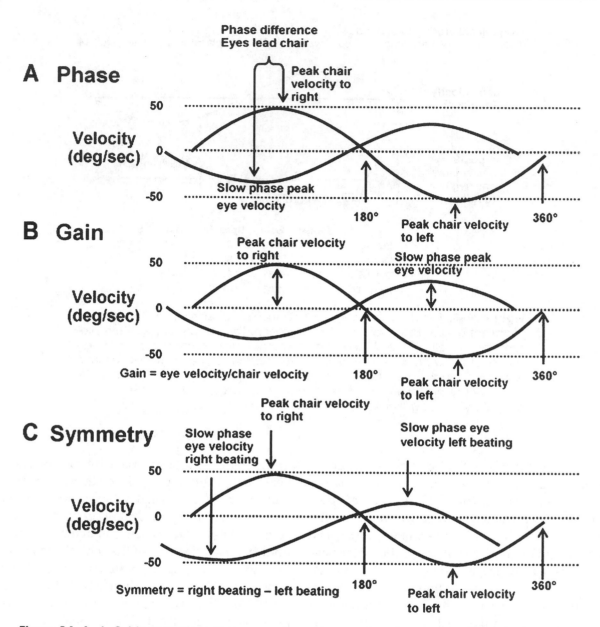

Figure 14-4. A–C. Measurement of phase, gain, and symmetry using a computerized rotary chair. Sine waves represent analysis of the velocity of the chair and slow-phase movement of the eyes as indicated. (From Brey, R. H. 2002. Vertigo and Balance. In J. R. Daube (Ed.), *Clinical neurophysiology* (pp. 431–433). By permission of Oxford University Press, Inc.)

compensatory eye velocity divided by the head velocity) of 1.0 and be out of phase 180 degrees (the eye in the opposite direction from the head velocity). Gain measurement then provides an indication of the overall responsiveness of the peripheral vestibular system (it is not related to the left or right but the combination of the two) and is particularly useful in documenting bilateral peripheral deficits over a range of test frequencies. Unfortunately, gain is influenced by a number of variables that must be considered by the examiner when evaluating test data. Gain values may be artifactually reduced by failure to adequately alert the patient, light leaks in the test room, disorders affecting the ability to generate eye movements, typically slowing of saccades (see Chapters 2 and 10 in this text for discussion of eye movements that can result in slowing of saccades) and calibration errors affecting the peak eye velocity measurements. Again, although one will occasionally evaluate a patient with a unilateral peripheral vestibular deficit who exhibits abnormally reduced gain (most typically at 0.01 Hz), a primary benefit of rotational testing is documenting the degree of bilateral vestibular weakness. Measurement of gain over a range of frequencies will allow for predictions to be made as to the degree and form of functional problems related to the loss of bilateral vestibular function as well as the likelihood of success in rehabilitation programs. The examiner must also keep in mind that when gain values are less than 0.1, phase and symmetry values at that same frequency are considered unreliable. It is generally accepted that until gain values exceed 0.15, these measurement parameters must be interpreted with caution (Shepard & Telian, 1996). For rotational peak velocities of 50 deg/s a gain of 0.10 is equivalent to a peak slow-phase eye velocity of 5 deg/s. Thus, low gains are associated with difficulty for the detection algorithms to identify nystagmus slow phases.

Spectral purity reflects how pure the sine wave is that is constructed from the slow-phase eye velocity. While ensuring the gain values have exceeded 0.15, it is also necessary to ensure the spectral purity is within the acceptable range. If spectral purity is poor, then the measurement parameters must also be interpreted with caution.

Symmetry of response to harmonic acceleration is measured as the difference between maximum left-beating and right-beating slow-phase average eye velocities divided by the total of left- and right-beating maximum slow-phase average eye velocities, multiplied by 100 to produce a percentage difference. Asymmetry assesses whether the right-beating or left-beating nystagmus is stronger but of importance is displayed as the percentage difference between the average maxium slow-phase velocity for the respective rotation to the right (right-beating nystagmus) and to the left (left-beating nystagmus). Analogous to the manner that directional preponderance is calculated for a caloric irrigation test with the use of the slow-phase velocity as the measure of the strength of the right or left-beating nystagmus, the same is done for chair asymmetry, the difference is that the chair results are typically reported by the slow component velocity being greater for the right versus the left. Therefore, when reporting the asymmetry results one would report the findings as right slow component velocity greater than the left or the left greater than the right or equivalent. If a negative value for asymmetry is observed, that suggests that the patient has greater gain for the slow component velocity to the left (rotation to the right), or a directional preponderance showing greater right-beating nystagmus compared to the left-beating nystagmus. If the asymmetry value is positive, then the patient would have demonstrated greater gain for the slow component velocity to the right (rotation to the left) or a left-beating directional preponderance. However, the examiner must always use caution when interpreting asymmetry values if measured gain values are low (<0.15), especially if spectral purity is below the normal range at the same frequency. An example of data collected for phase, gain, and symmetry is presented in Figure 14–3. The subject's scores are −7.7 degrees for phase (the eye is lagging behind the head and is normal), 0.88 for gain, and 85.8% for spectral purity (also both normal values). Symmetry is a −1% left greater than right slow-phase velocity asymmetry (i.e., right-beating directional preponderance on rotation to the right in comparison to rotation to the left with this value well within the normal range).

Saccade factor is a number under user control in many commercial systems that represents the limit of eye velocity accepted by the software for the slow phases. For example, a saccade factor of 1.0 implies that a multiplier of 1.0 times 50 deg/s would be used to determine the minimum velocity by which saccades would be identified. Thus, in a search for slow phases, fast phases greater than 50 deg/s would be discarded. With a saccade factor of 1.2 times 50, a value of 60 deg/s results. In this example, eye movements greater than 60 deg/s would be discarded. The purpose of the saccade factor is to eliminate nystagmus fast phases and retain nystagmus slow phases that are vestibular in origin. The fast phases represent the central component of nystagmus where the eyes are recentered in an attempt to maintain a stable image on the retina as the patient is rotated. This is the function of the VOR. In the example shown in Figure 14–3 the saccade factor was 1.20.

Analysis

The standard analysis technique for harmonic acceleration is to calculate the eye velocity as the patient oscillates back and forth from extractraction of the eye signal, specifically the vestibular component or slow-phase velocity. To accomplish this, nystagmus fast phases must be identified and discarded. After the fast phases are discarded, the remaining slow phases could be connected end-to-end thus creating a sine wave. This would create an eye position sine wave that could be compared to the input sine wave motion of the chair. Such an approach was proposed by Meiry (1971) and is displayed in Figure 14–5. Figure 14–6 shows eye motion for a patient generated during 0.16-Hz harmonic acceleration testing in the dark. The dashed line (A) at the top represents the chair oscillating back and forth and (B) the next line represents the eye position showing the nystagmus.

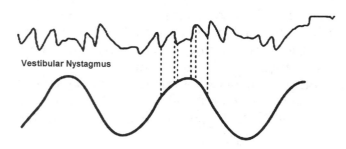

Figure 14-5. Rotational nystagmus analysis. A segment of rotation nystagmus is shown with slow components and quick components clearly marked. The slow components are pieced together to form a cumulative slow component eye position graph. (Adapted from Meiry, J. 1971. *Vestibular and Proprioceptive Stabilization of Eye Movements* (pp. 483–496). Copyright 1971, with permission from Elsevier.)

The fast phases during the first half-cycle are up-going producing right-beating nystagmus, consistent with the chair rotating to the right. Conversely, the vestibular slow phases are down-going or to the left. During the second half of that cycle, the fast phases are down-going (to the left) and the slow phases are up-going (to the right) resulting in a left-beating nystagmus. This is consistent with the chair turning to the left. The eye movement alternates back and forth through four cycles of harmonic acceleration at a frequency of 0.16 Hz. Line C shows the fast phases as solid lines and slow phases as dashed lines. Then using the slow phase (VOR phase), a sine wave is reconstructed (D). This patient's sine wave is actually fairly straight, that is, there is no drift of the sine wave. So, in Figure 14–6 the chair is rotating for four cycles at 0.16 Hz in the dark at a peak velocity of 50 deg/s. This patient has essentially no directional preponderance with an asymmetry of only –1% (i.e., mildly greater gain—average of the slow component velocity divided by the chair or head velocity—to the left, or a right-beating nystagmus).

Figure 14–7 displays similar data at 0.16 Hz for a second patient, except that the reconstructed lower line now has a downward drift from left to right, or a negative slope. The patient's data, displayed in Figure 14–7 represent four cycles of rotation at 0.16 Hz with the same peak velocity of 50 deg/s, but this time the patient has a –25% asymmetry which is

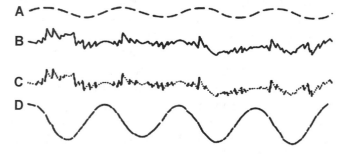

Figure 14-6. A summary of chair and eye position recordings during four cycles of harmonic acceleration at 0.16 Hz with a directional preponderance of –1.0%. The lines represent: chair rotation (**A**), right and left-beating nystagmus consistent with the chair rotation (**B**), dashed lines representing slow phases of the nystagmus and solid lines representing the fast phases of the nystagmus (**C**), and the reconstructed eye position sine wave from the slow-phase eye velocity vestibular components (**D**). Note that the reconstructed sine wave is relatively flat with no drift.

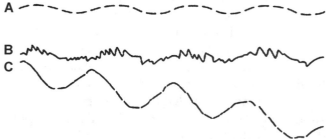

Figure 14-7. A summary of chair and eye position recordings during four cycles of harmonic acceleration at 0.16 Hz with a directional preponderance of –25%. The lines represent: chair rotation (**A**), right and left-beating nystagmus consistent with the chair rotation (**B**), and the reconstructed eye position sine wave using only the slow-phase vestibular components (**C**). Note that the reconstructed sine wave is not flat but has a negative slope or drift.

greater gain to the left or a right-beating directional preponderance.

These examples were provided to demonstrate how the eye movements are collected, deconstructed, and then reconstructed to provide the data needed clinically for assessment of the peripheral vestibular system for patients during rotational chair testing. This analysis procedure is completed with the use of computers; however, it is necessary for the clinician conducting rotational chair testing to understand how the data are obtained.

Secondary to the lack of a fully recognized standardized paradigm for sinusoidal rotary chair, there is no standardized set of normative data for the measured parameters for rotary chair. Therefore, each laboratory needs to develop their own or use ones developed by groups of laboratories as long as they are using the same features in the paradigm and settings for analysis. Shown in Table 14–1 are the normative ranges for the sinusoidal rotatory chair usage at Mayo Clinic in Rochester. These were developed from both the University of Michigan and Mayo Clinic. These are for the reader reference only without any recommendation for use and for these the saccade factor is set at 1.2 with peak chair velocity at 60 deg/s. The literature does contain other samples of normative ranges for various other protocols. The normative ranges in Table 14–1 were developed over age range from 20 to 80 but not with equal distribution of subjects in each age range. Although there is literature that shows a statistically significant change in phase angle with age (Peterka, Black, & Schoemhoff, 1990), the effect was not clinically significant enough to warrant an age-specific normative range for the parameters shown in the table.

Sinusoidal Harmonic Acceleration Paradigm

For some period of time there was interest in using a single-frequency sinusoidal stimulus for rotation (Cramer, 1963; Mathog, 1972). However, as the semicircular canal system acts as an angular accelerometer for head motion from very low frequencies such as those simulated with caloric stimulation (i.e., 0.004 to 0.008 Hz) to normal head motion (i.e., 0.5 to 5.0 Hz) (Leigh & Zee, 1991), it has become popular to evaluate output of the vestibular system over a wide portion of its operating range (Cyr, 1991).

Rotary chair test protocols vary somewhat but commonly clinicians use oscillation frequencies which are octaves of 0.01 Hz (i.e., 0.02, 0.04, 0.08, 0.16, 0.32, and 0.64 Hz) with peak fixed angular velocities of 50 to 60 deg/s at each frequency (Stockwell, 1988). The number of cycles used with each frequency increases with frequency as the time for each cycle shortens with the increase in frequency. Typical cycle repetitions would be as follows: 3 at 0.01 Hz, 3 at 0.02 Hz, 4 at 0.04 Hz, 8 at 0.08 Hz through 0.32 Hz, and 10 at 0.64 Hz. The slow component eye velocity is averaged over the number of cycles to reduce the noise in eye movement traces. It is advantageous to do as many cycles as possible, but this has to be balanced against the length of time it takes for multiple frequency testing. With this method, as frequency increases with the velocity fixed, acceleration increases and the excursions (i.e., rightward and leftward movement) of the chair decreases. Additionally, with the patient's body and head secured properly, 1.28 Hz and with newer torque chairs up to 2 Hz can be tested. However, the use of 1.28 Hz and

Table 14–1. Normative Data Two Standard Deviation Ranges for Sinusoidal Rotary Chair Systems Used at Mayo Clinic Rochester

	Sinusoidal Harmonic Acceleration Norms (Two Standard Deviations)						
	0.01 Hz	0.02 Hz	0.04 Hz	0.08 Hz	0.16 Hz	0.32 Hz	0.64 Hz
Gain	0.13–0.6	0.21–0.69	0.31–0.9	0.40–0.96	0.36–1.01	0.39–1.08	0.43–1.12
Phase (deg)	22–51.4	12–32	2.4–19.9	−2.8–10.7	−6.2–6.3	−16–5.7	−19–2.5
Asymmetry (%)	−14–18	−13.9–20.1	−14–17	−11–13	−16.5–16.5	−10–12.5	−12.3–13.8
Spectral purity (%)	63.8–99.9	68.4–99.9	81.3–99.9	85–99.9	85.3–99.9	90.3–99.9	90.3–99.9

above are now rarely if ever used as it is not possible to secure the head to the chair adequately and hence the head slips in its movement relative to the chair. In order to analyze such a situation a rate sensory would need to be added to the head to detect motion of the head compared to the chair and that factored into the analysis. This adds a level of complexity that is not practical, so the standard protocols stop at 0.64 Hz. A primary drawback to the use of multiple sinusoidal stimuli is the time it takes to test four to seven frequencies. This is particularly difficult when testing in the 0.01- to 0.08-Hz range (Shepard & Telian, 1996). For example, testing three cycles at 0.01 Hz requires 5 min to complete.

There have been numerous attempts to shorten the time required for testing. Both the pseudo-random impulse design (Wall, Black, & O'Leary, 1978) and the sum of sines method (Peterka, 2005; Wall, 1990) have been utilized with varying degrees of success to shorten the rotational test, but they have not found wide acceptance. More recently, a rotational chair manufacturer has proposed a protocol using a fixed acceleration instead of a fixed velocity. In theory, this would shorten the test time and increase the number of cycles obtained especially in the lower frequencies. The ability to obtain more cycles of data increases the reliability of the information obtained during testing. However, this is just a proposal and for it to become used clinically, further research needs to be completed to ensure the accuracy and reliability of the data obtained in this fashion.

When using the sinusoidal, fixed-velocity paradigm the most nauseating frequency by anecdotal report is 0.01 Hz. Also this is the one that lasts the longest and may provide the greater challenge for maintaining alertness for the subject, especially when we are testing infants to young children (this is discussed in Chapter 25). The authors therefore recommend that the order of frequency examination be 0.08, 0.04, 0.01, 0.16, 0.32, and 0.64 Hz (this would be with the number of cycles given above). Typically, for shortening the protocol in a patient with no indications of possible bilateral pathology a three-frequency approach of 0.08, 0.04, and 0.01 Hz is adequate. We will add in the other frequencies, typically 0.02 Hz for patients in whom there is a suspicion of bilateral peripheral involvement or indications of possible central vestibular system involvement

especially brainstem. The use in interpretation of the normative values and variations on the paradigm is discussed in Chapter 15.

VELOCITY STEP TESTING

The second form of rotational stimulus in general use is the velocity step or impulse stimulus. The primary advantage of step or impulse stimuli is the rapid measurement of gain and time constant of the VOR rotating in both a clockwise and counterclockwise direction (Baloh & Honrubia, 1990). Time constant and gain are the primary outcome parameters for the step test. Time constant is related to phase angle from the sinusoidal protocol, and this is discussed in detail below. The disadvantage of the step test is that this is not as comfortable for the patient as the sinusoidal testing and as a result only one test is usually performed in the CW and one in the CCW direction for each of the peak velocities used. The result is a reliability issue for the data obtained. In the sinusoidal protocol the repeated cycles at any of the frequencies are averaged to obtain the average slow component eye movements in which via the averaging technique, the noise in the eye trace has been reduced. There is typically no averaging scheme for the step testing protocol.

Figure 14–8 shows an example of the time course for step testing at 60 and 240 deg/s with acceleration and deceleration rates of 200 deg/s² (a more typical acceleration/deceleration rate currently would be 100 deg/s²). From this figure it can be seen that it requires 0.3 s to reach maximum velocity at 60 deg/s and 1.2 s to reach maximum velocity at 240 deg/s. Data are collected during the 60-s peak velocity times (per-rotatory nystagmus) as well as during the 60-s stop times (postrotatory nystagmus). Therefore, four estimates of time constants result. When the patient is spun to the right you stimulate the right periphery and once the acceleration is stopped, when the patient reaches the maximum velocity of 60 or 240 deg/s, the stimulation to the right peripheral system stops and the peripheral activity along with the resultant eye movements begin to decay (peripheral systems are responsive to acceleration/deceleration only). This is the per-rotatory nystagmus time constant for the right periphery. Once the chair is

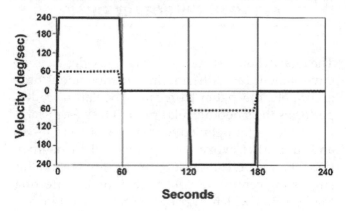

Figure 14–8. Time course for the 60 and 240 deg/s step tests. Acceleration and deceleration rates are 200 deg/s². Per-rotatory and postrotatory testing last 60 s in both right and left directions.

then decelerated rapidly to a stop, this produces stimulation of the left peripheral system and this is the postrotatory estimate of the time constant for the left periphery. When the patient is then spun to the left you get two additional estimates of the time constants for the left (per-rotatory) and the right (postrotatory). In general the per- and postrotatory time constant estimates for the right or left systems should be the same or very close. Therefore, for a final estimate of overall time constant for the right and left systems an average value of the two estimates is taken as the time constant for the right or left peripheral systems. The use of the time constants and the use of the estimates at the different speeds are discussed in detail in Chapter 15 under interpretations. Time constants, or the length of time it takes to go from peak nystagmus slow-phase velocity to 37% of that velocity in an exponential decay pattern, are calculated using a best-fit line, along with the initial peak velocity for comparisons of gain between the two ears.

Recording the vestibular system time constant allows the examiner to evaluate the combination of the peripheral vestibular (cupular) response to the velocity step, which has been reported to be approximately 6 s (Goldberg & Fernandez, 1971), as well as the central velocity storage influence over the duration of the eye movements (Raphan et al., 1979). These are reflected in the canal ocular reflex time constant which results from the slow compo-

nent eye velocity decay over time from the impulse stimulation to the right or the left. As noted earlier, the velocity storage system extends the eye movement response and sensation of motion beyond that of the peripheral labyrinth alone (the 6-s time constant to an average 14 to 16 s for the canal-ocular time constant).

There is a specific relationship between the time constant for the right and left periphery and the phase angle that is generated by the sinusoidal chair protocol. This relationship is grounded in the mathematical foundations that govern the workings of the peripheral vestibular system response to sinusoidal versus impulse stimulation. The simple form of this relationship is only valid for rotational frequencies below 0.04 Hz. In general, as the phase angle increases, the overall system time constant decreases. This time constant is a general one that is not specific to the left or the right but rather represents a combination of the sides. The conversion of phase angle to time constant is given as follows:

$$Tcor = 1/[\omega Tan\ \varphi]$$

Tcor is the canal ocular reflex time constant; ω is the angular frequency ($2\pi f$ where f is the frequency of rotation); and φ is the phase angle at that frequency of rotation.

The other measurements of interest during step testing are response gain and symmetry. The response gain is the peak slow-phase eye velocity divided by the peak chair (head) velocity (either 60 or 240 deg/s in this discussion). Like the time constant *s* there are two estimates of the response gain for step rotations to the right and two estimates of the response gain for the rotations to the left. These, like the time constants, are averaged for a response gain for the right and for the left. Symmetry of the response would be calculated by taking the averaged peak slow-phase eye velocity from the right and subtracting from that the average peak slow-phase eye velocity from the left, dividing by the sum of those two values, and multiplying by 100 to generate a percentage difference between the left and right similar to that used in the sinusoidal rotation paradigm and analogous to that used for calculating caloric irrigation symmetry. Typical normative values in the author's laboratory are response gain of 0.3 and above and symmetry of 30% or less with time constants between 10 and 26 s. These represent the lower of the two standard deviation values for the response gain, the upper of the two standard deviation values for symmetry, and the full two standard deviation ranges for the time constant. These have been developed from the author's laboratory at the University of Michigan and Mayo Clinic. There are no formally accepted normative ranges for step testing paradigms, but these agree with those used in other laboratories across the country. Variations in the equipment used in a laboratory and variations in protocols can make for differences in the normative ranges, and individual laboratories are encouraged to verify their normative ranges against those provided by manufactures and against individual laboratories such as that of the authors before adopting them for their personal use. The use of these values in regard to the meaning of values outside the normal range is discussed with patient examples in Chapter 15. This is done for both the step tests and the sinusoidal rotation test.

Step Test Paradigm

The primary purpose for the use of the 60 deg/s velocity is to provide an accurate estimate of the system time constant for both the right and left. As the velocity increases, especially above 200 deg/s, the estimate of time constant decreases. Most step test protocols use 60 to 100 deg/s as the peak low velocity with a 100 deg/s^2 acceleration/deceleration. As shown in Figure 14–8, a 60-s interval is used for recording the decay of the slow component velocity eye movements after the initial acceleration and the subsequent deceleration. The authors then strongly recommend that the testing be stopped for a 2- to 3-min break before proceeding to the other direction of rotation (this is not shown in the figure). By the use of the response gain values for the left and the right as well as the symmetry, one can suggest possible unilateral or bilateral hypofunction and a lack of physiologic compensation for the suspected peripheral insult. The use of the 240 deg/s step test is to try and drive a peripheral asymmetry that may be compensated well enough that the 60 deg/s step does not show abnormal gain or symmetry. Therefore, in the 240 deg/s step test time constant is ignored and only response gain and symmetry are used. Chapter 15 details the use of these parameters.

OPTOKINETIC AND OTHER TESTING IN THE ROTARY CHAIR

The rotary chair test enclosure also provides an ideal environment for gathering information about how accurately the patient produces ocular saccades, performs the smooth ocular pursuit task (see Chapters 9 and 10 for detailed discussions of these tests), and suppresses evoked nystagmus with visual fixation. The visual fixation suppression test is a tool for suggesting central nervous system deficit affecting this function which overlaps with the neurological substrate for smooth pursuit and gaze fixation (see Chapter 2 for discussion). The VOR cancellation or suppression test is noted with caloric irrigations (Chapters 12 and 13), and there is a bedside form of this same test (Chapter 7). This paradigm is the most similar to the bedside version of the test because in both cases, unlike that with caloric stimulation, natural stimulus of acceleration is being used. However, with the chair, the challenge to the patient's central vestibular system can be controlled in a precise manner. The patient rotates in the chair from 0.04 to 0.64 Hz and is asked to fix his or her gaze on the calibration light rotating with the patient. The gain ratio of slow component velocity to eyes fixed on the calibration light to the slow component velocity from the eyes while rotating in the dark is calculated. Because the stimulus is accurately controlled, this appears to be a much better measure than the fixation suppression test during caloric irrigation. Mayo Clinic normative data are presented in Table 14–2 (McPherson & Brey, 2005). Although all the frequencies can be used with increasing challenge to the central system, anecdotally a single frequency test of suppression is the most practical manner in which to perform the study and 0.08 Hz would be the frequency of choice.

Optokinetic stimulation, if performed, needs to be carried out in an environment where the stimulus will fill the entire visual field, together with the patient seated in a chair known to move, the patient is more likely to experience the phenomenon of circular vection (visually induced sensation of self-rotation) (Ito, 1999). The patient's field of vision must not be restricted if there is to be good perception of the chair turning with optokinetic stimulation. Therefore, either EOG measurement or video goggles with open sides would be ideal for this test. Optokinetic testing also provides a means of assessing central

Table 14–2. Normative Data for Fixation Suppression Testing in a Rotary Chair Environment for 0.04, 0.08, 0.16, 0.32, and 0.64 Hz

	Norms for Fixation Suppression[a]				
	.04	.08	.16	.32	.64
Mean grain ration	0.05	0.08	0.12	0.11	0.16
Plus 2 SD	0.11	0.18	0.23	0.18	0.26
Percent (%) reduction	89%	82%	77%	82%	74%

[a]Abnormal assumes deviation from normative data >2 SD.

velocity storage generated by the optokinetic signal called *optokinetic after nystagmus* (OKAN). Step testing as discussed previously, allows for the measurement of central velocity storage following rotation, whereas optokinetic testing only allows measurement of central velocity storage generated by a visual input. A more complete discussion of optokinetic testing (OKN) and the rationale behind the eye movements being dominated with smooth pursuit is provided in Chapter 10. There are two paradigms that can be used for studying OKN. First is the use of sinusoidal stimulus movement. The frequencies are typically ones in the range used for smooth pursuit tracking test (0.2 to 0.6 Hz). When this is done the velocity gain results (peak eye velocity divided by stimulus velocity) are compared to the velocity gain normative values shown in Chapter 10 for the standard smooth pursuit test given the significant dominance of the smooth pursuit system over the generation of the eye movements. This can be very useful in the evaluation of children between 2 and 6 months as they do not develop smooth pursuit abilities until around 4 to 5 months of age. The second, more traditional paradigm, is that of fixed velocity stimulus movement first in one direction and then in the reverse direction. Typically, target speeds of 20 and 40 deg/s are used. As in the discussion in Chapter 10, this would be the stimulus that would be used if an OKAN paradigm was to be used to tap into the true optokinetic system of central system neurologic substrate. For the fixed velocity paradigm, the visual field is fully filled with the stimulus but nonetheless the dominant system is still smooth pursuit and the test has poor performance and reliability attributes as described in Chapter 10. Mayo Clinic normative data for optokinetic fixed velocity testing are found in Table 14–3 (Baird, 2000).

Table 14–3. Normative Data for Slow-Phase Velocity During Optokinetic Testing in a Rotary Chair Environment at 20, 40, and 60 deg/s

	Optokinetics Test Norms[a]		
	20 deg/s	40 deg/s	60 deg/s
Mean velocities	22.52	42.48	61.91
Minus 2 SD	13.81	22.62	
Critical increase*	20 to 40 = 8.81	40 to 60 = –2.08	

[a]Abnormal assumes deviation from normative data >2 SD.

Off-Vertical Axis Testing

The topic of otolith-ocular function testing is addressed in subsequent chapters. However, off-vertical axis rotational test (OVAR) has been a method investigated for assessing otolith function (Furman & Baloh, 1992; Furman, Schor, & Kamerer, 1993; Kushiro et al., 2002). Figure 14–9 shows such a device.

In this test the patient's eye movements are evaluated during rotation about an axis that is tilted away from earth vertical (Darlot, Denise, Droulez, Cohen, & Berthoz, 1988; Guedry, 1965; Harris & Barnes 1987). A continuous nystagmus is evoked by relatively small angles of tilt having two components. A velocity drift of less than 10 deg/s in the direction opposite to rotation is referred to as *bias*, and a sinusoidal modulation of slow-phase velocity is referred to as *modulation* (Leigh & Zee, 1991). Although this test has found some degree of interest, off-vertical axis rotation does provoke nausea in many patients and has not gained wide acceptance clinically.

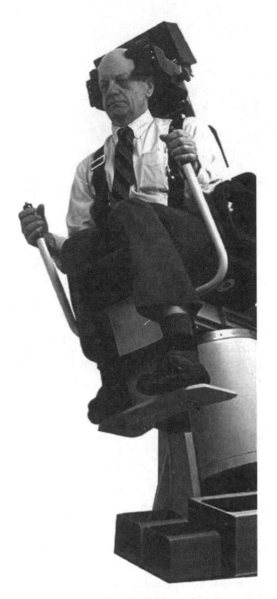

Figure 14–9. Jan C. Parmentier, EE, seated in a chair that not only rotates on earth axis, but also off earth axis by as much as 30 degrees of tilt. Photo courtesy of Neuro Kinetics, Inc.

Unilateral Centrifugation

A more recent development in otolith testing using rotation is the unilateral centrifugation test (UC) (Clarke & Engelhorn, 1998; Clarke, Schonfeld, Hamann, & Scherer, 2001; Wetzig, J., Hofstetter-Degen, K., Maurer, J., & von Baumgarten, 1992; Wetzig, Reiser, Martin, Bregenzer, & von Baumgarten, 1990; Wuyts, Hoppenbrouwers, Pauwels, & Van de Heyning, 2003). The goal of UC testing is to try to sepa-

rate populations with unilateral or bilateral utricular involvement from populations with normal utricular function. UC involves the assessment of the utricle by translating the rotational chair to the right or left so the axis of rotation, which is typically through the center of the head, is now through one of the utricles. For interested readers, this is discussed further in Chapter 22. Since the utricle is sensitivity to gravitational forces (linear acceleration), the utricle on axis is stimulated only by the pull of gravity but does not have any stimulation from centrifugal forces leaving the off-axis utricle isolated for individual assessment by the centrifugal force together with gravity. However, when translating the chair in order to isolate and test individual utricular function, the distance between utricles must be estimated for maximum effectiveness during testing.

Nowe et al. (2003) conducted research that showed the "mean distance between the medial margins of the vestibules was 7.22 cm with a 95% prediction interval of 6.38 to 8.06 cm." From this calculation, they determined the lateral displacement of the chair should be between 3.19 and 4.03 cm. Similarly, Figure 14–10 displays a high-resolution, computed tomography (CT) image of the temporal bones. Measurement of the anatomic features seen in this image allowed for description of the two vestibular systems and their relative positions in the head. From the center of the head to the utricle is 3.87 cm. When the patient is moved off-center axis by 3.87 cm to the right, the distance from the left utricle (now the center of rotation) to the right utricle that is now experiencing the centrifugal force will be twice the 3.87 cm or a distance of 7.74 cm. When it moves to the left, the opposite happens. The chair moves to the left placing the center of rotational axis through the right utricle, and the centrifugal force now at the left utricle will be based on a distance of 7.74 cm which is similar to the data reported by Nowe et al. (2003).

UC testing may be accomplished in two ways. In the first approach, the chair is locked and shifted to the right or left sufficient to place one utricle over the center of the axis of rotation so that the other utricle will have a horizontal centrifugal force placed on it as the chair rotates at 300 to 400 deg/s (Wetzig et al., 1990). The second approach differs in that the chair accelerates slowly up to 300 to 400 deg/s with the axis of rotation through the center of the head until the patient no longer senses rotation. Then,

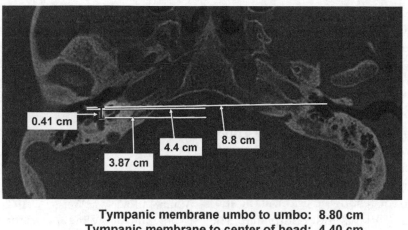

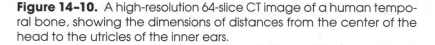

Tympanic membrane umbo to umbo: 8.80 cm
Tympanic membrane to center of head: 4.40 cm
Utricle to center of head: 3.87 cm
Reid's plane to utricle: 0.41 cm

Figure 14–10. A high-resolution 64-slice CT image of a human temporal bone, showing the dimensions of distances from the center of the head to the utricles of the inner ears.

maintaining this velocity of rotation, a motor drives the chair to the left or right creating the centrifugal force on the utricle away from the axis of rotation (Clarke & Engelhorn, 1998; Clarke et al., 2001; Wuyts et al., 2003).

For both methods, the patient's perceptions are that of tilting toward the ear that is off the axis of rotation. This result secondary to the horizontal force on the utricle away from the axis of rotation is the same as if the patient had physically tilted his or her head toward the shoulder on the side away from the axis of rotation. To quantify the response of the utricle getting the horizontal force, one can measure the ocular counter roll of the eyes back in the direction of the axis of rotation. This requires a three-dimensional eye movement recording system. The alternative is to have the patient perform a test called subjective visual vertical (SVV) while he or she is rotating at the fixed velocity of typically 300 deg/s off the axis of rotation. The SVV has the patient set a displayed line by remote control to what they perceive as vertical and to do this a number of times taking the average of their setting. The force on the eccentric utricle causes the eye to counter-roll in the opposite direction, and therefore they set the line off true vertical in the direction of the utricle that has the axis of rotation going through it. The actual torsion of the eye is difficult to measure reliably espe-

cially at a speed of 300 deg/s and in our and other's experience the patients do not tolerate 400 deg/s well secondary to a feeling of being thrown out of the chair. So the compromise is to use 300 deg/s and the SVV as the outcome measure.

Recently, Janky and Shepard (2010) examined both methods of completing UC (translate to the right or left first and then spin or spin and when at the final fixed velocity then translate to the right or left) with interest in how each method affected the outcome parameters of ocular torsion and SVV. Additionally, the level or nausea produced by each method was evaluated. The results of the study showed no significant difference in the use of either method in terms of ocular torsion, SVV deviation, and level of nausea.

UC Paradigm

For all rotational chair protocols, the patient is seated in light tight enclosed room in a chair mounted atop a computer controlled torque motor. The patient is secured using a five-point lap-belt torso harness and foot harnesses. Additionally, for UC and 240 deg/s step test, the between leg bolster should be raised (if available depending on the manufacturer of the chair) and the knee strap put in place. The patient's head is situated in a head rest that is tipped forward

30 degrees with the axis of rotation being through the center of the head. The head is stabilized using a head restraint system which is attached to the chair head rest. If for any reason the appropriate straps cannot be placed properly or the patient exceeds 350 lb, the test for UC or the 240 deg/s step test should not be performed.

In our laboratory, the first approach described above where the rotational chair is translated to the right or left first and then accelerated is what is utilized. However, after securing the patient and placing the patient in the testing position, static subjective visual vertical (SVV) is first completed. The patient is asked to adjust a 25-cm line, which is projected on the enclosure wall, to their perceived vertical using the hand controls on the chair. A minimum of five responses is needed to obtain the patient's static SVV.

The rotational chair is then translated to the right or left, which is a subjective choice given to the clinician. For example, if the right utricle is tested first the chair is translated 4 cm to the right, which takes roughly 32 s to complete. This would place the left utricle on-axis with the right utricle off-axis. The chair is then accelerated 3 deg/s² always in the direction of nose toward the direction of rotation (for the right utricle off axis the rotation is CCW and for the left utricle the rotation is CW) for 100 s while the patient is staring at a single fixation point projected onto the enclosure. The reason for the constant direction of rotation so that the ear off axis is positioned on the outside of the rotation circle is to avoid asymmetrical stimulation of the utricles that can result in biased results (Janky & Shepard, 2010). The chair accelerates to a constant velocity of 300 deg/s and remains at that constant velocity for 120 s. While at constant velocity, the patient is asked to again adjust the 25-cm projected line on the enclosure wall to their perceived vertical. The patient performs 12 trials, each 10 s in duration. After the 120 s has been completed, the chair then decelerates at a rate of 3 deg/s² for 100 s then comes to a stop. After stopping, the chair will then move back to center which again takes 32 s. The patient is then given a short break. The process is then repeated in similar fashion with the patient completing SVV in center sitting still prior to the chair being translated in the opposite direction. The average value of the tilt of the projected line away from true vertical during the two static trials (one prior to CCW and one prior to CW rotation) is used for comparison to the average value of the tilt of the line obtained during the rotations CCW and CW. A further discussion of the interpretation of these outcome parameters is given in Chapter 15.

REFERENCES

Allum, J., Tole, J., & Weiss, A. (1975). MITNYS-11-A digital program for on-line analysis of nystagmus. *IEEE Transactions on Biomedical Engineering, 22*, 196.

Baird, R. J. (2000). *Optokinetic response to 20, 40, 60, 80, and 100 deg/s full field drum and sphere stimulation* (Unpublished thesis). Brigham Young University, Provo, UT.

Baloh, R. H., & Honrubia, V. (1990). *Clinical neurophysiology of the vestibular system*. Philadelphia, PA: F. A. Davis.

Baloh, R. H., Kumley, W., Sills, A., & Honrubia, V. (1975). Quantitative measurement of saccade amplitude, duration and velocity. *Neurology, 25*, 1065.

Baloh, R. H., Langhofer, L., Honrubia, V., & Yee, R. D. (1980). On-line analysis of eye movements using a digital computer. *Aviation Space and Environmental Medicine, 51*(6), 563–567.

Bárány, R. (1907). *Physiologie und Pathologie des Bogengangsapparates beim Menchen*. Vienna, Austria: Deuticke.

Brey, R. H. (2002). Vertigo and balance. In J. R. Daube (Ed.), *Clinical neurophysiology* (pp. 431–433). New York, NY: Oxford University Press.

Clarke, A. H., & Engelhorn, A. (1998). Unilateral testing of utricular function. *Experimental Brain Research, 121*, 457–464.

Clarke, A. H., Schonfeld, U., Hamann, C., & Scherer, H. (2001). Measuring unilateral otolith function via the otolith-ocular response and the subjective visual vertical. *Acta Otolaryngology, Supplement 545*, 84–87.

Cohen, B., & Raphan, T. (2004). The physiology of the vestibuloocular reflex (VOR). In S. M. Highstein, R. R. Fay, & A. N. Popper (Eds.), *The vestibular system* (pp. 235–285). New York, NY: Springer-Verlag.

Cramer, R. (1963). The dynamic characteristics of the vestibulo-ocular reflex arc after prolonged stimulation. *Biomedical Scientific Instrumentation, 1*, 401–406.

Cyr, D. G. (1991). Vestibular system assessment. In W. Rintelmann (Ed.), *Hearing assessment* (pp. 739–804). Austin, TX: Pro-Ed.

Darlot, C., Denise, P., Droulez, J., Cohen, B., & Berthoz, A. (1988). Eye movements induced by off-vertical axis rotation (OVAR) at small angles of tilt. *Experimental Brain Research, 73*(1), 91–105.

Dodge, R. (1903). Five types of eye movements in the horizontal meridian plane of the field of regard. *American Journal of Physiology, 8*, 307–329.

DuBois-Reymond, E. (1849). Untersuchungen uber thiersche elektrizitat. *Verlag von G. Reimer*, pp. 256–270.

Engelken, E. J., & Wolfe, J. W. (1977). Analog signal processing of eye movements for on-line digital computer analysis. *Physiology and Behavior, 18*(1), 157–158.

Furman, J. M., & Baloh, R. W. (1992). Otolith-ocular testing in human subjects. *Annals of the New York Academy of Sciences, 656*, 431–451.

Furman, J. M., Schor, R. H., & Kamerer, D. B. (1993). Off-vertical axis rotational responses In patients with unilateral peripheral vestibular lesions. *Annals of Otology, Rhinology and Laryngology, 102*, 137–143.

Goldberg, J. M., & Fernandez, C. (1971). Physiology of peripheral neurons innervating semicircular canals of the squirrel monkey. I. Resting discharge and response to constant angular accelerations. *Journal of Neurophysiology, 34*(4), 635–660.

Guedry, F. E. (1965). Orientation of the rotation axis relative to gravity: Its influence on nystagmus and the sensation of rotation. *Acta Oto-Laryngologica, 60*, 30–48.

Harris, L. R., & Barnes, G. R. (1987). Orientation of vestibular nystagmus is modified by head tilt. In M. D. Graham & J. L. Kemink (Eds.), *The vestibular system: Neurophysiologic and clinical research* (pp. 539–548). New York, NY: Raven Press.

Honrubia, V., Katz, D., Strelioff, D., & Ward, P. (1971). Computer analysis of induced vestibular nystagmus rotatory stimulation of normal cats. *Annals of Otology, 80*(Suppl. 3), 7–25.

Ito, H. (1999). Motion direction distribution as a determinant of circular vection. *Perceptual Motor Skills, 89*(2), 564–570.

Janky, K. L., & Shepard, N. T. (2010). Unilateral centrifugation: Utricular assessment and protocol comparison. *Otology & Neurology, 32*, 116–121.

Jones, G. M., & Milsum, J. H. (1965). Spatial and dynamic aspects of visual fixation. *IEEE Transactions on Biomedical Engineering, 12*(2), 54–62.

Kushiro, K., Dai, M., Kunin, M., Yakushin, S. B., Cohen, B., & Raphan, T. (2002). Compensatory and orienting eye movements induced by off-vertical axis rotation (OVAR) in monkeys. *Journal of Neurophysiology, 88*(5), 2445–2462.

Leigh, R. J., & Zee, D. (1991). *The neurology of eye movements*. Philadelphia, PA: F. A. Davis.

Mathog, R. (1972). Testing of the vestibular system by sinusoidal angular acceleration. *Acta Otolaryngol (Stockholm), 74*, 96–103.

McPherson, J. H., & Brey, R. H. (2005). *Visual suppression of rotation induced nystagmus and perception of rotation:*

Significance in understanding patient symptoms. Paper presented at the Grand Rounds American Academy of Audiology, Annual Convention, Washington, DC.

Meiry, J. (1971). Vestibular and proprioceptive stabilization of eye movements. In P. Bachy-Rita, C. C. Collins, & J. E. Hyde (Eds.), *The control of eye movements* (pp. 483–496). New York, NY: Academic Press.

Niven, J. I., Hixom, W. C., & Correia, M. J. (1965). An experimental approach to the dynamics of the vestibular mechanisms. *NASA the role of the vestibular organs in the exploration of space, SP-77*, 43–56.

Nowe, V., Wuyts, F. L., Hoppenbrouwers, M., Van de Heyning, P. H., De Schepper, A. M., & Parizel, P. M. (2003). The interutricular distance determined from external landmarks. *Journal of Vestibular Research, 13*, 17–23.

Peterka, R. (2005). Pulse-step-sine rotation test for the identification of abnormal vestibular function. *Journal of Vestibular Research, 15*, 291–311.

Peterka, R., Black, F. O., & Schoemhoff, M. B. (1990). Age-related changes in human vestibulo-ocular reflexes: Sinusoidal rotation and caloric tests. *Journal of Vestibular Research, 1*, 49–59.

Ranacher, G. (1977). Nystagmus analysis by computer. *Archives Oto-Rhino-Laryngology, 215*, 257.

Raphan, T., Matsuo, V., & Cohen, B. (1979). Velocity storage in the vestibulo-ocular reflex arc (VOR). *Experimental Brain Research, 35*, 229–248.

Schilder, P., Pasik, P., & Pasik, T. (1973). On-line analysis of optokinetic nystagmus by small general purpose digital computer. *Acta Oto-Laryngologica, 76*, 443–449.

Shepard, N. T. (2001). Rotational chair testing. In J. A. Goebel (Ed.), *Practical management of the dizzy patient*. Philadelphia, PA: Lippincott Williams & Wilkins.

Shepard, N. T., & Telian, S. A. (1996). *Practical management of the balance disorder patient*. San Diego, CA: Singular.

Stockwell, C. W. (1988). Computerized vestibular function tests. *Hearing Journal, 41*, 20–29.

Van de Calseyde, P., & Dupondt, M. (1974). The damped torsion swing test. Quantitative and qualitative aspects of ENG patterns in normal subjects. *Archives of Otolaryngology, 100*, 449.

Van Egmond, A. A., Groen, J. J., & Jongkees, L. B. W. (1949). The mechanics of the semicircular canal. *Journal of Physiology, 110*, 1–17.

Waespe, W., Cohen, B., & Raphan, T. (1985). Dynamic modification of the vestibulo-ocular reflex by the nodulus and uvula. *Science, 228*(4696), 199–202.

Wall, C., 3rd. (1990). The sinusoidal harmonic acceleration rotary chair test. Theoretical and clinical basis. *Neurologic Clinics, 8*(2), 269–285.

Wall, C., 3rd, Black, F. O., & O'Leary, D. P. (1978). Clinical use of pseudorandom binary sequence white noise in assessment of the human vestibulo-ocular system. *Annals of Otology, Rhinology and Laryngology, 87*(6, Pt. 1), 845–852.

Wetzig, J., Hofstetter-Degen, K., Maurer, J., & von Baumgarten, R. J. (1992). Clinical verification of a unilateral otolith test. *Acta Astronautica, 27,* 19–24.

Wetzig, J., Reiser, M., Martin, E., Bregenzer, N., & von Baumgarten, R. J. (1990). Unilateral centrifugation of the otoliths as a new method to determine bilateral asymmetries of the otolith apparatus in man. *Acta Astronautica, 21*(6/7), 519–525.

Wuyts, F. L., Hoppenbrouwers, M., Pauwels, G., & Van de Heyning, P. H. (2003). Utricular sensitivity and preponderance assessed by the unilateral centrifugation test. *Journal of Vestibular Research, 13*(4–6), 227–234.

Clinical Utility and Interpretation of Whole-Body Rotation

Neil T. Shepard, Adam M. Goulson, and James H. McPherson

INTRODUCTION

In Chapter 14 the authors covered the history of the development of rotational chair testing and the majority of the technical aspects of the various protocols and the principal parameters used in the analysis. Chapter 15 concentrates less on the technical aspects of rotary chair and more on its clinical utility and the interpretation of the various outcome parameters typically used in the analysis of the various protocols. That said, there are some general technical issues that are worthy of reminding the reader. It is important to remember one of the differences between rotational testing and electronystagmography (ENG)/videonystagmography (VNG) is that both ears are involved simultaneously. Because the peripheral vestibular systems work in a *push-pull* manner, such that when one side is stimulated with angular or linear acceleration the opposite side is inhibited, the chair is not a tool that can be used to isolate one peripheral system from the other for evaluation but can be used to suggest possible localization.

As with many portions of the ENG/VNG, jerk nystagmus that is generated in response to the angular acceleration stimulus is the response of interest regardless of whether eye movements are recorded using EOG or digital video technology. Specifically, the slow component eye velocity of the VOR is the portion of the eye movement for which velocity is calculated for analysis. An assumption of rotational testing is that the head movement matches the movement of the chair. For that reason, the head must be secured to the chair with a restraint system. However, because of the potential for movement of the skin relative to the skull, this assumption becomes faulty at frequencies of 1 Hz or greater or acceleration/deceleration of greater than 300 degrees/s^2. Furthermore, the use of video technology creates the additional potential complication of camera movement relative to the head. Therefore, unless special restraint systems such as bite bars (not practical for routine clinical use) or systems such as accelerometers for measuring the head movement independent of the chair are used, testing above this range will provide erroneous results (personal experience—not from population studies). For those reasons, most commercial systems and clinical research have restricted the upper limit test frequencies to those approaching 1 Hz and upper limit of acceleration/deceleration of 100 degrees/s^2. Figure 15–1 illustrates a clinical rotary chair system consisting of a chair on a computer control electric torque motor pictured with binocular video cameras placed on the head. The head is held firm to the chair, and the

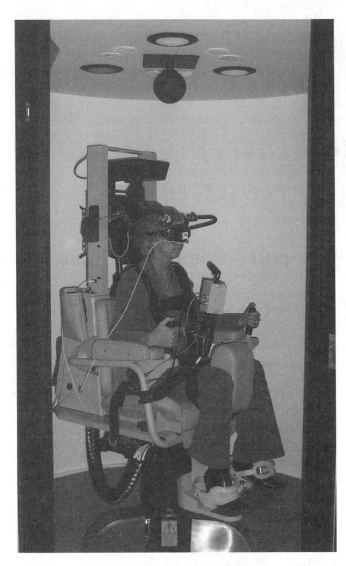

Figure 15–1. One of the commercial rotary chair systems used at Mayo-Rochester. This is a system that is capable of performing a UC protocol. The model in the chair demonstrates the manner in which a patient would be placed in the chair with the head and body restraints and the binocular video eye movement recording system.

system is in an enclosure to allow for testing in darkness with the eyes open.

Addressed briefly in Chapter 14 was the concept of the velocity storage system. In short constant velocity rotations of the head (<10 s), the direct VOR (that driven by the direct response from the vestibular end organ) compensates for the head velocity with appropriate eye velocity. However, for longer

constant velocity rotations the direct vestibular system and its eye movements are known to decay to zero, but compensatory eye movements for up to and beyond 10 s (out to around 15 s) continue. This prolongation of the compensatory eye movements beyond the decay of activity by the hair cells stimulated by the cupula (5 to 6 s) (Goldberg & Fernandez, 1971; Steinhausen, 1933) indicates that a central mechanism, the velocity storage integrator (Raphan & Cohen, 1980; Raphan, Matsuo, & Cohen, 1979) has stored the information from the peripheral system and discharged that over a longer time course than that of the peripheral mechanism. In other words, the velocity storage system has direct influence over the principal outcome parameters of phase and time constant discussed in Chapter 14. The velocity storage integrator is organized through neurologic substrate at the level of the vestibular nuclei in the brainstem (Katz, de Jong, Buttner-Ennever, & Cohen, 1991; Reisine & Raphan, 1992). Hence, lesions in the brainstem can affect the velocity storage system and result in an influence over phase and time constant like that of aberrant input from the VIIIth nerve, as a result of lesions in the VIIIth nerve, or the vestibular end organ. Lesions in both the brainstem and periphery can result in similar changes in the phase angle and the time constant estimates from rotary chair testing. We take this up in greater detail below.

SINUSOIDAL HARMONIC ACCELERATION (SHA) PROTOCOL

As introduced in Chapter 14, there are four outcome parameters related to the sinusoidal protocol used on a typical rotary chair analysis. These are be considered below and related to the interpretation of the study.

Spectral Purity

Spectral purity or similar measure (contingent on the commercial or homemade equipment being used) compares the quality of the sinusoidal nature of the chair movement to that of the eye movement at the frequency of rotation. The measure is not one of the principal outcome measures such as phase, gain, and symmetry. This measure increases or decreases the operator's confidence in the other three outcome measures. The measure looks at the strength of the fundamental frequency of the sinusoidal eye movement and chair movement and compares those in a percentage measure in some commercial systems. The closer to 100% the result, the purer the sinusoidal eye movement at the same frequency of the chair movement and the cleaner the eye movement signal from which to extract the other three principal outcome parameters. As the spectral purity declines, the more likely it is that the phase and symmetry values may be erroneous.

Phase Angle

Phase angle (in degrees) is the principal outcome parameter that signals abnormality of the chair findings. As briefly discussed in Chapter 14 this measure at the low frequencies (<0.04 Hz) is analogous with the parameter *time constant* which we get from the step test protocol. Also shown in Chapter 14 is the mathematical conversion from phase angle in degrees at 0.01 or 0.02 Hz to time constant. Because these are giving analogous information as we discuss phase angle (phase lead), the term *time constant* is used as well for introduction of the concept. Recall from Chapter 14 that if the phase angle shows an abnormally increased phase lead, the time constant will be abnormally low. Phase angle is not an intuitive concept; it is mathematical but can be thought of as a relationship between the head and eye movements. While in normal daily routine head movements the head will always lead the eye movements, this is not the case in sinusoidal head movements and the resultant compensatory eye movements. Refer to Figure 14–4 to visualize this relationship pictorially. The phase angle in degrees is the difference between when the head velocity trace is at its peak velocity and when the eye velocity trace is at its peak slow component eye velocity. In the example in Figure 14–4 the eye velocity trace is at its peak velocity prior to the head reaching its peak velocity, hence a phase lead—the eye is leading the head. As the chair frequency is increased from 0.01 to 0.64

Hz, the phase angle slowly decreases from a phase lead (represented in Table 14–1) as the normative range shifts from all positive to a mix of positive and lower limits being negative. This change in phase from a lead to a lag characterizes the normal function of the peripheral vestibular horizontal semicircular canal as an accelerometer with its inherent frequency dependent characteristics. This is shown in Figure 15–2 in the phase graph in the upper left and by the table of values for this patient in the lower right.

It is known through studies of patients with known peripheral dysfunction that as the vestibular portion of the VIII nerve or the vestibular labyrinth is damaged from a variety of pathologic insults, the resultant information that is sent to the velocity storage system and the eyes causes an abnormally increased phase lead (i.e., a larger than normal phase lead above the two standard deviation normal range) (Table 14–1) and an abnormally low time constant (<10 s) (Baloh, Jacobson, Beykirch, & Honrubia, 1989a; Baloh, Jacobson, & Honrubia, 1989b; Jenkins, Honrubia, & Baloh, 1982). Therefore, the primary clinical utility ascribed to the phase angle is the suggestion that there could be an abnormal input to the eyes and the velocity storage integrator from a lesion in the vestibular labyrinth or vestibular portion of the VIII nerve. Recall from the discussion above, the velocity storage integrator plays a major role in the setting of the normal range of the phase angle (time constant). Given that the neurologic substrate making up the velocity storage system is in the brainstem, lesions in the brainstem can also produce an increase in the phase angle (decrease in the time constant) value recorded, and this is especially true at frequencies below 0.16 Hz. The typical pattern for abnormally increased phase lead from a unilateral peripheral insult would be a decreasingly abnormal phase lead from 0.01 to 0.64 Hz typically returning to the normal range between 0.08 and 0.32 Hz. The magnitude of the abnormal phase angle will depend on the extent of the locus of the unilateral lesion (Figure 15–3). Another pattern that has been seen is a uniformly abnormal increase in phase lead from 0.01 to 0.32 or 0.64 Hz as opposed to the declining abnormal phase lead shown in Figure 15–3 for the patient with a known unilateral, peripheral vestibular system involvement. This pattern of

VESTIBULO OCULAR REFLEX (VOR)

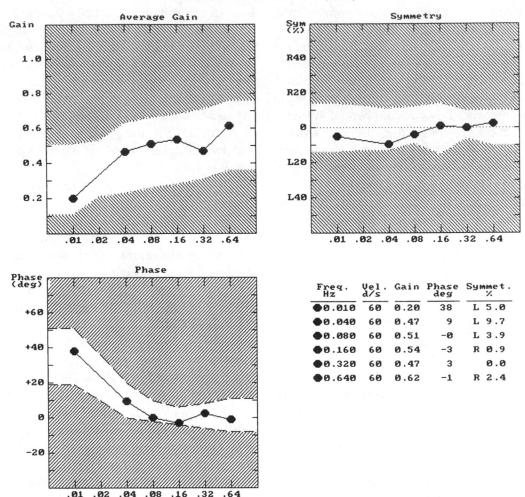

Freq. Hz	Vel. d/s	Gain	Phase deg	Symmet. %
●0.010	60	0.20	38	L 5.0
●0.040	60	0.47	9	L 9.7
●0.080	60	0.51	-0	L 3.9
●0.160	60	0.54	-3	R 0.9
●0.320	60	0.47	3	0.0
●0.640	60	0.62	-1	R 2.4

Figure 15-2. A normal SHA chair study on a patient—see text for details of the patient. The graphs in the upper left, upper right, and lower left show the values of gain, symmetry, and phase angle, respectively, as a function of frequency of chair rotation. The table in the lower right gives the value of the data points shown in the graphs as a function of rotational frequency. In each of the graphs, the two standard deviation range for normal for that parameter is shown in the nonstippled region.

uniformly, abnormal increased phase lead is more suggestive of a possible central vestibular system involvement (brainstem) rather than peripheral (Figure 15–4) (Baloh, Yee, Kimm, & Honrubia, 1981). In this figure the results are from a patient who showed other independent indications of possible brainstem involvement including direction changing gaze-evoked nystagmus (see Chapters 2 and 10).

As previously indicated the time constant for the peripheral vestibular system cupular movement is 5 to 6 s after a step response. The phase angle that corresponds to a time constant of this magnitude is 69 degrees at 0.01 Hz (see the conversion formula in Chapter 14). It is suggested that a time constant or abnormal phase lead of this magnitude represents a stable (lesion site has not recently changed), maximum peripheral vestibular lesion. There can be phase angles that will equal or exceed 69 degrees (a time constant ≤5 s). The implication is that to achieve a phase angle of ≥69 degrees you have to have an

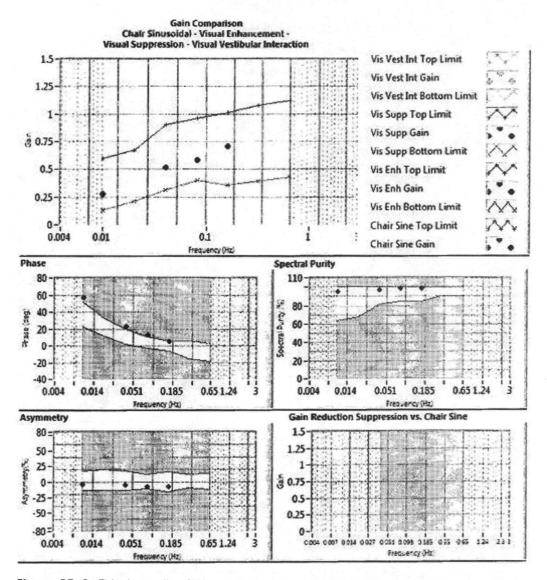

Figure 15–3. This shows the SHA results from a patient with classic peripheral vestibular involvement—see text for details. The graphs at the top, center left, center right, and lower left show the values of gain, phase angle, spectral purity, and symmetry, respectively, as a function of frequency of chair rotation. The graph in the lower right is not used for this or any other figures of similar configuration. The two standard deviation range for normal for each of the parameters is shown in the nonstippled region of each graph.

acute change in a unilateral peripheral lesion or a bilateral lesion. The clinician can take advantage of this pattern to help define a bilateral peripheral pathology. In the typical severe bilateral peripheral hypofunction, we would expect to see little or no response to caloric stimulation even from ice water and a rotary chair result like that shown in Figure 15–5. In this figure, gain values (discussed in detail below) are virtually zero. The spectral purity values are also very low indicating that the signal being recorded for eye movements is essential noise; therefore, no values for phase angle are calculated. In some of the manufacturer systems the operator can set a gain threshold such that no values for phase are calculated if gain falls below this value. However, not all bilateral hypofunction patients are

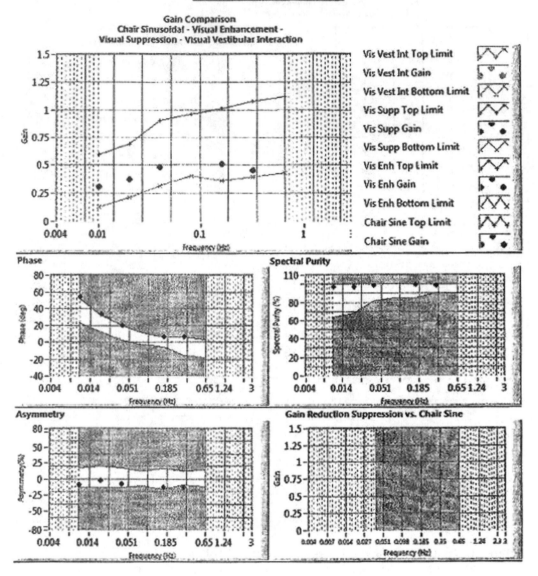

Figure 15–4. The SHA results from a patient with central system involvement—see text for details. Refer to Figure 15–3 legend for description of the figure layout.

this well defined. Figure 15–6 shows the rotary chair findings for a patient with four water caloric irrigations with absolute responses between 6 and 8 deg/s maximum average slow component velocity. The responses showed nystagmus in the correct directions for the temperature of irrigation used. Based on the criteria of possible bilateral hypofunction used in the author's laboratory of <10 deg/s for each of the irrigations, the patient could be a mild bilateral hypofunction. From the discussion above, if these responses represent bilateral peripheral pathology

then we would expect rotational chair phase lead results to show an abnormally large phase lead of greater than 68 degrees at 0.01 Hz, independent of the gain values. As seen in Figure 15–6 the phase lead is 82 degrees at 0.01 Hz but with fully normal gain. Therefore, these findings are interpreted as representing a mild, low frequency bilateral hypofunction. In another example the patient had all four caloric responses between 7 and 10 deg/s. Yet, the rotary chair findings are given in Figure 15–2 with fully normal results. In this case the lack of any

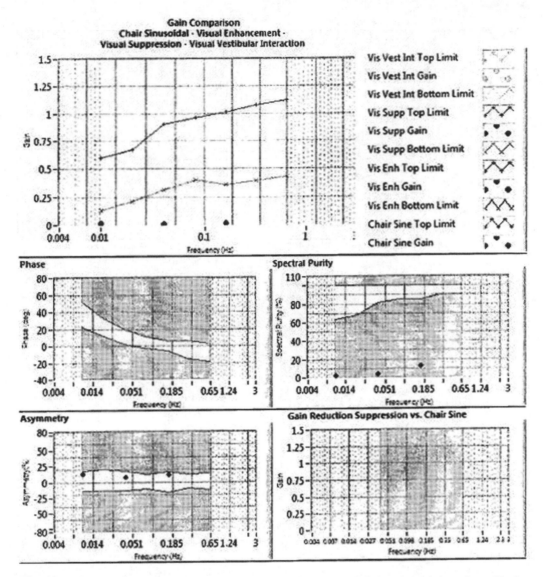

Figure 15-5. The SHA results from a patient with severe bilateral peripheral vestibular hypofunction—see text for details. Refer to Figure 15–3 legend for description of the figure layout.

abnormal phase lead would strongly argue against any bilateral peripheral pathology. This patient's findings were interpreted, as the level of the responsiveness on caloric irrigations is what is normal for this patient even though below the lower limit for the two standard deviation range—there are normal individuals who make up the group that represent the tails of the statistical range beyond two standard deviations.

The clinician needs to be aware that the findings on the sinusoidal rotary chair can be affected by alertness as are the caloric results. The patient rep-

resented in Figure 15–7 had warm and cool water caloric responses ranging from 3 to 5 deg/s for all four irrigations. The chair findings show very low gain values (all <0.15 from 0.01 to 0.32 Hz), and as a result phase angle while calculated is not reliable as the eye movements were in the noise floor and hence consistent with possible bilateral hypofunction of a significant nature. Yet, the ice water irrigations bilaterally were well within normal limits for 50 cc of 2 to 4°C temperature over 10- to 15-s irrigation (the protocol used in this laboratory). In this case the findings from the ice water irrigations do not match that

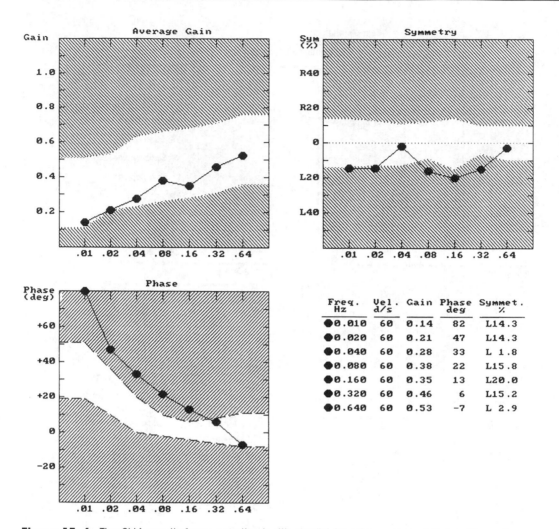

Figure 15–6. The SHA results from a patient with a mild, low-frequency, bilateral hypofunction—see text for details. Refer to Figure 15–2 legend for description of the figure layout.

of the rotary chair. The resolution of this dichotomy came with the realization that the patient was deaf and as a result was unable to be alerted properly with rotational stimulation even though the patient was kept talking with reciting multiplication tables throughout the testing. The same was true during the warm and cool water irrigations. However, the use of the ice water certainly aroused the patient and gave the robust response with the use of ice water. The point to this example is that there should be consistency between the rotary chair findings and the caloric response if bilateral hypofunction is suspected.

The question should be asked, what is the consistency between phase angle (time constant) and caloric irrigation asymmetry? As the asymmetry between the right and left caloric irrigation findings begins to exceed 25% should it be expected that an increasing phase angle would also be seen? A factor to remember when answering this question and related issues with gain and symmetry is that the caloric stimulation is the equivalent of a rotational stimulus of 0.002 to 0.004 Hz, and the rotational chair sinusoidal protocol has a range from 0.01 to 0.64 Hz. The peripheral vestibular system, both the otoliths and the semicircular canals, are, like our auditory system, frequency dependent systems. Therefore, it would not be unexpected to find differences in outcome parameters at different frequency ranges. In a study by Suzuki, Pulec, and Smith (1989), the mean

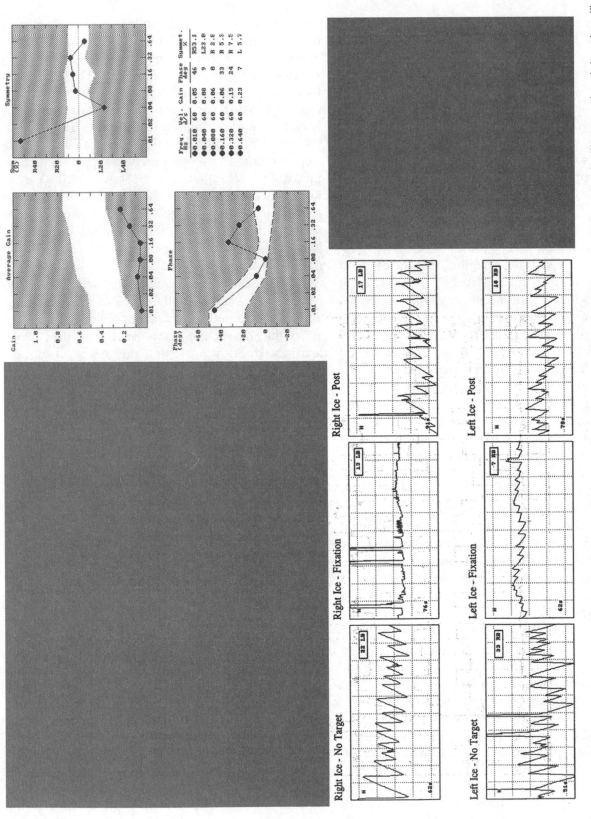

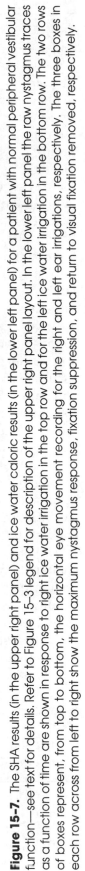

Figure 15-7. The SHA results (in the upper right panel) and ice water caloric results (in the lower left panel) for a patient with normal peripheral vestibular function—see text for details. Refer to Figure 15-3 legend for description of the upper right panel layout. In the lower left panel the raw nystagmus traces as a function of time are shown in response to right ice water irrigation in the top row and for the left ice water irrigation in the bottom row. The two rows of boxes represent, from top to bottom, the horizontal eye movement recording for the right and left ear irrigations, respectively. The three boxes in each row across from left to right show the maximum nystagmus response, fixation suppression, and return to visual fixation removed, respectively.

and standard deviation of the phase lag (phase lead = phase lag minus 180 degrees) were compared at frequencies of 0.01 to 0.16 in octaves for three groups of patients with peripheral vestibular disorders. The three groups were divided by the magnitude of the caloric asymmetry: group 1, asymmetry <19%; group 2, asymmetry between 20% and 49%; and group 3, asymmetry ≥50%. At all the frequencies there was no difference between the three groups in the magnitude of the phase lead. The implication from these results is that there was no greater likelihood of a larger phase lead with a larger caloric asymmetry. The two parameters of phase lead and caloric asymmetry, while loosely correlated, certainly did not predict the magnitude of the other. In more recent work (Ahmed, Goebel, & Sinks, 2009) an investigation of the sensitivity/specificity via receiver operator characteristics curve (ROC) and area under the curve value was used to compare rotary chair (both the SHA and step test protocols) and caloric asymmetry in the identification of 132 patients with peripheral vestibular involvement and 68 patients without any indication of vestibular system involvement. The results of their study showed that the single best predictor of peripheral involvement was that of the magnitude of the caloric asymmetry. The performance of phase lead alone at 0.025 Hz and in combination with 0.05 Hz was less effective but not a statistically significant difference. By use of logistic regression they investigated what combination of test was the best protocol for the prediction of peripheral vestibular involvement. The result was the combination of the magnitude of the caloric asymmetry, phase lead at 0.025 and 0.05 Hz with the estimate of time constant from the step test. The implication that can be drawn from this is that phase lead from the SHA test, the time constant from the step test and the magnitude of the caloric asymmetry are all positively correlated but less than 100%. This means that each of these studies identifies the same portion of the patients with peripheral involvement, but that each also identifies a unique subset of patients with peripheral vestibular system involvement. This would be especially true when using the tests in a protocol referred to as a series-negative protocol (Turner, Frazier, & Shepard, 1984) where you continue with the testing (caloric, step test, SHA) until you get a positive response

and then stop the testing in this combination protocol. Based on the work by Ahmed et al (2009) the order would be caloric first, if negative then on to step test, if negative then on to SHA. The problem is that you typically would not want to perform rotary chair after caloric as there can be a carryover effect from the caloric irrigation tests, and as discussed in Chapter 14 the difficulty with the reliability of the step test data. Therefore, practical aspects of using a protocol of this nature get in the way of the execution. One other aspect is the use of rotary chair to look for indications of lack of central compensation (discussed below under the symmetry parameter) is useful even if a caloric asymmetry of a positive nature has been identified.

The phase angle can be abnormally small (the time constant abnormally long) as well as being abnormally large (time constant abnormally short). When the phase angle is abnormally low (low phase lead) the implication is that the central vestibular cerebellum is likely involved (Baloh et al., 1981; Waespe, Hoppenbrouwers, Pauwels, & Vandeheyning, 1985). It is this neurologic substrate that restricts the level of nystagmus output of the vestibular system and influences the activity of the velocity storage system as to its governance of the phase angle. Therefore, a consequence of a lesion in this area can be a prolonged response from the vestibular system that results in an abnormally low phase lead and many times a hyperactive response for the slow component eye velocity both for caloric as well as for the rotational stimulation reflected in an abnormally high gain (see discussion of gain below).

Gain

Gain, output divided by input, is a dimensionless number that for the purposes of rotational chair movements is the slow component velocity eye movement (output) divided by the velocity of the head movement (input) that stimulated the VOR responses (refer to Figure 14–4). Therefore, the measure has to rely on the assumption that there is no slippage between the chair movement and the head movement. This way, knowing the velocity of the chair you know the velocity of the head. If there is slippage between the head and chair (if it occurs this is usually at the higher frequencies of rotation, 0.32 and 0.64 Hz) gain will drop many times outside the normal range. When this occurs you will typically notice an increase in the phase lead back into the abnormal range at the same frequencies. This combination of increased phase lead and trend for decrease in gain at only the higher frequencies is an indication that the head is not tightly coupled to the chair—this pattern is not reflective of a pathologic process (see example in Figure 15–8).

The gain values across frequency for the SHA test are a measure of the overall responsiveness at the frequency being tested. It reflects the responsiveness of the right and left horizontal canals in an additive manner. This is why it is unusual to see a decrease in gain for a unilateral peripheral vestibular system lesion (see Figure 15–3 that shows typical gain normal with the pattern of increased phase lead). It is not unusual to see a decrease in gain after an acute unilateral peripheral insult (within days after onset

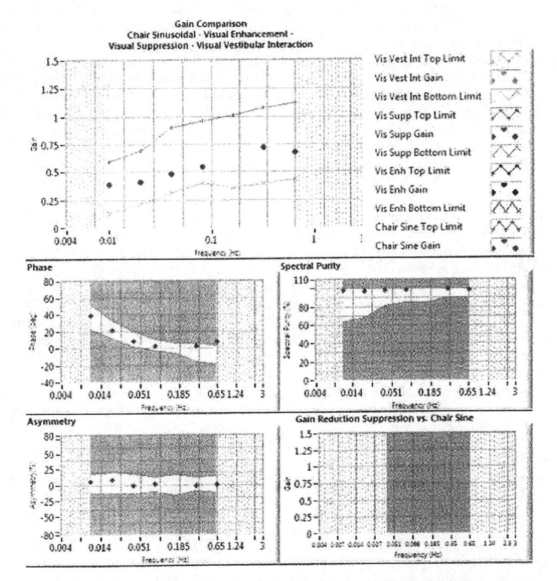

Figure 15–8. The SHA results of a normal subject whose head is not adequately coupled to the chair allowing for slippage of the head at the higher frequencies. See the text for further explanation of the figure. Refer to Figure 15–3 legend for details of the figure layout.

of the vertigo event) as the compensation process centrally results in a short-term bilateral reduction in responsiveness to effect a control over the patient's acute symptoms (Curthoys & Halmagyi, 2007). So, in stable, nonacute unilateral peripheral lesions the gain is normally well within the normal range. Also the gain value does not reflect differences in the response from the right versus the left; this is shown in the symmetry values discussed below. Therefore, the principal implication from abnormally low gain values is that of a bilateral reduction in the VOR from both the right and left horizontal canals. When this is seen in the absence of a significantly abnormal phase lead, then alternative explanations such as the patient being symptomatic with the rotational stimulus or lacking alertness, becoming drowsy are typically the cases. Shown in Figure 15–5 the gain in bilateral hypofunction can range from severely reduced with virtually no VOR to being in a normal range as shown in Figure 15–6. This is a result of differences in the locus of the lesion site in each of the horizontal canals—the greater the damage, the greater the reduction in the gain. This information can be useful in defining the extent of the bilateral hypofunction and to a limited extent how hard to push the patient in a vestibular and balance therapy program to regain functional stance when visual and foot support surface cues are both challenged.

One further example of an inconsistency between caloric results and that of the SHA test is given in Figure 15–9. This is a 74-year-old male who likely suffered an event of Ramsey Hunt syndrome with involvement in the hearing and vestibular end organ on the right. In July 2013, he reports sudden onset of severe unsteadiness without vertigo but with hearing loss. Two weeks prior he started with pain in the right ear that resolved after the first week of the unsteadiness. The unsteadiness continued to worsen in the next 2 weeks and by the end of 6 months his documented hearing loss had returned to its predizziness state. He presented in August 2014 with continuing unsteadiness with standing and walking and oscillopsia with head movements both of which would resolve with sitting. His chair findings shown in Figure 15–9 could be interpreted as indicating a mild bilateral pathology given the reduced gain and the phase lead at 81 degrees. His asymmetry (discussed below) showed a right greater than left slow

component velocity asymmetry that would indicate possible greater involvement on the right than the left. This would not be an acute insult as he is now 14 months away from the start but is likely a unilateral lesion on the right when his other test findings are reviewed. His other test results showed a normal warm water caloric response from the left (23 deg/s); no response to warm or ice water irrigations on the right; head impulse test was positive for all three canals on the right; and second-degree left-beating nystagmus with visual fixation removed and positional left-beating in the majority of the positions tested. These findings would be strongly suggestive of severe, uncompensated right unilateral hypofunction. His dynamic visual acuity (DVA) test (see Chapter 7) showed significantly abnormal DVA for head movements to the right but also abnormal results for head movements to the left, a finding like the chair findings that would be seen in bilateral hypofunction with greater involvement on the right. Collectively how can these findings be explained? Although rare, patients can get "stuck" in the initial phase of the central compensation process where the central actions are to reduce responsiveness from the noninvolved side. It is speculated that in this patient the compensation process is at work resulting in the reduction in chair gain, the exceptionally large phase lead, and the DVA results. He had not been started on any vestibular therapy to push the compensation process at the time of this evaluation. The remainder of his workup was negative for any central system involvement with a fully normal magnetic resonance image (MRI) of the brain without and with contrast and focused attention to the internal auditory canals. The use of the aphysiologic stimulus of the caloric, which is not typically affected in a situation of this nature, clearly showed that this was not a case of bilateral hypofunction.

Changes in gain can also be reflective of possible central vestibulo-cerebellar involvement. This interpretation would be most likely when gain is abnormally high, above the two standard deviation limit. As discussed above it is the vestibulo-cerebellum that controls the maximum slow component velocity output from stimulation of the VOR by the chair (Waespe et al., 1985) or caloric methods (see Chapter 2). Therefore, cerebellar damage can release that governor over the maximum output and allow

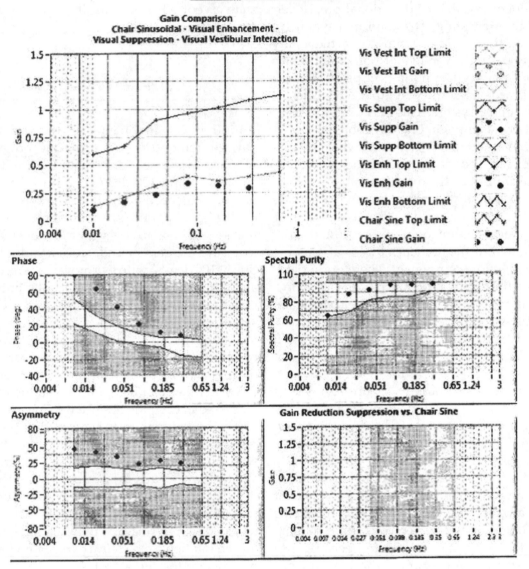

Figure 15-9. The SHA results from a patient where the chair and caloric results appear inconsistent. See text for details. Refer to Figure 15–3 legend for description of the figure layout.

gain to rise to better than one. What would be expected along with the abnormal high gain in the rotary chair results would be hyperactive caloric responses (Chapter 13) and disruption in pursuit tracking. Abnormally high gains in isolation without the hyperactive caloric or other abnormal ocular motor results should not be interpreted as central in origin.

Symmetry

This parameter investigates the percentage difference between the peak slow component eye velocity that is generated to the left from rotation to the right and the peak slow component eye velocity to the right generated from rotation to the left. As long as there are no indications of central system involvement, abnormal symmetry can be interpreted analogous to that of directional preponderance from caloric testing. The abnormal symmetry suggests that there is an asymmetry in the ability to stimulate the right versus left horizontal canals and that asymmetry has not as yet been compensated for at the level of the vestibular nuclei; hence, there is bias in the system. This bias makes it easier to stimulate nystagmus in one direction versus the other. It is important to recognize that when discussing directional preponderance from the caloric test, the nomenclature is by the direction of the fast component, even though the measurements are made based on the slow component velocities. In the chair the measurements are made from the slow component velocities, but the nomenclature is also by the direction of the slow component. Therefore, a right-beating directional preponderance from the caloric, if reflected in the chair results, would be a left greater than right slow component velocity asymmetry.

Since the SHA test inhibits one horizontal canal while stimulating the other with rotational acceleration, there are always two solutions to the meaning of an asymmetry. For example, Figure 15–9 shows a right greater than left slow component velocity asymmetry. This finding would be consistent with a right hypofunction or a left irritative lesion. We know from other findings for this patient that a right hypofunction is the result. Right slow component velocities are obtained by rotating the patient to the left, and because the right slow components are greater than the left, which come from rotation to the left, the implication is the stronger response was obtained by stimulation of the left horizontal canal compared to the right—hypofunction to the right.

When considering the state of central compensation physiologically relative to eye movements for a unilateral peripheral vestibular insult, the symmetry is one of the parameters that can be used to suggest lack of physiologic compensation. The other measures that can be used would be spontaneous, positional nystagmus and the directional preponderance from the caloric test. All of these measures would be expected to return to a normal value once central compensation is physiologically complete. Measures such as abnormal phase lead and a reduced vestibular response by caloric would

typically not return to normal in the compensated state except when the insult to the peripheral vestibular system is mild.

STEP TEST PROTOCOL

As introduced in Chapter 14 the step test (alternatively referred to as a trapezoid protocol) starts with a sudden acceleration to the right or left of usually around 100 deg/s² for duration to achieve one of two speeds. The speed is typically around 60 deg/s or 240 deg/s. The rotation is continued at that speed for 45 to 60 s with eye movement recordings, and the person undergoes a sudden deceleration at 100 deg/s² with eye movement recordings for an additional 45 to 60 s. This results in two sets of outcome parameters of time constant (TC) and two sets of gain for the rotation to the right and to the left. As described in Chapter 14 these two segments of the step test are referred to as per-rotary (while the chair is turning at the constant speed) and postrotary (after the chair has come to a sudden stop). Also discussed in Chapter 14 since we have two estimates of TC for stimulation to the right (per-rotary for a rotation to the right and postrotary for the sudden stop after the rotation to the left), we would average the two values for a single estimate of TC for the right. Analogously, the same is done for the two estimates of gain for the right. This is then all repeated for per-rotatory to the left and postrotatory for the rotation to the left. There are no formal fixed parameters for the step test; typical acceleration, deceleration is usually around 100 deg/s² with step test speeds of 60 and 240 deg/s. The duration of the rotatory and postrotatory segments will range from 45 to 60 s.

The purposes of the slow and fast speed protocols are distinctly different. The slow speed is used to obtain an estimate of the overall system time constant (TC) for stimulation of the right horizontal canal and a TC for stimulation to the left horizontal canal. This protocol also is used to estimate the gain of the VOR response for stimulation of the right and the left horizontal canals individually, and hence the percentage difference between the gains right versus left. The primary purpose for the fast speed protocol is to again estimate the gain for the VOR response for rotation to the right and the left and again develop a percentage difference between the VOR gain for right versus left. TC that is developed for this protocol is not as representative of the overall system protocol as with the slow speed step test. Therefore, this TC is typically ignored. As we increase the speed of the step test, we cause a decrease in the TC estimate secondary to the introduction of higher-frequency components to the overall stimulus with the higher speed.

Time Constant

As defined previously, TC is the time it takes for the peak slow component velocity eye to decay to 37% of the peak value after the acceleration (per-rotatory segment) and after the deceleration (postrotatory segment). The general interpretation of TC follows along the same line as the phase lead from the SHA test described above. The normal range used by the authors is 10 to 30 s as the two standard deviations away from the mean value for normal. There are other ranges published (Baloh & Honrubia, 1990) where the lower limit is 5 s, but now by consensus the lower limit has been accepted at 10 s. Therefore, if the TC is below 10 s, the implication is possible peripheral system involvement as long as brainstem involvement can be ruled out. If the TC is at or greater than 30 s, the concern would be for central vestibulo-cerebellar involvement. Unlike the use of phase angle, TCs representing the right horizontal canal and the left horizontal canal are returned from a full single step test. This information can be used to help localize a lesion to the left and the right especially with the information about gain (discussed below). Last, if the TC is approaching 5 s, then the implication is that there could be bilateral peripheral pathology, even if the gain values are within a normal range.

Gain

Although there is no established normative range for gain (peak VOR eye velocity divided by the peak chair [head] velocity) or for the asymmetry in

percentage, the values that the authors have established are gains of 0.4 or above as normal and percentage difference of less than 30% as normal. These represent the two standard deviation limits. There are estimates of normal ranges that place the gain at above 0.27 as normal for the two standard deviations below the mean (Baloh & Honrubia, 1990). As a result, when a step test is placed in service the laboratory needs to establish normative ranges for TC, gain, and asymmetry given their equipment and specifics of their protocol. The estimates of gain and percentage differences are compared between the two protocols to infer compensated versus uncompensated status. If the percentage difference for the slow speed is abnormal, then the implication is that there is a bias in the system most likely from asymmetrical peripheral vestibular performance that has not been compensated for at the vestibular nuclei level, similar to the discussion above about the symmetry values for the SHA test. We would then expect the fast speed to also show an abnormal percentage difference in the same direction for left versus right. The overall interpretation of these findings would be that of possible hypofunction on the side of the weaker response (could be an irritative lesion on the side of the greater of the response) that is uncompensated. If the slow speed step test returns a normal percentage difference and the high speed step shows an abnormal percentage difference, then the implication would be that of likely hypofunction on the weaker side (alternative is irritative lesion on the stronger side) that appears in a compensated state centrally. In other words, the slower speed step test is the one that is most likely to return to a normal percentage difference with central compensation, whereas the higher speed step test is designed to try and drive asymmetrical functioning between the horizontal canals if such exists, independent of compensation secondary to the speed of the stimulus. It will typically remain abnormal even with compensation. In this manner the high-speed step test continues to suggest localization to the right or left in the form of a hypofunction or irritative lesion. To distinguish between irritative or paretic lesion usually requires additional information unless the absolute gain for the right or the left is significantly less than 0.4, strongly suggesting that the weaker side is that of involvement in a hypofunction manner.

Gain from the step test, like that from the SHA protocol, is used to determine (with TC) indications for bilateral hypofunction. This would be reflected by right and left gain values less than 0.4 and as indicated above TC for the right and left of 5 to 7 s or less.

Gain values at 1.0 or above would be considered hyperactive and could suggest possible cerebellar involvement. But as in the discussion for SHA, this should not be interpreted as central in isolation. It should be seen with hyperactive caloric and/or hyperactive SHA gain or with ocular motor abnormalities.

As a representative example of the results of a normal step test, please refer to Figure 15–10 for the 60 deg/s step test and Figure 15–11 for the 240 deg/s step test. This is a 38-year-old male with normal TC and normal gain bilaterally. His full evaluation resulted in the diagnosis of right-side superior canal dehiscence that was resolved surgically. His SHA test was also normal. As can be seen in Figure 15–10, his 2TC for stimulation to the right and the 2 for stimulation to the left have all four within the normal range. Therefore, the average of those for the right and left would also fall well within the normal range. For gain there is a difference in the estimates for the right with the per-rotary being 0.5 and the post-rotary 0.35, but the average of 0.43 is within the normal limits. The gain for the left was normal for both estimates, and there is not a significant asymmetry for left versus right (6% difference). Figure 15–11 shows the results for the 240 deg/s step. As can be seen the TCs (that is not used for this protocol) show the expected reduction in value for all four estimates, all <10 s. Gain values show the average for the right stimulation to be 0.31, and this is a 23% weaker response compared to the left, normal.

Figures 15–12, 15–13, and 15–14 show the 60 deg/s step, the 240 deg/s step, and this same patient's SHA study. The patient was a 37-year-old female suspected to have had a posterior infererior cerebellar artery (PICA) distribution ischemic event that began with severe headache and within 2 hr she developed vertigo with nausea and vomiting and vertical diplopia. CT and MRI were both normal within the first 24 hr. Her symptoms slowly improved over 2 days resolving into head movement provoked unsteadiness with mild lightheadedness. She continued with vertical diplopia on gaze left. Her ocular motor studies of gaze, smooth pursuit, and saccade testing were all normal. There was no positional or spontaneous nystagmus, and caloric water irrigations were all normal. The question at hand was as follows: Was this a PICA ischemic event or could this have been a migraine event or simple vestibular neuronitis? The only abnormalities were from the chair testing. Figure 15–12 shows for the 60 deg/s step test that the TC for the right and the left is effectively at the TC for the cupula (5- to 8-s range) and the SHA test shows an abnormally large phase lead of 75 degrees at 0.01 Hz that would be consistent with a TC in the 5-s range. As discussed above these results could be suggestive of possible bilateral peripheral vestibular system involvement; however, all the gain values on both the 60 and 240 deg/s tests and the caloric values were all well within normal limits. Therefore, it is not likely that these findings represent peripheral vestibular system involvement. The one lesion that could produce increased phase lead and decreased TC with normal gain would be that of a brainstem lesion and, therefore, the suspicion of a transient vascular event in the brainstem in the region of the pons would be the most likely explanation for this patient's findings.

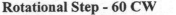

Rotational Step - 60 CW

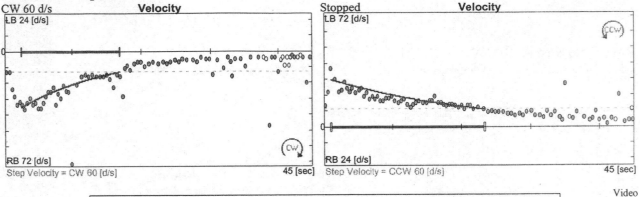

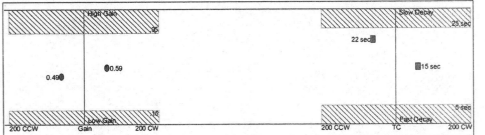

Rotational Step - 60 CCW

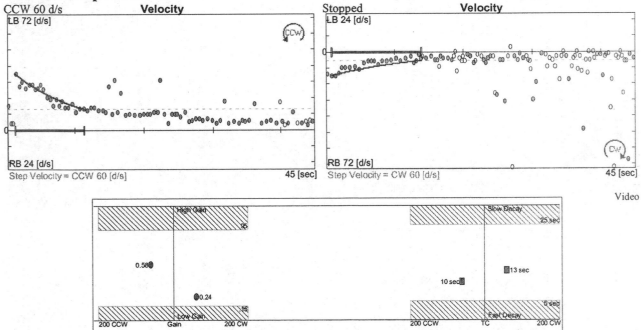

Figure 15–10. The results of a normal 60 deg/s step test for a patient. See the text for the details of the patient. The top two panels, left to right, show the decay of the slow component eye velocity (individual slow component eye velocities given in circle symbols) for the per-rotatory stimulation to the right horizontal canal (CW) and the postrotatory stimulation to the left horizontal canal (CCW) upon the stopping the chair. In both of the graphs the best-fit line through the individual slow component eye velocities is shown that was used to determine the estimate of the TCs for both the right and then the left and the gain values for the right and the left for the per- and postrotatory sections. The values of the gain for left canal stimulation (CCW) and the right (CW) are shown along with the TC estimates for the left (CCW) and the right (CW) in the panel beneath the graphs showing the eye movement decay. The three panels at the bottom of the figure give the same information but now for a per-rotatory rotation to the left (labeled CCW) and postrotatory stimulation to the right canal with the estimates of the gain and TC values in the very bottom panel.

Rotational Step - 240 CW

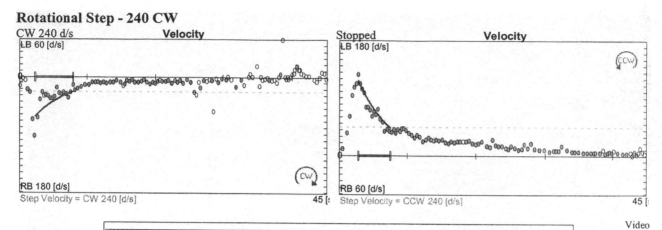

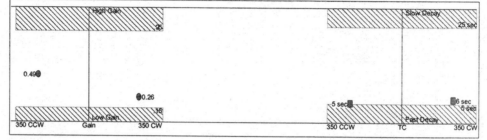

Rotational Step - 240 CCW

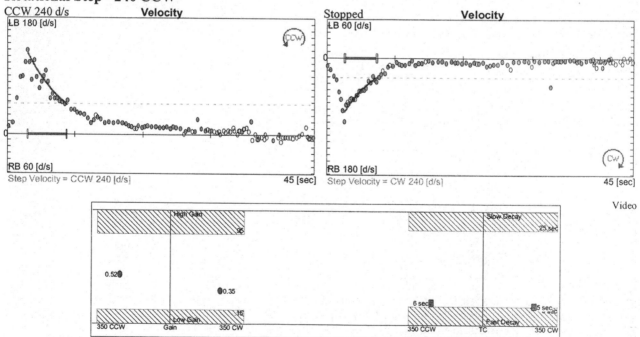

Figure 15-11. The 240 deg/s step test for the patient shown in Figure 15–10. Refer to Figure 15–10 legend for the description of the figure layout.

Rotational Step - 60 CW

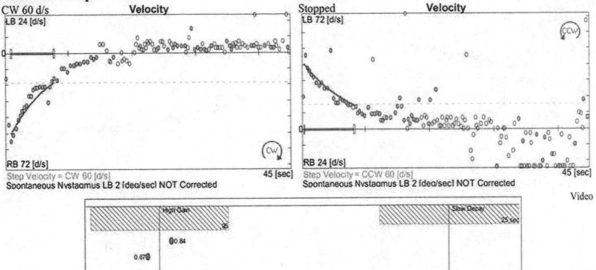

Rotational Step - 60 CCW

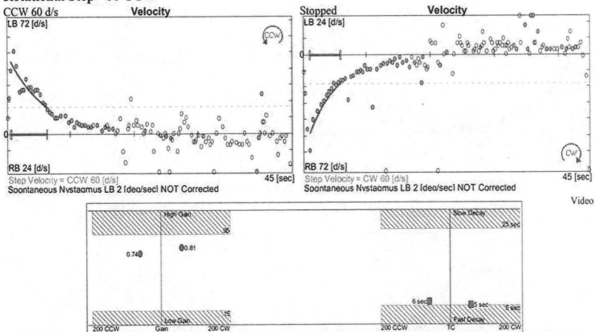

Figure 15–12. The 60 deg/s step test for the patient with a likely brainstem lesion. See the text for details. Refer to Figure 15–10 for the description of the layout.

Rotational Step - 240 CW

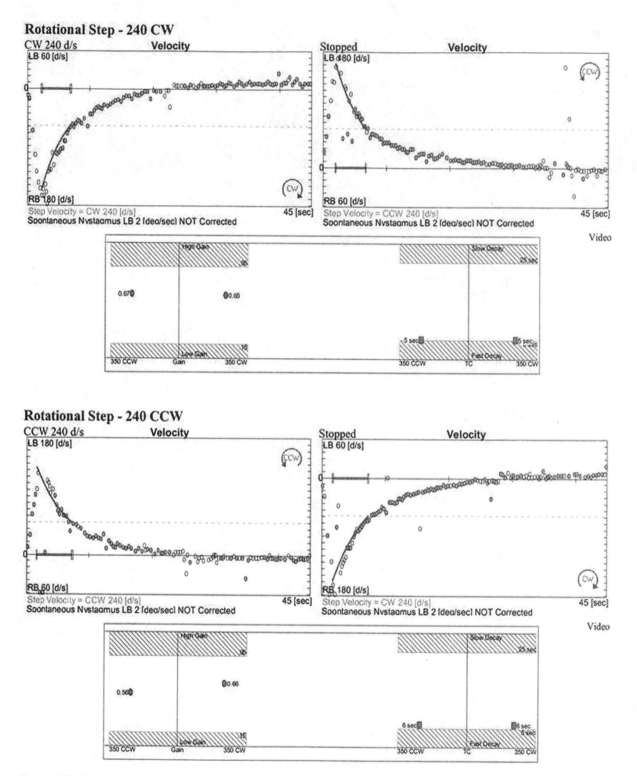

Figure 15–13. The 240 deg/s step test for the patient shown in Figure 15–12. Refer to Figure 15–10 legend for description of the layout.

VOR Summary

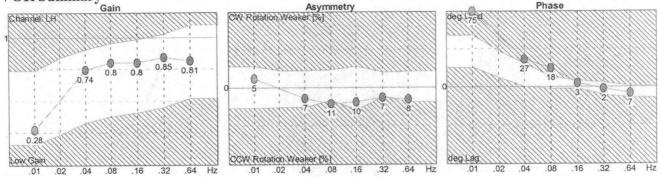

Figure 15-14. The SHA test results for the patient given in Figures 15–12 and 15–13. The three graphs shown from left to right give the values for gain, symmetry, and phase angle respectively. The values are shown as a function of frequency with the normal two standard deviation range in the nonstipple area.

UNILATERAL CENTRIFUGATION (UC)

In recent years there has been a focus on being able to assess the otolith organs, especially each of the four individually. Vestibular evoked myogenic potential testing has been one means for accomplishing this task (see Chapter 21 for full discussion). However, one question has been the use of a nonphysiologic stimulus (pressure waves such as loud sounds) instead of the use of linear acceleration which is the natural stimulus that the otolith organs are designed to detect. At least for the utricle this can be accomplished with the use of the UC protocol. Figures 15–15 and 15–16 demonstrate schematically how this can be accomplished by placing asymmetrical horizontal acceleration force on one of the utricular organs at a time. The reader is referred to Chapters 14 and 22 for more detailed discussions of the specifics of the protocols used for this procedure. As discussed in Chapter 14, we use the protocol that was investigated by Janky and Shepard (2011). Briefly, the patient is seated in the rotary chair, and as illustrated in Figure 15–16 the chair is first moved to the right or left (to the left in this figure) to align the axis of rotation with the position of the right utricle in the skull. After that movement is made, the chair starts a clockwise rotation at 3 deg/s^2 until the final velocity of 300 deg/s is achieved. This final speed is then maintained at a constant for 120 s while the subject performs the task of subjective visual vertical (SVV) setting a projected line on the wall of the booth to

their perception of vertical. They repeat this task with the line randomly reset between ±30 degrees of true vertical getting between 5 and 10 settings. The chair is then decelerated at 3 deg/s^2 until the chair comes to a stop. After a 5-min break the subject performs the SVV with the chair at rest and in its middle position as was done prior to the first lateral movement and rotation. Next the chair is again laterally moved this time to the right and the entire process is repeated. The average of the static SVV prior to the movement to the right and spin is used as the baseline for the utricular function for the right. The static SVV taken prior to placing the left utricle eccentric is used as the baseline for the left utricular function. In this manner any bias that is present prior to performing the dynamic SVV is noted in the baseline.

The outcome parameters for this test have not been fully worked out, but it is clear that the use of SVV is more reliable than the measurement of torsional eye movements given the small degree to which the eye undergoes torsional movement with the amount of force that can comfortably be placed on the individual utricle (Janky & Shepard, 2010). Based on this work, to be in the normal range for utricular function, the following two conditions need to be met. First, the average value of the dynamic SVV (that performed while the chair is at a constant velocity of 300 deg/s having been positioned by lateral translation to the left or right) should be outside the range of [−1.64° to 1.16°]. This range represents the mean ±1 standard deviation of normal static average SVV values (when the chair is not in motion).

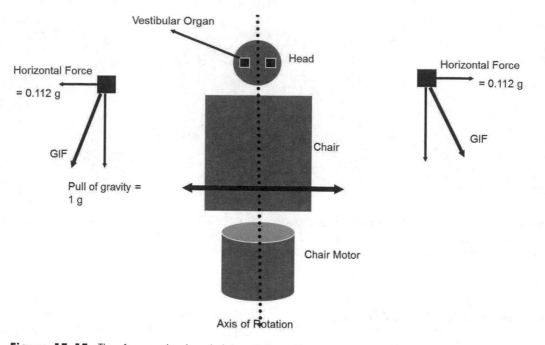

Figure 15–15. The forces, horizontal (centrifugal) and gravitational, that would be on each of the utricles in the normal orientation of the axis of rotation through the center of the head. Note that these forces would be equal left versus right.

Typically you would expect that when stimulating the right utricle the SVV should be set to the left of true vertical secondary to the ocular counter-roll of the eyes back to the left as the normal physiologic response to stimulation of the right greater than the left. This would be the same as tilting the head to the right (see Chapter 1 for further discussion on otolith function). The second condition that needs to be met is that the absolute value of the difference between the average dynamic SVV value and the average static SVV value taken prior to staring the stimulation to the right or left should be ≥2°. Let's consider the following example for better understanding of this analysis scheme. The patient while sitting still in the dark in the chair performs the SVV at least 10 times, and the static SVV is established prior to stimulation of the right utricle. The patient is then translated by 4 cm to the right, and the spin CCW is started with a fixation target point visible for fixation. (This is done to reduce any angular VOR response and to reduce any nausea.) Once 300 deg/s is reached, the fixation point changes to a line and the patient starts performing SVV for 120 s getting between 5 to 10 trials. The line returns to a fixation point and the chair starts its slow deceleration until

it comes to a stop. A short break is taken with the patient remaining in the chair (5 min at most). Next, another static SVV is performed, and the patient is then translated 4 cm to the left and the entire process is repeated. The following values were obtained for this patient: Static average SVV prior to right utricular stimulation = (−1.2°); dynamic average SVV for the right stimulation = (−8.5°) (note that the negative sign means the average line was set to the left of true vertical); static SVV prior to left = 0.6°; dynamic SVV with stimulation to the left = 2.3°. Therefore, for the right utricle the first condition is easily met with the right dynamic SVV of −8.5° being well outside the range of [−1.64° to 1.16°]. The second condition is also met with the following calculation: ABS[−8.5° − (−1.2°)] = 7.3°, well above 2. The conclusion for the right utricle is that it is functioning well within the normal range. The left utricle also meets Condition 1 as the dynamic SVV for the left is 2.3° that is outside the range of [−1.64° to 1.16°]. However, when the dynamic SVV is compared to static SVV prior to the left stimulation via the calculation: ABS[2.3° − 0.6°] = 1.7°, this value does not meet the criteria to satisfy Condition 2. Hence, for the left utricle there is a response, but it is minimal and this would be interpreted as being a

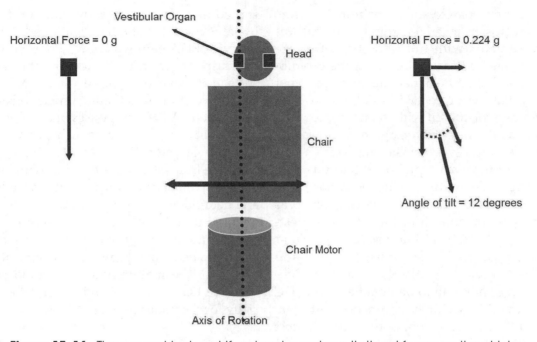

Figure 15–16. The symmetrical centrifugal and equal gravitational forces on the utricles with the chair now in an eccentric position with the axis of rotation through the right utricle.

hypofunction of the left utricle. There as yet has not been established a symmetry criteria for normal, so at this point determination is made based on each utricle in isolation and not by comparison right versus left. At present the criteria of any percentage difference between the values of the comparisons of dynamic and static SVV greater than 50% would be considered suspicious for asymmetrical performance.

Recognize that the paradigm described herein is different than that used in the literature, where for the majority of protocols once the chair is started spinning, the direction of the spin remains the same and only the translation to the right and back to the left changes without stopping between the spinning to the left and right (Clarke, Schönfeld, Hamann, & Scherer, 2001; Wuyts, Hoppenbrouwers, Pauwels, & Vandeheyning, 2003). The chapter authors have selected the protocol given above as it was shown to not have any significant difference in the actual ocular torsion or SVV values between the two methods (Janky & Shepard, 2010). The method described allows for taking the static values into account. Also this method was slightly less likely in normal subjects to provoke nausea.

The clinical utility of UC is that it allows for a more thorough investigation of the peripheral

vestibular system with the possibility of recognizing isolated utricular lesions (Schönfeld, Helling, & Clarke, 2010). Also UC allows for investigations of how diffuse peripheral involvement can be by investigating the utricles individually in patients with unilateral or bilateral hypofunction of horizontal and vertical canals (via video head impulse test or bedside head impulse test—see Chapters 7 and 16). An important question would be as follows: Can this investigation of the utricle be accomplished with ocular VEMP testing? In Chapter 21 this issue is discussed but a full answer to the question is not at this time available. There are no side-by-side data of UC and oVEMP testing on the same patient to investigate the extent of correlation between the two studies. This is especially needed given that the UC is a natural stimulus of linear acceleration while the oVEMP could be considered an artificial stimulus. Consider the following two patient examples that address these clinical utility issues.

Example 1 is a 40-year-old female who had a sudden onset of a mild acute vestibular syndrome with vertigo that was constant for 30 min with nausea without vomiting in December 2010. The symptoms then changed to head movement-provoked symptoms of vertigo that finally resolved into clear right-side benign paroxysmal positional vertigo (BPPV) of the posterior canal within weeks that was successfully treated with full resolution of symptoms. There was no hearing loss with these symptoms. In January 2011 the patient again had another acute vestibular syndrome with sudden onset of constant vertigo for 15 min with intensity described as the same as the first event. Again there was no hearing loss and the symptoms changed from persistent to head movement–provoked and this time she was diagnosed with left-side posterior canal BPPV. When seen for laboratory workup she was fully asymptomatic and all of the laboratory testing including caloric, head impulse testing, ocular motor tests, positional nystagmus, Hallpike and roll tests, and cervical VEMPs were normal. Ocular VEMPs were not able to be obtained while UC showed bilateral utricular hypofunction but were obtained with responses from both sides. The test results together with her presenting history would be most compatible with sequential, mild vestibular neuronitis with development of bilateral BPPV. The only marker for this diagnosis was that of bilateral utricular damage but not absence of utricular function. Work by Hong et al. (2008) showed reduced utricular responses from SVV by UC in patients with BPPV on the right and on the left consistent with the finding in this Example 1 patient. It is also important to realize that while the oVEMP was absent, the UC study did show bilateral utricular damage but not absence of function as would be interpreted from the oVEMP study.

Example 2, a female, presented in 2008 at age 79 with a history of slowly progressive unsteadiness only when standing and walking that had begun in 2000. By 2006 she had begun to notice oscillopsia and significant increase in her unsteadiness when walking in the dark or on uneven surfaces. At that time neither UC nor oVEMPs were in use. Her workup at that time showed normal ocular motor studies, weak warm water irrigations bilaterally (<9 deg/s slow component velocities), normal ice water caloric irrigations bilaterally (>15 deg/s slow component velocities), and SHA showed significantly abnormal phase lead (>70 degrees) and reduced gain. She had bilaterally abnormal bedside head impulse test for all three canals. She returned in 2010 with progression of her oscillopsia and generally the same complaints regarding unsteadiness (she had been

started on a specific therapy program for bilateral hypofunction that she had continued to utilize). At this visit SHA gain was now abnormal with minimal response from ice water irrigations, and now she had absent ocular and cervical VEMPs; however, UC showed fully functioning utricles bilaterally. The absent of the VEMP responses bilaterally could well be a result of age, not necessarily peripheral pathology (see Chapter 21) especially given the normal response from UC. These findings with her bilateral progressive hearing loss and fully normal imaging and neurological findings are strongly suggestive of bilateral peripheral auditory/vestibular degenerative disorder possibly of hereditary origin. It would be anticipated that if preservation of the otolith function could be maintained that would potentially improve her vestibular and balance therapy especially for the issues of unsteadiness.

PROTOCOLS FOR CENTRAL VESTIBULAR SYSTEM INVOLVEMENT

While the primary purpose for the clinical utilization of the rotary chair is the expansion of the investigation of peripheral vestibular system involvement, there are two less well-known protocols that are explicitly for the investigation of possible cerebellar involvement. For purposes of completeness, these are both briefly reviewed below.

VOR Cancelation Protocol

Analogous to fixation suppression in the caloric irrigations and for VOR cancelation in the bedside examination, the rotary chair, specifically using the SHA test, can be employed to investigate the patient's ability to suppress the VOR with a fixation target that moves with the chair. The test is described with the normative data in Chapter 14. Briefly, VOR gain is obtained at a sinusoidal frequency of 0.08 in the dark, as would be done if the SHA test was being used. Next a fixation light that moves with the chair is illuminated, and the test is repeated with the patient fixating on the light. Ratio of the VOR gain with the light to that in the dark is calculated and multiplied by 100 to obtain a measure of the percentage of reduction. As can be seen in Table 14–2, the effectiveness of the VOR cancelation shows a trend to decrease with increasing frequency. Abnormal responses on this test are interpreted as an indication of likely cerebellar involvement. This finding is typically highly correlated with saccadic disruptions in smooth pursuit tracking beyond that explainable with age (see Chapters 2 and 10 for further discussion). Recognize that since the neurological substrate for accomplishing this task crosses with that of smooth pursuit (Chapter 2), and smooth pursuit is highly sensitive to age, that VOR cancelation test would also reduce in performance with age (the normative data in Table 14–2 were not derived as a function of age).

Tilt Suppression Protocol

A last protocol for use with the rotational step test is applied to determine the effectiveness of being able to cancel the influence of the velocity storage system ("dump or short circuit") in the production of the typical canal-ocular TC. This is done by stimulation of otolith organs. The patient undergoes a standard step test as described above with the calculation of the per- and postrotatory TCs for the rotation to the right or left. Next the same step test is repeated, but this time as soon as the chair has come to a stop, the patient is to bend forward at the waist with head down toward the knees for 5 s and then slowly sit back up. The outcome parameter of interest is the postrotatory TC as this would be expected to decrease toward the value that would be seen if only the peripheral vestibular system cupular decay was responsible for the development of the canal-ocular TC. Normative data developed show that a minimum of at least a 40% reduction in the value of the postrotary TC from the normal step test should occur (Lockette, Shepard, Lyos, Boismier, & Mers, 1991). As described above and in Chapters 1, 2, and 14 as the peripheral system is stimulated with an acceleration or in this case deceleration, the velocity storage system "charges up" like that of an electronic capacitor and then drives the eyes for the prolongation of the VOR response beyond that resulting from the cupular stimulation decay. Stimulation of the otolith organs, by having the patient tilt his or her head forward, has the effect of dumping

the energy development in the velocity storage system while the cupula is undergoing its decay, like short-circuiting a capacitor that has been charged up. This effectively reduces the canal-ocular TC to that of, or close to, the TC of the cupular decay (Benson & Bodin, 1966). It has been shown that persons with essential hypertension and those with possible lesions of nodulus of the cerebellum have a failure of the tilt suppression test (Hain, Zee, & Maria, 1988; Waespe et al., 1985). The tilt suppression can also be accomplished with turning on a light immediately on stopping the chair movement, but anecdotally this is not as effective as the tilt. From a practical standpoint, this test can provoke nausea especially in patients with a tendency to motion sickness.

SUMMARY

Over the years, improvement in control over the drive motors and significant increase in the eye movement recording techniques and real-time analysis have led to rotary chair systems with greater clinical utility and reliability. Still, there are no ANSI standards for standard protocols, normative data across age, or manufacture specifications. This results in the need for these standards. As laboratories for vestibular function testing are set up, if protocols are adopted from texts and publications, the laboratory needs to verify the details of the movement parameters used on their systems and the normative data applied in the clinical investigation of patients.

REFERENCES

Ahmed, M. F., Goebel, J. A., & Sinks, B. C. (2009). Caloric test versus rotational sinusoidal harmonic acceleration and step-velocity tests in patients with and without suspected peripheral vestibulopathy. *Otology and Neurology, 30,* 800–805.

Baloh, R. W., & Honrubia, V. (1990). *Clinical neurophysiology of the vestibular system* (2nd ed.). Philadelphia, PA: F. A. Davis.

Baloh, R. W., Jacobson, K. M., Beykirch, K., & Honrubia, V. (1989a). Horizontal vestibulo-ocular reflex after acute peripheral lesions. *Acta Oto-Laryngologica Supplementum, 468,* 323–327.

Baloh, R. W., Jacobson, K. M., & Honrubia, V. (1989b). Idiopathic bilateral vestibulopathy. *Neurology, 39,* 272.

Baloh, B. W., Yee, R. D., Kimm, J., & Honrubia, V. (1981). The vestibulo-ocular reflex in patients with lesions of the vestibulocerebellum. *Experimental Neurology, 72,* 141.

Benson, A. J., & Bodin, M. A. (1966). Effect of orientation to gravitation vertical on nystagmus following rotation about a horizontal axis. *Acta Otolarynologica, 61,* 517.

Clarke, A. H., Schönfeld, U., Hamann, C., & Scherer, H. (2001). Measuring unilateral otolith function via the otolith-ocular response and the subjective visual vertical. *Acta Oto-Laryngologica Supplementum, 545,* 84–87.

Curthoys, I. S., & Halmagyi, G. M. (2007). Vestibular compensation: Clinical changes in vestibular function with time after unilateral vestibular loss. In S. J. Herdman (Ed.), *Vestibular rehabilitation* (2nd ed., pp. 76–97). Philadelphia, PA: F. A. Davis.

Goldberg, J. M., & Fernandez, C. (1971). Physiology of peripheral neurons innervating semicircular canals of the squirrel monkey. I. Resting discharge and response to constant angular accelerations. *Journal of Neurophysiology, 34*(4), 635–660.

Hain, T. C., Zee, D. S., & Maria, B. L. (1988). Tilt suppression of vestibulo-ocular reflex in patients with cerebellar lesions. *Acta Oto-Laryngologica (Stockholm), 105,* 13–20.

Hong, S. M., Park, M. S., Cha, C. I., Park, C. H., & Lee, J. H. (2008). Subjective visual vertical during eccentric rotation in patients with benign paroxysmal positional vertigo. *Otology Neurotology, 29,* 1167–1170.

Janky, K., & Shepard, N. T. (2011). Unilateral centrifugation: Protocol comparison. *Otology and Neurotology, 32*(1), 116–121.

Jenkins, H. R., Honrubia, V., & Baloh, R. W. (1982). Evaluation of multiple frequency rotatory testing in patients with peripheral labyrinthine weakness. *American Journal of Otolaryngology-Head and Neck Surgery, 3,* 182.

Katz, E., de Jong, J. M. B. V., Buttner-Ennever, J. A., & Cohen, B. (1991). Effects of midline medullary lesion on velocity storage and the vestibulo-ocular reflex. *Experimental Brain Research, 87,* 505–520.

Lockette, W., Shepard, N. T., Lyos, A., Boismier, T., & Mers, A. (1991). Altered Coriolis stress susceptibility in essential hypertension. *American Journal of Hypertension, 4*(8), 645–650.

Raphan, T., & Cohen, B. (1980). Integration and its relation to ocular compensatory movement. *Mt. Sinai Journal of Medicine, 47,* 410–417.

Raphan, T., Matsuo, V., & Cohen, B. (1979). Velocity storage in the vestibulo-ocular reflex arc (VOR). *Experimental Brain Research, 35,* 229–248.

Reisine, H., & Raphan, T. (1992). Neural basis for eye velocity generation in the vestibular nuclei during off-vertical axis rotation. *Experimental Brain Res.* 92:209–226.

Schönfeld, U., Helling, K., & Clarke, A. H. (2010). Evidence for unilateral isolated utricular hypofunction. *Acta Oto-Laryngologica, 130,* 702–707.

Steinhausen, W. (1933). Uber die beobachtung der cupula in den bogenansampullen des labyrinths des lebenden hechts. *Archive–European Journal of Physiology (Arch Ges Physiol), 232,* 500–512.

Suzuki, M., Pulec, J. L., & Smith, J. C. (1989). The sinusoidal harmonic acceleration test in vestibular disorders. *Acta Oto-Laryngologica Stockholm, 468,* 317–322.

Turner, R. G., Frazier, G., & Shepard, N. T. (1984). Formulating and evaluating audiological test protocols. *Ear and Hearing, 5,* 321.

Waespe, W., Cohen, B., & Raphan, T. (1985). Dynamic modification of vestibulo-ocular reflex by the nodulus and uvula. *Science, 228,* 199–202.

Wuyts, F. L., Hoppenbrouwers, M., Pauwels, G., & Vandeheyning, P. H. (2003). Utricular sensitivity and preponderance assessed by the unilateral centrifugation test. *Journal of Vestibular Research, 13,* 227–234.

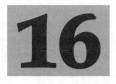

The Video Head Impulse Test (vHIT)

Ian S. Curthoys, Hamish G. MacDougall, Leigh A. McGarvie, Konrad P. Weber, David Szmulewicz, Leonardo Manzari, Ann M. Burgess, and G. Michael Halmagyi

ABBREVIATIONS

BVL bilateral vestibular loss

Contralesional, the side opposite to the actual or suspected lesion

Ipsilesional, on the same side as the actual or suspected lesion

LARP left anterior—right posterior

RALP right anterior—left posterior

UVL unilateral vestibular loss

vHIT video head impulse test

VOR vestibulo-ocular response

INTRODUCTION

The video head impulse test (vHIT) of semicircular canal function (MacDougall, Weber, McGarvie, Halmagyi, & Curthoys, 2009) is an important new development in vestibular testing. For interpreting the results, as well as carrying out the test, it is important to understand the rationale for the test. In this chapter we briefly set out the rationale, explain how the test should be conducted, explain how the test results should be interpreted, including a brief section on the neural basis of vHIT, and conclude with a FAQ section (Appendix 16–A). The main emphasis is on testing horizontal semicircular canal function, but in this chapter we also cover the very new tests

of vertical semicircular canal function (MacDougall, McGarvie, Halmagyi, Curthoys, & Weber, 2013a, 2013b). For readability we have kept references to a minimum but recent papers refer to the very extensive literature on head impulse testing. This chapter is focused on "how to do the test" and artifacts to beware of, rather than a review of the very extensive literature on the results of vHIT testing.

Why Measure Eye Movements to Test the Function of the Semicircular Canals of the Inner Ear?

A very basic reflex, called the vestibulo-ocular reflex (VOR), ensures a stable image on the retina and clear vision during head movements. Receptors in the semicircular canals of the vestibular system of the inner ear are activated by any head rotation, and neurons from those receptors drive the eyes via short fast neural pathways to move the eyes to correct for the head movement. The eye movement is equal and opposite to the head movement, so the image on the retina of the eye is stable and visual perception is clear. If this basic reflex does not operate properly, the eyes do not correct for the head movement, so the image of the visual world is smeared across the retina, and the patient experiences blurred or bouncing vision during head movement. Because of these visual problems, many patients with peripheral vestibular deficits are convinced that there is something wrong with their eyes, but the problem is in their inner ear which controls their eye movements.

Subjective visual problems are some of the first signs of peripheral vestibular disorders. Patients report blurring of the visual image during head movements. Patients with bilateral vestibular loss report that the visual world appears to be bouncing (a sensation called "oscillopsia") as they walk or turn their head. Patients with unilateral vestibular loss have the sensation that the visual world (or the patient) is turning (rotatory vertigo). These are the most common consequences of a peripheral vestibular loss and are usually accompanied by unsteadiness of posture and gait. These subjective sensations are frequently associated with asymmetrical function of the left and right inner ear vestibular systems, so a major goal of clinical vestibular testing is to quantify vestibular function and to identify functional asymmetry between the two vestibular labyrinths.

The functional state of the vestibular system can be assessed by measuring the corrective eye movement during an unpredictable head movement. Obviously this inference has to be made with care because there are many systems, apart from the semicircular canals, controlling eye movements (Leigh & Zee, 2006). Voluntary smooth pursuit, visual (optokinetic) input, or cervical input can all control eye movements and in order to test semicircular canal function specifically, the contribution of these additional sources of control must be excluded. We have shown that measures of the first 100 ms of the eye movement to an unpredictable, passive, small, abrupt, head turn exclude these other sources

of control (Halmagyi & Curthoys, 1987, 1988). But the clinician needs to be wary because other central disorders along the neural pathway from the inner ear to the eye muscles, or disease or dysfunction of the eye muscles themselves, can also affect the eye movement response. However, we showed that measurements of eye movements during the earliest part of the eye movement response to a vestibular stimulus—brief, small, abrupt, passive, unpredictable head movements with angular accelerations in the range experienced during normal head movements—are valuable in specifically assessing the functional state of each semicircular canal, and this test is called the head impulse test.

Natural head movements have brief but large angular accelerations that activate the semicircular canals. For example, as you turn your head to look left and right while driving, the angular acceleration of the head movement is around 3,000 to 4,000 deg/s (Grossman, Leigh, Abel, Lanska, & Thurston, 1988), which sounds enormous, but it is only very brief. Until recently it has not been possible to test vestibular function safely in the clinic using values of angular acceleration in this natural range. Thanks to the development of the video version of the head impulse test (vHIT), it is now possible.

Activation of the vestibular receptors occurs with any head movement—turning to the left or right (yaw head movements) as well as nodding the head forward or back (pitch head movements). There are six semicircular canals in the head (Figure 16–1) organized in pairs and the physiological evidence shows that in healthy individuals they work in three matched pairs: left horizontal—right horizontal, left anterior-right posterior (LARP), and right anterior-left posterior (RALP). Any head rotation causes a unique pattern of activation of the six semicircular canals (Curthoys, Blanks, & Markham, 1977a). Disease or dysfunction can range from affecting all canals in both ears (bilateral vestibular loss), to all the canals on one side (unilateral vestibular loss), to affecting just one individual canal. The ideal test of peripheral vestibular function is one that tests the function of all six semicircular canals specifically, using stimuli with the kind of magnitudes encountered in everyday life and excludes other sources of eye movement control. In this chapter we show that such a test is the video head impulse test (vHIT).

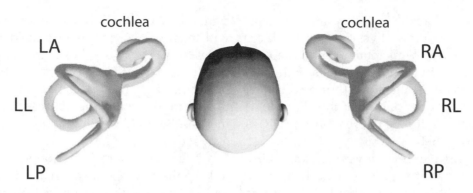

cochlea

cochlea

LA

RA

LL

RL

LP

RP

Figure 16–1. Orientations of the semicircular canals in the head. An enlarged reconstruction from a CT scan of a human patient and the head shows the point of view. The two labyrinths have been enlarged and translated so they are very close to one another. Each semicircular canal has a diameter of about 6 mm, and the two labyrinths are about 70 mm apart in the head (Curthoys, Blanks, et al., 1977a). The canals form three matched pairs. *LL*, left lateral; *LA*, left anterior; *LP*, left posterior; *RA*, right anterior; *RP*, right posterior; *RL*, right lateral. The matched pairs are LL-RL; LA-RP; RA-LP. These images are modified from the free educational iPhone or iPad app called "aVOR," developed by Hamish MacDougall and available on iTunes.

THE VHIT TEST—OVERVIEW

In clinical testing of hearing, precisely controlled stimuli are presented through carefully calibrated headphones, and the patient's responses are measured. In clinical testing of the vestibular system using natural values of head acceleration, this kind of presentation of controlled stimuli is just not clinically feasible. Instead vestibular stimuli are presented which are not well controlled—a head turn delivered by an operator can vary from one trial to the next, but in vHIT both the head movement stimulus and the eye movement response are measured exactly each time, and the analysis relates each response to the stimulus which caused it. The patient is given a small, unexpected, abrupt, head turn by the operator and this passive (involuntary) head movement stimulus and the eye movement response are measured. The patient does not actively turn his or her own head—it must be a passive, unpredictable head turn with an abrupt start and stop. Each head turn is called a head impulse or a trial. The head turn is carried out by the operator placing his or her hands on the top of the patient's head and turning the patient's head in an abrupt, unpredictable, horizontal head turn, and stopping abruptly so the patient's nose points to an imaginary

Typical Head Impulse metrics

- angular extent 5°–15°
- peak angular velocity 200°/s–300°/s
- peak angular acceleration 2000°/s²–4000°/s²

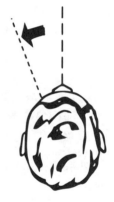

Figure 16–2. Approximate magnitudes of a head impulse: position, average velocity, average acceleration.

target within a range of about 10 deg to the left or right of the patient's straight ahead (Figure 16–2). The patient is instructed to keep staring at a fixation target on the wall in front of him or her during the head turn and to return his or her eyes to it as quickly as possible if the target is lost. The patient is also instructed to try not to blink ("keep your eyes wide open"), to relax the neck muscles ("like a rag doll"), and not to "help" with the head turns.

Such a head turn consists of an angular acceleration up to a peak head velocity, followed immediately by a deceleration back to rest. The semicircular canals of the inner ear are activated by angular acceleration, and that activation drives the eyes via short fast pathways from the semicircular canal receptors to the eye muscles. In healthy subjects both eyes move to compensate for the abrupt, unpredictable, passive head turn. A brief outline of the physiological basis for this vestibulo-ocular response (VOR) is given in Appendix 16–B.

Exact measures of the eye movement in a healthy subject in response to this passive head turn show that after a very short latency (about 10 ms) there is a smooth compensatory eye movement opposite in direction and almost equal in velocity to the head velocity, with the result that the subject's gaze remains fixed on the target irrespective of whether the head turn is to the left or right (Halmagyi & Curthoys, 1988; Halmagyi et al., 1990). This is a very fast and remarkably accurate response. Importantly, the velocity of the eye movement is equal and opposite to the velocity of the head movement, so in healthy subjects it is said that vestibulo-ocular response (VOR) gain is around 1.0, where VOR gain is defined as the ratio of eye velocity to head velocity.

How Can Eye Movements Be Used to Measure Vestibular Function Specifically in a Patient With a Vestibular Loss?

For patients with a unilateral vestibular loss, as their head is turned to their affected side, (an "ipsilesional" head turn), their eyes do not receive adequate neural drive from the semicircular canals on the affected side to compensate for the head turn, so their eyes do not correct for the head turn and so do not stay on the earth-fixed target but are moved with the head. At the end of the head turn the patient is looking away from the fixation target and must make a saccade to get back to the target as the instructions required (Figure 16–3). That corrective saccade is often clear to the clinician viewing the patient's eye movement; therefore, it is called an "overt" saccade. If such an overt saccade occurs in response to such a passive head turn, it is the tell-tale sign of deficient semicircular canal function on the side to which the head has been turned.

Be clear—a corrective saccade after a head turn to the left indicates a left horizontal canal loss. Similarly, a corrective saccade after a head turn to the right indicates a right horizontal canal loss. Patients with bilateral vestibular loss make corrective saccades for head turns in both directions.

If the patient's head is given a head turn to his or her healthy side (a "contralesional" head turn), the eye movement compensates for the head movement and the VOR gain is about 1.0 or is only modestly reduced.

The vHIT test requires cooperation by patients: to keep their eyes wide open and to try not to blink and to keep fixating the target on the wall and to relax their neck muscles to allow the operator to turn their head passively. Some people find it very difficult to relax their neck muscles and so the operator finds it difficult to turn their head abruptly, even through a very small angle. However, for this test to be a valid indicator of vestibular function the operator must be able to deliver a very small, abrupt movement which is a "turn and stop." The abrupt stop is every bit as important as the abrupt start. There should be as little overshooting or rebound as possible. It takes training and practice to be able to do acceptable head impulses and we explain how to practice them in a later section.

Recently our research showed that some patients with vestibular loss can actually generate a corrective saccade during the head turn itself, so the clinician viewing the patient's eye movements does not see an overt saccade at the end of the head turn and so may wrongly conclude that the patient has a healthy vestibular system (Halmagyi, Weber, & Curthoys, 2010; Weber et al., 2008; Weber, MacDougall, Halmagyi, & Curthoys, 2009). A corrective saccade generated during the head turn is called a covert saccade in contrast to the overt saccade made at the end of the head turn. It is called "covert" (hidden) because it cannot be detected by simple visual observation. These covert saccades mean that it is necessary to obtain objective measures of the eye movement during the head movement and that is what the video head impulse test (vHIT) does. Until 2009 the clinical head impulse test was conducted by a clinician simply visually observing the corrective (overt) saccade. But with the discovery of the covert saccade it was obvious that objective measures of eye movement and head movement were necessary for the head impulse test to be a valid indicator of vestibular function.

Obtaining objective, accurate, high-speed measures of eye movements during head movements

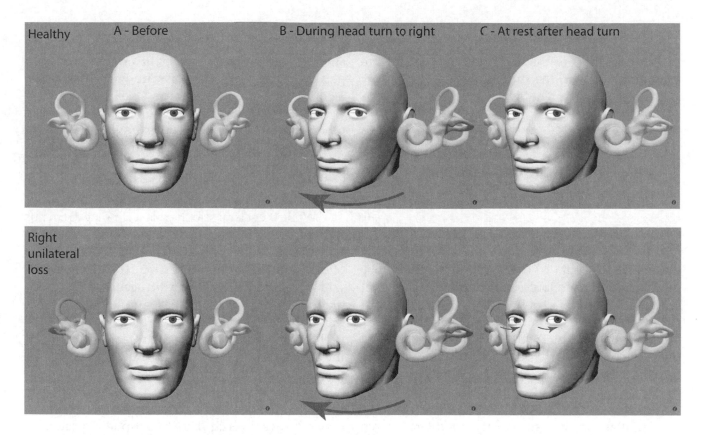

Figure 16–3. The difference between the response of a normal healthy subject (*top row*) and a patient after a unilateral vestibular loss on their right side (*bottom row*) during a rightward clinical head impulse (*large arrow in column B*). Before the head turn (*column A*) the person is instructed to look at the examiner's nose during the head turn and to try not to blink. During the head turn, the eyes of the healthy subject stay fixed on the examiner's nose (*column B*) and remain so at the end of the rotation (*column C*), so that no saccade is necessary. For the patient during the rotation to their affected side, the eyes do not move to compensate for the head rotation, so the eyes move in the same direction as the head rotation (i.e., to the right). At the end of the head turn (*column C*) the patient's eyes have been dragged off target and so they must make a corrective saccade back (*small arrows beneath the eyes*), to refixate on the examiner's nose That corrective saccade at the end of the head rotation to the affected side is usually easily detectable if the patient can refrain from blinking. A patient with right unilateral loss makes a corrective saccade after rightward head rotations, and a patient with a left unilateral vestibular loss makes a corrective saccade after leftward head rotations. (Figure from aVOR iPhone/iPad app.)

presented a significant challenge that has taken our group many years to solve. By using a miniature, very fast, video camera on lightweight, tightly fitting glasses, securely attached to the head, it is possible to measure the eye velocity and the head velocity during the head turn accurately and so quantify the VOR (MacDougall et al., 2009). The vHIT quantifies the VOR simply, quickly, and accurately and importantly shows the presence of covert or overt corrective saccades objectively. In particular, covert saccades are readily detected by the vHIT system. Similar systems now exist but vHIT, devised, developed, programmed, and validated by Hamish Mac-

Dougall is the original (MacDougall et al., 2009). Recently we have shown that the vHIT quantifies the VOR not only for horizontal but also for vertical semicircular canals (MacDougall et al., 2013a, 2013b), so providing objective evidence of the functional state of all six semicircular canals. In this chapter we focus mainly on the setup and testing of the horizontal VOR, since once this is understood it is a simple matter to transfer that knowledge to the vertical system as we do in a later section.

After we published the vHIT method and its validation (MacDougall et al., 2009), GN Otometrics developed a commercial version of vHIT, and markets

it as ICS Impulse. Some of the authors of this chapter are consultants to GN Otometrics. Throughout this chapter most of the vHIT data presented have been obtained with the prototype glasses made by Hamish MacDougall, but we also show some examples from ICS Impulse.

VALIDATION OF THE VIDEO HEAD IMPULSE TEST

Obviously it is necessary to verify that vHIT is valid, and that was accomplished by comparing the results of the vHIT test against the results of the laboratory gold standard of vestibulo-ocular testing—the scleral search coil method. These validation studies consisted of comparing simultaneous measures of the same eye by both methods (search coils and vHIT) in many healthy subjects and patients, and showing there was little systematic difference between results from these two measures (MacDougall et al., 2013a, 2013b; MacDougall et al., 2009) (Figure 16–4). In the simultaneous measurement with scleral search coils, it was shown that for horizontal head turns, the diagnostic accuracy of vHIT matched the diagnostic accuracy of the gold-standard scleral search coil method.

It should be noted that these validation data only pertain to vHIT equipment and software with a high-speed (250 Hz) frame rate, built on minimum slip glasses, run by very fast software with appropriate algorithms. While our system and the Impulse system meet these requirements, we are not sure any of the other systems do so. Few copies have been directly validated against simultaneous search coil recordings as vHIT has been. The validation of our vHIT system against search coils cannot be taken as a blanket certification of approval of all ersatz vHIT systems.

While the scleral search coils technology remains the reference standard, it is largely limited to the laboratory because of its very high cost and the complexity of data acquisition and processing. The vHIT system, with resolution and diagnostic accuracy comparable to scleral search coils, has simple data acquisition and processing and is completely portable. As such, it has found utility in the research laboratory, the clinic, the hospital ward, the outpatient clinic, or the ambulance. One very important use that we did not expect was the use of vHIT in the emergency room for distinguishing between patients presenting with severe vertigo due to peripheral vestibular loss as opposed to those with vertigo due to a stroke (Newman-Toker, Kattah, Alvernia, & Wang, 2008; Newman-Toker, Kerber, et al., 2013; Newman-Toker, Tehrani, et al., 2013).

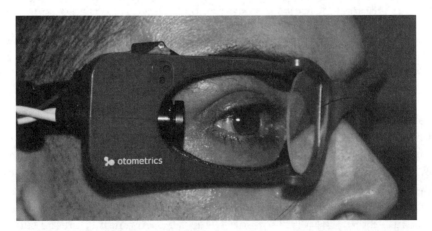

Figure 16-4. Simultaneous recording of the movements of one eye by vHIT and scleral search coils using the ICS Impulse vHIT goggles. The high-speed (250 Hz) video camera is mounted in the tightly fitting glasses. The image of the eye is reflected from a hot mirror onto the camera, allowing the subject to have an unobstructed visual field. The subject (HGM) is wearing a scleral search coil for simultaneously measuring the eye movement at 1,000 samples/s.

Examples of vHIT Results— Healthy Subjects

Before describing exactly how the test is conducted, let us consider how the results look. In carrying out vHIT it is absolutely crucial to ensure the results are acceptable (i.e., that the data are not noisy and the trajectory of the head turn stimulus is correct—close to "turn and stop" without significant overshoot or bounce, which is explained below). Figure 16–5 shows records from vHIT testing of a healthy subject. Figure 16–5A–B show the superimposed records over time (called time series) of the head velocity of every head turn and the eye velocity of the corresponding eye movement response. Figure 16–5A shows the results for leftward head turns (testing the function of the left horizontal canal). Figure 16–5B shows the results for rightward head turns testing the function of the right horizontal canal. The time series for all the impulses have been aligned. In this figure and later similar time series, the eye velocity records (light gray) have been inverted and superimposed on the head velocity records (dark gray) to show graphically how closely eye velocity matches head velocity. This method of presentation is especially valuable for detecting small but sys-

tematic departures of eye velocity from head velocity. The summary figure (Figure 16–5C) shows the VOR gains for rightward (open circles) and leftward head turns (filled circles) for the peak head velocity for every single head turn in both directions. In this example each head turn had about the same peak head velocity, and the repeatability of the stimulus and response is evident at a glance. As is clear from the closely matching eye and head velocity raw data, and the VOR gains close to 1.0, this person has normal semicircular canal function for both directions of head rotation, so we can conclude that the person's horizontal semicircular canal function is normal on both sides. This is a typical result for a healthy person.

Notice that although the eye velocity closely matches head velocity, this healthy subject makes some (very small) saccades for head turns in both directions. In fact these are tiny saccades (probably between the edges of the fixation dot), but even tiny saccades have relatively high peak eye velocity and so they are easily detected by vHIT. Many healthy people have small overt and covert saccades during head impulse testing. They can be just minor saccadic corrections to get back exactly to the center of the fixation dot. These small saccades are not

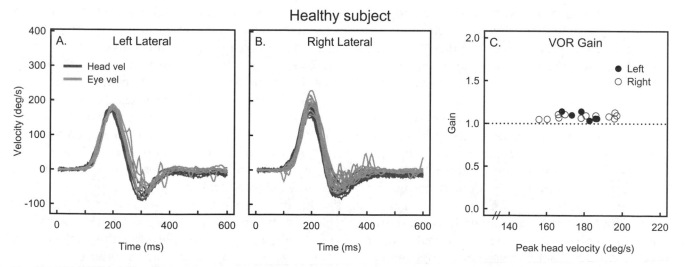

Figure 16–5. The time series results from testing a healthy subject. In this and the following similar figures of head and eye velocity, the convention is that eye velocity is light gray traces and head-velocity is dark gray traces. The time series is for leftward impulses (**A**) and rightward impulses (**B**). In this and the following similar figures, the signs of eye velocity for leftward impulses and of head velocity for rightward impulses have been inverted for easier comparison. The VOR gains (**C**) for both leftward (*filled circles*) and rightward impulses (*open circles*) are close to 1.0, as expected given that the head and eye traces in panels A and B are closely overlaid, and any corrective saccades are very small.

clinically important. The clinically important information is not the occurrence of a few saccades, such as are seen here, but whether the saccades occur systematically in combination with reduced slow phase eye velocity during the head impulse. That is not the case here—the VOR gain is obviously excellent so the tiny saccades have no clinical significance. In sum, the clinician's focus should be upon the slow eye velocity during the head impulse and how closely it matches the head velocity, not on the saccades. In patients the saccades are giving information that complements the evidence from the slow phase eye velocity—slow phase eye velocity and corrective saccades are two indicators of vestibular function, but the more important one is the slow phase eye velocity.

Notice also that in the example all the peak head velocities are about 150 to 200 deg/s. We now recommend that for routine vestibular testing the operator should aim to give a range of head velocities from relatively slow (around 100 deg/s) up to fast (about 300 deg/s). Many patients with unilateral vestibular loss may show normal VOR gain for ipsilesional head turns at low head velocities (50 deg/s), and their vestibular loss becomes apparent only at higher head velocities (above about 150 deg/s). (The physiological basis for this good response at low head velocities after unilateral loss is explained in Appendix 16–B.) For this reason it is recommended that wherever possible there should be trials where the head velocity is greater than 150 deg/s. Operators should be cautious about accepting any test result where this 150 deg/s velocity is not achieved. It is more difficult to achieve these higher head velocities, for example, in patients with stiff necks, so some operators tend not to achieve these higher values, but in that case the results are not an adequate test of semicircular canal function and can be positively misleading—suggesting a patient is normal when they have a unilateral deficit, undetected because the vestibular test is inadequate. In our experience achieving higher head velocities is a matter of practice. We consider that some recent strange published results using vHIT may be due to poor testing with inadequate peak head velocities using ersatz vHIT systems, and it is advisable to check the details of the stimulus and the system used before accepting vHIT results. The sole exception to this recommen-

dation for velocities above 150 deg/s is for testing patients during acute attacks of vertigo, where even low head velocities can be very valuable in verifying the cause of the attack (Manzari, Burgess, Macdougall, & Curthoys, 2012).

The video head impulse test requires high speed, high accuracy, minimal slip, and head-mounted cameras to record the eye movement during the brief passive, unpredictable head turns. But of equal importance are the instructions given to the subject or patient, the subject or patient's ability to understand the instructions and to carry them out, and the motivation of the subject to complete the test honestly. The instructions are to maintain fixation on an earth-fixed fixation target during the head turn, and to regain that fixation target promptly if that target is lost. It is most important to ensure that the subject can actually see the fixation target, since people must remove their spectacles for the test and this compromises the vision particularly of myopic patients. Also keeping looking at a target during any rapid head rotations is an unusual task, and some subjects have trouble understanding what they have to do. This is especially true of people who have language difficulties or senior subjects or subjects whose attention wanders. It helps to encourage the patient to do the task and even give the patient continual feedback on how he or she is doing.

The operator can usually detect if there is a problem on the first few trials. The tell-tale sign is that the subject makes an anticompensatory covert saccade during the head turn—the saccade goes in the direction of the head rotation during the head turn—and then the subject makes a corrective saccade (an overt saccade) back to the target at the end of the head impulse. This covert anticompensatory saccade in the direction of head rotation is the normal eye movement response to a head turn in healthy subjects, and in our first report we warned about how the subject or patient must suppress these anticompensatory saccades (Halmagyi & Curthoys, 1988). Fortunately, healthy subjects and patients who can see the target, who understand the instructions, and who are cooperative (i.e., not trying to falsify the test results) can quickly learn to suppress this anticompensatory saccade so the only eye movement during the head impulse is the slow phase eye movement, compensating for head rotation (or the compensatory covert saccade in patients with vestibular loss). Over the last 6 years in testing many thousands of patients using vHIT, the authors have found that covert anticompensatory saccades occur only rarely and when they do, they appear to be due to the person not seeing the fixation target or not understanding or not following the instructions, or malingering. The evidence for such a conclusion is that repeating the instructions and emphasizing how important it is for the person keep looking at the target causes the anticompensatory saccade to disappear.

Recently it has been asserted that the occurrence of these covert anticompensatory saccades (which the authors termed CAQEM) during a head impulse are common, and it was suggested that CAQEMs are indicators of vestibular disorders (Heuberger et al., 2014). In our view these claims are wrong. In our experience such saccades are very rare—experienced clinicians have only seen the occasional CAQEM saccade in many thousands of patients tested. They are not an indication of vestibular loss but of the fact that the subject cannot see the target or has not understood the instruction or allowed his or her attention to wander or is deliberately trying to give false results, possibly for financial reasons associated with an insurance claim. The operator should be aware of such possibilities. Heuberger et al. (2014) suggested that CAQEMs had been discovered because of video measures of eye movements and that they may be indicators of vestibular migraine or Ménière's disease. We do not accept this interpretation. Even perfectly healthy, asymptomatic subjects will make CAQEMs with video or search coils if they cannot see the target or do not understand that they must try to maintain fixation during the head turn. Indeed even healthy guinea pigs given unpredictable head rotations make exactly the same CAQEMs during head turns as the patients reported by Heuberger et al. (Gilchrist et al., 1998). Guinea pigs do not have a mechanism for fixation and cannot understand instructions so every horizontal head rotation produces an anticompensatory covert saccade (a CAQEM). We are confident that these guinea pigs did not have peripheral vestibular loss or Ménière's disease or vestibular migraine.

There is one proviso to this account. A central neural mechanism must be responsible for the sup-

pression of this anticompensatory saccade during a head impulse, and recently such an anticompensatory saccade has been reported in patients with cerebellar loss (Choi et al., 2014). It may be that the neural suppression mechanism for anticompensatory saccades originates in the cerebellum. Consistent anticompensatory covert saccades in patients who can see the target and who understand the instructions and are paying attention and are motivated could possibly indicate cerebellar loss rather than a vestibular deficit.

Example of Results—Patient With a Unilateral Loss of Horizontal Semicircular Canal Function

The results of vHIT for a patient with a right unilateral vestibular loss are shown in Figure 16–6.

The eye velocities for head turns toward the patient's healthy right ear (contralesional head turns) match head velocity and so are similar to that of the healthy subject, and the VOR gains for these head turns to the right ear are about 1.0 for every head impulse (Figure 16–6B). However, for leftward head turns toward the patient's affected ear ("ipsilesional" head turns) the pattern of results is very different; the peak eye velocity is much smaller than the peak head velocity on every single head impulse, and at the end of the leftward head turns there are large corrective (overt) saccades (Figure 16–6A). These are overt saccades because they occur after the head has stopped moving and so would probably be detectable by a trained eye. The objective records from vHIT show these saccades very clearly. The measured VOR gains for the ipsilesional leftward head turns are all around 0.3 which is substantially below the range of normal gains (0.79–1.20) (Table 16–1). For both directions of head turn, the VOR gains vary from impulse to impulse—the VOR gain is not always exactly 1.0 or always exactly 0.3. Notice in particular that the eye velocity during the head turn to the affected side is not 0.0—there is a small and inadequate eye velocity response and the physiological reason for such a weak response for head turns to the affected ear is explained in Appendix 16–B. Part of this is probably also due to small glasses slip. However, the overall pattern shown

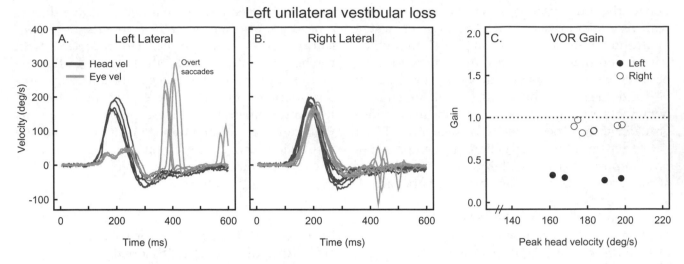

Figure 16–6. The time series results (**A–B**) and VOR gain (**C**) from testing a patient with a unilateral horizontal canal loss. During impulses toward the affected left side (**A**), the eye velocities reached are much lower than those during impulses toward the intact right side (**B**), and the VOR gains (**C**) for leftward impulses are correspondingly lower. Gains for impulses toward the right side have nearly normal value. After the end of the impulse, to the affected left side (**A**), strong overt saccades can be seen at around 400 ms.

Table 16-1. Normative Data: Average VOR Gains and Average Horizontal VOR Gain Asymmetry for Healthy Subjects From the Sydney Clinic

	Left Horizontal	Right Horizontal	Left Anterior	Left Posterior	Right Anterior	Right Posterior	Horizontal VOR Gain Asymmetry
N	28	28	29	29	29	29	28
Mean	0.92	1.00	0.96	0.92	0.95	0.98	5.9%
SD	0.06	0.07	0.12	0.17	0.12	0.15	3.7%
Lower cutoff	0.80	0.86	0.71	0.58	0.70	0.68	13.3%

Note: These numbers must be used with caution: they are only based on a relatively small sample of healthy subjects, and as Figure 16–14 shows, the measured VOR gain depends on the gain algorithm and the peak head velocity used. In the future, we plan to present the normative VOR gain as average values at different velocities. The VOR asymmetry values were calculated as

$$((VOR_{larger} - VOR_{smaller}) / (VOR_{larger} + VOR_{smaller})) \times 100$$

At high accelerations there is a systematic difference between the VOR gains in the two eyes dependent on the direction of the head turn (Weber, Aw, et al., 2008) and since vHIT only tests one eye this is a source of asymmetry. For most clinical testing this interocular source of asymmetry is small.

here is the common eye velocity response pattern for a patient with a unilateral loss of horizontal canal function, for example, a patient with an acute left vestibular neuritis (MacDougall et al., 2009; Manzari et al., 2012).

The objective evidence of the low VOR gain for ipsilesional head turns is corroborated by the objective evidence of the corrective saccades—these are two complementary indicators of vestibular loss. So this patient clearly has a substantial unilateral vestibular loss on the right side, shown by the reduced VOR gain and confirmed by the complementary corrective saccades.

Some patients show a rather different pattern— mixed overt and covert saccades during the ipsilesional head turn (Figure 16–7). This patient has a

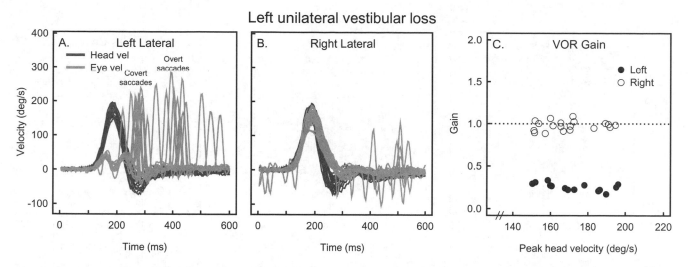

Figure 16–7. The time series results and VOR gains from testing a patient with a unilateral horizontal canal loss. This patient has reduced gain for impulses toward the affected left side, and strong overt saccades after the impulse, at around 400 ms. There are also covert saccades in the later part of the head impulse, at around 250 ms.

unilateral loss on the left side as shown very clearly by the reduced VOR gain for leftward head turns (see Figure 16–7A) and the patient generates both overt and covert saccades for leftward head turns, complementing the evidence of the reduced slow phase eye velocity. The covert saccades that occur while the head is still moving would be extremely difficult to detect by the naked eye. Again the low VOR gain (0.26) is confirmed by the presence of covert and overt saccades—the neural signals from the semicircular canal do not drive the eyes at a sufficient velocity to compensate for the head velocity.

Examples of Patient Results— Bilateral Vestibular Loss

Some patients have bilateral vestibular loss (BVL) possibly as a result, for example, of systemic gentamicin for the treatment of a previous serious infection (Weber, Aw, et al., 2009). Figure 16–8 shows the time series of head impulses to the left and right for a patient with BVL. The VOR gain is very small for both directions of head turn, and that is corroborated by the overt saccades after the head turn. The loss of vestibular function due to systemic gentamicin vestibulotoxicity (Halmagyi, Fattore, Curthoys, & Wade, 1994) cannot be quantified by caloric testing because of the great variability of the caloric

responses and because daily calorics are unacceptable to most patients. But we have demonstrated that such a progressive loss of semicircular canal function loss is measured objectively by the head impulse test (Weber, Aw, et al., 2009). vHIT demonstrates such a bilateral deficit objectively, even at the bedside in patients receiving a course of vestibulotoxic aminoglyocides, since vHIT runs on a laptop and does not require specialized conditions, such as absence of visual fixation. vHIT provides objective quantitative evidence, tracking changes in semicircular canal function even at intervals as short as a few minutes, if necessary. There is no evidence of adaptation or habituation to the head impulse stimulus.

Normal vHIT Gain and Cutoffs for Patients

We stress that before even considering the VOR gain values, *it is absolutely essential to look at the records first*. If the records are noisy the test should be repeated. This inspection of the data should occur while the patient is still wearing the glasses so if a re-test is needed it can be quickly done. As with all clinical investigations VOR gains need to be interpreted with care. A possible pitfall when interpreting the average VOR gain value occurs when there are outliers in the data set—that is, results from individual impulses that clearly lie outside the bulk of the rest

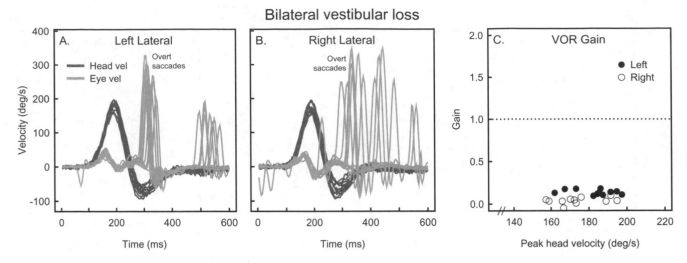

Figure 16–8. The time series results and VOR gains from testing a patient with a bilateral horizontal canal loss. Eye velocities during the impulse (**A–B**) and VOR gains (**C**) are well below normal values for impulses toward both sides. Strong overt saccades, beginning shortly before 300 ms, are present for impulses to both left and right sides.

of the test results. Such an outlying VOR gain value can occur if a partial blink or an eyelid droop occurs during the particular head impulse. In this case it is important to rely on the bulk of the actual traces and set aside the aberrant gain value. In some vHIT systems, the outlying results may be deleted from the calculation of average VOR gain in order to improve the accuracy of the calculated gain values. Remember that every head impulse is a separate test of the function of the semicircular canal (i.e., it is equivalent to half a caloric test). So in the usual vHIT test of 20 impulses, there are effectively 20 separate tests of semicircular canal function. To our knowledge no one has ever given 20 successive calorics to a patient to verify semicircular canal function (see section on VOR gain below).

with a modified pair of swimming goggles—see Appendix 16–C for a brief account of how vHIT was developed.) vHIT testing looks quick and easy, and indeed it is easy to perform, once the operator has had some training and practice. The video glasses are simply tightly fitting glasses. But vHIT is not "plug and play"; operators have to learn how to do the test properly. There are a number of subtle but very important factors that the operator needs to know in order to get acceptable data. With training and practice (using an easy technique described below), this test really does become as simple as it appears, but it does take attention to every detail, and practice and vigilant maintenance of the highest standards by the operator, for this to happen. This section discusses how to carry out the test.

HOW TO CARRY OUT THE vHIT TEST

Introduction and Instrumentation

Video systems have the huge advantage that they are noninvasive—no electrodes are attached to the person. vHIT is a deceptively simple system—a pair of glasses, the operator's hands, and some software. (Note that in this chapter we refer to them as glasses, but the term goggle is sometimes used and indeed the design for the vHIT system started

What Is Being Measured?

Overview: A small high-speed video camera in the glasses (see Figure 16–4) acquires images of the position of the eye in the head at a high frame rate (250 frames/s). The image of the eye is usually reflected from an infrared reflecting mirror (a "hot" mirror) into an infrared sensitive camera in the glasses which are attached by a tight strap to the subject's head. In this way the subject can see visual stimuli through the hot mirror while the image of the eye is reflected from the hot mirror and recorded by the camera. High-speed software processes each image to determine the position of the center of the pupil in relation to the camera. The position of that pupil center is tracked from one image to the next. Underlying all the data analysis is a robust well-defined geometrical coordinate frame since the mathematics of eye rotations are not trivial (Haslwanter, 1995). Even with the coordinate frame, a geometric correction is needed because the eye movement is measured from the image of a three-dimensional sphere projected onto a two-dimensional plane (Moore, Haslwanter, Curthoys, & Smith, 1996). These are a few of the development steps over many years by our team that have laid the foundations that led to the vHIT (Appendix 16–C). Software calculates the velocity of the eye movement and, for VOR gain calculations, identifies and removes any saccades that occur during the head impulse (i.e., the software "desaccades" the records). This is because the measure of VOR performance is calculated using the slow phase eye velocity, not using the velocity of the saccades or quick phases. The velocity sensor (a gyroscope) in the glasses signals the head velocity.

We emphasize what is being acquired is a video image—a sharp image of the pupil at high speed —so blinks, and so forth, prevent that image being acquired. What is measured by the software is the center of the pupil and how that center moves with respect to the head-fixed camera during the head movement. In fact, the image of the pupil usually moves only a few millimeters during the usual head impulse, so it is imperative to be as accurate as possible in every detail.

Where to Test?

To use vHIT it is recommended not to use a dark room because in low light levels the patient's pupil becomes very large and the video data acquisition is degraded because the eyelids tend to partly cover the large pupil. The ideal video image for vHIT is a small pupil, and so the testing should be done in a normally lit room with the seated patient facing an evenly illuminated wall about 1 m away from the patient (not closer). However, it is not advisable to conduct the test in a sunlit room because the infrared component of sunlight tends to cause reflections.

Perhaps surprisingly, the presence of visual stimuli does not affect the VOR measures from vHIT for targets at 1 m (Chim, Lasker, & Migliaccio, 2013). Of course this normally lit room is exactly the opposite of the conditions for the caloric test where any visual fixation stimulus causes visual suppression of the caloric nystagmus. In principle, visual suppression of the VOR also occurs for head impulses in vHIT, but with the accelerations used in the usual vHIT test, the latency to the initiation of VOR suppression is about 80 to 100 ms (Crane & Demer, 1999), so VOR suppression by visual stimuli would be just commencing at the very end of the head impulse.

Apart from the great convenience of testing in light, there is the added advantage that visual stimuli tend to suppress any spontaneous nystagmus that some patients have. In any case, spontaneous nystagmus with slow phase eye velocities of a few degrees per second or even tens of degrees per second is a relatively minor consideration in vHIT testing because the eye velocities to be measured are around 150 to 200 deg/s. This is in sharp contrast to the situation in caloric testing where the absence of visual fixation enhances the spontaneous nystagmus and this causes serious problems because the eye velocity of spontaneous nystagmus is large in relation to the velocity of caloric nystagmus.

Patient Position

The patient sits on a normal chair. The chair height should be adjustable since it is useful to have all patients at about the same head height during testing. There should be a small high-contrast fixation point (a brightly colored spot about 1 cm in diameter) on the wall directly in front of the patient at approximately eye height and about 1 m from the subject. The operator must ensure the patient can see this fixation point without wearing prescription spectacles because it is not possible for the patient to wear glasses during the vHIT test. Patients who wear contact lenses can continue to wear them during the test without affecting the results. Mascara must be removed.

Operator Position

For the test the operator stands behind the patient with his or her hands on the patient's head (Figure 16–9). The computer should be on an adjacent

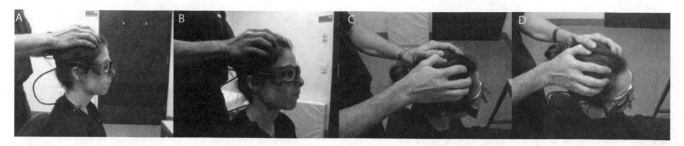

Figure 16-9. For testing horizontal head impulses, the operator's hands are placed on the vertex of the patient's head, well away from the glasses straps and by pushing down slightly on the patient's head, the operator can deliver the small head abrupt head "turn and stop" with minimum of glasses slip.

table, so the operator can deliver the stimulus and see the screen. In the ICS Impulse system, every acceptable head impulse is displayed and stored on the screen so the operator can see if it is acceptable or what they are doing wrong.

The Image

To get accurate measures of the pupil during the head movement, the camera must be stationary with respect to the head during the whole head movement, and the image of the pupil must be clear and sharp without shadows or a drooping eyelid obscuring the pupil (Figure 16–10). The following addresses how to get these results.

The Camera—Speed

The camera must be high speed. The vHIT cameras run much faster than standard video cameras—at around 250 frames/s, whereas the frame rate for standard video cameras is 30 frames/s. This high speed is necessary to measure a moving eye accurately. Saccades are the fastest eye movements, and they last only a very short time (Bahill & Troost, 1979). We know that 60 frames/s is too slow to give accurate measures of saccades, but that 250 frames/s does give accurate measures. We know from an unpublished direct comparison of fast and slow frame rates on the same data sets that low frame rates miss or greatly reduce the very saccades we are seeking to record. So in one patient at a low frame rate the eye movement of the patient with known unilateral vestibular loss looked normal, but with high speed the unilateral loss was clear, both because of the reduced

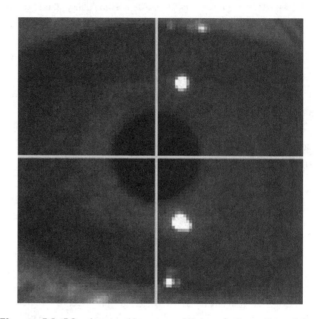

Figure 16-10. A good image of the eye from the video camera.

VOR gain and also the confirmatory covert saccades that the high-speed camera detected but the low-speed camera missed.

The camera used for vHIT measures must also have a high frame rate in order to measure eye velocity accurately. Our direct comparison of simultaneous measures of eye velocity by a video camera with a 250-Hz frame-rate to eye velocity from scleral search coil recordings sampled at 1000 Hz showed there was little systematic difference in measured eye velocity of the two systems (MacDougall et al., 2009), so we concluded that a 250 Hz frame rate is acceptable. Some vHIT copies use slower camera speeds and so miss saccades and give inadequate measures of eye velocity.

The Camera—Focus

The image of the pupil is small and the total movement of the eye across the camera plate during a head impulse is small, so a camera with poor focus will not be able to detect these small movements accurately.

Eye Illumination

Embedded in the ICS Impulse glasses are two low-power infrared illuminating (IR) light-emitting diodes (LEDs) for illuminating the eye uniformly. The glasses must be positioned so that the IR LEDS evenly illuminate the whole eye, with minimal shadows around the eye. Mascara should be removed. For the ICS Impulse system the level of IR illumination is very low and far below the internationally accepted infrared hazard criteria (Delori, Webb, & Sliney, 2007; Sliney et al., 2005). Because of these low levels of IR illumination, the ICS Impulse glasses can be worn for long periods without discomfort or danger to eye health. (That is yet another advantage of vHIT over scleral search coils.) The glasses (and camera) must be positioned on the head so that the eye is well illuminated and the image of the eye is clear (see Figure 16–10). This can be difficult in some people with deep-set eyes, and if the image is not satisfactory, reposition the glasses to get the very best result possible.

Any dark shadows around the eye should be minimized (Figure 16–11), since the algorithm for measuring the eye movement relies on finding the center of the pupil accurately. To get this center, the system inverts the contrast of the image in the region of interest (like a photographic negative), so all the black areas become white (see Figure 16–11). Then the center of the largest white object which does not touch the edge of the region of interest is determined and that center point is tracked during the head movement. Any shadows in the region of interest cause errors in the calculation of the pupil center and so errors in the calculation of eye position and eye velocity. The ideal is to have a sharp, round, white pupil (after thresholding) and the rest of the region of interest being black (see Figure 16–11A).

The Head Velocity Sensor

Also within the glasses is a sensor for measuring the angular velocity of the head in three dimensions directly. The head velocity sensor chip (a MEMs gyroscope) has long-term stability, and so there is no need for repeated calibration of head velocity.

Calibration Lasers

In the ICS Impulse glasses there are two tiny, very low power red lasers for projecting calibration spots

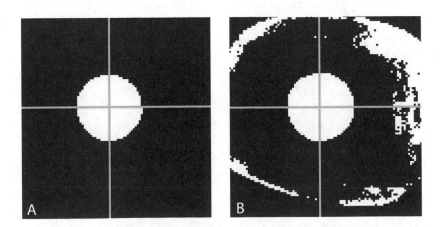

Figure 16–11. The pupil. **A.** The contrast threshold is ideal so the pupil is a small sharp circle. **B.** If the contrast threshold is not set properly, extraneous shadows are seen and pupil finding is degraded, resulting in noisy, unacceptable eye velocity records.

15 deg apart on the wall for the subject to stare at, to allow calibration of the eye movement measures (calibration is explained in detail below). If a patient is not able to see or to stare at these fixation spots (e.g., patients with acute vestibular neuritis and spontaneous nystagmus, or patients with congenital nystagmus), the operator can use a default calibration setting that is a good estimate for most subjects. Some color blind patients can have difficulty in seeing the projected laser spots if the wall illumination is too bright.

HOW TO CARRY OUT THE VHIT TEST— PERFORMING THE TEST

Fitting the Glasses to the Subject

The most important consideration in the vHIT test is stability of the glasses on the patient's head. Glasses slip occurs during a head impulse when the glasses slide on the patient's head and if the camera moves relative to the eye then the system erroneously records that camera slippage as an eye movement. And since the whole eye movement during a head impulse is very small, the camera only needs to slip by a very small amount to cause a big measurement error. It is almost impossible to eliminate glasses slip with a large, relatively heavy camera/glasses system used in some vHIT copies. The vHIT camera and glasses should be the lightest available so slippage is minimized. Also the camera should be as close to the center of the head as possible to minimize inertia. However, because the skin is flexible it is almost impossible to totally eliminate glasses slip, and in some obese subjects this will be a serious problem because the person may have so much skin between the glasses and the skull that major camera movement will occur. Every effort must be made to minimize glasses slip. The strap holding the glasses on the head should be very tight. This may be moderately uncomfortable for the patients, but the test usually takes only a few minutes so that discomfort does not last long. We find it useful to explain to the patient that the reason for the tight strap is to keep the glasses moving exactly with the head. Given that the patient's nose forms an anchoring point for the

glasses, it is important to check that, wherever possible, the glasses are sitting closely on the bridge of the nose. In some people the bridge of the nose is not well projected and so the glasses tend to slip without this nose "anchor." One solution is to construct a surrogate nose anchor out of wound-dressing tape, which is adhered to the bridge of the nose to create the anchor point on which the glasses nose-piece sits. How is it possible to identify if glasses slip has occurred? A tell-tale sign is the onset of an eye movement that precedes the onset of the head movement.

Optimizing the Image of the Eye

What is being measured is the center of the pupil, so anything that interferes with the image of the pupil is to be eliminated because it generates incorrect results. Drooping eyelids must be avoided. This can be achieved when fitting the glasses by lifting the glasses slightly off the face while manually raising the eyebrows and eyelids and then allowing the glasses to sit back on the face. This is not uncomfortable and it acts to ensure that the image of the pupil is not obstructed by a drooping eyelid. In some patients we have found that adhesive medical tape can be used to tape their eyelids up. Why is this necessary? If there is any droop of the eyelid during the head impulse, it can generate a double peak of eye velocity, which can be mistaken for a sign of pathology. The operator needs to be especially vigilant about the image of the pupil being unobstructed.

Once the image of the eye is obtained and displayed on the computer screen, the operator must optimize it: first by using the software controls to select a region of interest around the pupil, and then by setting the threshold so the pupil is a sharp white circle on an otherwise black field.

The Pupil

The vHIT system measures eye movement by tracking the movement of the center of the pupil. It is imperative that the image of the eye be of sufficient quality to allow an accurate determination of the pupil center. ICS Impulse has a graphical indication of whether or not the system is adequately tracking the pupil. Depending on the system being used, this may take the form of superimposed cross hairs over the image of the pupil (see Figure 16–10). Inadequate pupil tracking can be indicated by an absent or flashing cross-hair graphic. The consequences of poor pupil tracking are noisy eye velocity traces yielding spurious and unacceptable results.

Precise contrast threshold setting is needed for accurate pupil tracking. In setting the threshold, the objective is to maximize image contrast such that the pupil appears as different from the background as possible (see Figure 16–11). The noise level on the eye trace is at a minimum when the contrast and threshold are properly set. The high noise associated with a poor threshold means that the data are spurious and unusable.

Calibration

In order to measure eye velocity, the software requires information about the size of the pupil displacement caused by an eye movement through a known angle. Getting this information is called an in vivo calibration. It requires the understanding and cooperation of the patient. The usual procedure is to use two laser dots projected from the glasses onto the wall, and the patient is asked to look at each in turn and when he or she is doing so, the computer logs that data and uses it for calculating eye velocity. If there is an error in the calibration then all the eye velocity measures will be in error and so the VOR gain calculations will be in error. In the ICS Impulse vHIT system, the subject is asked to look between two points that are 15 deg apart projected on a wall at least 1 m distant by two very low power (safe)

lasers. Where a subject is unable to carry out this in vivo calibration (e.g., a patient with congenital nystagmus), a default calibration setting is available.

One simple technique we strongly recommend for verifying that calibration has been successful is, after the program has been started and is acquiring and displaying data, to slowly, passively rotate the subject's head horizontally from side to side through an angular range of about 20 deg at a very slow speed (about 0.5 Hz) while the subject is instructed to keep fixating on the earth-fixed fixation target. If the calibration is correct, the eye velocity trace should be exactly superimposed on the head velocity trace (Figure 16–12). The initial step in solving poor calibration is to repeat the calibration process, and if necessary, remove the glasses and start again.

Instructions

The operator must make it very clear to the patient that the patient's task is to try to keep looking at the exact center of the fixation spot the whole time during the head movement, to keep his or her eyes wide open, and if the gaze moves from that spot to get back to that fixation spot as quickly as possible. Make sure the patient can see the fixation spot and understands what they have to do. The patient should also be asked to try as hard as possible not to blink during the head movement and to keep his or her eyes wide open and to relax the neck muscles to the greatest extent possible. Many patients find this neck muscle relaxation difficult, and some gentle practice head turns by the operator are useful.

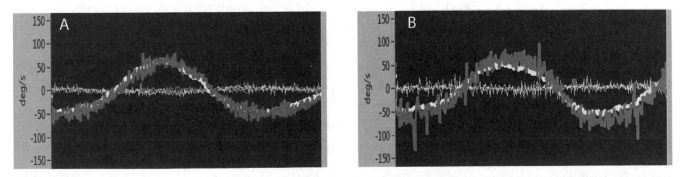

Figure 16–12. Calibration check. **A.** The eye calibration is correct, so during the low-frequency head rotation back and forth, the eye velocity record is almost exactly superimposed on the head velocity record. **B.** If the calibration is not correct, the eye velocity is systematically larger (or systematically smaller) than the head velocity record. In such a case the in vivo eye calibration should be done again.

Operator Hand Position

Careful positioning of the operator's hands assists in reducing the risk of glasses slip. Glasses movement may come about by direct contact of the operator's hands with the glasses themselves or with the glasses strap or indirectly, by movement of the patient's hair or headdress which indirectly moves the glasses strap. We have found a configuration of hand position to be useful in avoiding glasses slip: the hands are placed on the vertex of the patient's head, well away from the glasses straps (see Figure 16–9), and by pushing down slightly on the patient's head, the operator can deliver the small, abrupt head turns with minimal glasses slip.

The Head Movement

The key issues with the head movement are that the movement is only through a small angle (10 to 20 deg), and the start and the stop must be abrupt. The acceleration at the onset is activating the semicircular canal and so generating the eye movement response being measured. It is not the size of the head movement which is most important but the acceleration—how abrupt the start is. The actual extent of movement of the head is quite small, smaller than carried out by physiotherapists or chiropractors. If the patient has serious neck problems, then it would be wise not to test them. We recommend giving the patient a few practice head impulses before the actual data acquisition starts. This also helps the patient relax his or her neck muscles. The head turns should be unpredictable as to timing, direction, and speed. Many patients will try to predict what is coming next and will try to "help." But the operator is all the time trying to beat them at this prediction "game."

The Goal: The Ideal Head Impulse

Exactly how the operator moves the head is extremely important because if the head turn is not performed correctly, then even a patient with total bilateral vestibular loss will not make a corrective saccade. Many novice operators make the mistake of assuming that large head turns are required. This is wrong. In fact, small head turns are to be preferred since glasses slip is less of a factor with small head turns. Since eye velocity and head velocity are both being measured by low noise systems, it is not necessary to have very large head turns. The important thing is not how large the head turn is but how abruptly it starts and stops—the acceleration, not the displacement. The ideal head impulse is "turn and stop." A big advantage of vHIT is the instant feedback for the operator which improves the quality of the stimulus.

Delivering the Head Impulse

The operator stands behind the patient with his or her hands on the patient's head, but away from the glasses strap. The operator aims to turn the head to the left or right unpredictably, through a small angle and to aim the patient's nose at an imaginary target 10 to 20 deg to the left or right. The important part of the measurement is how the eye moves at the very early part of the head turn, so the start of the head turn should be abrupt—a small abrupt head turn is ideal. There should be as little overshoot (or rebound) as possible—the turn should conclude with an abrupt stop. By "rebound" we mean taking the head past the imaginary "stop" point and bringing it back toward the straight ahead. It is not a dead stop but an overshoot and a bounce back. Rebound is to be avoided. What is needed is a dead stop. This sounds very easy to do, but in fact it requires training and practice to do it properly since the tendency is to overshoot and then rebound the head back toward straight ahead, rather than stop the head abruptly at the imaginary target position. In a patient with a vestibular loss, the head turn will take the eyes with the head, off the target, and then the rebound will take the eyes back to the target so no corrective saccade will be necessary.

Where to Start From?

It is recommended to start with the head in a central position with the patient's nose pointing straight ahead at the fixation target, because from that central position the direction of the turn is unpredictable. Then the abrupt "turn and stop" head movement is carried out (see Video 16–1). In the ICS Impulse system, the computer signals whether the turn was an acceptable stimulus—very slow head turns are not accepted as being valid stimuli and doing all head turns with peak velocities less than 150 deg/s can be useless. After the end of the head turn, the head is slowly returned to the central position. It is important that the direction and the timing of the head turn are unpredictable. Falling into the habit of giving alternate left and right head turns at a regular interval, "metronoming," is to be avoided. All the time the operator should be playing the game of trying to prevent the patient from guessing which direction and speed the next head turn will be.

How Many Impulses?

Each head turn is a separate test of vestibular function of the semicircular canal on the side to which the head is turned. Each extra head turn in that direction just repeats the same test. In fact each head turn is equivalent to a whole caloric test of one ear, so repeated trials are effectively equivalent to repeated caloric tests on the same ear. This repetition is valuable for providing increased confidence to the operator about the functional state of the semicircular canal. We recommend about 20 to 30 head turns to each side, because in our experience that number for most patients gives a measure of VOR gain with an acceptably small confidence interval around the estimated VOR gain. But, as the data in Figure 16–13 show, with many patients it is not necessary to give 20. With many patients the results are very clear in the first two or three impulses, and the extra impulses just add to the operator's confidence.

In some patients—where it is very hard to get good results, for example, because of a stiff neck, or the patient "helping" too much—it is better to aim for a small number of quality head turns than religiously going after an impossible 20. It is the quality of the impulses, the abrupt start and stop, the peak head velocity, and not the number of impulses which is important. We emphasize that if possible the head velocity on some trials should exceed 150 deg/s, because if only small head velocities are used, a unilateral vestibular loss may not be revealed. We stress this because since the glasses have been widely used we find some operators always simply give a few unacceptably low velocity impulses (they are easier to deliver) and so finish up with a false diagnosis.

One good practice is to aim to give a range of head velocities, intermingled, for example, 10 less than 120 deg/s, 10 between 120 and 180 deg/s and 10 greater than 180 deg/s. This gives a range of stimulus velocities which is useful for accurately identifying vestibular loss and for monitoring recovery after neuritis (Figure 16–14). Intermingled velocities add to the unpredictability for the patient, and the computer program can sort these varied velocities easily. Figure 16–14 shows a representation of the results of this "range of velocity technique" for a healthy subject and a patient with a unilateral loss. Note in the patient's data that at low head velocities the VOR gain is relatively high and that it is the high head velocities that show the unilateral loss.

The Time Interval Between Successive Impulses

It is advisable to wait a variable interval of about a second or so between the end of one head impulse and the beginning of the next. It should not be a fixed interval. Usually a second is just a comfortable time interval to gently bring the head back to a straight-ahead position.

Blinks

Some patients frequently blink throughout the test and blinks can be very difficult for the patient to control. The vHIT software in ICS Impulse is usually able to exclude trials where there is a blink, and such trials are not captured as a valid impulse, and therefore are not used in the calculation of the average VOR gain. Such blink-prone patients must be strongly encouraged not to blink during the head turn—let them blink and then give them the impulse.

The Patient Who Tries to Help

Some patients have difficulty in relaxing their neck muscles. They may resist the operator turning their head or anticipate the head turn and actively try to help rotate their head. Both of these strategies are to be discouraged. Resistance means that it is not possible for the operator to deliver high head velocities. Why is "helping" by the patient discouraged?

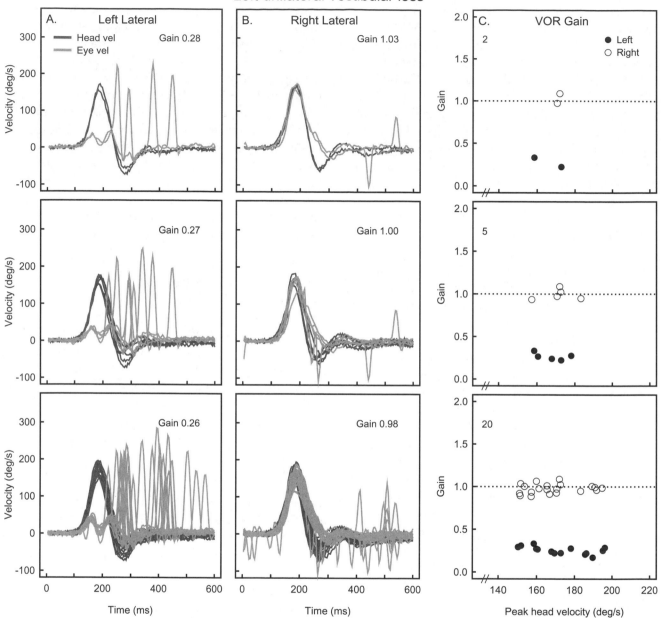

Figure 16–13. Traces of head and eye velocity, and VOR gain. Different numbers of impulses are shown in each row, to show that VOR gain can be measured reliably even with a small number of impulses. The first row shows results for two impulses, the second for five impulses, and the third for 20 impulses. Mean gains for both the affected left side and for the intact right side are hardly affected by the number of impulses included in the figure. This figure should not be taken as a reason to only give 2 or 3 impulses routinely—for acceptable reliability we recommend 20 impulses.

It is discouraged because we have shown that head impulses actively performed by the patient do not reveal the VOR deficit (Black, Halmagyi, Thurtell, Todd, & Curthoys, 2005), probably because the patients who actively generate the head turn can also actively generate the compensatory eye movement to correct for it. So the active contribution by the patient ("helping") is to be avoided in clinical vestibular testing—the head impulse should be a passive unpredictable head turn.

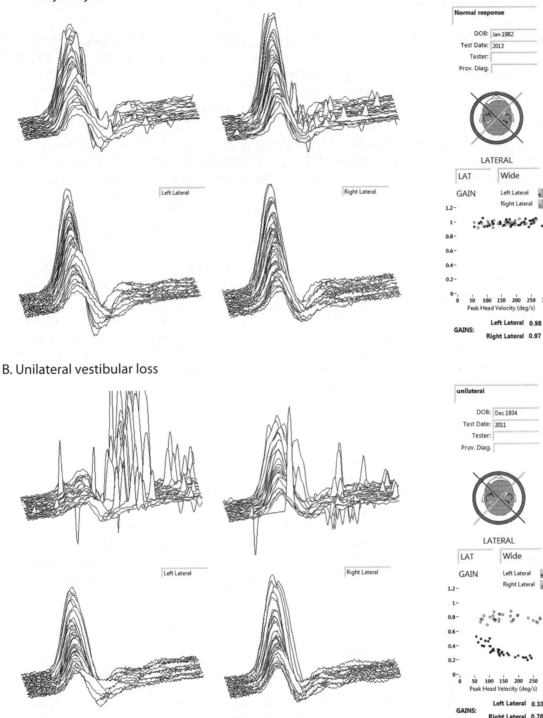

Figure 16–14. Instead of just giving one value of head velocity repeatedly, it is recommended to give a range of differing head velocities. The results are shown in a 3-d format (Weber et al., 2008). Each line is a separate head impulse and they have been plotted so that the head velocity progressively increases from very small to large. **A.** 3-d time series of eye velocity (*top row*) and corresponding head velocity (*bottom row*) and VOR gains (*inset graph*). The VOR gains for both leftward and rightward impulses (*filled and open circles respectively*) are close to 1 over the entire range of peak head velocity, and any corrective saccades are very small. **B.** Corresponding 3-d time series of eye and head velocity and VOR gains, for a patient with left unilateral vestibular loss. For impulses toward the affected left side, peak eye velocity during the impulse is lower than peak head velocity with many overt saccades, with this discrepancy being clearly greater for high-velocity impulses. The VOR gains for the leftward impulses (*filled circles*) decrease as head velocity increases.

When the Test Is Not Possible

Just as it is not possible to measure calorics in every patient, so there are a very few patients in whom it is not possible to measure their VOR with vHIT. They may have such stiff necks that it is not possible to turn their head with adequate velocity, or it may not be possible to get an adequate measure of their pupil, or the glasses slip may be too great to provide acceptable data. But such complete failures are rare.

Training

The operator should imagine a lateral target point and be aiming to turn the patient's head so that the patient's nose points exactly at this lateral, imagined point. Just as a technician carrying out a caloric test needs extensive training before the data are acceptable, so anyone using the vHIT technique needs training as well. It takes practice to deliver an optimum head impulse, and feedback is needed in order to see what you are doing wrong. One way of getting that feedback is by a training session using a laser or flashlight or headlight (used by hikers or cyclists) on the subject's head, projecting the headlight spot onto the wall. For this training session two adhesive dots should be placed (temporarily) on the wall about 20 cm on either side of the central fixation spot. These will be the targets for the operator. The headlight spot should start being superimposed on the central fixation point. Then the operator gives the subject an abrupt head turn and tries, in one smooth movement, to aim the headlight spot exactly on the left or right dot without any overshoot. By watching the headlight spot on the wall the operator can see exactly the trajectory of the head movement. At the first attempt the operator will get it wrong—the headlight spot will overshoot the dot, go past, and then come back again to the dot. That "bounce" or "rebound" is to be avoided. The head impulse is an abrupt, smooth turn and dead stop. The operator needs to practice the turn and stop so they can turn the head to put the headlight spot exactly on the target dot (or very close to it) every time, without overshoot or rebound. Having mastered that for wide targets, the operator should practice the "turn and stop" for a variety of sizes of head turns.

TESTING THE VERTICAL SEMICIRCULAR CANALS: LARPS AND RALPS

Introduction

So far this chapter has been focussed on testing horizontal semicircular canal function, but recently we have shown how it is possible to use vHIT to test the vertical canals (left anterior- right posterior, LARP; right anterior-left posterior, RALP) in similar fashion (MacDougall et al., 2013a, 2013b). Once again simultaneous recordings by vHIT and scleral search coils of the same eye, showed that vHIT detects vertical semicircular canal dysfunction as well as search coils.

The vertical canals are oriented in planes about 45 deg to the median plane of the head (see Figure 16–1) and form two matched pairs—left anterior-right posterior (LARP) and right anterior-left posterior (RALP) (Blanks, Curthoys, & Markham, 1975). If one attempts to measure the VOR in response to a head turn in the plane of a pair of vertical canals, with gaze straight ahead, then it is necessary to measure ocular torsion (rotation of the eye around the line of sight) at high sampling rates because the eye movement response to these diagonal head movements has both vertical and torsional components (Aw et al., 1996). High-speed, accurate measures of torsion require a very high-definition image of the iris which acts to slow down the acquisition speed. Moreover, moving the patient's head in these diagonal planes while the patient faces straight ahead, is awkward for the operator and uncomfortable for the patient.

Both of these problems can be overcome if, prior to the first impulse, the operator repositions the patient by turning the patient's body (using a swivel chair) so it is positioned so that the nose faces 30 to 40 deg to the left or right of straight ahead (see Figure 16–14). The subject must keep looking at the central fixation point out of the corner of his or her eyes. Then the head impulse is a pitch of the head forward and back in the direction of the fixation point. This is in the plane of the vertical canals (see Figure 16–14 and Video 16–2). This is relatively simple and comfortable for the patient and the operator, and tests the vertical canal response by measuring just the vertical eye movement component

(Migliaccio & Cremer, 2011). Head pitches like this activate the vertical canals and elicit corrective eye movements analogous to those for horizontal head turns (Figure 16–15).

To test the left anterior-right posterior pair of canals (LARPs) the patient is rotated so that the body and head are pointed 30 to 40 deg to the right of the fixation point. The subject still fixates the central fixation point, so the eye is shifted to the left in the orbit. A head pitch forward, toward the target, activates the left anterior canal, and a head pitch back away from the target activates the right posterior canal. To test the right anterior-left posterior (RALP) pair of canals, the patient is rotated so the head and body are pointed about 30 to 40 deg to the left of the target so the eye is shifted to the right of the orbit. A head pitch forward activates the right anterior canal, and a head pitch back activates the left posterior canal.

For testing LARPs and RALPs, the operator's hand position needs to be changed—it is best if one hand is placed under the patient's chin, and the other hand is on top of the patient's head (Figure 16–16). Be careful that the fingers of the hand under the chin do not wrap around and push the patient's cheek since that will lead to movement of the glasses. Both hands should be well away from the glasses and the strap.

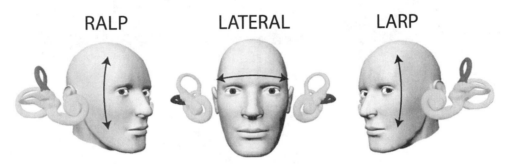

Figure 16–15. The head movements for LARP (left anterior-right posterior) and RALP (right anterior-left posterior) and lateral semicircular canal stimulation (*arrows*), as viewed from the fixation point. For testing the vertical canals, the person's head is turned as shown and the movement of the head is a pitch movement in the plane of the named canals as represented by the vertical arrows. For testing horizontal canals, the movement is in the plane of the horizontal canals as shown. These images are modified from the free educational iPhone or iPad app "aVOR," developed by Hamish MacDougall and available on iTunes. Reproduced with permission of Wolters Kluwer Health from H. G. MacDougall, L. A. McGarvie, G. M. Halmagyi, I. S. Curthoys, and K. P. Weber, 2013, Application of the video head impulse test to detect vertical semicircular canal dysfunction, *Otology and Neurotology, 34*(6), 974–979.

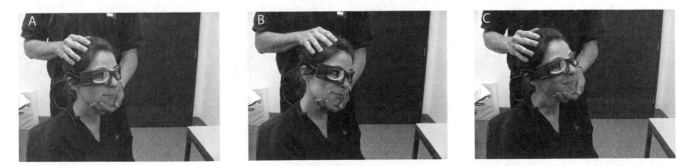

Figure 16–16. The positions of the hands for testing the vertical canals. One hand is placed under the chin and the other hand on top of the head, but well away from the glasses strap.

The results of testing all semicircular canals in a healthy subject are shown in Figure 16–17. The eye velocity matches head velocity for all directions. The advantage of testing the vertical as well as the horizontal canals is that in a patient with unilateral vestibular neuritis, it allows the clinician to identify whether the neuritis is total or just affects the

superior division of the vestibular nerve and so and leaves the posterior canal function, carried in the inferior division of the nerve, intact. In rare patients only the inferior vestibular nerve is affected.

The results of testing a patient with unilateral vestibular loss are shown in Figure 16–18. The patient's data show reduced eye velocity response

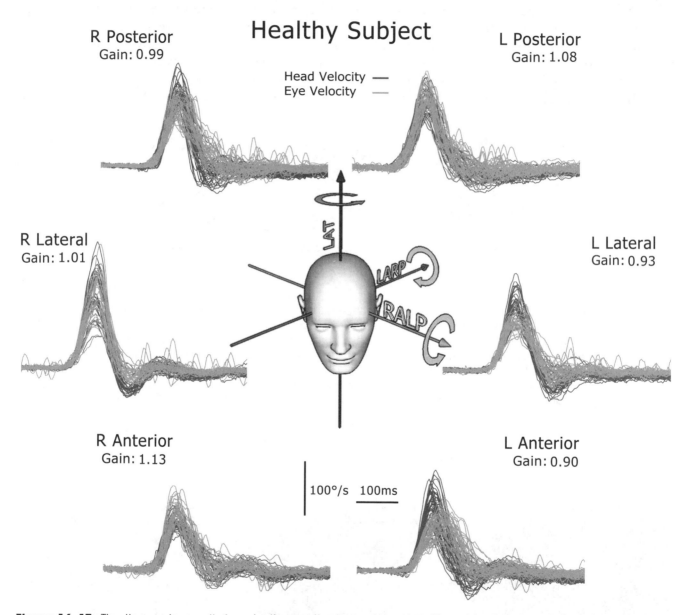

Figure 16–17. The time series results from testing vertical canals in a healthy subject. The plots show superimposed records of desaccaded eye velocity responses to head velocity stimuli in each plane. In a healthy subject the eye velocity matches head velocity so the head velocity traces and eye velocity traces are almost exactly superimposed in every plane. All gain values of the vestibulo-ocular reflex (VOR) are in the normal range. Reproduced with permission of Wolters Kluwer Health from H. G. MacDougall, L. A. McGarvie, G. M. Halmagyi, I. S. Curthoys, and K. P. Weber, 2013, Application of the video head impulse test to detect vertical semicircular canal dysfunction, *Otology and Neurotology, 34*(6), 974–979.

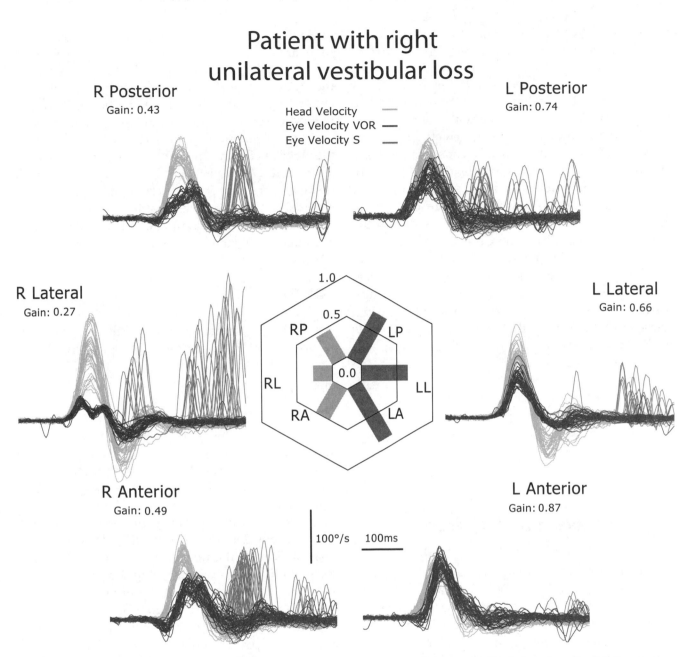

Patient with right unilateral vestibular loss

R Posterior
Gain: 0.43

Head Velocity —
Eye Velocity VOR —
Eye Velocity S —

L Posterior
Gain: 0.74

R Lateral
Gain: 0.27

1.0
0.5
RP — LP
RL — LL
RA — LA
0.0

L Lateral
Gain: 0.66

R Anterior
Gain: 0.49

100°/s 100ms

L Anterior
Gain: 0.87

Figure 16–18. The time series results from testing vertical canals in a patient with a unilateral vestibular loss. Super-imposed records of the head velocity stimulus and the eye velocity responses to brief unpredictable head turns in the direction of each semicircular canal. Eye velocity matches head velocity reasonably well for leftward head rotations (toward the healthy ear), but not for rightward head rotations (toward the affected ear). As is the case for the horizontal canal, reduced or absent slow phase eye velocity occurs during head turns toward the right anterior and right posterior canals. There are many overt saccades. The central graph shows the VOR gain for each canal in a variation of a radial or polar plot as explained in the text. The bars show the value of the VOR gain re the 1.0 or 0.5 scale shown by the hexagons. The bars are adjacent to the canal tested, so that it is quickly observed that all the right side canals have low gains relative to all the canals on the left side. Reproduced with permission of Wolters Kluwer Health from H. G. MacDougall, L. A. McGarvie, G. M. Halmagyi, I. S. Curthoys, and K. P. Weber, 2013, Application of the video head impulse test to detect vertical semicircular canal dysfunction, *Otology and Neurotology, 34*(6), 974–979.

and reduced VOR gains for head impulses activating all the canals in their affected right ear (right anterior, right posterior, and right horizontal head impulses). An impressive validation of vHIT for LARPs and RALPs is that it showed an isolated loss of one posterior canal in a patient whose isolated canal loss had previously been detected by search coils. vHIT showed reduced response for head impulses activating just the patient's affected right posterior canal (MacDougall et al., 2013b).

Vertical head impulses are more difficult to deliver than horizontal head impulses due to the fact that neck mobility is more limited for pitch head movements than for horizontal head movements. In addition, eccentric eye position and limited vertical range by the upper and lower eyelid make pupil tracking with video technically more demanding. These limitations mean that in testing vertical canals with vHIT, it is not usually possible to achieve a peak head velocity as large as that delivered in the plane of the horizontal canals. Again training with a subject wearing a headlight (aimed at the fixation point) will teach the operator how to do vertical head impulses with the usual turn and stop and minimum overshoot and ideally a peak velocity of around 150 deg/s.

INTERPRETING THE RESULTS

At the end of the test, many operators simply look at the average VOR gain number and base their diagnosis on that number. This is a serious mistake. What use is that number if the impulses have not been delivered properly? In such a case the VOR gain number will be meaningless, just as caloric data are meaningless unless the test has been carried out properly. It is vital to first ensure the records, the time series data, are acceptable—not too noisy, without large overshoot and rebound, and including impulses with peak head velocity at least 150 deg/s. We absolutely *insist* that the operator inspect the graphs of the time series of the results before putting any credence on the value of VOR gain. Ideally the operator should check the results while the patient still has the glasses on, so that if re-testing is necessary it will be quicker than starting from the very

beginning again. If the records are very noisy, or if there are large saccades, even before the peak head velocity, if the eye velocity leads the head velocity, then the operator should be very sceptical of the calculated VOR gain. The simple solution is to repeat the test ensuring the glasses are as tight as possible and the subject understands his or her task. Since the final results are available in a very short time after the test has finished, it is not difficult to repeat the test, correcting errors such as glasses slip, noisy records or unacceptable overshoot, or inadequate head velocity. Even a complete re-test will only take a fraction of the time for conducting a full caloric test.

VOR Gain

With vHIT, in contrast to calorics, the range of normality is tight: the average VOR gain for vHIT for healthy subjects in our clinic is 0.96 ± 0.12 (SD) so the mean gain ±2 SDs (including 95% of the population) (Zar, 2010) is 1.20 to 0.79 (see Table 16–1). In other words any VOR gain outside this range (e.g., less than 0.79 or greater than 1.20) is considered to be abnormal. The average vHIT gain asymmetry ratio (comparable to the canal paresis score) for high accelerations is 5.9% ± 3.7, so the normal range of vHIT gain asymmetry in this group of healthy subjects is from 0 to 13.3%, and a gain asymmetry greater than 13.3% is considered to be abnormal. This is smaller than the size of the normal range of canal paresis scores with calorics, which is of the order of 0 to 25%. Thus, vHIT can detect small asymmetries and also small deterioration in absolute bilateral semicircular canal function (i.e., whether VOR gains for both directions of rotation are below normal, as occurs in bilateral vestibular loss).

Even with good records our experience with vHIT has shown that the widely used measure—VOR gain—is not an adequate measure of vestibulo-ocular response. Why? VOR gain is a performance indicator usually taken at one point in time, or over a very narrow time window. VOR gain is usually defined as the ratio of eye velocity to head velocity, and it arose from an engineering analysis of the stimulus and the response. But the question becomes, which value of head velocity should be used for this calculation? In the past the VOR gain has been calculated using eye velocity at peak head acceleration, but peak head acceleration is exactly where the greatest artifact due to possible slippage of the glasses occurs.

As we have used the system on many thousands of patients, it has become clear that there should be a better use of all the response data rather than using just one isolated value—trying to quantify this entire complex response in a single number is a very inadequate representation of performance. For the present, VOR gain will continue to be used since it is so widely understood, but you should be aware that VOR gain has severe inadequacies. Our new method of calculating VOR gain (MacDougall et al., 2013b) uses all the data for an impulse to calculate VOR gain. This new method of calculating VOR gain for vHIT is much less susceptible to the glasses slip artifact in the eye velocity record, which we have referred to as the "bump." How is VOR gain calculated in the ICS Impulse system? First the eye velocity record is desaccaded: the data point at the beginning of the saccade is joined by a straight line to the data point at the end of the saccade, and the saccade eye velocity is removed. Then the area under the desaccaded eye velocity curve from the start of the head velocity to the end of the head velocity is calculated and compared to the area under the head velocity curve from the start of the head velocity until the moment when the head velocity returns to zero. VOR gain is defined as the ratio of these two areas. This is essentially a position gain, but our investigations have shown that this mode of calculating gain is very resistant to artifact due to glasses slip. It is a more functional measure of gain as the position error is the driver for the corrective saccade, so VOR gain and the corrective saccade are complementary.

The authors of some video systems claim that their goggles do not have goggle slip and imply that the "bump" in the eye velocity record is an artifact of the Otometrics Impulse system. That is because they have not measured the slippage of their goggles properly. Unless the glasses are bolted to the head, there will always be some slippage, and it is most important to recognize that fact, report it objectively, and correct for it, as we have done. VOR gain calculations done at peak head acceleration or peak head velocity are highly susceptible to the errors due to goggle slippage which our functional gain measure overcomes. Our extensive, exactly simultaneous, search coil and video measures on the *same* eye (rather than on different eyes as another group has done) confirm that our method of calculating VOR gain from vHIT records described above gives results that are statistically indistinguishable from the VOR gains from search-coil recordings of the same eye (MacDougall et al., 2009, 2013b). That is conclusive evidence that our functional method of measuring VOR gain has overcome the problem of goggle slippage.

Why Is VOR Gain Not Exactly 1.0?

Textbooks give the impression that the VOR gain should be exactly 1.0. In fact this is very rarely true. Perfectly healthy people who have no symptoms of visual blur or oscillopsia can gave gains much smaller than 1.0—for example, 0.85 or less—or gains much higher than 1.0 up to 1.2. These people do not complain of blur or oscillopsia during head movements. Why? There are probably a host of reasons. VOR gain is not a fixed immutable quantity but it can be changed by a variety of procedures. Subjects who have worn magnifying spectacles have increased VOR gain even when the spectacles are removed (Gonshor & Jones, 1976; Jones, 1985). VOR gain also increases above 1.0 if the fixation target is close (Chim et al., 2013; Viirre, Tweed, Milner, & Vilis, 1986). Cerebellar disorders can cause increased or decreased VOR gain (Shaikh et al., 2013).

VOR Gain Asymmetries

Clinicians carrying out vestibular tests are steeped in the tradition of looking at asymmetries of semicircular canal function between the two sides and the canal paresis score is the measure of asymmetry of horizontal semicircular canal function from caloric data. There are different ways of quantifying VOR gain asymmetries for vHIT data. One version is to uses a version of the Jongkees formula for calculating asymmetry (Weber, Aw, et al., 2008):

$$\text{VOR gain asymmetry (\%)} = [(\text{larger} - \text{smaller})/(\text{larger} + \text{smaller})] \times 100$$

Another version (Newman-Toker et al., 2013) uses the ratio of VOR gains:

$$\text{VOR Gain asymmetry (\%)} = [1 - (\text{lower VOR gain}/\text{higher VOR gain})] \times 100$$

Each of the asymmetry calculations can be carried on any pair of canals.

The Hex Plot of VOR Gain for Every Semicircular Canal

Now that testing of all six semicircular canals is routine with vHIT, we developed a simple, convenient, and intuitive way of communicating the results of these multiple tests. It is called a hex plot (MacDougall et al., 2013b), and it is a version of a polar plot. An example of a hex plot for all six canals is shown in Figure 16–18 for the data from a patient with a right unilateral vestibular loss. The data for each canal are shown on one face of a hexagon. So the results for the right anterior (RA), right horizontal (RH), and right posterior (RP) canals of one side are assigned three lateral hexagonal faces and similarly the left anterior (LA), left horizontal (LH) and left posterior (LP) canals are assigned three lateral hexagonal faces on the opposite side of the hexagon. (It is entirely arbitrary if the right canals are displayed on the right or left hexagonal faces.) The VOR gain for each canal is shown as a bar projecting from the center (VOR gain of 0.0) to the outermost level corresponding to a VOR gain of 1.0. As Figure 16–18 shows, this method shows the results, both the absolute value of VOR gains for all canals and the VOR asymmetry, intuitively, accurately, and immediately. This patient has suffered substantial loss of semicircular canal function for all canals on the right side.

Repeatability

In healthy subjects our unpublished data have shown that VOR gain is approximately constant from day to day but in patients this is not necessarily the case—it has been shown in early MD patients that there are fluctuations in VOR gain from occasion to occasion especially around the time of the attack (Manzari et al., 2011). These fluctuations may be occurring because of changes within the membranous labyrinth.

We now know that different patient conditions cause very different, but highly repeatable response profiles during a head turn. For example, some patients who may have endolymphatic hydrops show a greatly enhanced eye velocity at the onset of the head turn, but this enhanced eye velocity response very rapidly disappears during the turn and even reverses. As a result, these patients can have a measured VOR gain close to 1.0 but they have achieved this value by a totally different eye velocity profile compared to the eye velocity profile of healthy subjects. Only by examining the eye velocity records is it possible to identify this characteristic response pattern which is very different from that of a healthy subject but the cause of which is still uncertain.

DISCUSSION

Advantages of vHIT

Previous tests of semicircular canal function using rotation have used large rotatory chairs with carefully controlled angular accelerations. The maximum angular accelerations that could be achieved safely in this way are only of the order of 10 to 100 deg/s^2 and so are far below accelerations encountered in everyday life which are of the order of up to 2,000 to 5,000 deg/s^2. Also the rotary chair stimuli were often highly predictable, low frequency (0.2 to 0.5 Hz) sinusoidal horizontal rotations, to which even patients with bilateral loss can generate eye movement responses (probably by predictive pursuit) (Halmagyi & Curthoys, 1987). With a few very expensive and clinically impractical exceptions, it was not possible to test patients safely with very high accelerations using a mechanical device (Crane & Demer, 1998; Tian, Crane, & Demer, 2000).

We broke from that tradition when we showed that a patient with zero semicircular canal function following bilateral vestibular nerve surgical removal for the treatment of bilateral acoustic tumors could still generate compensatory eye movements to low frequency, low acceleration, predictable sinusoidal horizontal rotational stimuli (Halmagyi & Curthoys, 1987). But we found that this bilateral vestibular loss patient did not generate a compensatory eye movement response during the first 100 ms of an unpredictable, passive, high acceleration head turn, and so we concluded that such stimuli are specific probes of vestibular function. This was a very important result because it showed that even when all the other oculomotor control systems (e.g., pursuit, optokinetic, cervical input) were available, they were not capable of generating a compensatory eye movement during the very earliest part of the response to the head turn, so we concluded the eye movement response during this first 100 ms is a specific vestibular response (Halmagyi & Curthoys, 1987, 1988; Halmagyi et al., 1990).

VOR Suppression

Healthy people can almost totally override the vestibulo-ocular response. For example if you are reading a road map in a car as it goes around a corner, you want to keep your eyes on the map rather than have them driven off the map by the vestibular input automatically correcting for the angular turn by the car. In such a situation, descending cerebellar inhibition acts to suppress the drive from the vestibular receptors to the eye muscles, and this is referred to as VOR suppression (Crane & Demer, 1999). We considered that this may affect the vHIT result, but by restricting our measurements to just the start of these brief unpredictable high acceleration head turns we can selectively probe the function of the semicircular canals since with such stimuli it takes about 80 ms or more for VOR suppression to start to operate (Crane & Demer, 1999).

As a result our approach to vestibular testing has been totally different—to deliver passive head turns with natural values of angular acceleration using the safe means of the operator's hands, but to measure the stimulus and the response exactly and to relate the response on each trial to the stimulus on that trial. We have focused on the very earliest part of the response because the results from our bilateral loss patient shows that at later times other oculomotor control systems can operate and so the result is no longer a specific test of semicircular canal function. This has proved to be a very effective way of assessing semicircular canal function specifically and identifying deficits. Initially we used scleral

search coils for these tests but more recently we have used vHIT, having shown that vHIT results are similar to results using search coil recordings (MacDougall et al., 2009, 2013a, 2013b).

What Is the Sensitivity and Specificity of vHIT?

Some recent papers (Bartolomeo et al., 2014; Blodow, Blödow, Bloching, Helbig, & Walther, 2014; Mahringer & Rambold, 2014) report measures of the sensitivity and specificity of vHIT. Unfortunately these papers mistakenly refer to the caloric as the "gold standard" or the reference standard for the measure of the sensitivity and specificity of vHIT. There is a logical flaw in such an approach—both calorics and vHIT are tests of vestibular function. The caloric is *not* a definite indicator of vestibular loss—a "gold standard"—because some healthy people (such as skaters, dancers, and aviators, and one of the authors) have poor or even absent caloric responses but perfectly normal vHIT responses. A normal response on vHIT shows that in response to the physiological, adequate stimulus to the semicircular canal, the function is normal, whereas a small or absent caloric response may occur for a hosts of reasons, unrelated to horizontal semicircular canal function. Unsurprisingly, these two very different methods of testing semicircular canals do not always produce results which agree.

A further problem is that the patients who are tested in the studies referred to above are those with vestibular neuritis or unoperated vestibular schwannomas, so the actual level of vestibular function in these patients is unknown. The correct way of identifying the true sensitivity and specificity of vHIT is to assess how well vHIT can detect *known* unilateral vestibular loss, and the only group of patients in that category are those who have undergone surgical removal of one vestibular nerve to treat vestibular schwannoma. Our recent unpublished measures of 20 such patients and 37 healthy subjects showed that for detecting an objectively verified unilateral vestibular loss, the true sensitivity of vHIT was 1.0, the true specificity was 1.0, and the diagnostic accuracy was 100% (Habbema, Eijkemans, Krijnen, & Knotterus, 2008).

vHIT has the accuracy and the reliability to negate the need for scleral search coil testing in the majority of clinical situations. The ability to obtain objective results immediately in almost any context, be it at the bedside in an emergency department, in an intensive care unit or in the consulting room, far outweighs any marginal advantage that the highly specialized, expensive and complex gold standard scleral search coil technology might possess. The very rapid acceptance of vHIT since 2009, and the number of ersatz vHIT systems so far, has shown the value of the vHIT procedure. The future of balance disorder diagnosis is very likely to see objective bedside canal testing become far more commonplace.

vHIT Versus Calorics

The bithermal caloric test has remained the standard test of vestibular function. Warm or cool water (or air) is introduced into the external ear canal, and it is argued that the thermal stimulus causes small fluid flow in the horizontal semicircular canal and results in horizontal nystagmus. Obviously this is not a usual "physiological" stimulus—the natural stimulus for the canals is the angular acceleration from a head rotation, but nevertheless the caloric test continues to be used. To understand the significant value of vHIT it is useful to contrast vHIT with the standard test of semicircular canal function, the caloric test. With the caloric it is not possible to obtain an absolute measure of horizontal semicircular canal function from the stimulation of each ear. One reason is that there are such great variations between individuals in the pathways conveying the thermal stimulus from the external ear canal to the horizontal semicircular canal. So the magnitude of the stimulus delivered to the canal receptors is not known. Also unknown is exactly how the caloric stimulus stimulates the cupula of the semicircular canal. In the caloric test, the measure is slow phase eye velocity in relation to the temperature of the thermal stimulus—at best a very gross and indirect measure of horizontal semicircular canal function.

The functional state of the other four vertical canals cannot be evaluated by the caloric test. The vHIT test in contrast provides an absolute measure of the function level of every semicircular canal separately. This is possible because the stimulus, head rotation, is the adequate, natural, physiological stimulus for the semicircular canals, and this stimulus is measured exactly during the head turn.

Similarly, the response to this physiological stimulus—eye velocity—is measured exactly. These are accurate measures of the response to direct physiological stimuli, not just eye velocities to unknown thermal stimuli. These simultaneous measures of the stimulus and the response provide many significant advantages compared to the caloric test. Most importantly vHIT provides a measure of the gain of the vestibulo-ocular response for each canal individually. They allow inspection of the form of the temporal profile of the eye velocity response to every part of the stimulus during different stimulus magnitudes—different peak head velocities. One important aspect of the response profile is whether there are overt and covert saccades present. If these saccades are systematically present, they confirm the reduced or absent canal function, shown by the small VOR gain. They may also provide an indicator of the extent of compensation for vestibular loss (MacDougall & Curthoys, 2012). This allows the clinician to identify absolute loss of canal function, where there may be no asymmetry between the two sides but the canals on both sides show a loss of function. Such bilateral loss occurs with systemic gentamicin ototoxicity (Weber, Aw, et al., 2009). Caloric testing cannot provide this information with reliability.

With vHIT there is no question about the stimulus being degraded by the pathways from the external ear to the semicircular canal. With vHIT the stimulus is the natural stimulus for a semicircular canal—angular rotation—which is the natural, adequate, physiological stimulus so the results provide an accurate measure of the functional state of each canal. This is probably the most important advantage of vHIT testing compared to caloric testing.

Here we compare the relative merits of vHIT vs the caloric.

Many factors, apart from the functional state of the semicircular canals, affect caloric nystagmus:

- Wax in the external auditory canal
- Anatomic variations in the skull
- Variable meatal diameter
- Vascularization around the semicircular canal
- Middle ear pathology or surgery
- Patient alertness
- Medication
- Extraneous light (suppressing the caloric nystagmus)

Other problems with caloric testing are as follows:

- The caloric test is time consuming and unpleasant and is not well tolerated by patients.
- It only assesses the function of the two horizontal canals.
- It cannot be conducted with tympanic membrane perforation.
- It cannot be given at short testing intervals.
- It is highly variable from patient to patient.
- Some perfectly healthy subjects with normal semicircular canal function on vHIT have minimal or absent caloric responses.
- It usually requires a specialized testing area, to minimize stray light, which suppresses the nystagmus being measured.
- The caloric test has limited utility in assessing bilateral canal loss.
- It is very difficult, some say even impossible, to conduct caloric testing in very young children.
- The range of normality is wide, so it is difficult to detect small losses.
- Some patients decline to have this test or terminate testing halfway through.

In sharp contrast, vHIT measures of semicircular canal function

- can be performed in patients with acute vertigo, unlike calorics;
- does not rely on a high degree of patient alertness (although the patient should not be sleepy since a drooping eyelid obscures the pupil);
- uses a "physiological" stimulus—head turns with angular acceleration values similar to those encountered during everyday activities;
- is generally very well tolerated, even by patients with severe vertigo;
- should be conducted in a normally lit room;
- is fully portable and can be conducted at the bedside in the ward or the emergency room or at a patient's home;
- is very fast—it requires about 5 to 10 min of testing time;
- is able to assess the function of all six semicircular canals;
- can assess bilateral semicircular canal loss accurately (Weber, Aw, et al., 2009);

- can be conducted relatively easily in very young children (Manzari, Burgess, et al., 2012);
- find the range of normality of responses is much tighter than calorics;
- can be given repeatedly—even only minutes apart—and so is ideally suited to tracking changes in vestibular function (e.g., during disease or therapy or around the time of an acute attack in Ménière's disease) (Manzari, Burgess, MacDougall, Bradshaw, & Curthoys, 2011) , or during recovery (or otherwise) from vestibular neuritis;
- is complementary—with vestibular-evoked myogenic potentials and basic audiometry vHIT completes the ability to test the entire audiovestibular system (Curthoys, 2012).

Sometimes the results of vHIT do not agree with the results of calorics and that is to be expected, as we have listed above calorics can be affected by many parameters that do not affect the semicircular canal physiological response to the natural rotational stimuli used in vHIT. One of the authors of this chapter has no eye movement response to caloric stimulation but excellent responses to vHIT testing of all of his semicircular canals and is perfectly asymptomatic.

Special Patient Groups

Gentamicin Ototoxicity

The head impulse test can detect a small deterioration in absolute bilateral semicircular canal function, due for example to the vestibulotoxic effects of gentamicin on the vestibular receptors in both ears in patients receiving systemic antibiotic treatment (Halmagyi et al., 1994). The progressive loss of vestibular function due to systemic gentamicin cannot be quantified by calorics because of the great variability of the caloric responses and because daily calorics are unacceptable to most patients. A progressive bilateral loss is measured objectively even at the bedside by vHIT since vHIT is on a laptop and does not require specialized conditions. vHIT provides objective quantitative tracking of changes in semicircular canal function at the bedside during such treatment even at intervals as short as a few minutes if necessary. Similarly, vHIT can quantify semicircular canal function in patients receiving intratympanic gentamicin.

Ménière's Disease

Because it can be used at very short intervals, vHIT is now starting to be used to monitor semicircular canal function in patients with probable endolymphatic hydrops and patients with Ménière's disease even around the time of the attack.

CONCLUSION

Vestibular testing is being revolutionized by vHIT and when the results for vHIT are combined with the results of the new ocular and cervical vestibular evoked myogenic potential (oVEMP and cVEMP) tests it is possible to measure the function of all vestibular sense organs (Curthoys, 2012).

vHIT is very simple and does not require specialized conditions—testing is done with the patients sitting in an ordinary chair in a normally lit room. vHIT is undemanding and can be used on patients as young as three. vHIT is a fast, simple way of quickly, safely, and acceptably answering the question: Which side is affected? Is the canal function of each ear in the normal range? vHIT allows repeated testing even within a few minutes, whereas that would be out of the question with calorics. It is very well tolerated by patients and, unlike the calorics, it allows measurement of the function of all semicircular canals. The vHIT test is noninvasive, safe, simple, and quick (less than 10 min to test both sides), and very acceptable even to dizzy and nauseous patients. The analysis software provides objective, quantitative results in real time. In sharp contrast to caloric stimuli, with vHIT the magnitude of the stimulus at each instant in time is known and can be related directly to the response at that instant. vHIT is portable—it can be used in the clinic or at the bedside or the emergency room, or even in the patient's home. vHIT can be carried out even during acute attacks of vertigo (e.g., in a patient during a Ménière's attack or an attack of vestibular neuritis).

Acknowledgments. The vHIT test was developed with the continued support of the Garnett Passe and Rodney Williams Memorial Foundation and the National Health and Medical Research Council of Australia and we are grateful to those bodies. We thank Samanathi Goonetilleke for her comments.

VIDEOS ASSOCIATED WITH THIS CHAPTER

Video 16–1. How the horizontal head impulse test is carried out at RPA Hospital Sydney.

Video 16–2. How the standard LARP and RALP impulses are carried out at RPA Hospital Sydney.

REFERENCES

Aw, S. T., Haslwanter, T., Halmagyi, G. M., Curthoys, I. S., Yavor, R. A., & Todd, M. J. (1996). Three-dimensional vector analysis of the human vestibuloocular reflex in response to high-acceleration head rotations. I. Responses in normal subjects. *Journal of Neurophysiology, 76*(6), 4009–4020.

Bahill, A. T., & Troost, B. T. (1979). Types of saccadic eye-movements. *Neurology, 29*(8), 1150–1152.

Bartolomeo, M., Biboulet, R., Pierre, G., Mondain, M., Uziel, A., & Venail, F. (2014). Value of the video head impulse test in assessing vestibular deficits following vestibular neuritis. *European Archives of Oto-Rhino-Laryngology, 271*(4), 681–688.

Black, R. A., Halmagyi, G. M., Thurtell, M. J., Todd, M. J., & Curthoys, I. S. (2005). The active head-impulse test in unilateral peripheral vestibulopathy. *Archives of Neurology, 62*(2), 290–293. doi:10.1001/archneur.62.2.290

Blanks, R. H., Curthoys, I. S., & Markham, C. H. (1975). Planar Relationships of the semicircular canals in man. *Acta Oto-Laryngologica, 80*(3–4), 185–196.

Blödow, A., Blödow, J., Bloching, M. B., Helbig, R., & Walther, L. E. (2014, May 1). Horizontal VOR function shows frequency dynamics in vestibular schwannoma. *European Archives of Oto-Rhino-Laryngology.* doi:10.1007/s00405-014-3042-2 (Epub ahead of print).

Chim, D., Lasker, D. M., & Migliaccio, A. A. (2013). Visual contribution to the high-frequency human angular vestibulo-ocular reflex. *Experimental Brain Research, 230*(1), 127–135. doi:10.1007/s00221-013-3635-9

Choi, J. Y., Kim, J. S., Jung, J. M., Kwon, D. Y., Park, M. H., Kim, C., & Choi, J. (2014). Reversed corrective saccades during head impulse test in acute cerebellar dysfunction. *Cerebellum, 13*(2), 243–247. doi:10.1007/s12311-013-0535-2

Crane, B. T., & Demer, J. L. (1999). Latency of voluntary cancellation of the human vestibule-ocular reflex during transient yaw rotation. *Experimental Brain Research, 127*(1), 67–74. doi:10.1007/s002210050774

Crane, B. T., & Demer, J. L. (1998). Human horizontal vestibulo-ocular reflex initiation: Effects of acceleration, target distance, and unilateral deafferentation. *Journal of Neurophysiology, 80*(3), 1151–1166.

Curthoys, I. S. (2002). Generation of the quick phase of horizontal vestibular nystagmus. *Experimental Brain Research, 143*(4), 397–405. doi:10.1007/s00221-002-1022-z

Curthoys, I. S. (2012). The interpretation of clinical tests of peripheral vestibular function. *Laryngoscope, 122*(6), 1342–1352. doi:10.1002/lary.23258

Curthoys, I. S., Blanks, R. H., & Markham, C. H. (1977a). Semicircular canal functional anatomy in cat, guinea pig and man. *Acta Oto-Laryngologica, 83*(3–4), 258–265.

Curthoys, I. S., Blanks, R. H., & Markham, C. H. (1977b). Semicircular canal radii of curvature (R) in cat, guinea pig and man. *Journal of Morphology, 151*(1), 1–15. doi:10.1002/jmor.1051510102

Curthoys, I. S., & Halmagyi, G. M. (1995). Vestibular compensation: A review of the oculomotor, neural, and clinical consequences of unilateral vestibular loss. *Journal of Vestibular Research, 5*(2), 67–107. doi:095742719400026X [pii]

Curthoys, I. S., Markham, C. H., & Curthoys, E. J. (1977). Semicircular duct and ampulla dimensions in cat, guinea pig and man. *Journal of Morphology, 151*(1), 17–34. doi:10.1002/jmor.1051510103

Curthoys, I. S., & Oman, C. M. (1987). Dimensions of the horizontal semicircular duct, ampulla and utricle in the human. *Acta Oto-Laryngologica, 103*(5–6), 254–261. doi:10.3109/00016488709107791

Delori, F. C., Webb, R. H., & Sliney, D. H. (2007). Maximum permissible exposures for ocular safety (ANSI 2000), with emphasis on ophthalmic devices. *Journal of the Optical Society of America A-Optics Image Science and Vision, 24*(5), 1250–1265. doi:10.1364/josaa.24.001250

Gilchrist, D. P., Curthoys, I. S., Cartwright, A. D., Burgess, A. M., Topple, A. N., & Halmagyi, M. (1998). High acceleration impulsive rotations reveal severe long-term deficits of the horizontal vestibulo-ocular reflex in the guinea pig. *Experimental Brain Research, 123*(3), 242–254. doi:10.1007/s002210050566

Goldberg, J. M. (2012). *The vestibular system: A sixth sense.* New York, NY: Oxford University Press.

Gonshor, A., & Jones, G. M. (1976). Short-term adaptive-changes in human vestibulo-ocular reflex arc. *Journal of Physiology-London, 256*(2), 361–379.

Grossman, G. E., Leigh, R. J., Abel, L. A., Lanska, D. J., & Thurston, S. E. (1988). Frequency and velocity of rotational head perturbations during locomotion. *Experimental Brain Research, 70*(3), 470–476.

Habbema, J. D. F., Eijkemans, R., Krijnen, P., & Knotterus, J. A. (2008). Analysis of data on the accuracy of diagnostic tests. In J. A. Knotterus & F. Buntinx (Eds.), *The evidence base of clinical diagnosis* (2nd ed., pp. 118–145). Oxford, UK: Blackwell.

Halmagyi, G. M., & Curthoys, I. S. (1987). Human compensatory slow eye movements in the absence of vestibular function. In M. D. Graham & J. L. Kemink (Eds.), *The vestibular system: Neurophysiologic and clinical research* (pp. 471–478). New York, NY: Raven Press.

Halmagyi, G. M., & Curthoys, I. S. (1988). A clinical sign of canal paresis. *Archives of Neurology, 45*(7), 737–739.

Halmagyi, G. M., Curthoys, I. S., Cremer, P. D., Henderson, C. J., Todd, M. J., Staples, M. J., & D'Cruz, D. M. (1990). The human horizontal vestibulo-ocular reflex in response to high-acceleration stimulation before and after unilateral vestibular neurectomy. *Experimental Brain Research, 81*(3), 479–490.

Halmagyi, G. M., Fattore, C. M., Curthoys, I. S., & Wade, S. (1994). Gentamicin vestibulotoxicity. *Otolaryngology-Head and Neck Surgery, 111*(5), 571–574. doi:S0194599894001130 [pii]

Halmagyi, G. M., Weber, K. P., & Curthoys, I. S. (2010). Vestibular function after acute vestibular neuritis. *Restorative Neurology and Neuroscience, 28*(1), 37–46. doi:0536546LV2P752LW [pii]10.3233/RNN-2010-0533

Haslwanter, T. (1995). Mathematics of 3-dimensional eye rotations. *Vision Research, 35*(12), 1727–1739. doi:10.1016/0042-6989(94)00257-m

Heuberger, M., Saglam, M., Todd, N. S., Jahn, K., Schneider, E., & Lehnen, N. (2014). Covert anti-compensatory quick eye movements during head impulses. *PLoS One, 9*(4), e93086. doi:10.1371/journal.pone.0093086

Jones, G. M. (1985). Adaptive modulation of VOR parameters by vision. *Reviews of Oculomotor Research, 1*, 21–50.

Leigh, R. J., & Zee, D. S. (2006). *The neurology of eye movements.* Philadelphia, PA: F. A. Davis.

MacDougall, H. G., & Curthoys, I. S. (2012) Plasticity during vestibular compensation: The role of saccades. *Frontiers in Neurology, 3*, article 21, doi:10.3389/fneur.2012.00021

MacDougall, H. G., McGarvie, L. A., Halmagyi, G. M., Curthoys, I. S., & Weber, K. P. (2013a). Application of the video head impulse test to detect vertical semicircular canal dysfunction. *Otology and Neurotology.* doi:10.1097/MAO.0b013e31828d676d

MacDougall, H. G., McGarvie, L. A., Halmagyi, G. M., Curthoys, I. S., & Weber, K. P. (2013b). The video Head Impulse Test (vHIT) detects vertical semicircular canal dysfunction. *PLoS One, 8*(4), e61488. doi:10.1371/journal.pone.0061488

MacDougall, H. G., Weber, K. P., McGarvie, L. A., Halmagyi, G. M., & Curthoys, I. S. (2009). The video head impulse test. Diagnostic accuracy in peripheral vestibulopathy. *Neurology, 73*(14), 1134–1141. doi:10.1212/WNL.0b013e3181bacf85

Manzari, L., Burgess, A. M., MacDougall, H. G., Bradshaw, A. P., & Curthoys, I. S. (2011). Rapid fluctuations in dynamic semicircular canal function in early Meniere's disease. *European Archives of Oto-Rhino-Laryngology, 268*(4), 637–639. doi:10.1007/s00405-010-1442-5

Manzari, L., Burgess, A. M., Macdougall, H. G., & Curthoys, I. S. (2012). Objective measures of vestibular function during an acute vertigo attack in a very young child. *European Archives of Oto-Rhino-Laryngology, 269*(12), 2589–2592. doi:10.1007/s00405-012-2045-0

Markham, C. H., Yagi, T., & Curthoys, I. S. (1977). The contribution of the contralateral labyrinth to second order vestibular neuronal activity in the cat. *Brain Research, 138*(1), 99–109. doi:0006-8993(77)90786-7 [pii]

Migliaccio, A. A., & Cremer, P. D. (2011). The 2D modified head impulse test: A 2D technique for measuring function in all six semi-circular canals. *Journal of Vestibular Research-Equilibrium and Orientation, 21*(4), 227–234. doi:10.3233/ves-2011-0421

Moore, S. T., Haslwanter, T., Curthoys, I. S., & Smith, S. T. (1996). A geometric basis for measurement of three-dimensional eye position using image processing. *Vision Research, 36*(3), 445–459. doi:0042-6989(95)00130-1 [pii]

Newman-Toker, D. E., Kattah, J. C., Alvernia, J. E., & Wang, D. Z. (2008). Normal head impulse test differentiates acute cerebellar strokes from vestibular neuritis. *Neurology, 70*(24), 2378–2385. doi:10.1212/01.wnl.0000314685.01433.0d

Newman-Toker, D. E., Kerber, K. A., Hsieh, Y. H., Pula, J. H., Omron, R., Tehrani, A. S. S., . . . Kattah, J. C. (2013). HINTS outperforms ABCD2 to screen for stroke in acute vestibular syndrome. *Annals of Neurology, 74*, S9–S9.

Newman-Toker, D. E., Tehrani, A. S. S., Mantokoudis, G., Pula, J. H., Guede, C. I., Kerber, K. A., . . . Kattah, J. C. (2013). Quantitative video-oculography to help diagnose stroke in acute vertigo and dizziness. Toward an ECG for the eyes. *Stroke, 44*(4), 1158–1161. doi:10.1161/strokeaha.111.000033

Precht, W., Shimazu, H., & Markham, C. H. (1966). A mechanism of central compensation of vestibular function following hemilabyrinthectomy. *Journal of Neurophysiology, 29*(6), 996–1010.

Shaikh, A. G., Palla, A., Marti, S., Olasagasti, I., Optican, L. M., Zee, D. S., & Straumann, D. (2013). Role of cerebellum in motion perception and vestibulo-ocular reflex-similarities and disparities. *Cerebellum, 12*(1), 97–107. doi:10.1007/s12311-012-0401-7

Sliney, D., Aron-Rosa, D., DeLori, F., Fankhauser, F., Landry, R., Mainster, M., . . . Wolffe, M. (2005). Adjustment of guidelines for exposure of the eye to optical radiation from ocular instruments: Statement from a task group of the International Commission on Non-Ionizing Radiation Protection (ICNIRP). *Applied Optics, 44*(11), 2162–2176. doi:10.1364/ao.44.002162

Tian, J., Crane, B. T., & Demer, J. L. (2000). Vestibular catch-up saccades in labyrinthine deficiency. *Experimental Brain Research, 131*(10803413), 448–457.

Viirre, E., Tweed, D., Milner, K., & Vilis, T. (1986). A reexamination of the gain of the vestibuloocular reflex. *Journal of Neurophysiology, 56*(2), 439–450.

Weber, K. P., Aw, S. T., Todd, M. J., McGarvie, L. A., Curthoys, I. S., & Halmagyi, G. M. (2008). Head impulse test in unilateral vestibular loss: Vestibulo-ocular reflex and catch-up saccades. *Neurology, 70*(6), 454–463. doi:70/6/454 [pii] 10.1212/01.wnl.0000299117.48935.2e

Weber, K. P., Aw, S. T., Todd, M. J., McGarvie, L. A., Curthoys, I. S., & Halmagyi, G. M. (2009). Horizontal head impulse test detects gentamicin vestibulotoxicity. *Neurology, 72*(16), 1417–1424. doi:72/16/1417 [pii] 10.1212/WNL.0b013e3181a18652

Weber, K. P., Aw, S. T., Todd, M. J., McGarvie, L. A., Pratap, S., Curthoys, I. S., & Halmagyi, G. M. (2008). Inter-ocular differences of the horizontal vestibulo-ocular reflex during impulsive testing. *Progress in Brain Research, 171*, 195–198. doi:S0079-6123(08)00626-2 [pii] 10.1016/S0079-6123(08)00626-2

Weber, K. P., MacDougall, H. G., Halmagyi, G. M., & Curthoys, I. S. (2009). Impulsive testing of semicircular-canal function using video-oculography. *Annals of the New York Academy of Sciences, 1164*, 486–491. doi:NYAS03730 [pii]; 10.1111/j.1749-6632.2008.03730.x

Zar, J. H. (2010). *Biostatistical analysis* (5th ed.). Englewood Cliffs, NJ: Prentice Hall.

APPENDIX 16–A

18 FAQs

1. Why is the head impulse test a specific test of semicircular canal function?

2. Do healthy people have overt and covert saccades during head impulse testing?

3. How does vHIT measure eye movement?

4. What is an ideal head impulse?

5. Why is rebound during the head turn to be avoided?

6. What are five factors that should be avoided during head impulse testing?

7. Why are there some outlying data points on the VOR graph?

8. What can you do if the eye velocity record image is very noisy?

9. Where should the operator's hands be on the patient's head?

10. What is a normal VOR gain?

11. Do normal healthy subjects have overt and covert saccades?

12. In a healthy subject does the VOR gain vary from day to day?

13. What does a VOR gain greater than 1.0 mean?

14. In the vHIT test what is the indicator of reduced left peripheral vestibular function?

15. Why are drooping eyelids a problem?

16. Are the lasers in the ICS impulse system safe?

17. Why is a poor image of the eye a problem?

18. Once the test is over what is the very first thing to do?

ANSWERS TO 18 FAQS

1. Why is the head impulse test a specific test of semicircular canal function?

Because the evidence shows that the earliest part of the eye movement response to the head impulses is too early for other nonvestibular eye movement control mechanisms to be able to generate the slow phase eye velocity to correct for the head rotation (Halmagyi & Curthoys, 1987, 1988). In a rare patient with bilateral surgical vestibular loss, the influence of these other oculomotor control mechanisms only started to appear at about 80 ms after the onset of head rotation. That result has been confirmed in other patients with bilateral vestibular loss.

2. Do healthy people have overt and covert saccades during head impulse testing?

Yes, but they are usually very small and infrequent. The important thing is not the occurrence of an odd saccade, but whether the saccades systematically occur in combination with the reduced eye velocity during the head impulse.

3. How does vHIT measure eye movement?

By finding the center of the pupil and tracking the position of the pupil center at high speed during the head turn.

4. What is an ideal head impulse?

This is a small passive, unpredictable, abrupt turn and abrupt stop, with minimal overshoot.

5. Why is rebound during the head turn to be avoided?

Think about a head turn with total rebound —from nose straight ahead (0 deg), to nose 20-deg right and then rebounding back to nose straight ahead (0 deg)—in a patient with no vestibular function at all. Since the patient has no VOR, during the head turn their eyes moves with head, and come back with head, so that the end of the impulse the patient will be looking directly at the target just as they were at the beginning, so they do not need to make any corrective saccade at all even though they have absent vestibular function. In contrast with a turn and dead stop at the 20-deg nose right position, the eyes of the bilateral loss patient are taken many degrees off target during the head turn and do not come back, and so the patient needs to make a big corrective saccade at the end of the head turn to get back to target.

6. *What are five factors that should be avoided during head impulse testing?*
   1. Glasses slip
   2. Poor image of the pupil
   3. Touching the glasses strap
   4. Low peak velocity head rotations
   5. Overshoot and rebound

7. *Why are there some outlying data points on the VOR graph?*

This occurred because most likely because there were partial blinks or the pupil was partially obscured, or there was a reflection into the pupil so the pupil center was not correctly determined, or there was some glasses slip. These outliers should not be given undue weight because the other repeated trials show the real result and usually the outliers are obvious. If there is large scatter of all the data points, then the image of the pupil has probably not been obtained properly. Large scatter of VOR gain is usually due to a very noisy eye velocity record, possibly because the image of the pupil is poor or the threshold has not been set properly.

8. *What can you do if the eye velocity record image is very noisy?*

Check the illumination and the thresholding. If necessary re-fit the glasses.

9. *Where should the operator's hands be on the patient's head?*

They should be high up toward the top of the head and well away from the straps.

10. *What is a normal VOR gain?*

Theoretically it is 1.0 but it varies from trial to trial, and day to day, and even on fixation distance and whether the subject usually wears glasses. Normal VOR gain for the horizontal canals really is a range around 1.0. Gains from about 0.79 to 1.20 are considered to be in the normal range. (See Table 16–1 for the range of normal gains for all canals.)

11. *Do normal healthy subjects have overt and covert saccades?*

They are rare and infrequent.

12. *In a healthy subject does the VOR gain vary from day to day?*

The day to day variation in VOR gain is very small.

13. *What does a VOR gain greater than 1.0 mean?*

Many years of research have shown that VOR gain is modifiable—it changes in response to imposed demands, for example, wearing spectacles. Some healthy subjects have VOR gains greater than 1.0 due to their spectacle prescription. Also the VOR gain increases beyond 1.0 when the fixation distance is close. Ménière's patients are reported to show enhanced VOR gain around the time of the attack (Manzari, Burgess, MacDougall, Bradshaw, & Curthoys, 2011). Cerebellar disease can also cause increased VOR gain (Shaikh et al., 2013).

14. *In the vHIT test what is the indicator of reduced left peripheral vestibular function?*

For head turns to the left, the eye velocity is too slow. Therefore, it does not match head velocity, and there is a reduced VOR gain for leftward head turns, accompanied by corrective saccades (overt and/or covert).

15. *Why are drooping eyelids a problem?*

They obscure part of the pupil so the program for finding the center of the pupil will not yield a correct indication of eye position. The solution is a "lid lift" or a lid "tuck."

16. *Are the lasers in the ICS impulse system safe?*

Yes.

17. *Why is a poor image of the eye a problem?*

It is a problem because the analysis program calculates the geometric center of all the white area in the region of interest, and if there are shadows in that region then they will cause erroneous measures of the pupil center. The contrast of the image is inverted so all black regions become white (the pupil, but also any shadows in that region of interest), and the program calculates the center of all the largest white objects not touching the edge of the region of interest. Shadows generate false values.

18. *Once the test is over what is the very first thing to do?*

Inspect the raw data records—the eye and head traces for all the impulses. If these are not acceptable then the test should be repeated. It is wrong to use the numerical data from a test where the raw data are unacceptable. Unacceptable in what way? Too noisy, too variable.

APPENDIX 16–B

The Physiological Basis for the Head Impulse Test

Much of the following can be found interactively in the free app for iPhone 4 and later called aVOR. The work of Goldberg (2012) is the most recent detailed source of physiological information about canal function.

How can the vestibular system achieve the speed and precision of the VOR? The sensitivity

and the precision of the VOR are the outcomes of neural interaction between the signals from the two sets of semicircular canals on each side of the head. One way of thinking about this interaction is as follows: normally, with the head still, the neural output from the vestibular receptors and afferents on the two sides causes balanced (i.e., approximately equal) resting neural activity in the cells in the two vestibular nuclei in the brainstem (Figure 16–B–1). A head turn upsets that balance—canal neurons on the side toward the head turn are activated and canal neurons on the other side are inhibited. That imbalanced neural activity triggers the response—the corrective eye movement—and also sensations of turning and postural responses to ensure you do not fall.

ACCELERATION VERSUS VELOCITY

The mechanics of the semicircular canal convert the angular acceleration of the head into an angular velocity signal. Physiological recordings from primary semicircular canal afferents have shown that the mechanics of the semicircular canal-cupula system have effectively integrated the head acceleration stimulus to produce a neural signal corresponding to head velocity (Goldberg, 2012).

The passive head turn causes fluid flow in the membranous duct of the semicircular canal, deflecting the receptor hair cells on the crista in the ampulla in an excitatory direction, so that the primary afferent neurons are activated (see Figure 16–B–1) Simultaneously the same head turn causes fluid flow in the membranous duct of the semicircular canal on the opposite side of the head. However, because

of the orientation of the receptor hair cells in that opposite canal, this head turn causes these contralateral semicircular canal receptors to be bent in an inhibitory direction, so the afferent neurons on this opposite side of the head are inhibited. So the one head turn causes complementary neural events in the two vestibular labyrinths—excitation on one side and inhibition on the other (Figure 16–B–2). This reduction in their neural firing of these cells acts indirectly to reduce the inhibition exerted on central vestibular neurons. Reduced inhibition (called "disinhibition") is effectively excitatory. So in healthy subjects there are two sources of vestibular drive to the eye muscles—direct excitation and indirect excitation (disinhibition). These sum and drive the eyes to compensate for the head rotation with great speed and precision.

The contribution from the contralateral labyrinth by indirect activation from disinhibition is only effective over a small range of stimulus values since the neurons in the vestibular nuclei are relatively quickly inhibited to silence during a high acceleration head rotation. However, during a low acceleration head turn to the affected side in a patient with a unilateral loss, this source of indirect excitation from the remaining healthy ear can provide sufficient excitation to generate a compensatory eye movement response for ipsilesional head turns that looks normal. That is why low accelerations are to be avoided during clinical testing. This small indirect excitation component is generated during the low velocity part of the head impulse—at higher velocities this input probably does not contribute and that is why high-velocity head impulses are necessary to test canal function.

A big apparent advantage of calorics is that it specifically tests each ear separately. As the above shows vHIT also assesses each ear separately if the peak head velocity is large enough (>~150 deg/s) because the angular accelerations during high peak velocity head impulse stimulus are so large they effectively limit the contribution from the canals on the opposite side, so that essentially only one labyrinth drives the eye movement response. The result is

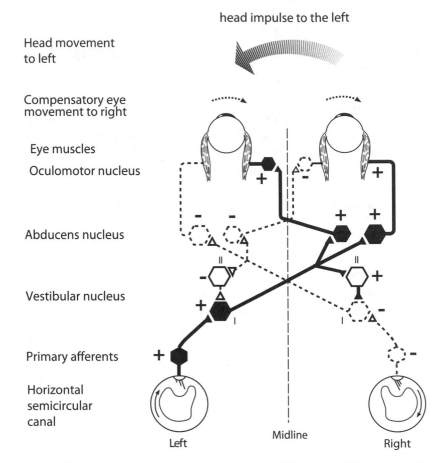

head impulse to the left

Head movement
to left

Compensatory eye
movement to right

Eye muscles
Oculomotor nucleus

Abducens nucleus

Vestibular nucleus

Primary afferents

Horizontal
semicircular
canal

Left   Midline   Right

Figure 16-B-1. Some of the neural mechanisms by which a head turn generates a compensatory eye movement response. The neural connections in the brainstem which have been extensively documented by physiological studies (references in Curthoys, 2002). Excitatory neurons are shown as filled hexagons; inhibitory neurons as open hexagons. Neurons that are activated (+) are shown as thick darker traces, neurons with reduced firing (–) are shown as light, dashed traces. The sequence is as follows: during a leftward head turn the receptors in the left horizontal canal are bent in an excitatory direction and so the primary afferent neurons from the left semicircular canal are activated. Simultaneously the receptors in the right horizontal canal are bent in an inhibitory direction so the primary afferent neurons from the right semicircular canal have reduced firing (*dashed lines*). The excitatory input from the left canal projects to the left vestibular nucleus and activates Type I neurons that are excitatory neurons which project to and excite neurons in the right abducens nucleus which project to the lateral rectus eye muscle and so act to generate the compensatory eye movement response to the right. This response of the Type I neurons in the vestibular nuclei is further increased because inhibition arising indirectly from the right horizontal canal via the Type II inhibitory neurons is reduced. This reduced inhibition is called disinhibition and it is functionally excitatory. It is a secondary source of an excitatory drive arising from the opposite labyrinth. So in healthy subjects there are two sources of vestibular drive to the eye muscles—direct excitation and indirect excitation (disinhibition). These sum and drive the eyes to compensate for the head rotation with great speed and precision. After a unilateral vestibular loss an ipsilesional head turn no longer causes the direct excitation but still causes the indirect excitation (the disinhibition) from the remaining healthy ear. For this reason the VOR for ipsilesional head turns is not zero. Transmission through the vestibular nucleus can be inhibited by cerebellar neurons, resulting in VOR suppression. It is stressed that this is a very basic figure showing just one of the many neural circuits controlling vestibulo-ocular responses.

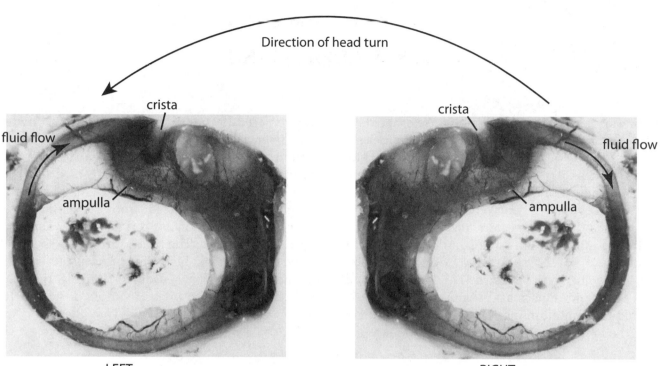

Figure 16–B–2. The semicircular canals are symmetrical on the two sides of the head (see Figure 16–1) so a horizontal head turn causes opposite effects in the semicircular canals on the two sides of the head. The figure shows a view directly downward onto enlarged and translated human horizontal canals (Curthoys & Oman, 1987). For the purposes of this illustration the one canal has been reflected around the median plane to show the symmetrical arrangement of the canals. The membranous semicircular duct (within the bony semicircular canal) has a tube diameter of about 0.3 mm and the diameter of the canal circle is about 6 mm (Curthoys, Blanks, & Markham, 1977b; Curthoys, Markham, & Curthoys, 1977). Within the swelling in the duct (the ampulla), there is a saddle-like crista (here viewed edge-on) which is covered by around 7,500 receptor hair cells, each projecting into a jelly-like structure (the cupula) that seals the membranous duct (the hair cells and the cupula are not shown in this figure). The one head rotation to the left in this example causes fluid flow in an excitatory direction (arrow in the duct) in the left semicircular canal. This deflects the cupula in the left canal and so all 7,500 receptors on the crista in the left canal are bent in an excitatory direction resulting in an increase of neural activity of all of the primary semicircular canal afferents in the left vestibular nerve. Simultaneously that leftward head turn causes endolymph flow in an inhibitory direction in the right semicircular canal (*arrow in the duct*), thus causing all the receptors on the right crista to be bent in an inhibitory direction and so the neural activity of all primary semicircular canal afferents on the right is reduced. The same "push-pull" principle for LLRL applies to accelerations in the planes of the pairs of vertical canals—LARP and RALP. Reproduced with permission of Informa Healthcare from I. S. Curthoys and C. M. Oman (1987). *Acta Oto-Laryngologica, 103*(3–4), 254–261, copyright © 1987, Informa Healthcare.

that high acceleration head turns to the left test the left horizontal semicircular canal. In patients with unilateral vestibular loss, the VOR gain for head turns to the healthy side is frequently systematically smaller than 1.0—it is lacking the (small) functionally excitatory drive from the affected side.

The detailed anatomical and physiological evidence underpinning this account is given in Curthoys and Halmagyi (1995) and Curthoys (2002). The relative importance of the intercommunication between the bilateral labyrinth inputs has been known since the physiological work of Precht, Shimazu, and Markham (1966) and Markham, Yagi, and Curthoys (1977). The most recent summary of vestibular physiology is by Goldberg (2012).

APPENDIX 16–C

A Brief History of vHIT

vHIT has been made possible because of the development of very fast, lightweight video glasses by Hamish MacDougall. It has been a long development process. The Vestibular Research Laboratory has been developing and validating video measures of human eye movements since 1990, and the vHIT glasses are the most recent realization of this work. It has required progressive solution of problems, and Figure 16–C–1 shows the development since 2004. The changes are instructive. Initially a modified Seal swimming mask was used, incorporating a unique aluminium insert to support the cameras. But the swimming mask slipped on the face so it was replaced by tightly fitting sunglasses frames. The cameras became smaller and were progressively mounted closer to the center of the head to minimize the inertia that generates glasses slip and artifactual data. Some recent ersatz vHIT systems have large heavy cameras mounted far from the center of the head rotation and so cause serious glasses slip during a head impulse. The headband beside the head in the early systems held the head velocity sensor, but more recently that sensor has been incorporated into the glasses. The present simple design is the outcome of a great amount of development.

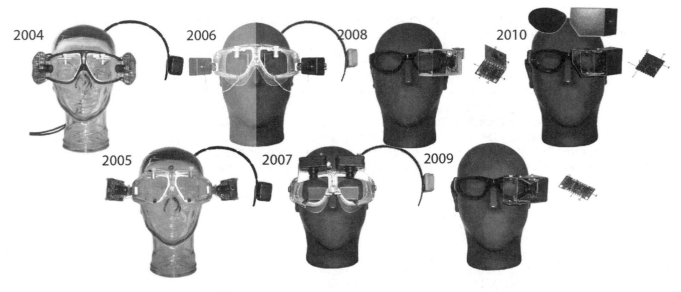

Figure 16-C-1. The evolution of vHIT.

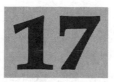

Practical Biomechanics and Physiology of Balance

Lewis M. Nashner

INTRODUCTION

Balance is a complex process involving the coordinated activities of multiple sensory, motor, and biomechanical components. The position of the body in relation to gravity and the surrounds is sensed by combining visual, vestibular, and somatosensory inputs. Balance movements involve motions of the ankle, knee, and hip joints, which are controlled by the coordinated actions of ankle, thigh, and lower trunk muscles. The aim of this chapter is to describe the principal biomechanical, sensory, and motor components of balance, and their interactions within a systematic model of balance control. Chapter 18 describes a method for assessing the sensory and motor components of balance based on this model.

BIOMECHANICS OF BALANCE

Definition of Balance

To balance with the feet in place, the position of the body's center of gravity (COG) must be maintained vertically over the base of support (Gurfinkel & Osevets, 1972; Koozekanni, Stockwell, McGhee, & Firoozmand, 1980; Nashner, 1981). When this condi-

tion is met, a person can both resist the destabilizing influence of gravity and actively move the COG. When a person moves slowly, the in-place limits of stability are exceeded whenever the COG position has been displaced beyond the perimeter of the base of support. At this point a rapid step or stumble to reestablish the base of support beneath the COG, or additional external support, is required to prevent a fall. When a person is moving more rapidly, the definition of balance is more complex, because momentum of the body motion must also be taken into consideration. For example, if the COG is displaced only slightly forward but moving forward rapidly, the person has lost balance because the forward momentum is sufficient to carry the COG beyond the forward stability limit.

The state of a person's balance is most simply described in terms of angular displacement of the COG from the gravitational vertical. Center of gravity sway is then defined as the angle formed by the intersection of a first line from the center of the base of support through the COG and a second line extending vertically from the center of support as shown in Figure 17–1. This definition of balance pertains, whether the person moves about the ankles, the hips, or about both joints, and also takes height into account (Nashner & McCollum, 1985). Thus, a given sway angle indicates a comparable state of balance for all body movement patterns and heights.

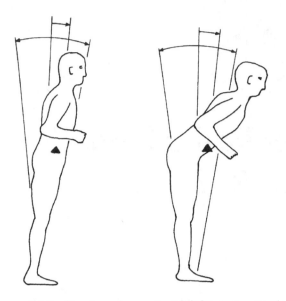

Figure 17-1. Center of gravity (COG) sway angle in relation to the "limits of stability" cone. The figure on the left is moving about the ankles; the figure on the right is moving about the hips. The COG sway angles of the two figures are approximately the same, although the joint motions are much larger using the hip strategy. Filled diamonds show the body COG positions. From Jacobson, *Handbook of balance function testing*, 1E. © 1998 Delmar Learning, a part of Cengage Learning, Inc. Reproduced by permission. http://www.cengage.com/permissions

This definition of balance is further discussed in the section on limits of stability. More recent studies have expanded the definition of balance to incorporate multiple joints of the body (Maurer & Peterka, 2005).

Base of Support

The base of support for standing on a flat, firm surface is defined as the area contained within the perimeter of contact between the surface and the two feet. The base of support area is nearly square when the feet are placed comfortably apart while the person is quietly standing. Similarly, a diagonal stance produces a parallelogram-shaped base of support extending forward on one side and backward on the other while a tandem stance position creates a long but very narrow base of support.

When the support surface area is smaller than the feet, or when surface irregularities limit the contact between the feet and the surface, the base of support is reduced. Standing sideways on a narrow beam, for example, provides a base with a normal width but very short length. Thus, the person's limits of stability are effectively reduced in the anterior-posterior (AP) but not the lateral dimensions.

Limits of Stability

The limits of stability (LOS) is a two-dimensional quantity defining the maximum possible COG sway angle as a function of sway direction from the center position (Koozekanni et al., 1980; McCollum & Leen (1989). The LOS depends on the placement of the feet and characteristics of the base of support. In normal adults standing on a flat, firm surface with feet spaced comfortably apart, the LOS perimeter can best be described as an ellipse as shown in Figures 17–1. The AP dimension of this ellipse is approximately 12.5° from the backward-most to the forward-most points on the perimeter (Nashner & McCollum, 1985). While height of the COG above the surface and foot length affect the AP limits of stability, these two features co-vary, resulting in approximately the same AP limits for people of various heights (Duncan, Weiner, Chandler, & Studenski, 1990).

The lateral LOS depends on the person's height relative to the spacing between the feet. When the feet of a person 70-inches tall are placed 4-inches apart, for example, the lateral dimension of the LOS ellipse is approximately 16° from the left to the right-most points on the perimeter. For taller individuals, a wider spacing between the feet is required to produce a 16° ellipse, whereas shorter people can place their feet closer together.

The biomechanical properties that determine the LOS are similar while standing in place, walking, and sitting without trunk support, as shown in Figure 17–2. During in-place standing the COG moves randomly within an LOS perimeter determined by the base of support and the placement of the feet. During walking, the COG progresses forward through the LOS in a smooth, rhythmic movement (Nashner, 1986; Nashner & Forssberg, 1986). At heel strike, a LOS is established with the COG positioned slightly behind the posterior perimeter but with sufficient forward momentum to carry it to the perimeter. As the step progresses, the COG moves

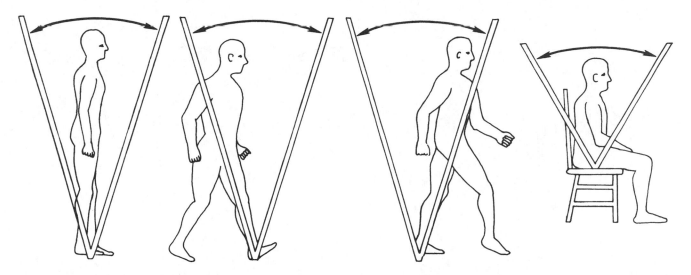

Figure 17-2. Limits of stability boundaries during standing, walking and sitting. From Jacobson, *Handbook of balance function testing*, 1E. © 1998 Delmar Learning, a part of Cengage Learning, Inc. Reproduced by permission. http://www.cengage.com/permissions

forward within the LOS. As the COG approaches and then exceeds the anterior perimeter of the LOS, the next step establishes a new LOS and the rhythmic process is repeated. When sitting without trunk support, the height of the COG above the support surface is considerably less and the base area is larger. Therefore, the LOS perimeter is larger in terms of COG sway angles when one is seated than in quiet standing.

Limits of Sway

It is impossible to maintain the COG motionless, because in-place standing is an inherently unstable task requiring periodic corrections to overcome the destabilizing influence of gravity (Begbie, 1967; Dichgans & Diener, 1986; Diener, Dichgans, Bacher, & Gompf, 1984; Scott & Dzendolet, 1972). Thus, a person attempting to maintain balance spontaneously sways back and forth and from side to side. The limits of sway is a two-dimensional quantity defining the maximum spontaneous COG sway angle as a function of the sway direction, as shown in Figure 17-3. A person's limits of spontaneous sway vary with the sensory conditions and the configuration of the base of support. But, unless the person loses balance, the limit of sway is always well within the LOS.

Center of Gravity Alignment

A point at the center of the area contained within the limits of sway perimeter defines the COG alignment, as shown in Figure 17-3. This definition of COG alignment is based on the assumption that a person is attempting to maintain a COG position which is at the center of the limits of sway perimeter. When a normal person is asked to stand erect, COG alignment is placed accurately above the center of the base of support.

Understanding the concepts of limits of sway and COG alignment is important, because each affects a person's balance differently. When the COG is aligned over the center of the base of support, the limits of sway can be as large as the LOS before balance is lost. A person whose COG alignment is offset forward, backward, or to one side of the center of support is not as stable as a person whose COG alignment is centered, even when the limits of sway are similar in the two. The person with the offset COG alignment is less stable, because smaller sway angles in the direction of the offset will move the COG beyond the LOS perimeter.

Limits of Stability and Sway Frequency

In addition to the base of support, the actual LOS is also influenced by COG sway velocity, which is

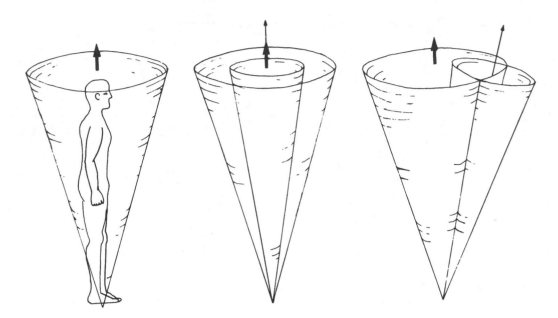

Figure 17–3. Relations between the LOS, the sway envelope, and the COG alignment. The middle figure shows the COG alignment within the LOS. The right figure shows the COG aligned forward relative to the center. From Jacobson, *Handbook of balance function testing*, 1E. © 1998 Delmar Learning, a part of Cengage Learning, Inc. Reproduced by permission. http://www.cengage.com/permissions

directly related to sway frequency (Nashner, Shupert, Horak, & Black, 1989). When the frequency of COG sway is low, gravity is the only significant destabilizing force that must be overcome, and the COG can be moved within the full range of the LOS. For the average adult, COG movements within the full range of the LOS are possible when a sway oscillation cycle (front to back or side to side and then back again) takes 2 to 3 s or longer. By contrast, when sway oscillation cycles take less than 1 s, momentum is an additional destabilizing force and the LOS perimeter can be reduced to as little as 3°.

Understanding the impact of COG sway frequency is important in assessing a person's balance. As higher frequencies reduce the effective LOS, a person using fast sway movements is closer to exceeding the LOS than an individual swaying slowly though a comparable arc. This principle is further explained by a theoretical multidimensional model of postural sway which demonstrates that 92% of the variance in sway is explained by two variables, one related to sway amplitude and the other to sway velocity (Maurer & Peterka, 2005; Pavol, 2005).

SENSING THE POSITION OF BALANCE

Sensory and Motor Components of Balance

To execute the constant corrections required to resist the destabilizing effect of gravity and the perturbing effects of purposeful motor actions while standing and walking, the balance system must determine the position of the COG relative to gravity and the base of support and then execute coordinated movements to correct any COG deviations. Although the neural processes for determining COG position and moving the COG are highly integrated, the two are separated here for purposes of developing a systematic model of balance control. From a clinical perspective, separating the sensory and motor processes of balance means that a patient may have impaired balance for one or a combination of two reasons: (1) the position of the COG relative to the base of support is not accurately sensed, and (2) the automatic movements required to bring the COG to a balanced position are not timely or effectively coordinated.

Visual, Vestibular, and Somatosensory Inputs

Sensing the position of the COG relative to gravity and the base of support requires a combination of visual, vestibular, and somatosensory (tactile, deep pressure, joint receptor, and muscle proprioceptor) inputs. Utilization of the three balance senses is reviewed in Table 17–1. Three senses are required because no single sense directly measures COG position. Somatosensory inputs provide information on the orientation of the body parts relative to one another and to the support surface. The vestibular system does not provide orientation information in relation to external objects. Rather, it measures gravitational, linear, and angular accelerations of the head in relation to inertial space. Vision measures the orientation of the eyes and head in relation to surrounding objects.

Neither is there a single combination of the three senses providing accurate COG information under all conditions. This is because one or more of the senses may provide information that is misleading or inaccurate for purposes of balance control. For example, when a person stands next to a large bus that suddenly begins to move forward, momentary disorientation or unsteadiness may result. A fraction of a second is required for the brain to determine whether the resulting visual stimulus indicates backward sway of the person or forward movement of the bus. If a downwardly tilted support surface is encountered, the brain must determine whether the surface is tilted downward or the surface is level and the body is tilted back. During sensory conflict situations, the brain must quickly select the sensory inputs providing accurate orientation information

and ignore the misleading ones. The process of selecting and combining appropriate sensory information is called sensory organization.

Somatosensory Input

Somatosensory input derived from the contact forces and motions between the feet and the support surface is the dominant sensory input to balance under normal (fixed) support surface conditions (Aggashyan, Gurfinkel, Mamsakhlisov, & Elner, 1973; Diener & Dichgans, 1988; Diener, Dichgans, & Guschlbauer, 1986; Dietz, Horstmann, & Berger, 1989; Gurfinkel, Lipshits, et al., 1976) . When a person stands on a firm, level surface, the extent of COG sway is very small relative to the LOS. Closing the eyes to eliminate vision causes little if any functionally significant increase in COG sway. Even a well-compensated patient with a bilateral vestibular loss sways well within the LOS with the eyes closed (Black & Nashner, 1984, 1985; Nashner, Black, & Wall, 1982, Shupert, Black, & Horak, 1988). In contrast, ischemic disruption of somatosensory input from the ankle muscles increases COG sway significantly when the eyes are closed (Diener, Dichgans, Guschlbauer, & Mau 1984; Horak, Nashner, & Diener, 1990).

Vestibular Input

When functionally useful somatosensory and visual inputs are available, vestibular inputs play a minor role in controlling COG position (Bles, deJong, & deWit, 1984; Nashner, Black, & Wall, 1982; Shupert, Black, Horak, et al. 1988). This is because the somatosensory and visual inputs are more sensitive to body

Table 17–1. Utilization of the Senses for Balance

Sense	Reference	Conditions Favoring Use	Conditions Disrupting Use
Somatosensory	Support surface	Fixed support surface	Irregular or moving support
Visual	Surrounding objects	Fixed visible surrounds and irregular or moving support	Moving surrounds, darkness
Vestibular	Gravity and inertial space	Irregular or moving support and moving surrounds or darkness	Unusual motion environments

sway than the vestibular system (Nashner, Shupert, Horak, & Black, 1989). The primary role of vestibular input under these conditions is most probably to allow independent and precise control of head and eye positions, and the direction of gaze. Precise head, eye, and gaze control are critical in the execution of many complex motor activities such as running and either kicking or catching a moving ball.

Vestibular input is, however, critical for balance when both the somatosensory and visual inputs are misleading or unavailable (Allum, Honegger, & Pfaltz, 1989; Bles & de Jong, 1986; Fregly, 1974). The patient with a profound bilateral vestibular loss, for example, is unsteady standing in darkness on a compliant or irregular surface. Because vestibular input is seldom if ever misleading (except in cases of disease or other disorder and unusual motion environments), vestibular information is critical for balance when conflicting visual and/or somatosensory information requires a person to identify and quickly ignore a misleading input (Black & Nashner, 1984, 1985). This is why patients with peripheral vestibular deficits frequently complain of dizziness and/or unsteadiness during exposure to conflicting visual and support surface stimuli.

Exposure to zero gravity or to a simulation of zero gravity is believed to cause changes in the way the brain interprets orientation input from the vestibular system. The utricular otoliths normally sense both the linear acceleration of the head and the tilt angle of the head with respect to gravity. Under zero-gravity conditions, the brain must adapt to an absence of the tilt angle component of the otolith input. The adaptive changes in interpretation of the vestibular input following zero-gravity exposure may be viewed as a temporary, environmentally induced pathologic condition (Paloski, Reschke, Doxey, & Harm, 1992; Young, Oman, Watt, Money, & Lichtenberg, 1984) These maladaptive changes are most potent immediately after return to normal terrestrial conditions and are most pronounced when the returning astronauts are exposed to conflicting visual conditions (Parker, Reschke, Arrott, Hormick, & Lichtenberg, 1985).

Visual Input

Among the three balance senses, vision is without doubt the richest and most varied in providing ori-entation and motion information. A comprehensive summary of visual orientation perception has been described by Gibson, 1979). Understanding the nature of visual perception is important for posture control, because the advent of modern computer animated virtual reality techniques allows assessment and training of the full range of visual influences on balance. Some of the key elements of visual motion perception that influence balance include visual field flow and changes in object size, both of which are influenced by the distance of objects from the observer, parallax effects influenced by the relative distances between near and far objects, and the spatial frequencies and contrast differences among objects in the surround. Recent virtual reality research demonstrates that individual elements of visual orientation perception differ in their influences on balance (Keshner & Kenyan, 2009; Streepey, Kenyan, & Keshner, 2007). For example, flow within the peripheral visual field has a stronger influence on balance control than the changing sizes of objects in the central visual field.

Vision plays a significant role in balance, especially when the support surface is unstable (Begbie, 1967; Diener, Dichgans, & Guschlbauer, 1986; Lee & Lishman, 1975; Paulus, Straube, & Brandt, 1984, 1987). For example, when toes-up and toes-down tilting of the surface in direct relation to the AP sway disrupts somatosensory input useful for balance, COG sway is significantly less with eyes open than with eyes closed (Black & Nashner, 1984, 1985; Nashner, Black, & Wall, 1982) . The stabilizing effect of vision is also illustrated by comparing eyes-open and eyes-closed sway while a person stands on a compliant foam rubber pad. Vision also influences COG alignment. When a person is exposed to a constant linear or rotational movement of the visual field, for example, the alignment of the COG over the base of support shifts in the direction of the visual field motion (Brandt, Paulus, & Straube, 1986; Lestienne, Soechting, & Berthoz, 1977).

The reader may have experienced the effect of vision on balance, for example, at the seashore when a wave causes a large area of the surrounding water to move in or out at constant velocity. If a person is attending to the moving water, there is a tendency to sway and sometimes even stumble in the direction of the moving water. Alterations in body alignment also occur when subjects are exposed to a room with tilted walls. Similar visual illusions are sometimes used in carnival fun-houses to throw participants off balance.

MOTOR CONTROL OF BALANCE

Anatomy and Physiology of Movement

During erect standing with the arms at the side or folded at the waist, the COG is located in the area of the lower abdomen, with the exact position at a given moment dependent on the relative positions of the ankle, knee, and hip joints (McCollum & Leen, 1989). Because there are three principal joint systems—ankles, knees, and hips—between the base of support and the COG during standing, a wide variety of different postures can be assumed with the COG over the center of the base of support, as illustrated in Figure 17–4. For similar reasons, a wide variety of active ankle, knee, and hip movement patterns can be used to produce similar shifts in COG position. Examples of this diversity of postures and balance movement patterns can be observed in individuals performing highly trained dance or martial arts routines.

A detailed description of the large number of muscles controlling ankle, knee, and hip joint motions is beyond the scope of this chapter. Instead, this section focuses on the key muscle groups involved in balance and on the general physiologic principles governing coordination of these muscles during postural movements.

Motions about a given joint are controlled by the combined actions of at least one pair of muscles working in opposition. All leg and lower trunk joints have multiple pairs of opposing muscles. Furthermore, many leg muscles act about two neighboring joints. At the ankle joint, the gastrocnemius and tibialis anterior are the major extensor (plantar flexor) and flexor (dorsiflexor) muscles, respectively. The quadriceps is the major knee extensor, while the hamstrings and gastrocnemius are both knee flexors. The hamstrings and lower back muscles are hip extensors, while hip flexion is controlled by quadriceps and abdominals.

An isolated muscle acts like a spring, tending to resist attempts to stretch the muscle beyond a resting length (Hill, 1953). The degree of the muscle's resistance to stretch is called muscle stiffness. Both the rest length of the muscle and the muscle stiffness vary depending on how strongly the muscle is being activated. An inactive muscle has an extended rest

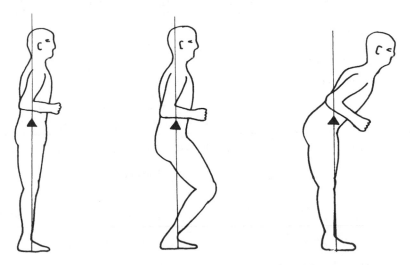

Figure 17–4. Examples of the variety of different postures during which the body COG is centered over the base of support. From Jacobson, *Handbook of balance function testing*, 1E. © 1998 Delmar Learning, a part of Cengage Learning, Inc. Reproduced by permission. http://www.cengage.com/permissions

length and offers little resistance to stretching. The rest length of a highly active muscle is shorter, and the muscle vigorously resists stretching.

When the forces exerted by pairs of opposing muscle about a joint are combined, the effect is to resist rotation of the joint relative to a resting position. The degree to which the joint resists rotation is called joint stiffness. The resting position and the stiffness of the joint are each altered independently by changing the activation levels of one or both muscles. Joint resting position and joint stiffness, however, are by themselves an inadequate basis for controlling postural movements. This is because the stiffness properties of muscle are highly nonlinear. While resistance to a small displacement from the resting position is strong, the resistance breaks down over larger displacements unless the activation level is increased (Houk, 1979).

The myotatic stretch reflex is the earliest mechanism for increasing the activation level of the muscles of a joint following an externally imposed rotation of the joint. This response component is initiated by inputs from muscle spindles, tiny stretch sensitive receptors embedded within the muscle. Output fibers from the muscle spindles enter the spinal cord and, by way of single synapses within the cord, activate muscle fibers within the same muscle originating the spindle inputs (Houk, 1979).

Current theory suggests that the myotatic stretch reflexes improve the nonlinear stiffness prop-

erties of muscle in controlling the effects of external disturbances during movement control (Houk, 1979). Thus, during larger joint displacements, reflexes rapidly increase activation of the stretching muscles, decrease activation of the shortening antagonists, and thereby prevent the breakdown of joint stiffness. There are, however, several reasons why the combined effects of the muscle stiffness properties and the stretch reflexes are still insufficient to maintain standing balance. First, the level of ankle joint stiffness resulting from these two mechanisms does not fully counteract the destabilizing force of gravity during sway (Elner, Popov, & Gurfinkel, 1972; Nashner, 1976). Second, because rotations of the support surface can elicit stretch reflexes inappropriate for balance control, other response mechanisms not dependent on local stretch inputs are required (Nashner, 1976).

Automatic and Volitional Movement Systems

The influences of stretch reflex, automatic movement system, and volitional movement system on standing balance are reviewed in Table 17–2. As described previously, the stretch reflexes regulate the stiffness properties of the joints involved in maintaining postural stability. Stretch reflexes, however, play little if any direct role in mediating a person's active pos-

Table 17-2. Properties of the Three Movement Systems

Property	Movement Systems		
	Reflex	Automatic	Voluntary
Mediating pathways	Spinal cord	Brainstem and subcortical	Brainstem and cortical
Mode of activation	External stimulus	External stimulus	Self-generated or external stimulus
Response properties	Localized to point of stimulus and highly stereotyped	Coordinated among leg and trunk muscles, and stereotyped but adaptable	Limitless variety
Role in posture control	Regulate muscle forces	Coordinate movements across joints	Generate purposeful behaviors
Response times	Fixed at 40 msec	Fixed at 100 msec	Varies with difficulty, 150+ msec

tural movements in response to external balance perturbations (Elner, Popov, & Gurfinkel, 1972; Gurfinkel, Lipshits, & Popov, 1974).

Automatic postural movements are the earliest functionally effective responses helping to maintain stability when a standing individual's balance is perturbed (Nashner, 1976, 1977; Nashner, Woollacott, & Tuma, 1979). Automatic postural movements resemble reflex responses in some respects, and voluntary movements in others. Like reflexes, automatic movements are triggered by external stimuli, occur at fixed latencies, and are relatively stereotyped. Like voluntary postural movements, automatic responses involve the coordinated actions of many leg and trunk muscles, and the amplitudes and patterns of automatic responses adapt to the task conditions. Although the pathways mediating automatic postural movements have not been fully elucidated, the 90- to 100-msec latencies of electromyographic (EMG) responses are sufficient to include significant brainstem and subcortical involvement (Evarts & Tajii, 1974; Marsden, Merton, & Morton, 1973; Melville Jones & Watt, 1971).

Voluntary postural movements can occur either in the presence or absence of external stimuli, and the variety of voluntary patterns is almost limitless, in theory at least. When elicited by external stimuli, voluntary movement latencies are 150 msec under the simplest and well-practiced task conditions, but can be or much longer when the task is more complex or novel and when the person's level of attention is reduced (Nashner & Cordo, 1981). When a freely standing person exerts a voluntary force against an external object, automatic and voluntary activities are closely coordinated to provide a stable base of support for the voluntary movement (Belenkii, Gurfinkel, & Paltsev, 1967; Nashner & Cordo, 1981). In these instances, automatic postural reactions occur first, and the onset of the voluntary component is delayed accordingly (Nashner & Cordo, 1981).

Automatic Postural Movements

When an automatic postural movement is initiated by an external stimulus, the onset of muscular EMG activity occurs within 90 to 100 msec, and the resulting patterns of activation among leg and lower trunk muscles are directionally specific and relatively stereotyped. The onset of active movement force is delayed an additional 20 to 40 msec, because there is a delay between electrical activation and force generation in a muscle (Bawa & Stein, 1976).

Local somatosensory input from the feet and ankle joints is by itself sufficient to trigger an automatic postural movement (Horak, Nashner, & Diener, 1990). The direction of the automatic movement is also determined by the triggering somatosensory stimulus (Horak & Nashner, 1986; Nashner, 1977; Nashner, Woollacott, & Tuma, 1979). A backward movement is triggered by forward displacement of the body's COG as, for example, when the support surface moves backward or when the subject pulls backward on a rigid object. A forward movement follows a backward COG displacement, caused by forward movement of the surface or pushing against a rigid object.

Although the amplitude of the automatic movement is related to the intensity of the triggering somatosensory stimulus (Diener, Horak, & Nashner, 1988), visual input, vestibular input, and the past experiences of the individual also influence the amplitude of the response (Nashner, 1976; Nashner & Berthoz, 1978; Shupert, Black, & Horak, 1988). The pattern of movement response among leg and lower trunk muscles, in contrast, is determined not by the triggering stimulus but by the configuration of the support surface and the previous experience of the individual.

COORDINATION OF AUTOMATIC POSTURAL MOVEMENTS

Biomechanics of Coordinated Movement

The major joint and muscle systems controlling the COG during standing are illustrated in Figure 17–5. Postural movements involve the coordinated actions of the ankle, knee, hip joints, and frequently also the neck. The motions about each of these joints, however, are not determined simply by the muscles acting directly about the joint. This is because leg and trunk muscles also exert indirect forces on neighboring joints through the inertial interaction forces among body segments (Nashner, 1985a; Nashner & McCollum, 1985). For example, when the ankle muscles contract to extend the lower leg segments backward, the hips will flex unless thigh and lower trunk muscles are activated to stabilize these joints. The hips will flex in the absence of additional stabilizing forces, because the inertia of the trunk tends to make its movements lag behind those of the legs.

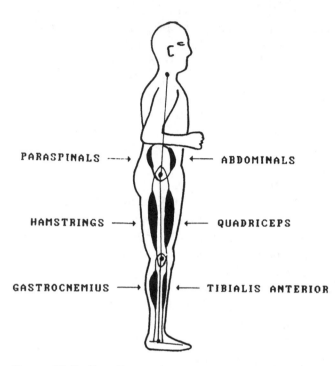

Figure 17–5. Functional anatomy of the major joint and muscle systems controlling movements of the body's COG during standing balance. From Jacobson, *Handbook of balance function testing*, 1E. © 1998 Delmar Learning, a part of Cengage Learning, Inc. Reproduced by permission. http://www.cengage.com/permissions

Because of the indirect inertial effects of muscular forces, the function of leg and trunk muscles during posture control can differ quite dramatically from their traditional anatomic classification, as summarized in Table 17–3. When a person is standing on a rigid surface, contraction of the tibialis anterior (anatomically classified as an ankle dorsiflexor) also causes knee flexion, even though there is no anatomic insertion of this muscle at the knee. As dorsiflexion of the ankle moves the lower leg forward, inertia causes the thigh to lag behind and the knee flexes as a result. Although the gastrocnemius is anatomically classified as an ankle extensor and knee flexor, its functional effect on the knee during standing is extension rather than flexion. The knee extends because of inertial interactions similar to the others mentioned.

Contractions of thigh and lower trunk muscles exert similar indirect effects on the knee and ankle joints. The quadriceps muscle is not only a hip flexor and knee extensor by direct action, but also an ankle extensor by indirect action. The hamstrings muscle is an indirect ankle flexor in addition to its direct knee flexor and hip extensor functions.

One common example of an abnormal movement pattern is the destabilization of a proximal knee or hip joint during postural movement. This problem is often called proximal joint instability. While it is tempting to attribute an unstable knee or hip joint to weakness or inactivity in the muscles acting directly about these joints, the instability can also be caused by the indirect effects of delayed

Table 17–3. Functional Anatomy of Muscles Involved in Balance Movements

Joint	Extension		Flexion	
	Anatomic	Functional	Anatomic	Functional
Hip	Paraspinals Hamstrings	Paraspinals Hamstrings Tibialis	Abdominal Quadriceps	Abdominals Quadriceps Gastrocnemius
Knee	Quadriceps	Paraspinals Quadriceps Gastrocnemius	Hamstrings Gastrocnemius	Abdominals Hamstrings Tibialis
Ankle	Gastrocnemius	Abdominals Quadriceps Gastrocnemius	Tibialis	Paraspinals Hamstrings Tibialis

ankle muscle activation (Nashner, Shumway-Cook, & Marin, 1983).

Coordination of Postural Movements Into Strategies

When a person's balance is disrupted by an external perturbation, one or a combination of three different strategies can be used to coordinate movement of the COG back to a balanced position. Properties of the three strategies are reviewed in Figure 17–6. A step or stumbling reaction is the only movement strategy effective in preventing a fall when the perturbation displaces the COG beyond the LOS perimeter. When the COG remains within the LOS, two different strategies or combinations of strategies can be used to move the COG while maintaining the initial placement of the feet on the support surface. The following sections describe the biomechanical and physiologic properties of these two in-place movement strategies.

Ankle Strategy

The ankle strategy shifts the COG while maintaining the placement of the feet by rotating the body as an approximately rigid mass about the ankle joints, as shown in Figure 17–6. This is accomplished by contracting the ankle joint muscles to generate torque about the ankle joints. At the same time, contractions of thigh and lower trunk muscles are required to resist the destabilization of these proximal joints due to the indirect effects of the ankle muscles on the proximal joints (see Table 17–3).

Ankle movements are generated by EMG responses which begin at 90 to 100 msec in the directionally appropriate ankle joint muscles (Horak & Nashner, 1986; Nashner, 1977; Nashner, Woollacott, & Tuma, 1979). The gastrocnemius muscles are activated for backward postural movements, while contractions of the tibialis anterior produce forward movements. Electromyographic activity then radiates in sequence to the thigh and then the lower trunk muscles on the same dorsal or ventral aspect of the body. Activation of the thigh and lower trunk muscles stabilizes the knees and hips, allowing the body to move as a unit about the ankles. Thigh and trunk muscle EMG onsets average 10 to 30 msec later than those of the ankle. Activation of the ankle muscles first provides proximal muscles with a stable movement base.

Hip Strategy

Movements organized into the hip strategy are centered about the hip joints with smaller opposing ankle joint rotations, as shown in Figure 17–6. The COG shifts in the direction opposite to the hip because of the inertia of the trunk (moving in one direction),

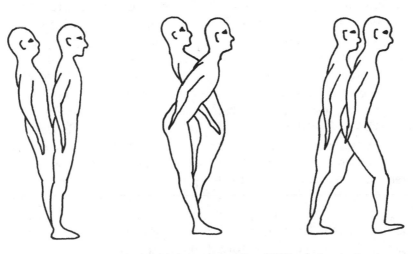

Figure 17–6. Three strategies for moving the COG relative to the base of support during postural sway, and their functional properties. From Jacobson, *Handbook of balance function testing*, 1E. © 1998 Delmar Learning, a part of Cengage Learning, Inc. Reproduced by permission. http://www.cengage.com/permissions

generating an opposite horizontal (shear) reaction force against the support surface. The tendency for destabilization of the knee joints is resisted by coordination of the muscular actions about the ankle, knee, and hip joints.

Hip strategy movements are generated by activation of the directionally appropriate thigh and lower trunk muscles at 85- to 95-msec latencies (Horak & Nashner, 1986). Quadriceps and abdominal muscles are activated to flex the hips and move the COG backward. The knee remains relatively stable because these two muscles have opposite functional effects about this joint (see Table 17–3). Paraspinal and hamstring activation extends the hips and moves the COG backward. Opposing functional effects of these two muscles also stabilize the knees. During movements in both directions, the ankle muscles are relatively inactive.

Appropriate Use of Postural Movement Strategies

The relative effectiveness of ankle, hip, and stepping strategies in repositioning the COG over the base of support depends on the configuration of the base of support, the COG alignment in relation to the LOS, and the speed (frequency) of the postural movement (Horak & Nashner, 1986; McCollum, Horak, & Nashner, 1984; Nashner & McCollum, 1985). For example, the ankle strategy is most effective in executing relatively slow, low-frequency COG movements when the base of support is firm and the COG is well within the LOS perimeter. The ankle strategy is also effective in maintaining a static posture with the COG offset from the center.

The amplitude and speed of ankle movements are biomechanically limited by the torque that can be exerted about the ankles before the feet lift off the support surface (Nashner, Shupert, & Horak, 1989). The reader can experience this biomechanical constraint by increasing the amplitude and frequency of sway about the ankles to the point where the feet begin to lift off the floor. The strengths of the ankle joint muscles are not the limiting factors. Gastrocnemius strength is determined by the force requirements for running and jumping, and therefore far exceeds the requirements for executing ankle movements. The maximum force capabilities of the tibialis anterior muscles, in contrast, are more closely

matched to the requirements for balance. Thus, reductions in ankle muscle strength are more likely to impair a person's use of ankle movements to recover from backward displacements of the COG.

Hip movements rely on horizontal shear forces rather than ankle torques to shift the COG and are therefore not limited by constraints on ability to exert torque about the ankles. Thus, hip movements are effective when the COG is positioned near the LOS perimeter, the LOS boundaries are contracted by a narrowed base of support, or the body is swaying at higher frequencies. The reader can experience the conditions requiring the use of hip movements by attempting to shift posture slowly while standing on tiptoes or rapidly on a firm, flat surface.

Hip movements also have biomechanical limitations in that they cannot produce large shifts in COG position. In addition, because hip movements rely on inertial reaction forces, they cannot be used to maintain balance effectively with the COG offset from the center.

When the COG is displaced beyond the LOS, a step or stumble is the only effective strategy for preventing a fall. While stepping and stumbling are subject to fewer biomechanical limitations, they are inefficient, disruptive, and usually inappropriate when simpler ankle or hip movements are effective.

Selecting the Postural Movement Strategy

The strategy selected for responding to an external perturbation is set in advance depending on the person's immediate past experience, not on a conscious decision made at the time of response (Horak & Nashner, 1986; McCollum, Horak, & Nashner, 1984). When a person is well practiced at standing on a particular support surface, a relatively pure example of the appropriate movement strategy described in the preceding sections is observed. In contrast, a more complex movement combining the two pure strategies is observed during the initial practice trials following a change in support surface conditions. After 10 to 15 practice trials on the new surface, however, the less appropriate component is progressively reduced, and reliance on the well-practiced pure strategy increases. Movement strategies are not voluntarily changed by instruction alone, even if a person is familiar with and motivated to change the pattern quickly.

COORDINATION OF HEAD AND BODY MOVEMENTS

Head Movement Strategies

Movements of the head relative to the trunk have a relatively minor effect on the COG position during standing. This is because the mass of the head is sub-stantially smaller than that of the trunk. Motions of the head during postural sway are important, never-theless, because they have a strong influence on two of the three principal senses of balance: vision and the vestibular system. The head and body move-ment strategies reviewed in Figure 17–7 can affect the ability to determine the position of the COG accurately during postural sway (Nashner, 1985b; Shupert, Black, & Horak, 1988).

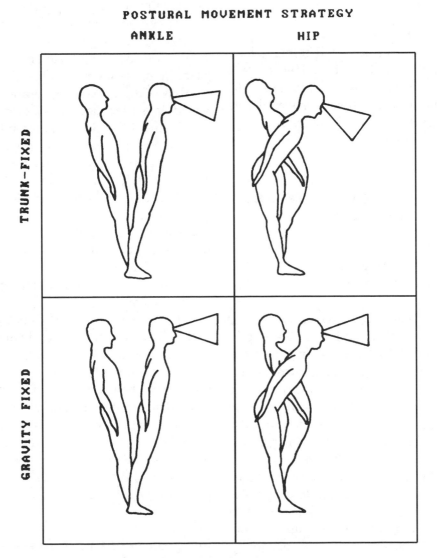

POSTURAL MOVEMENT STRATEGY

ANKLE   HIP

TRUNK-FIXED

GRAVITY FIXED

Figure 17–7. Strategies for moving the head relative to the trunk dur-ing postural sway, and their functional properties. Visual "rays" show the direction of the gaze. Note that when the head position is trunk-fixed, the gaze direction is disturbed substantially more by the hip than the ankle strategy. When head position is gravity-fixed, gaze direction is not dis-turbed by either strategy. From Jacobson, *Handbook of balance func-tion testing*, 1E. © 1998 Delmar Learning, a part of Cengage Learning, Inc. Reproduced by permission. http://www.cengage.com/permissions

Trunk-Fixed Strategy

Strategies for coordinating movements of the head relative to the trunk can be classified in three categories: trunk fixed, gravity fixed, and combinations of the two. In the trunk-fixed strategy, the head and trunk move as a unit. The neck muscles stiffen to resist the inertial and gravitational forces tending to rotate the head opposite to the trunk. Thus, this strategy fixes movements of the head to those of the trunk.

Gravity-Fixed Strategy

The gravity-fixed strategy rotates the head in opposition to the trunk so that the head remains level relative to the gravitational vertical. This strategy requires coordinated neck and trunk muscular actions to eliminate head rotations correlated with COG sway, while preserving the linear translational components of head motion.

INTERACTIONS BETWEEN SENSORY AND MOTOR COMPONENTS OF BALANCE

Sensory Effects of Body and Head Movement Strategies

The pattern of ankle, knee, hip, and head movements strongly influences the visual and vestibular inputs to balance (Nashner, 1985a). If a person is swaying about the ankles while holding the head fixed to the trunk, for example, the head and body move as a unit and the linear and rotational motions of the head and the body COG are similar. In theory at least, this strategy simplifies the brain's task of interpreting input from the visual and vestibular systems.

Moving the head and body as a unit, however, is disadvantageous whenever independent head and eye movements are required, such as maintaining gaze on an object or scanning the terrain. Without the ability to move the head and eyes independently, backward or forward sway will move the head and eyes up or down, respectively, and thus away from a desired visual target. The negative impact on vision of the body-fixed strategy of head control is particularly great during hip movements, when motions of the trunk are large and rapid.

Fixing the rotational position of the head relative to gravity has two potential benefits. First, the eyes are freer to maintain gaze on objects in the visual surround with the head fixed in relation to gravity. Second, the gravity-fixed strategy of head coordination has the potential for reducing the confusion between linear and angular accelerations, a shortcoming of all inertial-gravitational systems including the vestibular system. An example of this type of confusion can be experienced when a wide-bodied jet brakes immediately after touching down on the runway. A passenger looking straight ahead will sometimes sense that the cabin is tilting downward, even to the point of dipping below the level of the runway. This illusion occurs even though the plane remains level, because the brain incorrectly interprets the linear deceleration inputs from the vestibular system as being caused by forward tilting.

There is the potential for misinterpretation of tilt and linear acceleration inputs to the vestibular system during sway, because the head both tilts and moves linearly (Parker et al., 1985). Fixing the rotational position of the head relative to gravity reduces the confusion between tilting and linear motions, because this strategy eliminates the tilt component of the vestibular input. When a gravity-fixed strategy is used, linear acceleration input from the vestibular system can be safely interpreted as actual linear head acceleration.

This theoretical analysis of the senses suggests that selection of head and body movement strategies is based not only on surface conditions and COG position within the LOS, as described previously, but also on the need to simplify the interpretation of vestibular input to balance. There is no conclusive experimental proof that sensory processes influence a person's choice of head and body movement strategies. The following section describes results with healthy individuals and patients with sensory balance problems which are consistent with this conclusion.

Integration of Head and Body Movement Strategies

In normal individuals, movements of the head and body are coordinated when a hip strategy is used during in-place standing, and when running, jumping, and hopping (Nashner et al., 1988; Pozzo, Berthoz, & Lefort, 1989). During these tasks, the head is approximately stabilized relative to the gravitational vertical, as shown in Figure 17–7. Analysis of leg, lower trunk, and neck muscle EMG activity during automatic postural movements indicates that the motions of the head and body are coordinated at the automatic level of control. During forward automatic hip movements, for example, rectus abdominus (hip flexor) and sternocleidomastoid (neck flexor) are simultaneously activated at 90 to 100 msec. The sternocleidomastoid activation prevents the large nose-up rotation of the head that would occur in the absence of active head control.

When normal individuals use the ankle strategy, head and body movements are not tightly coordinated. Instead, the head moves passively in the direction opposite to the body, rotating nose up and then nose down in relation to gravity over a range of approximately 10°. These opposing head rotations occur as predicted by biomechanics in the absence of active head control. Analysis of leg, lower trunk, and neck muscle EMG activities during automatic ankle movement confirms that neck muscle actions are not correlated with those of the legs and lower trunk (Shupert et al., 1988).

In contrast to normal individuals, patients with bilateral loss of vestibular inputs avoid hip movements under all conditions, even though they have no motor deficits that impair their hip motor control (Shupert et al., 1988). These patients also tend to fix the position of the head relative to the trunk. Subjects deprived of somatosensory inputs from the feet by transient ischemia prefer hip movements under all support surface conditions, even though the sensory loss does not impair their ability to execute ankle movements.

Head-body coordination during in-place hip movements and during running, hopping, and jumping is consistent with the need for head stabilization during complex movements. As suggested in the section on sensory effects of head and body movement strategies, the COG position is more difficult to determine from vestibular and visual inputs during complex movements. This process is simplified by stabilizing the position of the head relative to gravity.

Voluntary Movements Influence Balance

A standing person's voluntary motor activities, as well as gravity and external perturbing forces, can destabilize balance. Excluding movements having a direct effect on the base of support (shifting weight, raising or changing the placement of a foot), the voluntary actions summarized in Table 17–4 are classified in two categories based on their effects on balance.

The first category of voluntary actions includes movements involving manipulation of external objects. These actions have the greatest destabilizing effects on balance. For example, when pulling open a heavy door, the backward force required to move the door generates an equal and opposite forward force on COG of the body. If this destabilizing force is not compensated by an appropriate postural reaction, the person falls forward into the opening door.

Table 17-4. Functional Properties of Two Types of Voluntary Actions

Property	Voluntary Actions	
	Object Manipulations	**Free Body Movements**
Effect on center of gravity	Direct equal and opposite force	Little if any direct force
Coordination during free standing	Anticipatory postural response and delayed voluntary onset	Less postural activity and rapid voluntary onset
Coordination with the body supported	Little postural activity and rapid voluntary onset	Little postural activity and rapid voluntary onset
Examples	Pull or push on object, grasp and lift object	Lift arm, reach or point

The second category includes voluntary actions not involving external objects. These actions change body posture but have only indirect and relatively minor effects on COG position. Raising an arm from the side to a forward pointing position, for example, does not substantially alter the COG position, because the force required to accelerate the arm forward produces an equal and opposite force accelerating the trunk slightly backward. The net result is little if any change in balance.

Students of physics will recognize that voluntary actions are distinguished based on the presence or absence of external and internal forces. External forces have a direct effect on the COG position of a body, while internal forces acting between body parts tend to reorient the parts relative to one another with little net effect on COG position. "Real-world" situations, however, are never quite so simple. Because the body is supported by contact with a surface, rapid elevations of an arm can have minor effects on balance.

Coordination of Voluntary and Automatic Postural Movements

When a freely standing person performs a voluntary action involving external forces (e.g., pulling on a heavy external object), an automatic postural movement is initiated in advance of the voluntary arm movement to compensate for the disturbance in balance (Belenkii et al., 1967; Cordo & Nashner, 1982; Nashner & Cordo, 1981). The anticipatory automatic postural movement minimizes any disturbance to balance and provides a stable base for the voluntary action.

The properties of an anticipatory postural movement depend on the requirements for balance at the time of the voluntary action. Removing the need to maintain balance by providing trunk support during a voluntary action, for example, abolishes the anticipatory postural movement. In this instance, the voluntary action itself can actually be initiated sooner. This later observation indicates that, to meet the requirements of balance in a freestanding task, voluntary actions with the potential for disrupting balance are actively delayed so that a stable base of support is established first.

CONCLUSIONS

Balance is a multicomponent and highly adaptable control process. When the balance of a healthy individual is challenged, the sensory inputs determining the COG position and the pattern of movement correcting the perturbation depend on the task conditions and the person's immediate past experience. An individual with one or more impaired sensory input or motor output component will attempt to compensate by adapting both the impaired and normally functioning components to best meet the demands of the balance task.

When a patient complains of unsteadiness, the problem is seldom caused by the absence of balance-related activities. More frequently, some components are functioning normally and others abnormally, the interactions of which lead to functionally inappropriate or ineffective balance responses. Because of these multiple interactions, focusing the diagnostic assessment or treatment on isolated component(s) of the balance system is frequently ineffective. In these cases, understanding the patient's abnormality requires an assessment approach that systematically examines all components and their interactions under a variety of task conditions. A test battery designed to generate a systematic description of the patient's balance problem, called computerized dynamic posturography, is described in Chapter 18.

REFERENCES

Aggashyan, R. V., Gurfinkel, V. S., Mamasakhlisov, G. V., & Elner, A. M. (1973). Changes in spectral and correlation characteristics of human stabilograms at muscle afferentation disturbance. *Agressologie, 14,* 5–9.

Allum, J. H. J., Honegger, F., & Pfaltz, C. R. (1989). The role of stretch and vestibulo-spinal reflexes in the generation of human equilibrating reactions. In J. H. J. Allum & M. Hulliger (Eds.), *Progress in brain research* (Vol. 80, pp. 399–409). New York, NY: Elsevier.

Bawa, P., & Stein, R. B. (1976). Frequency response of human soleus muscle. *Journal of Neurophysiology, 39,* 788–793.

Begbie, J. V. (1967). Some problems of postural sway. In A. V. S. deReuck & J. Knight (Eds.), *CIBA Foundation Sym-*

posium on myotatic, kinesthetic and vestibular mechanisms (pp. 80–92). London, UK: Churchill.

Belenkii, V. Y., Gurfinkel, V. S., & Paltsev, Y. I. (1967). On the elements of voluntary movement control. *Biophysics, 12,* 135–141.

Black, F. O., & Nashner, L. M. (1984). Vestibulospinal control differs in patients with reduced versus distorted vestibular function. *Acta Oto-Laryngologica, 406,* 110–114.

Black, F. O., & Nashner, L. M. (1985). Postural control in four classes of vestibular abnormalities. In M. Igarashi & F. O. Black (Eds.), *Vestibular and visual control of posture and locomotor equilibrium* (pp. 271–281). Basel, Switzerland: S Karger.

Bles, W., & de Jong, J. M. B. V. (1986). Uni and bilateral loss of vestibular function. In W. Bles & T. Brandt (Eds.), *Disorders of posture and gait* (pp. 127–139). New York, NY: Elsevier.

Bles, W., de Jong, J. M. B. V., & de Wit, G. (1984). Somatosensory compensation for loss of labyrinthine function. *Acta Oto-Laryngologica, 97,* 213–221.

Brandt, T., Paulus, W., & Straube, A. (1986). Vision and posture. In W. Bles & T. Brandt (Eds.), *Disorders of posture and gait* (pp. 157–175). New York, NY: Elsevier.

Cordo, P. J., & Nashner, L. M. (1982). Properties of postural adjustments associated with rapid arm movements. *Neurophysiology, 47,* 287–302.

Dichgans, J., Held, R., Young, L. R., & Brandt, T. (1972). The moving visual scenes influence the apparent direction of gravity. *Science, 178,* 1217–1219.

Diener, H. C., & Dichgans, J. (1988). On the role of vestibular, visual, and somatosensory information for dynamic postural control in humans. In O. Pompeiano & J. H. J. Allum (Eds.), *Progress in brain research* (Vol. 76, 253–262). New York, NY: Elsevier.

Diener, H. C., Dichgans, J., Bacher, B., & Gompf, B. (1984). Quantification of postural sway in normals and patients with cerebellar diseases. *Electroencephalography Clinical Neurophysiology, 157,* 134–142.

Diener, H. C., Dichgans, J., & Guschlbauer, B. (1986). Role of visual and static vestibular influences on dynamic posture control. *Human Neurobiology, 5,* 105–113.

Diener, H. C., Dichgans, J., Guschlbauer, B., & Mau, H. (1984). The significance of proprioception on postural stabilization as assessed by ischemia. *Experimental Brain Research, 296,* 103–109.

Diener, H. C., Horak, F. B., & Nashner, L. M. (1988). Influence of stimulus parameters on human postural responses. *Journal of Neurophysiology, 59,* 1888–1895.

Dietz, V., Horstmann, G. A., & Berger, W. (1989). Significance of proprioceptive mechanisms in the regulation of stance. In J. H. J. Allum & M. Hulliger (Eds.), *Progress in brain research* (Vol. 80, pp. 419–423). New York, NY: Elsevier.

Duncan, P. W., Weiner, D. K., Chandler, J., & Studenski, S. (1990). Functional reach: A new clinical measure of balance. *Gerentology, 45,* 192–197.

Elner, A. M., Popov, K. E., & Gurfinkel, V. S. (1972). Changes in stretch reflex system concerned with the control of postural activity of human muscle. *Agressologie, 13,* 19–23.

Evarts, E. V., & Tanjii, J. (1974). Gating of motor cortex reflexes by prior instruction. *Brain Research, 71,* 479–494.

Fregly, A. R. (1974). Vestibular ataxia and its measurement in man. In H. H. Kornhuber (Ed.), *Handbook of sensory physiology* (Vol. 6, No. 2, pp. 321–360). Berlin, Germany: Springer-Verlag.

Gibsin, J. J. (1979). *The Ecological Approach to Visual Perception.* Boston, MA: Houghton Mifflin Company.

Gurfinkel, V. S., Lipshits, M. I., Mori, S., & Popov, K. E. (1976). The state of the stretch reflex during quiet standing in man. In H. Homma (Ed.), *Progress in brain research* (Vol. 44, pp. 473–490). New York, NY: Elsevier.

Gurfinkel, V. S., Lipshits, M. I., & Popov, K. Y. (1974). Is the stretch reflex the main mechanism in the system of regulation of the vertical posture of man? *Biophysics, 19,* 744–748.

Gurfinkel, V. S., & Osevets, M. (1972). Dynamics of the vertical posture in man. *Biophysics, 17,* 496–506.

Hill, V. (1953). The mechanics of active muscle. *Proceedings of the Royal Society of London, 141B,* 104–117.

Horak, F. B., & Nashner, L. M. (1986). Central programming of postural movements: Adaptation to altered support surface configurations. *Neurophysiology, 55,* 1369–1381.

Horak, F. B., Nashner, L. M., & Diener, H. C. (1990). Postural strategies associated with somatosensory and vestibular loss. *Experimental Brain Research, 82,* 167–177.

Houk, J. C. (1979). Regulation of stiffness by skeletomotor reflexes. *Annual Review of Physiology, 41,* 99–114.

Keshner, E. A., & Kenyan, R. V. (2009). Postural and spatial orientation driven by virtual reality. *Studies in Health Technology and Informatics, 145,* 209–228.

Koozekaani, S. H., Stockwell, C. W., McGhee, R. B., & Firoozmand, F. (1980). On the role of dynamic models in quantitative posturography. *IEEE Transactions Biomedical Engineering, 27,* 605–609.

Lee, D. N., & Lishman, J. R. (1975). Visual proprioceptive control of stance. *Journal of Human Movement Studies, 1,* 87–95.

Lestienne, F., Soechting, J., & Berthoz, A. (1977). Postural readjustments induced by linear motion of visual scenes. *Experimental Brain Research, 28,* 363–384.

Marsden, C. D., Merton, P. A., & Morton, H. B. (1973). Latency measurements compatible with a cortical pathway for the stretch reflex in man. *Journal of Physiology, 230,* 58–59.

Maurer, C., & Peterka, R. J. (2005). A new interpretation of spontaneous sway measures based on a simple model of human postural sway. *Journal of Neurophysiology, 93,* 189–200.

McCollum, G., Horak, F. B., & Nashner, L. M. (1984). Parsimony in neural calculations for postural movements. In J. Bloedel, J. Dichgans, & W. Precht (Eds.), *Cerebellar functions* (pp. 52–66). Berlin, Germany: Springer-Verlag.

McCollum, G., & Leen, T. K. (1989). Form and exploration of mechanical stability limits in erect stance. *Journal of Motor Behavior, 21,* 225–244.

Melville Jones, G., & Watt, D. G. D. (1971). Observations on the control of stepping and hopping movements in man. *Journal of Physiology, 219,* 709–727.

Nashner, L. M. (1976). Adapting reflexes controlling the human posture. *Experimental Brain Research, 26,* 59–72.

Nashner, L. M. (1977). Fixed patterns of rapid postural responses among leg muscles during stance. *Experimental Brain Research, 150,* 403–407.

Nashner, L. M. (1981). Analysis of stance posture in humans. In A. L. Towe & E. S. Luschei (Eds.), *Handbook of behavioral neurobiology* (Vol. 5, pp. 527–565). New York, NY: Plenum Press.

Nashner, L. M. (1985a). Strategies for organization of human posture. In M. Igarashi & F. O. Black (Eds.), *Vestibular and visual control of posture and locomotor equilibrium* (pp. 1–8). Basel, Switzerland: S Karger.

Nashner, L. M. (1985b). A functional approach to understanding spasticity. In A. Struppler & A. Weindl (Eds.), *Electromyography and evoked potentials* (pp. 22–29). Berlin, Germany: Springer-Verlag.

Nashner, L. M. (1986). The organization of human postural movements during standing and walking. In S. Grillner, P. S. G. Stein, & D. G. Stewart (Eds.), *Neurobiology of posture and locomotion* (pp. 637–648). London, UK: MacMillan.

Nashner, L. M., & Berthoz, A. (1978). Visual contribution to rapid motor responses during posture control. *Brain Research, 150,* 403–407.

Nashner, L. M., Black, F. O., & Wall, C. (1982). Adaptation to altered support and visual conditions during stance: Patients with vestibular deficits. *Journal of Neuroscience, 2,* 536–544.

Nashner, L. M., & Cordo, P. J. (1981). Relation of automatic postural responses and reaction-time voluntary movements of human leg muscles. *Experimental Brain Research, 43,* 395–405.

Nashner, L. M., & Forssberg, H. (1986). Phase-dependent organization of postural adjustments associated with arm movements while walking. *Journal of Neurophysiology, 55,* 538–548.

Nashner, L. M., & McCollum, G. (1985). The organization of human postural movements: A formal basis and experimental synthesis. *Behavioral and Brain Sciences, 8,* 135–172.

Nashner, L. M., Shumway-Cook, A., & Marin, O. (1983). Stance posture control in select groups of children with cerebral palsy: Deficits in sensory organization and muscular coordination. *Experimental Brain Research, 49,* 393–409.

Nashner, L. M., Shupert, C. L., & Horak, F. B. (1988). Headtrunk coordination in the standing posture. In O. Pompeiano & J. H. J. Allum (Eds.), *Progress in brain research* (Vol. 76, pp. 243–251). New York, NY: Elsevier.

Nashner, L. M., Shupert, C. L., Horak, F. B., & Black, F. O. (1989). Organization of posture controls: An analysis of sensory and mechanical constraints. In J. H. J. Allum & M. Hulliger (Eds.), *Progress in brain research* (Vol. 80, pp. 411–418). New York, NY: Elsevier.

Nashner, L. M., Woollacott, M., & Tuma, G. (1979). Organization of rapid responses to postural and locomotor-like perturbations of standing man. *Experimental Brain Research, 36,* 463–476.

Paloski., W. H., Reschke, M. F., Doxey, D. D., & Harm, D. L. (1992). Neurosensory adaptation associated with postural ataxia following space flight. In M. Woollacott & F. Horak (Eds.), *Posture and gait: Control mechanisms* (Vol. I, pp. 311–314). Eugene, OR: University of Oregon Books.

Parker, D. E., Reschke, M. F., Arrott, A. P., Hormick, J. L., & Lichtenberg, B. K. (1985). Otolith tilt-translation reinterpretation following prolonged weightlessness: Implications for preflight training. *Aviation and Space Environmental Medicine, 56,* 601–606.

Paulus, W. M., Straube, A., & Brandt, T. (1984). Visual stabilization of posture: Physiological stimulus characteristics and clinical aspects. *Brain, 107,* 1143–1163.

Paulus, W. M., Straube, A., & Brandt, T. (1987). Visual postural performance after loss of somatosensory and vestibular function. *Journal of Neurology Neurosurgery and Psychiatry, 50,* 1542–1545.

Pavol, M. J. (2005). Detecting and understanding differences in postural sway. *Journal of Neurophysiology, 93,* 20–21.

Pozzo, T., Berthoz, A., & Lefort, L. (1989). Head kinematics during various motor tasks in humans. In J. H. J. Allum & M. Hulliger (Eds.), *Progress in brain research* (Vol. 80, pp. 377–383). New York, NY: Elsevier.

Scott, D. E., & Dzendolet, E. (1972). Quantification of sway in standing humans. *Agressologie, 13,* 35–40.

Shupert, C. L., Black, F. O., & Horak, F. B. (1988). Coordination of head and body in response to support surface translations in normals and patients with bilaterally reduced vestibular function. In B. Amblard, A. Berthoz, & F. Clarac (Eds.), *Posture and gait: Development, adaptation and modulation* (pp. 281–289). New York, NY: Elsevier.

Streepey, J. W., Kenyan, R. V., & Keshner, E. A. (2007). Field of view and base of support width influence postural responses to visual stimuli during quiet stance. *Gait and Posture, 25,* 49–55.

Young, L. R., Oman, C. M., Watt, D. G. D., Money, K. E., & Lichtenberg, B. K. (1984). Spatial orientation in weightlessness and readaptation to earth's gravity. *Science, 225,* 202–208.

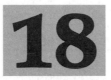

Computerized Dynamic Posturography

Lewis M. Nashner

BACKGROUND

Historical Development of Posturography

Computerized dynamic posturography (CDP) is a quantitative method for assessing upright and in-place balance function under a variety of tasks that effectively simulate the conditions encountered in daily life. The test protocols are designed to isolate the principle sensory, motor, and biomechanical components contributing to balance, and to analyze the patient's ability to effectively use these components singularly and in concert to maintain balance. The protocols and data analysis techniques employed in CDP are based on a systems model of human posture derived from the experimental research on normal and abnormal human balance and movement control reviewed in Chapter 17.

In recent years, advances in measurement and display technologies promise to expand the capabilities of CDP within the systems model of human postural control. Expanded capabilities include the use of miniature inertial devices to provide more comprehensive measures of body movement patterns and the incorporation of more dynamic balance tasks, and computer animated immersive visual displays to provide a wider variety of dynamic visual conditions.

Performance Measures of Posture Control

Historically, assessment of human posture control has developed using two complementary methodologies summarized in Table 18–1. The first method had its beginning with the 19th century work of Romberg (1853), who compared spontaneous sway under eyes-open and eyes-closed body conditions to identify peripheral somatosensory system deficits. Implicit in Romberg's interpretation of the eyes-open and eyes-closed performance of the patient is the assumption that the somatosensory input should dominate the control of balance whenever one is standing on a fixed support surface, and that visual input is the primary backup whenever the somatosensory input is disrupted. Based on this assumption, a substantial increase in sway under eyes closed relative to eyes open conditions is indicative of impairment of the dominant somatosensory input.

With the advent of forceplate technology, the use of "static" posturography expanded Romberg's original concept to enable examiners to acquire quantitative measurements and impose more rigorous analysis of the patient's postural sway (Black, Wall, & O'Leary, 1978; Black & Wall, 1982; Dichgans, Mauritz, Allum, & Brandt, 1976; Kapteyn & de Wit, 1972; Njiokikjien & De Rijke, 1972; Terekhov, 1976). The typical forceplate consists of a flat, rigid surface supported on three or more points by independent

Table 18-1. Methodologies for Assessing Human Posture Control

Method	Data Obtained	Advantages	Disadvantages
Performance tests	Postural stability Movement strategies	Correlates with daily life functional capabilities Quantifies adaptive capabilities	Influenced by conscious effort Dependent on patient cooperation
Posture-evoked response tests	Latency Pattern Strength	Provides diagnostic information Unaffected by patient motivation	Uncorrelated with daily life functional capabilities No adaptive capability information

force-measuring devices. As the patient stands on the forceplate, the distribution of vertical forces recorded by the measuring devices are used to calculate the position of the center of the vertical forces exerted on the forceplate surface over time.

The centers of vertical force movements provide an indirect measure of postural sway activity. This measure, however, is limited by the fact that motions of the center of vertical force produced by an equivalent angle of sway are larger in taller and/or heavier individuals than in shorter and lighter persons. Furthermore, as frequencies of sway increase, amplitudes of center of vertical force excursions produced by a given amplitude of sway increase dramatically and increasingly lead the sway angle in time (Nashner, Woollacott, & Tuma, 1979).

When the height and weight of the patient on the forceplate is known, a computer model of body dynamics can be used to estimate the center of gravity (COG) sway angle over time from the center of vertical force (COF) movements. To produce a near perfect measure of COG sway using the COF requires considerable computational complexity and time. Therefore, sway angle estimates are highly accurate when sway frequencies are low. During higher frequency sway movements, knee and hip motions come increasingly into play and forceplate-based measures tend to lag behind the actual COG motions.

The forceplate can also be used to measure the horizontal shear forces exerted by the patient's feet against the support surface. Horizontal shear forces measure the accelerations of the body COG in the antero-posterior (AP) and lateral directions. These

acceleration forces are extremely small when the body moves slowly, but increase dramatically as the frequency of COG sway increases. For this reason, horizontal shear forces are useful in identifying when knee and hip joint motions are contributing to COG sway.

The recent introduction of miniaturized inertial measurement units (IMU) and video motion technologies when combined with forceplate-based COG sway measures promise to substantially improve the accuracy of sway measures during high-frequency movements. These newer technologies can be used to directly measure the knee and hip joint motions.

Measurement of Discrete Postural Responses

A second approach used by investigators to study posture control has involved the use of brief and unexpected disturbances in balance to quantify the characteristics of the resulting discrete postural responses. With this method, balance is disturbed by briefly translating the support surface in the anterior or posterior direction (Nashner, 1976, 1977; Nashner et al., 1979) or by rotating the surface about the ankle joints, toes up or toes down (Allum & Keshner, 1986; Diener, Bootz, Dichgans, & Bruzek, 1983; Diener, Dichgans, Bootz, & Bacher, 1984; Dietz, Quintern, Berger, & Schenck, 1985; Nashner, 1976). The major emphasis of these studies has been analyzing the latency, strength, and pattern of response to variations in disturbance size and direction.

Relative Value of Discrete and Performance Measures

Computerized dynamic posturography combines the discrete response and continuous performance methods for assessing balance function. The motor control test (MCT) includes protocols that use various types of brief displacements in the support surface to evoke discrete postural responses. In the standard MCT protocol, the patient's postural responses are recorded with forceplate technology and comprise the classic "motor control test" of CDP. When combined with surface electromyography (EMG) recordings, the data set is expanded to include the posture-evoked responses (PER) which directly reflect activation of the segmental, spinal, and long-loop response pathways as well as the coordination of ankle, thigh, and lower trunk muscles.

In general, the MCT protocols offer two distinct advantages. First, the approach is similar to that used in traditional clinical "reflex" tests and is therefore conceptually familiar to most clinicians. Second, because evoked postural responses are not under conscious control, the test results are relatively unaffected by patient motivation and effort. The MCT protocols, however, have limitations. First, they do not characterize a patient's functional status relative to daily life tasks. Second, because the evoked postural responses are discrete events, they do not reveal the patient's adaptive ability to combine the various individual components under more complex task conditions.

The sensory organization test (SOT) assesses the patient's continuous balance performance during a sequence of progressively more difficult sensory task conditions. Continuous performance measures of balance have several advantages. First, performance measures correlate more closely with a patient's functional status. Second, knowledge of the task conditions leading to poor performance help isolate the cause of instability to an individual balance component (or components) and document a patient's strategy for utilizing the components of balance under varying task conditions. Third, improvements in balance performance with repeated practice can help identify those patients for whom a course of balance therapy may be appropriate.

The disadvantage of measuring balance performance is the potential influence of both competing cognitive demands and "nonphysiologic" factors such as patient motivation, cooperation, and anxiety. Computerized dynamic posturography overcomes this limitation by combining the evoked response and performance methodologies. "Nonphysiologic" influences such as poor motivation, anxiety, and deliberate exaggeration of symptoms lead to inconsistencies in the results generated by the two types of protocols and can therefore be readily identified. The addition of protocols to measure the effect of competing cognitive demands on balance promises to provide another venue for documenting the impairments associated with aging and brain injuries (McNevin, Weir, & Quinn, 2013).

SELECTION, INSTRUCTION, AND PREPARATION OF PATIENTS FOR CDP TESTING

Minimum Physical Requirements for CDP Testing

Patients must be able to stand erect with eyes open and unassisted for periods of at least 1 min. Little useful information will be obtained from those who spontaneously lose their balance in less than a minute while standing eyes open on a fixed support surface. Special care should be taken with patients who have severe arthritic or orthopedic conditions affecting the ankles, knees, hips, or back. These conditions might be aggravated by the abrupt movements associated with "falls" into the supporting harness. The test administrator should take note of any musculoskeletal abnormalities affecting the relative lengths of the two legs; the ranges of ankle, knee, and hip joint motion; the strengths of leg and lower trunk musculature; and the postural orientation of limb and or trunk. While these types of musculoskeletal disorders do not preclude CDP testing, the interpretation of, especially, the motor coordination results relative to central nervous system and peripheral sensory functions must be qualified in these cases.

Patient Instructions

Prior to the day of testing, patients should be instructed to abstain from drugs that may affect their balance function. Ideally, drugs should be withheld for a period of 24 to 48 hr. Patients should also refrain from alcohol and caffeine during this period. Of course, the treating physician should be consulted to assure that the patient continues life-sustaining drugs such as insulin, blood pressure, heart, and seizure control medications. Women should be asked to wear loose-fitting slacks to permit easier mounting of the safety harness.

On the day of testing, the aim of pretest instructions is to minimize anxiety and assure the best possible patient performance. The purpose and general features of the test should be explained to the patient. The patient should be reassured that testing begins with easy tasks and only slowly progresses to more difficult tasks and that the safety harness is available in case one's balance is lost. Also it should be explained that CDP is a sensitive test which best documents the extent of any abnormality when the patient gives his or her best performance.

Preparation for Testing

To eliminate the risk of falls when balance is lost, the patient is fitted with a parachute-type safety harness connected to an overhead bar, as shown in Figure 18–1. The shoulder, waist, and leg straps of the harness are adjusted to ensure that any patient weight on the harness is transferred through the lower trunk rather than the upper trunk and shoulders. It is essential that the straps connecting the harness to the overhead bar are adjusted to allow complete freedom of motion within the normal limits of stability. An overly tight harness may provide the patient with external postural support and result in inappropriately high scores under the more difficult SOT conditions. An overly tight harness also will interfere with the forceplate measurements of the patient's movement strategy.

Proper placement of the feet on the forceplates is essential for accurate scoring of COG alignment during the SOT and MCT. To assure proper scoring of AP alignment, the medial maleolis of the ankle joint (the protruding ankle bone on the inside of the foot) is centered directly over a marking stripe that laterally transects the two forceplates. Accurate scoring of lateral alignment requires that the feet are laterally centered relative to the line dividing the left

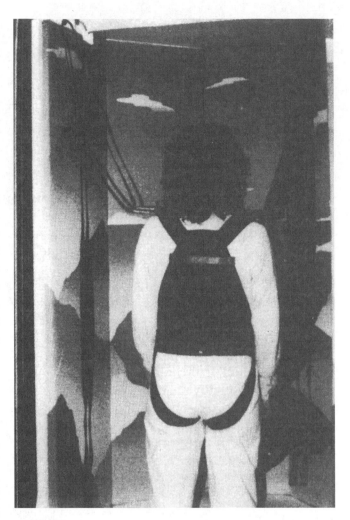

Figure 18–1. Fitting the overhead harness. From Jacobson, *Handbook of balance function testing*, 1E. © 1998 Delmar Learning, a part of Cengage Learning, Inc. Reproduced by permission. http://www.cengage.com/permissions

and right forceplates. Although the SOT equilibrium and strategy scores, and all MCT scores, are unaffected by foot placement, proper alignment of the ankle joints with the platform rotation axis gives the most accurate results.

Operator Administration of Testing

During administration of the test, the operator should observe the patient for signs of anxiety and fatigue. If either of these problems arise, the test can be interrupted for brief rest periods. In some cases of anxiety, the patient should be calmed by the operator who should describe each test protocol more thoroughly. Because the automatic posture control system is relatively unaffected by the patient's conscious efforts, results are not compromised by providing the patient a detailed description of the test protocol. When the patient is suspected of exaggerating symptoms for secondary gain, one preferred approach is to repeat the test and look for inconsistent results. When inconsistent CDP results are obtained, the finding can be further supported by repeating the test components in a random order.

The operator is provided a continuous display of the position of the patient's COG relative to the center of the support surface during all CDP protocols. During the SOT, the patient must be properly aligned on the forceplate and should be encouraged to stand as vertically as possible. The patient, however, should not be given feedback by the operator when the COG position is displaced from the center. Under no circumstances should the patient's foot placement on the forceplate be adjusted to center the COG curser. This is because abnormalities in COG alignment relative to center are one of the clinically useful measures provided by the SOT.

The purpose of the MCT and the PER tests is to detect abnormalities in the long-loop automatic pathways controlling balance movements. In contrast to the SOT, COG alignment errors in these tests can introduce artifacts in the results. Specifically, automatic responses may be suppressed in a leg bearing substantially less than the normal one-half share of body weight. Furthermore, forward or backward motor responses can be suppressed when the patient's COG is aligned substantially forward or backward of the center, respectively. For these reasons, the operator should determine that the patient is centered during administration of the MCT and PER tests. If the patient is forward, backward, or to one side, the operator can inform the patient and encourage him or her to correct the error. Again, however, the COG curser should not be centered by adjusting the placements of the patient's feet on the forceplate.

CDP RESULTS IN A CLINICALLY NORMAL POPULATION

A number of independent studies have gathered CDP results in samples of asymptomatic normal individuals. In the original study sponsored by Neurocom, Inc., a sample of 145 individuals, 58 distributed between 20 and 59 years of age, 54 between 60 and 69 years, and 28 between 70 and 79 years, received the complete SOT and MCT battery. An additional 54 individuals between 20 and 59 years of age were included only in the SOT portion of the assessment. A sample of 49 adult individuals between the ages of 20 and 69 received the complete PER test battery.[1]

The clinically normal samples consisted of unpaid volunteers recruited by ordinary means. Each subject was examined by a trained audiologist or neurotologist prior to testing. All subjects had normal vision (corrected with lenses, if necessary) and normal oculomotor function. No clinical vestibular or neurologic signs were present. Subjects with a history of vestibular, neurologic, or orthopedic disorders were excluded. Any subject taking medication affecting the central nervous system or known to affect balance and coordination were also excluded. Individuals above 65 years of age were also screened to exclude those with diabetes; symptoms of depression; and those with history of falls, blackouts, head or back injury, or joint surgery.

For all age ranges and CDP measures, the limits of clinically normal performance are defined to include the scores achieved by 95% of the asymptomatic sample. In the subsequent presentations of results, the reader will note that some CDP scores are considered clinically abnormal only when they deviate in one direction from the population average (one-sided distributions), while deviations of other scores in either direction from the average are considered clinically abnormal (two-sided distributions). For scores considered clinically abnormal in one direction from the mean, the normal limit is established at ±1.67 SD from the sample average. For

---

[1]The MCT and SOT data from samples of asymptomatic normal subjects were provided to NeuroCom International Inc., by Jules Friedman, M.D., Braintree Hospital, Braintree, MA; Susan Herdman, Ph.D., Johns Hopkins University Hospital, Baltimore, MD; David Cyr, Ph.D., Boys Town National Institute, Omaha, NE; and Neil Shepard, Ph.D., University of Michigan Hospitals, Ann Arbor, MI.

scores considered clinically abnormal in either direction from the mean, or upper and lower normal limits, are established at ±2 SD from the sample average.

The CDP results of the above asymptomatic normal samples are statistically summarized in the Appendices. A number of other laboratories have collected SOT, MCT, and PER results on independent samples of asymptomatic normal individuals (Beckley et al. 1991; Diener, Ackermann, Dichgans, & Guschlbauer, 1985; Huttunen & Romberg, 1990; Jackson & Epstein, 1991; Nardone, Giordano, Corra, & Schieppati, 1990; Peterka & Black, 1990a, 1990b; Wolfson et al., 1992). These studies used similar criteria for defining the clinically normal range, for adults and children, and in all cases their results compare favorably with those presented in this chapter.

POSTURE-EVOKED RESPONSE

Test

Support Surface Rotation as Stimulus

When the support surface rotates significantly faster than the body can move, the COG initially remains stationary and the ankle joints rotate. For example, rapid toes-up rotation of the support surface dorsiflexes the ankles and stretches the gastrocnemius muscles. Rapid toes-down rotation plantarflexes the ankles and stretches the tibialis anterior muscles. Brief and rapid rotations of the support surface are commonly used to elicit the PER.

In the standardized PER protocol, responses are elicited by a series of 10 to 20 toes-up or toes-down surface rotations. To ensure that the segmental reflex and automatic systems are saturated by the ankle "stretch" stimuli, high-velocity support surface rotations (50°/s for 80 ms) are used (Diener et al., 1984; Nardone et al., 1990). The addition of a random time interval between rotations serves to minimize anticipation by the patient and further enhance response amplitude. Because forward and backward leaning postures can influence the results, care must be taken to ensure that the patient is tested in an approximately centered stance position (Diener et al., 1983).

Presentation of PER Results

During support surface rotations, the relation between the directions of induced COG sway and ankle rotation is opposite that which occurs in physiologic sway while a subject is standing on a fixed support surface, as illustrated in Figure 18–2. The earliest two components of response to support surface rotation, termed *short latency* (SL) and *medium latency* (ML) responses, occur in the stretching ankle joint muscles. Rather than having a stabilizing effect on posture, in the stretching ankle joint these two responses serve to exaggerate the COG sway disturbance (Nardone et al., 1990). However, healthy subjects do not lose balance. This is because a later stabilizing component, termed the *long latency* (LL) response, occurs in the ankle muscles initially shortened by the rotations (Allum & Keshner, 1986; Diener, Dichgans, & Scholz, 1985).

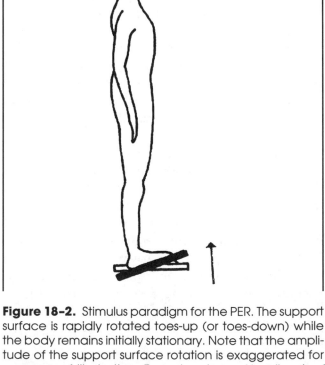

Figure 18–2. Stimulus paradigm for the PER. The support surface is rapidly rotated toes-up (or toes-down) while the body remains initially stationary. Note that the amplitude of the support surface rotation is exaggerated for purposes of illustration. From Jacobson, *Handbook of balance function testing*, 1E. © 1998 Delmar Learning, a part of Cengage Learning, Inc. Reproduced by permission. http://www.cengage.com/permissions

To measure the three response components, surface EMG signals are recorded simultaneously from the gastrocnemius and tibialis anterior muscles of the two legs. Each of the four raw EMG signals is full-wave rectified, low-pass filtered, and then averaged over the 10 to 20 trials relative to the onset times of the individual rotational stimuli. Figure 18–3 shows the graphical and raw data components obtained from a typical PER test in which a sequence of 10 toes-up rotations of the support surface was imposed. The top trace shows the rotational stimulus waveform. The subsequent four traces show the EMG waveforms of the four ankle muscles, each averaged relative to the stimulus onset times.

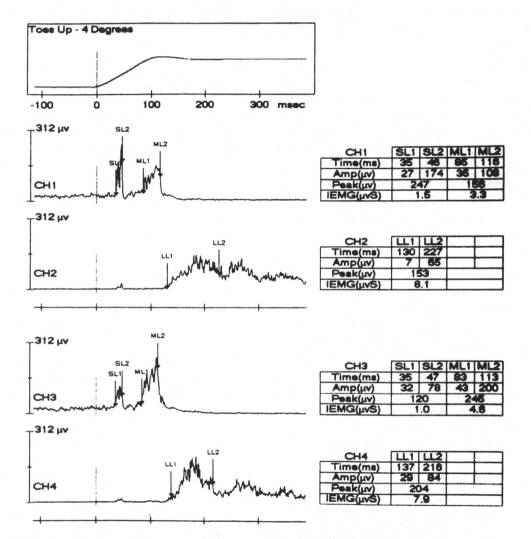

Figure 18-3. Averaged data summaries of the toes up PER test of a clinically normal 28-year-old man. The EMG traces are full-wave rectified EMG signals averaged over 20 trials. Channel 1 is right gastrocnemius; channel 2, right tibialis; channel 3, left gastrocnemius; and channel 4, left tibialis. Arrows show the marked beginning (1) and ending (2) times of the SL, ML, and LL components. Numerical data use similar labels to show beginning and ending times of the three components. Additional numerical data show the signal amplitude at each marker, the signal peak between pairs of markers, and the integrated area (IEMG) between pairs of markers. From Jacobson, *Handbook of balance function testing*, 1E. © 1998 Delmar Learning, a part of Cengage Learning, Inc. Reproduced by permission. http://www.cengage.com/permissions

PER Results in Clinically Normal Subjects

In asymptomatic normal subjects, toes-up rotations of the support surface elicit the SL and ML responses in the gastrocnemius muscles of both legs (see Figure 18–3). The average latencies of the SL responses are approximately 32 ms. Latency variations among individuals are less than a few milliseconds. These SL responses are attributed to the monosynaptic stretch reflex system (Dichgans & Diener, 1985; Nardone et al., 1990).

Medium latency responses are identifiable in some but not all clinically asymptomatic subjects. In those subjects with identifiable ML components, average latencies in the gastrocnumius muscles are approximately 80 ms. ML responses are attributed to polysynaptic segmental reflex mechanisms (Dietz, Quintern, & Berger, 1984; Dietz, Quintern, Berger, & Schenck, 1985). Because the SL and ML responses both resist the rotation of the ankle joints, they exaggerate rather than help compensate for the associated COG sway disturbances.

Following toes-up rotation, well-defined LL responses are recorded in the tibialis anterior muscles of both legs of all subjects. Average LL response latencies are approximately 110 ms. The LL responses are mediated by requirements for postural stability rather than local stretch inputs (Diener, Dichgans, Bacher, & Guschlbauer, 1984; Nardone et al., 1990; Nashner, 1976). Long latency responses observed during PER testing are thought to be equivalent to the automatic postural responses that are the main line of defense against many types of unexpected postural disturbances (Horak & Nashner, 1986; Nardone et al., 1990; Nashner et al., 1979).

Toes-down rotations of the support surface stretch the tibialis anterior muscles and displace the COG forward. Because myotatic stretch reflexes are relatively inactive in the flexor leg muscles of humans, SL responses are typically not observed in the stretching tibialis anterior muscles. However, the ML and LL components in the tibialis anterior and gastrocnemius muscles, respectively, are observed with latencies similar to those reported for toes-up rotations.

The short, medium, and long response latencies reported for asymptomatic normal samples are summarized in Appendix 18–A. Similar PER results in clinically normal samples of subjects have been reported by other laboratories (Beckley, Bloem, van Dijk, Roos, & Remier, 1991; Diener, Ackermann, Dichgans, & Guschlbauer, 1985; Huttunen & Romberg, 1990; Nardone et al., 1990). Because only delayed response latencies are considered abnormal, one-sided distributions are used to identify the upper limits of clinically normal latencies for the SL, ML, and LL components.

Except for one factor, the results presented in Appendix 18–A are consistent. In three of the older studies the latencies reported for all three components were approximately 10 to 15 ms greater in comparison to those in more recent investigations. The probable cause for the 10 to 15 ms differences in latencies was the use of the command signal onset, rather than the actual onset time of the surface rotation, as the benchmark time.

Potential Problems With PER Testing

The principal technical problem with PER testing is obtaining accurate and reliable EMG recordings from the ankle joint musculature. Sources of EMG inaccuracy include electrical resistance between skin and electrodes too high to be compatible with the recording amplifiers, external electrical noise contamination, and inaccurate placement of the electrodes. The first two sources can be minimized by thorough skin preparation for EMG recording, proper placement and spacing of electrodes, differential amplifiers with high common mode rejection, and adequate patient grounding. Errors in electrode placement can be minimized by palpating the skin to ensure electrode placement over the belly of the muscle rather than neighboring bony areas.

A potential physiologic problem with PER testing is suppression of the LL response component. Suppression will occur only when the patient is not actively controlling balance during the test. To minimize this source of error, the safety harness must not be overly tight. In addition, the operator must motivate the patient to avoid falls into the harness if at all possible.

In many patients, identification of the ML component is difficult. This component is absent in some patients and is combined with the SL component in others. Although there are no technical remedies for this problem, the test results are valid without the

ML component. This is because most of the diagnostic value of the PEP is obtained by determining the latency characteristics of the SL and LL components.

STANDARD MOTOR CONTROL TEST

Horizontal Support Surface Displacement

In the MCT, automatic postural responses are elicited by translating the support surface in the horizontal direction. When the support surface translates horizontally more rapidly than the body COG, the COG remains approximately stationary and becomes offset relative to the base of support as illustrated in Figure 18–4 (Beckley et al., 1991; Nashner, 1977).

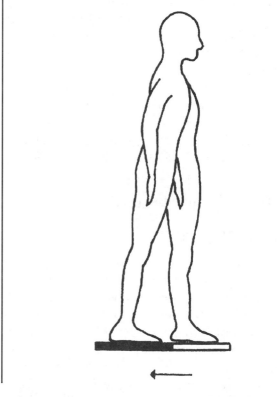

Figure 18-4. Stimulus paradigm for the MCT. The support surface is translated backward (or forward) while the position of the upper body remains initially stationary. Note that the amplitude of the translation is exaggerated for purposes of illustration. From Jacobson, *Handbook of balance function testing,* 1E. © 1998 Delmar Learning, a part of Cengage Learning, Inc. Reproduced by permission. http://www.cengage.com/permissions

Backward translation stretches the gastrocnemius muscles and displaces the COG forward in relation to the base of support. The COG is re-centered over the base of support by a backward-directed automatic postural response. Similarly, forward surface translation stretches the tibialis anterior muscles and displaces the COG backward. This disturbance to posture is corrected by a forward-directed automatic postural response.

In contrast to the responses elicited by surface rotations during the PER, activation of the stretching ankle joint muscles in response to horizontal translation is helpful in compensating for the COG sway disturbance. Compared to the rapid rotation used in PER testing, support surface translation rotates the body about the ankle joints at a significantly much slower speed ranging between 3°/s and 8°/s. At these slower rotational speeds SL responses in the stretching ankle muscles are seldom observed (Nashner, 1976, 1977; Nashner et al., 1979). Rather, the earliest responses occur in the stretching ankle joint muscles and correspond in time to the LL responses observed in the PER. These compensatory postural movements are termed *automatic postural responses*. This is because their latencies are too long to be mediated by the segmental stretch reflex pathways but too short to be initiated under voluntary control of the subject (Nashner & Cordo, 1981).

The MCT protocol is summarized in Table 18–2. In the protocol, the automatic postural response system is analyzed over a range of velocities and directions using forward and backward translations varying in magnitude (threshold, intermediate, and saturating) and timing (random intervals between stimuli). Translations of the same direction and size are always imposed in groups of three. Results from the three trials are then averaged to obtain a stable characterization of the active force responses.

Responses to forward and backward translations are analyzed separately, because the flexor and extensor pathways mediating automatic postural responses are anatomically separate and may be effected differently by a disease process. Responses of the left and right legs are analyzed separately, because the pathways mediating responses on the two sides can also be selectively effected by disease. The random intervals between trials minimize the likelihood that the patient can anticipate the onset of displacements.

Table 18–2. Protocol for the Motor Control Test

Stimulus	Number of Trials	Measurements
Backward translation 1.25 em in 250 ms (height scaled)	3	
Backward translation 3.15 em in 300 ms (height scaled)	3	Active force responses: latency, strength symmetry
Backward translation 5.7 em in 400 ms (height scaled)	3	
Toes-up rotation 4.0° in 500 ms	5	Sway energy
Forward translation 1.25 em in 250 ms (height scaled)	3	
Forward translation 3.15 em in 300 ms (height scaled)	3	Active force responses: latency, strength symmetry
Forward translation 5.7 em in 400 ms (height scaled)	3	
Toes-up rotation 4.0° in 500 ms	5	Sway energy

In the standard MCT protocol, the support surface translates at a constant velocity over a fixed interval of time to achieve a predetermined velocity and amplitude of COG displacement. Using a 180-cm-tall patient as an example, a small translation of 1.25 cm over a 250-ms interval rotates the COG about the ankle joints at 2.8°/s for a total distance of 0.7°. This is approximately the threshold displacement required to elicit an automatic postural response. A medium translation of 3.15 cm over a 300-ms interval rotates the COG about the ankle joints at 6°/s for a total distance of 1.8°. Finally, a large translation of 5.70 cm over a 400-ms interval rotates the COG about the ankle joints at 8°/s for a total distance of 3.2°. This stimulus produces an approximately maximum amplitude automatic response in the healthy subject (Horak, Diener, & Nashner, 1989).

For individuals shorter or taller than 180 cm, the translation amplitude is automatically adjusted to produce the same velocity and amplitude of COG sway. For individuals shorter or taller than 180 cm, the distance the surface translates is proportionately smaller or larger, respectively, while the durations of the translations are the same.

Recording Active Force Responses

Automatic postural responses to support surface translations are recorded using separate forceplates for each foot, each of which measures the active compensatory force exerted by the foot against the support surface. When each foot is properly positioned on the forceplate, the forceplate measures the portion of total body weight carried by the foot and the position of the center of vertical force exerted by the foot relative to the ankle joint position. The weight and position quantities are used to calculate the active torque exerted by the musculature of leg about the ankle joint (Nashner, 1977; Nashner et al., 1979).

Presentation of MCT Results

Real-Time MCT Display

The computer displays a real-time summary of the raw COG sway data and the resulting active force latency scores during administration of the MCT. The latency plot on the left side of the display indicates the current movement direction, amplitude, and trial number, and also plots the latency scores of all completed trials. In the actual system printouts, green bars show latencies falling within the normal range, and red bars show latencies falling above the normal limits established for the age-matched clinically normal sample. Numbers on each bar indicate the confidence level of the automatic scoring algorithm. If the operator chooses to repeat a previously executed and scored trial, the replacement bar is striped.

The right section of the display charts the AP and lateral positions of the COG in real time. This display accurately indicates COG position relative to the center of the base of support when the patient's feet are properly placed on the support surface. Because accurate scoring of MCT latencies and strengths depends on weight bearing within the normal range, alignment of the COG (lateral, forward, or backward) should be corrected if possible with the following procedure. The positions of the patient's feet should be checked first to assure that inaccurate foot placement is not the cause. Each foot should not be positioned away from the proper position on the forceplate as the means to correct the

COG misalignment. Instead, the patient should be encouraged by the operator to shift the upper body to center the COG.

Weight Symmetry

The graphic and raw data components of a typical MCT result are shown for one movement direction in Figure 18–5. In the complete MCT printout, an identical series of plots are included for backward and forward movement responses on the left and right sides of the page, respectively. For each movement direction, separate plots show weight symmetry, active force response latency, and active force

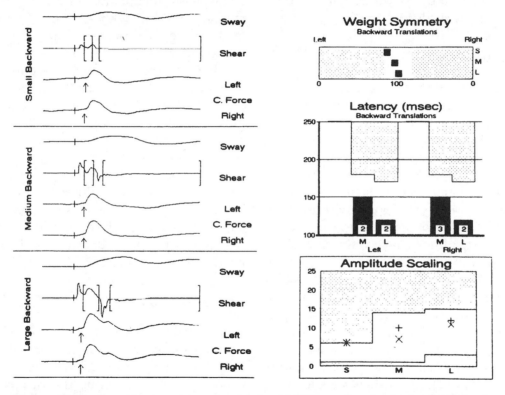

Figure 18–5. Graphical and raw summaries of MCT results of a typically clinically normal adult for backward support surface translations. Traces on the left show COG sway, horizontal shear force, and left and right center of vertical force (COF) (torque) responses averaged over three trials each for the three sizes of perturbations. Vertical lines show onset of surface translations. Arrows on the COF traces show onset times of the active force responses. Plots on the right show the relative bearing of weight between the two legs (100 equals perfect symmetry), the active force response latencies for left and right legs and the two larger sized translations, and the active force response strengths for the left (x) and right (+) legs. Shaded areas show scores falling outside the clinically normal limits, based on the normal population study. From Jacobson, *Handbook of balance function testing*, 1E. © 1998 Delmar Learning, a part of Cengage Learning, Inc. Reproduced by permission. http://www .cengage.com/permissions

response strength scores. In all of the plots, open areas encompass the range of scores considered to be within the clinically normal limits based on results from the asymptomatic sample.

A weight symmetry plot for each movement direction indicates the percentage of total body weight borne by each leg during the automatic postural response. Weight symmetry is displayed as a nondimensional quantity, with a score of 100 indicating that weight is borne equally by the two legs. The weight symmetry score decreases to zero or increases to 200 when all the weight is borne by the left or right leg, respectively. Weight symmetry scores are important, because the onset latencies and the strengths of automatic postural responses in each leg are influenced by the fraction of total body weight supported by the leg.

Active Force Latency

The automatic postural response elicited by a support surface translation compensates for COG sway by exerting active torque about the ankle joints. As the patient's COG moves forward (or backward) in response to horizontal surface translation, the initial resistance due to the inherent stiffness of the ankle joints is small and insufficient to stabilize the COG sway (Gurfinkel, Lipshits, & Popov, 1974; Nashner, 1976). The myotatic reflexes are either too weak or inhibited during standing to have a significant overall impact on the active force response (El'ner, Popov, & Gurfinkel, 1972; Gurfinkel et al., 1974). Active force increases abruptly within 30 to 40 ms following onset of the automatic component of the postural response at 90 to 100 ms latencies as recorded by EMG (Dichgans & Diener, 1985; Nashner, 1977; Nashner et al., 1979)? This is indicated by an abrupt and rapid increase in force resistance as measured by the forceplates. This sequence of events is illustrated in the raw data components of Figure 18–5.

The active force response latencies are calculated automatically for each leg and for each direction and magnitude of displacement, along with a quality factor indicating the reliability of the latency score. To produce each latency score, four separate slope detection algorithms are used to identify the active force "takeoff point." The four results are then compared. If results of none of the algorithms agree within a 10-ms tolerance, the longest of the four latency scores is used, and a quality factor of 1 is indicated.

If two or more scores are within 10 ms, the longest of these scores is used, and a quality factor of 2 to 4 indicates the number scores within the tolerance. Thus, a quality factor of 4 indicates the highest level of consistency, while a 1 indicates the least consistency. Latency scores for each leg and translation size are presented as separate bars in the latency plot.

The second page of the MCT printout shows the active force response traces of each leg and the COG sway averaged over the three trials. The latency takeoff points identified by the computer for the left and right leg active force responses are marked with arrows as shown in Figure 18–5. If the operator disagrees with the placement of one or more arrows, a magnified view of the force traces in question can be displayed on the monitor and the takeoff points manually marked by the operator. In these cases the quality factor is displayed as an "M" on the graphic printout page.

Because the active force response elicited by a small translation is near the automatic response threshold, the associated latency is quite variable and in some instances impossible to identify. Medium and large translations, in contrast, elicit vigorous active force responses with a high degree of latency symmetry between left and right legs, and between forward and backward translations of the same magnitude. Thus, latency results from medium and large translations can be of significant value in identifying motor system abnormalities in patients with imbalance or postural instability.

Active Force Strength

Adjusting the size of support surface translations for variations in patient height assures that the velocity and amplitude of COG sway is the same for all patients. In physical terms, this means that a given size translation imparts the same sway momentum to all patients, regardless of individual variations in body height and weight. To counteract the sway momentum produced by the translation, the patient must exert a restoring force that imparts approximately twice the momentum in the opposite direction. Half of the restoring momentum is required to stop the COG sway; the other half, to return the body to the original equilibrium position. For this reason, the magnitude (strength) of the active force response is best characterized by the momentum generated by the active force.

Following onset of the active force response, the support surface continues to translate, displace the COG, and stretch the ankle joint muscles. This requires the continued exertion of active force by the two legs to regain balance. The magnitude (strength) of this active force is quantified relative to the rate of increase of ankle torque exerted by each leg over a 150-ms interval following the latency onset by dividing the raw scores by patient height and weight compensates for differences in patient stature and produces strength scores with the appropriate units of (sway) angular momentum.

For each movement direction, active force strength is plotted as a function of translation size for each leg and translation size. In the clinically normal individual, strength scores for equivalent-sized translations in the two directions are similar. In addition, lateral strength symmetry is demonstrated when the active force responses for a given size translation are similar in the two legs. When differences in strength between the two legs exceed the normal range, the data points in question are enclosed by a box.

MCT Results in a Clinically Normal Sample

Selected results from the asymptomatic normal sample of individuals are described in Appendix 18–A. Latency scores in normal children are similar to those of the adults (Hassan & Azzam, 2012). For all age ranges, the average weight symmetry scores are near 100, indicating that weight is borne equally by the two legs. Because scores both significantly above and below 100 (weight bearing to the right and left of center, respectively) are considered abnormal, the clinically normal limits for symmetry are set at ±2 SD from the average.

In all age groups and in both movement directions, onset latencies are slightly longer for the medium than for the large translations. Furthermore, the response latencies show the expected slight increases with age. Other research studies have also shown subtle variations in EMG latencies that are dependent on the velocity and magnitude of the evoking translation (Diener et al., 1984; Nardone et al., 1990). These latencies have been shown to increase with age (Peterka & Black, 1990b; Wolfson et al., 1992). Only those latency scores significantly longer than the averages of the asymptomatic

normal sample are considered clinically abnormal. Thus, the upper limits for clinically normal latencies are set at 1.67 SD above the sample averages.

In all age groups, the height and weight compensated response strengths are symmetrical for the two legs and movement directions. For all translation magnitudes, the average strength scores are sufficient to return the COG to the centered position without excessive undershoot or overshoot. Specifically, the angular momenta imparted to the body by the small, medium, and large translations are 2.8°/s, 6.0°/s, and 8.0°/s, respectively. To return the COG to center, the total angular momentum generated by the two legs must be twice that produced by the translation. One half of the response momentum is needed to arrest the sway, the other half to return the body COG to the center position. This is accomplished when each leg generates angular momentum equal to that of the translation. Figure 18–6 shows that, on average, asymptomatic normal individuals produce the amount of active force necessary to accurately

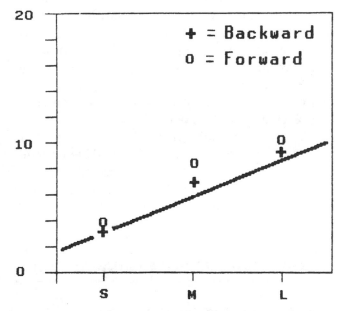

Figure 18-6. Active force strengths in a clinically normal sample of persons 20 to 59 years of age as functions of translation size and direction. The heavy line shows the response strengths needed to exactly re-center the COG. Vertical units of measurement refer to angular momentum per unit of body mass (deg/s/kg). Horizontal notations refer to amplitude of displacement (S = small; M = medium; L = large). From Jacobson, *Handbook of balance function testing*, 1E. © 1998 Delmar Learning, a part of Cengage Learning, Inc. Reproduced by permission. http://www.cengage.com/permissions

return the body COG to the original centered position. Response strengths significantly weaker or stronger than the averages of the asymptomatic normal sample are considered clinically abnormal. Thus, the normal limits of the strengths for each age group are set at ±2 SD from the sample averages.

Potential Problems With MCT Results

The greatest potential sources of error in the MCT are latency and strength changes in one leg caused by a substantial unweighting of that leg during testing. Errors in one leg are readily recognized by the combination of delayed latencies, low response strengths, and weight bearing toward the opposite leg. The problem can only be remedied during testing. The operator should monitor the real time COG cursor during MCT testing and instruct the patient to center the COG cursor within the normal limits whenever a substantial lateral displacement of the cursor is noted.

Weak response strengths create the potential for latency scoring errors. This problem is minimized by reviewing the raw data and determining that the marker arrows are appropriately placed at the active force response takeoff points. Questionable scores can be manually rescored by the operator. In the case of a very weak response, an accurate determination of latency may not be possible.

The response takeoff point and strength may be difficult to identify in highly unstable patients, because responses are obscured by the high level of background sway activity. Manual review of the raw data is sometimes helpful in these cases.

AUTOMATIC RESPONSE ADAPTATION

Slow Support Surface Rotations

The adaptation protocol exposes the patient to a series of five identical toes-up or toes-down rotations of the support surface. In contrast to the PER test, the rotations are imposed at a relatively slow 8°/s. These relatively slower stimulus velocities rotate the ankle joints at velocities similar to those generated by the large support surface translations during the MCT. Because these slower stimulus velocities do not satu-

rate the automatic posture control system, it is possible to measure adaptive changes in the patient's responses over the course of the five rotations.

A series of five identical rotations is typically interposed between sets of support surface translations. When the first unexpected surface rotation is imposed after a set of surface translations, the automatic posture control system is initially prepared to actively resist ankle joint rotation as a means to stabilize COG sway. Because resisting the ankle joint rotation is destabilizing when the surface rotates, the COG sway is frequently increased during the recovery period following the first surface rotation. Asymptomatic subjects, however, do not typically lose their balance. By the fourth and fifth rotations of the series, the automatic system attenuates the ankle joint resistance. This adaptive change enhances the subject's stability during the recovery period (Nashner, 1976).

The adaptive mechanisms responsible for attenuating ankle joint resistance and reducing COG sway during the recovery period following support surface rotation are complex and probably involve both reduction in the amplitude of the stretch-evoked (destabilizing) responses and enhancement of the later stabilizing responses. Nevertheless, when the patient makes these adaptive changes, COG sway is reduced during the recovery periods following the last few rotational trials of the series.

Presentation of Adaptation Results

Sway energy is used as a nonspecific but quantitative measure of the magnitude of COG sway during the recovery period following a support surface rotation. Sway energy is a weighted sum of the root mean square COG sway velocity and sway acceleration measured over the 2.5-s interval immediately following rotation. While this measure does not reflect changes within the individual response components described previously, it is an accurate measure of the overall functional effect of these adaptive changes.

Adaptation results are presented by plotting a separate sway energy score for each of the five rotations. The display of results of toes-up rotation, which elicits a backward COG displacement, is displayed under the backward movement response results of the MCT. Similarly, the results of toes-down rotations are displayed under the forward movement results of the MCT.

Adaptation Results in the Clinically Normal Sample

Asymptomatic normal individuals show progressive reductions in sway energy over the course of five repeated exposures to toes-up or toes-down rotations, as shown in Figure 18–7. Adaptation scores are

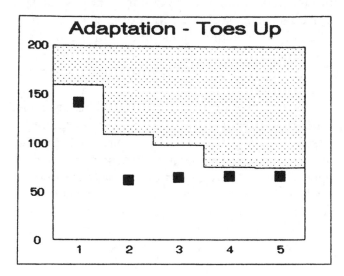

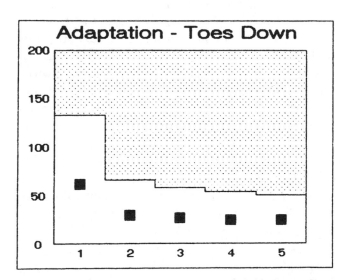

Figure 18-7. Graphical summary of the adaptation results of a typical clinically normal subject. The vertical axes show the sway energy expended during corrective responses. The horizontal axes show trial numbers. Shaded areas show scores falling outside the clinically normal limits, based on the normal population study. From Jacobson, *Handbook of balance function testing*, 1E. © 1998 Delmar Learning, a part of Cengage Learning, Inc. Reproduced by permission. http://www.cengage .com/permissions

similar in children (Hassan & Azzam, 2012). Even though the sway energy scores of younger and older subjects are similar during the first toes-up and toes-down trials, improvements in stability are significantly greater in the younger subjects by the fourth and fifth trials. Poorer adaptation in the elderly may be caused by a slowing of central adaptation, musculoskeletal factors which increase mechanical stiffness and/or reduce muscle strength at the ankles, or a combination of these factors (Horak, Shupert, & Mirka, 1989; Wolfson et al., 1992).

The upper limits for clinically normal sway energies are set at 1.67 SD above the sample averages. This is because only significantly increased sway energies are considered abnormal.

Potential Problems With Adaptation Testing

Sway energy scores may be inaccurate when a patient falls, steps back, or stumbles on the platform rather than maintaining balance with the feet in place. When the patient's response to a rotation is a free-fall, step, or stumble, the operator should mark the trial as a fall. The maximum sway energy score is assigned to these trials. If a free fall is not marked as a fall by the operator, a deceptively low sway energy score will usually result. In contrast, unmarked steps and stumbles usually result in more appropriately high sway energy scores.

SENSORY ORGANIZATION TESTING

Sensory Conditions

The six conditions of the SOT protocol are designed to assess the patient's ability to effectively use visual, vestibular, and somatosensory inputs to maintain balance, and to select the input(s) providing the functionally most appropriate orientation information under a variety of conditions. Sensory organization is evaluated by selectively disrupting somatosensory and/or visual information regarding body COG orientation in relation to vertical and then measuring the patient's ability to maintain balance.

Somatosensory and/or visual information is disrupted by a method commonly referred to as *sway-referencing*. This method involves the tilting of the support surface and/or the visual surround about an axis colinear with the ankle joints to directly follow the patient's COG sway in the AP direction (Nashner, Black, & Wall, 1982). Under sway-referenced conditions, the orientation of the support surface and/or the visual surround remains constant in relation to the COG sway angle. Although the somatosensory and visual systems continue to provide information during sway-referenced conditions, these inputs contain no functionally useful information relating the orientation of the body COG relative to the gravity vertical.

Information derived from a sense subjected to sway-referencing (vision/proprioception) indicates that the orientation of the body COG relative to gravity is not changing when in fact it is. Healthy subjects ignore a sway-referenced sensory input that is functionally inaccurate and maintain balance using other sensory inputs. In addition to sway-referencing, eyes-closed conditions are used to further isolate the somatosensory and vestibular systems. Unfortunately, there is no noninvasive way to selectively disrupt vestibular orientation information.

In the classical version of the SOT, the visual surround is a "mechanical" enclosure that can be tilted forward or backward about the ankle joints under continuous control of a servomotor. The visual scene within the enclosure is fixed and rotational motions are limited to ±10 degrees about the ankle joint axis only. A recent development is the "virtual reality" version of the SOT in which computer animated visual images are projected onto a fixed enclosure which fully surrounds the patient's field of view. The virtual reality approach has the distinct advantage of allowing not only sway-referenced vision in the forward-backwards direction but also lateral sway-referencing, continuous and random visual flow motions in any combination of linear and angular dimensions as well as control over critical elements of visual orientation perception including differentiating between peripheral and central field effects, parallax effects and the relative distance of objects, and the effects of spatial frequencies and contrast. Recent research has already demonstrated some of the potential improvements in assessment and training capabilities (Keshner & Kenyan, 2009; Lange et al., 2010; Streepey, Kenyan, & Keshner, 2007).

Protocol for the Sensory Organization Test

The classical SOT exposes the patient to the six sensory conditions illustrated in Figure 18–8. The six conditions consist of all combinations of normal (fixed), eyes closed, and sway-referenced visual and support surface sensory conditions (Black et al., 1978; Nashner et al., 1982). The six conditions are presented beginning with the simplest, eyes open on a fixed support surface, and ending with the most challenging in which the support surface and the visual surround are both sway-referenced.

During sensory conditions 1 and 2, the support surface and visual surround are fixed, and the patient stands with eyes open and eyes closed, respectively. These trials provide baseline measures of the patient's postural stability. Under sensory condition 3, the surface remains fixed while the patient stands with eyes open within a sway-referenced visual surround. In the last three test conditions, the support surface is sway-referenced while the patient stands with eyes open and with the visual surround fixed (condition 4), eyes closed (condition 5), and eyes open and the visual surround sway-referenced (condition 6).

The complete protocol consists of eighteen 20-s trials, three consecutive trials for each of the six sensory conditions. During each trial, the patient is instructed to ignore any surface or visual surround motion and remain upright and as steady as possible. Three trials for each sensory condition improve the reliability of the resulting measures. The repeated measures also provide an opportunity to determine whether the patient's performance improves under a given condition with practice.

Potential additions to the original six sensory conditions include a visual surround flowing continuously in one or a combination of dimensions while the patient stands under fixed and sway-referenced support surface conditions.

Equilibrium Scores

During each trial, the COG sway angle is calculated in real time based on the biomechanical relations between the position of the center of vertical force (COF) exerted by the feet against the support surface, the position of the COG, and the limits of stability (Koles & Castelein, 1980; Riley, Mann, & Hodge,

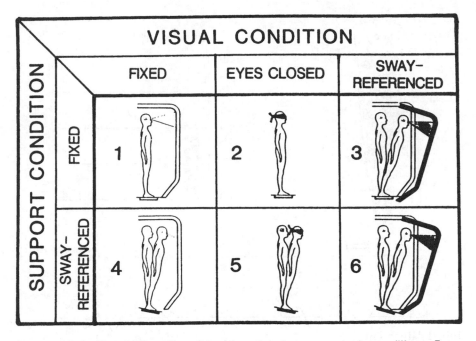

Figure 18-8. The SOT protocol showing the six sensory test conditions. From Jacobson, *Handbook of balance function testing*, 1E. © 1998 Delmar Learning, a part of Cengage Learning, Inc. Reproduced by permission. http://www.cengage.com/permissions

1990). When the frequency of COG sway is below 0.5 Hz, the COG is located vertically above the COF. As COG sway frequency increases, movements of the COG lag behind the COF and decrease in relative size (Nashner et al., 1989; Riley et al., 1990). A real-time, multiple pole digital filter is used to approximate these amplitude and frequency relations between the COF and COG motions.

A separate measure of stability, called the *equilibrium score*, is calculated for each trial. As shown in Figure 18–9, the equilibrium score is a nondimensional percentage that compares the patient's peak amplitude of AP sway to the theoretical AP limits of stability (LOS). The patient's theoretical LOS is the maximum forward and backward COG sway angles that can be achieved by a normal individual of similar height and weight. Equilibrium scores near 100% indicate little sway, while scores approaching zero indicate that sway is nearing the LOS. Trials in which the patient exceeds the LOS and loses balance are arbitrarily assigned equilibrium scores of zero.

Recent research indicates that postural sway is a complex process that is best characterized by at least two measures, one related to sway amplitude and the other to sway velocity (Maurer & Peterka, 2005;

Pavol, 2005). These studies suggest that the sensitivity of SOT measures can be used by calculating a second RMS sway velocity score for each trial.

Center of Gravity Alignment

For each SOT trial, separate AP and lateral alignment scores are calculated by averaging the AP and lateral positions of the COG sway angle over the 20-s test interval. These calculations are based on the assumption that the patient's spontaneous COG swaying over the course of the trial occurs symmetrically about the point of COG alignment.

Ankle Versus Hip Movements

When ankle movements are used to control sway, the associated low-frequency motions of the COG generate relatively little horizontal shear force against the support surface. Higher-frequency hip and upper body movements, in contrast, generate small but rapid shifts in COG position and much larger horizontal shear forces (Horak & Nashner, 1986; Nashner & McCollum, 1985). Based on this biomechanical

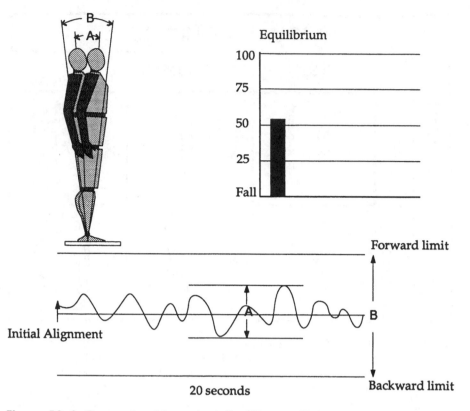

Figure 18–9. The method for calculating the equilibrium score from the raw COG sway data of a 20-s trial. The equilibrium score compares the maximum patient anteroposterior sway angle (A) to the patient's theoretical limits of stability (B). As A increases from 0 toward B, the equilibrium score decreases from 100 (perfect stability) toward 0 (loss of balance). From Jacobson, *Handbook of balance function testing*, 1E. © 1998 Delmar Learning, a part of Cengage Learning, Inc. Reproduced by permission. http://www.cengage.com/permissions

principle, the relative amounts of ankle and hip movement are determined by comparing the peak-to-peak amplitude of the horizontal shear force to a theoretical limit for normal of similar weight. Although this method provides an accurate measure of the extent of hip and upper body movement activity, this score does not measure the time-dependent trajectory of the actual body motion. The accuracy and time-dependent trajectory of upper body movement activity can be substantially improved with the addition of one or more body mounted IMUs.

Presentation of Sensory Organization Test Results

Real-Time Display of Results

The CRT display presents a real-time summary of the raw COG sway data and the resulting equilibrium

scores during administration of the SOT. The left side of the display indicates the currently selected sensory condition and trial number, and also plots the equilibrium scores of all completed trials. In the actual system printouts, green bars show scores of completed trials falling within the normal range, while red bars show scores below the fifth percentile relative to the age-matched clinically normal sample. If the operator chooses to repeat a previously executed and scored trial, the replacement bar is striped.

The right section of the CRT provides a real-time plot of the AP and lateral positions of the COG. This display accurately indicates COG position relative to the center of the base of support when the patient's feet are properly placed on the support surface. If lateral, forward, or backward alignment of the COG is noted during testing, the positions of the patient's feet should be rechecked for accurate placement. Under no circumstances, however, should the patient be coached to reposition the feet away from their proper positions or to shift the COG, as these procedures will invalidate the COG alignment scores.

Raw Sway Data and Equilibrium Scores

The raw data and graphic components of a typical SOT result are shown in Figures 18–10 and 18–11,

respectively. The first graphic plot summarizes the equilibrium scores obtained from a maximum of three trials under each of the six sensory conditions. Each equilibrium score is presented as a bar. All areas of the plot in which equilibrium scores fall below the fifth percentile relative to the age-matched clinically normal sample are indicated by stippling.

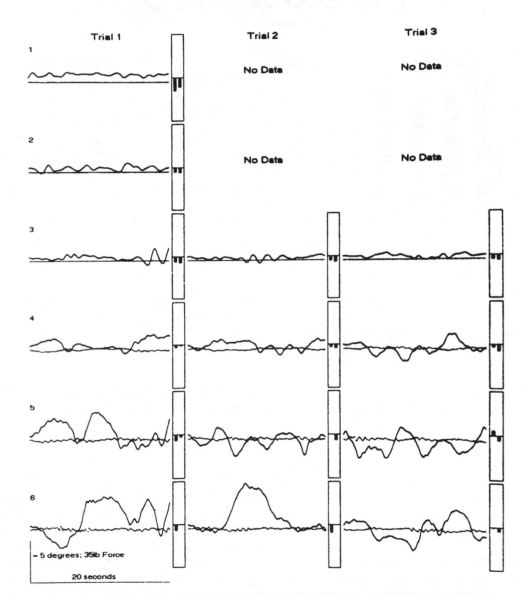

Figure 18-10. Raw data summary of the SOT results shown in Figure 18–9. The numbered rows show COG sway responses for each sensory test condition. Note that conditions 1 and 2 were tested at only one trial each. Heavy traces show the COG sway (up indicates forward and down indicates backward). Fine traces show the horizontal shear force. Bars to the right of each table show COG alignment. Shaded areas show scores falling outside the clinically normal limits, based on the normal population study. From Jacobson, *Handbook of balance function testing*, 1E. © 1998 Delmar Learning, a part of Cengage Learning, Inc. Reproduced by permission. http://www.cengage.com/permissions

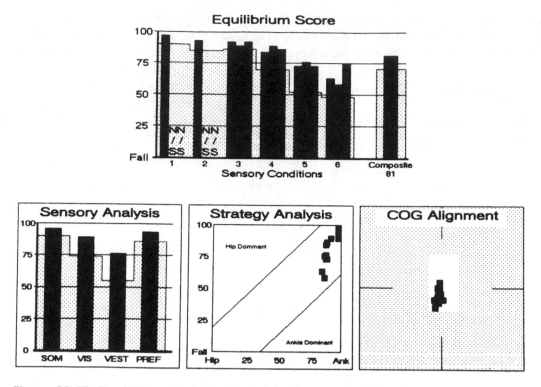

Figure 18–11. The SOT results of a typical clinically normal subject. The upper plot shows the equilibrium scores for the six sensory conditions (up to three trials per condition) and the composite equilibrium score. The lower plots show the four sensory analysis ratios, the analysis of movement pattern versus equilibrium score, and COG alignment. Shaded areas show scores falling outside the clinically normal limits, based on the normal population study. From Jacobson, *Handbook of balance function testing*, 1E. © 1998 Delmar Learning, a part of Cengage Learning, Inc. Reproduced by permission. http://www.cengage.com/permissions

The raw data traces for each 20-s trial are presented using the two formats (see Figure 18–10). One format plots the AP sway angle (heavy trace) and the horizontal shear force (light trace) signals as concurrent functions of time. The second format (not illustrated) plots the AP versus the lateral component of the COG sway angle.

Composite Equilibrium Score

A patient's overall level of performance on the SOT is best characterized by the composite equilibrium score, which is the average of the following 14 equilibrium scores: the condition 1 average score, the condition 2 average score, and the three scores from each of the conditions 3 through 6 trials. Note that the resulting composite score is a weighted average that emphasizes the equilibrium scores for conditions 3 through 6. This weighting is used because sensory balance deficits are more readily reflected under the more difficult sensory conditions.

Sensory Organization Analysis

The specific nature of a patient's sensory balance problem is best characterized by quantifying relative differences in the equilibrium scores among the six sensory conditions. Differences in equilibrium scores are shown in the sensory organization analysis plot of Figure 18–11. Relative differences in scores are quantified using ratios in which the three-trial average equilibrium score of one sensory condition is divided by the three-trial average score of another condition. The four equilibrium score ratios and their physiologic meaning are summarized in Figure 18–12.

The somatosensory ratio, which compares the condition 2 to the condition 1 equilibrium score, quantifies the extent of stability loss when the patient closes

SENSORY ANALYSIS			
RATIO NAME	**TEST CONDITIONS**	**RATIO PAIR**	**SIGNIFICANCE**
SOM Somatosensory	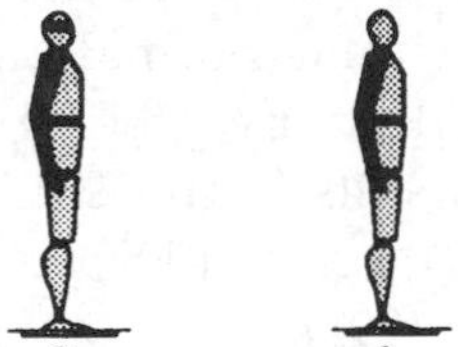 2 1	Condition 2 / Condition 1	**Question:** Does sway increase when visual cues are removed? **Low scores:** Patient makes poor use of somatosensory references.
VIS Visual	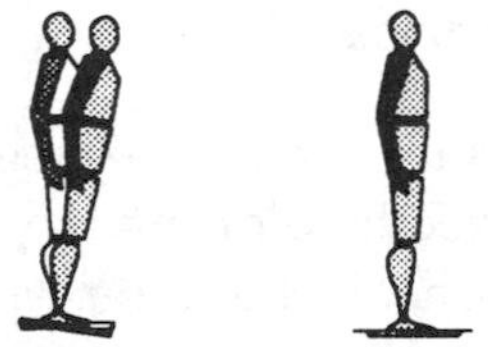 4 1	Condition 4 / Condition 1	**Question:** Does sway increase when somatosensory cues are inaccurate? **Low scores:** Patient makes poor use of visual references.
VEST Vestibular	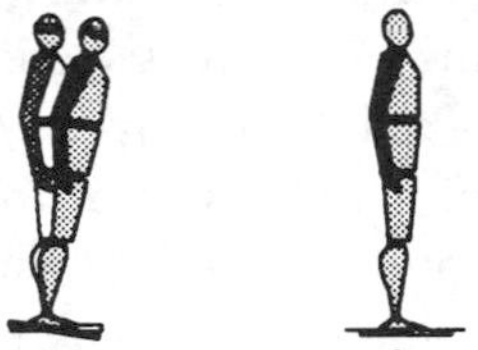 5 1	Condition 5 / Condition 1	**Question:** Does sway increase when visual cues are removed and somatosensory cues are inaccurate? **Low scores:** Patient makes poor use of vestibular cues, or vestibular cues unavailable.
PREF Visual Preference	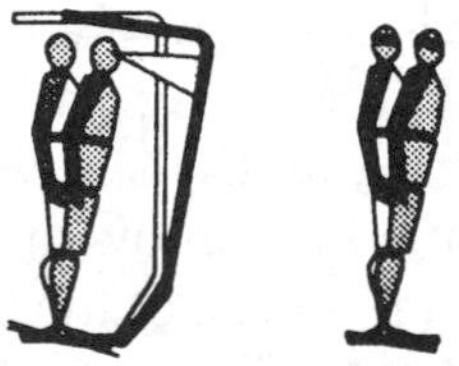 3 + 6 2 + 5	Condition 3 + 6 / Condition 2 + 5	**Question:** Do inaccurate visual cues result in increased sway compared to no visual cues? **Low scores:** Patient relies on visual cues even when they are inaccurate.

Figure 18-12. Sensory analysis ratios and their normal functioning. From Jacobson, *Handbook of balance function testing*, 1E. © 1998 Delmar Learning, a part of Cengage Learning, Inc. Reproduced by permission. http://www.cengage.com/permissions

the eyes. Since eye closure eliminates the visual input, an atypically low ratio is interpreted as dysfunction of the remaining somatosensory input, which normally dominates the control of balance during stance on a fixed support surface. Although the vestibular input is potentially a second alternative to vision during eye closure, this alternative is substantially less sensitive than the somatosensory input in a controlling sway. Therefore, use of the vestibular input rather than the somatosensory input during eye closure on a fixed surface significantly increases the COG sway. This is the same interpretation originally proposed by Romberg (Dichgans et al., 1976; Horak et al., 1989).

The visual ratio compares the condition 4 score with the condition 1 score. This ratio quantifies the extent of stability loss when the normally dominant somatosensory input is disrupted by sway-referencing of the support surface. Although COG sway usually increases slightly when the somatosensory input is disrupted, the increase in sway is small when the alternative visual input is functioning normally. For reasons similar to those presented previously, sway increases will be abnormally large if the vestibular input rather than the visual input is used. Therefore, a lower than normal ratio in this case is interpreted as dysfunction of the visual sense of balance.

The vestibular ratio comparing the condition 5 score with the condition 1 score reflects a relative reduction in stability when visual and somatosensory inputs are simultaneously disrupted. Although COG sway increases significantly under condition 5 for the reasons described previously, clinically normal individuals maintain their balance well within the LOS using the remaining vestibular inputs. A lower than normal ratio is therefore interpreted as a dysfunctional vestibular sense of balance.

The vision preference ratio comparing the sum of conditions 3 and 6 scores to the sum of conditions 2 and 5 scores reflects a relative reduction of stability under sway-referenced visual conditions compared with the equivalent eyes closed conditions. The stability of clinically normal individual is similar when eyes are closed and when presented with a functionally inappropriate visual input. In both cases, no visual information useful for controlling balance is available. Thus, a lower than normal ratio in this case is interpreted as an abnormal preference for using vision. In other words, the patient attempts to orient himself or herself to the sway-referenced (conflicting) visual input and sways more in comparison to the equivalent eyes closed conditions.

COG Alignment

Center of gravity alignment is analyzed by plotting for each of the 18 SOT trials the average AP and lateral positions of the COG (see Figure 18–9). When the patient's COG is aligned over the center of the base of support, the points corresponding to each trial are clustered near the center of the plot. Points above the center indicate an alignment forward of center, while points below the center of the plot indicate a backward COG alignment. Points to the left or right of the center indicate a laterally misaligned COG in the corresponding direction. Areas of the alignment plot falling outside the fifth percentile relative to the clinically normal sample are indicated by stippling.

SOT Results in the Clinically Normal Sample

Equilibrium Scores and Sensory Analysis Ratios

In the appendix to this chapter, Tables 18–A1 through 18–A6 show the ranges of equilibrium scores, com-

posite scores, and sensory organization ratios for the sample of asymptomatic subjects. Equilibrium scores for each sensory condition are based on the average of scores for the three trials. Equilibrium scores of zero are used for trials in which subjects lost balance. Sizable normal population studies in children to elderly by other groups have yielded similar SOT results (Hang & Lipsitz, 2010; Jackson & Epstein, 1991; Ledin, 1992; Peterka & Black, 1990a; Wolfson et al., 1992).

Strategy Analysis

The patient's movement strategy during each SOT trial is analyzed by plotting the resulting movement strategy score against the corresponding equilibrium score as shown in Figure 18–9. Points falling in the upper left quadrant of the strategy plot indicate trials in which the COG sway excursions are small but the amplitude of hip and upper body movements is large. This region of the plot is therefore labeled "hip dominant." Points in the lower right quadrant indicate trials in which COG sway excursions are large, but the movements are primarily about the ankle joints. This region is therefore labeled "ankle dominant." Points falling along an upper right to lower left diagonal indicate trials in which the amplitude of hip and upper body movements increase in proportion to the amplitude of the COG sway.

Because the distributions of equilibrium scores are skewed toward the higher values, the limits for clinically normal scores are determined by calculating the lowest fifth percentile of equilibrium scores for each age range and condition. Because the sensory analysis ratio scores are normally distributed, scores below 1.67 SD of the population means define the lower limits of the clinically normal range.

The equilibrium scores of clinically normal subjects of all ages are the highest for the first three sensory conditions. This is because somatosensory inputs dominate balance when the support surface is fixed, regardless of the status of visual and vestibular inputs. Although equilibrium scores decrease when the functionally useful somatosensory input is disrupted (sway-referenced support surface) during conditions 4 through 6, clinically normal subjects continue to maintain balance well within the LOS. The sensory condition 4 scores are the highest of these three conditions, because normal visual inputs are available. The lowest equilibrium scores occur under conditions 5 and 6, when both somatosensory and visual inputs are disrupted and subjects must rely on vestibular inputs alone to maintain balance.

Center of Gravity Alignment

Clinically normal subjects align the COG very near to the center of the base of support under all six sensory conditions. Even though sway amplitudes increase significantly under conditions 5 and 6, the average COG positions remain very nearly centered. Because offset positions in all directions are considered abnormal, alignment values beyond ±2 SD in lateral and AP directions are considered abnormal.

Strategy Analysis

In the strategy analysis plots of our normal subject population, points corresponding to individual trials fall along a diagonal. This is because normal subjects use ankle movements when the COG is well within the limits of stability (high equilibrium scores) and will increase their use of hip movements as the COG approaches the limits of stability (low equilibrium scores). When points in the strategy analysis plot fall along a nearly vertical line, the patient is abnormally dependent on ankle movements. Points along a horizontal line indicate that the patient is abnormally dependent on hip movements.

Repeatability of Sensory Organization Test Results

A number of investigators have performed multiple SOT evaluations on samples of clinically normal individuals to answer two questions: specifically, are test results reliable and do subjects tested repeatedly learn to improve their test scores (Barin, Seitz, & Welling, 1992; Coogler & Wolf, 1992; Epstein & Jackson, 1992). For example, Coogler and Wolf (1992) evaluated 45 subjects who received SOT evaluations on three separate days. A comparison of the mean equilibrium scores from each session showed small but statistically significant improvements in equilibrium scores between the first to the third session on the more difficult sensory conditions. The mean equilibrium score improved approximately 5% for sensory condition 4, while improvements in sensory condition 5 and 6 scores were less than 10%. Most

improvements were noted between the first and second sessions. This result suggests that the SOT is reliable and that multiple administrations of the SOT can be used to follow progressive improvements of greater than 10% over time.

As part of an ongoing study of space motion sickness, astronauts participating in the NASA space shuttle program received preflight SOT evaluations at regular intervals, and then received serial postflight evaluations beginning within hours of their return from zero gravity (Paloski, Reschke, Doxey, & Harm, 1992). The average equilibrium scores on SOT condition 6 for the first 10 returning astronauts dropped from the preflight range of 70% to 80% ("supernormal" values relative to the sample of asymptomatic normal individuals) to the 35% to 45% range immediately after flight (considered borderline "abnormal" compared to the clinically normal sample). Although not specifically documented in the report, results of the first five sensory conditions were reported to show much smaller postflight reductions. In all cases, equilibrium scores improved to their preflight values within several days.

The returning astronauts demonstrated a significant and specific reduction in sensory balance control, despite the fact that they were familiar with the SOT prior to space flight, and despite the fact that they were also highly motivated individuals. This suggests that the SOT can be used to track progress during treatment, because prior knowledge of the test will not mask a sensory organization abnormality.

A more recent study demonstrated that the SOT is also reliable in a population of elderly patients with unilateral transtibial amputation (Jayakaran, Johnson, & Sullivan, 2011).

Potential Problems With the SOT

Equilibrium scores may be higher than the actual functional capabilities when a tight safety harness "catches" a patient who would otherwise have fallen. Falls into the safety harness, however, can be identified on the raw shear force trace. While the shear forces generated by free swaying are very brief and symmetrical about zero axis, harness bumps cause large and prolonged deflections of the sheer force trace in one direction.

As already discussed for the PER and MCT, results are most accurate when the patient gives his or her best performance without outside help. Poorly motivated patients, or patients who exaggerate symptoms, may produce equilibrium scores below their best functional capabilities. In these cases, the equilibrium scores are frequently inconsistent. Surprised and overly anxious patients also perform below their maximum functional capabilities. In these cases, the test protocols can be carefully explained to reassure the patient. As already discussed in relation to repeatability and reliability, detailed knowledge of the test is generally not a problem, because the functions being assessed are automatic rather than consciously controlled.

As is also true with the MCT, inaccurate placement of the feet on the forceplates affects the COG alignment and weight symmetry scores. However, as long as both feet are completely on the forceplates, the equilibrium and strategy scores will not be affected.

Finally, small movements and changes in position by the patient can artificially lower the equilibrium score on a trial. This problem is especially true during the first three sensory conditions, when scores are normally very high. The operator should watch the patient for evidence of head turns, postural shifts, coughs, and sneezes. Data obtained on these trials should be deleted and the trials repeated.

SUMMARY

Computerized dynamic posturography uses a multiplicity of independent test protocols to objectively assess the major sensory and motor components of balance. All protocols are based on documented physiologic principles of human balance. Some protocols provide information relative to the patient's functional capacity within a variety of daily life tasks. Others provide information that can help localize the cause of a balance system disorder. The ability to identify inconsistencies among independent test results is an additional advantage in identifying nonphysiologic causes of unsteadiness such as anxiety and deliberate exaggeration of symptoms. Experimental studies with various populations of clinically normal individuals indicate that CDP can provide reliable and repeatable test results.

REFERENCES

Allum, J. H. J., & Keshner, E. A. (1986). Vestibular and proprioceptive control of sway stabilization. In W. Bles & T. Brandt (Eds.), *Disorders of posture and gait* (pp. 19–40). New York, NY: Elsevier.

Barin, K., Seitz, C. M., & Welling, D. B. (1992). Effect of head orientation on the diagnostic sensitivity of posturography in patients with compensated unilateral lesions. *Otolaryngology-Head and Neck Surgery, 106,* 355–362.

Beckley, D. J., Bloem, B. R., van Dijk, J. G., Roos, R. A., & Remier, M. P. (1991). Electrophysiological correlates of postural instability in Parkinson's disease. *Electroencephalography and Clinical Neurophysiology, 81,* 263–268.

Black, F. O., & Wall, C. III. (1982). Normal subject postural sway during the Romberg test. *American Journal of Otolaryngology, 3,* 309–318.

Black, F. O., Wall C. III., & O'Leary, D. P. (1978). Computerized screening of the human vestibulospinal system. *Annals of Otology, Rhinology, & Laryngology, 87,* 853–861.

Coogler, C. E., & Wolf, S. (1992). Consistency of postural responses in elderly individuals. In M. Woollacott & F. Horak (Eds.), *Posture and gait: Control mechanisms* (Vol. II, pp. 239–242). Eugene, OR: University of Oregon Books.

Dichgans, J., & Diener, H. C. (1985). Clinical evidence for functional compartmentalization of the cerebellum. In J. R. Bloedel, J. Dichgans, & W. Precht (Eds.), *Cerebellar functions* (pp. 126–147). New York, NY: Springer-Verlag.

Dichgans, J., Mauritz, K. H., Allum, J. H. J., & Brandt, T. (1976). Postural sway in normals and ataxic patients: Analysis of the stabilizing and destabilizing effects of vision. *Agressologie, 17,* 15–24.

Diener, H. C., Ackermann, H., Dichgans, J., & Guschlbauer, B. (1985). Medium- and long-latency responses to displacements of the ankle joint in patients with spinal and central lesions. *Electroencephalography and Clinical Neurophysiology, 60,* 407–416.

Diener, H. C., Bootz, F., Dichgans, J., & Bruzek, W. (1983). Variability of postural "reflexes" in humans. *Experimental Brain Research, 52,* 423–428.

Diener, H. C., Dichgans, J., Bacher, M. & Guschlbauer, B. (1984). Characteristic alterations of long-loop "reflexes" in patients with Friedreich's disease and late atrophy of the cerebellar anterior lobe. *Journal of Neurology, Neurosurgery, and Psychiatry, 47,* 679–685.

Diener, H. C., Dichgans, J., Bootz, F., & Bacher, M. (1984). Early stabilization of human posture after sudden disturbance: Influence of rate and amplitude of displacement. *Experimental Brain Research, 56,* 126–134.

Diener, H. C., Dichgans, J., & Scholz, E. (1985). Long loop reflexes in a standing subject and their use for clinical diagnosis. In M. Igarashi & F. O. Black (Eds.), *Vestibular and visual control on posture and locomotor equilibrium* (pp. 290–294). Basel, Switzerland: S Karger,

Dietz, V., Quintern, J., & Berger, W. (1984). Corrective reactions to stumbling in man: Functional significance of spinal and transcortical reflexes. *Neuroscience Letters, 44*, 131–135.

Dietz, V., Quintern, J., Berger, W., & Schenck, E. (1985). Cerebral potentials and leg muscle EMG responses associated with stance perturbation. *Experimental Brain Research, 57*, 348–354.

El 'ner, A. M., Popov, K. E., & Gurfinkel, V. S. (1972). Changes in stretch reflex system concerned with the control of postural activity of human muscle. *Agressologie, 13*, 19–23.

Epstein, C. M., & Jackson, R. T. (1992). Head extension and sway in normal volunteers. In M. Woollacott & F. Horak (Eds.), *Posture and gait: Control mechanisms* (Vol. I, pp. 171–174). Eugene, OR: University of Oregon Books.

Gurfinkel, V. S., Lipshits, M. I., & Popov, K. Y. (1974). Is the stretch reflex the main mechanism in the system of regulation of the vertical posture of man? *Biophysics, 19*, 744–748.

Hang, H. G., & Lipsitz, L. A. (2010). Stiffness control of balance during quiet standing and dual task in older adults: The MOBILIZE Boston study. *Journal of Neurophysiology, 104*, 10–17.

Hassan, D. M., & Azzam, H. (2012). Sensory integration in attention deficit hyperactivity disorder: Implications to postural control. In J. M. Norvilitis (Ed.), *Contemporary trends in ADHD research*. Rijeka, Croatia: InTech. Retrieved from http://www.intechopen.com/books/contemporary-trends-in-adhd-research/sensory-integration-in-attention-deficit-hyperactivity-disorder-implications-to-postural-control

Horak, F. B., Diener, H. C., & Nashner, L. M. (1989). Influence of central set on human postural responses. *Journal of Neurophysiology, 62*, 841–853.

Horak, F. B., & Nashner, L. M. (1986). Central programming of postural movements: Adaptation to altered support surface configurations. *Journal of Neurophysiology, 55*, 1369–1981.

Horak, F. B., Shupert, C. L., & Mirka, A. (1989). Components of postural dyscontrol in the elderly: A review. *Neurobiology of Aging, 10*, 727–738.

Huttunen, J., & Romberg, V. (1990). EMG responses in leg muscles to postural perturbations in Huntington's disease. *Journal of Neurology, Neurosurgery, and Psychiatry, 53*, 55–62.

Jackson, R. T., & Epstein, C. M. (1991). Effect of head extension on equilibrium in normal subjects. *Annals of Otology, Rhinology, and Laryngology, 100*, 63–67.

Jayakaran, P., Johnson, G. M., & Sullivan, S. J. (2011). Test-retest reliability of the sensory organization test in older persons with a transtibial amputation. *Physical Medicine and Rehabilitation, 3*, 723–729.

Kapteyn, T. S., & de Wit, G. (1972). Posturography as an auxiliary in vestibular investigation. *Acta Oto-Laryngologica, 73*, 104–111.

Keshner, E. A., & Kenyan, R. V. (2009). Postural and spatial orientation driven by virtual reality. *Studies in Health Technology and Informatics, 145*, 209–228.

Koles, Z. J., & Castelein, R. D. (1980). The relationship between body sway and foot pressure in normal man. *Journal of Medical Engineering and Technology, 4*, 279–285.

Lange, B. S., Requejo, P., Flynn, S. M., Rizzo, A. A., Valero-Cuevas, F. J., Baker, L., & Winstein, C. (2010). The potential of virtual reality and gaming to assist successful aging with disability. *Physical Medicine and Rehabilitation Clinics of North America, 21*, 339–356.

Ledin, T. (1992). Dynamic posturography in childhood and senescence. In M. Woollacott & F. Horak (Eds.), *Posture and gait: Control mechanisms* (Vol. II, pp. 279–282). Eugene, OR: University of Oregon Books.

Maurer, C., & Peterka, R. J. (2005). A new interpretation of spontaneous sway measures based on a simple model of human postural sway. *Journal of Neurophysiology, 93*, 189–200.

McNevin, N., Weir, P., & Quinn, T. (2013). Effects of attentional focus and age on suprapostural task performance and postural control. *Research Quarterly for Exercise Sport, 84*, 96–103.

Nardone, A., Giordano, O., Corra, T., & Schieppati, M. (1990). Responses of leg muscles in humans displaced while standing. *Brain, 113*, 65–84.

Nashner, L. M. (1976). Adapting reflexes controlling the human posture. *Experimental Brain Research, 26*, 59–72.

Nashner, L. M. (1977). Fixed patterns of rapid postural responses among leg muscles during stance. *Experimental Brain Research, 150*, 403–407.

Nashner, L. M., Black, F. O., & Wall, C. (1982). Adaptation to altered support and visual conditions during stance: Patients with vestibular deficits. *Journal of Neuroscience, 2*, 536–544.

Nashner, L. M., & Cordo, P. G. (1981). Relation of automatic postural responses and reaction-time voluntary movements of human leg muscles. *Experimental Brain Research, 43*, 395–405.

Nashner, L. M., & McCollum, G. (1985). The organization of human postural movements: A formal basis and experimental synthesis. *Behavioral and Brain Sciences, 8*, 135–172.

Nashner, L. M., Shupert, C. L., & Horak, F. B. (1989). Organization of posture controls: An analysis of sensory and mechanical constraints. In J. H. J. Allum & M. Hulliger (Eds.), *Progress in brain research* (Vol. 80, pp. 411–418). New York, NY: Elsevier.

Nashner, L. M., Woollacott, M., & Tuma, G. (1979). Organization of rapid responses to postural and locomotor-like perturbations of standing man. *Experimental Brain Research, 36*, 463–476.

Njiokiktjien, C., & De Rijke, W. (1972). The recording of Romberg's test and its application in neurology. *Agressologie, 13*(C), 1–7.

Paloski, W. H., Reschke, M. F., Doxey, D. D., & Harm, D. L. (1992). Neurosensory adaptation associated with postural ataxia following spaceflight. In M. Woollacott & F. Horak (Eds.), *Posture and gait: Control mechanisms* (Vol. I, pp. 311–314). Eugene, OR: University of Oregon Books.

Pavol, M. J. (2005). Detecting and understanding differences in postural sway. *Journal of Neurophysiology, 93*, 20–21.

Peterka, R. J., & Black, F. O. (1990a). Age-related changes in human posture control: Sensory organization tests. *Journal of Vestibular Research, 1*, 73–85.

Peterka, R. J., & Black, F. O. (1990b). Age-related changes in human posture control: Motor coordination tests. *Journal of Vestibular Research, 1*, 87–96.

Riley, P., Mann, R. W., & Hodge, A. (1990). Modelling of the biomechanics of posture and balance. *Journal of Biomechanics, 23*, 503–506.

Romberg, M. H. (1853). *Manual of nervous system disease of man* (pp. 395–401). London, UK: Sydenham Society.

Streepey, J. W., Kenyan, R. V., & Keshner, E. A. (2007). Field of view and base of support width influence postural responses to visual stimuli during quiet stance. *Gait and Posture, 25*, 49–55.

Terekhov, Y. (1976). Stabilometry as a diagnostic tool in clinical medicine. *Journal of the Canadian Medical Association, 115*, 631–633.

Wolfson, L., Whipple, R., Derby, C., Amerman, P., Murphy, T., Tobin, J. N., & Nashner, L. M. (1992). A dynamic posturography study of balance in healthy elderly. *Neurology, 42*, 2069–2075.

APPENDIX 18–A

Table 18-A1. Normal Subject Posture-Evoked Response Latencies*

Reference	Number of Subjects	Short Latency	Medium Latency	Long Latency
2	10	42.9 ± 3.3	86.6 ± 6.4	128.6 ± 10.1
8	50	43.5 ± 4.2	89.5 ± 10.0	125.3 ± 17.8
21†	26	34 ± 3	86 ± 6	114 ± 16
† and ∴	74	30.0 ± 4.6	73.3 ± 11.2	104.2 ± 17.0

*All studies used 50-deg/s 4-degree toes-up rotations. In these studies, time was determined by the actual platform movement onset rather than the movement command, reducing latencies by 10 to 15 ms.

Source: Data provided to NeuroCom International, Inc. by Chris Diener, Universitat Essen, Germany.

Table 18-A2. Mean (+1.67 SO) Latency Scores as Functions of Translation Size, Direction, and Subject Age

Movement	Population Latency Scores (ms)		
	20–59 Years (*n* = 58)	60–69 Years (*n* = 54)	70–79 Years (*n* = 28)
Medium back	156 (182)	160 (187)	168 (200)
Large back	137 (168)	148 (171)	155 (178)
Medium forward	164 (194)	164 (184)	170 (196)
Large forward	153 (167)	155 (173)	159 (177)

Table 18-A3. Mean (±2 SD) Active Force Strengths as Functions of Translation Direction, Size, and Subject Age*

Movement	Population Strength Scores		
	20–59 Years (*n* = 29)	60–69 Years (*n* = 54)	70–79 Years (*n* = 28)
Small back	03.4 ± (1.4)	04.1 ± (4.6)	04.2 ± (4.5)
Medium back	07.1 ± (5.8)	07.8 ± (5.5)	07.9 ± (7.0)
Large back	08.7 ± (5.2)	09.9 ± (5.5)	10.4 ± (7.4)
Small forward	03.6 ± (3.9)	05.1 ± (4.5)	05.2 ± (4.2)
Medium forward	08.4 ± (4.9)	09.0 ± (5.0)	08.6 ± (4.2)
Large forward	10.0 ± (5.7)	10.1 ± (5.3)	09.7 ± (6.0)

*All values are in units of angular momentum normalized for differences in body mass.

Table 18-A4. Mean (+1.67 SO) Sway Energy Scores as Functions of Toes-Up and Toes-Down Trial Numbers and Subject Age*

Motion	Population Adaptation Scores		
	20–59 Years (*n* = 64)	60–69 Years (*n* = 54)	70–79 Years (*n* = 28)
Toes up			
1	85 (160)	76 (125)	75 (132)
2	67 (109)	68 (97)	74 (118)
3	62 (99)	62 (91)	74 (103)
4	54 (76)	59 (81)	72 (111)
5	53 (75)	60 (83)	66 (91)
Toes down			
1	76 (134)	75 (120)	72 (113)
2	45 (66)	59 (88)	66 (112)
3	40 (58)	52 (81)	61 (95)
4	37 (54)	49 (77)	60 (99)
5	36 (50)	49 (76)	60 (99)

*All values are in units of sway energy normalized for differences in body mass.

Table 18-A5. Mean (Fifth Percentile) Equilibrium Scores as Functions of Age and Sensory Test Condition

Condition	Population Equilibrium Scores		
	20–59 Years (*n* = 112)	60–69 Years (*n* = 54)	70–79 Years (*n* = 28)
1	94 (90)	94 (90)	89 (70)
2	92 (85)	91 (86)	86 (63)
3 Average	91 (86)	89 (80)	88 (82)
4 Average	82 (70)	85 (77)	78 (69)
5 Average	69 (52)	65 (51)	61 (45)
6 Average	67 (48)	65 (49)	53 (27)
Composite	798 (704)	776 (676)	729 (638)

Table 18-A6. Mean(±2 SO) COG Alignment Scores as Functions of Sensory Test Conditions and Age*

Condition	Population Alignment Scores		
	20–59 Years (*n* = 77)	60–69 Years (*n* = 54)	70–79 Years (*n* = 28)
Initial dynamic	0.3 ± (1.8)	−0.1 ± (2.0)	0.0 ± (1.8)
1	0.2 ± (2.0)	−0.3 ± (1.9)	−0.2 ± (1.9)
2	0.3 ± (1.6)	−0.1 ± (2.0)	0.0 ± (1.7)
3	0.3 ± (1.6)	0.0 ± (2.1)	−0.2 ± (1.7)
4	0.3 ± (1.6)	−0.1 ± (2.1)	−0.1 ± (1.7)
5	0.7 ± (1.8)	0.1 ± (2.2)	0.2 ± (2.2)
6	0.8 ± (1.9)	0.4 ± (2.3)	0.3 ± (1.7)

*All values are in units of degrees from the center position.

Interpretation and Usefulness of Computerized Dynamic Posturography[1]

Neil T. Shepard

INTRODUCTION

The development of clinically practical methods of static and dynamic postural control evaluation were discussed in Chapter 18 with the basics of the biomechanics of postural control in Chapter 17. The focus of this chapter is the clinical utility of the tests of postural control and their clinical interpretations. This is provided in a series of patient case studies that present the use of computerized dynamic posturography (CDP) within the construct of the patient's signs and symptoms represented by the patient history and results from the other clinical evaluations of VNG, rotational chair, and otolith function testing. The presentation of the material is provided in this manner as the principal use of CDP is not in isolation.

CLINICAL UTILIZATION

When considering the clinical utility of formal postural control assessment, the primary discussion becomes focused on when specific tests should be performed and the reliability and validity of the tests.

Staged Protocol

In addressing when the tests should be performed, one can make the argument that some level of assessment should be used on all patients complaining of dizziness even if imbalance or falls are not part of the principal symptoms. This argument is supported by the increased likelihood of a fall at all ages with the identification of peripheral vestibular involvement (Herdman, Blatt, Schubert, & Tusa, 2000). Further support is the evidence that if identified as being at risk for a fall, even if no falls have yet occurred, the use of vestibular and balance rehabilitation therapy can reduce the risk of falls and specific programs have been successful in reducing the rate of falls with young and older populations (Gillespie et al., 2007; Hall, Schubert, & Herdman, 2004; McClure et al., 2007). It has been shown that tests other than those dealing with postural control can also predict a falls risk. These involve the use of functional evaluations of gaze stability (i.e., dynamic visual acuity and the gaze stabilization test) (Honaker & Shepard, 2012; Honaker, Lee, & Shepard, 2013). Within this context it can be questioned as to whether all patients require a full formal postural control analysis. Given the ability to make a reasonable prediction as to whether

[1]Significant portions of this chapter also appear, by the same author with permission from Shepard (2007).

the sensory organization test (SOT; see Chapter 18) will be abnormal by first performing the clinical test of sensory interaction on balance (CTSIB or modified CTSIB) (el-Kashlan, Shepard, Asher, Smith-Wheelock, & Telian, 1998; Shumway-Cook & Horak, 1986; Wrisley & Whitney, 2004) and then setting specific criteria for use of postural-evoked responses (PERs), a staged protocol can be used. By clinical experience only and not through an experimental clinical trial study, the author finds the motor control test (MCT; see Chapter 18) assistive in helping to interpret complex patterns of abnormality that can occur on the SOT and therefore recommends its use (if available) whenever formal SOT is performed.

As an example of the staged protocol concept, one used by the author is provided. The criteria were developed based on (1) a study comparing the CTSIB to SOT (el-Kashlan et al., 1998); (2) a large retrospective study of findings in over 2,000 patients when all tests were used on all patients (Shepard & Telian, 1996); and (3) two prospective studies—one on false-positive findings of the MCT and one on sensitivity/specificity of PERs (Shepard, 2000); a retrospective study on informational overlap between MCT and PERs (Shepard et al., 2010)

Indications for when to use SOT and MCT (both performed together) are given below. These are applied in a parallel loose format such that if any one of the criteria is met, the patient goes on for a full postural control evaluation. SOT and MCT are indicated by the following:

1. Abnormal performance on the modified CTSIB. Normative data across age exist for this study performed in a semiqualitative manner or via the use of a fixed forceplate (el-Kashlan et al., 1998; Rose & Clark, 2000; Shumway-Cook & Horak, 1986; Weber & Cass, 1993).
2. A major complaint in the presenting symptoms is unsteadiness or imbalance in standing and/or walking (constant or episodic) in the absence of vertigo at the same time.
3. Known or suggested pathologic involvement of the pyramidal/extrapyramidal tracks, involvement in spinal tracks, or suggestion of sensory and/or motor neuropathy via the patient's presenting symptoms or past medical history.

The basis for the criteria for performing postural-evoked responses and the normative data for this

procedure are provided in published studies and are not reviewed in this chapter (Lawson, Shepard, Oviatt, & Wang, 1994; Shepard & Telian, 1996; Shepard et al., 2010). However, the criteria are as follows:

1. Abnormally increased composite scores for latencies on motor control test—this is focused on the latency to active recovery from the forward translation of the support surface independent of the results of the backward translation.
2. Report of two or more unexplained falls within the 12 months prior to the laboratory assessment.

As with the criteria for SOT/MCT, these are also applied in a parallel loose format such that either being positive is sufficient for going on for PERs.

Validity and Reliability

Validity of the SOT and MCT protocols has been partially approached in a study comparing normal young and older adult's performance on the clinical protocols to performance in a basic laboratory situation using an optoelectric, two-dimensional, three camera, motion analysis system (Shepard et al., 1993). The findings of this work showed that the impressions of hip versus ankle-dominant strategies and the ability to predict the movement of the upper body and whole body sway from the forceplate data were consistent with the detailed analysis used under similar conditions with the motion analysis system.

In the desire to use serial sensory organization testing to monitor patient progress, test-retest reliability becomes important. Studies looking at this issue in normal volunteers retested on different days had mixed results, some suggesting no learning effect with test repetition (Black, Pabski, Reschke, Calkins, & Shupert, 1993; Kubo & Wall, 1990) and another giving results implying that a learning effect is present (Ford-Smith, Wyman, Elswick, Fernandez, & Newton, 1995). An additional study investigating the test-retest reliability when testing was repeated within the same day on patients (Shepard & Boismier, 1992) suggested that a learning effect is present. In the study where interclass correlation coefficients (ICCs) were used as part of the outcome evaluation (Ford-Smith et al., 1995), the values for all six conditions were found to be less than the recommended value for routine clinical use (Portney &

Watkins, 1993). Findings of this nature should not be interpreted as rendering the equipment inappropriate for serial monitoring. Given the novel nature of the task at hand, it would be surprising if there was not some minimal learning effect. In the work using the ICC statistic, the magnitude of the improvement suggesting a learning effect was within the known range for the variance given in the normative data used to develop clinical cutoff criteria for abnormal performance. Therefore, although a learning effect likely does exist for normal subjects, the magnitude of the effect is relatively small which introduces the issue of its clinical relevance.

Although the work on normal subjects is important in studying the reliability, it is also important to know if the same result occurs in patients who start with abnormal performance. Clinical experience suggests that patients have an increased likelihood for improvement on a second test administration if they meet either of the following conditions: (1) show a pattern of improving performance across three trials of a given condition; or (2) suspect an unreliable test result secondary to significant anxiety noted by the examiner. A pilot study investigating this issue prospectively showed that greater than 50% of the patients meeting one or both of the above criteria changed to a normal pattern with repeat testing on the same day (Boismier & Shepard, 1991). To study this issue in the average balance disorder patient not suspected for retest improvement, a prospective, random, 20% sample of 650 consecutive patients were subjected to repeat dynamic posturography within 120 min of the original testing (Shepard & Boismier, 1992). The study did demonstrate statistically significant improvement in sensory organization test scores for several of the test conditions and for the overall composite score, suggesting a learning effect. However, only 10% of those with abnormal sensory organization test composite scores initially changed to a normal score with repeat testing. All of those changing to a normal score were initially outside the normal range by an amount less than the variance in normal subjects for the conditions in question. Therefore, our current clinical protocol suggests repeat testing of an abnormal sensory organization test on patients only if they meet one of the following three conditions:

- The patient shows a pattern of improving performance across three trials of a given condition.

- The test result is suspected to be unreliable secondary to significant anxiety noted by the examiner. (Typically this would involve a pattern that appears functional with improved performance on the more difficult tests. This is discussed further below.)
- The composite score is outside the normal range by 20 or less points.

The same concerns about test-retest reliability and validity are discussed elsewhere and are only summarized herein (Shepard, 2000; Shepard & Telian, 1996). To consider the MCT results being a reliable indication of abnormality, the following three conditions need to be considered:

- The latencies following the medium translation must be longer than those for the large translation, unless the latencies for both responses are greater than 190 ms.
- If the latencies are abnormal by 50 ms or less, the condition must be repeated and the results replicated. If the latencies remain in the abnormal range, the data can be considered abnormal. If the latencies fall within the normal limits on the repeat test, then the results should be considered as normal findings.
- Complaints of pain in the lower back, lower limb, or hip joints are a likely source of abnormality in latency on the backward translation studies.

The PER study utilizes the techniques of rectifying and averaging multiple trials of the EMG responses to assist in delineating the onset and offset of the three responses of the short (SLR), medium (MLR), and long latency responses (LLR) (EMGs from gastrocnemius and tibialis anterior). This can be a principal factor in the test-retest reliability of the study. This was addressed in a prospective study using a double-blinded format having two separate facilities with experienced and inexperienced interpreters marking the sets of data with the results compiled by a third party (Fortin, Shepard, Diener, & Lawson, 1996). Details of the study are provided in another publication and are not repeated here (Shepard, 2000).

The conclusions regarding the reliability of determining the onset and offset points for each of the muscle responses based on Cronbach's alpha reliability index follow:

- Overall reliability of latency markings were good (index >0.73) for between laboratories and for within a single laboratory.
- Several specific conditions led to errors in the markings and poor reliability. These were
  - separation of offset of SLR and onset of MLR when the trace was noisy;
  - determination of true offset time for MLR when cross-talk from the tibialis anterior was reflected in the gastrocnemius response; and
  - the above two conditions were exacerbated in error production when the examiner was inexperienced.
- The most highly reliable latency markings were with the onset time of the SLR and LLR (index >0.9).

VOLITIONAL REDUCTION IN LIMITS OF STABILITY

As described in Chapter 18 the equilibrium score is a percentage representing the magnitude of sway in the sagittal plane for each trial of each condition. This score is based on a normal value of 12.5 degrees of anterior/posterior sway about the ankle joint, typically 8 degrees forward and 4.5 degrees backward. It is assumed that this range of sway is available to all patients during the test. Some patients may not have this normal range because of physical restrictions at the ankle, or because of limits the patient has adopted secondary to his or her sense of imbalance and fear of a potential fall. Recognizing the patient who has a reduction in his or her volitional limits of sway can be helpful in the interpretation of the SOT results and may be able to be addressed with a vestibular and balance rehabilitation program. Therefore, testing the limits of volitional limits of sway for each patient as part of the sensory organization test protocol can provide useful additional information.

Prior to testing under condition 1, patients are asked to lean as far forward onto their toes as possible without taking a step or reaching out, and then as far back on their heels as possible. This is done

with the eyes open, stressing that the movements are to be done about the ankle joint rather than bending at the hip. Following this practice trial of allowing the patient to explore the limits of sway, the equipment is activated under condition 1. Rather than maintaining stable stance at first, the patient is asked to repeat the limits of sway task again during the 20-s trial. When completed, the equilibrium score on the screen can be interpreted roughly as the percent reduction in limits of sway in the sagittal plane. A score of 35% or less is interpreted as no significant reduction, knowing that the range of movement only increases if repeated practice is allowed. Then, the actual condition 1 test is repeated, so that the limits of sway test results do not enter into the calculation of the cumulative equilibrium score at the end of the test. An example of the use of this procedure to help explain an inconsistent test result is given in Figure 19–1. The SOT results shown are from a patient with severe bilateral vestibular hypofunction. His average performance (the numeric average of the three trials) for conditions 1 through 3 are well within normal limits. This is also reflected in the raw data shown in the bottom portion of the slide with little or no calculated center-of-mass (COM) sway on any of the trials for conditions 1 through 3. On condition 4 in the summary plot giving the equilibrium score, he shows a fall reaction on trial 1, performs significantly better on trial 2, yet has another fall reaction on trial 3. Both conditions 5 and 6 show repeated fall reactions (indicated as free falls from inspection of the raw COM trace—no attempt to correct the falls) on all three trials of each condition. From the COM traces for condition 4 it is seen that he starts with a free fall on trial 1, maintains stance with increased sway for the entire 20 s on trial 2, and has a fall reaction within the last 4 s of trial 3. In testing his reduction in volitional limits of sway his result was 55%. Therefore, the 0 or fall line on the equilibrium score plot, it could be argued, should be at 55% equilibrium score (position of the dashed black line) as that represents his range of anterior-posterior move. He has no physical limitations in range of motion or strength that would explain the limited range of motion. It is likely an artificial limit that makes him feel secure during stance. Given this reduction in limits of sway, it is easy to explain the apparent inconsistency in performance on condition 4. As his sway magnitude is so close to his perceived limits

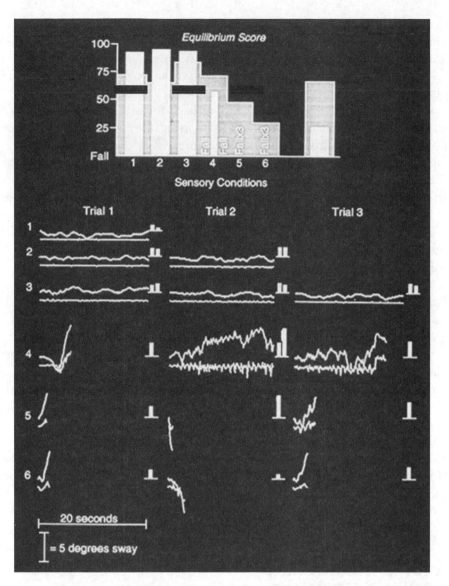

Figure 19–1. The SOT EquiTest summary of the equilibrium scores and the corresponding raw data results for each of the trials for each of the six SOT conditions tested. For conditions 1 through 3, the single bar on the Equilibrium Score graph represents the average of the three individual trials. For conditions 4 through 6 the individual results for each trial are shown as a fall reaction (word Fall) or the equilibrium score by the single bar on condition 4. In the lower section of the figure the thicker line represents the calculated COM anterior/posterior excursion over the 20-s trials. The thinner line represents the force activity on the shear force transducer sensing horizontal force applied to the dual platforms. See text for further explanations of the figure.

of movement and when those limits are exceeded, he simply takes a step to prevent what he perceives as an impending fall risk. His performance on conditions 5 and 6 would be expected and explainable given the severity of his bilateral hypofunction. Yet

the hypofunction would not provide an explanation for the performance on condition 4. He was treated with a vestibular and balance rehabilitation program with no change in performance on conditions 5 and 6 (not unexpected given the bilateral loss) but within

3 weeks of the onset of the program condition 4, well within normal limits on all three trials, and his reduction in volitional limits of sway was reduced to 35%.

An additional measurement that may also be important in explaining results that appear to be inconsistent is that of the average position of the center of mass during each trial. Normal distribution would have the weight positioned 2 to 3 degrees in front of the ankle joint. The interactive display can give the examiner an indication as to whether the patient appears to be standing with his or her weight distributed significantly over the heel of the foot. When this situation is noted during condition 1 testing, correct patient foot placement and a normal comfortable posture should be confirmed prior to continuing. If the COM continues positioned far to the rear with correct foot position and the patient reporting what he or she perceives as his or her normal posture, the range of motion in the posterior direction is severely limited. Therefore, if they start to sway backward from their neutral position, they are very likely to have to quickly take a step or make another fall reaction to prevent further posterior sway. This type of performance can result in an appearance of inconsistency, especially on the more difficult conditions 4 through 6, though they may be able to maintain their COM in their neutral or a forward position on one of the trials within normal limits, but on another trial a slight sway backward causes the fall reaction.

DETERMINATION OF EXAGGERATED (APHYSIOLOGIC) PERFORMANCE

Dynamic posturography is useful for identification of patients who may be, for whatever reason, exaggerating their condition. Works by several investigators (not all with EquiTest) have attempted to quantify the use of this tool to identify these patients and list qualitative factors that would raise questions in this dimension (Allum, Huwiler, & Honegger, 1994; Cevette, Puetz, Marion, Wertz, & Muenter, 1995; Goebel et al., 1997). Among the most common factors is the improvement of performance as the person being tested proceeds from condition 1 through condition 6. In a situation of this nature the equilibrium score is outside the normative range for the age of the patient on the easier conditions (1 through 3), yet as the task significantly increases in

difficulty the performance returns to normal or near normal. Another common feature is that of a regular sway pattern seen in the raw COM traces. This typically is sinusoidal in nature at a closely maintained frequency across the conditions with only the amplitude of the sway varying. Both of these conditions are indications of influences beyond a peripheral or central vestibular system lesion. However, the term *aphysiologic* may be inappropriate as some of these features are seen regularly in patients with anxiety disorders. Therefore, these types of performance may be a physiologic reaction to the anxiety disorder. A thorough discussion of this issue is given in Chapter 30 in this text.

CASES

The remainder of this chapter presents a group of cases that illustrate many of the interpretation points and clinical uses of dynamic posturography together with the other studies that have been discussed up to this point in this text including the office exam, ENG/VNG, and rotational chair testing. It is important for the clinician to understand the interaction of the tests on the final interpretation of the laboratory studies in the context of the patient's presenting signs and symptoms for final determination of the patient's condition. The majority of these cases are presented here, with permission from Shepard (2007).

Case 1

Case 1 is a male, who was 35 years of age, seen for complaints of sudden-onset vertigo, 6 months prior, with nausea and vomiting in a crisis event (acute vestibular syndrome) with continuous symptoms lasting 3 days, steadily showing slow improvement and no accompanying auditory symptoms. The continuous vertigo resolved into head movement provoked spells of light-headedness with imbalance and occasional vertigo lasting seconds to a minute after a movement. All planes of motion were provocative. Symptoms had continued to improve but still occurred on an infrequent daily basis. He presented with no neurologic focal complaints and past medical history was noncontributory. Audiometric evaluation was completely normal bilaterally as was his contrasted magnetic resonance imaging (MRI) study of the head. His detailed vestibular examination both with and without visual fixation was remarkable for a positive head thrust test to the left, right-beating post-head-shake nystagmus, and spontaneous right-beating nystagmus with visual fixation removed. The full neurologic and ocular motor components of the examination together with Hallpike testing were normal. His CTSIB was well within normal limits, and together with his history formal postural control testing was not needed in this case. The history with the examination was strongly suggestive of uncompensated left peripheral vestibular hypofunction, secondary to vestibular neuritis. Laboratory vestibular function testing revealed spontaneous right-beating nystagmus with visual fixation removed and a 76% left reduced vestibular response with ocular motor testing and postural control assessment normal. In this case the tests were, as is typical in most cases, confirmatory of the clinic suspicions from the history and direct examination. Management decisions made at the time of the office visit to initiate treatment with vestibular and balance rehabilitation therapy (VBRT) and to discontinue vestibular suppressive medication were not in any manner altered with obtaining the laboratory findings. The vestibular function and balance tests were well justified given the length of symptoms and the fact that the testing has better sensitivity for some ocular motor findings than the direct examination, specifically saccade velocity testing and quantification of smooth pursuit. Sensitivity to mild peripheral vestibular function asymmetry is also better with the laboratory testing. In this case the magnitude of the peripheral asymmetry made it detectable by both the direct examination and the caloric irrigation studies. This patient's vestibular rehabilitation program consisted primarily of exercises focused on improvement of the vestibulo-ocular reflex (VOR exercises, X1 and X2) and habituation exercises to reduce symptom production with head movements in the horizontal and vertical planes. No specific balance or gait activities were needed for this patient; however, he was put on a general walking program with casual head movements to increase his overall level of activity. Given that the primary reason for his lack of compensation was avoidance of head movements, he responded rapidly to the use of the rehabilitation program becoming virtually asymptomatic with a 6- to 8-week interval.

Case 2

A 31-year-old male presented with onset of head motion-provoked vertigo with more or less constant imbalance with standing and walking. He denied any vestibular crisis event or auditory complaints. His symptoms were more concentrated in sagittal plane movement and when rolling left or right from a supine position. These symptoms had been ongoing for several years with intervals when the vertigo was resolved and the imbalance was reduced but not absent. He reported an MRI from several years prior to this evaluation that was normal with a cervical MRI positive for mild disk abnormalities. Audiologic examination was normal. Other than the development of mild paresthesia of the right hand and arm over the last year, he had no other neurologic complaints and his past medical history was noncontributory. His direct office examination was remarkable for anterior semicircular canal benign paroxysmal positional vertigo (BPPV) canalithiasis, and inability to maintain quiet stance on foam with his eyes closed during the CTSIB. The remainder of the examination was normal. He was treated in the office with a canalith repositioning procedure and referred for a formal VBRT program. Secondary to the length of time of the symptoms and the complaints of persistent imbalance (although this is a common report with BPPV), vestibular and balance function testing was requested. The laboratory studies continued to show anterior canal BPPV with no other indications of peripheral vestibular system involvement. Pursuit tracking tests were normal, but saccade testing was positive for mild right internuclear ophthalmoplegia (INO). Postural control abnormalities were collectively consistent with that seen in demyelinating disorders, increased latency on the MCT test together with prolonged onset to the long latency response during postural-evoked response testing. The MCT test abnormality, although nonspecific to the cause of his symptoms was completely unexpected and difficult to explain on the basis of BPPV alone. However, given the ocular motor results and the PER findings, the prolonged latencies to active recovery fit with the overall suspicion of central nervous system involvement. His SOT results showed an increase in sway under conditions 5 and 6 without fall reactions. The SOT results are nonspecific to the disorder underlying the condition but reflective of his functional ability to maintain quiet stance when challenged. The SOT results simply reflect the fact that he was having difficulty using vestibular system information when visual and proprioceptive/somatosensory cues were absent or disrupted. Secondary to these findings and his report of paresthesia starting in the left foot a new MRI was obtained that showed multiple hyperintense spots throughout the brainstem region. He was referred on to neurology and is being followed with a diagnosis of probable multiple sclerosis with BPPV. Unlike Case 1, the management of this case was driven strongly by the results of the ocular motor and collective results of the dynamic postural control tests. The test results revealed abnormalities too subtle to be detected in a direct examination, the ocular motor abnormality of INO. Although the CTSIB and the SOT results were consistent, they were nonspecific and could have realistically been caused by the ongoing BPPV. It was the MCT and PER tests that reinforced the ocular motor findings

with strong presumptive diagnosis of MS. This is an exception to the impact that the testing has on a more routine basis in the decisions regarding management of the dizzy patient where confirmation is the more common roll of the laboratory testing of the dizzy patient.

Case 3

A 44-year-old female presented with spontaneous spells of light-headedness and imbalance lasting hours. Frequency of occurrence was 1 per every 8 weeks but increasing. Typically, she would return to her normal baseline between events. The core studies involving ENG and ocular motor tests were normal. Her CTSIB was normal, but as her history was that of unsteadiness, episodic without vertigo, full SOT/ MCT were indicated. The results of these evaluations are given in Figure 19–2. This figure dem-

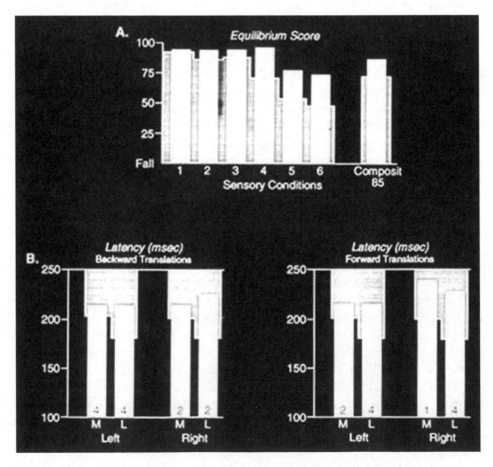

Figure 19–2. SOT and MCT results, respectively, for the patient in Case 3.

onstrates normal SOT with significantly prolonged latencies on the MCT. Secondary to the prolonged latency for the forward support surface translation, the protocol indicated the use of PER. Results of the PER are given in Figure 19–3. This demonstrates a

pattern of absent middle latency component and, when taken with the abnormally long MCT latencies for both limbs, is suggestive of possible demyelinating disease. Therefore, this patient's care was directed to neurology from otolaryngology, and she

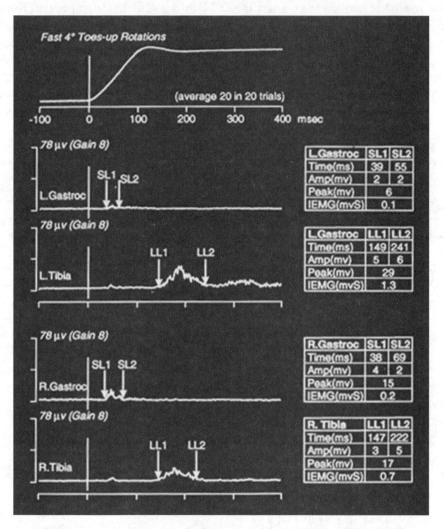

Figure 19-3. Postural-evoked response (PER) study for Case 3 is shown. CH1 and CH3 show the response for the gastrocnemius of the left and right legs, respectively, with CH2 and CH4 showing the response from the tibialis anterior from the left and right legs, respectively. *SL1*—onset time for the short latency response; *SL2*—offset time for the short latency response; *LL1*—onset time for the long latency response; and *LL2*—offset time for the long latency response. Latencies for onset and offset times are given in the grids at the right of each trace in milliseconds. The grids also provide for the absolute amplitude of the trace at the time of the onset and offset marks and peak amplitude of the short, medium, and long responses in microvolts. Integrated amplitude (IEMG) is given in microvolt-seconds for each response. The trace in the panel at the top left shows the timing of the toe-up rotation of the support surface. Zero time indicates the time of actual start of the platform movement. Note the striking absence of a medium latency response bilaterally.

was followed for possible demyelinating disease as a result of the test findings guiding the management.

Case 4

A 70-year-old male reported with a working diagnosis of right-side Ménière's disease. Laboratory testing was to be used to establish a baseline against which to compare for monitoring his disorder and possible treatment. His history was classic with regard to Ménière's disease with spontaneous spells of true vertigo with nausea and emesis production lasting 1 to 4 hr. Spells had been ongoing for a year beginning with one event every 2 months increasing in frequency to one to two times per week at the time of his evaluation. Conservative treatment with a low-sodium diet and diuretic were being used with no effect. He reported fluctuant hearing on the right with bilateral tinnitus and significant past noise exposure (Figure 19–4). Between the events he was free of dizziness symptoms. He did admit to increasing falls with his events but not between. The remainder of his past medical/surgical history

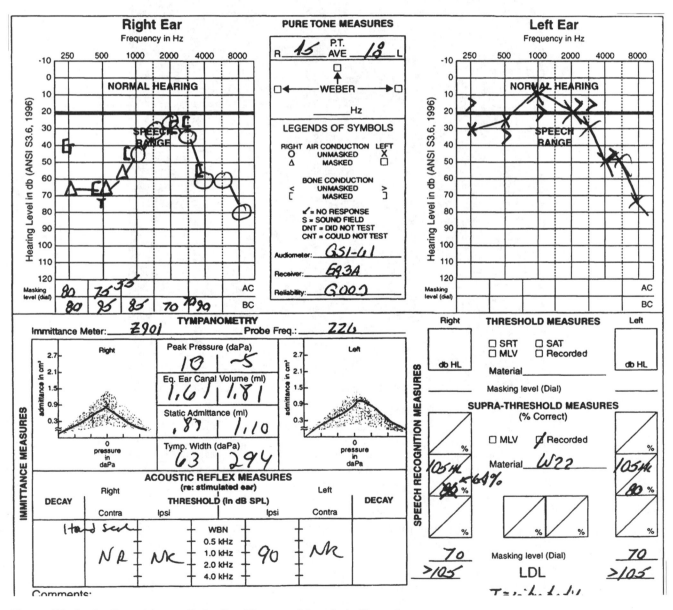

Figure 19-4. Audiometric results for the 70-year-old male in Case 4.

was noncontributory. Results from his VNG showed ocular motor findings that were normal or consistent with his age. Spontaneous right-beating nystagmus with a slow component velocity of 1 to 3 deg/s was noted in sitting with fixation removed. No exacerbation with head-shake testing and no positional nystagmus were seen. His caloric irrigation test revealed a surprising bilateral reduction with warm, cool, and ice water irrigations producing nystagmus with slow component velocity less than 4 deg/s for both right and left stimulations. The immediate question that required an answer was what was the degree of his bilateral involvement? If significant, it could limit more aggressive treatment options.

To attempt an answer to the issue of the degree of bilateral involvement rotational chair, the SOT of dynamic posturography and dynamic visual acuity testing (Herdman et al., 1998; Hillman, Bloomberg, McDonald, & Cohen, 1999; Peters & Bloomberg, 2005; Chapter 7, this text) were combined to provide a collective estimate of involvement. Rotational chair results to sinusoidal harmonic acceleration testing (see Chapters 14 and 15) and the SOT results of posturography are given in Figures 19–5 and 19–6, respectively. In summary, the chair results demonstrated an abnormally high phase lead in the lower frequencies with a left greater than right slow component velocity asymmetry. These findings, given the negative ocular motor testing, would suggest peripheral involvement of either a left paretic or right irritative style lesion. Given his spontaneous right-beating nystagmus and documented asymmetric hearing loss worse on the right, the right irritative lesion would be considered more likely. Of importance were the overall gain values within normal limits, although trending to the lower limit of normal as the test frequencies approached 0.01 Hz. This suggested that the extent of the bilateral involvement was minimal and restricted to the very low-frequency region of the peripheral system. The magnitude of the phase lead at 0.01 Hz was also supportive of this impression. If this impression from rotary chair is correct, then the functional impact of his bilateral involvement should also be minimal regarding maintenance of quiet upright stance and his ability to maintain visual clarity with his head in motion. The results of the SOT shown in Figure 19–6, although showing difficulty when he was forced to rely on vestibular system cues alone, demonstrates

his ability with practice to maintain stance within a normal range for his age by the second or third trial of test conditions 5 and 6. This SOT result would be consistent functionally with minimal bilateral vestibular involvement. Last, the DVA test performed using the clinical office technique with horizontal reciprocal head movements at 2 Hz was within normal limits. Overall, the collective results of the laboratory studies demonstrated peripheral vestibular system involvement bilaterally, but were mild in degree and restricted to the very low-frequency region of function of the peripheral system with greater involvement on the right than the left. These findings including the SOT and DVA provided a firm baseline physiologically and functionally for monitoring of the patient's slowly titrated transtympanic gentamicin treatment for his right-side Ménière's disease. This was successful in stopping the spontaneous events without causing him to experience any further functional deficits of significance related to his bilateral peripheral system involvement.

Case 5

This 55-year-old female was referred for evaluation with complaints of oscillopsia and imbalance with ambulation especially in darkened environments or on walking surfaces that were uneven or soft. Her history was that of diagnosis of non-Hodgkin's lymphoma and started on chemotherapeutic agents including cisplatin 1.5 years prior to her laboratory evaluation. Shortly after starting treatment she experienced a vestibular crisis event (acute vestibular syndrome) with sudden onset true vertigo, nausea, and vomiting without hearing change. Symptoms were continuous over a 3-day interval, improving into head movement–provoked symptoms and resolving completely within 2 weeks. She was without dizziness until 1 year later when she experienced another vestibular crisis event, equal in intensity to the first and again without auditory symptoms. This began after a second chemotherapy treatment with cisplatin. This event had a similar time course to the first crisis event; however, she developed left-side benign paroxysmal positional vertigo (BPPV) of the posterior semicircular canal that finally responded to treatment maneuvers and resolved after 1 month. Since the resolution of the BPPV, she has had the

VESTIBULO OCULAR REFLEX (VOR)

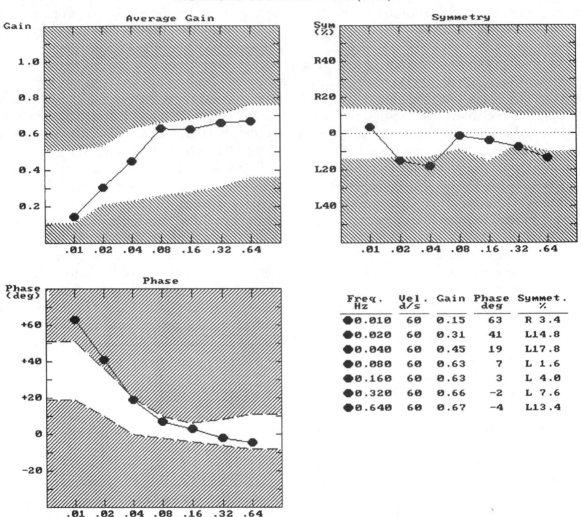

Freq. Hz	Vel. d/s	Gain	Phase deg	Symmet. %
●0.010	60	0.15	63	R 3.4
●0.020	60	0.31	41	L14.8
●0.040	60	0.45	19	L17.8
●0.080	60	0.63	7	L 1.6
●0.160	60	0.63	3	L 4.0
●0.320	60	0.66	-2	L 7.6
●0.640	60	0.67	-4	L13.4

Figure 19-5. Rotational chair results from the sinusoidal harmonic acceleration test for the male in Case 4. The graph in the upper left shows overall gain values of the slow component velocity of the eye referenced to the velocity of the head as a function of test frequency. The graph in the upper right provides the percentage difference in the average strength of the slow component eye velocity stimulated during rotations to the right versus rotations to the left as a function of frequency. At several frequencies the slow component velocities to the left (produced by rotation to the right) were significantly greater then the slow component eye velocities to the right (produced by rotation to the left). The resulting asymmetry could therefore be a result of a left paretic horizontal canal system or an irritative right horizontal peripheral system (an irritative status is not unusual in Ménière's disease). The graphical result in the lower left of the figure presents the phase angle (timing relationship of eye velocity versus head velocity) as a function of test frequency. This graph shows phase angle to be within normal limits progressing to an abnormal phase angle lead as the test frequency is lowered to 0.01 Hz. The table in the figure provides for the numerical results of gain, phase angle, and asymmetry at each of the frequencies tested.

complaints of oscillopsia and imbalance that she presented with for evaluation. The physicians working with the patient strongly suspected that she was now a bilateral peripheral paresis patient but wanted to know if there was any evidence that could suggest whether this was as a result of the use of the cisplatin. Her history would suggest otherwise given the two sequential crisis events, but ototoxic drugs have been

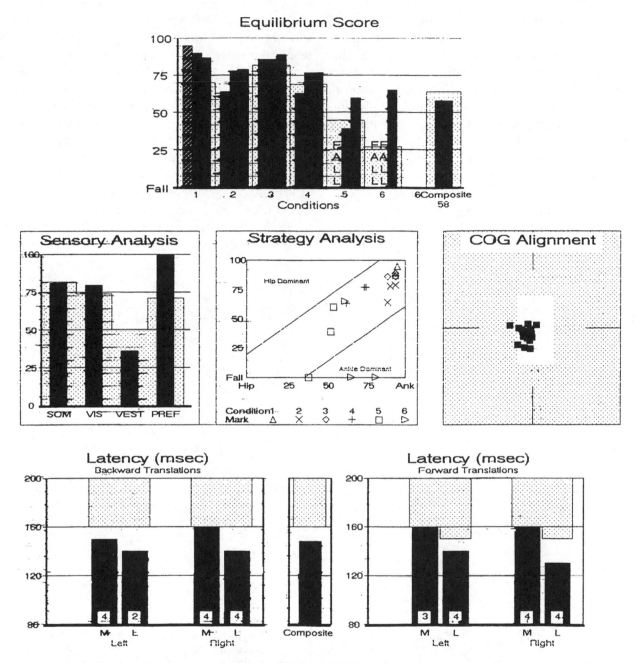

Figure 19-6. The graphical summary of the SOT and MCT tests for the gentleman in Case 4. The six conditions of the SOT test are shown in the graph at the top of the figure. This shows performance on conditions 1 through 4 to be within a normal range given the patient's age. Conditions 5 and 6 demonstrate fall reactions on the first trial with performance normal and improving on trials 2 and 3 for condition 5 and normal on trial 3 for condition 6. The graphs at the bottom of the figure demonstrate normal MCT findings for posterior (*graph on the left*) and anterior (*graph on the right*) translations of the surface on which the patient was standing.

known to produce other than symmetric effects on the vestibular system. Of importance in the history is the identification of left-side BPPV after the second crisis event. This verified report tells us that the pos-

terior semicircular canal on the left was indeed functioning normally as to the neuroephithelial tissues but had abnormal mechanical reaction to changes in a gravitational field. The possibility of differential damage to a labyrinth would not be the pattern of damage expected if caused by cisplatin. The laboratory challenge was to objectively investigate this issue. The VNG study demonstrated normal ocular motor results; no spontaneous, hyperventilation, or post-head-shake nystagmus; but clinically significant left-beating positional nystagmus with slow component velocity ranging from 3 to 6 deg/s was noted. Caloric irrigation with warm, cool, and ice water produced right- and left-side responses less than 4 deg/s. Formal hearing evaluation was well within normal limits through 8 kHz bilaterally. Her rotational chair and SOT/MCT findings are given in Figures 19–7 and 19–8.

In contrast to those of Case 4, these findings show none to minimal vestibulo-ocular reflex (VOR) responses to chair rotations across the entire frequency range tested and a profound functional impact on postural control when forced to rely on vestibular system cues alone with repeated true free falls (see tracings in Figure 19–8B) on all trials of conditions 5 and 6 with normal MCT findings. The functional impact of the loss of horizontal VOR was reflected in a dramatic DVA result of a five-line loss of visual acuity with reciprocal head movements at 2 Hz in the horizontal plane. The collective findings to this point demonstrated, as suspected, bilateral peripheral horizontal canal paresis of a moderate to

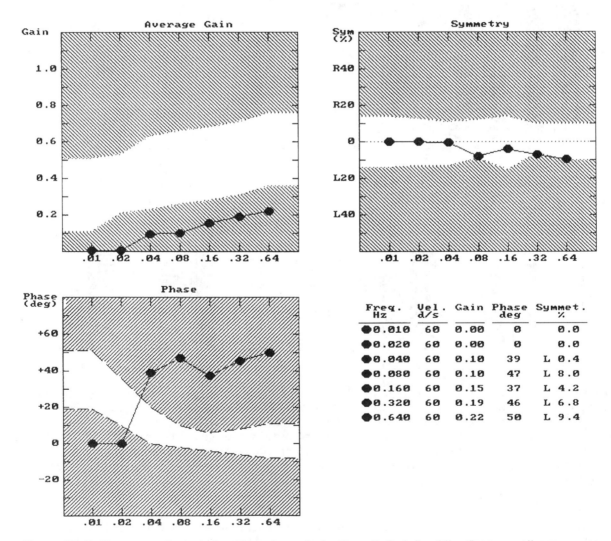

Figure 19-7. Shown are the rotational chair results for Case 5. Details of the figure are the same as given in Figure 19–4.

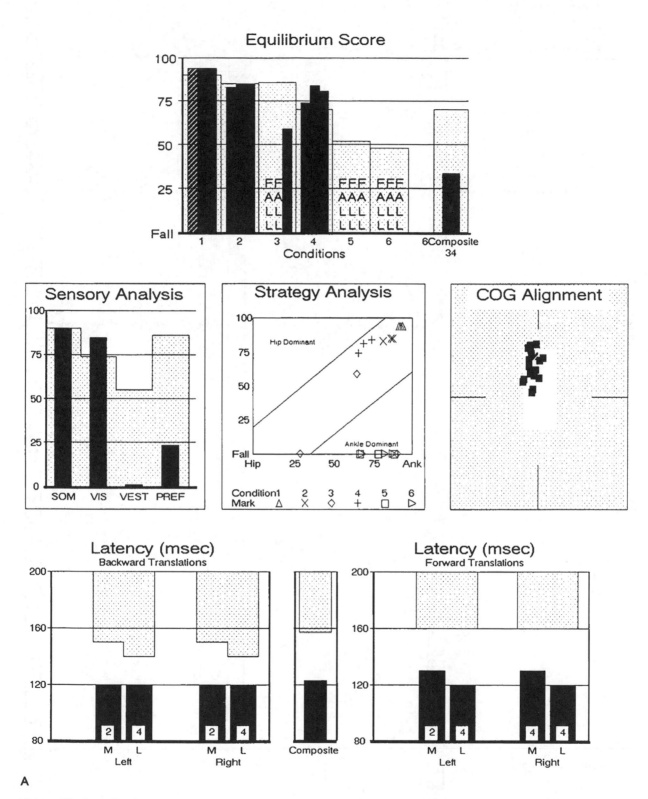

Figure 19-8. A. For Case 5 results of the sensory organization test and motor control tests are given. *continues*

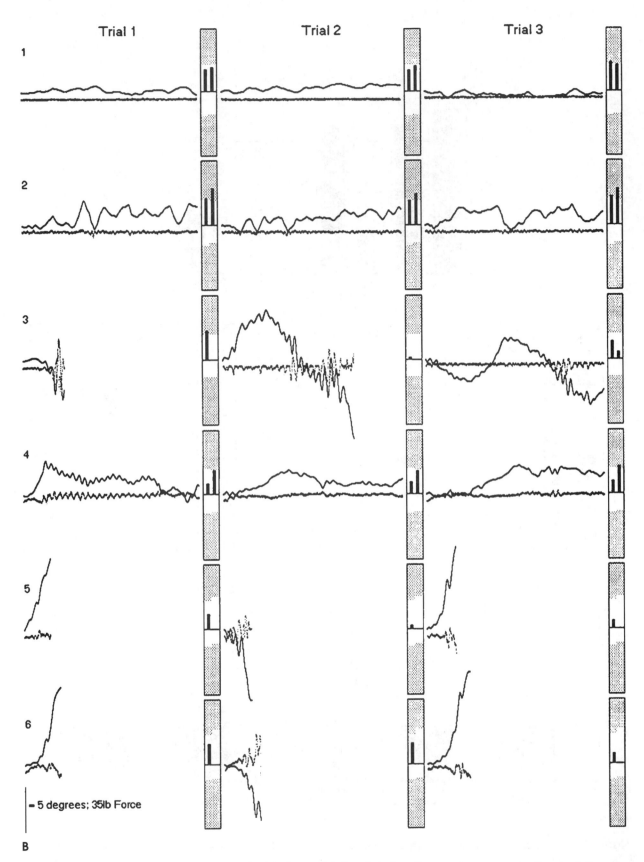

Trial 1 Trial 2 Trial 3

Figure 19-8. *continued* **B.** The raw data tracings obtained during the sensory organization test. See the text for explanation of the findings.

= 5 degrees; 35lb Force

B

496

severe degree. However, nothing has been done to directly evaluate components of the peripheral vestibular system other than the horizontal canal.

To investigate the vertical semicircular canals clinical head thrusts were performed with video-oculography in the planes of the right anterior/left posterior canals (called the RALP thrust), and the left anterior/right posterior (called the LARP thrust) (Aw et al., 1999; Chapter 7, this text). In both of these thrust tests, the patient was able to maintain her vision steady on the target during a thrust upward (assessing posterior canals) but made repeated corrective saccades for downward (assessing anterior canals) movements. For assessment of the utricular otolith organs, video-oculography was used to assess the ocular counter-roll (static position of the eye as an orienting response relative to the pull of gravity mediated by the utricular organs causing the eye to make a static torsional position change away from the ear that is down) when the head was tilted in the coronal plane from upright toward the left or right shoulders (Raphan & Cohen, 2002). For movements in toward either shoulder no counter-roll of the eyes was observed. Collectively, these clinical findings suggest involvement in both anterior canals and the utricular systems but preservation of function in the posterior canals, a pattern seen commonly in vestibular neuronitis (Aw, Fetter, Cremer, Karlberg, & Halmagyi, 2001). Finally, to investigate the saccular system, vestibular-evoked myogenic potential (VEMP) testing was performed using a click stimulus for the auditory signal (see Chapter 21 this text). Figure 19–9 shows the potential recorded from the left and right sternocleidomastoid muscles resulting from stimulation to the left and right ears, respectively. The presence of these responses confirmed functioning on at least a partial basis of both saccular organs and the integrity of the inferior division of the vestibular portion of the VIIIth cranial nerve.

In summary, the overall results for the patient in Case 5 clearly demonstrated differential damage to the vestibular labyrinthine systems bilaterally in a pattern of lesion site and by history of events most consistent with sequential vestibular neuronitis not damaged as a result of the use of the ototoxic agent cisplatin. This cleared the way for a third round of chemotherapy that would include cisplatin.

Case 6

A 42-year-old female reported for evaluation after multiple episodes of 1 to 3 days of head movement sensitivity. These intervals of time had been going on for about 6 months prior to the evaluation. She denied any changes in hearing and denies any spontaneous events of vertigo. On the days when she was sensitive to head movements, it was dominantly movements in the pitch plane or when rolling in bed that would provoke vertigo that would last for less than 1 min after a provocative movement. Her direct examination and all of her laboratory studies including SOT and MCT were all normal other than a positive Hallpike maneuver on the left. She also scored high on the Hospital Anxiety and Depression Scale for anxiety. She was treated with a left Canalith repositioning maneuver and symptoms resolved completely. She was instructed as to how she could treat herself if the symptoms were to return. A year later she returned reporting she had several recurrences of the symptoms but was able to manage the symptoms with the home maneuver she had been taught up until about 5 months ago. She reports that about 5 months ago she had a severe recurrence and the home exercise had reduced the symptoms as in the past but had not resolved the symptoms. She reported that repeated use of the treatment at home and by her local physical therapist had not helped. She was now having symptoms that were a constant sensation of vague movement in the head with unsteadiness that worsened with head movements. Symptoms were best when lying down and increased with sitting and going to standing and walking. She also reported that her symptoms would be exacerbated with visual motion, visual complexity such as stores, walking over or past visual patterns, and reading.

On re-evaluation she was again high on the Anxiety scale but all of her VNG, rotary chair, VEMP, both ocular and cervical testing, were normal. Her Hallpike to the left and right provoked equal symptoms, but there were was no nystagmus. The Hallpike was repeated a second time after about 30 min with the same results. She also reported that the symptoms with the Hallpike were that of unsteadiness, vague motion in her head but no true vertigo that had been present at the start of this recurrence

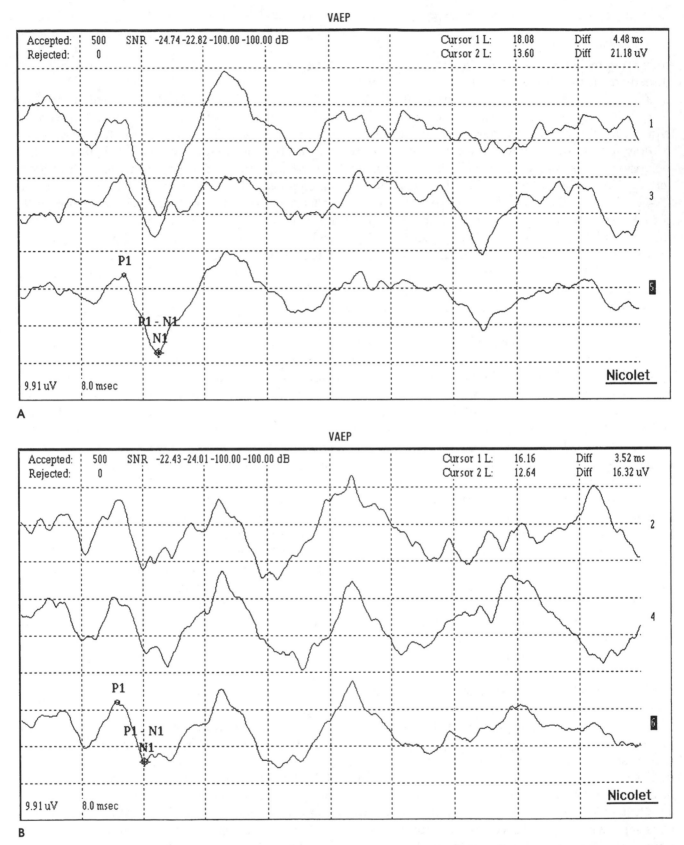

Figure 19-9. A. Results of the vestibular-evoked myogenic potential test are provided for stimulation to the left saccule. **B.** Stimulation to the right saccule in. The acoustic stimulus was a click presented at 105 dB nHL to each ear individually. In each panel the top two average responses are for two different recording trials. The third trace is the average of the two individual trials. The response of interest is marked in each panel as PI, N I.

of symptoms. Her MCT was well within normal limits, but her SOT showed abnormally increase sway magnitude without fall reactions on conditions 1, 2, and 3 with normal performance on conditions 4 to 6. While this pattern has been reported as aphysiologic per the discussion above, we interpreted the pattern as showing an anxiety reaction to the testing situation. The combination of her persistent symptoms and the development of the visual sensitivities along with the anxiety reaction on SOT collectively supported the diagnosis of chronic subjective dizziness syndrome (CSD) (see Chapter 30 for a full detailed discussion of CSD). As is described in Chapter 30 typical treatment was to start a medication for anxiety and depression and to start on habituation therapy for the sensitivities to visual and head movement stimuli that exacerbate her symptoms. She had developed CSD secondary to the severity of the recurrence of the BPPV and to the length of time that the symptoms lasted (1 to 2 weeks) compared to the other times with symptoms for only 1 to 4 days. At follow-up in 3 months she was virtually free of symptoms and had not had any recurrence of the BPPV. At the second follow-up she called to cancel informing us that she was now fully without any of the symptoms. She was slowly tapered off the medication and told she could stop the therapy exercises.

In this case the findings on SOT had changed from the initial symptoms to those consistent with CSD. The findings that are seen on SOT that imply an "aphysiologic pattern" should be interpreted in the context of the overall presentation as in more cases than not this appears as an anxiety reaction to the testing situation.

CONCLUSION

This chapter aimed to discuss the clinical utilization of dynamic posturography by presenting a series of illustrative cases. It is important, as shown in the cases, to understand how posturography can be used in the overall assessment of the patient with dizziness and balance complaints with other studies for a full picture of the patient's status. It is also important to realize that dynamic posturography has multiple uses ranging from a dominantly functional assess-

ment to site-of-lesion work contingent on the protocol used and the outcome parameters obtained.

As computerized dynamic postural control assessment moves into its next phase of technology with the use of virtual reality as substitute for the mechanical visual surround, it is hoped that new uses of the device clinically will become apparent. These may focus on using the device for recognizing and performing therapy for visual motion sensitivity that is seen in migraine patients and in those with CSD.

REFERENCES

Allum, J. H. J., Huwiler, M., & Honegger, F. (1994). Objective measures of non-organic vertigo using dynamic posturography. In K. Taguchi, M. Igarashi, & S. Mori (Eds.), *Vestibular and neural front: Proceedings of the 12th International Symposium on Posture and Gait* (pp. 51–55). Amsterdam, the Netherlands: Elsevier.

Aw, S. T., Fetter, M., Cremer, P. D., Karlberg, M., & Halmagyi, G. M. (2001). Individual semicircular canal function in superior and inferior vestibular neuritis. *Neurology, 57,* 768–774.

Aw, S. T., Halmagyi, G. M., Black, R. A., Curthoys, I. S., Yavor, R. A., & Todd, M. J. (1999). Head impulses reveal loss of individual semicircular canal function. *Journal of Vestibular Research, 9,* 173–180.

Black, F. O., Pabski, W. H., Reschke, M. F., Calkins, D. S., & Shupert, C. L. (1993). Vestibular ataxia following shuttle flights: Effects of microgravity on otolith-mediated sensorimotor control of posture. *American Journal of Otology, 14,* 9–17.

Boismier, T. E., & Shepard, N. T. (1991). *Test-retest variability of dynamic posturography in a patient population.* Abstracts for Association for Research in Otolaryngology, Fourteenth Midwinter meeting (p. 91). St. Petersburg Beach, FL.

Cevette, M. J., Puetz, B., Marion, M. S., Wertz, M. L., & Muenter, M. D. (1995). A physiologic performance on dynamic posturography. *Otolaryngology-Head and Neck Surgery, 112,* 676–688.

el-Kashlan, H. K., Shepard, N. T., Asher, A., Smith-Wheelock, M., & Telian, S. A. (1998). Evaluation of clinical measures of equilibrium. *Laryngoscope, 108*(3), 311–319.

Ford-Smith, C. D., Wyman, J. F., Elswick, R. K., Fernandez, T., & Newton, R. A. (1995). Test–retest reliability of the sensory organization test in noninstitutionalized older adults. *Archives of Physical Medicine and Rehabilitation, 76,* 77–81.

Fortin, M., Shepard, N. T., Diener, H. C., & Lawson, G. D. (1996). *Reliability of latency markings for the postural-evoked response test.* Abstracts for Association for Research in Otolaryngology, Fourteenth Midwinter meeting. St. Petersburg Beach, FL.

Gillespie, L. D., Gillespie, W. J., Robertson, M. C., Lamb, S. E., Cumming, R. G., & Rowe, B. H. (2007). Interventions for preventing falls in elderly people. *Cochrane Database of Systematic Reviews.*

Goebel, J. A., Sataloff, R. T., Hanson, J. M., Nashner, L. M., Hirshout, D. S., & Sokolow, C. C. (1997). Posturographic evidence of nonorganic sway patterns in normal subjects, patients and suspected malingerers. *Otolaryngology-Head and Neck Surgery, 117*(4), 293–302.

Hall, C. D., Schubert, M. C., & Herdman, S. J. (2004). Prediction of fall risk reduction as measured by dynamic gait index in individuals with unilateral vestibular hypofunction. *Otology and Neuro-otology, 25*(5), 746–751.

Herdman, S. J., Blatt, P., Schubert, M. C., & Tusa, R. J. (2000). Falls in patients with vestibular deficits. *American Journal of Otology, 21*(6), 847–851.

Herdman, S. J., Tusa, R. J., Blatt, P., Suzuki, A., Venuto, P. J., & Roberts, D. (1998). Computerized dynamic visual acuity test in the assessment of vestibular deficits. *American Journal of Otology, 19,* 790.

Hillman, E. J., Bloomberg, J. J., McDonald, P. V., & Cohen, H. S. (1999). Dynamic visual acuity while walking in normals and labyrinthine-deficient patients. *Journal of Vestibular Research, 9,* 49–57.

Honaker, J. A., Lee, C., & Shepard, N. T. (2013). Clinical use of the Gaze Stabilization Test for screening falling risk in community-dwelling older adults. *Otology and Neurotology, 34,* 729–735.

Honaker, J. A., & Shepard, N. T. (2012). Performance of Fukuda stepping test as a function of the severity of caloric weakness in chronic dizzy patients. *Journal of the American Academy of Audiology, 23*(8), 616–622.

Kubo, N., & Wall, C. (1990). Serial data variation in the dynamic posturography. *Abstracts for Association for Research in Otolaryngology,* Thirteenth Midwinter meeting (p. 350). St. Petersburg Beach, FL.

Lawson, G. D., Shepard, N. T., Oviatt, D. L., & Wang, Y. (1994). Electromyographic responses of lower leg muscles to upward toe tilts as a function of age. *Journal of Vestibular Research, 4*(3), 203–214.

McClure, R., Turner, C., Peel, N., Spinks, A., Eakin, E., & Hughes, K. (2007). Population based interventions for the prevention of fall-related injuries in older people. *Cochrane Review Library.*

Peters, B. T., & Bloomberg, J. J. (2005). Dynamic visual acuity using "far" and "near" targets. *Acta Oto-Laryngologica, 125,* 353–357.

Portney, L. G., & Watkins, M. P. (1993). *Foundations of clinical research: Applications to practice.* Norwalk CT: Appleton & Lange.

Raphan, T., & Cohen, B. (2002). The vestibulo-ocular reflex (VOR) in three dimensions. *Experimental Brain Research, 145,* 1–27.

Rose, D. J., & Clark, S. (2000). Can the control of bodily orientation be significantly improved in a group of older adults with a history of falls? *Journal of the American Geriatric Society, 48*(3), 275–282.

Shepard, N. T. (2000). *Clinical utility of the Motor Control Test (MCT) and Postural Evoked Responses (PER)* (pp. 1–20). Clackamas, OR: NeuroCom.

Shepard, N. T. (2007). *Management of the chronic patient with complaints of dizziness: An overview of laboratory studies* (pp. 1–17). Clackamas, OR: NeuroCom.

Shepard, N. T., & Boismier, T. E. (1992). *Variability of dynamic posturography in randomly sampled balance disorder patients.* Abstracts for Association for Research in Otolaryngology Fifteenth Midwinter meeting (p. 82). St. Petersburg Beach, FL.

Shepard, N., Boismier, T., & Anderson, A. (2010). Prediction of abnormalities of Postural Evoked Responses (PER) with Motor Control Test (MCT) results. Twenty-sixth Bárány Society Meeting, Reykjavik, Iceland, August 18–21. *Journal of Vestibular Research, 20*(3&4), 312.

Shepard, N. T., Schultz, A. B., Alexander, N. B., Gu, M. J., & Boismier, T. (1993). Postural control in young and elderly adults when stance is perturbed: Clinical versus laboratory measurements. *Annals of Otology, Rhinology, and Laryngology, 102*(7), 508–517.

Shepard, N. T., & Telian, S. A. (1996). *Practical management of the balance disorder patient.* San Diego, CA: Singular.

Shumway-Cook, A., & Horak, F. B. (1986). Assessing the influence of sensory interaction of balance. Suggestion from the field. *Physical Therapy, 66*(10), 1548–1550.

Weber, P. C., & Cass, S. P. (1993). Clinical assessment of postural stability. *American Journal of Otology, 14*(6), 566–569.

Wrisley, D. M., & Whitney, S. (2004). The effect of foot position on the modified clinical test of sensory interaction and balance. *Archives of Physical Medicine and Rehabilitation, 85*(2), 335–338.

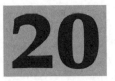

20

Vestibular Sensory-Evoked Potentials

Sherri M. Jones and Timothy A. Jones

INTRODUCTION

The clinician has many tests currently available to assess vestibular function. The material covered in this text demonstrates the ever-expanding options that the clinician should be familiar with when working with patients who are dizzy. Many clinics have the equipment and expertise to perform standard oculomotor, positioning, positional, and caloric testing. Beyond the classic test battery, one might utilize vestibular autorotation testing, head impulse test, vestibular myogenic potentials, and rotary chair testing. Dynamic visual acuity, eccentric and off-vertical rotation, subjective visual vertical and visual-vestibular interaction testing are also among the growing list of available vestibular assessment strategies. Computerized dynamic posturography includes a variety of tasks to measure sway or postural motor reflexes in response to changes in visual, somatosensory, or vestibular input. All of these techniques rely on the sequential activation of the periphery, central brainstem relay neurons, and alpha motor neuron pools innervating neck, extraocular or postural musculature. Common to all of these assessment approaches is the fact that one is observing or quantifying a motor output response, be it eye movements, head movements, or whole-body posture or sway. These measurements provide a view of the entire input-output system and are of critical importance in assessing motor control across entire reflex loops; however, they are all indirect measures of the inner ear. If one wishes to assess the peripheral sensors directly, then it is necessary to use other approaches.

Direct assessment of sensory function requires some means to stimulate the sensory receptor adequately and record the response of the sensory receptor and/or the neural pathway. Such assessment can be accomplished with invasive recordings of single cells (e.g., microelectrode or patch clamp recordings) or by utilizing far-field evoked potential recording strategies. Although the former methodology is useful for basic science research, the latter method has far more clinical utility. Evoked potential electrophysiology has been applied to assessment of the auditory sensory system for many years. Short, middle, and long latency auditory-evoked potentials (AEPs) have been utilized for basic and clinical studies and allow one to make a direct examination of the sensitivity, timing, and synchrony of the auditory periphery and afferent neural pathway. Theoretically, such direct evaluation should also be possible for the vestibular system. A noninvasive, direct assessment of the vestibular periphery and central relays might offer tremendous advantages in the clinical assessment of dizziness and imbalance.

This chapter reviews the scientific literature applying evoked potential electrophysiology to directly assess the vestibular system. Such sensory-evoked potentials have been broadly labeled in the literature as vestibular-evoked responses (VER or VsER), vestibular-evoked potentials (VsEP, VbEP, or VESTEP), or neurogenic vestibular-evoked potentials

(NVsEP). Throughout the chapter, we use the acronym VsEP as the general label for all vestibular-evoked potentials discussed. It is important to distinguish vestibular-evoked myogenic potentials (VEMP covered in Chapter 21) with VsEPs. VEMP recording strategies also utilize evoked potential electrophysiology; however, VEMPs are motor output responses (sternocleidomastoid or extraocular muscles) elicited by intense sound stimuli (e.g., Cody & Bickford, 1969; Welgampola & Colebatch, 2005) or by head movements driven by a minishaker (Paillard, Kluk, & Todd, 2014; Todd, Rosengren, & Colebatch, 2008). VsEPs, particularly short latency VsEPs, are compound action potentials generated by the peripheral vestibular nerve and its central pathways. Even though VsEPs reportedly have been elicited with intense sound stimuli, electrical pulses, or caloric irrigations (e.g., Bordure, Desmadryl, Uziel, & Sans, 1989; Kato et al., 1998; Molinari & Mingrino, 1974; Papathanasiou, Piperidou, Iliopoulos, et al., 2005; Papathanasiou, Piperidou, Pantzaris, et al., 2005; Rosengren & Colebatch, 2006; Todd, Rosengren, & Colebatch, 2003), the discussion here is limited to VsEPs elicited by adequate vestibular stimuli (i.e., head motion).

The goals for this chapter are to (1) consider the elements necessary for one to record VsEPs; (2) review studies that have reportedly recorded VsEPs; and (3) briefly consider the future development of clinical VsEPs. As there is not yet a widespread clinical measure of VsEPs for human vestibular assessment (several reasons for this are presented later), both human and animal studies are considered. We begin with a description of the general principles of evoked potential electrophysiology followed by a discussion of the adequate stimuli for eliciting VsEPs. Investigations of ampullar and macular sensory systems are discussed with regard to long, middle, and short latency epochs.

EVOKED POTENTIAL ELECTROPHYSIOLOGY

Far-field sensory-evoked potentials are compound action potentials recorded via electrodes placed some distance from the neural generators. Adequate stimuli that synchronously activate the neuronal population of interest are presented to elicit neural

responses that are time locked to the stimulus. Signal averaging is used to resolve the tiny neural evoked potential from the much larger ongoing electroencephalographic (EEG) activity. VsEPs, therefore, are compound action potentials of the vestibular nerve and/or central relays. VsEPs are elicited by stimuli that activate vestibular sensors and vestibular neurons and are recorded via electrodes placed on the surface of the scalp.

Three general areas are important for evoked potential electrophysiology: (1) stimulus parameters; (2) hardware/recording parameters; and (3) subject variables. References that discuss these issues with regard to AEPs are available (e.g., Burkard, Don, & Eggermont, 2007; Hall, 2007) and will not be discussed in great detail here. Consideration of these factors, however, is important for VsEPs. Throughout the VsEP literature, there is a tremendous variability in stimulus and hardware/recording parameters. No standard set of parameters has yet been adopted. Therefore, these issues will be discussed generally with relevant examples highlighted. Here we focus briefly on salient hardware and recording parameters beginning with a look at just what VsEP waveforms look like.

Some examples of VsEP waveforms reported in the literature appear in Figures 20–1 and 20–2. As with all evoked potentials, VsEP waveforms consist of a series of positive and negative peaks that occur at sequentially increasing time intervals. Most short latency potentials occur within 10 ms after the stimulus onset (see Figures 20–1A and 20–2). Middle latency responses have been reported between 15 and 50 ms (see Figure 20–1B), and we consider long latency responses to occur at 75 ms or later (see Figure 20–1C). Such responses have been elicited with rotary (i.e., angular) or linear stimuli. Table 20–1 lists many of the studies that have examined VsEPs to rotary or linear stimuli in humans. Table 20–2 lists animal studies. While the majority of human studies have focused on long latency responses (greater than 75 ms) to rotational stimuli (Bertora & Bergmann, 1995; Bodó, Rózsa, & Antal, 1981; Hansen, Zangemeister, & Kunze, 1988; Hofferberth, 1984, 1995; Hood, 1983; Hood & Kayan, 1985; Kast & Lankford, 1986; Keck, 1990; Kenmochi, Ohashi, Nishino, & Sato, 2003; Loose et al., 2002; Mergner, Schrenk, & Muller, 1989; Molinari & Mingrino, 1974; Munoz-Gamboa & Jimenez-Cruz, 1994; Pirodda, Ghedini, & Zanetti,

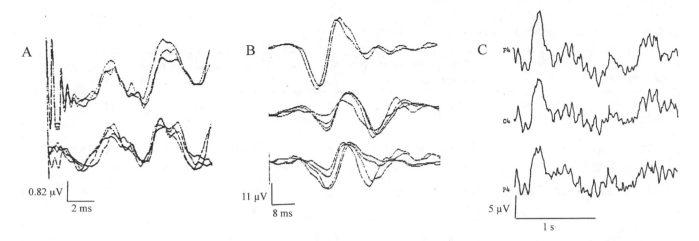

Figure 20-1. Representative VsEPs from the published literature for short (**A**), middle (**B**), and long (**C**) latency time epochs for human and animal studies. Amplitude and time calibration marks were taken from the original publications. Various waveform morphologies are notable across the varying time scales. Different stimuli and recording parameters were used to elicit these waveforms (see Table 20–1 as well as original references). Other examples of short latency linear VsEPs are found in the remaining figures in this chapter. A and B: Reprinted from Liebner et al. (1990, pp. 121, 122) with permission from Elsevier; C: Reprinted from Salamy et al. (1975, p. 58) with permission from Blackwell Publishing.

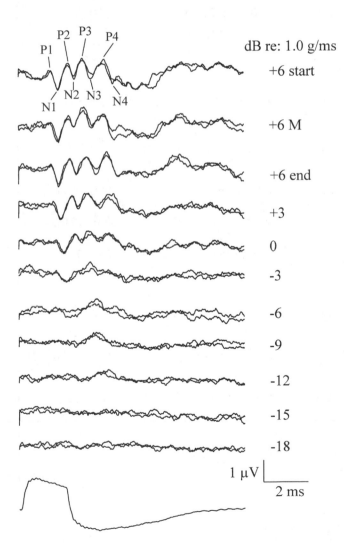

Figure 20-2. Representative short latency VsEP waveforms recorded at decreasing stimulus levels from a mouse. Stimulus level (in dB re: 1.0 g/ms) is shown on the right for each trace pair. The first three trace pairs were collected at the maximum stimulus intensity (+6 dB). The first two pairs were collected at the beginning of the recording session with (M) and without (NM) a broadband forward masker confirming the absence of any auditory components. The third pair was recorded at the end of the session approximately 30 min after the first two pairs confirming the stability of the response and the experimental preparation. The first four positive and negative response peaks are labeled. Total time shown for each trace is 10 ms. The bottom tracing reflects the stimulus that was applied to the head in order to elicit the responses shown.

Table 20-1. Representative Studies Reporting VsEPs for Human Subjects

Publication	Stimulus and Stimulus Shape	Stimulus Axis	Stimulus Levels and Rise Time	Response Latencies
Spiegel, Szekely, & Moffet (1968)	Rotary; bell shape	Yaw	120°/s deceleration	600–1000 ms
Salamy, Potyin, Jones, & Landreth (1975)	Rotary spring loaded manually released	Yaw	50°/s² at release	200–400 ms
Bodó, Rozsa, & Antal (1981)	Rotary; not stated	Yaw	125°/s² Time not stated	60 ms
Hood (1983)	Rotary; bell shape	Yaw	120°/s in 1 s	500–1000 ms
Hofferberth (1984, 1995)	Rotary; velocity ramp	Yaw	2.5, 5, 7.5, or 10°/s² for 1 s then stopped	220 ms
Hood & Kayan (1985)	Rotary; bell shape	Yaw	88°/s in 2 s; 51°/s in 1 s, 23 °/s in 0.5 s	800–1000 ms
Kast & Lankford (1986)	Rotary; manual drop	Pitch	20 cm over 200 ms	50–200 ms
Pirodda, Ghedini, & Zanetti (1987)	Rotary; sinusoidal	Yaw	800°/s² in 250 ms 3400°/s² in 125 ms	200–800 ms
Hansen, Zangemeister, & Kunze (1988)	Active head rotation	Yaw	10,000 to 20,000°/s²	68–424 ms
Trinus (1988)	Rotary and linear; not given	Not given	0 to 30°/s² 0 to 40 cm/s²	Not presented 30–150 ms
Mergner, Schrenk, & Muller (1989)	Rotary; bell shape and sinusoidal	Yaw	20, 84, 188°/s² (Bell); 15 and 30°/s (sinusoidal)	800–1000 ms
Keck (1990)	Rotary; bell shape	Yaw	3 to 20°/s² in 0.5 s	500–1000 ms
Zangemeister & Hansen (1990)	Active head rotation	Yaw	8,500 to 12,000°/s²	68–424 ms
Liebner et al. (1990); Elidan et al. (1991); Elidan, Sela, Liebner, & Sohmer (1991)	Rotary transient accel. sigmoid onset	Yaw	12,500 °/s² in 3.3 ms	3.5–27 ms
Knox, Isaacs, Woodard, Johnson, & Jordan (1993)	Linear deceleration	Gx	1.5 g (g = 9.8 m/s²)	3–10 ms
Claussen & Koltschev (1993); Claussen (1995)	Rotary; velocity ramp	Yaw	53°/s² for 1 s	65–800 ms
Munoz-Gamboa & Jiménez-Cruz (1994)	Rotary; position step	Yaw	Not stated	18–60 ms
Bertora & Bergman (1995)	Rotary; velocity ramp	Yaw	120°/s² for 500 ms 240°/s² for 250 ms	90–450 ms
Probst, Katterbach, & Wist (1995)	Rotary; bell shape	Yaw	100°/s² in 2.106 s	340 ms

Table 20–1. *continued*

Publication	Stimulus and Stimulus Shape	Stimulus Axis	Stimulus Levels and Rise Time	Response Latencies
Rodionov, Elidan, Sela, Nitzan, & Sohmer (1996)	Rotary transient accel. sigmoid onset	Pitch	$10,000°/s^2$ in 3 ms	2.2–31 ms
Probst, Ayan, Loose, & Skrandies (1997)	Rotary; bell shape	Yaw	$74°/s^2$ in 2 s	1–2 s
Trinus (1997)	Rotary and linear; not given	Not given	0 to $20°/s^2$ 0 to $20 cm/s^2$	40–150 ms 30–150 ms
Baudonnière, Belkhenchir, Lepecq, & Mertz (1999)	Linear; velocity ramp	Gz	0.1, 0.2, or 0.4 g for 30 ms ($g = 9.8 m/s^2$)	86 ms
Schneider, Schneider, Claussen, & Kolchev (2001)	Rotary; velocity ramp	Yaw	$15°/s^2$ for 1 s	50–850 ms
Loose et al. (2002)	Rotary; bell shape	Roll	64 or $66°/s$ in 2 s	500–1500 ms
Kenmochi, Ohashi, Nishino, & Sato (2003)	Rotary; velocity ramp	Yaw	20, 15, $10°/s^2$ for 1, 1.3, 2 s, respectively	250–400 ms

Table 20–2. Studies Reporting VsEPs Using Animal Models

Publication	Animal	Stimulus and Stimulus Shape	Stimulus Axis	Stimulus Levels and Rise Time	Response Latency
Elidan, Sohmer, & Nitzan (1982)	Rat	Rotary transient, not described	Yaw	$5000°/s^2$ in 1.5 ms	7–12 ms
Bohmer, Henn, & Lehmann (1983)	Monkey	Rotary sinusoid	Yaw	$2000°/s^2$	44 ms
Hoffman & Horowitz (1984)	Rat	Rotary, not described	Yaw	$1.3°$ in <15.5 ms	Not given
Elidan, Lev, Sohmer, & Gay (1984), Elidan, Sohmer, & Nitzan (1985)	Cat	Rotary transient, sigmoid onset	Yaw	$7000°/s^2$ in 2 ms	4–4.7 ms
Elidan et al. (1987a), Elidan, Li, & Sohmer (1995), Li, Elidan, & Sohmer (1993, 1995), Li, Elidan, Meyler, & Sohmer (1997)	Cat	Rotary transient, sigmoid onset	Yaw	$20,000°/s^2$ or $30,000°/s^2$ in 1.5–3 ms	2–4 ms for P1 and P2
T. A. Jones & Pederson (1989)	Chicken	Linear accel., transient	Gx	3 g in 3 ms 1 g in 1.5 ms	1.3–5 ms
Latkowski & Puzio (1989)	Guinea pig	Rotary	Yaw	Not defined	5.8–7.5 ms

continues

Table 20-2. *continued*

Publication	Animal	Stimulus and Stimulus Shape	Stimulus Axis	Stimulus Levels and Rise Time	Response Latency
Weisleder, Jones, & Rubel (1990), T. A. Jones (1992), T. A. Jones et al. (1993), S. M. Jones & Jones (1996), Nazareth & Jones (1998)	Chicken	Linear accel., sigmoid transient	Gx	1 g in 0.5 ms 0.031 to 1 g peak in 0.5 ms	1–5 ms
Inokuchi, Yamamoto, & Uemura (1991)	Guinea pig	Triangular velocity change	Yaw	$50°/s^2$ in 2 s	1.7–5.6 ms
Bohmer (1994)	Guinea pig	Linear accel., sigmoid transient	+Gz	2 g in 0.7 ms	0.6 ms for N1
Bohmer (1995), Bohmer, Hoffman, & Honrubia (1995)	Chinchilla	Linear accel., sigmoid transient	+Gz	0.5 to 8 g in 1 ms	0.6 ms for N1 1.5 ms for N1
S. M. Jones, Jones, & Shukla (1997)	Japanese quail	Linear accel., ramp transient	Gx	−30 to 0 dB re: 1 g/ms for 2 ms	1.2–5 ms
Plotnik, Elidan, Mager, & Sohmer (1997), Plotnik, Freeman, Sohmer, & Elidan (1999), Freeman, Plotnik, Elidan, Rosen, & Sohmer (1999)	Rat	Linear accel., sigmoid transient	Gx	0.1 to 12 g in 1 ms	2–10 ms
S. M. Jones, Ryals, & Colbert (1998)	Canary	Linear accel., ramp transient	Gx	−30 to 0 dB re: 1 g/ms for 2 ms	1.2–5 ms
T. A. Jones, Jones, & Colbert (1998)	Chicken	Linear accel., ramp transient	Gx	−30 to 0 dB re: 1 g or −30 to 0 dB re: 1 g/ms for 0.5, 1, 2, 4, 8 ms	1.1 ms for P1
S. M. Jones, Erway, Bergstrom, Schimenti, & Jones (1999), S. M. Jones et al. (2002), S. M. Jones, Erway, Yu, Johnson, & Jones (2004), S. M. Jones et al. (2005, 2006)	Mouse	Linear accel., ramp transient	Gx	−18 to +6 dB re: 1.0 g/ms for 2 ms	1.2–5 ms
T. A. Jones & Jones (1999)	Mouse, rat, gerbil, guinea pig	Linear accel., ramp transient	Gx	−18 to +6 dB re: 1.0 g/ms for 2 ms	1.2–5 ms
S. M. Jones & Jones (2000)	Chicken	Linear accel., ramp transient	Gx	−30 to 0 dB re: 1 g/ms for 2 ms	1.3–5 ms
S. M. Jones, Jones, Bell, & Taylor (2001)	Chicken	Linear accel., ramp transient	Gy, Gz	0 dB re: 1 g/ms for 2 ms	1.1–1.2 ms for P1
Oei, Segenhout, Wit, & Albers (2001)	Guinea pig	Linear accel., Gaussian transient	Gz	4 g in 0.5 ms	1.16–3 ms

1987; Probst, Ayan, Loose, & Skrandies, 1997; Probst, Katterbach, & Wist, 1995; Salamy, Potvin, Jones, & Landreth, 1975; Schneider, Schneider, Claussen, & Kolchev, 2001; Spiegel, Szekely, & Moffet, 1968; Trinus, 1988, 1997; Zangemeister & Hansen, 1990), some human studies have reported middle and short latency potentials (Elidan, Leibner, et al., 1991; Elidan, Sela, Liebner, & Sohmer, 1991; Knox, Isaacs, Woodard, Johnson, & Jordan, 1993; Leibner et al., 1990; Rodionov, Elidan, Sela, Nitzan, & Sohmer, 1996; Trinus, 1988). Much of the research in animal models has focused on short latency potentials. Indeed, short latency VsEPs to angular acceleration stimuli have been reported for monkeys (Bohmer, Henn, & Lehmann, 1983), rats (e.g. Elidan, Sohmer, & Nitzan, 1982; Hoffman & Horowitz, 1984), guinea pigs (Inokuchi, Yamamoto, & Uemura, 1991; Latkowski & Puzio, 1989), and cats (e.g., Elidan, Li, & Sohmer, 1995; Elidan, Lin, & Honrubia, 1987; Li, Elidan, Meyler, & Sohmer, 1997; Li, Elidan, & Sohmer, 1993, 1995). VsEPs elicited with linear stimuli have been described for several bird species including chickens (Fermin et al., 1996; T. A. Jones & Pedersen, 1989; S. M. Jones & Jones, 1996, 2000; S. M. Jones et al., 2000; S. M. Jones, Jones, Bell, & Taylor, 2001; T. A. Jones et al. 1993; T. A. Jones, Jones, & Colbert,

1998; Nazareth & Jones, 1998; Weisleder, Jones, & Rubel, 1990), quail (S. M. Jones, Jones, & Shukla, 1997), canary (S. M. Jones, Ryals, & Colbert, 1998), and mammalian species such as guinea pig (Bohmer, 1994; T. A. Jones & Jones, 1999; Oei, Segenhout, Wit, & Albers, 2001), chinchilla (Bohmer, 1995; Bohmer, Hoffman, & Honrubia, 1995), rat (Freeman, Plotnik, Elidan, & Sohmer, 1999a, 199b; T. A. Jones & Jones, 1999; Plotnik, Elidan, Mager, & Sohmer, 1997; Plotnik, Freeman, Sohmer, & Elidan, 1999), gerbil (T. A. Jones & Jones, 1999), and mouse (S. M. Jones, Erway, Bergstrom, Schimenti, & Jones, 1999; S. M. Jones, Erway, Yu, Johnson, & Jones, 2004; S. M. Jones et al., 2002, 2005, 2006; T. A. Jones & Jones, 1999).

In order to obtain waveforms from each of the time epochs (short, middle, and long), shown in Figures 20–1 and 20–2, repetitive stimuli to move the head were presented. Often short latency responses require that a greater number of stimuli be presented than that required for long latency responses and the nature of the stimulus, particularly the rise time, is critical. Stimuli can be delivered via whole-body motion or direct stimulation of the head. Direct stimulation to the head can be accomplished with commercially available mechanical shakers (e.g., Figure 20–3) or via custom systems

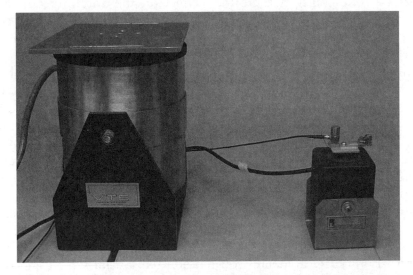

Figure 20–3. Two commercially available mechanical shakers that have been used for human (*left*) or small animal (*right*) linear VsEP studies. For both shakers, the center post moves in a vertical direction when a controlled voltage ramp is applied to the shaker. The shaker on the right also shows a stimulus platform that includes an accelerometer for monitoring platform motion and a clip for securing the animal's head to the stimulus platform.

(e.g., helmet bite bar system, see Elidan, Sela, et al., 1991; Sohmer, Elidan, Rodionov, & Plotnik, 1999). Coupling the stimulus to the head is critical in order to transfer the stimulus energy effectively to the inner ear sensory receptors.

Several coupling strategies have been used for delivering stimuli to the whole body or directly to the head. In human studies, whole-body motion (rotational or linear) has been delivered via a standard or modified rotary chair. For example, Schneider et al. (2001) used a rotary chair to present consecutive trials of clockwise and counterclockwise whole-body rotations about the Earth vertical (or yaw) axis. Probst et al. (1997) also used a rotary chair to present an angular stimulus profile in the yaw axis. Trinus (1988, 1997) modified a rotary chair so that it could be lifted, thereby producing a whole-body motion that was linearly directed in the Earth vertical (or Gz) plane. Knox et al. (1993) seated their subjects on a spring-loaded track to produce a whole-body linear motion in the naso-occipital (or Gx) translational axis. With whole-body stimulation, presumably the head is restrained via straps or a headband that is coupled to the chair (or other stimulating device), thereby limiting extraneous head movement and allowing one to assume that head motion (i.e., velocity or acceleration) is identical to the chair (or sled) kinematics. Alternatively, one could measure the head motion directly with an accelerometer located on the head. Knox et al., for example, utilized just such a strategy.

Rotating the human head directly has most often been accomplished with a custom helmet and bite bar system that is driven by a servo-controlled motor (Elidan, Sela, et al., 1991; Sohmer, Elidan, Rodionov, & Plotnik, 1999). Presumably, such a system can deliver high levels of angular acceleration in a short period of time with relatively minimal displacement. Such a short duration stimulus is termed a transient, which should be an optimal stimulus for eliciting short latency VsEPs. Direct application of linear acceleration stimuli has been delivered to the head of animal models via surgical mounts coupled to the skull (e.g., T. A. Jones & Jones, 1999; S. M. Jones et al., 2002, 2004, 2006), noninvasive clamp placed over the animal's snout (e.g., Oei et al., 2001; Plotnik et al., 1997; Plotnik, Sichel, Elidan, Honrubia, & Sohmer, 1999), or a noninvasive head clip encircling the cranium.

If the stimulus is applied directly to the head, it is important that the stimuli be monitored using precision calibrated accelerometers. Monitoring the stimulus at the head should also be considered an important strategy for whole-body motion. The placement of the accelerometer on the head may be limited by available space and it may not be possible to monitor skull movement directly (as in studies of small animals). In this case, the accelerometer is often mounted on the stimulus platform or the device that is delivering the stimulus to the head. If one is monitoring acceleration at the head, then other kinematic elements can be derived by routing the accelerometer output to an electronic differentiator or integrator.

Once the stimulus is effectively coupled to the cranium and monitored adequately, then stimuli can be delivered in a controlled manner. How then do we record VsEP waveforms from the surface of the scalp? EEG recordings typically involve placement of many electrodes over the surface of the scalp so that the investigator can examine the neural activity occurring between several pairs of electrode sites. For evoked potentials, electrodes must be placed strategically to maximize detection of the neural activity that is time-locked to the presented stimulus. Electrode position can have a profound effect on the amplitude of the evoked potential that is recorded. For eighth nerve compound action potentials, electrodes are typically placed with the noninverting lead at the vertex (Cz according to the International 10-20 system), the inverting lead at the mastoid (M1 and/or M2) and a ground at the forehead or other "neutral" site. Electrode placement for VsEPs generally follows this montage. Some investigators examining long latency VsEPs have recorded from additional sites on the scalp (frontal and parietal areas on both the left and right hemispheres) in order to look at the pattern of long latency evoked activity across the surface of the scalp and to demonstrate which electrode montages revealed the largest VsEPs. Of course, the more electrode pairs from which one wants to accumulate data, the more recording channels one must have available. Although the vertex to mastoid (pinna or post external acoustic meatus in the case of animal studies) has often been used for short latency VsEP recordings, S. M. Jones et al. (2002) demonstrated that a more caudal location for the noninverting electrode (nuchal crest) yielded larger amplitudes for short latency VsEPs in mammalian species. The vertex or Cz position appears to be optimal for avian models.

Hardware parameters (filter cutoffs, amplifier gain) and signal averaging parameters (sampling rate, number of responses averaged) can all influence the VsEP. Recording parameters for short latency VsEPs are similar to those for short latency AEPs (e.g., auditory brainstem response [ABR]). It is customary to use differential amplifier gains of 100,000 to 200,000 and filtering from 300 to 3000 Hz to amplify and bandpass filter electrophysiological activity recorded from electrodes. The processed signals are then led to a signal averager where they are digitized. In the author's laboratory, the amplified signals for short latency VsEPs are typically converted to digital waveforms by sampling at 10 μs/point for 1,024 points (sampling rate of 100,000 Hz). Middle and long latency VsEPs may require less gain (perhaps 50,000 or less), lower cutoff frequencies for the bandpass filter (e.g., 30 to 300 Hz for middle latency responses, 0.1 to 100 Hz for cortical potentials) and a lower sampling rate (e.g., 50,000 Hz down to 500 Hz used by Munoz-Gamboa & Jimenez-Cruz, 1994). S. M. Jones et al. (2002) demonstrated that the low-pass setting had the most significant influence on short latency linear VsEP amplitudes. The largest response amplitudes were obtained with the low-pass cutoff set to 10,000 Hz; however, these settings can result in increased high frequency noise. In general, one should always attempt to use the broadest bandpass possible, and it is important to specify the settings regardless of the filter bands used.

Standard signal averaging techniques are used to resolve response waveforms out of the background noise. Sampling of responses and initiation of the stimulus often occur simultaneously, but many signal averagers can be triggered pre- or poststimulus if needed or desired. Stimuli can be presented at various rates, which will affect the time it takes to average and display the final response waveform. For short latency VsEPs in animal models, stimulus rates of 2 to 17 stimuli per second are common and 128 to 256 individual primary responses are averaged to produce a final VsEP trace (e.g., T. A. Jones & Jones, 1999; Plotnik, Sichel, et al., 1999). Human studies of short latency rotary VsEPs have presented stimuli at slower rates (e.g., 0.5 to 2 stimuli per second) and averaged a larger number of primary responses (e.g., 500 to 2000, see Elidan, Sela, et al., 1991). Middle and long latency VsEP studies have used similar slow rates (0.2 to 0.5 Hz) but have averaged fewer responses (as few as 30 responses averaged by Probst et al., 1995).

The effects of stimulus rate on short latency VsEPs have been studied to some extent. The short latency rotary VsEP reportedly is stable at stimulus rates below 10 per second, but diminishes at stimulus rates between 10 and 15 per second (Elidan et al., 1984, 1985, 1986, 1987). This is considerably different than short latency linear VsEPs, which are highly resistant to stimulus rates showing little change in the VsEP response up to rates of 20 stimuli per second in rats (Plotnik et al., 1997) and up to 40 per second in mice (S. M. Jones et al., 2002). S. M. Jones et al. also showed that at a stimulus rate of 80 per second the linear VsEP response begins to deteriorate. The basis for differences between rotary and linear VsEPs in sensitivity to stimulus rate is not known, but it may reflect differences in the mechanical dynamics of the end organs. Effects of stimulus rate have not been studied systematically in human subjects or for middle or longer latency VsEPs.

Two additional stimulus features that will affect the final averaged waveform are the stimulus polarity and the axis in which the rotary or linear stimulus is applied. Stimulus polarity implies which way the head is being rotated (clockwise or counterclockwise) or translated (e.g., upward, downward, forward, backward). The axis of stimulation indicates the plane in which the rotation or translation is occurring. Conventions used to describe the rotational or translational axes are based on traditional anatomical axes (Hixson, Niven, & Correia, 1966) including naso-occipital (Gx, roll axis), interaural (Gy, pitch axis), and rostro-caudal (Gz, yaw axis). For rotational stimuli, the center of the head is typically placed on the axis of rotation and the direction of stimulation is indicated as clockwise or counterclockwise rotation in the axis under study. Most investigations have used angular rotation about the yaw axis, presumably providing maximal stimulation in the plane of the horizontal semicircular canals. Stimulation in the planes of other canals has also been described (see Table 20–1). For linear stimuli, the most common stimulus axis used has been the naso-occipital (Gx), which provides an effective stimulus to both the utricle and the saccule.

Once the stimulation axis is defined, VsEPs can be recorded to each direction of motion about the axis of interest (e.g., clockwise and counterclockwise about the yaw axis, forward and backward in the Gx axis) or responses can be averaged to motion in both directions. Alternatively, the orientation of the axis of interest may be altered systematically placing the subject in various alignments relative to Earth's gravity vector or relative to the neutral position of the stimulation axis. Several investigators have evaluated the effects of altering the direction of cranial linear translation or the plane of rotation on the VsEP (Elidan et al., 1982; S. M. Jones et al., 1999; Plotnik, Freeman, Sohmer, & Elidan, 1999; Probst et al., 1995). As described above, it is often convenient to average VsEP traces produced by opposite stimulus polarities to generate final response waveforms as such an approach reduces mechanical artifact from electrode movement. Again, this information needs to be clearly defined in the VsEP recording protocol.

It is important to have a means to remove, from the response average, individual response sweeps that contain significant electrical artifacts. In small animals, the electrocardiogram often is superposed on EEG activity, and its magnitude can be several times that of the background activity. In addition, both animals and humans can display occasional transient bursts of muscle activity, which will also introduce noise to traces, obscure responses, and make threshold determinations difficult. Signal averaging hardware or software often includes an artifact rejection process where acceptance levels for recording voltages can be set to prevent excessive voltage events from being included in trace averages.

One additional recording procedure should be used in a VsEP protocol. When recording VsEPs, particularly with stimuli coupled directly to the cranium, it is important to rule out auditory components or, if present, eliminate unwanted auditory contributions. On rare occasions, the applied stimulus may produce an audible stimulus that is conducted to the cochlea via air or bone conduction. When this occurs, the VsEP waveform also includes AEP components. An effective means to eliminate cochlear contributions is to present a broadband masker (encompassing the frequency range of the subject's hearing) along with the vestibular stimulus while recording the waveforms. If the VsEP obtained while the masker is present is identical to the unmasked condition, then one can be certain that there are no auditory components in the VsEP response. If, however, auditory contamination is a concern, the masker may be left on throughout the VsEP protocol. Figure 20–2 displays results from the unmasked (NM) and masked (M) conditions used in the standard protocol at the author's laboratory. The masker is a broadband (50 to 50,000 Hz), intense (90 to 100 dB SPL) forward masker that is presented during the averaging of two traces at the maximum stimulus amplitude. If no changes are seen in the VsEP, then the masker is turned off for the remainder of the protocol. This is the case for the data collected in Figure 20–2. If the VsEP had been altered in the masked condition, then the masker would be left on throughout the intensity series. It is important that the masker levels are no higher than 100 dB SPL as more intense levels have been shown to affect the vestibular sensors and hence affect the VsEP directly (T. A. Jones & Jones, 1999; Sohmer et al., 1999).

ADEQUATE STIMULUS FOR VSEPS

The adequate stimulus for any sensory system is defined as that stimulus requiring the least amount of energy to activate a response. VEMPs and some reported VsEPs (presumably of vestibular origin) (Kato et al., 1998; Papathanasiou, Piperidou, Iliopoulos, et al., 2005; Papathanasiou, Piperidou, Pantzaris, et al., 2005; Rosengren & Colebatch, 2006; Todd, Rosengren, & Colebatch., 2003) utilize auditory stimuli to elicit responses; however, the auditory stimulus levels must be intense (often greater than 90 dB nHL) to elicit these types of vestibular responses because sound is not the adequate stimulus for vestibular sensors.

Vestibular sensors are normally activated by head motion and gravity. The cristae of the semicircular canals are most sensitive to rotational or angular head motion, whereas the maculae located in the vestibule are most sensitive to linear or translational motion and gravity. Vestibular sensors are capable of selectively detecting and encoding a number of kinematic elements during head motion including position (the location of an object in space, x), velocity (the change in position per unit time, dx/dt), acceleration (the change in velocity with time, dv/dt) and jerk (the change in acceleration with time, da/dt). Studies of individual primary afferent neurons indicate that discharge activity in a particular afferent may be proportional to one or more kinematic elements depending on the frequency or dynamic characteristics of the stimulus (for review see Lysakowski & Goldberg, 2004). Presumably this sensory information enhances the brain's ability to control motor systems and maintain balance and posture during complex locomotion. When characterizing a VsEP it is important to understand which kinematic element has been used or monitored during testing.

As you can see from Tables 20–1 and 20–2, many different stimulus kinematics have been described across all of the studies listed. Figure 20–4 schematically represents some of the common stimulus profiles that have been used in VsEP studies. For rotary stimuli, angular acceleration is most often characterized. In several studies, a velocity ramp is used where a constant acceleration is presented for some specified period of time. With this information (i.e., acceleration and time) one can calculate peak velocity if desired. In other studies, a bell-shaped stimulus was used where acceleration or velocity

reached some peak value in a specified amount of time. In this case, acceleration or velocity is changing over time but not in a linear manner. A few studies used rotary transients with a sigmoid onset, which achieve specified peak acceleration in a period of time that is much shorter than the time required to achieve peak acceleration for the bell-shaped stimulus. Similar to the bell-shaped stimulus, however, rotary transients have acceleration increasing nonlinearly. Nonlinear changes in acceleration create complex onset kinematics that can be difficult if not impossible to replicate and interpret. For linear stimuli, studies are divided between those that characterized a constant linear acceleration (often specified in g where $1.0 \text{ g} = 9.81 \text{ m/s}^2$) for a specified time period (velocity ramp) and those that monitored stimulus levels in terms of jerk specified in g/ms presented for a specified duration. Describing stimuli in terms of jerk could also be characterized as an acceleration ramp where acceleration is changing linearly between zero and some peak level over the time period of the ramp. Because vestibular neurons

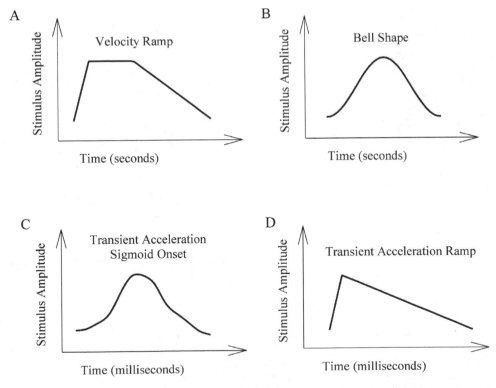

Figure 20-4. Stimulus profiles used in VsEP studies. Panels **A** and **B** reflect stimuli used in long latency VsEP studies (primarily human) where the stimulus reaches some peak value (be it velocity or acceleration) in several seconds. Panels **C** and **D** represent stimuli used for short latency VsEP studies where the peak level of acceleration is achieved in a matter of milliseconds.

encode motion it is extremely important that stimuli used in VsEP recordings be well characterized, precisely controlled, and consistent in amplitude and kinematic makeup.

Natural stimuli with sharply rising onsets (i.e., transients) are generally required to record well-formed short latency compound action potential responses from peripheral neurons. This is due to the requirement that the neurons be activated in a relatively synchronous fashion. Systematic study of kinematic elements and rotary VsEPs has not been reported and thus standardized adequate stimuli in terms of kinematic elements have not been defined for the rotary VsEP. T. A. Jones et al. (1999) studied the adequate stimulus for short latency VsEPs to linear stimuli in the chicken and demonstrated that

the peak acceleration of the linear stimulus could change quite dramatically, but if jerk were held constant, linear VsEPs were unchanged. Figure 20–5 demonstrates this for the bird and one mammalian species. These data indicate that the peripheral neurons generating linear VsEPs are keying in on the jerk component of the motion rather than displacement, velocity, or acceleration. Of course, if jerk is encoded by some vestibular neurons, then all of the other kinematic features are "available" to the central nervous system as it integrates peripheral input over time. In addition, it is well established that vestibular primary afferents encode other kinematic elements (see review by Lysakowski & Goldberg, 2004).

The specific kinematic features of the stimulus are key determinants of response amplitudes and

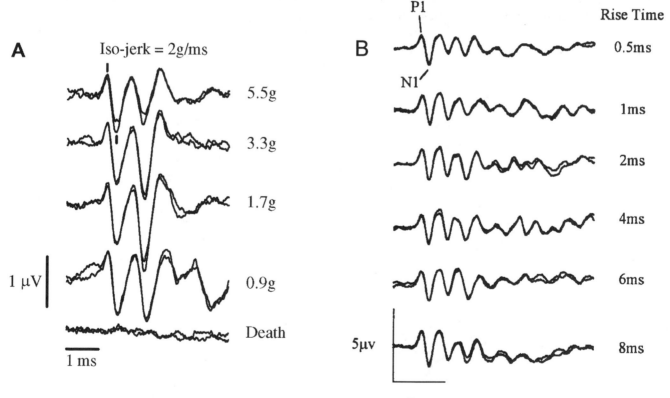

Figure 20–5. A. Mammalian VsEPs elicited with iso-jerk stimuli. Each trace pair was elicited with jerk amplitude at 2 g/ms presented at four different durations to produce a peak acceleration ranging from 0.9 to 5.5 g. Despite the broad range of acceleration, the earliest VsEP response peak (P1–N1) remains stable (i.e., consistent amplitude) if jerk level is held constant. **B.** Isojerk responses from the bird recorded with stimuli where jerk was held constant at 1.0 g/ms. Peak acceleration varied from 0.5 g (for 0.5 ms rise time) to 8.0 g (for 8 ms rise time). As with the mammal, VsEPs for the bird remain stable as long as jerk is held constant. A: Reprinted from T. A. Jones et al. (2011, p. 135) with permission from Elsevier. B: Reprinted from T. A. Jones et al. (1998, p. 265) with permission of IOS Press.

latencies for the short latency VsEP. In the author's laboratory, a common convention is to express stimulus amplitude in dB relative to a reference amplitude (i.e., jerk amplitude), where X dB re: 1.0 g/ms = 20 log [(Y g/ms)/(1.0 g/ms)] where Y is the stimulus level in g/ms and X is the numerical equivalent in dB re: 1.0 g/ms. This convention uses a reference level of 1.0 g/ms, where 0 dB re: 1.0 g/ms = 1.0 g/ms. Expressing stimulus levels in dB facilitates the use of precision attenuators and the characterization of vestibular responses over a wide dynamic range. The absolute magnitude can be extracted from levels expressed in dB by computing Y g/ms = 1.0 g/ms × $10^{(X dB/20)}$.

QUESTIONS REGARDING VSEPS

Several questions regarding VsEPs have been raised including: Are VsEPs real or an artifact? If real, are VsEPs generated by the inner ear? If generated by the inner ear, do vestibular organs generate the VsEP waveform? What neural generators contribute to the various response peaks? Finally, what can VsEPs tell us about inner ear vestibular function? These are important concerns with any far-field evoked potential; therefore, let's look at the evidence available to answer these questions. The most convincing data have been documented with short latency VsEPs in animal models so most of the data we will consider come from such studies. However, relevant human work will also be presented.

Virtually all animal studies have shown that short latency VsEPs are not electrical or mechanical artifacts since the VsEP waveform does not replicate the form of the stimulus and it disappears following death. Numerous studies have shown that the VsEP cannot be generated by the visual, somatosensory, olfactory, or gustatory systems. Instead, VsEPs are dependent on the labyrinth since bilateral labyrinthectomy or pharmacological blockade of the peripheral eighth nerve eliminates response components (Figure 20–6) (Elidan et al., 1984, 1985, 1987; Hoffman, 1987; S. M. Jones, & Jones, 1996; S. M. Jones et al., 1997; T. A. Jones, 1992; T. A. Jones & Pederson, 1989; Plotnik et al., 1997, Plotnik, Sichel, et al., 1999; Weisleder et al., 1990). The earliest peaks are clearly generated by vestibular neurons since VsEPs

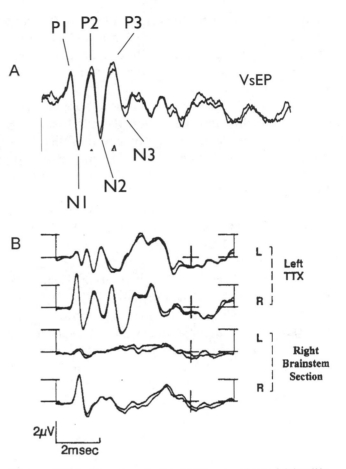

Figure 20–6. Representative VsEP waveform **A** identifying P1 and N1, which are generated by the peripheral vestibular nerve as shown in the data in panel **B**. In this study, function from the left side was eliminated using a neuropharmacological blocking agent (TTX). Responses after TTX therefore reflect activity from only the intact right side. Sectioning the right peripheral vestibular nerve from the brainstem leaves P1 and N1 intact while P2 and later peaks disappear. Response peaks after N1 are generated by relays within the central nervous system, but specific generator sites have yet to be confirmed. B: Reprinted from T. A. Jones and Nazareth (1998, p. 243) with permission from IOS Press.

are not affected substantially by intense, broadband auditory maskers (see Figure 20–2) (Freeman, Plotnik, Elidan, Rosen, & Sohmer, 1999; T. A. Jones, 1992; T. A. Jones & Pederson, 1989; T. A. Jones & Jones, 1999) nor are VsEPs eliminated following selective cochlear extirpation (see Figure 20–6) (S. M. Jones et al., 1997, 2001; S. M. Jones & Jones, 1996; T. A. Jones, 1992; T. A. Jones & Jones, 1999; Weisleder et al., 1990) or selective pharmacological blockade of cochlear dendrites (Irons-Brown & Jones, 2004). The evidence for the vestibular origins of the rotary VsEP has been most extensively studied in the cat and it is also compelling (Elidan, Lin, & Honrubia, 1986; Elidan, Langhofer, & Honrubia, 1987a, 1987b; Li et al., 1993, 1995).

Human VsEP studies have used subjects with unilateral or bilateral vestibular deficits to attempt to demonstrate the vestibular origins of VsEPs. Several studies demonstrate or describe the absence or alteration of VsEPs in individuals with presumed bilateral vestibular deficits (Baudonniere et al., 1999; Elidan, Liebner, et al., 1991; Elidan, Sela, et al., 1991; Hood, 1983; Hood & Kayan, 1985; Keck, 1990; Schneider et al., 2001); however, a few studies report inconsistent or nonspecific findings from normal subjects as well as those with bilateral vestibular dysfunction (Durrant & Furman, 1988; Hamid & Hughes, 1986; Mergner et al., 1989). Kenmochi et al. (2003) reported that long latency potentials to whole-body rotation in individuals with bilateral vestibular deficits required a larger acceleration stimulus (>20°/s²) than that required for normal subjects, which they suggested may have invoked somatosensory stimulation. Somatosensory, vestibulo-ocular reflex and optokinetic stimulation are major sources of artifact that have not always been well-controlled in human rotary VsEP studies. (Hood, 1983, Hood & Kayan, 1985, and Zangemeister & Hansen, 1990, addressed these issues specifically with regard to long latency human VsEPs. Probst et al. (1997) suggested that one should not expect the long latency VsEP to have purely vestibular origins because of multimodal inputs to cortical vestibular areas.

The findings from animal studies noted above have clearly demonstrated that the VsEP is a vestibular response in both birds and mammals. Which vestibular organs are contributing to linear and rotary VsEPs? S. M. Jones et al. (1999, 2004) investigated two genetic mutant mouse strains [head tilt (*Nox3het*) and tilted (*Otop1tlt*)] that completely lack otoconia in the utricle and saccule but have normal cochlea and semicircular canals. Otoconia ensure that the membrane overlying the macular hair cells will undergo movement relative to the surrounding tissue when placed in a linear acceleration field, therefore stimulating the underlying sensory receptors. When otoconia are absent there is no density difference between the otoconial membrane and the surrounding endolymph making it impossible for the otoconial layer to be moved with an accel-

eration force. Studies in otoconia-deficient mice demonstrated explicitly that VsEPs elicited with linear acceleration stimuli are dependent only on the otolithic organs, that is, the utricle and the saccule (Figure 20–7). Moreover, data from lethal milk mice (*Slc30a4lm*, a genetic mutant that lacks otoconia in the utricle but has a variable loss of otoconia in the saccule) showed that the amplitude of the earliest VsEP response peak (P1–N1) was correlated with the graded loss of otoconia. Indeed, linear VsEP amplitudes for P1–N1 are linearly proportional to the amount of otoconia present in the saccule (S. M. Jones et al., 2004).

While VsEPs to linear stimuli reflect selective activation of otolith organs, rotary VsEPs may be more complex. With rotary VsEPs, it is likely that macular and ampullar end organs are contributing to the responses due to coactivation. The onset of any motion, including rotation, has a linear kinematic component, and if sufficient, coactivation of the otolithic organs with an angular stimulus is possible. There is also the possibility of centrifugal forces activating otolith organs during some rotation profiles,

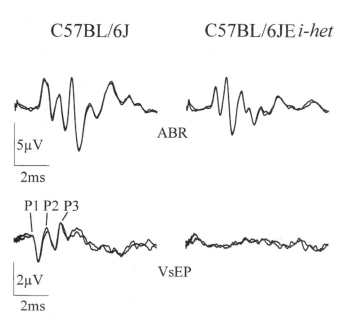

C57BL/6J   C57BL/6JE *i-het*

ABR

5µV
2ms

P1 P2 P3

2µV
2ms

VsEP

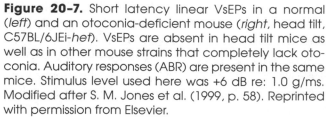

Figure 20–7. Short latency linear VsEPs in a normal (*left*) and an otoconia-deficient mouse (*right*, head tilt, C57BL/6JEi-*het*). VsEPs are absent in head tilt mice as well as in other mouse strains that completely lack otoconia. Auditory responses (ABR) are present in the same mice. Stimulus level used here was +6 dB re: 1.0 g/ms. Modified after S. M. Jones et al. (1999, p. 58). Reprinted with permission from Elsevier.

such as eccentric or off-axis rotation. Figure 20–8 shows linear and rotary VsEPs recorded from an otoconia-deficient mouse and a control mouse that has a normal complement of otoconia. Note the normal linear VsEP for the control mouse and the absent linear VsEP in the otoconia-deficient mouse. The rotary stimulus in this example was a pulsed angular acceleration ramp adjusted to approximately 57,500 degrees/s^2. Corresponding peak angular velocity and displacement were 77 degrees/s and 0.09 degrees in the yaw axis with the animal's head placed at the center of the rotational axis (Trimble & Jones, 2001). The rotary VsEP obtained from the normal mouse is larger in amplitude than that from the otoconia-deficient mouse, which suggests that coactivation of canal and otolith organs likely occurred in the normal mouse. Evidence for coactivation and a combined canal-otolith response in the rotary VsEP has also been reported by Li et al. (1995).

With regard to generators of the short latency VsEP, the earliest VsEP response components (P1 and N1) reflect activity of the peripheral vestibular nerve while later response peaks reflect activity of vestibular relays within the brainstem and higher centers (Figure 20–9) (Elidan, Langhofer, et al., 1987a, 1987b, 1989; Elidan, Li, & Sohmer, 1995; T. A. Jones, 1992; Li et al., 1997; Nazareth & Jones, 1998). Gaines (2012) showed that linear VsEPs were not altered by removal of the flocculus and cerebellum suggesting no role for these central relays in gener-

ating VsEP response peaks. The current hypothesis is that P2 is generated by the vestibular nucleus. Li et al. (1997) suggested that peaks beyond P2 for the rotary VsEP were generated by oculomotor, abducens, and vagus nerve nuclei. The precise origins of later central response peaks of the short latency VsEP remain to be convincingly discerned. Not in doubt are the distinction between peripheral and central response components, the peripheral origins of the earliest response peak, and the utility of the short latency linear VsEP in assessing peripheral vestibular function.

While generators for short latency VsEPs have been well studied, generators for middle and long latency VsEPs are unknown. Indeed, as previously discussed, the vestibular origins for long latency VsEPs have not been fully accepted. The latencies of these responses (>75 ms) may suggest brainstem or cortical regions are likely involved. Baudonniere et al. (1999) recorded from 21 surface electrodes placed across the human scalp and used a modeling strategy to define potential "active" areas contributing to their middle to long latency linear VsEP. The active areas they defined included the medial frontal gyrus, precentral gyrus (supplemental motor area), and the medial occipital gyrus. Probst et al. (1997) also recorded from 21 electrode sites for rotary VsEPs demonstrating large potentials over temporoparietal regions (T3 and T4 according to the International 10-20 system) that also showed direction

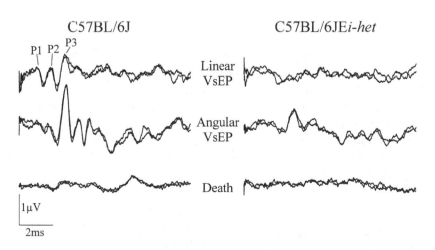

Figure 20–8. Linear and rotary (angular) VsEPs recorded from normal (*left*) and otoconia-deficient head tilt mice (*right*). Note the absence of a linear VsEP and the small amplitude of the angular VsEP in the head tilt mouse. The larger amplitudes visible for the angular VsEP from the normal mouse suggest coactivation of otolith and canal systems.

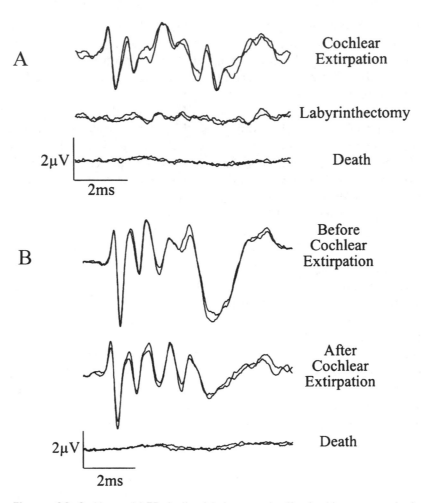

Figure 20-9. Linear VsEPs in the bird are not affected by removal of the cochlea (panels **A** and **B**), but are eliminated after labyrinthectomy (**A**) and death. Reprinted from S. M. Jones et al. (1997, p. 635) with permission from Springer Science and Business Media.

specific cortical activity between the two hemispheres. Schneider et al. (2001) reported that the largest amplitudes for their middle to long latency rotary VsEPs were at sites corresponding to the primary motor field (Brodmann's area 4) and the primary somatosensory cortex (Brodmann's areas 1, 2, and 3), areas consistent with the electrode alignment from T3 to T4 (i.e., T3-C3-Cz-C4-T4).

VSEP RESPONSE PARAMETERS

Figure 20–2 shows the linear VsEP recorded from a mouse using a linear jerk pulse stimulus (transient linear acceleration ramp) with duration of 2 ms, a repetition rate of 17 stimuli per second, and a magnitude ranging from 2 g/ms (+6 dB re: 1.0 g/ms) to 0.125 g/ms (−18 dB re: 1.0 g/ms). Stimuli were presented in the naso-occipital axis (Gx) in two directions of motion (+/−Gx) and the anesthetized animal was placed in a noninvasive head holder, positioned supine with the nose up so that the naso-occipital axis was oriented vertically (T. A. Jones & Jones, 1999). Electrodes were placed subcutaneously over the nuchal crest (noninverting or active electrode), postauricular (inverting or reference electrode), and at the ventral neck (ground). The electrical activity recorded by the electrodes was amplified (200,000 times), bandpass filtered (300 to 3000 Hz), and digitized (10 μs per point for 1,024 points). Averaging began at stimulus onset and two responses were averaged per final trace, one to 128 upward pulses (+Gx) and another to 128 downward pulses (−Gx). The upward and downward waveforms were averaged offline to produce the final response average representing 256 stimuli. A pair of such response averages is superposed at each stimulus level in Figure 20–2 to demonstrate the reproducibility of the response. It can be seen that the linear VsEP recorded in this manner consists of three to five posi-

tive and negative response peaks occurring within the first 6 ms after stimulus onset. One can also see that the peaks occur at approximately 1-ms intervals and have peak-to-peak amplitudes of approximately 1.0 µV at a stimulus level of +6 dB re: 1.0 g/ms. The quantitative changes in latency and amplitude as a function of stimulus level are shown in Figures 20–10 and 20–11, respectively. The data shown in Figures 20–10 and 20–11 reflect birds and mammals,

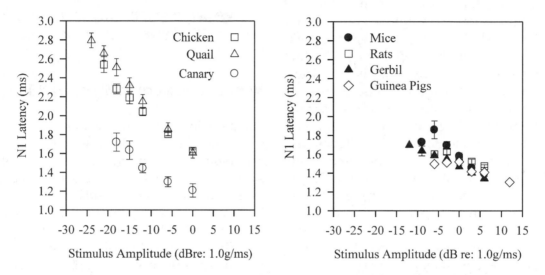

Figure 20–10. Latency intensity functions for short latency linear VsEPs from avian (*left*) and mammalian (*right*) species. Means and standard errors are shown. Birds have a larger dynamic range than mammals and steeper LI slopes. Mammalian data reprinted from T. A. Jones and S. M. Jones (1999, p. 79) with permission from Elsevier.

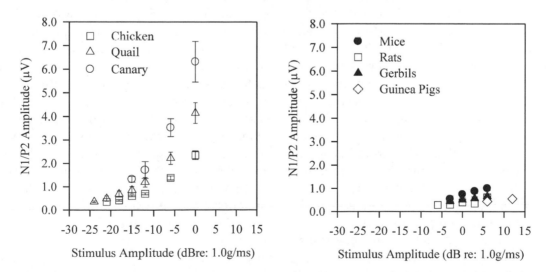

Figure 20–11. Amplitude intensity functions for short latency linear VsEPs from avian (*left*) and mammalian (*right*) species. Means and standard errors are shown. Birds have larger VsEP amplitudes, larger dynamic range and steeper AI slopes. Mammalian data reprinted from T. A. Jones and S. M. Jones (1999, p. 80) with permission from Elsevier.

and one can see that response latencies increase systematically as stimulus level decreases and peak-to-peak amplitudes decrease with decreasing stimulus level.

The VsEP response parameters most often reported are response threshold, peak latencies, and peak-to-peak or peak amplitudes. Response threshold provides an estimate of general sensitivity of the end organ and neural relays. In order to obtain a VsEP response threshold, one must record VsEPs to stimuli varying in level as shown in Figure 20–2. Threshold can be defined a number of ways and can be determined objectively or subjectively. For example, threshold might be defined as the lowest stimulus level where a response is just visible, or the highest level where no response is visible or the lowest stimulus level that produces a specified response magnitude. Regardless of how threshold is defined, it is important to state the criterion used to determine threshold and be consistent. In the author's laboratory, threshold is consistently defined as the stimulus level midway between the maximum level failing to produce a visible response and the minimum level generating a reproducible response. Using this definition, one can see that the threshold in Figure 20–2 is −13.5 dB re: 1.0 g/ms.

VsEP latencies and amplitudes may be used to quantify dynamic features of the sensory response to vestibular stimuli. Response peak latencies are defined as the time, in microseconds (µs) or milliseconds (ms), from stimulus onset to the occurrence of each respective positive (P1, P2, and P3) and/or negative (N1, N2, N3) peak. Peak-to-peak amplitudes (P1–N1, P2–N2, and P3–N3), often measured in microvolts (µV), represent the difference in amplitude between each positive peak and its subsequent negative peak. Latencies provide a measure of the timing of neural activation and conduction through vestibular relays. Amplitudes reflect the general number of cells responding to the stimulus and the degree of synchronization among the discharging neurons. We look more at latency and amplitude in the next section. Tables 20–1 and 20–2 identify the latency range encompassing all response peaks measured in each study or the latency for one specific peak if only one peak was reported.

By recording waveforms at various stimulus levels, one may obtain input-output functions for latency and amplitude. Latency-intensity (LI) and amplitude-intensity (AI) functions also provide a view of the dynamic aspects of response parameters. LI slopes, often described in ms/dB give some idea about how the neural timing and conduction of neural firing changes with stimulus level. Similarly, AI slopes, typically expressed in µV/dB, provide insight into the neural population and synchronicity with changes in stimulus level.

WHAT VSEPS DEMONSTRATE ABOUT VESTIBULAR FUNCTION

Nonpathological Subject Variables

Nonpathological subject variables that have been shown to affect VsEPs include general physiological conditions, core temperature, and level of anesthesia. Gender is a subject variable that has been shown to affect other evoked potential response parameters (AEP latencies, for example), but it does not appear to influence VsEP response parameters.

The general physiological status of an individual can influence the VsEP. The VsEP is stable over time, as indicated in repeated testing over many hours in anesthetized animals (Irons-Brown, Jones, & Jones, 2003) and indeed over months in the same animals provided the animals and the inner ear remain in good physiological condition (T. A. Jones & Nelson, 1992). Like many evoked potentials, the VsEP is sensitive to temperature. Quantitative measurements in birds and mammals indicate that latencies are prolonged with lower temperatures. Latency-temperature slopes reported for the bird were on the order of 15 to 23 µs/°C for the earliest response peaks (P1, N1) with progressively steeper slopes for later peaks (39 to 80 µs/°C) (Nazareth & Jones, 1998). Comparable values have been reported for the mammalian VsEP (Hoffman, 1987).

Some components of the short latency VsEP are affected by anesthesia. Studies of anesthetized and unanesthetized animals have shown that early response peaks are minimally affected by barbiturate anesthesia, whereas later peaks (those greater than 6 ms), presumed to be myogenic, were abolished upon induction of anesthesia (T. A. Jones, 1992). This is likely to be similar in mammals, although there have been no reports comparing anesthetized and unanesthetized mammals. Similar late myogenic potentials have been reported in the rotary VsEP, where neuromuscular junction blockers eliminated such response peaks (Elidan et al., 1984, 1985, 1986).

Comparative Physiology

Animal studies have used both birds and mammals, and comparisons between the two classes have revealed some interesting results. While comparisons across laboratories are difficult due to widely varying stimulus parameters, a few studies have examined several species within each class utilizing the same parameters (S. M. Jones et al., 1997, 1998; S. M. Jones & Jones, 2000; T. A. Jones & Jones, 1999). Figures 20–10, 20–11, and 20–12 show LI functions, AI functions, and VsEP thresholds, respectively, for three bird and four mammalian species. Visible in these figures is the fact that birds have considerably lower thresholds and a larger dynamic range (25 to 30 dB) than mammals (10 to 15 dB), larger VsEP amplitudes, similar peak latencies at 0 dB re: 1.0 g/ms, but steeper LI and AI functions overall. The reasons for these differences between birds and mammals are not yet clear, but one might be led to ponder (along with this author) what the VsEP results for a flying mammal (e.g., bat) might reveal.

Ototoxicity and Neuropharmacology

Studies of ototoxic antibiotic agents have consistently shown that the VsEP is sensitive to and disappears following administration of aminoglycosides (Elidan et al., 1987; T. A. Jones & Nelson, 1992; Perez, Freeman, Sohmer, & Sichel, 2000). The ototoxicity of a variety of other agents has also been assessed using VsEPs (Perez, Freeman, Cohen, Sichel, & Sohmer, 2003; Perez, Freeman, Sohmer, & Sichel, 2000). In addition, the linear VsEP has been used to characterize the disappearance and subsequent recovery of macular function in birds treated with streptomycin. Hair cells in the avian cochlea and labyrinth have long been known to regenerate following damage to the sensory epithelia (e.g., Cruz, Lambert, & Rubel, 1987; Corwin & Cotanche, 1988; Ryals & Rubel, 1988; Weisleder & Rubel, 1992). T. A. Jones and Nelson (1992) showed that avian gravity receptor function recovered virtually completely during the regeneration of hair cells and repair of the epithelium over a period of approximately 60 days following drug injury (Figure 20–13). Studies of the loop diuretics furosemide and ethacrynic acid as well as the cochleotoxic aminoglycoside amikacin have emphasized the resistance of VsEPs to systemic or local administration of these drugs, whereas AEPs recorded simultaneously were reduced in amplitude or eliminated (Elidan et al., 1986; Freeman, Plotnik,

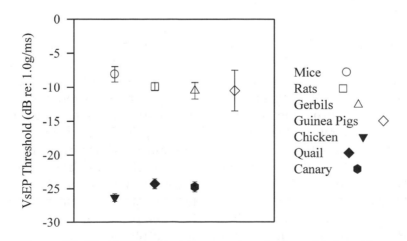

Figure 20–12. VsEP threshold comparison for three bird and four mammalian species. The bird species tested to date have significantly lower VsEP thresholds compared to mammals. Reprinted from T. A. Jones and S. M. Jones (2000, p. P43) with permission from The Galileo Foundation.

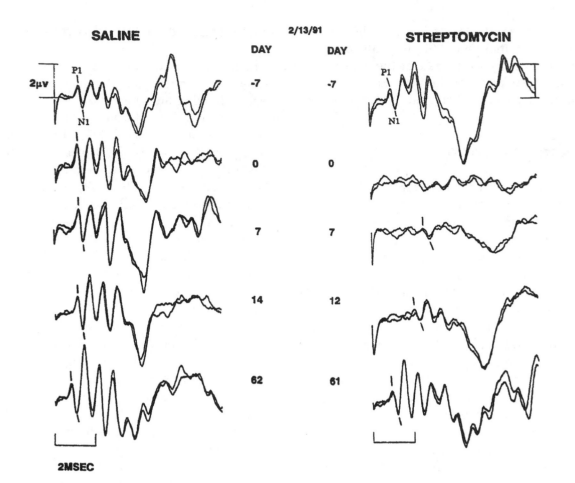

Figure 20-13. Linear VsEPS are eliminated after treatment with the ototoxic drug streptomycin (*right*). A control group treated with saline (*left*) show no changes in VsEPs. With sufficient time, the inner ear hair cells in the bird are capable of regenerating and the VsEP fully recovers as well approximately 60 days after treatment. Reprinted from T. A. Jones and Nelson (1992, p. 183) with permission from Elsevier.

Elidan, & Sohmer, 1999a; Freeman, Priner, Elidan, & Sohmer, 2001) illustrating that AEPs and VsEPs may be used together to study modality specific characteristics of the cochlea and vestibular labyrinth.

Auditory and vestibular information must pass from hair cells to primary afferents across the first relay synapse during its transmission to the brain. This first synaptic junction is located in the peripheral sensory epithelia, it is bathed by extracellular and perilymphatic fluids, and it is critical to the generation of compound action potentials for both the VsEP and the AEP. Irons-Brown and Jones (2004) evaluated the pharmacology of this synapse in the chicken by delivering selective receptor blockers to the neuroepithelium using perilymphatic perfusion (Irons-Brown et al., 2003) and simultaneously measuring the linear VsEP and the short latency AEP. The results demonstrated that the AEP, and hence auditory transmission, was exquisitely sensitive to non-NMDA glutamate receptor antagonists; however, the VsEP was remarkably resistant to all selective blockers including non-NMDA agonists and antagonists. Irons-Brown and Jones concluded that there was some dependence on non-NMDA receptors by macular systems; however, the VsEP findings demonstrated that either the vestibular sensors were protected from the agents perfused into the perilymph or that vestibular transmission was dominated by different receptors or processes than those found in auditory transmission.

Development and Aging

Age is an important subject variable. The VsEP begins to appear on postnatal days 6 to 10 in mice and rats (Freeman, Plotnik, Elidan & Sohmner, 1999b). In the chicken, the linear VsEP appears in the embryo at approximately 19 days of incubation and thresholds and latencies decrease while amplitudes increase and approach mature values over the next 10 days (S. M. Jones & Jones, 1996, 2000). S. M. Jones and Jones (2000) were able to distinguish and characterize maturational processes for peripheral and central pathways by evaluating early and late VsEP response components. For example, peripheral response components as well as thresholds reached mature values by 6 to 9 days post-hatch. Central response components matured much faster reaching adult-like values by 3 days post-hatch. These results suggest some distinct maturational profiles exist for peripheral and central vestibular relays.

Figure 20–14 shows linear VsEPs from young ages to senescence in two mouse strains (Mock, Jones, & Jones, 2009). The normal life span for mice is approximately 2 yr, which makes them an ideal model for aging studies. Qualitatively, the waveforms from the C57BL/6J strain suggest little change in the VsEP even at advanced ages. Interestingly, the C57 strain carries a genetic mutation that leads to age-related hearing loss (Johnson, Zheng, & Erway, 2000). By 12 months of age, C57 mice are severely

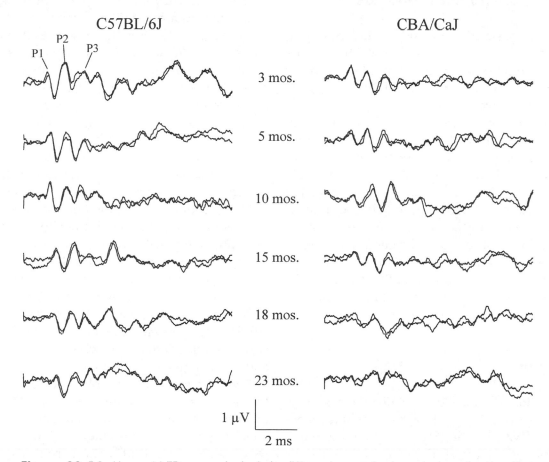

Figure 20-14. Linear VsEPs recorded at six different ages for two strains of mice. The C57BL/6J strain (*left*) carries a mutation in the cadherin23 gene (*Cdh23^753A/G*) that results in age related hearing loss. The CBA/CaJ strain (*right*) has no known mutations for hearing loss. Visible here is the deterioration of the VsEP with age for the CBA/CaJ strain while the C57 strain appears to maintain gravity receptor function into advanced age even though severe hearing loss is present in C57 mice by 12 months of age.

hearing impaired yet the data in Figure 20–14 suggest that there may be no appreciable loss of gravity receptor function at 12 months or beyond. The CBA/CaJ strain, with no known hearing loss mutations shows more deterioration in VsEPs with age. VsEP thresholds, latencies, and amplitudes as well as AEPs and otoacoustic emissions collected in aging mice demonstrate that vestibular and auditory functional aging varies with the genetic background (Mock, Jones, & Jones, 2009; Mock, Jones, & Jones, 2011). Further studies of genetic influences on auditory and vestibular sensory modalities should improve our understanding of cochlear and vestibular aging and may alter our expectations for the aging inner ear.

Other Nonpathological Variables

These include basic studies aimed at understanding the gravitational environment or exposures to various dynamic environments that may alter vestibular ontogeny or induce adaptation and ultimately alter VsEPs. In hypergravity or microgravity environments, peripheral response peaks of the short latency VsEP have been shown to remain stable while central VsEP response peaks were reduced (Fermin et al.,1996; S. M. Jones et al., 2000; T. A. Jones et al., 1993; T. A. Jones & Jones, 2000). Loose et al. (2002) also described reductions in the long latency human VsEP for human subjects during parabolic flights. Exposures to vibration and chronic intense noise environments have not altered VsEPs substantially (Jones et al., 2000; Sohmer et al., 1999; Trinus, 1997). While the animal data are compelling, the human studies have limited data for review.

Pathologies

Various pathologies have been evaluated in animals and humans using VsEPs. Disorders include diabetes (Perez, Ziv, Freeman, Sichel, & Sohmer, 2001), endolymphatic hydrops (Bohmer, 1993, 1994) or Ménière's disease (Trinus, 1997), demyelinating disorders, unilateral and bilateral peripheral vestibular deficits (e.g., Baudonniere et al., 1995; Elidan et al., 1991; Keck, 1990; Pirodda et al., 1987), cerebral infarctions (Hofferberth, 1995), and genetic mutations (including those that lead to syndromic and

nonsyndromic hearing loss) (Alagramam, Stahl, Jones, Pawlowski, & Wright, 2005; Geng et al., 2009; Goodyear, Jones, Sharifi, Forge, & Richardson, 2012; S. M. Jones et al., 2005, 2011; S. M. Jones & Jones, 2014; Lee et al., 2013). Unfortunately, many of the human studies describe results from patients with pathology, but have not published waveforms or quantifiable data to a great extent. We consider a few examples where data are available from the author's laboratory to demonstrate what one might see in VsEP response components due to pathology.

Demyelinating disorders affect neural timing and conduction and as such one expects to see prolongation of peak latencies and/or deterioration of waveform morphology with increasing stimulation of the neurons (as with higher stimulus rates). Figure 20–15 shows the dramatic prolongation of peak latencies for two mutant mouse strain known as quaking (Qk^{qk}; Sidman, Dickie, & Appel, 1964) and shiverer (Mbp^{shi}; Chernoff, 1981). These mouse strains have mutations in completely different genes, but both mutations affect the myelin sheath that surrounds neurons in the peripheral and central nervous system. Both peripheral (P1) and central response peaks (P2 and beyond) are prolonged in homozygous mice (−/− homozygote, i.e., mice that have two copies of the defective gene). AEP peak latencies are also prolonged in these mouse strains. VsEP thresholds for quaking homozygotes are typically not affected, but VsEP threshold for shiverer mice are significantly elevated by four months of age compared to normal controls (in this case the C3HeB/FeJ strain is the background control strain). Amplitudes for both quaking and shiverer tend to be larger than controls as well. According to Trinus (1997), Koltchev and colleagues studied patients with multiple sclerosis (a disease that affects myelin) and found larger amplitudes for long latency VsEPs.

VsEP testing in a number of genetic mutant mouse strains has demonstrated that the severity of vestibular functional abnormalities varies widely including elevated thresholds, prolonged latencies, reduced peak amplitudes and absent responses (S. M. Jones et al., 1999, 2004, 2005; S. M. Jones & Jones, 2014). The inner ear vestibular structural deficits leading to VsEP abnormalities include otoconia deficiencies, stereociliary abnormalities, hair cell structural deficits, ion transport deficits in various cell types and abnormal inner ear morphogenesis. Sev-

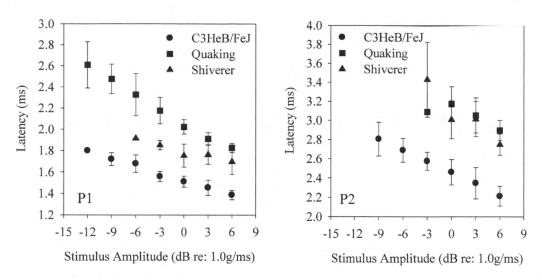

Figure 20–15. Mean latencies and standard deviations for VsEP response peaks P1 (*top*) and P2 (*bottom*) for two mouse strains with significant demyelination: quaking (*squares*) and shiverer (*triangles*). Both response peaks are significantly prolonged in comparison to control mice with normal myelin (C3HeB/FeJ, *circles*).

eral of the mouse strains evaluated are animal models for human syndromic and nonsyndromic hearing impairment. Figure 20–16 shows VsEP waveforms for several such mutants and their control strains. The human hereditary hearing impairment(s) is also represented for each genetic mutation in Figure 20–16. Do the VsEP results from the animal models have implications for the status of vestibular function in human hereditary hearing loss? It is well known that Usher syndrome type 1 has vestibular areflexia (i.e., absent caloric responses) and the absent VsEPs for the mouse strains $Myo7a^{sh1}$ (Usher 1B), $Cdh23^{v-2J}$ (Usher 1D), $Pcdh15^{av}$ (Usher 1F), and $Sans^{js}$ (Usher 1G) are consistent with the human data. In contrast, $Kcne1$ mutations in a mouse model of Jervell Lange Nielsen syndrome consistently show absent VsEPs, yet vestibular dysfunction is not generally included as a common phenotype of Jervell Lange Nielsen syndrome in humans. There could be several reasons for differences in the vestibular findings between the mouse models and human disorders, but in reality little human vestibular data have been published for most genetic forms of hearing loss (particularly nonsyndromic forms); therefore, comparison between mice and humans with regard to genetic vestibular dysfunction is difficult at present.

Despite the lack of human data regarding the genetics of vestibular function, we have learned

a good deal from genetic mouse models. VsEPs obtained from a broad range of inbred and mutant mouse strains have shown that gravity receptor function varies across strains and genetic mutations that alter various structural elements in the vestibular labyrinth. Figure 20–17 shows variations in VsEP thresholds, latencies, and amplitudes across 12 inbred strains of mice. Figure 20–18 shows VsEP threshold variations across several mutant mouse strains (S. M. Jones et al., 2005). In the near future, we are poised to learn a great deal about genetics of vestibular dysfunction and the role(s) that genes may play in the vestibular system.

Bohmer (1994) examined short latency VsEPs in guinea pigs with experimentally induced endolymphatic hydrops. Endolymphatic hydrops is thought to be one pathological condition underlying Ménière's disease. Bohmer obliterated the endolymphatic sac on one side to produce unilateral hydrops and recorded linear VsEPs up to 11 months postoperatively. His results demonstrated little to no postoperative changes in VsEPs at 1 month (a time interval considered to be early hydrops). At 11 postoperative months (described as late hydrops), however, the operated side produced VsEPs with elevated thresholds whereas the unoperated ear continued to reveal normal VsEPs. In some cases, the VsEP was absent for the operated side at the late hydrops

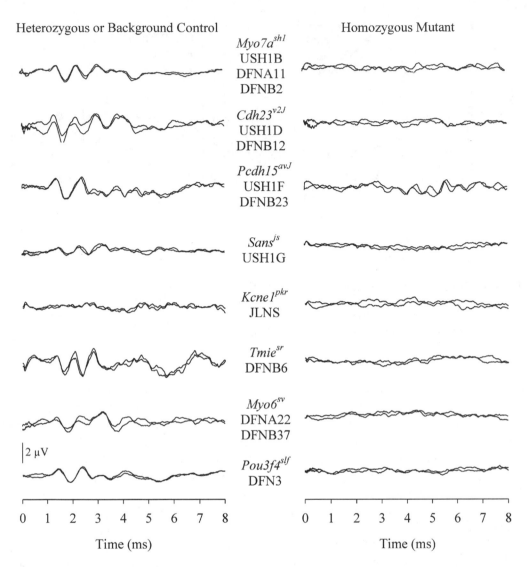

Figure 20–16. Examples of VsEPs recorded from a number of mutant mouse strains that are considered models for human hereditary hearing loss. The gene for each mouse strain is italicized. The human hereditary hearing loss that may result from mutations in the identified gene is shown in capital letters. Three forms of nonsyndromic hearing loss are shown: DFNA# signifies autosomal dominant, DFNB# designates autosomal recessive and DFN# identifies an X-linked hearing loss. Four genes leading to Usher syndrome Type I (USH1B, C, F and G) have been studied as well as the gene for Jervell Lange Nielsen syndrome (JLNS). The mutants shown here are homozygous for the particular gene mutation (–/–) and the corresponding control animals are heterozygote (+/–) animals that carry the mutation on one allele or are inbred background strains. Clearly visible is the profound loss of gravity receptor function in each of the homozygous animals. In some cases, abnormalities may manifest to some degree in the heterozygote.

stage. Bohmer demonstrated that the VsEP could be used to monitor a slowly deteriorating condition of the inner ear and is a useful measure to understand mechanisms that may lead to decreased inner ear function. More recently, Kingma and Wit (2009) induced acute endolympahic hydrops in guinea pigs by injecting artificial endoylmph into scala media. Linear VsEPs recorded for 5 hr postinjection showed a slow deterioration in VsEP amplitude associated with the perforation produced by the injection. No changes could be directly attributed to the acute increase in endolymphatic pressure.

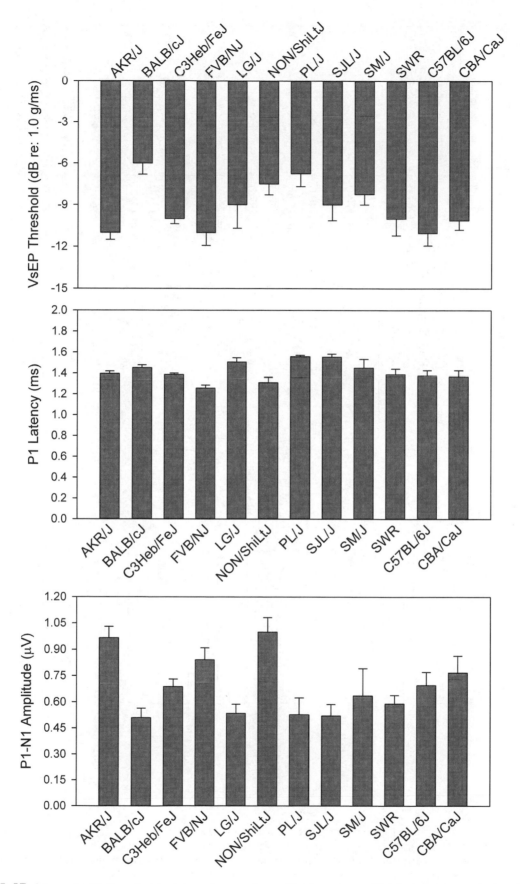

Figure 20-17. Mean VsEP thresholds, latencies, and amplitudes across 12 inbred mouse strains. Error bars show standard errors. Statistically significant variation among strains is evident for all response parameters.

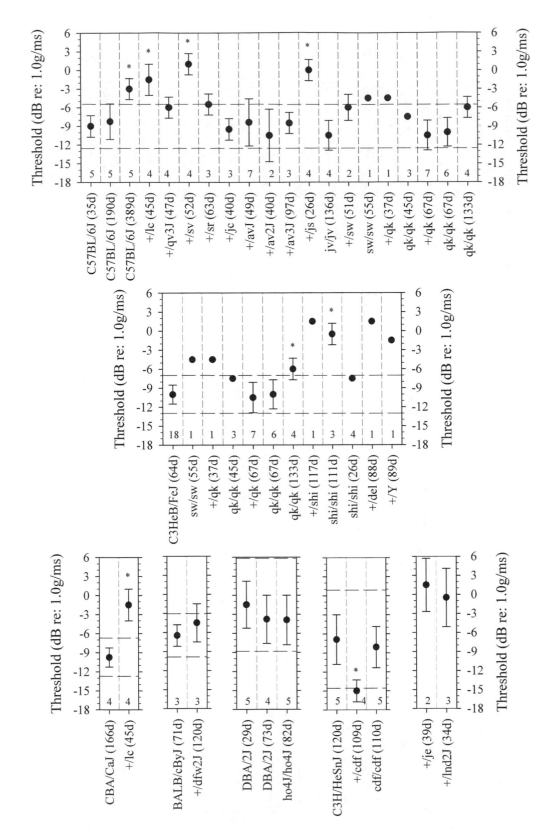

Figure 20-18. Mean VsEP thresholds (*errors bars* show standard deviation) for homozygote and heterozygote mutations. The number of observations contributing to each mean is shown. Homozygote data can be compared with the heterozygote counterparts, the respective background strain, or the normative range (the range for two standard deviations for each background strain shown as *dashed lines*). Asterisks represent those strains whose thresholds were significantly higher than the background strain threshold or the respective heterozygote group. Reprinted from S. M. Jones et al. (2005, p. 304) with permission from Springer Science and Business Media.

A BRIEF LOOK TO THE FUTURE

The material presented in this chapter provides evidence that direct measures of inner ear vestibular function are possible. Such measures have allowed investigators to evaluate ampullar and macular function with respect to various aspects of the stimulus (e.g., stimulus level, direction of motion), the dynamic environment as well as normal and abnormal vestibular physiology. In the research laboratory, the utility of VsEPs is clear and these methods have not yet been applied to many areas of new research. The clinical implications and potential for such a measure may be obvious, but the real issue remains whether human VsEPs will become a clinical reality.

There are a number of reasons why VsEPs are not used for human clinical vestibular assessment. Different laboratories have used different stimulating devices and different stimuli with vastly different kinematic profiles. The various recording paradigms have made it difficult to compare various results and develop a "standard" protocol for use across laboratories. In addition, several published reports provide insufficient detail for critical evaluation or replication. Moreover, human studies have been inconsistent and somewhat controversial. Some studies have described response reproducibility and others have demonstrated equivocal findings from normal and vestibular disordered patients (Durrant & Furman, 1988; Hamid & Hughes, 1986). The complexity and broad distribution of the central vestibular nervous system has been identified as a limiting factor for clinical utility of long latency vestibular-evoked potentials.

The animal studies to date provide strong evidence that short latency linear VsEPs provide a valuable, objective perspective into vestibular function, particularly gravity receptor function. Extending such a measure to the human is an important and worthy objective. The transient nature of the required stimulus, the obligate stimulus intensities, and secure coupling to the head represent difficult problems to overcome. However, once again, basic research may provide some keen insights into how such issues might be resolved.

Acknowledgments. The authors gratefully acknowledge research funding from the National Institutes on Deafness and Other Communication Disorders, Deafness Research Foundation, National Organization for Hearing Research, and National Aeronautics and Space Administration that contributed to the work reported here from the authors' laboratories.

REFERENCES

Alagramam, K. N., Stahl, J. S., Jones, S. M., Pawlowski, K. S. & Wright, C. G. (2005). Characterization of vestibular dysfunction in the mouse model for Usher syndrome 1F. *Journal of the Association for Research in Otolaryngology, 6*(2), 106–118.

Baudonniere, P. M., Belkhenchir, S., Lepecq, J. C. & Mertz, S. (1999). Otolith-vestibular-evoked potentials in humans. *Annals of the New York Academy of Sciences, 871,* 384–386.

Bertora, G., & Bergmann, J. M. (1995). Cortical responses of vestibular reactions measured by topographic brain mapping and vestibular evoked potentials. *Acta Oto-Laryngologica Supplement, 520,* 126–129.

Bodo, G., Rozsa, L., & Antal, P. (1981). Scalp electrical response evoked by acceleration in young healthy men. In L. Surjan & G. Bodo (Eds.), *Borderline Problems in Otorhinolaryngology: Proceedings of the XIIth World Congress in Otorhinolaryngology* (pp. 389–392). Amsterdam, the Netherlands: Excerpta Medica.

Bohmer, A. (1993). Hydrostatic pressure in the inner ear fluid compartments and its effects on inner ear function. *Acta Oto-Laryngologica Supplement, 507,* 1–24.

Bohmer, A. (1994). Vestibular evoked potentials and auditory electrophysiological parameters of increased inner-ear pressure in experimental endolymphatic hydrops. In R. Filipo & M. Barbara (Eds.), *Meniere's disease: Perspectives in the '90s* (pp. 347–351). Amsterdam, the Netherlands: Kugler.

Bohmer, A. (1995). Short latency vestibular evoked responses to linear acceleration stimuli in small mammals: Masking effects and experimental applications. *Acta Oto-Laryngologica Supplement, 520,* 120–123.

Bohmer, A., Henn, V., & Lehmann, D. (1983). Vestibular evoked potentials in the awake rhesus monkey. *Advances in Oto-Rhino-Laryngology, 30,* 54–57.

Bohmer, A., Hoffman, L. F., & Honrubia, V. (1995). Characterization of vestibular potentials evoked by linear acceleration pulses in the chinchilla. *American Journal of Otology, 16*(4), 498–504.

Bordure, P., Desmadryl, G., Uziel, A., & Sans, A. (1989). Short latency vestibular potentials evoked by electrical round window stimulation in the guinea pig. *Electroencephaolography and Clinical Neurophysiology, 73,* 464–469.

Burkard, R. F., Don, M., & Eggermont, J. J. (2007). *Auditory evoked potentials: Basic principles and clinical application.* Philadelphia, PA: Lippincott, Williams & Wilkins.

Chernoff, G. F. 1981. Shiverer: An autosomal recessive mutant mouse with myelin deficiency. *Journal of Heredity, 72*(2), 128.

Claussen, C. F. (1995). Vestibular evoked responses: A new frontier in equilibriometry. *Acta Oto-Laryngologica Supplement, 520,* 113–116.

Claussen, C. F., & Koltschev, C. (1993). Vestibular evoked potentials. In I. Kaufman-Arenberg (Ed.), *Dizziness and balance disorders* (pp. 413–428). New York, NY: Kugler.

Cody, D. T., & Bickford, R. G. (1969). Averaged evoked myogenic responses in man. *Laryngoscope, 79*(3), 400–416.

Corwin, J. T., & Cotanche, D. A. (1988). Regeneration of sensory hair cells after acoustic trauma. *Science, 240,* 1772–1774.

Cruz, R. M., Lambert, P. R., & Rubel, E. W. (1987). Light microscopic evidence of hair cell regeneration after gentamicin toxicity in chick cochlea. *Archives of Otolaryngology-Head and Neck Surgery, 113*(10), 1058–1062.

Durrant, J. D., & Furman, J. M. R. (1988). Long-latency rotational evoked potentials in subjects with and without bilateral vestibular loss. *Electroencephalography and Clinical Neurophysiology, 71,* 251–256.

Elidan, J., Langhofer, L., & Honrubia, V. (1987a). Recording of short-latency vestibular evoked potentials induced by acceleration impulses in experimental animals: Current status of the method and its application. *Electroencephalography and Clinical Neurophysiology, 68,* 58–69.

Elidan, J., Langhofer, L., & Honrubia, V. (1987b). The neural generators of the vestibular evoked response. *Brain Research, 423,* 385–390.

Elidan, J., Langhofer, J., & Honrubia, V. (1989). The firing properties of second-order vestibular neurons in correlation with the far-field recorded vestibular-evoked responses. *Laryngoscope, 99*(1), 92–99.

Elidan, J., Leibner, E., Freeman, S., Sela, M., Nitzan, M., & Sohmer, H. (1991). Short and middle latency vestibular evoked responses to acceleration in man. *Electroencephalography and Clinical Neurophysiology, 80,* 140–145.

Elidan, J., Lev, S., Sohmer, H., & Gay, I. (1984). Short latency vestibular evoked response to acceleration stimuli recorded by skin electrodes. *Annals of Otology, Rhinology & Laryngology, 93*(3), 257–261.

Elidan, J., Li, G., & Sohmer, H. (1995). The contribution of cranial-nerve nuclei to the short latency vestibular evoked potentials in cat. *Acta Oto-Laryngologica, 115,* 141–144.

Elidan, J., Lin, J., & Honrubia, V. (1986). The effect of loop diuretics on the vestibular system. Assessment by recording the vestibular evoked response. *Archives of Otolaryngology-Head and Neck Surgery, 112,* 836–839.

Elidan, J., Lin, J., & Honrubia, V. (1987). Vestibular ototoxicity of gentamicin assessed by the recording of a short-latency vestibular-evoked response in cats. *Laryngoscope, 97*(7), 865–870.

Elidan, J., Sela, M., Liebner, E., & Sohmer, H. (1991). Short latency vestibular evoked response to angular acceleration impulse in human beings. *Otolaryngology-Head and Neck Surgery, 105,* 353–359.

Elidan, J., Sohmer, H., & Nitzan, M. (1982). Recording of short latency vestibular evoked potentials to acceleration in rats by means of skin electrodes. *Electroencephalography and Clinical Neurophysiology, 53,* 501–505.

Elidan, J., Sohmer, H., & Nitzan, M. (1985). A surface recorded vestibular evoked response to acceleration in cats. *Journal of Laryngology and Otology Supplement, 9,* 111–119.

Fermin, C. D., Martin, D., Jones, T. A., Vellinger, J., Deuser, M., Hester, P., & Hullinger, R. (1996). Microgravity in the STS-29 space shuttle Discovery affected the vestibular system of chick embryos. *Histology and Histopathology, 11*(2), 407–426.

Freeman, S., Plotnik, M., Elidan, J., Rosen, L. J., & Sohmer, H. (1999). Effect of white noise "masking" on vestibular evoked potentials recorded using different stimulus modalities. *Acta Oto-Laryngologica, 119,* 311–315.

Freeman, S., Plotnik, M., Elidan, J., & Sohmer, H. (1999a). Differential effect of the loop diuretic furosemide on short latency auditory and vestibular-evoked potentials. *American Journal of Otology, 20,* 41–45.

Freeman, S., Plotnik, M., Elidan, J., & Sohmer, H. (1999b). Development of short latency vestibular evoked potentials in the neonatal rat. *Hearing Research, 137,* 51–58.

Freeman, S., Priner, R., Elidan, J., & Sohmer, H. (2001). Objective method for differentiating between drug-induced vestibulotoxicity and cochleotoxicity. *Otology & Neurotology, 22*(1), 70–75.

Gaines, C. (2012). *Generators of mammalian vestibular surface responses to head motion.* Dissertation. East Carolina University, Greenville, NC.

Geng, R., Geller, S. F., Hayashi, T., Ray, C., Reh, T. A., Bermingham-McDonogh, O., . . . Flannery, J. G. (2009). Usher syndrome IIIA gene clarin-1 is essential for hair cell function and associated neural activation. *Human Molecular Genetics, 18*(15), 2748–2760.

Goodyear, R. J., Jones, S. M., Sharifi, L., Forge, A., & Richardson, G. (2012). Hair-bundle defects and loss of function in the vestibular end organs of mice lacking the receptor-like inositol lipid phosphatase, PTPRQ. *Journal of Neuroscience, 32*(8), 2762–2772.

Hall, J. W. (2007). *New handbook of auditory evoked responses.* Boston, MA: Allyn & Bacon.

Hamid, M. A., & Hughes, G. B. (1986). Vestibular evoked potentials in man: An overview. *Otolaryngology-Head and Neck Surgery, 95,* 347–348.

Hansen, H. C., Zangemeister, W. H., & Kunze, K. (1988). Head rotation evoked EEG responses are governed by rate of angular acceleration change. *Advances in Otorhinolaryngology, 41,* 210–215.

Hixson, W. C., Niven, J. I., & Correia, M. J. (1966). Kinematics nomenclature for physiological accelerations with special reference to vestibular applications. *Monograph 14.* Pensacola, FL: Naval Aerospace Medical Institute.

Hofferberth, B. (1984). Evoked potentials to rotatory stimulation. *Acta Oto-Laryngologica Supplement, 406,* 134–136.

Hofferberth, B. (1995). The clinical significance of vestibular evoked potentials (REP). *Acta Oto-Laryngologica Supplement, 520,* 124–125.

Hoffman, L. F. (1987). *Evoked potentials from inner ear sensory systems: Effects of hypothermia and masking* (Unpublished doctoral dissertation). University of California, Davis.

Hoffman, L. F., & Horowitz, J. M. (1984). Far-field brainstem responses evoked by vestibular and auditory stimuli exhibit increases in interpeak latency as brain temperature is decreased. *Physiologist, 27*(6), S89–S90.

Hood, J. D. (1983). Vestibular and optokinetic evoked potentials. *Acta Oto-Laryngologica, 95,* 589–593.

Hood, J. D., & Kayan, A. (1985). Observations upon the evoked responses to natural vestibular stimulation. *Electroencephalography and Clinical Neurophysiology, 62,* 266–276.

Inokuchi, A., Yamamoto, T., & Uemura, T. (1991). Vestibular evoked potentials to angular acceleration in the guinea pig. *Acta Oto-Laryngologica Supplement, 481,* 477–480.

Irons-Brown, S., & Jones, T. A. (2004). Effects of selected pharmacological agents on avian auditory and vestibular compound action potentials. *Hearing Research, 195,* 54–66.

Irons-Brown, S. R., Jones S. M., & Jones, T. A. (2003). The simultaneous in vivo perilymphatic perfusion of avian auditory and vestibular end organs. *Journal of Neuroscience Methods, 131*(1–2), 57–64.

Johnson, K. R., Zheng, Q. Y., & Erway, L. C. (2000). A major gene affecting age-related hearing loss is common to at least ten inbred strains of mice. *Genomics, 70*(2), 171–180.

Jones, S. M., Erway, L. C., Bergstrom, R. A., Schimenti, J. C., & Jones, T. A. (1999). Vestibular responses to linear acceleration are absent in otoconia-deficient C57BL/6JEi-*het* mice. *Hearing Research, 135,* 56–60.

Jones, S. M., Erway, L. C., Yu, H., Johnson, K. R., & Jones, T. A. (2004). Gravity receptor function in mice with graded otoconial deficiencies. *Hearing Research, 191,* 34–40.

Jones, S. M., Johnson, K. R., Yu, H., Erway, L. C., Alagramam, K. N., Pollak, N., & Jones, T. A. (2005). A quantitative survey of gravity receptor function in mutant mouse strains. *Journal of the Association for Research in Otolarlyngology, 6*(4), 297–310.

Jones, S. M., & Jones, T. A. (1996). Short latency vestibular evoked potentials in the chicken embryo. *Journal of Vestibular Research, 6*(2), 71–83.

Jones, S. M., & Jones, T. A. (2000). Ontogeny of vestibular compound action potentials in the domestic chicken. *Journal of the Association for Research in Otolaryngology, 1*(3), 232–242.

Jones, S. M., & Jones, T. A. (2014). Genetics of peripheral vestibular dysfunction: Lessons from mutant mouse strains. *Journal of the American Academy of Audiology, 25*(3), 289–301.

Jones, S. M., Jones, T. A., Bell, P. L., & Taylor, M. J. (2001). Compound gravity receptor polarization vectors evidenced by linear vestibular evoked potentials. *Hearing Research, 154,* 54–61.

Jones, S. M., Jones, T. A., Johnson, K. R., Yu, H., Erway, L. C., & Zheng, Q. Y. (2006). A comparison of vestibular and auditory phenotypes in inbred mouse strains. *Brain Research, 1091,* 40–46.

Jones, S. M., Jones, T. A., & Shukla, R. (1997). Short latency vestibular evoked potentials in the Japanese quail (*Coturnix coturnix japonica*). *Journal of Comparative Physiology A, 180,* 631–638.

Jones, S. M., Robertson, N. G., Given, S., Heisch, A. B. S., Liberman, M. C., & Morton, C. C. (2011). Hearing and vestibular deficits in the *Coch* null mouse model: Comparison to the *Coch*$^{G88E/G88E}$ mouse and to DFNA9 hearing and balance disorder. *Hearing Research, 272,* 42–48.

Jones, S. M., Ryals, B. M., & Colbert, S. M. (1998). Vestibular function in Belgian Waterslager canaries (*Serinus canaries*). *Hearing Research, 121,* 161–169.

Jones, S. M., Subramanian, G., Avniel, W., Guo, Y., Burkard, R. F., & Jones, T. A. (2002). Stimulus and recording variables and their effects on mammalian vestibular evoked potentials. *Journal of Neuroscience Methods, 118,* 23–31.

Jones, S. M., Warren, L., Shukla, R., Browning, A., Fuller, C. A., & Jones, T. A. (2000). The effects of hypergravity and substrate vibration on vestibular function in developing chickens. *Journal of Gravitational Physiology, 7*(3), 31–44.

Jones, T. A. (1992). Vestibular short latency responses to pulsed linear acceleration in unanesthetized animals. *Electroencephalography and Clinical Neurophysiology, 82*(5), 377–386.

Jones, T. A., Fermin, C. D., Hester, P. Y., & Vellinger, J. (1993). Effects of microgravity on vestibular ontogeny: Direct physiological and anatomical measurements following space flight [STS-29]. *Acta Veterinaria BRNO, 62*(6), S35–S42.

Jones, T. A., & Jones, S. M. (1999). Short latency compound action potentials from mammalian gravity receptor organs. *Hearing Research, 136,* 75–85.

Jones, T. A., & Jones, S. M. (2000). Vestibular ontogeny in warm-blooded vertebrates: Four models for study in altered gravitational fields. *Journal of Gravitational Physiology, 7*(2), 43–46.

Jones, T. A., Jones, S. M., & Colbert, S. M. (1998). The adequate stimulus for avian short latency vestibular responses to linear translation. *Journal of Vestibular Research, 8*(3), 253–272.

Jones, T. A., Jones, S. M., Vijayakumar, S., Brugeaud, A., Bothwell, M., & Chabbert, C. (2011). The adequate stimulus for mammalian linear vestibular evoked potentials (VsEPs). *Hearing Research, 280,* 133–140.

Jones, T. A., & Nelson, R. C. (1992). Recovery of vestibular function following hair cell destruction by streptomycin. *Hearing Research, 62,* 181–186.

Jones, T. A., & Pederson, T. L. (1989). Short latency vestibular responses to pulsed linear acceleration. *American Journal of Otolaryngology, 10,* 327–335.

Kast, R., & Lankford, J. E. (1986). Otolithic evoked potentials: A new technique for vestibular studies. *Acta Oto-Laryngologica, 102,* 175–178.

Kato, T., Shiraishi, K., Eura, Y., Shibata K., Kakata T., Morizono T., & Soda, T. (1998). A "neural" response with 3-ms latency evoked by loud sound in profoundly deaf patients. *Audiology and Neuro Otology, 3,* 253–264.

Keck, W. (1990). Rotatory evoked cortical potentials in normal subjects and patients with unilateral and bilateral vestibular loss. *European Archives of Otorhinolaryngology, 247,* 222–225.

Kenmochi, M., Ohashi, T., Nishino, H., & Sato, S. (2003). Cortical potentials evoked by horizontal rotatory stimulation: The effects of angular acceleration. *Acta Oto-Laryngologica, 123,* 923–927.

Kingma, C. M., & Wit, H. P. (2009). Acute endolymphatic hydrops has no acute effect on the vestibular evoked potential in the guinea pig. *Journal of Vestibular Research, 19,* 27–32.

Knox, G. W., Isaacs, J., Woodard, D., Johnson, L., & Jordan, D. (1993). Short latency vestibular evoked potentials. *Otolaryngology-Head and Neck Surgery, 108,* 265–269.

Latkowski, B., & Puzio, J. (1989). Recording of electrical-evoked responses from a remote field in the vestibular part of the eighth nerve. *Audiology, 28,* 111–116.

Lee, S. I., Conrad, T., Jones, S. M., Lagziel, A., Starost, A. F., Belyantseva, I., . . . Morell, R. J. (2013). A null mutation of mouse *Kcna10* causes significant vestibular and mild hearing dysfunction. *Hearing Research, 300,* 1–9.

Leibner, E., Elidan, J., Freeman, S., Sela, M., Nitzan, M., & Sohmer, H. (1990). Vestibular evoked potentials with short and middle latencies recorded in humans. In P. M. Rossini & F. Mauguiere (Eds.), *New trends and advanced techniques in clinical neurophysiology* (pp. 119–123). Amsterdam, the Netherlands: Elsevier.

Li, G., Elidan, J., Meyler, Y., & Sohmer, H. (1997). Contribution of the eighth nerve and cranial nerve nuclei to the short-latency vestibular evoked potentials in cats. *Otolaryngology-Head and Neck Surgery, 116,* 181–188.

Li, G., Elidan, J., & Sohmer, H. (1993). The contribution of the lateral semicircular canal to the short latency vestibular evoked potentials in cat. *Electroencephalography and Clinical Neurophysiology, 88,* 225–228.

Li, G., Elidan, J., & Sohmer, H. (1995). Peripheral generators of the vestibular evoked potentials in the cat. *Archives of Otolaryngology-Head and Neck Surgery, 121,* 34–38.

Loose, R., Probst, R., Tucha, O., Bablok, E., Aschenbrenner, S., & Lange, K. W. (2002). Vestibular evoked potentials from the vertical semicircular canals in humans evoked by roll-axis rotation in microgravity and under 1-G. *Behavioural Brain Research, 134,* 131–137.

Lysakowski, A., & Goldberg, J. M. (2004). Morphology of the vestibular periphery. In S. M. Highstein, R. R. Fay, & A. N. Popper (Eds.), *The vestibular system* (pp. 57–152). New York, NY: Springer-Verlag.

Mergner, T., Schrenk, R., & Muller, C. (1989). Human DC scalp potentials during vestibular and optokinetic stimulation: Non-specific responses. *Electroencephalography and Clinical Neurophysiology, 73,* 322–333.

Mock, B. E., Jones, T. A., & Jones, S. M. (2009). Cdh23[753A] does not impact functional aging of gravity receptors in C57BL/6J mice [Abstract]. *Association for Research in Otolaryngology Abstracts, 32,* 198.

Mock, B. E., Jones, T. A., & Jones, S. M. (2011). Gravity receptor aging in CBA/CaJ: A comparison to auditory aging. *Journal of the Association for Research in Otolaryngology, 12,* 173–183.

Molinari, G. A., & Mingrino, S. (1974). Cortical evoked responses to vestibular stimulation in man. *Journal of Laryngology and Otology, 88,* 515–521.

Munoz-Gamboa, C., & Jimenez-Cruz, J. (1994). Human vestibular evoked responses. *Medical Progress Through Technology, 20,* 31–35.

Nazareth, A. M., & Jones, T. A. (1998). Central and peripheral components of short latency vestibular responses in the chicken. *Journal of Vestibular Research, 8*(3), 233–252.

Oei, M. L. Y. M., Segenhout, J. M., Wit, H. P., & Albers F. W. J. (2001). The vestibular evoked response to linear, alternating, acceleration pulses without acoustic masking as a parameter of vestibular function. *Acta Oto-Laryngologica, 121,* 62–67.

Paillard, A. C., Kluk, K., & Todd, N. P. (2014). Thresholds for vestibular evoked myogenic potentials (VEMPS) produced by impulsive transmastoid acceleration. *International Journal of Audiology, 53*(2), 138–141.

Papathanasiou, E. S., Piperidou, C., Iliopoulos, I., Maleki-dou, A., Katelari-Theocharidou, E., Kyriakides, T., . . . Papacostas, S. S. (2005). Neurogenic vestibular evoked potentials in three cases of vestibular system dysfunction. *Electromyography and Clinical Neurophysiology, 45*, 39–45.

Papathanasiou, E. S., Piperidou, C., Pantzaris, M., Iliopoulos, I., Petsa, M., Kyriakides, T., . . . Papacostas, S. S. (2005). Vestibular symptoms and signs are correlated with abnormal neurogenic vestibular evoked potentials in patients with multiple sclerosis. *Electromyography and Clinical Neurophysiology, 45*, 195–201.

Perez, R., Freeman, S., Cohen, D., Sichel, J. Y., & Sohmer, H. (2003). The effect of hydrogen peroxide applied to the middle ear on inner ear function. *Laryngoscope, 113*(11), 2042–2046.

Perez, R., Freeman, S., Sohmer, H., & Sichel, J. Y. (2000). Vestibular and cochlear ototoxicity of topical antiseptics assessed by evoked potentials. *Laryngoscope, 110*(9), 1522–1527.

Perez, R., Ziv, E., Freeman, S., Sichel, J., & Sohmer, H. (2001). Vestibular end-organ impairment in an animal model of type 2 diabetes mellitus. *Laryngoscope, 111*(1), 110–113.

Pirodda, E., Ghedini, S., & Zanetti, M. A. (1987). Investigations into vestibular evoked responses. *Acta Oto-Laryngologica, 104*, 77–84.

Plotnik, M., Elidan, J., Mager, M., & Sohmer, H. (1997). Short latency vestibular evoked potentials (VsEPs) to linear acceleration impulses in rats. *Electroencephalography and Clinical Neurophysiology, 104*, 522–530.

Plotnik, M., Freeman, S., Sohmer, H., & Elidan, J. (1999). The effect of head orientation on the vestibular evoked potentials to linear acceleration impulses in rats. *American Journal of Otology, 20*, 735–740.

Plotnik, M., Sichel, J. Y., Elidan, J., Honrubia, V., & Sohmer, H. (1999). Origins of the short latency vestibular evoked potentials (VsEPs) to linear acceleration impulses. *American Journal of Otology, 20*, 238–243.

Probst, T., Ayan, T., Loose, R., & Skrandies, W. (1997). Electrophysiological evidence for direction-specific rotary evoked potentials in human subjects—A topographical study. *Neuroscience Letters, 239*, 97–100.

Probst, T., Katterbach, T., & Wist, E. R. (1995). Vestibularly evoked potentials (VESTEPs) of the horizontal semicircular canals under different body positions in space. *Journal of Vestibular Research, 5*, 253–263.

Rodionov, V., Elidan, J., Sela, M., Nitzan, M., & Sohmer, H. (1996). Vertical plane short and middle latency vestibular evoked potentials in humans. *Annals of Otology Rhinology & Laryngology, 105*, 43–48.

Rosengren, S. M., & Colebatch, J. G. (2006). Vestibular evoked potentials (VsEPs) in patients with severe to profound bilateral hearing loss. *Clinical Neurophysiology, 117*, 1145–1153.

Ryals, B. M., & Rubel, E. W. (1988). Hair cell regeneration after acoustic trauma in the adult Coturnix quail. *Science, 240*, 1774–1776.

Salamy, J., Potvin, A., Jones, K., & Landreth, J. (1975). Cortical evoked responses to labyrinthine stimulation in man. *Psychophysiology, 12*, 55–61.

Schneider, D., Schneider, L., Claussen, C. F., & Kolchev, C. (2001). Cortical representation of the vestibular system as evidenced by brain electrical activity mapping of vestibular late evoked potentials. *Ear Nose and Throat Journal, 80*, 251–252, 255–258, 260.

Sidman, R., Dickie, M., & Appel, S. (1964). Mutant mice (quaking and jumpy) with deficient myelination in the central nervous system. *Science, 144*, 309–311.

Sohmer, H., Elidan, J., Plotnik, M., Freeman, S., Sockalingam, R., Berkowitz, Z., & Mager, M. (1999). Effect of noise on the vestibular system—Vestibular evoked potential studies in rats. *Noise & Health, 2*(5), 41–52.

Sohmer, H., Elidan, J., Rodionov, V., & Plotnik, M. (1999). Short and middle latency vestibular evoked potentials to angular and linear acceleration. In G. Comi, C. H. Lucking, J. Kimura, & P. M. Rossini (Eds.), *Clinical neurophysiology: From receptors to perception* (pp. 226–234). Amsterdam, the Netherlands: Elsevier.

Spiegel, E. A., Szekely, E. G., & Moffet, R. (1968). Cortical responses to rotation: 1. Responses recorded after cessation of rotation. *Acta Oto-Laryngologica, 66*, 81–88.

Todd, N. P. M., Rosengren, S. M., & Colebatch, J. G. (2003). A short latency vestibular evoked potential (VsEP) produced by bone-conducted acoustic stimulation. *Journal of the Acoustical Society of America, 114*(6), 3264–3272.

Todd, N. P., Rosengren, S. M., & Colebatch, J. G. (2008). Ocular vestibular evoked myogenic potentials (OVEMPS) produced by impulsive transmastoid accelerations. *Clinical Neurophysiology, 119*(5), 1638–1651.

Trimble, M. V., & Jones, S. M. (2001). Vestibular evoked potentials to rotary stimulation in the head tilt (*het*) mouse [Abstract]. *Association for Research in Otolaryngology Abstracts, 24*, 19.

Trinus, K. F. (1988). Vestibular evoked potentials—A new method for study of the combined effects of environmental factors. In O. Manninen (Ed.), *Combined effects of environmental factors* (pp. 143–152). Finland: Keskupino Central Print House.

Trinus, K. F. (1997). Vestibular evoked potentials. *Advances in Oto-Rhino-Laryngology, 53*, 155–181.

Weisleder, P., Jones, T. A., & Rubel, E. W. (1990). Peripheral generators of the vestibular evoked potentials (VsEP) in the chick. *Electroencephalography and Clinical Neurophysiology, 76*, 362–369.

Weisleder, P., & Rubel, E. W. (1992). Hair cell regeneration in the avian vestibular epithelium. *Experimental Neurology, 115*(1), 2–6.

Welgampola, M. S., & Colebatch, J. G. (2005). Charcteristics and clinical applications of vestibular evoked myogenic potentials. *Neurology, 64*(10), 1682–1688.

Zangemeister, W. H., & Hansen, H. C. (1990). Cerebral potentials evoked by fast head accelerations. *Neurological Research, 12,* 137–146.

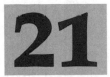

21

Vestibular-Evoked Myogenic Potentials (VEMPs)

Devin L. McCaslin and Gary P. Jacobson

HISTORY AND SIGNIFICANCE OF THE VESTIBULAR-EVOKED MYOGENIC POTENTIALS (VEMPS)

It is now well known that the vestibular system can be stimulated using sound. In 1929, Pietro Tullio initiated the original investigations demonstrating the vestibular system's sensitivity to auditory stimuli. Tullio's experiments consisted of fenestrating the bony labyrinth of pigeons, subjecting them to sound produced by a flute, and observing the motion of the labyrinthine fluids (the frequency of the notes produced by the flute matched the frequency of the movement of the endolymph) and eye movements. From these experiments Tullio was able to determine that the vestibular system could be stimulated using sound (Tullio, 1929). Von Békésy (1935) built on the findings of Tullio and observed that when human subjects were exposed to a high-intensity stimulus (122 to 134 dB SPL) there was a corresponding head displacement toward the stimulated ear. Von Békésy argued that this reflexive movement of the head in response to an auditory stimulus was likely due to movement of the endolymph stimulating the vestibular system.

In the mid-1960s, Bickford, Jacobson, and Cody (1964) reported the presence of a sound-evoked electrical potential (negative waveform peaking at approximately 30 ms) that could be recorded from an active electrode placed on the inion. Initially, this response was believed to be "neurogenic." However, the investigators demonstrated that the earlier components of the response were significantly reduced in amplitude following administration of a muscle paralyzing agent. Additionally, it was noted that the response grew in amplitude with increases in the tonic level of electromyography (EMG) in the neck extensors. This evoked-potential response was subsequently named the *inion potential*. Further studies by this group of investigators led to the theory that the vestibular system (i.e., the saccule) was the peripheral origin of the inion potential (Cody, Jacobson, Walker, & Bickford, 1964; Townsend & Cody, 1971). Finding no good clinical application for these responses, they were abandoned for almost 30 years. Then, in 1992 when Colebatch and Halmagyi reported the presence of another short-latency large amplitude myogenic potential recorded in response to a loud click with an electrode (noninverting) placed over the belly of a contracted sternocleidomastoid muscle (SCM). This response was characterized by a positive wave (P1) followed by a negative wave (N1) occurring ipsilateral to the ear that received the stimulus (Colebatch & Halmagyi, 1992; Colebatch, Halmagyi, & Skuse, 1994). Compelling evidence suggesting a vestibular origin was derived from studies showing that the response could be recorded in patients who were completely deaf, yet had intact vestibular function (Colebatch & Halmagyi, 1992;

Colebatch et al., 1994). As with the inion potential, this sonomotor response represented a sound-evoked attenuation of tonic EMG activity in the SCM (Bickford et al., 1964; Colebatch & Halmagyi, 1992). It has been suggested that the sound-synchronized decrease in the tonic level of EMG that occurs during the response is interpreted by the central nervous system as a sudden loss in postural tone. The reflexive response from the vestibular system to compensate for this perceived decrease in muscle activity is to increase extensor muscle tone and decrease flexor muscle tone (Carey & Amin, 2006). Therefore, amplitude of this inhibitory muscle response represents an interaction between the level of tonic EMG and the size of the inhibitory postsynaptic potential (IPSP) initiated at the end organ (Colebatch & Rothwell, 2004) (Figure 21–1). Colebatch and Halmagyi (1992) referred to this response as a *vestibular-evoked myogenic potential* (VEMP). In this case the response was recorded from the SCM and is now referred to as the *cervical VEMP* (cVEMP).

The cVEMP that is recorded using an evoked-potential system is the measurable output from the effector organ (SCM) of the activated vestibulocolic reflex (VCR) (Colebatch & Halmagyi, 1992; Colebatch et al., 1994). The VCR is an involuntary muscle contraction that occurs when stimuli are introduced that are capable of translating the otolith organs. The corresponding changes in the tonic background EMG level in the neck extensors that are observed during head movements represent a vestibular-driven muscle coordination in the neck used to stabilize the head (Lysakowski, McCrea, & Tomlinson, 1998). The afferent and efferent limbs of the VCR have been described by several groups and are considered to represent the pathway for the clinical response we know as the cVEMP.

There have been many sound-evoked, signal-averaged muscle responses described in the literature, and they may represent either sound-evoked *onsets* or *offsets* of EMG activity. Examples of sound-evoked EMG onset responses (or sonomotor responses) are the stapedial reflex, the postauricular muscle potential (PAM) and the ocular vestibular-evoked myogenic potential (oVEMP), that are discussed later. Examples of sound-evoked attenuation

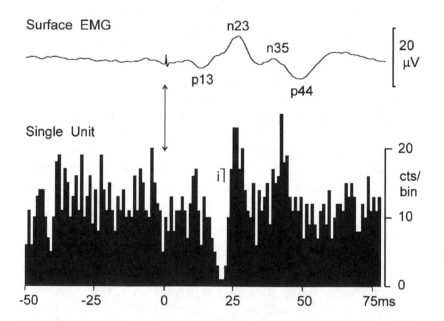

Figure 21–1. Surface and single motor unit (intramuscular-sternocleidomastoid muscle) recordings simultaneously recorded in response to click stimuli. The initial response is a decrease in single unit activity and is represented by "il." From Colebatch, J. G., and Rothwell. R. (2004). Motor unit excitability changes mediating vestibulocollic reflexes in the sternocleidomastoid muscle. *Clinical Neurophysiology, 115*(11), 2567–2573. Used with permission from the International Federation of Clinical Neurophysiology.

of existing EMG activity include the inion potential, the acoustic jaw reflex, and the cervical vestibular-evoked myogenic potential (cVEMP) that are discussed in this chapter. It is our objective to describe the anatomy and physiology underlying the cVEMP and oVEMP. Additionally, we describe how each of these responses are recorded and measured, and how normal and abnormal responses appear. A discussion of the common patterns of abnormality and the diagnostic significance of these patterns is addressed in Chapter 24.

CLINICAL PHYSIOLOGY OF THE SACCULE AND UTRICLE

The macula utriculi and sacculi are one of the two types of sensory epithelia in the vestibular system (the other is the semicircular canals). The macula of the saccule and utricle have a specialized sensory epithelium that enables them to sense linear acceleration. The otoliths are positioned in the otic capsule in such a way that they respond to movements in the horizontal and vertical planes. Calcium carbonate crystals with a specific gravity of 2.71 g/mL are embedded in a gelatinous matrix known as the otolithic membrane (Gacek, 1982). The two primary components of the otolithic membrane are the mass (i.e., otoconia) and the neurosensory cells (Type I and Type II). The macula has an elastic connection to the skull, making the system sensitive to acceleration and gravitational forces during head movement.

The saccule is located in the vestibule directly beneath the stapes in the sagittal plane. This proximity to the middle ear space makes the saccule sensitive to high-intensity air-conducted stimuli (ACS). In fact, in several animal species the saccule acts as a hearing receptor (Popper & Fay, 1973). However, the functional significance of the ability to stimulate the saccule acoustically is still not completely understood.

Convincing physiologic evidence from animal studies investigating the origin of the cVEMP now implicates the saccule as the primary end-organ generator of the response (Colebatch and Halmagyi, 1992; Colebatch et al., 1994; Curthoys, 2010). In 1999, Kushiro, Zakir, Ogawa, Sato, and Uchino published a report describing the neural connec-

tions between the saccule and the SCM in cats. Using electrical stimulation, the authors showed that when the vestibular afferents originating at the saccule were stimulated, an inhibitory postsynaptic potential (IPSP) in the ipsilateral SCM motor neurons was initiated. Following transection of the medial vestibulo-spinal tract (MVST) in the brainstem at the level of the obex, electrical stimulation of the saccular nerve failed to generate IPSPs that were present prior to the surgery. This classic series of animal studies laid the groundwork for understanding the functional significance of the sacculocollic reflex pathway.

The orientation of the utricle is not quite horizontal, but rather tilted down and back approximately 25 to 30 degrees (Schwarz & Tomlinson, 2005). The structure of the utricle is identical to that of the saccule with two notable exceptions. First, the utricle is two times larger than the saccule (Rosenhall, 1973; Wright, Hubbard, & Clark, 1979). Additionally, the utricle is not affixed to the temporal bone in its entirety (Jaeger & Haslwanter, 2004; Uzun-Coruhlu, Curthoys, & Jones, 2007). These differences in size and stiffness would be expected to effect differences in the tuning characteristics of the utricle and saccule. As observed for the saccule, the utricle consists of an otolith membrane whose porous characteristics enable otolith crystals to remain in place acting as a mass. Stereocilia and kinocilia project from the sensory cells and supporting cells up into the otolith membrane. In effect, Newton's first law of motion which states "an object either remains at rest or continues to move at a constant _velocity_, unless acted upon by an external _force_." As such, linear, tangential, or centrifugal acceleration in the lateral (i.e., left to right, or right to left) and vertical planes (i.e., anterior/posterior planes) causes the otolith mass to lag behind the movement of the head. This results in shearing of the kinocilia and neural transduction. Like the saccule and unlike the semicircular canals, the utricle is polarized in such a way that each utricle is capable of responding to linear horizontal acceleration and deceleration. This provides a degree of redundancy should disease result in the loss of one utricle.

Studies of the neural response properties of otolith projections have also been investigated. Murofushi et al., (1995) recorded extracellular responses from single neurons in the vestibular nerves in guinea pigs in an effort to show that primary vestibular neurons were capable of being activated by air-conducted stimuli. When stimulated using sound, vestibular afferents projecting from the otolith organs were shown to manifest a variety of tonic resting discharge rates based on the type of hair cell they originated from (i.e., Type I or Type II). Vestibular afferents projecting from Type I hair cells demonstrated irregular firing rates while those that synapsed on Type II hair cells typically produced a more regular firing rate (Gresty & Lempert, 2001; Minor & Goldberg, 1991). It is now known that the majority of projections sent from the saccule's macula demonstrate irregular firing rates and are highly sensitive to air-conducted stimuli (Curthoys, Kim, McPhedran, & Camp, 2006; Murofushi & Curthoys, 1997) (Figure 21–2).

The fact that the saccule, utricle, and cochlea are in close proximity to one another led to an entire line of research showing that the early components of the VEMP response were largely independent of auditory function. Many of the early investigations involved studying patients with specific impairments in the vestibular and auditory system. For example, the cVEMP was abolished in patients who had undergone a vestibular nerve section (i.e., inferior vestibular nerve) yet had normal auditory function (Brantberg & Mathiesen, 2004). Conversely, the cVEMP was shown to be present in patients with normal vestibular function but had profound sensorineural hearing impairment (Colebatch & Halmagyi, 1992). Normal VEMP responses can be recorded from patients who have undergone semicircular canal ablations, and who have severe deformation or absence of the cochlea but a functioning saccule (Sheykholeslami & Kaga, 2002). Additionally, if the air-conducted auditory stimulus is masked with a bone-conducted stimulus, the cVEMP response still persists although there is an observed decrease in amplitude (McNerney & Burkard, 2011).

DESCRIPTION OF THE cVEMP RESPONSE

Early on in the literature, almost any muscle response that was recorded following sound or vibration was termed a *vestibular-evoked myogenic potential* (VEMP). However, at the time of this writing, the cVEMP is

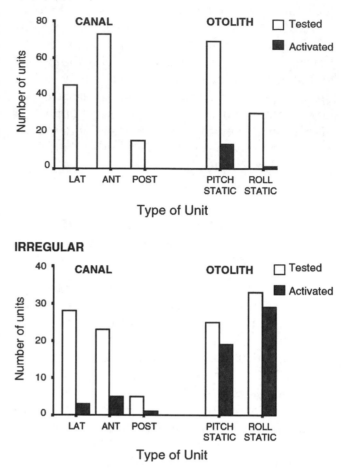

Figure 21–2. Number of animal canal and otolith primary afferent vestibular neurons tested (*white*) and activated (*gray*) using low-frequency vibratory stimuli. Only a small number of canal neurons were found to respond. Otolith regular neurons were occasionally responsive; however, the vast majority of otolith irregular neurons were activated at low stimulus levels. From Curthoys, I. S. (2010). A critical review of the neurophysiological evidence underlying clinical vestibular testing using sound, vibration and galvanic stimuli. *Clinical Neurophysiology, 121*, 132–144. Used with permission from the International Federation of Clinical Neurophysiology.

now considered an evoked potential that is recorded from an activated SCM. The cVEMP is characterized by a biphasic waveform that begins with a primary positive waveform followed by a negative waveform (Figure 21–3). The mean latency of the positive deflection in response to a click stimulus is ~13 ms and is referred to in the literature as either P1 or p13. The negative deflection occurs at ~23 ms and

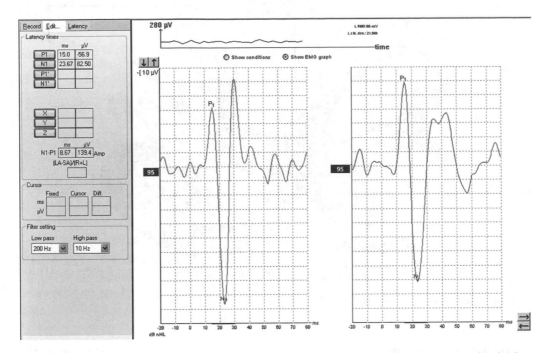

Figure 21–3. Left and right cervical evoked myogenic potential waveform evoked using a 95 dB nHL 500 tone-burst.

is commonly referred to as N1 or n23 (Colebatch & Halmagyi, 1992). The direction of the initial deflection (i.e., positive) suggests that the cVEMP is an inhibitory response (i.e., moving from a state where there is increased EMG activity to a state where there is decreased EMG activity) (Colebatch & Rothwell, 2004; Wit & Kingma, 2006). The response is primarily ipsilateral.

cVEMP PATHWAY

The saccullo-collic response is a reflexive adjustment of the musculature in the neck triggered by activation of the saccule. By definition a reflex consists of an afferent limb (i.e., representing the activation of the peripheral end organ and ending at the brain center where these signals are received), central processing (i.e., where the afferent activity is routed to the central origin of the efferent limb), and an efferent limb (i.e., where the efferent activity terminates at an end muscle). Based on the work described in the previous section, the pathway associated with the cVEMP

reflex has been thoroughly described. The afferent limb of the cVEMP extends from the saccule (i.e., receptor organ) to Scarpa's ganglion where neural projections course through the inferior branch of the vestibular nerve (McCue & Guinan, 1995; Murofushi & Curthoys, 1997) (Figure 21–4). The inferior vestibular nerve becomes part of the VIIIth cranial nerve and the fibers projecting from the saccule terminate on interneurons within the medial and lateral vestibular nuclei. The efferent limb of the cVEMP reflex descends from the vestibular nucleus and courses through the vestibulo-spinal tract to the motonucleus of CNXI. From there the activity is routed through CNXI to terminate on the SCM (Fitzgerald, Comerfiord, & Tuffery, 1982). CNXI originates in the anterior horn of the first five cervical segments of the spinal column and is the solitary motor input to the SCM (Krause, Bremerich, & Herrmann, 1991) (Figure 21–5). This neural pathway has been confirmed by attenuation or ablation of the VEMP response following selective neurectomies, neural pathologies, or local anesthetic delivered to SCM (Colebatch & Halmagyi, 1992; Murofushi, Matsuzaki, & Wu, 1999).

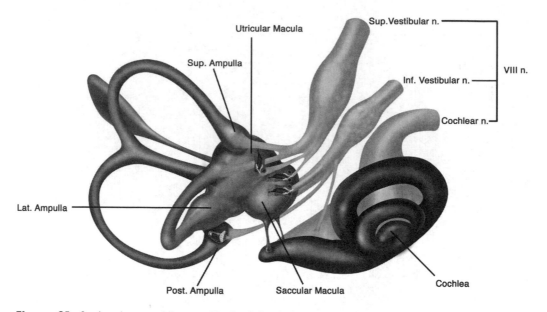

Figure 21-4. Anatomy of the vestibular labyrinth.

STIMULUS VARIABLES

Type of Stimuli

Typically, when the head is moved in everyday life the process of otolithic stimulation is continual and largely goes unnoticed. For clinical assessment, activation of the saccule can be accomplished in a number of ways without a corresponding head movement (Welgampola & Colebatch, 2005). For example, cVEMPs can be recorded when a calibrated amount of sound, vibration, or force is delivered to the head that is sufficient to translate the otoliths (Colebatch et al., 1994; Sheykholeslami, Murofushi, Kermany, & Kaga, 2000). A summary of cVEMP stimulus parameters is presented in Table 21–1 and Table 21–2.

Air-Conducted Stimuli

At the time of this writing, an acoustical stimulus (click or tone burst) is most commonly used in the clinic (Papathanasiou, Murofushi, Akin, & Colebatch, 2014). When a high-intensity, low-frequency, acoustical transient is introduced to the ear canal, the sound pressure is routed through the middle ear system to the oval window into the vestibule (Lysakowski et al., 1998). This creates a situation where the endolymph in the vestibule is moved and the

vestibular hair cells (Type I and Type II) are sheared resulting in transduction (Murofushi et al., 1995). It is worth reiterating that the patient need not have hearing for sound to be used as the evoking stimulus. In this case, the acoustical transient serves as a hydromechanical force that translates the otoliths (of the saccule in this case) and stimulates the VCR. A requirement for recording a robust response is that the sound conducting system (i.e., middle ear mechanism) be intact. When a conductive impairment is present, the magnitude of the stimulus reaching the vestibule may be attenuated to a degree where the response is eliminated. In situations such as this, the preferred stimulus is vibratory or mechanical (i.e., vibration produced by a Bruel and Kjaer 4810 "minshaker" or a mechanical stimulus produced by a specially outfitted tendon hammer). Calibration of acoustic stimuli for cVEMP testing should be accomplished using dB peak SPL (Papathanasiou et al., 2014).

Bone-Conducted Vibration

As previously mentioned, one of the issues encountered using an air-conducted stimulus is that impairments in the middle ear conductive mechanism can reduce or abolish the cVEMP response (Bath, Harris, McEwan, & Yardley, 1999). Bone-conducted vibration (BCV) is an alternative stimulus to air-conducted stimuli that has been used successfully

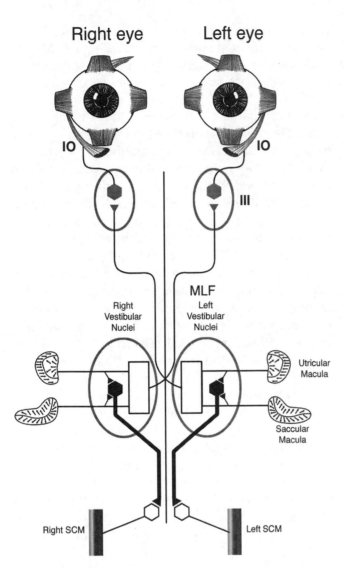

Figure 21–5. Presumed pathways responsible for generating the cervical and ocular vestibular-evoked myogenic potential. *Note. IO* = Inferior oblique; *MLF* = Medial longitudinal fasciculus; *SCM* = Sternocleidomastoid muscle.

Table 21–1. cVEMP Air-Conducted Stimulus Protocol

Frequency	400–700 Hz or click
Level	120 dB pSPL or greater, caution above 140 dB pSPL
Gating	Blackman-weighted, 7 ms maximum duration
Rate	5 per second

Table 21–2. cVEMP Bone-Conducted Stimulus Protocol

Frequency	100–500 Hz
Level	31.6 newtons peak
Gating	Blackman-weighted, 7 ms maximum duration
Rate	5 per second

and colleagues (2003) showed that cVEMP responses using BCV stimulation were present bilaterally with the ipsilateral (bone vibrator placed on one side of the head) response being larger. The authors also reported that the contralateral response occurred, on average, 1 ms later than the ipsilateral cVEMP. Thresholds for cVEMPs generated using BCV were better than those obtained using air-conducted stimuli (i.e., 114-dB SPL versus 97.5-dB SPL) (Welgampola et al., 2003). The authors also reported that the optimal placement for delivery of BCV was 3 cm posterior and 2 cm superior to the external auditory canal because this location produced the largest amplitude cVEMPs. In a similar study investigating BCV, Sheykholeslami and associates (2000) recorded cVEMPs using BCV applied to the mastoid. Tone bursts (i.e., 100, 200, 400, 800, 1600, and 3200 Hz) were used with a stimulus intensity of 70 dB nHL. The investigators reported that the largest amplitude VEMPs were in response to 200-Hz stimuli. Reliable cVEMP responses were unable to be obtained when 1600- and 3200-Hz stimuli were used.

Mechanical Stimuli

The otolith mass also can be translated by lightly tapping the head. cVEMP responses can be obtained using a commercially available tendon hammer that

to stimulate the otolith organs and subsequently activate vestibular afferents (i.e., irregular neurons) (Goldberg, 2000). Vibratory stimuli can be delivered to the skull via a bone vibrator and may be either a click or a tone burst (McNerney & Burkard, 2011). In this regard, bone-conducted tone bursts have been shown to be capable of generating consistent cVEMP responses (Sheykholeslami et al., 2000; Yang & Young, 2003). Interestingly, cVEMPs in response to BCV have larger amplitudes when lower-frequency stimuli are used (i.e., 200 to 250 Hz) (Sheykholeslami et al., 2000; Welgampola et al., 2003). Welgampola connects to an evoked potential machine (Brantberg, Löfqvist, Westin, & Tribukait, 2008; Jacobson & McCaslin, 2007) (Figure 21–6). The hammer (e.g., Nicolet Biomedical Inc., Wisconsin) has an inertial trigger in the head and each time the patient is tapped, a triggering signal is sent to the evoked potential system to record an epoch (e.g., 100 ms). Halmagyi, Yavor, and Colebatch (1995) reported that cVEMPs could be consistently recorded by tapping the head in the frontal region using a similar hammer. The investigators showed that cVEMP responses generated using taps could be recorded bilaterally, had larger amplitudes than air-conducted stimuli, and were measurable in the presence of conductive hearing loss. In a similar study, Yang and Young

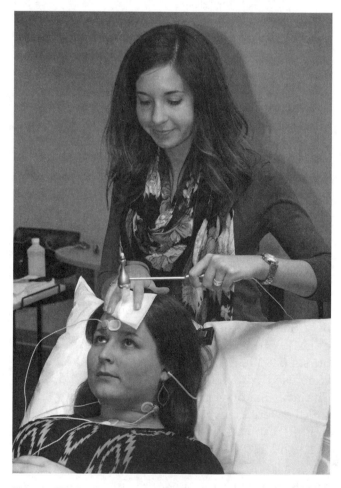

Figure 21–6. A patient prepared for a cVEMP recording using frontal skull taps. The mechanical stimulus is an inertial reflex hammer that generates a trigger pulse when the hammer strikes the head. The pulse triggers a recording epoch and the signal averager records the response.

(2003) compared the clinical utility of skull taps and air-conducted stimuli for recording cVEMPs in patients with otitis media. As expected, only 59% of the subjects with middle ear disease generated measurable cVEMPs in response to the air-conducted stimuli compared to 91% when light skull taps were used. The patients who failed to generate responses to skull taps had larger conductive impairments. Skull taps have also been shown to be useful in identifying peripheral vestibular end-organ impairments. Brantberg and colleagues (2003) evaluated cVEMP responses using forehead skull taps and air-conducted stimuli in patients diagnosed with vestibular neuritis. cVEMPs recorded using air-conducted clicks and skull taps were similar. It is noteworthy that the location (e.g., lateral versus forehead) of the tapping on the skull can produce different responses. Brantberg and Tribukait (2002) showed that taps to the forehead produced bilateral cVEMP waveforms similar to those generated by air-conducted stimuli. However, cVEMPs in response to lateral skull taps generated a typical looking cVEMP (i.e., P1–N1) from the contralateral side but an antiphasic waveform from the ipsilateral side. The authors suggested that this bilateral response represented synchronized EMG activity from the SCMs analogous to what would occur during a natural translation of the head. Figure 21–7 illustrates cVEMP responses obtained in the author's lab using a customized "skull tapper" delivered to the midline of the skull.

Stimulus Frequency

The effect of stimulus frequency on the cVEMP has been systematically described by several groups of investigators (Akin, Murnane, & Proffitt, 2003; Murofushi et al., 1999; Piker, Jacobson, Burkard, McCaslin, & Hood, 2013). The consensus of these investigations and others has been that although the cVEMP can be recorded using unfiltered click stimuli, maximum cVEMP amplitude is obtained using short-duration, low-frequency tone bursts. In one of the first studies describing the effects of stimulus frequency on the cVEMP, Murofushi and colleagues (1999) compared cVEMP amplitudes in response to low-frequency tone-bursts and clicks. The frequency-specific stimuli were 500, 1000, and 2000 Hz tone-bursts. The authors showed responses recorded

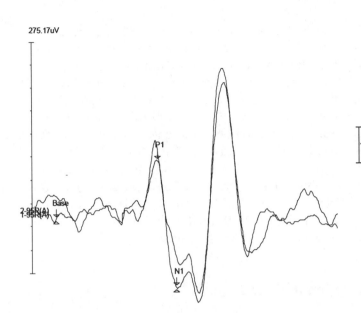

Figure 21–7. A cVEMP recorded in response to frontal skull taps using a novel bone tapper device (Intelligent Hearing Systems). *Note.* x-axis is time in ms.

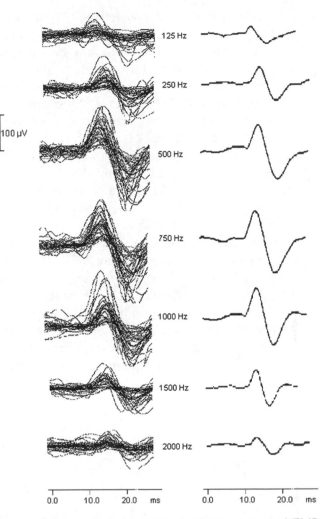

Figure 21–8. The effect of stimulus frequency on cVEMP amplitude. Stimulus level was 127 dB pSPL. The tracings on the left represent individual runs and the recordings on the right represent the average of responses. From Piker, E. G., Jacobson, G. P., Burkard, R. F., McCaslin, D. L., and Hood, L. J. (2013). Effects of age on the tuning of the cVEMP and oVEMP. *Ear and Hearing, 34*(6), 65–73. Used with permission.

with 500-Hz tone-bursts and clicks were similar in amplitude while the 2000 Hz cVEMPs were the smallest (Figure 21–8). Similarly, Todd, Cody, and Banks (2000) investigated the differences in the amplitude of cVEMPs recorded with 100-, 200-, 400-, 800-, 1600-, and 3200-Hz tone-bursts while keeping the intensity stable (100 dB SPL). The authors applied a curve-fitting algorithm to the data and determined that the stimulus frequency that maximized cVEMP amplitude was between 300 and 650 Hz. Akin, Murnane, and Proffitt (2003) also investigated the effect of stimulus frequency (i.e., 500 to 750 Hz) on latency and threshold of the cVEMP response. Changing the frequency of the stimulus does not appear to have an effect on latency when the rise and fall time of the stimulus remained constant (Akin et al., 2003; Welgampola & Colebatch, 2001a). Welgampola & Colebatch (2001a) recorded cVEMP responses using tone-bursts between 200 and 1000 Hz using 100-Hz increments. The investigators reported that cVEMPs with the largest amplitudes were generated in response to stimuli between 600 and 1000 Hz. The finding that low frequency tone-bursts between 500 and 1000 Hz are the optimal auditory stimuli to generate a cVEMP has been replicated by numerous groups of investigators (Akin et al., 2003; Lin et al., 2006; Murofushi, et al., 1999). These findings are in

agreement with neurophysiological recordings from the inferior vestibular nerve afferents in cats where tuning is most sensitive from 500 to 1000 Hz (McCue & Guinan, 1995).

Stimulus Intensity

The level of the stimulus used to elicit a cVEMP response directly influences the amplitude of the cVEMP. Recording a cVEMP response requires a high-intensity stimulus with a short onset time (e.g., 95 to 100 dB nHL) (Colebatch et al., 1994; Ochi, Ohashi, & Nishino, 2001). In fact, stimulus intensities near or below 75 dB HL are not sufficient to generate a cVEMP in most individuals with normal vestibular function (Akin et al. 2003; Papathanasiou, Murofushi, Akin, & Colebatch, 2014). Most commercial evoked potential systems that are employed to record cVEMPs are capable of generating stimuli of sufficient intensity to consistently record cVEMPs. However, it is important to ensure that the system generating the stimulus is calibrated using peak-to-peak equivalent SPL (sound pressure level) so that peak and cumulative sound exposure can be measured and calculated (Papathanasiou et al., 2014; Rosengren, Govender, & Colebatch, 2009). The stimulus generator should be routinely calibrated in dB peak SPL using a sound-level meter. Stimulus level is one of the key factors that modulates the amplitude of the cVEMP response. The relationship between oVMEP amplitude and intensity is maintained with click stimuli as well as frequency-specific stimuli

such as tone-bursts (Akin et al., 2003; Colebatch et al., 1994; Ochi et al., 2001). In a comprehensive look at the effect of stimulus level on cVEMP amplitude, Ochi and colleagues reported significant changes in the amplitude of the cVEMP with increasing stimulus level (i.e., 85, 95, and 105 dB). Specifically, the authors reported peak-to-peak amplitudes of 203.96 µV, 264.10 µV, and 293.35 µV for cVEMPs evoked using clicks at 95-, 100-, and 105 dB nHL, respectively. However, this relationship between stimulus intensity and cVEMP amplitude is not completely linear. Figure 21–9 illustrates the effect of stimulus intensity on cVEMP amplitude.

Stimulus Rate

The effects of presentation rate/stimulus presentation rate on the cVEMP have been described (Brantberg & Fransson, 2001; Wu & Murofushi, 1999). Brantberg and Fransson (2001) presented stimuli

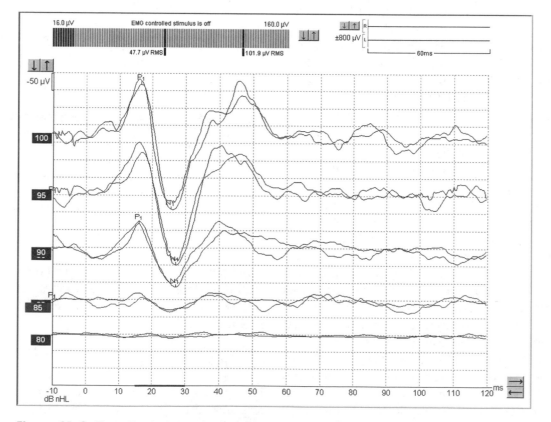

Figure 21–9. The effect of stimulus level on cVEMP amplitude.

using presentation rates of 4, 6, 8, and 20 per second. The authors evaluated waveform reproducibility and used a specific set of criteria to register whether a cVEMP response was present or absent. In order for a response to be classified as present, the peak-to-peak amplitude of the cVEMP had to significantly exceed the voltage variation of the first 5 ms following stimulus onset. Furthermore, the initial component of the cVEMP needed to be identifiable in the 15- to 20-ms poststimulus period and had to be reproducible. The authors reported that as stimulus rate was increased from 6 to 20 Hz, cVEMP responses that met the preset criterion decreased from 87% (six per second) to 56% (20 per second). Furthermore, the cVEMP peak-to-peak amplitude was shown to decrease significantly as stimulus rate was increased.

In a similar study, Wu and Murofushi (1999) evaluated the effects of five repetition rates (1, 5, 10, 15, and 20 Hz) on the response characteristics of the cVEMP. They reported that responses could be recorded using repetition rates of 10 Hz and below. cVEMP responses were recorded in only 63% of subjects when the rate of stimulus presentation was 20 Hz. The investigators also reported that the largest VEMP amplitudes were recorded using stimulation rates of 5 Hz and below (Figure 21–10). Based on this investigation, the authors recommended a stimulus repetition rate of 5 Hz to maximize amplitude and reproducibility.

Stimulus Gating and Duration

The envelope of a tone burst refers to how the onset and offset of the stimulus are shaped. Different gating parameters can change the spectral characteristics of a frequency-specific stimulus. It has been shown that the cVEMP parameters of amplitude and latency are affected by the characteristics of the stimulus (Cheng & Murofushi, 2001b; Welgampola & Colebatcha, 2001a). Cheng and Murofushi (2001a) evaluated the effect of stimulus rise/fall time on the latency of the VEMP. The investigators reported their observations of the effects of four rise and fall times on the latency of the P1 and N1, and the time separating the two peaks. The investigators reported that P1 latency increased as the rise fall time increased. A similar trend of increasing latency with increasing stimulus rise and fall time was reported for N1.

Welgampola and Colebatch (2001a) evaluated the optimal duration for frequency-specific stimuli using stimuli with durations of 1, 3, 5, 7, 10, and 20 ms delivered at a rate of five per second. The investigators reported that the largest cVEMP responses were

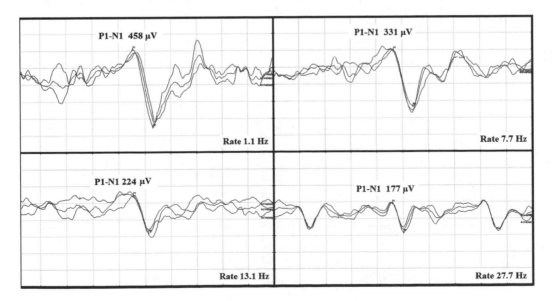

Figure 21–10. The effect of stimulus rate (500 Hz tone-burst) on cVEMP response amplitude.

obtained when stimuli of approximately 7-ms duration were used (Figure 21–11).

Stimulus Monaural/Binaural

The clinical utility of monaural versus binaural stimulation for recording cVEMPs has been described. Yang and Young (2003) described the characteristics of cVEMPs in response to monaural and binaural stimulation. The authors were particularly interested in determining if cVEMP latencies, amplitudes, and response rates recorded using binaural stimulation were similar to those recoded when two monaural responses were recorded and analyzed separately. In fact, there were no significant differences found when response metrics were compared between the two stimulation paradigms. The authors concluded that it was appropriate to use bilateral stimulation and recordings. Bilateral testing has the potential to reduce the amount of recording time by 50%. This procedure has merit where patients may be unable to sustain the required muscle contraction for the time it would take to record two monaural recording (e.g., elderly patients).

RECORDING VARIABLES

Electrode Placement

cVEMP recording requires that the noninverting electrode (i.e., active electrode) be placed at the midpoint between the termination of the muscle at the mastoid and its origin at the sternum. The resulting response is a positive peak (P1) followed by a negative peak (N1) (Jacobson & McCaslin, 2007). Sheykholeslami, Murofushi, and Kaga (2001) examined the effect of electrode position on cVEMP amplitude and latency by recording from several different locations along the length of the SCM (Figure 21–12). The investigators showed that response latency was most stable when the response was recorded from the belly (i.e., middle) of the muscle. The inverting electrode (i.e., reference) should be placed in an electrically indifferent position. Several investigations have reported placing the inverting electrode near the sternal tendons or at the sternoclavicular junction (Rosengen, Welgampola, & Colebatch, 2010). However, in our experience, these locations are not always free from reference contamination. The chin has been shown

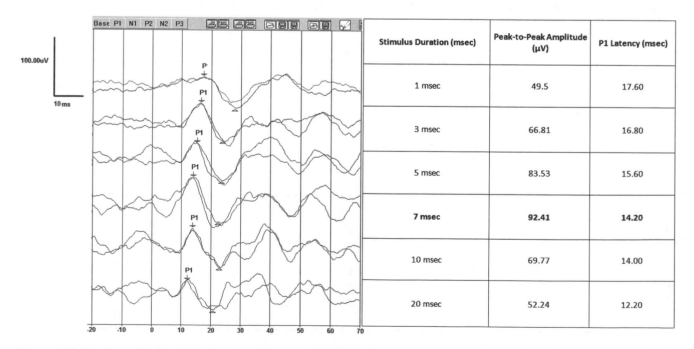

Stimulus Duration (msec)	Peak-to-Peak Amplitude (µV)	P1 Latency (msec)
1 msec	49.5	17.60
3 msec	66.81	16.80
5 msec	83.53	15.60
7 msec	92.41	14.20
10 msec	69.77	14.00
20 msec	52.24	12.20

Figure 21–11. The effect of stimulus duration on cVEMP response amplitude. Latency is shown to increase with increasing stimulus duration.

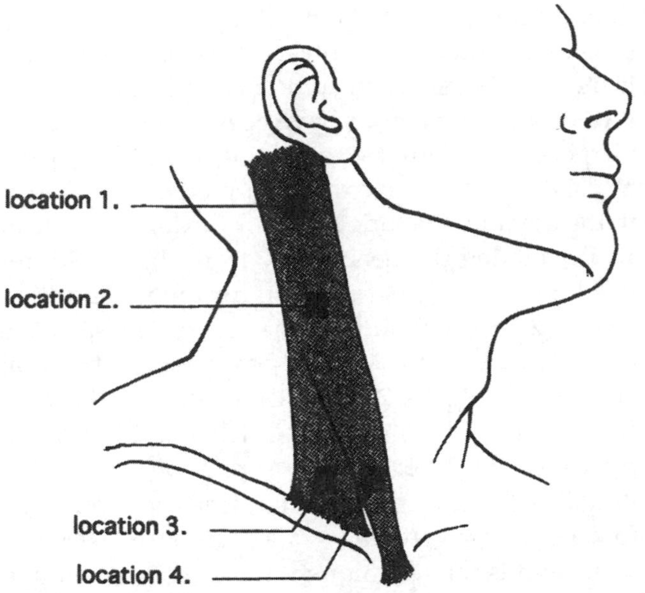

Figure 21-12. Electrode locations used to determine the optimal placement for recording the cVEMP. The middle part of the SCM muscle is the optimal location for recording cVEMPs. From Sheykholeslami, K., Murofushi, T., and Kaga, K. (2001). The effect of sternocleidomastoid electrode location on vestibular-evoked myogenic potential. *Auris Nasus Larynx, 28*(1), 41–43. Used with permission.

to provide consistent cVEMP responses that are free of any reference contamination (Jacobson & McCaslin, 2007; McCaslin et al., 2013; McCaslin et al., 2014). The common or ground electrode can be affixed to the forehead. This electrode configuration results in positive potentials represented as upward deflections. The cVEMP response is predominantly a unilateral response although in some instances contralateral responses have been shown to be present. Accordingly, a one- or two-channel evoked potential system is appropriate for recording the response because only the ipsilateral response is typically measured for diagnostic purposes.

Amplification and Filtering

The cVEMP is one to two orders of magnitude larger than a typical neurogenic auditory evoked potential. This means that amplification values of only approximately 5,000 are necessary to record the cVEMP. Because the response is a synchronized attenuation of tonic EMG activity, it is necessary to ensure that

artifact rejection is disabled. If artifact rejection is disabled, it is incumbent on the examiner to monitor the amplifier input to the signal average to ensure that saturation of the amplitude has not occurred (i.e., clipping of the raw EMG). Where amplifier saturation has occurred, it is simple to reduce the amplifier gain (e.g., 5000× to 3000×).

There has been variability in the reported optimal bandpass filter (BPF) settings (Burkard, McCaslin, Jacobson, & McNeerney, 2010; McCaslin, Jacobson, Hatton, Fowler, & Delong, 2013; Ochi et al., 2001; Vanspauwen, Wuyts, & Va de Henning, 2006). BPF is a process that rejects unwanted bioelectrical activity and electrical activity originating from outside sources (e.g., 60-Hz electrical interference) (Jones et al., 2002). The decision of how wide to set the BPF to record the response of interest is based on (1) the spectral characteristics of the response, (2) the spectral characteristics of the unwanted noise, and (3) the "skirt" of the filter (Wang, Jaw, & Young, 2013). In an effort to describe the optimal BPF for the cVEMP, Burkard, McCaslin, Jacobson, and McNeerney (2010) recorded cVEMPs from eight subjects, using a NeuroScan Evoked potential system. VEMPs were obtained using 120 dB pSPL 500 Hz tone-bursts (2-1-2 cycle, Blackman window) and presented at a rate of 5 Hz (Jacobson & McCaslin, 2007). Responses were averaged to ~250 stimuli, and each response was replicated one time. The authors reported that the dominant energy composing the cVEMP response was in the range of 15 and 70 Hz. Therefore, authors recommended a minimum high-pass cutoff of ~5 to 15 Hz and a minimum low-pass cutoff of ~100 to 150 Hz.

SUBJECT VARIABLES

EMG Activity and Monitoring

Even though the absolute latency of P1 and interaural P1 latency differences are routinely measured during the cVEMP recording, amplitude has become the standard parameter for detecting most abnormalities affecting the end-organs in clinical populations (Jacobson & McCaslin, 2007; McCaslin et al., 2013). An issue that arises when assessing absolute cVEMP amplitude measures is that there is high intersubject variability. One method to account for the intersubject amplitude variability is to use relative amplitude measures through the use of amplitude asymmetry calculations. A confounding factor associated with using amplitude measures is the known relationship between the tonic background EMG and the peak-to-peak amplitude of the cVEMP. In this regard, Lim, Clouston, Sheean, and Yiannikas (1995) reported that cVEMP amplitude was positively correlated with the level of tonic muscle activity (Lim et al., 1995). That is, as the level of tonic EMG increases the amplitude of the response increases (Akin et al., 2004; Karino et al., 2005; Lim et al., 1995; Lee et al., 2008; McCaslin et al., 2014; Welgampola & Colebatch, 2001b) (Figure 21–13). Because the cVEMP represents a synchronized *attenuation* of tonic EMG activity, patients must activate the SCM (i.e., pro-

duce a criterion level of tonic EMG above the resting baseline) in order to resolve a response (i.e., which is the sound-synchronized reduction in background EMG). Several methods have been described for the purpose of maximally activating the SCM during cVEMP recording. Two proven methods described in the literature include superior flexion of the head while rotating the head away from the ear stimulated with the patient in a semirecumbent position (Figure 21–14), and lifting the head at midline while the patient is in the supine position (i.e., bilateral activation) (Figure 21–15) (Colebatch et al., 1994; Rosengren, Welgampola, & Colebatch, 2010; Vanspauwen et al., 2006; Wang & Young, 2006; Zapala & Brey, 2004). The former technique has been reported to consistently generate cVEMP in normal participants and is the technique we currently employ in

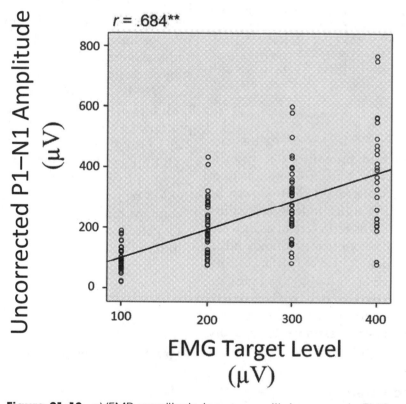

Figure 21–13. cVEMP amplitude increases with increases in EMG amplitude. Each subject was instructed to keep their tonic EMG as close to a fixed point as possible on the monitor. From McCaslin, D. L., Fowler, A., and Jacobson, G. P. (2014). Amplitude normalization reduces cervical vestibular evoked myogenic potential (cVEMP) amplitude asymmetries in normal subjects: Proof of concept. *Journal of the American Academy of Audiology, 25*(3), 268–277. doi: 10.3766/jaaa.25.3.6. Used with permission.

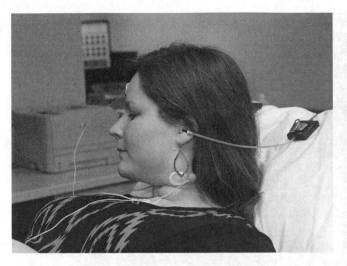

Figure 21-14. A model prepared for a two-channel cVEMP recording using the sternoclavicular junction as the inverting (reference) electrode. The head is rotated away from the ear stimulated while in the semirecumbent position.

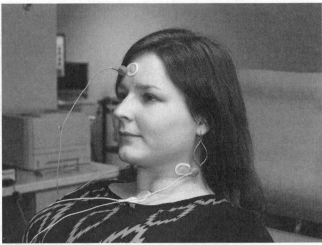

Figure 21-15. A model prepared for a two-channel cVEMP recording using the sternoclavicular junction as the inverting (reference) electrode. The head is lifted in the midline while the patient is in the supine position. This technique can be used for bilateral activation and recording.

our laboratory (Isaradisaikul et al., 2008; McCaslin et al., 2013; Wang & Young, 2006).

Accounting for the level of SCM activation is critical for both the reliability of cVEMP measures as well as validity of interaural measures. Occasionally, patients are unable to generate equal amounts of background EMG for testing the left and right sides (e.g., patients with cervical spondylosis). Two primary methods have been shown to be valid for use in controlling for the level of background tonic EMG activity. These include: (1) self-monitoring of the EMG activity by the patient through the use of a visual EMG target (Colebatch & Halmagyi, 1992) and (2) mathematical correction (i.e., amplitude normalization) of evoked potential amplitude for the magnitude of EMG that occurred during signal averaging (Brantberg et al., 2008; McCaslin et al., 2014; Welgampola & Colebatch, 2001b).

Patient Self-Monitoring (Biofeedback)

Self-monitoring of EMG involves the use of biofeedback. That is, the patient is provided an ongoing measure of his or her rectified continuous tonic EMG activity. The EMG is transformed into a visual target and displayed on a screen for the patient to observe in real time during the recording. In most instances,

EMG magnitude is represented on the vertical axis and recording time displayed along the horizontal axis (Figure 21–16).

This form of feedback enables the patient to compare his or her current level of EMG to the preset target level window (i.e., minimum and maximum amount of allowable EMG). The patient must continually maintain a specified level of EMG activity and either increase or decrease his or her ongoing EMG activity to stay within the predefined target window. When the level of EMG in a particular recording epoch exceeds the ceiling of the window or falls below the minimum allowable EMG, the individual sweep is rejected. In this way the variability of the EMG is controlled to a degree that the tester predetermines. Viewing the ongoing EMG activity during the recording also provides the patient with a threshold to exceed in order to ensure that an adequate level of SCM contraction is achieved to produce a cVEMP (e.g., 50 µV). What must be known before a target window for the EMG can be created is what the variability is when a subject is asked to maintain a certain level of EMG at a target level (McCaslin et al., 2014). In order to answer this question, McCaslin and colleagues (2014) instructed study participants to contract their SCMs in such a way as to maintain the level of EMG at one of four target levels (i.e.,

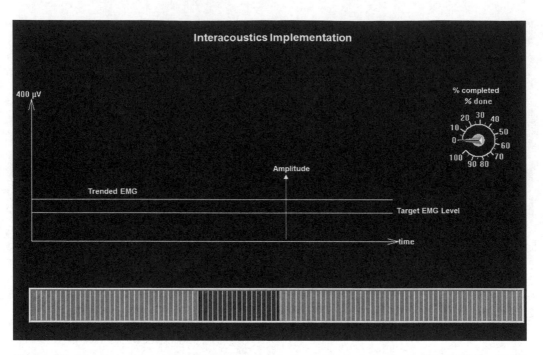

Figure 21–16. A representative EMG monitor (Interacoustics) for recording cVEMPs. EMG magnitude is represented on the vertical axis and time represented on the horizontal axis. The percent completed dial allows the patient see how much time remains for the recording.

of 100, 200, 300, and 400 μV). A visual target was provided via a video monitor for the subjects to observe. At the end of each recording, a mean (SD) of the EMG activity was calculated. EMG variability (i.e., window width) was calculated using two standard deviations from the mean. Figure 21–17 shows that as the EMG target increases, background muscle activity variability increases and the window should be widened (McCaslin et al., 2014). Because of the variability in commercial EMG monitors, it is recommended that normative data be obtained that quantify the variability associated with different target levels before setting the target window width.

There is now consensus that controlling for the level of EMG during a cVEMP recording is critical (Akin et al., 2004; Akin, Murnane, Tampas, & Clinard, 2011; McCaslin et al., 2014). In one of the first articles demonstrating the relationship between EMG and cVEMP amplitude, Akin and associates (2004) systematically described how cVEMP amplitude increased with corresponding increases in EMG. The authors employed an EMG monitor to quantify the amplitude of the background muscle activity and concluded that the optimal amount of tonic EMG for recording a cVEMP fell between 30

and 50 μV. The results of the study concluded that the close relationship between EMG and cVEMP amplitude make monitoring the EMG during a cVEMP recording necessary. Without the ability to monitor background SCM EMG, the cVEMP responses from the left and right sides cannot be reliably compared. However, some investigators have failed to find statistically significant differences in grouped data between unmonitored and self-monitoring conditions when optimal muscle activation techniques were used (Isaradisaikul et al., 2008; McCaslin et al., 2013). Isaradisaikul and associates (2008) acknowledged that there were a number of patients that did benefit from monitoring (although it did not reach statistical significance) and suggested that EMG monitoring is beneficial for a subset of patients receiving a less than perfectly administered test procedure (e.g., in the case of a severely asymmetrical SCM activation).

cVEMP Amplitude Normalization

A second technique for controlling for the effects of asymmetrical tonic EMG activity during the cVEMP recording is through the use of a mathematical

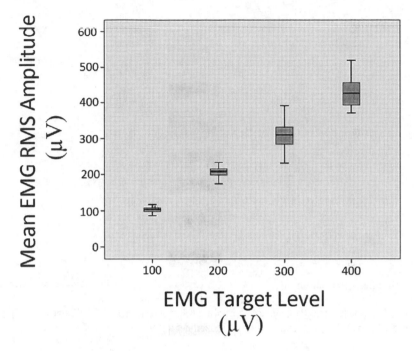

Figure 21-17. Mean RMS EMG variability increases with increases in EMG amplitude. Each subject was instructed to keep his or her tonic EMG as close to a fixed point as possible on the monitor. The upper ends of the boxplots represent the 75th percentile (upper quartile), and the lower ends of the boxplots represent the 25th percentile (lower quartile). The median of the data is represented by the line in the center of the boxplot. From McCaslin, D. L., Fowler, A., and Jacobson, G. P. (2014). Amplitude normalization reduces cervical vestibular evoked myogenic potential (cVEMP) amplitude asymmetries in normal subjects: Proof of concept. *Journal of the American Academy of Audiology, 25*(3), 268–277. doi:10.3766/jaaa.25.3.6. Used with permission.

correction known as *amplitude normalization* (Colebatch et al., 1994; Lee, Cha, Jung, Park, & Yeo, 2008; McCaslin et al., 2013; McCaslin et al., 2014). Colebatch and colleagues (1994) described a method to correct for asymmetrical muscle contraction that utilized a calculation of the magnitude of the rectified EMG that occurred in the prestimulus period. The method consists of collecting a sample of tonic EMG activity preceding the stimulus onset (e.g., 100 ms in duration) during each recording epoch and then calculating the mean RMS value of the rectified prestimulus EMG to derive an average. This prestimulus EMG average theoretically represents an estimate of the EMG produced by the contraction of the SCM during the overall recording. A derived waveform that accounts for the level of EMG during the recording is then calculated by dividing the

mean RMS of the EMG into each data point of the final signal averaged cVEMP waveform. In this way the amplitude of P1–N1 is "normalized" so that side-to-side amplitude comparisons can be calculated and the variability of side-to-side differences in muscle contraction (reflected by EMG amplitude) can be controlled (Figure 21–18).

Several investigators have studied the clinical utility of amplitude normalization with mixed results (Bogle, Zapala, Criter, & Burkard, 2013; Kim, Jung, Lee, & Suh, 2013; McCaslin et al., 2013). McCaslin and associates (2013) reported that in a group of normal subjects (i.e., pediatric and adult) amplitude normalization did not reduce significantly the variability in the interaural amplitude asymmetry when a single EMG target was employed. In some instances, amplitude normalization converted

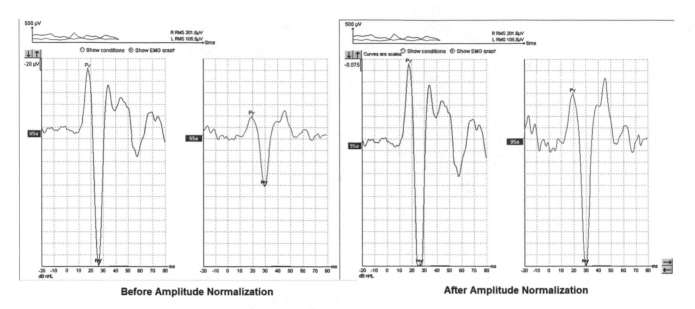

Before Amplitude Normalization   **After Amplitude Normalization**

Figure 21–18. Example of a subject with asymmetrical EMG during the cVEMP recording and whose interaural asymmetry value was transformed by amplitude normalization.

an "abnormal" cVEMP into a "normal" cVEMP although the opposite effect occurred as well, suggesting that the amplitude normalization technique was valuable in a subset of patients in their sample but not enough to reach statistical significance. In a follow-up study designed to further investigate the effectiveness of amplitude normalization on asymmetrical EMG, the investigators recorded cVEMPs while having patients maintain four different levels of EMG (i.e., 100, 200, 300, and 400 μV) amplitude for each ear. This method enabled the investigators to compare cVEMP responses obtained with varying levels of background EMG and evaluate the effectiveness of amplitude normalization. For each ear in each condition the P1 to N1 IAA ratios were calculated. As was expected, when responses obtained using dramatically different EMG target levels were compared (e.g., 100 μV target versus 400 μV target), large asymmetries were noted (Figure 21–19). Following the application of amplitude normalization, cVEMP amplitude did not change significantly with changes in RMS EMG or EMG target levels for any condition (see Table 21–2). This study confirmed the benefits of using amplitude normalization and also helped determine the degree of tonic EMG asymmetry that is required in order to generate an abnormal amplitude asymmetry result in normal subjects.

One fact that has come to light recently is that the relationship between EMG amplitude and P1–N1 amplitude is not entirely linear. That is, the input-output growth function for cVEMP peak-to-peak amplitude has been shown to saturate at supramaximal SCM contraction levels (Bogle et al., 2013, McCaslin et al., 2014). The point where further increases in background SCM EMG do not yield corresponding increases in P1–N1 amplitude is important to know when amplitude normalization techniques are being applied to responses. The underlying assumption that is used when employing amplitude normalization is that EMG level and peak-to-peak amplitude of the cVEMP are linearly correlated. However, McCaslin et al. (2014) reported that when increasing the EMG target level from 300 μV to 400 μV, there continue to be significant differences in tonic SCM EMG amplitude with no observable differences in cVEMP peak-to-peak amplitude. Although amplitude normalization techniques have been shown to be highly effective at controlling for moderate levels of EMG, collecting cVEMP responses at supramaximal levels and then using amplitude correction may produce invalid responses and lead to misinterpretation. We suggested that it is safe to use an EMG target that is between 50 μV and 300 μV RMS (McCaslin, Fowler, & Jacobson, 2014). A summary of cVEMP recording parameters is presented in Table 21–3.

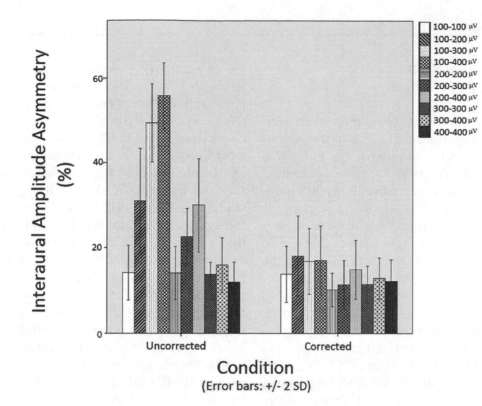

Figure 21-19. Effect of amplitude correction on cVEMP interaural amplitude asymmetry with varying degrees of EMG amplitude asymmetry. Following amplitude correction, mean group amplitude asymmetry data for all conditions did not exceed 18%. From McCaslin, D. L., Fowler, A., and Jacobson, G. P. (2014). Amplitude normalization reduces cervical vestibular evoked myogenic potential (cVEMP) amplitude asymmetries in normal subjects: Proof of concept. *Journal of the American Academy of Audiology, 25*(3), 268–277. doi:10.3766/jaaa.25.3.6. Used with permission.

Table 21-3. cVEMP Recording Protocol

Inverting electrode (reference)	Sternoclavicular junction
Noninverting electrode (active)	Midpoint or upper third of SCM mastoid muscle
Ground (Earth)	Forehead (chest if using skull taps)
Electrode impedances	<10,000 ohms
Channels	Two channels (left and right SCM)
Amplification (gain)	5,000
Artifact rejection	Disabled
Filter bandpass	10 to 1000 Hz
Epoch	100 ms
Number of accepted samples	100 to 200
Number of completed averages	Two minimum to ensure repeatability

Effect of Age on cVEMP Measurement Parameters

Beginning early on in the life span, there are significant maturational changes that occur in the peripheral and central vestibular systems. Therefore, it is critically important to account for these age-related differences in laboratory normative data when judgments are being made as to whether a response is normal or abnormal. Numerous studies have been published describing the age-related changes in cVEMP measurement parameters. To date, the majority of cVEMP studies have focused on describing the degenerative changes that occur, as patients grow older. A few of the findings that are consistently reported are an overall decrease in peak-to-peak cVEMP amplitude, decreased EMG amplitude, and higher thresholds (Akin et al., 2011; Lee, Cha, et al., 2008; McCaslin et al., 2013; Su, Huang, Young, & Cheng, 2004; Welgampola & Colebatch, 2001b; Zapala & Brey, 2004). An additional finding that has been reported is the high percentage of bilaterally absent cVEMP responses in some patient populations. In fact, it has been reported that up to 40% of neurologically and otologically intact people between 60 and 75 years of age do not generate a cVEMP

(Su et al., 2004). This inability to record cVEMPs has also been reported in very young subjects. For example, Chen, Wang, Wang, Hsieh, and Young (2007) reported that cVEMPs recorded from newborns were absent in 33% of the ears evaluated. This most likely occurred because unlike adults, infants are unable to follow the commands that are necessary to activate the SCM. Even though both of these studies highlight findings from the extreme ends of the aging continuum, it is important to remember that an absent cVEMP response may not simply be due to pathology affecting the peripheral components of the system (i.e., saccule and/or inferior vestibular nerve). Rather, the absence of recordable cVEMP responses may represent impairment occurring anywhere along the cVEMP pathway.

In an attempt to describe the effects of age on cVEMP response metrics, McCaslin et al. (2013) compared cVEMP findings in three different groups of neurologically and otologically healthy participants (i.e., 5 to 17 years of age, 18 to 40 years of age, and 41 to 70 years of age). The authors compared P1 latency, peak-to-peak amplitude, RMS EMG, and EMG variability in the various groups. The authors reported that there were significant increases in p13 latency associated with increased age (Figure 21–20). The

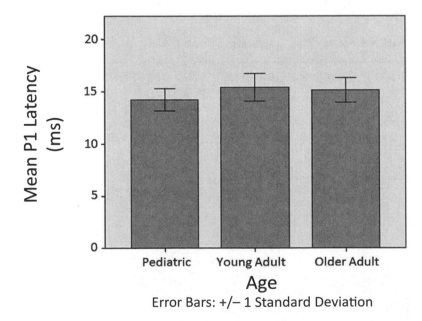

Figure 21-20. Effect of age on cVEMP p13 latency. p13 latency significant increased with age. From McCaslin, D. L., Jacobson, G. P., Hatton, K., Fowler, A. P., and DeLong, A. P. (2013). The effects of amplitude normalization and EMG targets on cVEMP interaural amplitude asymmetry. *Ear and Hearing, 34*(4), 482–490. Used with permission.

finding that P1 occurs earlier in younger subjects has been reported by other investigators (Kelsch, Schaefer, & Esquivel, 2006; Phillips & Backous, 2002; Sheykholeslami, Megerian, Arnold, & Kaga, 2005). It has been suggested that the finding of shorter latencies in younger individuals may be a result of structural differences. In this regard, P1 latencies in children have been significantly correlated with the length of the participant's neck (Chang, Yang, Wang, & Young, 2007). Additionally, N23 latency has also been shown to occur at longer latencies as age increases (Lee, Cha, et al., 2008; Su, Huang, Young, & Cheng, 2004). The latency of P1 and N1 represent central nervous system transmission through the afferent and efferent limbs of the reflex. Thus, these prolonged latencies may represent age-related slowing in the conduction velocity of the response through the cVEMP pathway (e.g., age-related degenerative changes in sensory and motor neural conduction).

In addition to the finding of significantly longer latencies with increasing age, the investigators reported significantly different cVEMP peak-to-peak amplitudes between all three groups (McCaslin et al., 2013). The amplitudes were largest for the pediatric group and smallest for the oldest group (Figure 21–21). The authors hypothesized that one contributor to the larger amplitudes in the younger populations could be related to the decreased amount of tissue interposed between the muscle and the recording electrode. Chang et al. (2007) showed that cVEMP amplitudes in adults were negatively correlated with subcutaneous thickness (i.e., how much tissue was between the muscle and the electrode). The authors also suggested that other anatomical factors such as head size could potentially contribute to the finding of larger amplitudes in younger individuals. Others have also documented decreased cVEMP amplitude with aging (Akin, Murnane, Tampas, & Clinard, 2011; Basta, Todt, & Ernst, 2007; Su et al., 2004; Welgampola & Colebatch, 2001b). Akin et al. (2011) reported that when cVEMP responses were obtained from a younger and an older group using similar EMG targets, the younger group generated significantly larger amplitudes. The authors suggested that the reduced amplitudes observed in

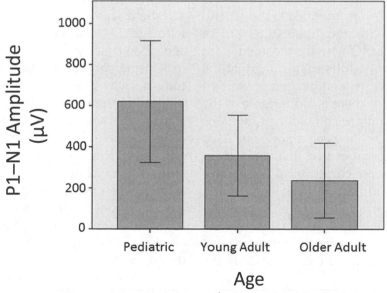

Figure 21–21. Grouped P1–N1 amplitudes as a function of age. Cervical vestibular evoked myogenic potential amplitude decreased with increases in subject age when similar EMG targets were employed. From McCaslin, D. L., Jacobson, G. P., Hatton, K., Fowler, A. P., and DeLong, A. P. (2013). The effects of amplitude normalization and EMG targets on cVEMP interaural amplitude asymmetry. *Ear and Hearing, 34*(4), 482–490. Used with permission.

the older group were a result of the degenerative effects on the vestibular system and not the muscle tonus since similar EMG targets were employed (i.e., 30 and 50 µV).

One of the key questions regarding reported age-related decrements in cVEMP amplitude is whether the observed changes are caused by degeneration of structures that are part of the afferent limb, efferent limb, or both limbs of the reflex. One approach that has been used to answer this question is to use a standard EMG target and then measure both the tonic activity of the SCM EMG and P1–N1 amplitude in subjects of different ages (Akin et al., 2011; McCaslin et al., 2013). Using this methodology, McCaslin and colleagues (2013) reported decreased SCM EMG amplitude with increasing age across the three age groups when a similar EMG target level was used. The investigators designed the study to determine whether the significantly increased peak-to-peak amplitudes observed in the younger groups were a direct effect of the tonic EMG that was recorded during the cVEMP recording. The results, in fact, showed that there were significant differences in SCM RMS tonic EMG activity between the pediatric and older adult groups, and between the young adult and older adult groups. That is, even when the visual target (i.e., 50 µV) was provided to the patient, level of EMG varied with age. Interestingly, there was no difference in EMG activity recorded from the pediatric and young adults suggesting that the SCM tonic activity is largely equivalent in the two groups. The finding that there is a difference in the SCM EMG between younger and older populations using the same target has also been reported by Akin et al. (2011). The authors reported that when older and younger groups were compared using a similar EMG target, EMG amplitude was significantly smaller for the older group. The results of these two studies support the idea that the smaller cVEMP amplitudes noted throughout the literature are most likely a function of age-related changes in both the SCM and vestibular system.

Age Effects of cVEMP Tuning

The frequency "tuning" of the otolith system has been the subject of a number of recent investigations. In healthy subjects, when VEMP responses are elicited with different frequency acoustic sig-

nals, some stimuli elicit larger amplitude VEMPs than others (Chihara et al., 2009; McCue & Guinan, 1995; Piker et al., 2013; Rauch, Zhou, Kujawa, Guinan, & Herrmann, 2004; Todd, Rosengren, Govender, & Colebatch, 2009; Welgampola & Colebatch, 2001a). In the majority of studies, it is a stimulus frequency close to 500 Hz that produces the largest VEMP amplitude and lowest VEMP threshold (Akin et al., 2003; Murofushi et al., 1999; Timmer et al., 2006). It is precisely for this reason that a 500-Hz tone-burst has been selected as the stimulus of choice in most clinics. However, there is speculation that age-related changes in the vestibular system may change the "best" frequency. As such, studies have been conducted evaluating how the tuning of the vestibular system changes as we age. In 2009, Janky and Shepard described the age-related changes in the tuning of the vestibular system using cVEMPs. Subjects enrolled in the study consisted of five age categories spanning 20 to 60+ years of age. The investigators used clicks, 250-, 500-, 750-, and 1000-Hz tone-bursts and reported on changes in cVEMP response amplitude, threshold, and latency. There were no differences detected between ears for any of the metrics tested, but significant differences were identified for latency and threshold. cVEMP threshold was reported to be positively correlated with age (i.e., thresholds increased with increasing age). However, peak-to-peak amplitude was shown to be negatively correlated with age (i.e., p13 amplitude decreased with increasing age). The lowest threshold responses were obtained using the 500-Hz stimuli and, as mentioned previously, the presence of measurable responses were found to decrease with increasing age. These findings prompted the authors to conclude that age should always be considered when interpreting cVEMP thresholds. This has important implications for the identification of disorders that manifest themselves with significantly low cVEMP thresholds (e.g., superior canal dehiscence).

In a similar study, Piker, Jacobson, Burkard, McCaslin, and Hood (2013), characterized the effects of age on the optimal frequency, or frequencies, used to record the cVEMP. Thirty-nine study participants were divided into three groups based on age (i.e., 18 to 39 years, 40 to 59 years, >60 years of age). As had been shown in previous studies, the vestibular system in all three age groups showed broad tuning unlike the auditory system that is finely tuned.

The investigators reported that stimulus frequencies 500, 750, and 1000 Hz produced significantly larger amplitudes than 125-, 250-, 1500-, and 2000-Hz stimulus frequencies. However, no significant differences in mean amplitude were observed between 500, 750, and 1000 Hz. In the youngest group of subjects, the "best" frequency was 750 Hz (i.e., the tip of the tuning curve), while in the oldest group the "best" frequency was 1000 Hz (Figure 21–22). It was the author's contention that these findings represented evidence of age-related tuning shifts in the vestibular system. That is, the "best" frequency shifted to a higher frequency for the oldest group. The clinical utility of this finding is that 500 Hz may not always be the ideal frequency to elicit a cVEMP, especially when age is considered. When assessing patients who are older, 750- or 1000-Hz tone-burst stimuli may yield better responses.

cVEMP ANALYSIS AND NORMATIVE DATA

Amplitude

Traditionally, the analysis of cVEMP responses consists of four key measures: interaural latency difference, peak latency, response threshold, and the amplitude asymmetry ratio (AR). The data presented in this chapter represent normative data from several different laboratories. Each clinical site should have its own age- and gender-adjusted normative data with upper and lower limits (e.g., 2.5 standard deviations). It has been recently recommended that normative data should be collected using recordings from at least 10 healthy subjects from each decade of life (Papathanasiou et al., 2014).

Investigators have evaluated the use of absolute amplitude of P1–N1 response, but the large degree of interindividual variability has limited the clinical utility of absolute amplitude measures (Li, Houlden, & Tomlinson, 1999). In order to control for the intersubject variability in the amplitude of cVEMP responses, side-to-side differences can be expressed as percent asymmetry (Welgampola & Colebatch, 2001a). This is a similar approach to how caloric responses are analyzed using the Jongkees formula (Jongkees, 1964). The VEMP asymmetry ratio is determined by the following equation:

$$\frac{(\text{Amplitude right cVEMP} - \text{Amplitude left cVEMP})}{(\text{Amplitude right cVEMP} + \text{Amplitude left cVEMP})}$$
$$\times 100$$

Table 21–4 shows our laboratory upper limits of percent cVEMP asymmetry (mean + 2 SD) by age in healthy subjects. When the cVEMP asymmetry exceeds the upper limit for the appropriate age

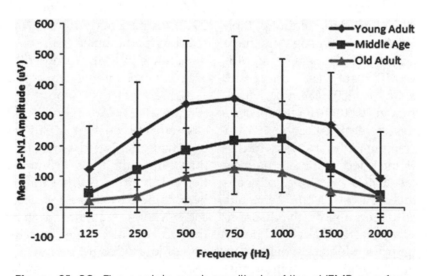

Figure 21–22. The peak-to-peak amplitude of the cVEMP as a function of stimulus frequency for different age groups. From Piker, E. G., Jacobson, G. P., Burkard, R. F., McCaslin, D. L., and Hood, L. J. (2013). Effects of age on the tuning of the cVEMP and oVEMP. *Ear and Hearing, 34*(6), e65–73. Used with permission.

Table 21-4. cVEMP Interaural Amplitude Asymmetry (Vanderbilt Normative Data)

Age Group (years)	Asymmetry %	Mean + 2 SD
5 to 17	12.87	33.75
18 to 40	16.72	42.84
>41	20.72	47.86

group, we consider the examination to be abnormal. The weaker side (i.e., side with the smaller response) is typically considered the impaired side but not in all cases (e.g., superior canal dehiscence). Interaural asymmetry measures can also be calculated following a correction for the EMG level (McCaslin et al., 2014; Miyamoto, Seo, Node, Hashimoto, & Sakagami, 2006; Welgampola & Colebatch, 2001a). Side-to-side amplitude differences in healthy subjects have typically been reported to be in the range of ~20% to ~45% depending on the technique used (e.g., monoraural or binaural stimulation) and whether or not EMG amplitude correction was used (Brantberg & Frannson, 2001; Li et al., 1999; McCaslin et al., 2013; Welgampola & Colebatch, 2001a; Zapala & Brey, 2004).

Latency

Peak latency has also been used to identify pathology in the cVEMP pathway. Investigators have reported on the diagnostic usefulness of significantly prolonged cVEMP responses (Murofushi, Shimizu, Takegoshi, & Cheng, 2001; Shimizu, Murofushi, Sakurai, & Halmagyi, 2000). In a retrospective study, cVEMP latencies were measured in 134 (61 men and 73 women) patients with a variety of disorders. The diagnoses included vestibular neuritis (VN), Ménière's disease (MD), vestibular schwannoma (VS), and multiple sclerosis (MS). The results of latency were varied depending on the disorder. Specifically, there was very little change in latency for patients suffering from Ménière's disease or vestibular neuritis. Only four patients with acoustic neuromas showed a significantly prolonged P1. Interestingly, all of the patients diagnosed with MS demonstrated significantly late P1 responses. It was

the contention of the authors based on these findings that prolonged cVEMP latencies are suggestive of retrolabyrinthine impairments localized to the vestibulospinal tract. Findings from studies such as these have led to the recommendation that the latency of P1 and N1 be reported. Prolonged latencies can be suggestive of retrolabyrinthine or central impairments.

Threshold

cVEMP thresholds are also an important measurement parameter when interpreting the response, and can add greatly to the differential diagnosis. The cVEMP threshold is the lowest level that a cVEMP response can be measured and reproduced. In our clinic, the practice is to reduce the intensity of the stimulus in 10-dB steps until there is no longer a reproducible response and then increase by 5 dB until the response is identified. This effectively becomes the threshold. In normal patients, cVEMPs will typically not be measurable below 75 to 80 dB nHL (Streubel, Cremer, Carey, Weg, & Minor, 2001). The presence of a cVEMP below these intensity levels is often suggestive of the presence of pathology such as superior canal dehiscence (SCD). The cVEMP is now known to be highly sensitive to the presence of SCD (Aw et al., 2010; Brantberg, Bergenius, & Tribukait, 1999; Cremer, Minor, Carey, & Della Santina, 2000; Zuniga, Janky, Nguyen, Welgampola, & Carey, 2013). In patients with SCD and any other third-window pathologies (e.g., fistulas or lateral canal dehiscence), VEMPs recorded from the affected side are often measurable at a significantly lower sound pressure level than would normally be expected (Figure 21-23). Additionally, when stimulus intensity remains constant, VEMP recordings from SCD ears will often yield larger P1 and N1 amplitudes than ears without SCD (Brantberg et al., 1999). It is noteworthy to stress that thresholds should always be obtained when performing cVEMP testing. In cases where a patient may have a unilateral SCD, the presence of a larger amplitude response on the impaired side could be interpreted as impairment on the intact side (i.e., the smaller response from the normal ear). Tables 21-5 and 21-6 show cVEMP and oVEMP sensitivity and specificity for patients diagnosed with SCD.

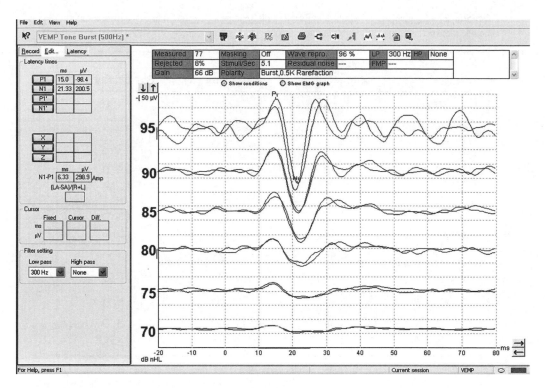

Figure 21-23. Example of a patient with reduced cVEMP thresholds and a confirmed superior canal dehiscence.

Table 21-5. Cervical Vestibular-Evoked Myogenic Potential Sensitivity and Specificity for Patients with Superior Canal Dehiscence

		Cutoff Value	Sensitivity (%)	Specificity (%)
Tone-burst-oVEMP	Peak-to-peak amplitudes	>11.7	100	88
		>17.1	100	98
		>20.3	97	100
Tone-burst-oVEMP	N1 amplitudes	>7.5	100	94
		>9.3	100	100
		>9.9	93	100
Click-oVEMP	Peak-to-peak amplitudes	>9.9	100	100
Click-oVEMP	N1 amplitudes	>2.5	100	68
		>6.6	94	100

Source: Data from Zuniga, M. G., Janky, K. L., Nguyen, K. D., Welgampola, M. S., and Carey, J. P. (2013). Ocular versus cervical VEMPs in the diagnosis of superior semicircular canal dehiscence syndrome. *Otology and Neurotology, 34,* 121–126.

Table 21–6. Ocular Vestibular-Evoked Myogenic Potential Sensitivity and Specificity for Patients with Superior Canal Dehiscence

Age Decade	Cutoff Value (µv) (threshold)	Sensitivity (%)	Specificity (%)
30s	<75	80	100
	<85	80	73
	<90	100	46
40s	<75	45	100
	<85	73	87
	<90	90	54
50s	<75	45	100
	<85	73	100
	<90	90	60
60s	<75	50	100
	<85	100	100
	<90	100	75

Source: Data from Zuniga, M. G., Janky, K. L., Nguyen, K. D., Welgampola, M. S., and Carey, J. P. (2013). Ocular versus cervical VEMPs in the diagnosis of superior semicircular canal dehiscence syndrome. *Otology and Neurotology, 34,* 121–126.

OCULAR VESTIBULAR-EVOKED MYOGENIC POTENTIAL (oVEMP)

Description of the Response

The response is dominated by a negative peak that is followed by a positive peak. The negative peak in response to click stimuli has a mean latency of ~11 ms and is referred to as N1 or n11. The following positivity shows a mean peak latency of ~15 ms and is referred to as either P1 or p15. The direction of the initial deflection suggests that the oVEMP is an onset response (i.e., moving from a state where there is no EMG activity to a state where there is an onset of stimulus-synchronized EMG activity). An ipsilateral response also can be recorded; however, it is inconsistently present. The mean latencies of N1 and P1 are significantly longer, and the peak-to-peak amplitude is significantly smaller, recorded ipsilaterally compared to contralaterally.

Data culled from oVEMP waveforms include the peak latencies of n11 and p15, the n11 threshold (in dB nHL or peak SPL), the interaural N1/n11 latency difference, and the percent interaural peak-to-peak amplitude asymmetry.

oVEMP Pathway

The oVEMP is recorded from extraocular muscles with skin surface electrodes. The predominate peripheral generator of the oVEMP is now known to be the ipsilateral utricular macula (Curthoys, 2010; Iwasaki et al., 2009). The first-order neurons are activated by shearing of the kinocilia that occurs when a low-frequency, high-intensity acoustical transient is routed through the oval window into the vestibule. In this way the acoustical energy is transformed into hydromechanical energy. Transduction also can occur when the skull is vibrated with a calibrated vibratory device (e.g., Bruel and Kjaer #4810, Mini-Shaker) or tapped in the forehead with a reflex hammer that has been modified so that a trigger pulse is produced each time the hammer strikes the skin. The activity from the utricle is routed through the utricular branch of the superior vestibular nerve. The superior vestibular nerve becomes part of the VIIIth cranial nerve that terminates at its root entry zone at the junction of the pons and the medulla (Curthoys et al., 2011). The signal is then routed to the vestibular nuclei, and that is the end of the afferent limb of the VOR.

The efferent limb begins when the activity from the vestibular nuclei is routed ipsilaterally and contralaterally through the medial longitudinal fasciculus (MLF) to the motor nuclei of cranial nerves III and VI. The cranial nerves emanating from those cranial nerve nuclei terminate on the extraocular muscles. For the contralateral oVEMP the cranial nerves terminate on the inferior oblique muscle. For the ipsilateral oVEMP the cranial nerve terminates on the superior rectus muscle (see Figure 21–5 for schematic diagram of the oVEMP pathway).

The VOR is a crossed and bilateral pathway. This means that in response to vibration, or a high-intensity and low-frequency acoustical transient, a response can be recorded from beneath both the ipsilateral and contralateral eyes (Figure 21–24).

Stimulus Variables

Type of Stimuli

The oVEMP can be evoked by any stimulus that will produce translation of the otoliths. The stimuli include high-intensity sound or direct vibration of the skull (i.e., using a B&K #4810 Minishaker, or a tendon hammer outfitted with an inertial trigger). Last, the oVEMP can be recorded following anodal electrical stimulation (e.g., galvanic stimulus of ~5 mA) of the mastoid and vestibular nerves.

The acoustical stimulus is the one most commonly used partially because it is most easily obtained. It is interesting that in at least one report (Cheng, Chen, Wang, & Young, 2009) the response rates were reported to be superior for bone-conducted sound and galvanic stimulation (i.e., 100% presence) and good in response to air-conducted stimuli (i.e., 80% presence). Not surprising was the shorter latency of the oVEMP in response to galvanic stimulation because the driving signal was delivered directly to the VIIIth nerve.

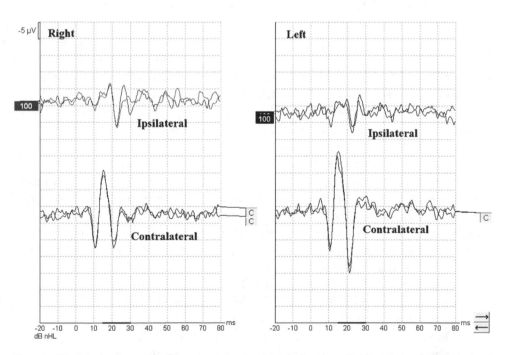

Figure 21–24. Left and right ocular-evoked myogenic potential waveform evoked using a 95 dB nHL 500 tone-burst. The initial positive waveform occurs at approximately 11 ms and the following negativity at 15 ms.

The patient need not have hearing for sound to be used as the evoking stimulus. However, the sound-conducting system must be intact if acoustical stimuli are used. When there exists a conductive impairment, acoustical stimulation may not produce a VEMP (i.e., since the magnitude of the stimulus is attenuated by the conductive impairment). In that situation the preferred stimulus is vibration. For vibratory stimulation the waveform routed to the stimulator is identical to that routed to an earphone for acoustical stimulation.

Most clinicians evoke oVEMPs using tone-burst stimuli. In this situation the tone-burst acts as a hydromechanical force to translate the otoliths that rest in the otolith membrane. The best acoustical stimulus to evoke the oVEMP is a low-frequency tone-burst (e.g., 500-Hz tone-burst) that is presented at supramaximal stimulation levels (e.g., 95 dB nHL). A vibratory stimulus is indiscriminate in the manner it activates the vestibular end organs. That is, a vibratory stimulus applied to the skull activates both vestibular end organs in much the same way that a bone vibrator activates both cochlea. The skull tap acts as a short duration vibratory stimulus. As a general rule, the vibratory and mechanical stimuli yield the largest amplitude oVEMPs.

Stimulus Frequency

When stimulus intensity is held constant, the oVEMP is larger in response to some acoustical tone burst frequencies and is smaller in response to others. In this way the oVEMP can be described with respect to its "tuning." Several investigators have attempted to define the optimal stimulus frequency to record the oVEMP.

The determination of what is the best frequency for evoking the oVEMP is based on what frequency produces the largest oVEMP at maximal stimulus intensity and persists at the lowest stimulus intensity. What constitutes the best frequency is determined, in part, by the physical characteristics of the end organ including its mass and stiffness. For example, the utricle is larger than the saccule and is less rigidly attached to the temporal bone (i.e., the utricle is floppier and more compliant). Because of this the utricle responds preferentially to lower frequencies than does the saccule (Todd et al., 2009).

Several attempts have been made to measure the tuning properties of the oVEMP. These studies have varied in the level of precision by which the best frequency was determined, in how the stimuli were delivered (i.e., by air or bone conduction), and what age groups were examined.

The discussion of tuning in the peripheral vestibular system is very different than that of the auditory system. Auditory physiologists are accustomed to the description of tuning as a result of active processes in the cochlea. The resulting tuning curves are quite sharp with clear "tips." Tuning is very different in the vestibular system. There are no known active tuning processes in the peripheral vestibular system, and there is no need for the same level of frequency selectivity that is found in the auditory system.

Donnellan et al. (2010) examined the tuning characteristics of the bone-conducted oVEMP. The examiners used tone-bursts with frequencies between 250 and 2000 Hz. The stimuli were routed to a bone oscillator placed on the mastoid process. The investigators reported a best frequency for N1 that was 383 Hz. Lewis, Mustain, Xu, Eby, and Zhou (2010) evaluated 12 subjects with 9 tone-bursts between 125 and 4000 Hz. The stimuli were 130 dB pSPL, had a 1-ms rise/fall time and a 10-ms plateau. The investigators reported a best oVEMP frequency of 1000 Hz

Murnane, Akin, Kelly, and Byrd (2011) investigated the effect of stimulus frequency on oVEMP amplitude and latency. Their stimuli were tone-bursts at octave frequencies 250 to 4000 Hz. The authors reported the greatest response amplitudes occurred for the 500-Hz stimulus.

Winters, Berg, Grolman, and Klis (2012) examined the tuning properties of the acoustical oVEMP in normals and in patients suspected of having Ménière's syndrome. Stimuli were 250-, 500-, and 1000-Hz tone-bursts delivered by air conduction. The investigators reported that normal subjects showed a best frequency of 500 Hz.

Zhang, Govender, and Colebatch (2011) attempted to examine the effects of stimulus frequency on both air-conducted and bone-conducted tone-bursts. Their assumption was that the peripheral origins of the oVEMP were in both the utricle and the saccule. The result of their investigation showed that in response to air-conducted sound, there were two peaks in the tuning curve. One peak occurred at

600 Hz and was felt to originate from the saccule, and there was a second peak occurring at 100 Hz that was believed to originate from the utricle. In a subsequent investigation Zhang, Govender, and Colebatch (2012) evaluated the bone-conducted oVEMP using vibratory stimuli ranging in frequency from 50 to 1000 Hz. The stimuli were delivered to both the forehead and mastoid. In response to vibratory stimulation the oVEMP showed a best frequency of 100 Hz.

Last, Piker et al. (2013) examined the tuning characteristics of the oVEMP using acoustical stimuli from 125 to 2000 Hz in octave and interoctave steps. The stimuli had a 2-ms rise/fall time and a 2-ms plateau. One interesting wrinkle in this study is that all seven stimulus frequencies were presented in a randomized fashion in each run. By doing this, fatigue effects were distributed evenly across the responses to all seven stimuli. The VEMPs for each frequency were differentiated and signal-averaged after data collection. Furthermore, the investigators determined whether the tuning characteristics differed significantly for young adults (18 to 39 years), middle age adults (40 to 59 years), or old adults (≥60 years). The results suggested that there were no significant differences in responses to the frequencies 500, 750, or 1000 Hz across all age groups. However, 500 Hz probably is the best frequency for most subjects. The investigators reported a significant interaction between stimulus frequency and age suggesting that the oVEMP might occur more frequently at 750 or 1000 Hz for older subjects due to age-related changes in the physical characteristics of the utricle (i.e., possibly making the system stiffer) (Figure 21–25).

Stimulus Intensity

The oVEMP is not a graded response like the ABR but instead is an "all or nothing" response. This means that the oVEMP is absent until the threshold intensity is reached when the response is present but small in amplitude. In normal, otologically and neurologically intact subjects the response is present at 85 to 95 dB nHL (Piker et al., 2011). Once threshold has been exceeded the response grows quickly in amplitude. The test normally is conducted using a stimulus magnitude that is "supramaximal" which is usually ~95 dB nHL.

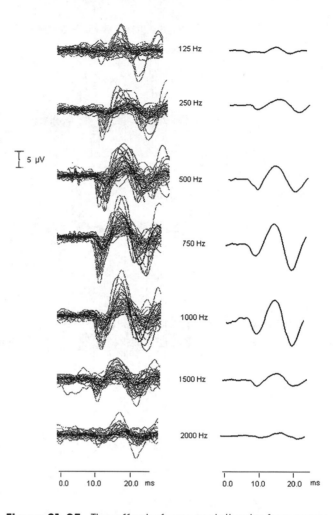

Figure 21–25. The effect of age and stimulus frequency on peak-to-peak amplitude of the oVEMP. The tracings on the left represent individual runs and the recordings on the right represent the average of responses. From Piker, E. G., Jacobson, G. P., Burkard, R. F., McCaslin, D. L., and Hood, L. J. (2013). Effects of age on the tuning of the cVEMP and oVEMP. *Ear and Hearing, 34*(6), e65–73. Used with permission.

Murnane et al. (2011) assessed the effects of stimulus intensity on the oVEMP elicited with a 500-Hz tone-burst (Figure 21–26). The authors reported oVEMP thresholds occurred at ~119 dB peak SPL (± ~6.1 dB) or ~85 dB nHL. Once the response threshold was exceeded the response grew with increases in stimulus intensity. There were few responses at intensities of 105 dB peak SPL. For the remaining intensities (110 dB peak SPL and greater) oVEMP amplitudes significantly differed for all post hoc comparisons. Interestingly, the latency of N1 and P1

INDIVIDUAL WAVEFORMS   GRAND AVERAGE

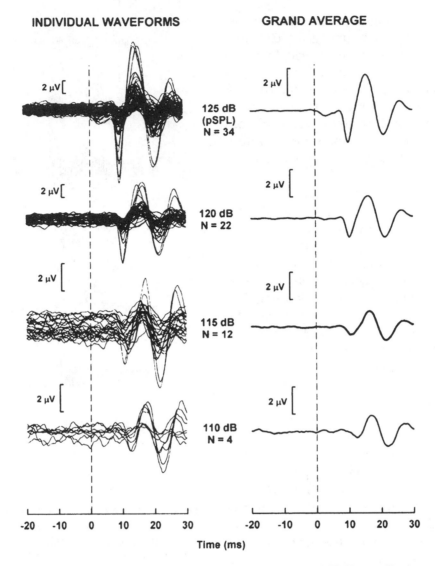

Figure 21–26. The effect of stimulus intensity on the oVEMP amplitude. From Murnane, O. D., Akin, F. W., Kelly, K. J., and Byrd, S. (2011). Effects of stimulus and recording parameters on the air conduction ocular vestibular-evoked myogenic potential. *Journal of the American Academy of Audiology, 22, 469–480.* Used with permission.

decreased as stimulus intensity was increased. That is, the absolute latency of N1 occurring in response to a 120 dB peak SPL was significantly longer than that occurring at 125 dB peak SPL.

Stimulus Rate

The optimal stimulus rates (i.e., producing superior amplitudes with no effect on latency) for bone-conducted oVEMP recordings have been reported to be between 5 and 20 Hz (Chang, Cheng, Wang,

& Young, 2010). As such, the investigators recommended a stimulus rate of 20 Hz for bone-conducted oVEMP testing. For air conduction stimuli, the superior rate is 5 Hz, and in fact, that is the stimulus rate used in our balance function laboratory (Figure 21–27).

Stimulus Gating

Stimulus gating has been studied systematically for both air-conducted and bone-conducted stimuli (Kantner, Hapfelmeier, Drexl, & Gurkov, 2013). The

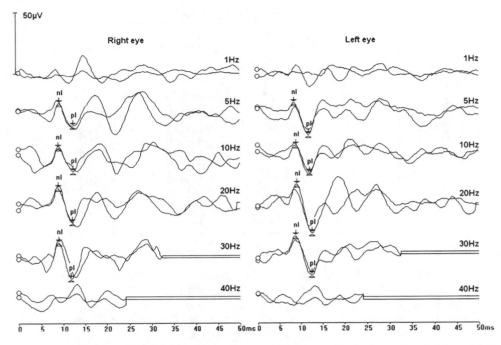

Figure 21–27. The effect of stimulus rate on oVEMP amplitude from the right and left eye. Negative is up in this figure. From Chang, C. M., Cheng, P. W., Wang, S. J., and Young, Y. H. (2010). Effects of repetition rate of bone-conducted vibration on ocular and cervical vestibular-evoked myogenic potentials. *Clinical Neurophysiology, 121,* 2121–2127. Used with permission.

effect of stimulus rise/fall and plateau time (i.e., duration, see below) on the oVEMP was examined by Cheng, Wu, and Lee (2012). oVEMPs were recorded in response to clicks (i.e., with an instantaneous rise/fall time), and 500-Hz tone-bursts with rise times, plateau times, and fall times of 0.5-2-0.5 ms, 0.5-4-0.5 ms, 2-2-2 ms, and, 2-4-2 ms. The authors reported that the oVEMP could be recorded to click stimuli (i.e., instantaneous onset) 66% of the time but was recorded 100% of the time to tone-bursts. Although the latency of the N1 increased with rise/fall time, there were no significant differences in the N1 amplitude with differences in plateau time. Burgess et al. (2013) reported that for bone-conducted pure tones, the best stimulus had a frequency of 250 or 500 Hz and a 0-ms rise time. Figure 21–28 illustrates the effect of stimulus rise/fall time and plateau on oVEMP amplitude.

Stimulus Duration

The effects of tone-burst stimulus duration on the oVEMP were evaluated by Lim, Dennis, Govender, and Colebatch (2013). The stimuli were delivered by both air and bone conduction. The investigators examined the effects of increasing stimulus duration from 2 to 10 ms for an air-conducted 500-Hz tone-burst. The investigators reported that increasing the stimulus duration produced a reduction of oVEMP amplitude. There was no benefit to increasing stimulus duration beyond 2 ms.

Stimulus Monaural/Binaural

Wang, Jaw, and Young (2009) reported their experience recording oVEMPs in response to monaural and binaural 500-Hz tone-burst stimulation (i.e., 95 dB nHL). The authors reported no significant differences in response threshold, latencies, or amplitudes when data obtained from the two modes of stimulation were compared. The investigators suggested that binaural stimulation produced significant time savings over monaural stimulation.

Despite the oVEMP being represented intermittently ipsilateral to the stimulus ear, Kim and Ban (2012) examined what effect, if any, binaural stimulation would have on the oVEMP. The investigators presented 500-Hz tone-burst stimuli monaurally

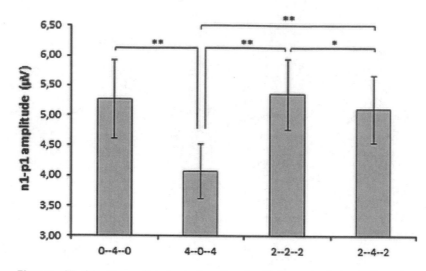

Figure 21–28. The effect of stimulus rise/fall and plateau time on oVEMP amplitude. From Kantner, C., Hapfelmeier, A., Drexl, M., and Gürkov, R. (2013). The effects of rise/fall time and plateau time on ocular vestibular-evoked myogenic potentials. *European Archives of Oto-Rhino-Laryngology.* Used with permission.

and binaurally on three occasions. The investigators measured peak latency of N1, amplitude of N1–P1, and the interaural differences in these data points. The authors reported no significant differences in the peak-to-peak amplitude and amplitude asymmetry ratios when monaural and binaural data were compared. The interclass correlation coefficients ranged from 0.68 to 0.98. Latency of N1 was significantly later for the binaural presentation compared to monaural stimulation. This latency delay occurred possibly because the response to binaural stimulation represents a combination of ipsilateral and contralateral waveforms, and the ipsilaterally recorded oVEMP occurs later than the contralaterally recorded oVEMP. The greatest effect was the reduction in test time that occurred for binaural stimulation (Figure 21–29). The oVEMP air-conducted and bone-conducted stimulus protocols are presented in Tables 21–7 and 21–8.

Recording Variables

Electrode Placement

Electrodes are silver/silver chloride disposable electrodes. The locations of the recording electrodes are shown in Figures 21–29 and 21–30.

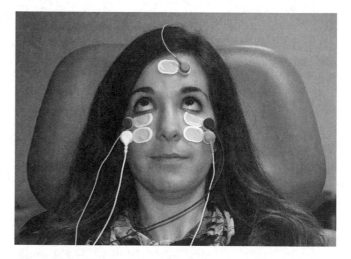

Figure 21–29. A model prepared for a two-channel oVEMP recording using the active electrode (infraorbital 1cm) referenced to the infraorbital 3-cm electrode.

The skin should be degreased with rubbing alcohol at the left and right infraorbital midlines (i.e., the electrodes should be placed as close to the middle bottom of the lower eyelid as possible). These electrodes serve as active (or noninverting) inputs to channels 1 (left eye) and 2 (right eye) of the differential amplifier. The reference (or inverting) inputs for channels 1 and 2 are a single electrode placed on the chin (i.e., common reference in our protocol)

Table 21-7. oVEMP Air-Conducted Stimulus Protocol

Frequency	500 Hz
Level	95 dB nHL
Gating	Blackman
Rate	5.1/s

Table 21-8. oVEMP Bone-Conducted Stimulus Protocol

Frequency	500 Hz
Level	150 dB peak FL (31.6 N peak) (Papathanasiou et al., 2014)
Gating	6 ms duration (2 ms rise/fall)
Rate	5 Hz
Location of stimulator	Mastoid or Glabella

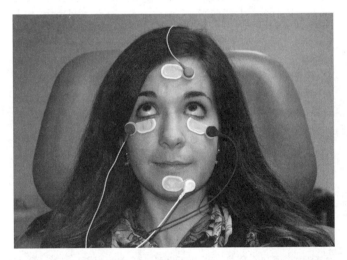

Figure 21-30. A model prepared for a two-channel oVEMP recording using the active electrode (infraorbital 1cm) referenced to the chin.

that is "jumped" into the reference electrode inputs for channels 1 and 2 (Figure 21–30). Alternately, the reference can be two electrodes placed 2 to 3 cm inferior to each of the near infraorbital electrodes (Figure 21–29). This is the protocol followed by most clinicians. The ground electrode is placed at FPz or Fz for the sake of convenience but could be placed anywhere on the body (Colebatch, 2013). Closely spaced

bipolar electrodes are very sensitive to signals occurring between the two electrodes and relatively insensitive to other signals generated on the face/body. However, we found (Piker et al., 2011) that the near infraorbital reference electrodes were recording, on average, 30% of the oVEMP amplitude recorded by the active electrode creating a problem called *reference contamination*.

When reference contamination occurs, the oVEMP recorded by the reference electrode is subtracted in the differential amplifier from the oVEMP recorded by the active electrode. The net effect is an "artificial" reduction or phase cancellation of part or all of the oVEMP recorded by the active electrode. In our experience very little of the oVEMP is volume conducted to the chin. The advantage of the referential technique (i.e., as opposed to the bipolar recording method) is the enhancement of the N1–P1 amplitude. The single disadvantage of this technique is the potential for EMG generated at the chin to be "injected" into the signal-averaged responses recorded from the infraorbital electrodes.

An interesting recent report by Sandhu, George, and Rea (2013) was a reexamination of the effects of the location of the active electrode. The investigators placed the reference electrode at its normal location (i.e., below the contralateral eye at midline) but placed a series of five active electrodes infraorbitally and equidistant from the inner canthus to the outer canthus. The ground electrode was placed on the sternum. The investigators reported the largest oVEMP was recorded from the electrode just lateral to the infraorbital midline electrode when it was referenced to the electrode placed at the inner canthus. The investigators reasoned that that electrode montage optimized the recording of the oVEMP since the active electrode was placed over the belly of the inferior oblique muscle (i.e., where the maximum response is recorded) and the reference was placed over its tendon which is electrically neutral (i.e., theoretically none of the evoked potential is recorded from that location).

Amplification

The oVEMP is one to two orders of magnitude smaller than the cVEMP and therefore requires 10 to 100 times more amplification to bring the signal within range of the signal averager. This means that amplification values of 50,000× to 100,000× are necessary to increase the magnitude of the raw EMG signal to be within the range of the signal averaging computer so that the oVEMP can be recorded. Since this is a much smaller response than the cVEMP and because this is not entirely a stimulus-synchronized attenuation of evoked EMG from the IO muscle, it is necessary to reject EMG artifacts. This means artifact rejection must be enabled to record the oVEMP.

Filtering

The subject of optimal bandpass filtering has been addressed in the recent literature. Wang, Jaw, and Young (2013) recorded the oVEMP to acoustical stimuli using high-pass filter settings of 1, 10, and 100 Hz, and, low-pass filter settings of 500, 1000, and 2000 Hz. The investigators reported that the bandpass yielding the best amplitude oVEMP without affecting its latency was 1 to 1000 Hz.

Burkard and colleagues (2013, personal communication) also have examined systematically the effect of filter bandpass on oVEMP amplitude. They observed that the critical frequencies that must be available for signal averaging are ~20 Hz for the high-pass filter and 200 Hz for the low-pass filter. The spectra of the oVEMP shows little energy in the response beyond 140 Hz (Burkard 2013, personal communication).

Subject Factors

Gaze Effects

Although it has been reported that the oVEMP can be recorded with the patient's eyes at center gaze (Huang, Yang, & Young, 2012) and in patients with closed eyes (i.e., although the waveforms looked quite different from the conventional oVEMP, Huang et al., 2012), the oVEMP is best recorded with the patient gazing upward ~20 degrees or more (Govender, Rosengren, & Colebatch, 2009; Hsu, Wang, & Young, 2009). Moving the eye from center gaze to upward gaze is believed to position the contralateral inferior oblique muscle closer to the active (noninverting) infraorbital electrode. This observa-

tion about gaze position effects on the oVEMP was also supported by the results of Murnane et al. (2011) who reported maximal amplitude of the oVEMP was recorded with subjects gazing at 30 degrees vertically (i.e., the study examined the effects of gaze angles from 5 to 30 degrees) (Figure 21–31).

It is significant that Rosengren, Colebatch, Straumann, and Weber (2013) who systematically examined gaze effects, reported that the increase in oVEMP amplitude with upward gaze could not be explained entirely by the reduction in the distance of the contralateral infraorbital recording electrode to the IO muscle. Instead, it was the investigator's contention that upward gaze increased the tonic activity in the IO muscle and, much like occurs with the SCM, the onset of the tone burst results in a stimulus-initiated reduction in that tonic activity. If this is in fact true, what is not clear is why the oVEMP is a negative-positive waveform instead of a positive-negative waveform. One possible explanation might be that this reflects a dipole effect. That is, the active electrode might be viewing the negative pole of the IO muscle dipole. Thus, as of this writing (Fall 2013) it is believed that the effect of upward gaze accomplishes two things that collectively increase the amplitude of the oVEMP over the amplitude when the eyes are staring at center gaze: (1) upward gaze moves the contralateral inferior oblique muscle closer to the active electrode, and (2) it increases the tonic EMG activity in the contralateral IO muscle that is then either attenuated or augmented by the driving acoustical stimulus. The oVEMP recording protocol is shown in Table 21–9.

Age Effects

A number of processes occur as we age that have an effect on the normal function of the peripheral and central vestibular systems. These age-related changes are addressed in detail elsewhere in this text (Chapter 32); however, we address a few of the age-related changes here.

There have been documented age-related effects at the hair cell level and also at the level of the afferent neurons (Ishiyama, 2009). The loss of both hair cells and first-order afferents has been documented in the cristae, the utricle, and the saccule. A decrease in hair cell density occurs after age 50 years. The

INDIVIDUAL WAVEFORMS   GRAND AVERAGE

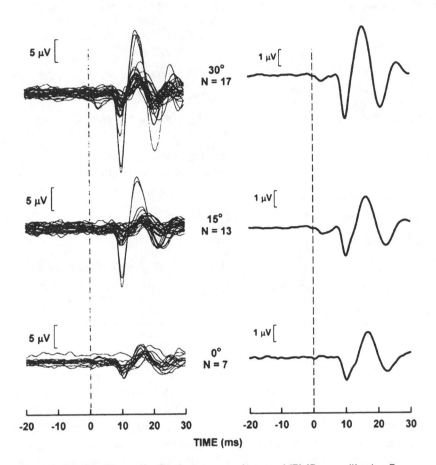

Figure 21–31. The effect of gaze angle on oVEMP amplitude. From Murnane, O. D., Akin, F. W., Kelly, K. J., and Byrd, S. (2011). Effects of stimulus and recording parameters on the air conduction ocular vestibular-evoked myogenic potential. *Journal of the American Academy of Audiology, 22,* 469–480.

greatest effects may be observed in the saccules and the cristae with less age-related damage occurring for the utricle. That is, when young and older individuals were compared, hair cell density was reduced by 40% at the cristae, 24% at the saccule, and 21% at the utricle (Rosenhall, 1973). More specifically the fetal cristae contain ~7,800 hair cells and this is reduced to 4,700 for adults between the ages of 71 and 95 years (i.e., a reduction of 38% on average). A reduction of 30% in hair cell density in the senescent mouse produces a reduction of VOR gain at 0.8 Hz. That gain reduction produces retinal smear during movements of the head or head and body. In

the human, VOR gain shows significant reductions beyond age 70 years.

There are age effects specific to the utricle and saccule. Many of the changes affect the otolith crystals. The density of the crystals is reduced and the normal regeneration of the crystals is impaired with age. This results in reduced otoconial volume, fractured otoconia (i.e., producing debris in the canal and an increasing the likelihood of BPPV), and even the generation of "giant" otoconia. In parallel with structural changes affecting the end organ there can be impaired perfusion of the end organ. Over and above these changes there has been reported a 25% reduction in neurons

Table 21–9. oVEMP Recording Protocol

Inverting electrode (reference)	3 cm infraorbital or chin (conventional reference electrode placement is immediately below the infraorbital midline electrode)
Noninverting electrode (active)	Infraorbital midline
Ground (Earth)	Forehead (i.e., Fz)
Electrode impedances	≤10,000 ohms, with interelectrode impedance differences ≤2000 ohms
Channels	Two (ipsilateral and contralateral infraorbital midline responses)
Amplification (gain)	× 30,000 to 50,000
Artifact rejection	Enabled
Filter bandpass	1–10 Hz to 500–1000 Hz
Epoch	100 ms (with a 20-ms prestimulus period)
Number of accepted samples	150
Number of completed averages	2

at Scarpa's ganglion, and a 37% loss of afferents when comparing younger adults to older adults.

Hsu et al. (2009) evaluated age-related differences in oVEMP latency and amplitude. Subjects were adults ($N = 15$, 24 to 33 years of age) and children ($N = 15$, 3 to 13 years of age). The stimulus was a tone burst presented at 105 dBnHL. The authors did not report age-related differences in N1 latency, P1 latency, or the N1–P1 interval or the peak to peak amplitude of the oVEMP.

Chang et al. (2012) evaluated the effect of age on oVEMPs recorded in response to bone-conducted vibration and galvanic stimulation. Since the galvanic stimulus bypasses the end organ and stimulates the afferent nerve fibers directly, an abnormal or absent BC oVEMP with a normal galvanic oVEMP would suggest an end organ impairment, whereas a unilaterally delayed galvanic oVEMP would suggest an impairment in neural conduction. The investigators reported significant N1 latency delays for a group of subjects older than 60 years of age compared to groups younger than 60 years of age. There were nonsignificant differences in the prevalence of the galvanic oVEMP suggesting that age differences observed in the prevalence of bone-conducted oVEMPs reflected age changes in the peripheral ves-

tibular system. The effect of age and stimulus type on the prevalence of the oVEMP is shown in Table 21–10.

The study of age effects on the oVEMP is complicated by the differing stimuli used by investigators to evoke the response (e.g., electrical/galvanic, bone conduction, skull tap, acoustical click, acoustical tone burst) and the methods used to obtain the data (e.g., threshold versus suprathreshold stimulation for evaluation of effects of stimulus frequency).

Tseng, Chou, and Young (2010) examined 70 subjects with an age range of 24 to 76 years. They placed the subjects into six groups representing six age decades. The stimuli were delivered by bone conduction stimulation. All subjects from ages 20 to 59 years generated oVEMPs. Conversely 55% of those subjects aged 60 to 69 years and 40% 70 years and older failed to generate an oVEMP. With age treated as a continuous variable both N1 latency ($r = 0.54$) and N1–P1 amplitude ($r = -0.37$) showed age effects. The investigators reported a positive correlation between N1 latency and age and a significant negative correlation between age and N1–P1 amplitude.

Nguyen, Welgampola, and Carey (2010) evaluated 53 subjects between the ages of 20 and 70 years. Stimuli were acoustical clicks and 500-Hz tone-

Table 21–10. Prevalence of the oVEMP in Response to Galvanic and Bone-Conducted Stimuli

Age Group	Galvanic oVEMP % Prevalence	BC oVEMP % Prevalence
20 to 29 years	100	100
30 to 39 years	100	100
40 to 49 years	100	100
50 to 59 years	100	86
60 to 69 years	84	63

bursts, skull taps (i.e., delivered with a specially modified tendon hammer) and skull vibration (i.e., delivered with a Bruel and Kjaer mini shaker). The interclass correlation coefficients between subject age and oVEMP for tone-burst stimuli ranged from 0.81 (N10 amplitude) to 0.79 (N10–P15 peak-to-peak amplitude) to 0.50 (for the amplitude asymmetry of the N10–P15 peak-to-peak amplitude). Unlike reported by Tseng, when age and oVEMP amplitudes were plotted as continuous variables there was no significant relationship. This finding was also at odds with the findings of Iwasaki et al. (2007) who reported a linear decrease in oVEMP amplitude with age when the stimuli were skull taps and skull vibration (i.e., minishaker).

Rosengren et al. (2011) examined age effects on the oVEMP in response to forehead taps, lateral (mastoid) vibration, and both air- and bone-conducted tone bursts. Subjects were 61 normal individuals aged 18 to 80 years of age. The oVEMPs evoked with taps and vibration did not demonstrate age effects. The authors reported a moderate correlation between oVEMP and age for acoustical clicks and bone-conducted tone bursts. The authors reported elevated oVEMP thresholds by 6 dB on average when oVEMP threshold intensities were compared to cVEMP threshold intensities for 500-Hz tone-burst stimuli. Response prevalence was 93% for stimuli of an intensity of 110 dB L_{Aeq}. oVEMPs demonstrated latencies that were significantly longer with age for air-conducted clicks and 500-Hz tone-bursts.

Piker et al. (2011) examined the effects of age on N1 and P1 latency, N1–P1 peak to peak amplitude, N1 interaural latency difference, and interaural N1–P1 amplitude asymmetry. Subjects were young indi-

viduals (mean age 12.5 years), middle-aged adult (mean age 34 years) and old adults (mean age 63 years). The authors reported significant decreases in N1–P1 peak-to-peak amplitude when young subjects and middle-age subjects were compared to older subjects. With age treated as a continuous variable the correlation coefficient for oVEMP peak-to-peak amplitude was negative and statistically significant ($r^2 = .14, p < .001$). Further, there were significant age differences in N1 threshold intensity (see below).

Age Effects of oVEMP Threshold. Increased age results in elevated oVEMP thresholds. When treated as a continuous variable oVEMP threshold correlated positively with subject age ($r^2 = .11, p = .002$). In fact, there was a 3.4 dB difference in N1 thresholds when data from young adults and old adults were compared (i.e., threshold occurred at higher intensities for old adult subjects) (Piker et al., 2011).

Age Effects of oVEMP Tuning. The effects of age on the "tuning" of the oVEMP was addressed by Piker and colleagues (2013). Stimuli consisted of acoustical tone bursts of frequencies 125, 250, 500, 1000, 1500, and 2000 Hz that were presented at 127 dB pSPL. All stimuli were presented in a pseudo-randomized manner for each run so that the effects of fatigue might be distributed evenly across all stimuli. Subjects ranged in age from 22 to 78 years ($N = 39$, mean age 46 years, ±15.7 years). Subjects were placed into three age groups consisting of young, middle, and older adults. The investigators reported a best frequency occurred for 500- and 750-Hz tone-bursts (i.e., stimulus yielding the greatest amplitude oVEMP), although there were no significant differences in oVEMP amplitude across age groups for each frequency. Whereas the best frequency to evoke the oVEMP for young adult subjects was 750 Hz, the best frequency increased to 1000-Hz stimulus for older adult subjects. Armed with this information the authors cautioned that clinicians might choose different evoking stimuli depending on the age of their patients (e.g., 500-Hz tone-bursts for younger adults and 1000 Hz for older adults if they failed to generate an oVEMP in response to the 500-Hz stimulus).

It is our practice to first record the oVEMP in response to 95 dB nHL, 500-Hz tone-bursts delivered monaurally. Responses are replicated at least one time so that reproducibility of the data can be assessed. Where the response exists we then use a bracketing technique to estimate oVEMP threshold separately for the left and right ears.

When a negative waveform is plotted as a downward deflection, the normal oVEMP appears as a "W" with the first negative peak occurring at ~11 ms. The variables we quantify include: N1 latency, P1 latency, N1–P1 peak-to-peak amplitude, interaural N1 latency differences, and interaural differences in N1–P1 amplitude (in percent). The most common abnormality encountered is either a unilaterally or bilaterally absent oVEMP, or a unilaterally abnormal reduction in oVEMP amplitude. Rarely does a latency prolongation occur. When a latency prolongation occurs, it usually occurs bilaterally and signifies an impairment in central transmission occurring either in the afferent or efferent limbs of the reflex arc. Table 21–11 shows normative data for the oVEMP gathered in our laboratory.

cVEMP AND oVEMP IN SELECT DISEASES

Superior Semicircular Canal Dehiscence Syndrome (SSCDS)

The approach to the identification of SSCDS with the oVEMP has gone in two directions. The underlying assumption for each approach is that the dehiscence results in an abnormal "amplification" of the normal response to either air-conducted or bone-conducted stimuli. For example, subjects/patients as a general rule do not generate oVEMPs in response to 4000-Hz tone-bursts. However, Manzari, Burgess, McGarview, and Curthoys (2013) observed in a very clever investigation that patients with SSCDS clearly generated oVEMPs in response to either an air- or bone-conducted 4000-Hz tone-burst. None of their normal controls generated oVEMPs to the same stimulus. In this way the investigators suggested that they had created a one-trial protocol for the identification of SSCDS.

In a slightly different implementation Zuniga, Janky, Nguyen, Welgampola, and Carey (2013) recorded both oVEMPs and cVEMPs in response to air-conducted and bone-conducted clicks and 500-Hz tone-bursts. They recorded responses from patients that were placed in different age groups. The authors reported that the absolute peak-to-peak amplitude of N1–P1 discriminated well between patients with (sensitivity) and without (specificity) SSCDS. In fact, using their absolute amplitude criterion both sensitivity and specificity values exceeded 90%. For example, the investigators reported that using an upper limit of 17.1 µV yielded sensitivity and specificity of 100% and 98% respectively This absolute N1 amplitude upper limit varied by age (Tables 21–12 and 21–13 from Zuniga et al., 2013).

It would appear that there now exist two methods that have been offered by investigators for the identification of SSCDS that do not rely on the

Table 21–11. Comparison of Characteristic Parameters of oVEMP Among the Three Age Groups

Age Group (yr)	N (ears)	N1 Latency, ms	P1 Latency, ms	N1–P1 Latency, ms	Interaural N1 Latency Difference, ms	N1–P1 Amplitude, µV	Interaural Amplitude Asymmetry Ratio, %	Threshold, dB nHL
1 (<18)	20	12.1 (1.1)	17.1 (1.3)	5.2 (1.1)	1.2 (.9)	5.3 (2.8)	14 (10)	90.7 (3.7)
2 (18–49)	58	12.5 (.88)	17.6 (1.1)	5.0 (.84)	.61 (.59)	5.1 (3.1)	13 (10)	92.8 (2.9)
3 (≥ 50)	22	12.7 (1.3)	17.2 (2.3)	4.0 (2.3)	1.4 (1.1)	1.5* (1.4)	16 (12)	94.1* (1.9)
Total	100	12.4 (1.0)	17.4 (1.3)	5.0 (1.3)	.85 (.81)	4.4 (3.1)	14 (10)	92.5 (3.2)
p value		0.116	0.346	0.077	0.019	<0.001	0.755	0.007

Note. p value = one-way analysis of variance test. Data are expressed as mean (sd).

*p <.05, Bonferroni-adjusted t-test.

Source: Data from Piker, E. G., Jacobson, G. P., McCaslin, D. L., and Hood, L. J. (2011). Normal characteristics of the ocular vestibular evoked myogenic potential. *Journal of the American Academy of Audiology, 22,* 222–230.

Table 21–12. oVEMP Sensitivity and Specificity for the Diagnosis of Superior Canal Dehiscence Syndrome

		Cutoff Value	Sensitivity (%)	Specificity (%)
Tone-burst oVEMP	Peak-to-peak amplitudes	>11.7	100	88
		>17.1	100	98
		>20.3	97	100
Tone-burst oVEMP	N1 amplitudes	>7.5	100	94
		>9.3	100	100
		>9.9	93	100
Click oVEMP	Peak-to-peak amplitudes	>9.9	100	100
Click oVEMP	N1 amplitudes	>2.5	100	68
		>6.6	94	100

Source: Data from Zuniga, M. G., Janky, K. L., Nguyen, K. D., Welgampola, M. S., and Carey, J. P. (2013). Ocular versus cervical VEMPs in the diagnosis of superior semicircular canal dehiscence syndrome. *Otology and Neurotology, 34,* 121–126.

Table 21–13. Ocular Vestibular Evoked Myogenic Potential Sensitivity and Specificity for Patients with Superior Canal Dehiscence

Age Decade	Cutoff Value (µv) (Peak-to-Peak-Amplitude)	Sensitivity (%)	Specificity (%)
30s	17.5	100	100
40s	22	100	100
50s	16.6	100	94
	21.3	90	100
60s	14.8	100	100

Source: Data from Zuniga, M. G., Janky, K. L., Nguyen, K. D., Welgampola, M. S., and Carey, J. P. (2013). Ocular versus cervical VEMPs in the diagnosis of superior semicircular canal dehiscence syndrome. *Otology and Neurotology, 34,* 121–126.

tedious activity of oVEMP threshold estimation. The authors of this chapter suggest that the examiner might create a two stage criteria for the identification of SSCDS patients: (1) "Does there exist an oVEMP in response to a 4000-Hz, air-conducted, tone-burst stimulus?" and (2) "Does the amplitude of the oVEMP in response to a 500-Hz, 95 dBnHL, air-conducted tone-burst stimulus equal or exceed 17.1 µV?" If the answer to either or both of these questions is "Yes," the likelihood is high that the patient has a dehiscent or even a "near dehiscent" (Ward et al., 2013) superior semicircular canal.

Large Vestibular Aqueduct Syndrome (LVAS)

In a related investigation, Taylor et al. (2012) evaluated the oVEMP in a patient with bilateral LVAS. The investigators recorded both oVEMPs and cVEMPs in response to tone-bursts at octave frequencies between 250 and 2000 Hz. The VEMP amplitudes were compared to that of a control group. As in SCDS the investigators reported abnormally reduced oVEMP thresholds and augmented amplitudes at supramaximal stimulating levels.

Brainstem Disease

A description of changes in the oVEMP that occur for patients with brainstem disease, including multiple sclerosis (MS), have been reported (Ivankovic et al., 2013). There has been variability in how frequently the oVEMP has been abnormal, and how the abnormality is manifested. This is not surprising since the nature of MS is the occurrence of plaques at any point of the central nervous system. This means that a patient with MS affecting the spinal cord might demonstrate an abnormal cVEMP and have a normal oVEMP, whereas a patient with an internuclear opthalmoplegia (INO) might demonstrate an abnormal oVEMP and have a normal cVEMP. It is likely that VEMP testing (i.e., coupled with multimodal sensory-evoked potentials) could supplement MRI and spinal fluid analysis to help semi-objectively demonstrate the presence of multiple CNS lesions occurring at different locations over time.

In this regard, Rosengren and Colebatch (2011) conducted both oVEMP and cVEMP examinations on 13 patients with MS. oVEMPs showed abnormalities more often than cVEMPs (i.e., 69% abnormal for oVEMP and 8% abnormal for cVEMP). oVEMPs were absent 50% of the time and demonstrated latency prolongations ~20% of the time. Normal oVEMPs occurred only 30% of the time.

Gazioglu and Boz (2012) recorded oVEMPs from 62 patients with MS and 35 controls. The investigators reported that the N1 and P1 potentials were significantly prolonged in the patient sample. In fact, the oVEMP latencies were positively correlated with values on a disability status scale.

Gabelic et al. (2013) assessed the oVEMP findings in normal controls and in patients with an MS diagnosis. The stimulus was an acoustical click of 130 dB SPL. The investigators reported N1 latency prolongations in 30% and absent responses (i.e., referred to by the investigators as a "conduction block") in 40% of the MS patients. When paired with the cVEMP a total of 80% of the patients demonstrated an abnormal VEMP test.

Ivankovic et al. (2013) reported oVEMP findings from a cohort of 32 patients with diagnoses of MS where plaques affected the brainstem. Results showed that oVEMP abnormalities were present in 37.5% of the sample. In a similar vein, Oh et al. (2013)

reported their observations recording oVEMPs in response to air-conducted tone-bursts from a sample of 52 patients with acute brainstem lesions. The investigators reported that 53.8% of the patients demonstrated oVEMP abnormalities and these patients had MRI confirmed lesions affecting the medial longitudinal fasciculus (MLF), the crossed ventral tegmental tract and ocular motor nuclei, and their cranial nerves. The oVEMP abnormalities consisted of N1 latency prolongations.

Bilateral Vestibulopathy

Agrawal, Bremova, Kremmyda, and Strupp (2013) examined peripheral vestibular system function in patients with bilateral vestibular system impairment due to aminoglycoside ototoxicity and bilateral Ménière's disease. Caloric and vHIT tests were used to assess function in the semicircular canals. The oVEMP and cVEMP tests were used to assess the otolith organs. A general finding was that damage was most severe for semicircular canals (100% of sample) compared to the saccule (61%) or the utricle (64%). Damage to the utricle was greatest for patients with ototoxicity and was least for patients with Ménière's disease. The investigators reported that the VEMP test results correlated best with a self-report dizziness disability/handicap. This is a finding the present authors have been unable to demonstrate in their own investigations.

Benign Paroxysmal Positional Vertigo (BPPV)

Lee and colleagues reported tone-burst–evoked cervical and ocular VEMP findings in 16 patients with recurrent BPPV and 20 patients with nonrecurrent BPPV. The investigators reported significant differences in the proportion of patients with abnormal VEMP test results. That is, VEMP abnormalities occurred in 50% of the patients with recurrent BPPV and 15% of patients with nonrecurrent BPPV. The implication is that the utricle is the most likely source of the stray otoliths and it would follow that an abnormal oVEMP would suggest a utricular impairment and the source of the canaliths.

Vestibular Neuritis

Shin et al. (2012) examined 30 patients with superior vestibular neuritisneuritis (SVN), 3 patients with inferior vestibular neuritis (IVN), and 8 patients with both branches impaired, then compared them to data obtained from 60 normal controls. The investigators reported absent oVEMPs and caloric responses and normal cVEMPs for patients with SVN. They reported normal caloric responses and oVEMPs and absent cVEMPs in patients with IVN, and absent c- and oVEMPs and caloric responses for patients with both vestibular nerve branches affected.

Migraine

Gozke, Erdal, and Ozkarakas (2010) assessed oVEMP in a sample of 43 patients who had migraine without aura and no dizziness complaints, and a sample of 29 healthy controls. The stimulus was a high-intensity click. The migraine sample generated bilateral responses 46% of the time, unilateral responses 35% of the time, and absent responses 19% of the time. Alternately, the normal group generated responses bilaterally 87% of the time and unilaterally 13% of the time. The investigator interpreted the evidence to suggest subclinical vestibular disease was present in the migraine patients.

Ménière's Disease (MD)

The investigators Huang, Wang, and Young (2011) assessed the effect of MD on oVEMPs and cVEMPS recorded in response to air-conducted sound and bone-conducted vibration. The number of patients with abnormal sound-evoked oVEMPs, vibration-evoked oVEMPs, sound-evoked cVEMPs, and vibration-evoked cVEMPs was 65%, 25%, 45%, and 25%, respectively, in the affected ears and 40%, 0%, 15%, and 0%, respectively, in the unaffected ears of patients. When the existence of hearing loss was added as a variable, the proportion of patients with hearing loss, abnormal air-conducted cVEMP, bone-conducted oVEMP, and caloric tests in affected ears was 65%, 45%, 25%, and 20%, respectively, and these proportions are similar to the frequency that hydrops affects the cochlea, saccule, utricle, and semicircular canals.

In an interesting study, Manzari, Tedesco, Burgess, and Curthoys (2010) recorded cVEMP and oVEMP on two occasions in 16 controls. Additionally, the investigators recorded the same responses in patients with MD both ictally (i.e., during a spell) and interictally (i.e., during the quiescent period). The investigators reported no significant test-retest differences in responses from the control group. The investigators reported a significant increase in the amplitude of oVEMP N10 and a significant decrease in the amplitude of P13 during the spell. The authors concluded that the MD attacks affected the utricles and saccules differently.

SUMMARY: CAVEATS REGARDING VEMP TESTING

It would be misleading to end this chapter without stating briefly a few caveats about pathologies affecting the oVEMPs and cVEMPs (adapted from Curthoys, Manzari, Smulders, & Burgess, 2009). Abnormal oVEMP and cVEMP certainly can occur in the presence of significant impairments affecting either or both the saccules, utricles, and superior and/or inferior vestibular nerves. However, abnormal VEMP tests can occur when there is a conductive hearing impairment that reduces the sound intensity reaching the vestibular end organs. So it is essential to obtain a recent audiogram and immittance test before acoustical stimuli are used to evoke a VEMP. When a conductive impairment significantly reduces the intensity of the acoustical stimulus the examiner must use an alternative method to translate the otoliths (e.g., mechanical stimulation or vibratory stimulation). Additionally, significant neuromuscular disease (e.g., myasthenia gravis) can produce an abnormal VEMP even when the vestibular end organs are intact. Diseases of the central nervous system (e.g., multiple sclerosis) can also produce abnormal VEMP tests where the end organs are normally functioning. Last, and certainly not least, there are a myriad of technical mistakes that young and seasoned clinicians can make that can reduce or eliminate the likelihood of recording a VEMP. These errors included: incorrect placement of electrodes, over- or underamplification of the bioelectrical activity, incorrect routing of the stimulus (i.e., sending the stimulus to the right ear for a left ear VEMP test), and testing an ear that is occluded with cerumen. This is only the beginning of a long list of possible technical errors. Given these assumptions it is best to approach each patient as "normal until proven otherwise."

REFERENCES

Agrawal, Y., Bremova, T., Kremmyda, O., & Strupp, M. (2013). Semicircular canal, saccular and utricular function in patients with bilateral vestibulopathy: Analysis based on etiology. *Journal of Neurology, 260*(3), 876–883.

Akin, F. W., Murnane, O. D., Panus, P. C., Caruthers, S. K., Wilkinson, A. E., & Proffitt, T. M. (2004). The influence of voluntary tonic EMG level on the vestibular-evoked myogenic potential. *Journal of Rehabilitation Research and Development, 41*(3B), 473–480.

Akin, F. W., Murnane, O. D., & Proffitt, T. M. (2003). The effects of click and tone-burst stimulus parameters on the vestibular evoked myogenic potential (VEMP). *Journal of the American Academy of Audiology, 14*(9), 500–509; quiz 534–505.

Akin, F. W., Murnane, O. D., Tampas, J. W., & Clinard, C. G. (2011). The effect of age on the vestibular evoked myogenic potential and sternocleidomastoid muscle tonic electromyogram level. *Ear and Hearing, 32*(5), 617–622.

Aw, S. T., Welgampola, M. S., Bradshaw, A. P., Todd, M. J., Magnussen, J. S., & Halmagyi, G. M. (2010). Click-evoked vestibulo-ocular reflex distinguishes posterior from superior canal dehiscence. *Neurology, 75*(10), 933–935.

Basta, D., Todt, I., & Ernst, A. (2007). Characterization of age-related changes in vestibular evoked myogenic potentials. *Journal of Vestibular Research, 17*(2–3), 93–98.

Bath, A. P., Harris, N., McEwan, J., & Yardley, M. P. (1999). Effect of conductive hearing loss on the vestibulo-collic reflex. *Clinical Otolaryngology and Allied Sciences, 24*(3), 181–183.

Bickford, R. G., Jacobson, J. L., & Cody, T. R. (1964). Nature of average evoked potentials to sound and other stimuli in man. *Annals of the New York Academy of Sciences, 112*, 204–223.

Bogle, J. M., Zapala, D. A., Criter, R., & Burkard, R. (2013). The effect of muscle contraction level on the cervical vestibular evoked myogenic potential (cVEMP): Usefulness of amplitude normalization. *Journal of the American Academy of Audiology, 24*(2), 77–88.

Brantberg, K., Bergenius, J., & Tribukait, A. (1999). Vestibular-evoked myogenic potentials in patients with dehiscence of the superior semicircular canal. *Acta Oto-Laryngologica, 119*(6), 633–640.

Brantberg, K., & Fransson, P. A. (2001). Symmetry measures of vestibular evoked myogenic potentials using objective detection criteria. *Scandinavian Audiology, 30*(3), 189–196.

Brantberg, K., Löfqvist, L., Westin, M., & Tribukait, A. (2008). Skull tap induced vestibular evoked myogenic potentials: An ipsilateral vibration response and a bilateral head acceleration response? *Clinical Neurophysiology, 119*(10), 2363–2369.

Brantberg, K., & Mathiesen, T. (2004). Preservation of tap vestibular evoked myogenic potentials despite resection of the inferior vestibular nerve. *Journal of Vestibular Research, 14*(4), 347–351.

Brantberg, K., & Tribukait, A. (2002). Vestibular evoked myogenic potentials in response to laterally directed skull taps. *Journal of Vestibular Research, 12*(1), 35–45.

Burgess, A. M., Mezey, L. E., Manzari, L., Macdougall, H. Q., McGarvie, L. A., & Curthoys, I. S. (2013). Effect of stimulus rise-time on the ocular vestibular evoked myogenic potential to bone conducted vibration. *Ear and Hearing, 34*(6), 799–805.

Burkard, R. F., McCaslin, D. L., Jacobson, G. P., & McNeerney, K. M. (2010). *Spectral analyses of the vestibular evoked myogenic potential (VEMP)*. Poster session presented at the International Evoked Response Auditory Study Group: 29, Moscow, Russia.

Carey, J., & Amin, N. (2006). Evolutionary changes in the cochlea and labyrinth: Solving the problem of sound transmission to the balance organs of the inner ear. *Anatomical Record, Part A: Discoveries in Molecular, Cellular, and Evolutionary Biology, 288*(4), 482–489.

Chang, C. H., Yang, T. L., Wang, C. T., & Young, Y. H. (2007). Measuring neck structures in relation to vestibular evoked myogenic potentials. *Clinical Neurophysiology, 118*(5), 1105–1109.

Chang, C. M., Cheng, P. W., Wang, S. J., & Young, Y. H. (2010). Effects of repetition rate of bone-conducted vibration on ocular and cervical vestibular-evoked myogenic potentials. *Clinical Neurophysiology, 121*, 2121–2127.

Chang, C. M., Young, Y. H., & Cheng, P. W. (2012). Age-related changes in ocular vestibular-evoked myogenic potentials via galvanic vestibular stimulation and bone-conducted vibration modes. *Acta Oto-Laryngologica, 132*(12), 1295–1300. doi:10.3109/00016489.2012.708437

Chen, C. N., Wang, S. J., Wang, C. T., Hsieh, W. S., & Young, Y. H. (2007). Vestibular evoked myogenic potentials in newborns. *Audiology and Neurotology, 12*(1), 59–63.

Cheng, P. W., Chen, C. C., Wang, S. J., & Young, Y. H. (2009). Acoustic, mechanical and galvanic stimulation modes elicit ocular vestibular-evoked myogenic potentials. *Clinical Neurophysiology, 120,* 1841–1844.

Cheng, P. W., & Murofushi, T. (2001a). The effect of rise/fall time on vestibular-evoked myogenic potential triggered by short tone bursts. *Acta Oto-Laryngologica, 121*(6), 696–699.

Cheng, P. W., & Murofushi, T. (2001b). The effects of plateau time on vestibular-evoked myogenic potentials triggered by tone bursts. *Acta Oto-Laryngologica, 121*(8), 935–938.

Cheng, Y. L., Wu, H. J., & Lee, G. S. (2012). Effects of plateau time and ramp time on ocular vestibular evoked myogenic potentials. *Journal of Vestibular Research, 22,* 33–39.

Chihara, Y., Iwasaki, S., Fujimoto, C., Ushio, M., Yamasoba, T., & Murofushi, T. (2009). Frequency tuning properties of ocular vestibular evoked myogenic potentials. *Neuroreport, 20*(16), 1491–1495.

Cody, D. T., Jacobson, J. L., Walker, J. C., & Bickford, R. G. (1964). Averaged evoked myogenic and cortical potentials to sound in man. *Transactions of the American Otological Society, 52,* 159–176.

Colebatch, J. G. (2013). Exploring the oVEMP montage. *Clinical Neurphysiology, 124,* 1051–1052.

Colebatch, J. G., & Halmagyi, G. M. (1992). Vestibular evoked potentials in human neck muscles before and after unilateral vestibular deafferentation. *Neurology, 42*(8), 1635–1636.

Colebatch, J. G., Halmagyi, G. M., & Skuse, N. F. (1994). Myogenic potentials generated by a click evoked vestibulocollic reflex. *Journal of Neurology, Neurosurgery, and Psychiatry, 57*(2), 190–197.

Colebatch, J. G., & Rothwell, J. C. (2004). Motor unit excitability changes mediating vestibulocollic reflexes in the sternocleidomastoid muscle. *Clinical Neurophysiology, 115*(11), 2567–2573.

Cremer, P. D., Minor, L. B., Carey, J. P., & Della Santina, C. C. (2000). Eye movements in patients with superior canal dehiscence syndrome align with the abnormal canal. *Neurology, 55*(12), 1833–1841.

Curthoys, I. S. (2010). A critical review of the neurophysiological evidence underlying clinical vestibular testing using sound, vibration and galvanic stimuli. *Clinical Neurophysiology, 121*(2), 132–144.

Curthoys, I. S., Iwasaki, S., Chihara, Y., Ushio, M., McGarvie, L. A., & Burgess, A. M. (2011). The ocular vestibular evoked myogenic potential to air-conducted sound: Probable superior vestibular nerve origin. *Clinical Neurophysiology, 122,* 611–616.

Curthoys, I. S., Kim, J., McPhedran, S. K., & Camp, A. J. (2006). Bone conducted vibration selectivity activates irregular primary otolith vestibular neurons in the guinea pig. *Experimental Brain Research, 175,* 256–267.

Curthoys, I. S., Manzari, L., Smulders, Y. E., & Burgess, A. M. (2009). A review of the scientific basis and practical application of a new test of utricular function—ocular vestibular-evoked myogenic potentials to bone-conducted vibration. *Acta Otorhinolaryngologica Italica, 29*(4), 179–186.

Donnellan, K., Wei, W., Jeffcoat, B., Mustain, W., Xu, Y., Eby, T., & Phd, W. Z. (2010). Frequency tuning of bone-conducted tone burst-evoked myogenic potentials recorded from extraocular muscles (BOVEMP) in normal human subjects. *Laryngoscope, 120*(12), 2555–2560.

Fitzgerald, M. J., Comerford, P. T., & Tuffery, A. R. (1982). Sources of innervation of the neuromuscular spindles in sternomastoid and trapezius. *Journal of Anatomy, 134*(3), 471–490.

Gabelić, T., Krbot, M., Šefer, A. B., Išqum, V., Adamec, I., & Habek, M. (2013). Ocular and cervical vestibular evoked myogenic potentials in patients with multiple sclerosis. *Journal of Clinical Neurophysiology, 30,* 86–91.

Gacek, R. R. (1982). The anatomical-physiological basis for vestibular function. In V. Honrubia & M. A. B. Brazier (Eds.), *Nystagmus and vertigo: Clinical approaches to the patient with dizziness* (pp. 3–23). New York NY: Academic Press.

Gazioglu, S., & Boz, C. (2012). Ocular and cervical vestibular evoked myogenic potentials in multiple sclerosis patients. *Clinical Neurophysiology, 123,* 1872–1879.

Goldberg, J. (2000). Afferent diversity and the organization of central vestibular pathways. *Experimental Brain Research, 130,* 277–297.

Govender, S., Rosengren, S. M., & Colebatch, J. G. (2009). The effect of gaze direction on the ocular vestibular evoked myogenic potential produced by air-conducted sound. *Clinical Neurophysiology, 120,* 1386–1391.

Gozke, E., Erdal, N., & Ozkarakas, H. (2010). Ocular vestibular evoked myogenic potentials in patients with migraine. *Acta Neurologica Belgica, 110,* 321–324.

Gresty, M. A., & Lempert, T. (2001). Pathophysiology and clinical testing of otolith dysfunction. In P. Tran Ba Huy & M. Toupet (Eds.), *Otolith function and disorders* (pp. 15–33). New York, NY: Karger.

Halmagyi, G. M., Yavor, R. A., & Colebatch, J. G. (1995). Tapping the head activates the vestibular system: A new use for the clinical reflex hammer. *Neurology, 45*(10), 1927–1929.

Hsu, Y. S., Wang, S. J., & Young, Y. H. (2009). Ocular vestibular-evoked myogenic potentials in children using air conducted sound stimulation. *Clinical Neurophysiology, 120,* 1381–1385.

Huang, C. H., Wang, S. G., & Young, Y. H. (2011). Localization and prevalence of hydrops formation in Meniere's disease using a test battery. *Audiology and Neurotology, 16,* 41–48.

Huang, Y. C., Yang, T. L., & Young, Y. H. (2012). Feasibility of ocular vestibular-evoked myogenic potentials (oVEMPS) recorded with eyes closed. *Clinical Neurophysiology, 123,* 376–381.

Isaradisaikul, S., Strong, D. A., Moushey, J. M., Gabbard, S. A., Ackley, S. R., & Jenkins, H. A. (2008). Reliability of vestibular evoked myogenic potentials in healthy subjects. *Otology and Neurotology, 29*(4), 542–544.

Ishiyama, G. (2009). Imbalance and vertigo: The aging human vestibular periphery. *Seminars in Neurology, 29*(5), 491–499. doi:10.1055/s-0029-1241039

Ivankovic, A., Nesek, M., Starcevic, K., Krbot, S., Gabelic, T., Adamec, I., & Habek, M. (2013). Auditory evoked potentials and vestibular evoked myogenic potentials in evaluation of brainstem lesions in multiple sclerosis. *Journal of Neurological Sciences, 328,* 24–27.

Iwasaki, S., Chihara, Y., Smulders, Y. E., Burgess, S. M., Halmagyi, G. M., Curthoys, I. S., & Murofushi, T. (2009). The role of the superior vestibular nerve in generating ocular vestibular-evoked myogenic potentials to bone conducted vibration at Fz. *Clinical Neurophysiology, 120,* 588–593

Iwasaki, S., McGarvie, L. A., Halmagyi, G. M., Burgess, A. M., Kim, J., Colebatch, J. G., & Curthoys, I. S. (2007). Head taps evoke a crossed vestibulo-ocular reflex. *Neurology, 68*(15), 1227–1229.

Jacobson, G. P., & McCaslin, D. L. (2007). The vestibular evoked myogenic potential and other sonomotor evoked potentials. In R. F. Burkard, M. Don, & J. J. Eggermont (Eds.), *Auditory evoked potentials: Basic principles and clinical application* (pp. 572–598). Baltimore, MD: Lippincott Williams & Wilkins.

Jaeger, R., & Haslwanter, T. (2004). Otolith responses to dynamical stimuli: Results of a numerical investigation. *Biological Cybernetics, 90,* 165–175.

Janky, K. L., & Shepard, N. (2009). Vestibular evoked myogenic potential (VEMP) testing: Normative threshold response curves and effects of age. *Journal of the American Academy of Audiology, 20*(8), 514–522.

Jones, S. M., Subramanian, G., Avniel, W., Guo, Y., Burkard, R. F., & Jones, T. A. (2002). Stimulus and recording variables and their effects on mammalian vestibular evoked potentials. *Journal of Neuroscience Methods, 118*(1), 23–31.

Jongkees, L. B., & Philipszoon, A. J. (1964). Electronystagmorgaphy. *Acta Oto-Larngologica,* (Suppl. 189), 189–191.

Kantner, C., Hapfelmeier, A., Drexl, M., & Gürkov, R. (2013). The effects of rise/fall time and plateau time on ocular vestibular evoked myogenic potentials. *European Archives of Oto-Rhino-Laryngology.* doi:10.1007/s00405-013-2697-4

Karino, S., Ito, K., Ochiai, A., & Murofushi, T. (2005). Independent effects of simultaneous inputs from the saccule and lateral semicircular canal. Evaluation using VEMPs. *Clinical Neurophysiology, 116*(7), 1707–1715. doi:10.1016/j.clinph.2005.04.007

Kelsch, T. A., Schaefer, L. A., & Esquivel, C. R. (2006). Vestibular evoked myogenic potentials in young children: Test parameters and normative data. *Laryngoscope, 116*(6), 895–900.

Kim, K. W., Jung, J. Y., Lee, J. H., & Suh, M. W. (2013). Capacity of rectified vestibular evoked myogenic potential in correcting asymmetric muscle contraction power. *Clinical and Experimental Otorhinolaryngology, 6*(4), 209–213.

Kim, M. B., & Ban, J. H. (2012). The efficiency of simultaneous binaural ocular vestibular evoked myogenic potentials: A comparative study with monaural acoustic stimulation in healthy subjects. *Clinical and Experimental Otorhinolaryngology, 5,* 188–193.

Krause, H. R., Bremerich, A., & Herrmann, M. (1991). The innervation of the trapezius muscle in connection with radical neck-dissection. An anatomical study. *Journal of Craniomaxillofacial Surgery, 19*(2), 87–89.

Kushiro, K., Zakir, M., Ogawa, Y., Sato, H., & Uchino, Y. (1999). Saccular and utricular inputs to sternocleidomastoid motoneurons of decerebrate cats. *Experimental Brain Research, 126*(3), 410–416.

Lee, K. J., Kim, M. S., Son, E. J., Lim, H. J., Bang, J. H., & Kang, J. G. (2008). The usefulness of rectified VEMP. *Clinical and Experimental Otorhinolaryngology, 1*(3), 143–147.

Lee, S. K., Cha, C. I., Jung, T. S., Park, D. C., & Yeo, S. G. (2008). Age-related differences in parameters of vestibular evoked myogenic potentials. *Acta Oto-Laryngologica, 128*(1), 66–72.

Lewis, A., Mustain, W., Xu, Y., Eby, T., & Zhou, W. (2010). Frequency tuning in the tone burst-evoked myogenic potentials in extraocular muscles in normal human subjects. *Journal of Otolaryngology-Head and Neck Surgery, 39,* 491–497.

Li, M. W., Houlden, D., & Tomlinson, R. D. (1999). Click evoked EMG responses in sternocleidomastoid muscles: characteristics in normal subjects. *Journal of Vestibular Research, 9*(5), 327–334.

Lim, C. L., Clouston, P., Sheean, G., & Yiannikas, C. (1995). The influence of voluntary EMG activity and click intensity on the vestibular click evoked myogenic potential. *Muscle and Nerve, 18*(10), 1210–1213.

Lim, L. J., Dennis, D. L., Govender, S., & Colebatch, J. G. (2013). Differential effects of duration for ocular and cervical vestibular evoked myogenic potentials evoked by air- and bone- conducted stimuli. *Experimental Brain Research, 224,* 437–445.

Lin, M. Y., Timmer, F. C., Oriel, B. S., Zhou, G., Guinan, J. J., Kujawa, S. G., . . . Rauch, S. D. (2006). Vestibular evoked myogenic potentials (VEMP) can detect asymptomatic saccular hydrops. *Laryngoscope, 116*(6), 987–992.

Lysakowski, A., McCrea, R. A., & Tomlinson, R. D. (1998). Anatomy of vestibular end organs and neural pathways. In C. W. Cummings, J. M. Fredrickson, L. A. Harker, C. J. Krause, M. A. Richardson, & D. E. Schuller (Eds.), *Otolaryngology-Head and Neck Surgery* (3rd ed., 2561–2583). St. Louis, MO: Mosby.

Manzari, L., Burgess, A. M., McGarview, L. A., & Curthoys, I. S. (2013). An indicator of probable semicircular canal dehiscence: Ocular vestibular evoked myogenic potentials to high frequencies. *Otolaryngology-Head and Neck Surgery, 149,* 142–145.

Manzari, L., Tedesco, A. R., Burgess, A, M., & Curthoys, I. S. (2010). Ocular and cervical vestibular-evoked myogenic potentials to bone conducted vibration in Meniere's disease during quiescence vs during acute attacks. *Clinical Neurophysiology, 121,* 1092–1100.

McCaslin, D. L., Fowler, A., & Jacobson, G. P. (2014). Amplitude normalization reduces cervical vestibular evoked myogenic potential (cVEMP) amplitude asymmetries in normal subjects: Proof of concept. *Journal of the American Academy of Audiology, 25*(3), 268–277. doi:10.3766/jaaa.25.3.6

McCaslin, D. L., Jacobson, G. P., Hatton, K., Fowler, A. P., & DeLong, A. P. (2013). The effects of amplitude normalization and EMG targets on cVEMP interaural amplitude asymmetry. *Ear and Hearing, 34*(4), 482–490.

McCue, M. P., & Guinan, J. J. (1995). Spontaneous activity and frequency selectivity of acoustically responsive vestibular afferents in the cat. *Journal of Neurophysiology, 74*(4), 1563–1572.

McNerney, K. M., & Burkard, R. F. (2011). The vestibular evoked myogenic potential (VEMP): Air- versus bone-conducted stimuli. *Ear and Hearing, 32*(6), e6–e15.

Minor, L. B., & Goldberg, J. M. (1991). Vestibular-nerve inputs to the vestibulo-ocular reflex: A functional-ablation study in the squirrel monkey. *Journal of Neuroscience, 11*(6), 1636–1648.

Miyamoto, A., Seo, T., Node, M., Hashimoto, M., & Sakagami, M. (2006). Preliminary study on vestibular-evoked myogenic potential induced by bone-conducted stimuli. *Otology and Neurotology, 27*(8), 1110–1114.

Murnane, O. D., Akin, F. W., Kelly, K. J., & Byrd, S. (2011). Effects of stimulus and recording parameters on the air conduction ocular vestibular evoked myogenic potential. *Journal of the American Academy of Audiology, 22,* 469–480.

Murofushi, T., & Curthoys, I. S. (1997). Physiological and anatomical study of click-sensitive primary vestibular afferents in the guinea pig. *Acta Oto-Laryngologica, 117*(1), 66–72.

Murofushi, T., Curthoys, I. S., Topple, A. N., Colebatch, J. G., & Halmagyi, G. M. (1995). Responses of guinea pig primary vestibular neurons to clicks. *Experimental Brain Research, 103*(1), 174–178.

Murofushi, T., Matsuzaki, M., & Wu, C. H. (1999). Short tone burst-evoked myogenic potentials on the sternocleidomastoid muscle: Are these potentials also of vestibular origin? *Archives of Otolaryngology-Head and Neck Surgery, 125*(6), 660–664.

Murofushi, T., Shimizu, K., Takegoshi, H., & Cheng, P. W. (2001). Diagnostic value of prolonged latencies in the vestibular evoked myogenic potential. *Archives of Otolaryngology-Head and Neck Surgery, 127*(9), 1069–1072.

Nguyen, K. D., Welgampola, M. S., & Carey, J. P. (2010). Test-retest reliability and age-related characteristics of the ocular and cervical vestibular evoked myogenic potential tests. *Otology and Neurotology, 31,* 793–802.

Ochi, K., Ohashi, T., & Nishino, H. (2001). Variance of vestibular-evoked myogenic potentials. *Laryngoscope, 111,* 522–527.

Oh, S. Y., Kim, J. S., Lee, J. M., Shin, B. S., Hwang, S. B., Kwak, K. C., . . . Kim, T. W. (2013). Ocular vestibular evoked myogenic potentials induced by air-conducted sound in patients with acute brainstem lesions. *Clinical Neurophysiology, 124,* 770–778.

Papathanasiou, E. S., Murofushi, T., Akin, F. W., & Colebatch, J. G. (2014). International guidelines for the clinical application of cervical vestibular evoked myogenic potentials: An expert consensus report. *Clinical Neurophysiology, 125*(4), 658–666.

Phillips, J. O., & Backous, D. D. (2002). Evaluation of vestibular function in young children. *Otolaryngologic Clinics of North America, 35*(4), 765–790.

Piker, E. G., Jacobson, G. P., Burkard, R. F., McCaslin, D. L., & Hood, L. J. (2013). Effects of age on the tuning of the cVEMP and oVEMP. *Ear and Hearing, 34*(6), e65–e73.

Piker, E. G., Jacobson, G. P., McCaslin, D. L., & Hood, L. J. (2011). Normal characteristics of the ocular vestibular evoked myogenic potential. *Journal of the American Academy of Audiology, 22,* 222–230.

Popper, A. N., & Fay, R. R. (1993). Sound detection and processing by fish: Critical review and major research questions. *Brain, Behavior and Evolution, 41*(1), 14–38.

Rauch, S. D., Zhou, G., Kujawa, S. G., Guinan, J. J., & Hermann, B. S. (2004). Vestibular evoked myogenic potentials show altered tuning in patients with Meniere's disease. *Otology and Neurotology, 25*(3), 333–338.

Rosengren, S. M., Aw, S. T., Halmagyi, G. M., Todd, N. P., & Colebatch, J. G. (2008). Ocular vestibular evoked myogenic potentials in superior canal dehiscence. *Journal of Neurology, Neurosurgery and Psychiatry, 79,* 559–568.

Rosengren, S. M., & Colebatch, J. G. (2011). Ocular vestibular evoked myogenic potentials are abnormal in internuclear ophthalmoplegia. *Clinical Neurophysiology, 122,* 1264–1267.

Rosengren, S. M., Colebatch, J. G., Straumann, D., & Weber, P. (2013). Why do oVEMPs become larger when you look up? Explaining the effect of gaze elevation on the ocular vestibular evoked myogenic potential. *Clinical Neurophysiology, 124,* 785–791.

Rosengren, S. M., Govender, S., & Colebatch, J. G. (2009). The relative effectiveness of different stimulus waveforms in evoking VEMPs: significance of stimulus energy and frequency. *Journal of Vestibular Research, 19*(1-2), 33–40. doi:10.3233/VES-2009-0345

Rosengren, S. M., Govender, S., & Colebatch, J. G. (2011). Ocular and cervical vestibular evoked myogenic potentials produced by air- and bone-conducted stimuli: comparative properties and effects of age. *Clinical Neurophysiology, 122*(11), 2282–2289. doi:10.1016/j.clinph.2011.04.001

Rosengren, S. M., Welgampola, M. S., & Colebatch, J. G. (2010). Vestibular evoked myogenic potentials: Past, present and future. *Clinical Neurophysiology, 121*(5), 636–651. doi:10.1016/j.clinph.2009.10.016

Rosenhall, U. (1973). Degenerative patterns in the aging human vestibular neuro-epithelia. *Acta Oto-Laryngologica, 76*(2), 208–220.

Sandhu, J. S., George, S. R., & Rea, P. A. (2013). The effect of electrode position on the ocular vestibular evoked myogenic potential to air-conducted sound. *Clinical Neurophysiology, 124,* 1232–1236.

Schwarz, D. W. F., & Tomlinson, R. D. (2005). Physiology of the vestibular system. In R. K. Jackler & D. E. Brackman (Eds.), *Neurotology* (2nd ed., pp. 91–121). Philadelphia, PA: Elsevier Mosby.

Sheykholeslami, K., Habiby Kermany, M., & Kaga, K. (2001). Frequency sensitivity range of the saccule to bone-conducted stimuli measured by vestibular evoked myogenic potentials. *Hearing Research, 160*(1–2), 58–62.

Sheykholeslami, K., & Kaga, K. (2002). The otolithic organ as a receptor of vestibular hearing revealed by vestibular-evoked myogenic potentials in patients with inner ear anomalies. *Hearing Research, 165*(1–2), 62–67.

Sheykholeslami, K., Megerian, C. A., Arnold, J. E., & Kaga, K. (2005). Vestibular-evoked myogenic potentials in infancy and early childhood. *Laryngoscope, 115*(8), 1440–1444.

Sheykholeslami, K., Murofushi, T., & Kaga, K. (2001). The effect of sternocleidomastoid electrode location on vestibular evoked myogenic potential. *Auris Nasus Larynx, 28*(1), 41–43.

Sheykholeslami, K., Murofushi, T., Kermany, M. H., & Kaga, K. (2000). Bone-conducted evoked myogenic potentials from the sternocleidomastoid muscle. *Acta Oto-Laryngologica, 120*(6), 731–734.

Shimizu, K., Murofushi, T., Sakurai, M., & Halmagyi, M. (2000). Vestibular evoked myogenic potentials in multiple sclerosis. *Journal of Neurology, Neurosurgery and Psychiatry, 69*(2), 276–277.

Shin, B. S., Oh, S. Y., Kim, J. S., Kim, T. W., Seo, M. W., Lee, H., & Park, Y. A. (2012). Cervical and ocular vestibular-evoked myogenic potentials in acute vestibular neuritis. *Clinical Neurophysiology, 123,* 369–375.

Streubel, S. O., Cremer, P. D., Carey, J. P., Weg, N., & Minor, L. B. (2001). Vestibular-evoked myogenic potentials in the diagnosis of superior canal dehiscence syndrome. *Acta Oto-Laryngologica Supplementum, 545,* 41–49.

Su, H. C., Huang, T. W., Young, Y. H., & Cheng, P. W. (2004). Aging effect on vestibular evoked myogenic potential. *Otology and Neurotology, 25*(6), 977–980.

Timmer, F. C., Zhou, G., Guinan, J. J., Kujawa, S. G., Herrmann, B. S., & Rauch, S. D. (2006). Vestibular evoked myogenic potential (VEMP) in patients with Ménière's disease with drop attacks. *Laryngoscope, 116*(5), 776–779.

Todd, N. P., Cody, F. W., & Banks, J. R. (2000). A saccular origin of frequency tuning in myogenic vestibular evoked potentials: Implications for human responses to loud sounds. *Hearing Research, 141*(1–2), 180–188.

Todd, N. P., Rosengren, S. M., Govender, S., & Colebatch, J. G. (2009). Low-frequency tuning in the human vestibular ocular projection is determined by both peripheral and central mechanisms. *Neuroscience Letters, 458*(1), 43–47.

Townsend, G. L., & Cody, D. T. (1971). The averaged inion response evoked by acoustic stimulation: Its relation to the saccule. *Annals of Otology, Rhinology, and Laryngology, 80*(1), 121–131.

Tseng, C. L., Chou, C. H., & Young, Y. H. (2010). Aging effect on the ocular vestibular evoked myogenic potentials. *Otology and Neurotology, 31,* 659–663.

Tullio, P. (1929). *Some experiments and considerations on experimental otology and phonetics.* Bologna, Italy: Licinio Capelli.

Uzun-Coruhlu, H., Curthoys, I. S., & Jones, A. S. (2007). Attachment of the utricular and saccular maculae to the temporal bone. *Hearing Research, 233*, 77–85.

Vanspauwen, R., Wuyts, F. L., & Va de Henning, P. H. (2006). Validity of a new feedback method for the VEMP test. *Acta Oto-Laryngologica, 162*(8), 796–800.

von Békésy, G. (1935). Über akustishe Reizung des Vestibularapparates. *Arch. F D Ges Physiol., 236*, 59.

Wang, C. T., & Young, Y. H. (2006). Comparison of the head elevation versus rotation methods in eliciting vestibular evoked myogenic potentials. *Ear and Hearing, 27*(4), 376–381. doi:10.1097/01.aud.0000224126.24604.db

Wang, S. J., Jaw, F. S., & Young, Y. H. (2009). Ocular vestibular-evoked myogenic potentials elicited from monaural versus binaural acoustic stimulations. *Clinical Neurophysiology, 120*, 420–423.

Wang, S. J., Jaw, F. S., & Young, Y. H. (2013). Optimizing the bandpass filter for acoustic stimuli in recording ocular vestibular-evoked myogenic potentials. *Neuroscience Letters, 542*, 12–16.

Wang, S. J., & Young, Y. H. (2003). Vestibular evoked myogenic potentials using simultaneous binaural acoustic stimulation. *Hearing Research, 185*(1–2), 43–48.

Ward, B. K., Wenzel, A., Ritzl, E. K., Gutierrez-Hernandez, S., Della Sartina, C. C., Minor, L. B., & Carey, L. P. (2013). Near-dehiscence: clinical findings in patients with thin bone over the superior semi-circular canal. *Otology and Neurotology, 34*(8), 1421–1428.

Welgampola, M. S., & Colebatch, J. G. (2001a). Characteristics of tone burst-evoked myogenic potentials in the sternocleidomastoid muscles. *Otology and Neurotology, 22*(6), 796–802.

Welgampola, M. S., & Colebatch, J. G. (2001b). Vestibulocollic reflexes: Normal values and the effect of age. *Clinical Neurophysiology, 112*(11), 1971–1979.

Welgampola, M. S., & Colebatch, J. G. (2005). Characteristics and clinical applications of vestibular-evoked myogenic potentials. *Neurology, 64*, 1682–1688.

Welgampola, M. S., Rosengren, S. M., Halmagyi, G. M., & Colebatch, J. G. (2003). Vestibular activation by bone conducted sound. *Journal of Neurology, Neurosurgery,* *and Psychiatry, 74*(6), 771–778. Erratum in: *Journal of Neurology, Neurosurgery, and Psychiatry, 76*(9), 1312.

Winters, S. M., Berg, I. T., Grolman, W., & Klis, S. F. (2012). Ocular vestibular evoked myogenic potentials: Frequency tuning to air-conducted acoustic stimuli in healthy subjects and Meniere's disease. *Audiology and Neurotology, 17*, 12–19.

Wit, H. P., & Kingma, C. M. (2006). A simple model for the generation of the vestibular evoked myogenic potential (VEMP). *Clinical Neurophysiology, 117*(6), 1354–1358.

Wright, C. G., Hubbard, D. G., & Clark, G. M. (1979). Observations of human fetal otoconial membranes. *Annals of Otology, 88*, 267–274.

Wu, C. H., & Murofushi, T. (1999). The effect of click repetition rate on vestibular evoked myogenic potential. *Acta Oto-Laryngologica, 119*, 29–32.

Yang, T. L., & Young, Y. H. (2003). Comparison of tone burst and tapping evocation of myogenic potentials in patients with chronic otitis media. *Ear and Hearing, 24*(3), 191–194.

Zapala, D. A., & Brey, R. H. (2004). Clinical experience with the vestibular evoked myogenic potential. *Journal of the American Academy of Audiology, 15*(3), 198–215.

Zhang, A. S., Govender, S., & Colebatch, J. G. (1985). Tuning of the ocular vestibular evoked myogenic potential to bone-conducted sound stimulation. *Journal of Applied Physiology, 112*, 1279–1290.

Zhang, A. S., Govender, S., & Colebatch, J. G. (2011). Tuning of the ocular vestibular evoked myogenic potential (oVEMP) to AC sound shows two separate peaks. *Experimental Brain Research, 213*, 111–116.

Zhang, A. S., Govender, S., & Colebatch, J. G. (2012). Tuning of the ocular vestibular evoked myogenic potential (oVEMP) to air- and bone-conducted sound stimulation in superior canal dehiscence. *Experimental Brain Research, 223*(1), 51–64.

Zuniga, M. G., Janky, K. L., Nguyen, K. D., Welgampola, M. S., & Carey, J. P. (2013). Ocular versus cervical VEMPs in the diagnosis of superior semicircular canal dehiscence syndrome. *Otology and Neurotology, 34*, 121–126.

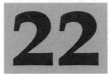

Tests of Otolith Function and Vestibular Perception

Adolfo M. Bronstein

In this chapter we review two different topics: tests of otolith function and how to assess a relatively neglected component of the vestibular output, namely, vestibulo-perceptual function.

TESTS OF OTOLITH FUNCTION

A chapter on tests of otolith function in a textbook aimed at clinicians inevitably is brief. This is not a reflection of the scientific interest and effort invested by the basic and clinical vestibular community into this topic. Rather, it reflects the technical difficulties encountered when attempting to document otolith function. These procedures are currently evolving and therefore are rarely available as routine tests in clinical departments. The topics to be discussed include: (1) linear acceleration tests of otolith function and (2) perceptual tests of vestibular function, with an emphasis on the procedure known as the subjective visual vertical (SVV). In the last 5 to 10 years day-to-day clinical assessment of otolith function has been transformed by the clinical neurophysiologic test known as vestibular myogenic potentials (VEMP), but this is reviewed in Chapter 21.

Linear Acceleration Tests

The otoliths are selectively stimulated by linear acceleration, including gravity (Fernandez & Goldberg, 1976). Due to their morphology and curved trajectory of the polarization vectors of the hair cells, both the utricular and saccular maculae are sensitive to multiple axes of linear acceleration (see Chapter 1). The predominantly horizontal orientation of the utricules, however, makes them mostly sensitive to accelerations in this plane (right-left, fore-aft) or tilt away from the horizontal plane. The predominantly parasagittal orientation of the sacculi makes them more sensitive to sagittal plane tilt (pitch tilt) and acceleration (fore-aft, rostro-caudal). Accordingly, linear acceleration that can only be detected by the utricles would be interaural (right-left), whereas acceleration only sensed by the sacculi would be caudorostral (up-down). One should remember that linear acceleration is also generated during rotatory motion, that is, centrifugal and tangential acceleration, and this has been exploited in the field of otolith testing. This chapter discusses principles of otolith testing but interested readers are encouraged to follow the original articles.

Otolith testing is technically challenging. The generation of pure linear acceleration of sufficient magnitude (>0.2 g; 1 g = gravitational acceleration) under controlled conditions requires motorized sleds running on precision tracks. In our laboratory the system is driven by two electrically powered linear motors (Figure 22–1).

Centrifugal and tangential accelerations (Figure 22–2) can be generated with rotating devices but these have to be powerful and sturdy to carry the weight of a human subject placed eccentrically from the rotational axis. The simpler way to obtain tangential acceleration of the head and stimulate otolith-ocular reflexes is the procedure described by Gresty and Bronstein (1986) in which the subject leans forward onto an eccentric chin or head rest, while seated on a conventional rotating chair (head eccentric rotation) (Gresty & Bronstein, 1986; Gresty et al., 1987). As in all otolith-ocular procedures, the subject's head has to be rigidly secured to avoid contamination with unwanted head movements. Figure 22–2 shows how the subject's head is positioned forward on an adapted conventional rotating chair in order to stimulate the utricles.

The concurrent otolith (utricular) stimulation increases the slow phase velocity of the VOR by approximately one-third, depending on stimulus parameters and ocular convergence (Figure 22–3). This technique shows asymmetries in the otolith contribution to the VOR response (Barratt, Bronstein, & Gresty, 1987) and some of these findings are long-lasting, for instance after unilateral vestibular lesions (Tian, Ishiyama, & Demer, 2007).

Following a similar principle, one can rotate a person around an earth-vertical axis passing through one of the labyrinths, thus positioning one labyrinth centrally and the other eccentrically (Figure 22–4). In this way only the eccentric labyrinth is subjected to tangential and centrifugal acceleration and this test is the only conventional test capable of providing information on each individual utricle (eccentric centrifugation or unilateral utricular centrifugation) (Clarke & Engelhorn, 1998; Wuyts, Hoppenbrouwers, & Van de Heyning, 2001). Responses can be recorded as ocular torsion, for example, with three-dimensional video-oculography or as subjective

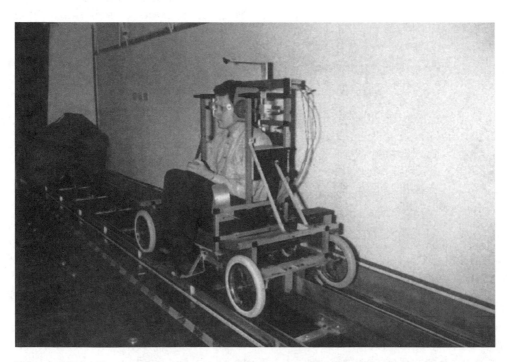

Figure 22–1. Linear motor-powered sled for acceleration of a subject along the interaural axis for utricular testing. The subject has EOG electrodes for horizontal eye movement recordings.

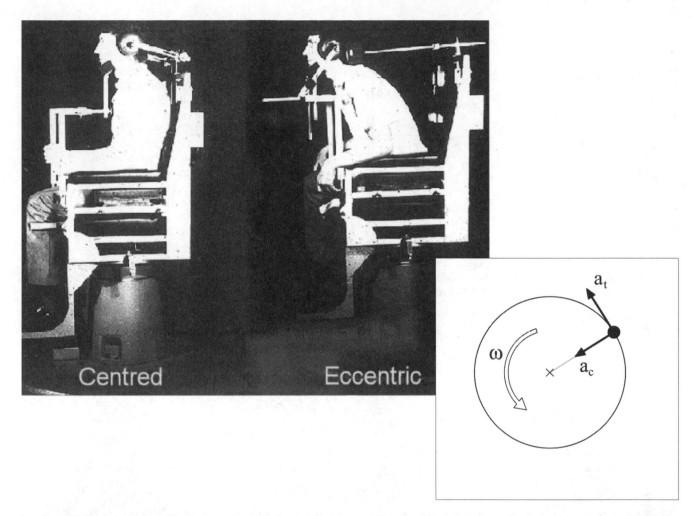

Figure 22–2. Subject positioned on the rotating chair for canal VOR testing (centered) or combined canal-utricular VOR testing (eccentric). The eccentric position of the head adds a component of tangential linear acceleration along the inter-aural axis of the head. Subtraction of centered from eccentric ocular responses provides the utricular contribution. Inset: Linear accelerations generated during rotation: x = axis of rotation, ω = angular velocity, at = tangential acceleration (which equals the rate of change of tangential velocity), ac = centripetal acceleration (which is proportional to the radius of the rotation and the square of the angular velocity). Tangential acceleration for testing otolith function is shown at the top. Centripetal acceleration is used in centrifuge studies—a specific case (unilateral utricular centrifugation) is illustrated in Figure 22–4.

visual tilt with a chair-mounted subjective visual vertical system (see below).

Another way of obtaining controlled stimulation of the otolith is to rotate the subject about an axis which is tilted ("off-vertical axis" rotation or OVAR) (Figure 22–5) or orthogonal ("barbeque-spit" rotation, not shown) with respect to the gravitational vector. In these tests the otolithic stimulus is provided by the continuous reorientation of the head with respect to gravity (Furman & Redfern, 2002;

Koizuka, 2003). It is important to note that when the linear acceleration is generated by rotation, the otolith response can only be assessed either by subtracting the component due to angular motion (e.g., subtracting head eccentric response from head-centered response, in the head eccentric test) or by waiting until the angular VOR has ceased (e.g., in OVAR or barbeque rotation). Finally, a way of stimulating the otoliths is simple, static head tilt with respect to gravity, thus eliciting static ocular counter-rolling.

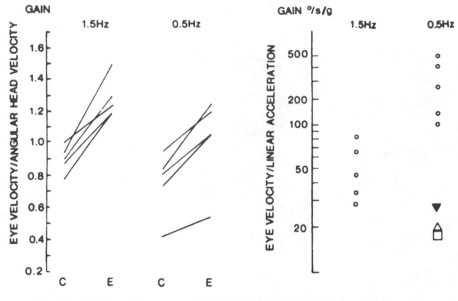

Figure 22-3. *Left:* ratio of slow phase eye velocity/angular head velocity in centered (C) and eccentric (E) positions on the rotating chair as shown in Figure 22–2. Note the increase in eye velocity in the eccentric position due to additional otolith (utricle) stimulation. Also note the increase at higher frequency of oscillation. *Right:* shows the ratio of eye velocity attributed to otolith stimulation (i.e., having subtracted the angular VOR) per unit of linear acceleration (deg/sec/g). For comparisons gains obtained during pure linear acceleration in the dark are provided (Steer, 1967, filled triangle; Correia and Guedry, 1966, open triangle; Nyven et al., 1966, square) at frequencies of about 0.5 to 0.8 Hz. Taken from Gresty and Bronstein (1986) with permission.

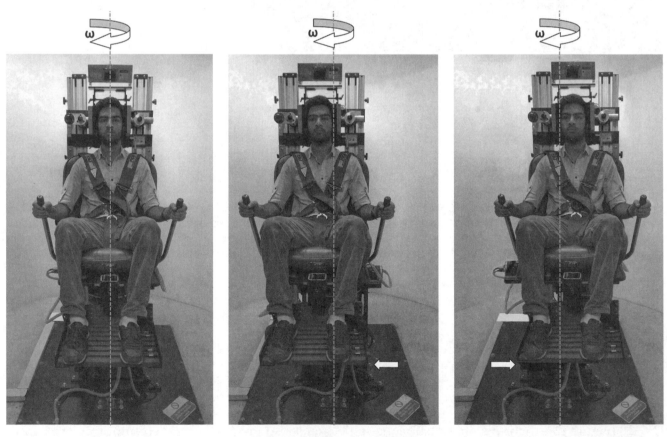

| Central rotation | Right Utricular Centrifugation | Left Utricular Centrifugation |

Figure 22-4. Unilateral utricular centrifugation test. Subject seated on a yaw axis rotating chair. The chair is fitted with a linear actuator that allows translation of the subject sideways to position one utricle on the rotational axis. Rotation at constant velocity through an earth-vertical axis passing through one of the labyrinths, delivers centrifugal acceleration to the eccentrically placed utricle.

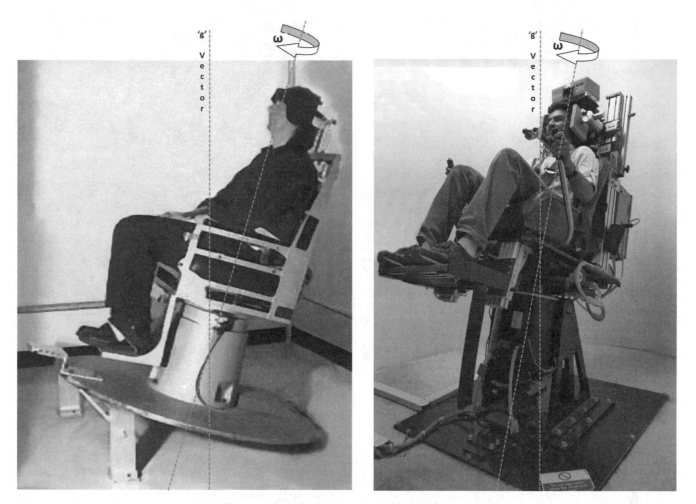

Off Axis Vertical Rotation (OVAR)

Figure 22–5. Off-vertical axis rotation (OVAR): Subject seated on a yaw axis rotating chair. The chair rotates at constant velocity (ω) about an axis that is tilted with respect to earth-vertical (dotted line "G vector"). During rotation, the otoliths are continuously stimulated as they are dynamically reoriented with respect to the gravity vector. The figure shows a commercial chair that can be tilted with a motorized actuator (*right*) and a conventional rotating chair tilted with a wedge (*left*).

This technique can be refined with precision gimbals systems and ocular torsion recordings (Figure 22–6) (Diammond & Markham, 1983). In order to minimize semicircular canal stimulation during the tilt, subjects can be tilted slowly at threshold velocities for the canals.

What physiologic responses can be measured to assess otolith function? The more common measure is the slow phase eye movement response, called linear or translational VOR or, more generally, otolith-ocular reflex (Lempert, Gianni, Gresty, & Bronstein, 1997). Recording of eye movements during otolith testing also poses technical problems. The forces involved usually generate more movement artifact than during conventional rotational or caloric procedures. In addition, the smaller size of the otolith-ocular response (with respect to the canal-ocular response) and the fact that an important component of the otolith response is ocular torsion (not recorded by EOG) often requires three-dimensional oculography (3-D video-oculography or scleral search coil technique) (Clarke & Engelhorn, 1998). Another response, which can be measured during linear acceleration, particularly in centrifugation tests (Bohmer & Mast, 1999), is the subjective visual vertical (SVV) which largely follows ocular torsional position (Curthoys,

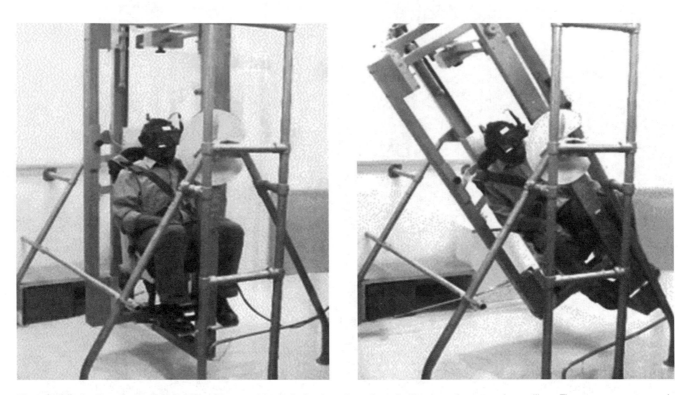

Figure 22-6. Controlled static tilt with precision gimbals system for eliciting ocular counter-rolling. The eye movements are usually recorded with 3-D VOG. Similar systems can also be used to measure the subjective postural vertical.

Dai, & Halmagyi, 1991) (see below). Dynamic visual acuity, a measure of how much vision degrades, in this case, during linear acceleration, has also been used in bilateral vestibular patients but is unlikely to be helpful in unilateral lesions (Lempert et al., 1997).

More recently, by analogy with the angular head impulse or head thrust test, there have been attempts at delivering high-frequency, high linear acceleration head movements in order to measure unilateral utricular vestibular function by clinical observation or laboratory recording of the eye movements. This procedure, often referred to as the head heave test, can demonstrate clinical abnormalities (Kessler et al., 2007; Nuti, Mandala, Broman, & Zee, 2005; Tian, Crane, & Demer, 2003) but clearly is in need of further validation. The responses to head acceleration as delivered by a head vibrator or "shaker," which are not well controlled as they inevitably include angular as well as linear acceleration, are used to elicit ocular VEMPs and are therefore found in Chapter 21.

Difficulties in testing the otoliths are not only technical. Anatomic and physiologic properties of the otolith system conspire as well. The orientation

of the hair cells is such that a single utricle (or sacculus) is capable of sensing linear accelerations in many directions. Thus, deficits due to unilateral otolith lesions are usually only acute and transient. For instance, the horizontal otolith-ocular reflex in response to interaural linear acceleration remains abnormally asymmetric for only approximately 4 weeks after a unilateral vestibular nerve section (Lempert, Gianna, Brookes, Bronstein, & Gresty, 1998). Also, as the magnitude of otolith-ocular responses depends on the angle of ocular convergence, tests have to be carried out while controlling for vergence angle (Paige, 2002). This can be either achieved by accelerating the subject during actual visual fixation (Bronstein & Gresty, 1988; Paige, 1989) (in which case precautions have to be taken so that the response is not contaminated by visuomotor mechanisms) or during "fixation" of imaginary targets (in which case vergence has to be measured with separate-eye oculography).

In summary, there are many tests of otolith function and most have been validated in a few patients with acute vestibular lesions (spontaneous or surgical). Such lesions are not selective and destroy not only the otoliths but actually most of the vestibular labyrinth. In such circumstances there is little clinical doubt that a patient has sustained unilateral vestibular damage; thus, documenting otolith involvement in such cases is just a research exercise. The challenge of devising a test of otolith function in a patient who lacks independent evidence of vestibular lesion still remains. Currently, there is very little evidence that any test can confirm that a patient has a selective unilateral otolith lesion. Research in this area must therefore continue as clinicians encounter patients reporting symptoms of tilt, lateropulsion, or rocking sensations that are compatible with otolith dysfunction and normal canal VOR testing (Gresty, Bronstein, Brandt, & Dieterich, 1992).

Subjective Visual Vertical (SVV)

Intuitively, the perception of verticality must relate to the otoliths organs as these sense linear acceleration, and by extension, gravity. However, common sense and introspection indicate that it is easy to deduce that one is lying sideways by the unambiguous asymmetry in pressure/contact cues between the two sides of the body, and/or by seeing that buildings or trees appear to be tilted to our eyes. This trivial example makes it clear that the perception of verticality cannot be viewed as exclusively otolith based. Other extravestibular senses, in particular contact (tactile), proprioceptive, and visual inputs, participate as well.

In the clinical setting, the test of verticality more commonly used is the subjective visual vertical (SVV). The technique is easy, low cost, simple, and reliable. Essentially, a subject seats in front of an adjustable straight luminous line (Figure 22–7A). The line may be viewed either in the dark or against a verticality cue-free background (e.g., all white or covered in dots). The subject's task is to set the line to what he or she thinks is real (gravitational) vertical. Normal subjects are quite accurate, all settings being within one to two degrees of real vertical (Friedmann, 1970). The line either can be remote controlled by the subject or an assistant adjusts the line according to the subject's instructions.

Initial excitement with this test was justified as vestibular lesions produce definite abnormalities of the SVV. Acute unilateral peripheral vestibular

lesions produce tilt of the subject's SVV settings ipsilaterally (Friedman, 1970). Initially, in the acute stage, the tilt is large, of the order of 8 to 10 degrees, but gradually disappears within a few weeks or months as compensation develops (Curthoys et al., 1991). Central vestibular lesions, particularly in the brainstem, can cause larger and longer-lasting SVV tilts (Dieterich & Brandt, 1993). Lesions involving the vestibular nuclei create ipsilateral SVV tilt (usually with an ocular-tilt reaction or skewed eye deviation with the lower eye ipsilesional). Lesions in the upper brainstem induce contralateral SVV tilts and skewed deviations with the upper eye ipsilesional, indicating a central vestibular pathway decussation at pontine level. It is likely that the interstitial nucleus of Cajal is responsible for the midbrain effects observed.

Initially these findings were thought to represent the direct contribution of the otoliths to the overall perception of verticality. However, patients with large tilts of the SVV usually show normal perception of verticality to other modalities, for example, the haptic or tactile vertical or the perception of whole-body verticality (subjective postural vertical) (Bisdorff, Wolsley, Anastasopoulos, Bronstein, & Gresty, 1996; Bronstein, Perennou, Guerraz, Playford, & Rudge, 2003). Furthermore, 3-D oculography has demonstrated an almost one-to-one correlation between torsional eye position measurements and SVV tilts (Curthoys et al., 1991). Therefore, all evidence indicates that generally, the tilt of the SVV is secondary to torsional VOR bias (i.e., the tilt of the eye) not a primary perceptual defect.

The SVV would still be useful as a simple test of otolith function if the ocular torsional tilt (and usually associated skew) were due to an otolith-ocular pathway asymmetry. However, it has been shown that sustained ocular torsion, skewed deviation, and SVV tilts can all be induced by selective stimulation of the vertical semicircular canals (Jauregui-Renaud, Faldon, Gresty, & Bronstein, 2001; Pavlou, Wijnberg, Faldon, & Bronstein, 2003). In summary, SVV tilts of labyrinthine or brainstem origin can be taken to indicate an imbalance in the torsional ocular system. Claims of any specificity to otolith function (peripheral or central) are not tenable but a combined otolith-vertical canal effect is more likely.

Hemisphere lesions can also induce tilts of the SVV but the magnitude is smaller; when the

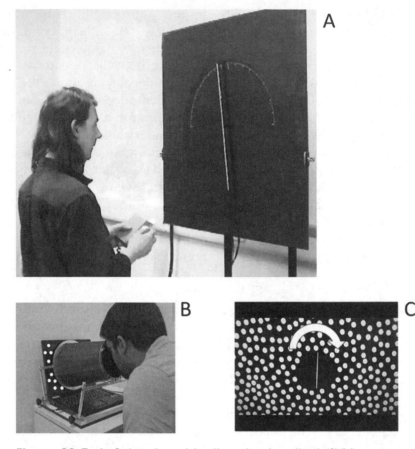

Figure 22–7. A. Setup for subjective visual vertical (SVV) measurements. The subject views the fluorescent luminous line (in otherwise total darkness) and controls its position with a hand-held device. The chin rest has been removed for illustration purposes. **B.** Laptop based SVV system. The subject views the luminous rod either through a cone, as illustrated, or in a dark room in order to reduce peripheral visual cues. **C.** SVV assessments in the presence of a static or rotating visual background, with the system illustrated in B, allows measurement of the degree of visual dependence. The software can be downloaded from http://www.imperial.ac.uk/medicine/dizzinesssandvertigo

tilt is large, this is due to involvement of mesodi-encephalic subcortical areas which are also likely to induce ocular torsional tilt (Dieterich & Brandt, 1993). The polarity is also variable. Interpretation of a cortical tilt is further confounded by the fact that proprioceptive input can also influence the SVV (Anastasopoulos & Bronstein, 1999). It is therefore safer at this stage to consider any SVV tilt of cortical origin as due to disruption of central multisensory integration rather than to involvement of central vestibular pathways (Brandt, Dieterich, & Danek, 1994; Perennou et al., 2008).

Investigation of the subjective visual vertical these days is achieved with computer-based systems, in which the orientation of the target line is controlled by the patient with a mouse or the arrow keys. The system illustrated in Figure 22–7B is laptop based so it can be easily carried around for examination of acutely ill patients. Figure 22–7C also shows a rotating visual background which allows examination of visual dependence, by probing how much the SVV readings can be influenced by the rotating visual stimulus (the rod-and-disk test). Research has shown that patients with refractory chronic vestibular symptoms and visual vertigo (Bronstein, 1995; Guerraz et al., 2001), have increased visual dependence (i.e., larger visually induced tilts of the SVV). Determining the presence of visual vertigo and increased visual dependence, either by simple questionnaires (Pavlou, Davies, & Bronstein, 2006) or with the rod-and-disk test (Cousins et al., 2014) as shown in Figure 22–7B–C, is of considerable clinical importance as effective treatments are available to improve the dizziness that vestibular patients experience in visually disorienting environments (Pavlou, Lingeswaran, Davies, Gresty, & Bronstein, 2004).

Subjective Postural Vertical

Verticality perception mediated by nonvisual sensory channels can also be explored. We all have a natural ability to know when we are truly upright and the subjective postural vertical, can be measured with whole-body tilt devices of the type shown in Figure 22–6 (Bisdorff et al., 1996). Subjects are tilted slowly, if possible below the threshold of the semicircular canals, and they indicate when they feel that they are upright. Biases (tilts) in the perception of the subjective postural vertical cannot easily be induced experimentally by stimulation of the vestibular or visual (optokinetic) systems. Similarly, unilateral peripheral vestibular lesions do not create a significant bias (Anastasopoulos et al., 1997; Bisdorff et al., 1996) unless simultaneous masking by whole-body vibration is added (Aoki, Ito, Burchill, Brookes, & Gresty, 1997). These findings indicate that the input from an intact somatosensory system tends to override any tilted perception of body verticality arising from a unilateral vestibular lesion. In turn, this implies that the somatosensory input appears to be dominant for the perception of verticality, at least in the seated position. In fact, even patients with bilateral vestibular lesions are able to perceive body verticality fairly normally although with a slight decrement in accuracy (Bisdorff et al., 1996). More recent studies in three patients with complete vestibular ablation show threshold abnormality during roll tilt but, as with linear acceleration thresholds, the separation between normal data and vestibularly deprived patients is marginal, compared to the separation for angular (semicircular canals)

experiments (Valko, Lewis, Priesol, & Merfeld, 2012). This, again, testifies to the prominent role of the somatosensory contribution in linear acceleration and tilt perception.

Overall, there is no clear practical role in clinical neuro-otology for subjective postural vertical measurements. Patients with stroke, however, can show a tilted perception of body verticality along with tilts in other modalities of verticality perception. Verticality measurements in these patients can be useful to understand underlying mechanisms of unusually tilted body postures (e.g., as in the "pusher" syndrome) and may help to guide rehabilitation (Perennou & Bronstein, 2005; Perennou et al., 2008).

PERCEPTUAL ASSESSMENT OF VESTIBULAR FUNCTION

Perceptual tests of vestibular function were in use before oculography came along with the advancement of electronics in the 1950s. Perceptual tests underwent a revival in the last 15 to 20 years once the vestibular community realized that vestibulo-ocular test results often do not correlate well with patients' symptoms. We must not forget that dizziness is a symptom, a percept, and therefore, assessing how a patient perceives vestibular sensation may be more clinically relevant than just measuring oculomotor responses. However, perceptual tests should not attempt to replace but rather complement eye movement tests, as oculography provides a more objective measure of vestibular function. In patients with long-standing blindness (Seemungal, Glasauer, Gresty, & Bronstein, 2007) or eye movement disorders, typically in congenital nystagmus (Okada, Grunfeld, Shallo-Hoffmann, & Bronstein, 1999) or chronic external ophthalmoplegia (Grunfeld et al., 2003), perceptual tests are the only vestibular tests possible.

The simplest perceptual test is to ask the patient to compare subjectively the quality and intensity of the vestibular sensation for right and left stimuli. The stimuli can be the ones used in routine vestibular tests. Extremely useful information can be gained from simply asking a patient with a large congenital nystagmus or a complete ophthalmoplegia if the patient experienced vertigo from caloric irrigation on both ears. The information can be improved by timing the duration of the vertigo or asking the patient to consider the subjectively better ear as 100%, and then estimate how much the other ear's vertigo is reduced. No formal normative data are available for this test, but the author personally has full confidence in the result when a patient says that one ear is down 50% or more (naturally, most patients wrongly believe that the "sick" ear is the one producing more, not less, vertigo). Caloric-induced sensation asymmetries of 15% to 25% between the two ears are not clinically meaningful. Patients with directional preponderance can also report asymmetry in the perception of rotationally induced sensation. In the appropriate clinical context this information can help in the diagnosis of a dizzy patient, specifically when the patient suffers from preexisting visual or oculomotor disorders.

Even in patients undergoing conventional eye movement tests of vestibular function, enquiring about the quality of the sensation experienced during the caloric or rotational test can be extremely useful. One must not forget that a fundamental problem in the clinic is finding out if a patient's complaint of dizziness is of vestibular origin or not. In this scenario, a patient's equating the calorically elicited sensation to that of his own dizzy spells brings in considerable support for a diagnosis of vestibular disorder. And vice versa, when a patient says that his or her own dizziness does not resemble at all the caloric-induced vertigo, a vestibular explanation for the patient's symptoms is unlikely.

Vestibular perceptual tests can be divided into those investigating threshold or steady-state (suprathreshold) function. Rotational thresholds investigating semicircular canal function were popular before the advent of oculography. One technique consisted of delivering a range of constant accelerations for a period of time and noting the particular acceleration that is just sufficient to elicit a sensation of rotation; such methods, for instance, were used to detect early ototoxicity (Hood, 1984). It was then observed that thresholds obtained while fixating a chair-fixed target light were lower than those investigated in total darkness. With the target on subjects perceive the light as moving (the oculogyral illusion) with accelerations as small as 0.10 deg/s². Recent work has shown that rotational thresholds in total darkness are higher for sensation than for eliciting nystagmus (Seemungal, Gunaratne, Fleming, Gresty, & Bronstein, 2004), which probably explains the lower thresholds observed during the oculogyral procedure. Rotational thresholds studies are not part of the routine assessment of vestibular patients these days, although abnormalities in unilateral (Cousins et al., 2013) and bilateral peripheral vestibular lesions (Cutfield, Cousins, Seemungal, Gresty, & Bronstein, 2011; Priesol, Valko, Merfeld, & Lewis, 2014; Valko et al., 2102) have been recently documented. An interesting finding that patients with vestibular migraine have lower ("better") thresholds than normal controls (Lewis, Priesol, Nicoucar, Lim, & Merfeld, 2011) awaits confirmation.

Thresholds studies have also been applied to the assessment of otolith function. In contrast to rotation, the situation here is complicated by the fact that linear acceleration is detected by contact/tactile cues and that vibration-free linear acceleration devices suitable for threshold studies are expensive and difficult to build. These factors almost certainly account for the lack of convincing differences between normal and bilaterally labyrinthine defective subjects for thresholds to linear acceleration or tilt (Bringoux et al., 2002; Gianna, Heimbrand, & Gresty, 1996; Priesol et al., 2014; Valko et al., 2012).

Regarding suprathreshold vestibular perceptual tests, the main quantitative vestibular perceptual test in use before the advent of electro-oculography was cupulometry (Hulk & Jongkees, 1948). This test consists of measuring the duration of the postrotational (stopping) sensation to a range of velocities, so that the sensitivity and time constant of decay of the sensation could be measured. The procedure could also be conducted with direct observation of the nystagmus with Frenzel's lenses. In either case, the procedure took far too long to complete and was tiring for the subject and, as a consequence, it is no longer in use. Not many studies reporting patient data with this technique are available.

Quantitative and fast-to-deliver perceptual protocols have been applied more recently to the investigation of vestibular function in visually or eye movement impaired patients. Some of these tests measure the ability of subjects to angularly navigate in space; typically subjects on a rotating chair are given a rotational displacement and their task is to return to the origin using the joystick control in total darkness (the "self-rotation" test). The positional error between stimulus and response is plotted, and clear right-left asymmetries in peripheral unilateral vestibular lesions are observed (von Brevern, Faldon, Brookes, & Gresty, 1977).

In the "velocity perception test" or "wheel test" subjects on a rotating chair turn the wheel of a tachometer according to their online perceived angular velocity during velocity steps in the dark (Figure 22–8A). The output of the tachometer, an indication of the subject's rotational sensation, follows quite closely the exponential decay of recordings of slow phase eye velocity in normal subjects (Figure 22–8B). Use of this paradigm has established that absent (blindness) (Seemungal et al., 2007) or deranged visual input leads to shortening of the vestibular time constant mediated by the velocity storage vestibular integrator (ophthalmoplegia, Grunfeld, Okada, Jáuregui-Renaud, & Bronstein, 2003; congenital nystagmus, Okada et al., 1999). This technique has been recently applied to patients with vestibular neuritis and showed that in the acute vertiginous phase an intriguing ocular-perceptual dissociation takes place (Cousins et al., 2013). Although vestibulo-ocular time constants are, as expected, asymmetric (shorter during rotation toward the lesion sides), vestibulo-perceptual time constants are quite drastically shortened but in a symmetric fashion (ipsi- and contralesionally). This finding suggests a cortical suppression of vestibular sensation—a kind of a central acute antivertiginous effect (Cousins et al., 2013).

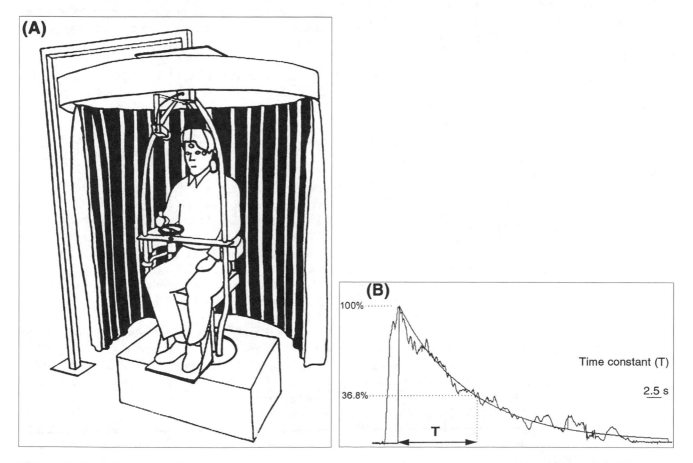

Figure 22–8. **A.** Technique for measurement of perceived angular velocity by means of a rotating chair fitted with a tacho-wheel (*top*). The subject turns the wheel manually according to his subjective rotational feeling. **B.** The output of this tachometer in a subject after stopping from a velocity step at 90 deg/sec in the dark is shown in the bottom trace. Note the exponential decay, from which the time constant can be measured (Okada et al., 1999). There is usually a good agreement between slow phase velocity recordings of vestibular nystagmus and perceived angular velocity, both with yaw plane time constants of about 15 sec.

A useful aspect of most perceptual tests is that they can be easily conducted with the head placed in different positions, thus providing potentially useful information on vertical canal function (Grunfeld et al., 2000; von Brevern et al., 1997). Another encouraging aspect is that perceptual tests of vestibular function appear to correlate better with patients' symptoms than do conventional vestibulo-ocular tests (Kanayama, Bronstein, Gresty, & Brookes, 1995).

Within this chapter various means of testing otolith function have been explored, as well as some of the inherent difficulties contained within them. These considerations highlight the challenges present in the continued development of otolith specific testing. An evaluation of the SVV as a test of otolith functioning has been carried out and addresses some of the factors that must be taken into account when interpreting outcomes—in particular, the fact that both semicircular canal and proprioceptive stimuli can also influence the verticality perception. A promising test has been developed which, by eccentric rotation, is capable of testing unilateral utricular function. The clinical relevance of various perceptual tests of vestibular sensation has also been reviewed here. Interest in vestibulo-perceptual tests has been recently revived as clinicians often find discrepancy between patients' symptoms and results from vestibulo-ocular tests.

REFERENCES

Anastasopoulos, D., & Bronstein, A. M. (1999). A case of thalamic syndrome: Somatosensory influences on visual orientation. *Journal of Neurology, Neurosurgery, & Psychiatry, 67,* 390–394.

Anastasopoulos, D., Haslwanter, T., Bronstein, A., Fetter, M., & Dichgans, J. (1997). Dissociation between the perception of body verticality and the visual vertical in acute peripheral vestibular disorder in humans. *Neuroscience Letters, 19,* 151–153.

Aoki, M., Ito, Y., Burchill, P., Brookes, G. B., & Gresty, M. A. (1997). Tilted perception of the subjective "upright" in unilateral loss of vestibular function. *American Journal of Otology, 18,* 484–493.

Barratt, H., Bronstein, A. M., & Gresty, M. A. (1987). Testing the vestibular-ocular reflexes: Abnormalities of the otolith contribution in patients with neuro-otological disease. *Journal of Neurology, Neurosurgery, and Psychiatry, 50*(8), 1029–1035.

Bisdorff, A. R., Wolsley, C. J., Anastasopoulos, D., Bronstein, A. M., & Gresty, M. A. (1996). The perception of body verticality (subjective postural vertical) in peripheral and central vestibular disorders. *Brain, 119,* 1523–1534.

Bohmer, A., & Mast, F. (1999). Chronic unilateral loss of otolith function revealed by the subjective visual vertical during off center yaw rotation. *Journal of Vestibular Research, 9,* 413–422.

Brandt, T., Dieterich, M., & Danek, A. (1994). Vestibular cortex lesions affect the perception of verticality. *Annals of Neurology, 35,* 403–412.

Bringoux, L., Schmerber, S., Nougier, V., Dumas, G., Barraud, P. A., & Raphel, C. (2002). Perception of slow pitch and roll body tilts in bilateral labyrinthine-defective subjects. *Neuropsychologia, 40,* 367–372.

Bronstein, A. M. (1995). The visual vertigo syndrome. *Acta Oto-Laryngologica Supplementum, 520*(1), 45–48.

Bronstein, A. M., & Gresty, M. A. (1988). Short latency compensatory eye movement responses to transient linear head acceleration: A specific function of the otolith-ocular reflexes. *Experimental Brain Research, 71,* 406–410.

Bronstein, A. M., Perennou, D. A., Guerraz, M., Playford, D., & Rudge P. (2003). Dissociation of visual and haptic vertical in two patients with vestibular nuclear lesions. *Neurology, 61*(9), 1172–1173.

Clarke, A. H., & Engelhorn, A. (1998). Unilateral testing of utricular function. *Experimental Brain Research, 121,* 457–464.

Correia, M. J., & Guedry, F. E. (1966). Modification of vestibular responses as a function of rate of rotation about an earth horizontal axis. *Acta Otolaryngolica, 62,* 297–308.

Cousins, S., Cutfield, N. J., Kaski, D., Palla, A., Seemungal, B. M., Golding, J. F., . . . Bronstein, A. M. (2014). Visual dependency and dizziness after vestibular neuritis. *PLoS One, 9*(9), e105426. doi:10.1371/journal.pone.0105426

Cousins, S., Kaski, D., Cutfield, N., Seemungal, B., Golding, J. F., Gresty, M., . . . Bronstein, A. M. (2013). Vestibular perception following acute unilateral vestibular lesions. *PLoS One. 8*(5), e61862. doi:10.1371/journal.pone.0061862

Curthoys, I. S., Dai, M. J., & Halmagyi, G. M. (1991). Human ocular torsional position before and after unilateral vestibular neurectomy. *Experimental Brain Research, 85,* 218–225.

Cutfield, N. J., Cousins, S., Seemungal, B. M., Gresty, M. A., & Bronstein, A. M. (2011). Vestibular perceptual thresholds to angular rotation in acute unilateral vestibular paresis and with galvanic stimulation. *Annals of the New York Academy of Sciences, 1233,* 256–262.

Diammond, S. G., & Markham, C. H. (1983). Ocular counter-rolling as an indicator of vestibular otolith function. *Neurology, 33,* 1460–1469.

Dieterich, M., & Brandt, T. (1993). Ocular torsion and perceived vertical in oculomotor, trochlear and abducens nerve palsies. *Brain, 116,* 1095–1104.

Fernandez, C., & Goldberg, M. J. (1976). Physiology of peripheral neurons innervating otolith organs of the squirrel monkey. II. Directional selectivity and force response relations. *Journal of Neurophysiology, 39,* 985–995.

Friedmann, G. (1970). The judgement of the visual vertical and horizontal with peripheral and central vestibular lesions. *Brain, 93,* 313–328.

Furman, J. M., & Redfern, M. S. (2002). Visual-vestibular interaction during OVAR in the elderly. *Journal of Vestibular Research, 11,* 365–370.

Gianna, C. C., Heimbrand, S., & Gresty, M. A. (1996). Thresholds for perception of lateral motion in normal subjects and patients with bilateral loss of vestibular function. *Brain Research Bulletin, 56,* 443–449.

Gresty, M. A., & Bronstein, A. M. (1986). Otolith stimulation evokes compensatory reflex eye movements of high velocity when linear motion of the head is combined with concurrent angular motion. *Neuroscience Letters, 65,* 149–154.

Gresty, M. A., Bronstein, A. M., & Barratt, H. (1987). Eye-movement responses to combined linear and angular head movement. *Experimental Brain Research, 65,* 377–384.

Gresty, M. A., Bronstein, A. M., Brandt, T., & Dieterich, M. (1992). Neurology of otolith function. Peripheral and central disorders. *Brain, 115,* 647–673.

Grunfeld, E. A., Okada, T., Jáuregui-Renaud, K., & Bronstein, A. M. (2000). The effect of habituation and plane of rotation on vestibular perceptual responses. *Journal of Vestibular Research, 10,* 193–200.

Grunfeld, E. A., Shallo-Hoffmann, J. A., Cassidy, L., Okada, T., Faldon, M., Acheson, J. F., & Bronstein, A. M. (2003). Vestibular perception in patients with acquired ophthalmoplegia. *Neurology, 60,* 1993–1995.

Guerraz, M., Gianna, C. C., Burchill, P. M., Gresty, M. A., & Bronstein, A. M. (2001). Effect of visual surrounding motion on body sway in a three-dimensional environment. *Perception & Psychophysics, 63*(1), 47–58.

Hood, J. D. (1984). Tests of vestibular function. In M. R. Dix & J. D. Hood (Eds.), *Vertigo* (pp. 55–90). Chichester, UK: Wiley.

Hulk, J., & Jongkees, L. B. W. (1948). The turning test with small regulable stimuli: II. The normal cupulogram. *Journal of Laryngology and Otology, 62,* 70–75.

Jauregui-Renaud, K., Faldon, M. E., Gresty, M. A., & Bronstein, A. M. (2001). Horizontal ocular vergency and the three-dimensional response to whole body roll motion. *Experimental Brain Research, 136,* 79–92.

Kanayama, R., Bronstein, A. M., Gresty, M. A., & Brookes, G. B. (1995). Vertical and torsional VOR in posterior canal occlusion. *Acta Oto-Laryngologica Supplementum, 520,* 405–407.

Kessler, P., Tomlinson, D., Blakeman, A., Rutka, J., Ranalli, P., & Wong, A. (2007). The high-frequency/acceleration head heave test in detecting otolith diseases. *Otology and Neurotology. 28*(7), 896–904.

Koizuka , I. (2003). Adaptive plasticity in the otolith-ocular reflex. *Auris Nasus Larynx,* (30 Suppl.) 3–6.

Lempert, T., Gianna, C., Brookes, G., Bronstein, A., & Gresty, M. (1998). Horizontal otolith-ocular responses in humans after unilateral vestibular deafferentation. *Experimental Brain Research, 118,* 533–540.

Lempert, T., Gianni, C. C., Gresty, M. A., & Bronstein, A. M. (1997). Effect of otolith dysfunction. Impairment of visual acuity during linear head motion in labyrinthine defective subjects. *Brain, 120*(6), 1005–1013.

Lewis, R. F., Priesol, A. J., Nicoucar, K., Lim, K., & Merfeld, D. M. (2011). Dynamic tilt thresholds are reduced in vestibular migraine. *Journal of Vestibular Research, 21*(6), 323–330.

Nuti, D., Mandalà, M., Broman, A. T., & Zee, D. S. (2005). Acute vestibular neuritis: Prognosis based upon bedside clinical tests (thrusts and heaves). *Annals of the New York Academy of Sciences, 1039,* 359–367.

Nyven, J. I., Hixson, W. C., & Correia, J. J. (1966). Elicitation of horizontal nystagmus by periodic linear acceleration. *Acta Otolaryngolica, 62,* 429–441.

Okada, T., Grunfeld, E., Shallo-Hoffmann, J., & Bronstein, A. M. (1999). Vestibular perception of angular velocity in normal subjects and in patients with congenital nystagmus. *Brain, 122*(7), 1293–1303.

Paige, G. D. (1989). The influence of target distance on eye movement responses during vertical linear motion. *Experimental Brain Research, 77*(3), 585–593.

Paige, G. D. (2002). Otolith function: Basis for modern testing. *Annals of the New York Academy of Sciences, 956,* 314–323.

Pavlou, M., Davies, R. A., & Bronstein, A. M. (2006). The assessment of increased sensitivity to visual stimuli in patients with chronic dizziness. *Journal of Vestibular Research, 16*(4–5), 223–231.

Pavlou, M., Lingeswaran, A., Davies, R. A., Gresty, M. A., & Bronstein, A. M. (2004). Simulator based rehabilitation in refractory dizziness. *Journal of Neurology, 251*(8), 983–995.

Pavlou, M., Wijnberg, N., Faldon, M., & Bronstein, A. M. (2003). Effect of semicircular canal stimulation on the visual vertical. *Journal of Neurophysiology, 90,* 622–630.

Perennou, D., & Bronstein, A. M. (2005). Balance disorders after stroke: Assessment and rehabilitation. In M. P. Barnes, B. C. Dobkin, & J. Bogousslavsky (Eds.), *Recovery after stroke*. New York, NY: Cambridge University Press.

Pérennou, D. A., Mazibrada, G., Chauvineau, V., Greenwood, R., Rothwell, J., Gresty, M. A., & Bronstein, A. M. (2008). Lateropulsion, pushing and verticality perception in hemisphere stroke: A causal relationship? *Brain, 131*, 2401–2413.

Priesol, A. J., Valko, Y., Merfeld, D. M., & Lewis, R. F. (2014). Motion perception in patients with idiopathic bilateral vestibular hypofunction. *Otolaryngology-Head and Neck Surgery, 150*(6), 1040–1042.

Seemungal, B. M., Glasauer, S., Gresty, M., & Bronstein, A. M. (2007) Vestibular perception and navigation in the congenitally blind. *Journal of Neurophysiology, 97*, 4341–4356.

Seemungal, B. M., Gunaratne, I. A., Fleming, I. O., Gresty, M. A., & Bronstein, A.M. (2004). Perceptual and nystagmic thresholds of vestibular function in yaw. *Journal of Vestibular Research, 14*, 461–466.

Steer, R. W., Jr. (1967). *The influence of angular and linear accelerations and thermal stimuli on the human semi-circular canal*. ScD. Thesis, Massachusetts Institute of Technology (MIT–67–63).

Tian, J. R., Crane, B. T., & Demer, J. L. (2003). Vestibular catch-up saccades augmenting the human transient heave linear vestibulo-ocular reflex. *Experimental Brain Research, 151*(4), 435–445.

Tian, J. R., Ishiyama, A., & Demer, J. L. (2007). Temporal dynamics of semicircular canal and otolith function following acute unilateral vestibular deafferentation in humans. *Experimental Brain Research, 178*, 529–541.

Valko, Y. I., Lewis, R. F., Priesol, A. J., & Merfeld, D. M. (2012). Vestibular labyrinth contributions to human whole-body motion discrimination. *Journal of Neuroscience, 32*(39), 13537–13542.

von Brevern, M., Faldon, M. E., Brookes, G. B., & Gresty, M. A. (1997). Evaluating 3D semicircular canal function by perception of rotation. *American Journal of Otology, 18*, 484–493.

Wuyts, F. L., Hoppenbrouwers, M., & Van de Heyning, P. H. (2001). Unilateral otolith function testing. In M. Lacour (Ed.), *Dysfonctionnements du systeme vestibulaire Compensation et reeducation* (pp. 257–265). Marseille, France: Solal.

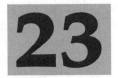

Electrocochleography (ECochG)

Paul R. Kileny

INTRODUCTION

Electrophysiology terminology does not always refer to the same neurophysiologic phenomenon or the same application. In one form or another the term *electrocochleography* has preceded the majority of the current terms referring to auditory neurodiagnostic procedures. An early reference and description of clinical applications of the "cochleogram" is provided in an article authored by noted otologist, Julius Lempert and noted auditory physiologists, Ernst Glen Weaver and Merle Lawrence, published in the *Archives of Otolaryngology* in 1947. In one of the first documented translational studies, this team recorded electrical potentials from the exposed round window of patients undergoing surgeries for otosclerosis, tinnitus, or Ménière's disease. They envisioned the use of these potentials for diagnosis and for surgical guidance—an early precursor of intraoperative monitoring. They referred to the response they recorded as the *cochleogram*. Today we would refer to it as the cochlear microphonic. They stated that "the cochlear potentials are representative of end organ activity not of the behavior of the auditory nerve or the more central processes." They cited a study published in 1934 (Guttmann & Barrera, 1934) in which "sectioning the cochlear nerve in cats but sparing the blood supply to the cochlea, these cochlear potentials are spared as they depend only on the integrity of the sensory cells."

In the 1970s there was a significant increase in research and publications related to auditory electrophysiologic measures obtained from human subjects and patients. This was in part prompted by the discovery of the auditory brainstem response by Jewett and Williston (1971), and by advances in the technology used for recording electrophysiologic phenomena. While the term *electrocochleography* (ECochG) was at the time used to refer to what we would call today the auditory brainstem response (Terkildsen, Osterhammel, & Huis in't Veld, 1973), the term began to be used to describe the simultaneous recording of electrical potentials generated by cochlear receptors and cochlear nerve in response to acoustic stimulation, and recorded relatively near-field (i.e., the promontory or the round window). In 1976, the proceedings of a symposium on ECochG held in June 1974 at Yeshiva University, New York, were published as a book (Ruben, Elberling, & Salomon, 1976). This book contained both experimental work in animals as well as clinical studies in patients using ECochG, including studies dealing with recording techniques and sites, specific pathologies such as Ménière's disease, and a comparison of threshold estimation using ECochG versus cortical-evoked responses, to name just a few.

Since then, the level of interest and frequency of diagnostic utilization of ECochG has fluctuated somewhat. It never really lost popularity among our European colleagues; however, here in the United States the advent of noninvasive, tympanic membrane surface recording techniques has definitely had a positive effect on the clinical utilization and clinical diagnostic innovations using ECochG.

THE NEUROPHYSIOLOGY OF ELECTROCOCHLEOGRAPHY

The auditory-evoked response is a continuum of neurophysiological responses that begin very soon following the delivery of an effective auditory stimulus to the ear, and extend in time as far as 1 s, reflecting the primary auditory cortex, association cortex, and cognitive potentials associated with auditory discrimination abilities. In the clinic, we attempt to limit the response duration range based on specific clinical applications and auditory-evoked response components of interest. For instance, when we are recording auditory brainstem responses, we tend to limit recording sweep duration to no more than 20 ms, as the components of interest occur within approximately 10 ms following the presentation of a stimulus.

Recording in this fashion we ascertain we can capture responses such as Wave V of the auditory brainstem response, known to be generated by the nucleus of the lateral lemniscus, as it is the most relevant component for threshold of hearing estimation. If one wishes to focus on cochlear and cochlear nerve potentials, we can limit the recording epoch to no more than 10 ms, as the essential components in this category occur within 5 ms following stimulation.

What is ECochG? It is the recording of cochlear potentials such as the cochlear microphonic and the summating potential, and the whole-nerve action potential generated by the cochlear nerve, using recording techniques that emphasize these particular components. Stated earlier, based on animal studies, our basic science and clinical forbearers already understood in the 1930s the differences between cochlear and cochlear nerve potentials, and the effects of the recording electrode placement on emphasizing these responses. It is now of course clear to all of us that the cochlear nerve action potential also referred to as N1, is in fact one and the same as the Wave I of the auditory brainstem response.

For the purpose of this chapter, ECochG is defined as the measurement of a combination of inner ear and cochlear nerve generated potentials elicited by a transient acoustic stimulus. In order to emphasize the responses of interest from cochlear and auditory nerve structures, the active electrode is placed in relative proximity of the respective generator sources. This electrode placement can be either a transtympanic needle electrode placed on the promontory, or a tympanic membrane surface electrode introduced by microscopic visualization of the ear canal and tympanic membrane. The components that make up the ECochG (depending upon stimulus polarity) are the cochlear microphonic, the summating potential, and the cohlear nerve compound action potential. Given that we record with a time base of 10 ms, it is also possible to identify other auditory-evoked potential components pertaining to the auditory brainstem response. To summarize, the neural-generator sources and the nature of the ECochG components are as follows.

The cochlear microphonic (CM) is an alternating current (AC) potential that closely resembles the wave form of the acoustic stimulus used to elicit the response. Thus, if the acoustic stimulus consists of a brief one to two cycle tone, the cochlear microphonic will have a similar sinusoidal configuration with an identical period as the acoustic stimulus. This response is related to changes in resistance of predominately outer hair cells during stimulation.

The summating potential (SP) is a direct current (DC) potential that follows the stimulus envelope and when coexisting with the cochlear microphonic, appears as a baseline shift of the cochlear microphonic. Typically, in a normal ear this baseline shift is minimal; therefore, the summating potential is not very prominent. The summating potential arises from direct current intracellular potentials and is generated predominantly by inner hair cells. While it is typically described as following the stimulus envelope, more accurately, the summating potential is related to a rectified and smoothed version of the basilar membrane displacement pattern (Dallos, 1976). When using a very brief stimulus, like a click, the summating potential is also very brief, as it precedes the action potential (AP), or at times it blends into the leading edge of the AP.

The AP or N1 (the cochlear nerve compound action potential) represents the summed activity of synchronously firing cochlear nerve fibers, in other words, the auditory-evoked potential of the cochlear nerve synonymous to Wave I of the auditory brainstem response. In order to obtain these responses, certain recording techniques need to be employed.

RECORDING METHODS

In this section I will attempt to provide detailed instructions to optimize the recording of an ECochG. This information is based on personal experience with close to 2,000 ECochGs recorded from patients of various ages, with various auditory thresholds and normal-hearing subjects.

First, the type, location, and placement of the active electrode play a very important role in determining the quality of the recording, and the resolution of the ECochG waveform. One of the main principles underlying all forms of electrophysiologic recording is that the utility of the response is only as good as the quality of the waveform. Therefore, substantial attention needs to be paid to the technical aspects of recording a response, in particular the nature and placement of the electrode. In order to emphasize the components of interest (the summating potential, the action potential, and at times the cochlear microphonic), the electrode needs to be as much as possible in the proximity of the genera-

tor sources. Much of the experimental work involving ECochG was done in animals models where the electrode was placed directly on the exposed round window or even penetrating the round window into the distal portion of the basal turn of the cochlea. Clearly, such placement would result in large and easy-to-identify potentials that necessitate very little signal averaging. In clinical applications, for many years, the electrode of choice was a transtympanic needle placed onto the cochlear promontory in the vicinity of the round window niche. This will also result in large amplitude responses as shown in Figure 23–1. Figure 23–1 is an illustration of a simultaneous surface recording of the auditory brainstem response with the reference or inverting electrode placed on the medial surface of the earlobe along with a transtympanic recording using a needle placed on the promontory.

This figure illustrates the identical latency of the surface recorded Wave I and the N1 or action potential (AP) of the cochlear nerve. The difference between the two recordings is obvious: the amplitude of the promontory recorded AP is substantially larger than the surface-recorded Wave I; however, the later waves of the auditory brainstem response are not as prominent with the promontory recording as they are with the standard surface recording. It is of note that the amplitude calibration of the two

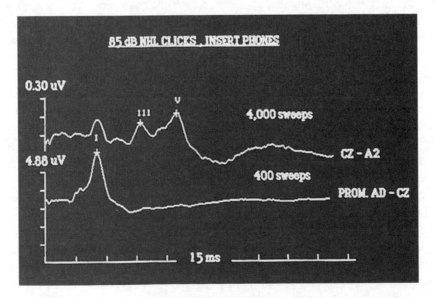

Figure 23–1. Simultaneous standard surface (*upper trace*) and promontory needle (*lower trace*) recording of ABR and EcochG, respectively, from otologically normal subject with normal hearing.

traces is different, and this gives the illusion that the promontory recorded response is only slightly larger than the surface recorded auditory brainstem response. Over the years, a variety of extra-tympanic recording methods were attempted and recommended, such as the Coats Leaf electrode consisting of strip of plastic carrying a ball electrode at the tip, which was folded and introduced into the ear canal, and it would stabilize within the bony portion of the ear canal when deployed. This was uncomfortable for patients. Other extra-tympanic options were the tip-trodes, consisting of a foil wrapped around a standard foam earplug used for insert earphones. This foil was connected to a lead by means of a type of alligator clip. This required scrubbing the lumen of the external ear canal and then inserting the tip-trode. The resolution of the summating potential and the action potential recorded with this type of electrode was not much more prominent than when recording with a surface electrode placed on the medial surface of the earlobe. Another solution promoted by several colleagues was to place an electrode on the surface of the tympanic membrane. This could be either a foam or cotton wick or a hydrogel tip dipped into a conductive medium, connected to a silver wire which is insulated except where connects to the wick or hydrogel, and contained in a soft polyethylene tube. This electrode can be guided down the ear canal under microscopic visualization, and introduced so that the tip would adhere to the tympanic membrane. This method does not provide a response amplitude quite like one obtained with a transtympanic needle, but it provides superior resolution when compared to a tip-trode, and is much more comfortable that the Coats Leaf Electrode. Currently there are two commercial versions of the tympanic membrane surface electrode, one ending in a cotton wick dipped into a conductive medium, the other following a similar concept except that the tip is an elastic hydrogel encasing the looped end of a silver wire. Both of these electrodes need to be dipped into saline for a few minutes, and then just prior to introducing it into the ear canal and on to the tympanic membrane, immersed into a conductive cream for a few minutes. It is important to place these electrodes under direct visualization of the ear canal and the tympanic membrane with an oto-microscope to ascertain that in fact the proximal end of the electrode rests against the tympanic membrane, as shown in Figure 23–2. The use of a small nasal or Lempert speculum is recommended as opposed to a standard ear speculum, to allow the removal of the speculum without disturbing the electrode tip location on the tympanic membrane.

Once the electrode is visually confirmed to be in place, the clinician needs to hold the distal end of the electrode with a steady hand, remove the speculum, followed by the introduction of a standard foam insert tip along the lead of the electrode. This stabilizes the electrode in the ear canal and no further fixation is necessary, except perhaps taping the extension lead to the patient's cheek so that there is no inadvertent movement when it is in place. Contact with the tympanic membrane is further verified by examining the electrode impedance. The typical impedance of such electrodes ranges between 25 and 100 kΩ. This range of impedances is acceptable and results in noise-free recording. It is important to note that the impedance measurement alone does not confirm or ascertain contact with the tympanic membrane. Contact with the external ear canal can also result in low impedances; therefore, it is necessary to both visualize the electrode making contact with the tympanic membrane as well as measuring its impedance. This technique is tolerated well by patients. Approximately 25% to 30% of patients report a brief episode of discomfort that some describe as an earache that might occur during electrode placement. However, once the electrode and foam ear plug are in place, the discomfort goes away. The majority of patients report a fullness sensation, a pressure sensation as well as a dull sound when the electrode touches the tympanic membrane. It is recommended to use the pediatric version of the foam tip in most adult ear canals as the lead occupies some space within the ear canal and the smaller, pediatric tip is easier to place and can be placed more medially in most ear canals.

Some fellow professionals recommend the use of the tip-trode electrode option to record the ECochG, stating that it is a reliable modality to record the SP and the AP. This has not been our experience. The resolution of the response is not much better than when recording with a reference electrode attached to the medial surface of the earlobe. The presence and magnitude of the SP and the AP tend to be incon-

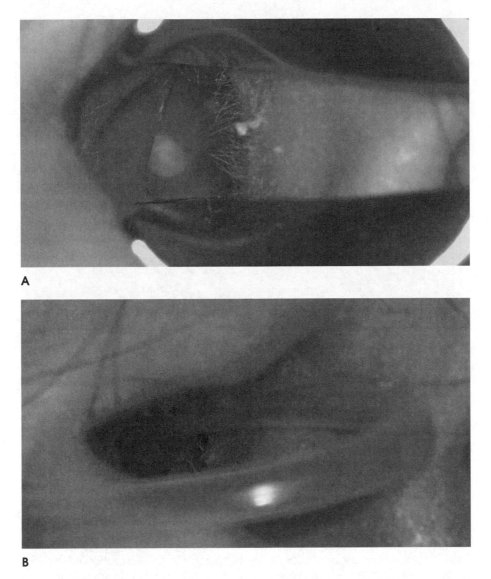

Figure 23–2. A. Tympanic membrane electrode placement: right ear, patient supine, microscope view using small nasal speculum. **B.** View following placement of the tympanic membrane electrode, the speculum has been withdrawn.

sistent and variable. This is especially problematic when carrying out follow-up evaluations to determine the efficacy of a specific treatment, or monitoring the status of a condition such as endolymphatic hydrops, or superior semicircular canal dehiscence. Figure 23–3 illustrates the difference in response resolution and configuration between simultaneously recorded ECochGs with a tympanic membrane electrode (top trace) and a tip-trode (bottom trace). These responses were obtained simultaneously with a two-channel recording from the same ear with identical recording parameters. While the top trace recorded with a TM electrode exhibits prominent and clearly identifiable SP and AP components, the bottom trace obtained with the tip-trode exhibits an overall reduced amplitude of the AP, and an uncertain SP. It is interesting to note that both traces exhibit identical wave V amplitudes. This is not surprising, as relative to the neural generators of wave V, these two are identical far-field recordings. As for the earlier components, the tympanic membrane recording is relatively near-field as opposed to the tip-trode

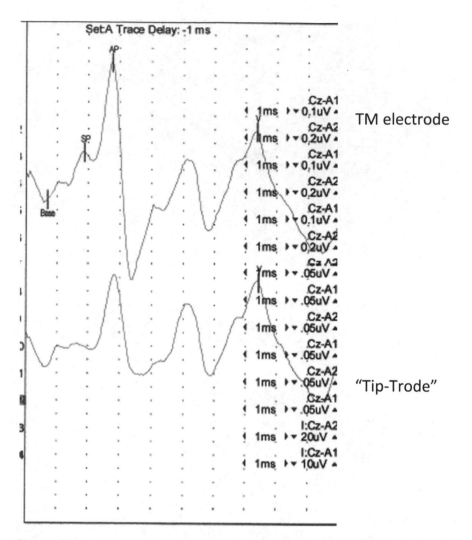

Figure 23–3. Tympanic membrane electrode (*top trace*) versus tip-trode electrode (*second trace*): significant difference in the resolution of the SP and the AP. These were recorded simultaneously from a normal subject.

recording which is relatively far field for the SP and AP generators, and thus the significant differences, in favor of the tympanic membrane recording when it comes to the identification of the components that make up the ECochG.

Stimuli and Recording Parameters

The configuration of the response and its diagnostic utility also depend significantly on the stimulus choice and recording parameters. In general, regardless of the specific stimulus used, it is recommended to use relatively high stimulus intensities, such as 80 to 95 dB nHL in order to promote a good response resolution. This is not different from stimulus intensities used for neurodiagnostic ABR applications. The summating potential, cochlear microphonic, and the action potential can be elicited by both tone-burst stimuli and clicks. Each has advantages and disadvantages, and in addition to the specific stimulus, the delivery using constant versus alternating polarity changes the configuration of the response. When using tone-bursts, the dominant component recorded is the cochlear microphonic. It is typically difficult to identify or discern the cochlear nerve action potential. In particular, if the summating potential is relatively large, it can be identified and it combines with the cochlear microphonic. As it grows, it "displaces" the cochlear microphonic baseline, giving the impression that the cochlear microphonic "rides" on top of a rectangular ramp (Figure 23–4).

One way to eliminate the cochlear microphonic and be left with the summating potential is to elicit responses with alternating polarity tone bursts, or sum responses obtained with rarefaction and condensation polarity. This will cancel out the cochlear microphonic and leave the summating potential, especially in cases where it is relatively prominent.

When using clicks, constant polarity stimulation will result in a cochlear microphonic followed by the cochlear nerve action potential, when adding responses elicited by rarefaction and condensation clicks, or eliciting a response with alternating polarity clicks, the cochlear microphonic (which is very brief due to the nature of the stimulus) will be canceled and the cochlear nerve action potential (AP) will be preceded by a summating potential, as illustrated in Figure 23–5.

The recording parameters need to also be adjusted to optimize the identification of the components of interest. Primarily, it is important to utilize appropriate bandpass filtering, keeping in mind that the summating potential is very low frequency in nature; in fact, it is often referred to as a direct current (DC) component. Therefore, the usual high-pass filters used for neurodiagnostic auditory brainstem response testing are not adequate for this recording. The high-pass filter needs to be between 10 and 20 Hz with a low slope, such as 6 dB per octave in order to avoid distortion and ringing that can alter

the response and make it difficult to interpret. The low-pass filter is somewhat less important, however, if desired to also include the typical components of the ABR, the low-pass filter should not be any lower than 1500 Hz.

Beyond stimulus characteristics and electrode placement, the specifics of the recording protocol also play an important role in the response presentation and resolution. The specific components of

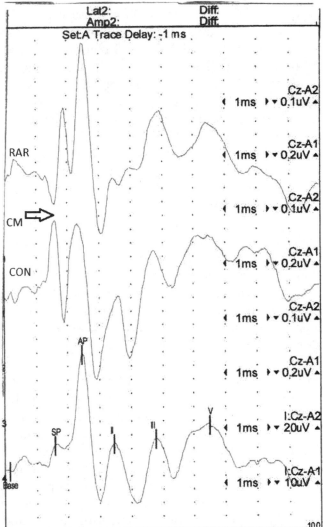

Figure 23–5. Constant polarity (rarefaction and condensation) click-evoked responses result in the definition of the corresponding cochlear microphonic preceding the cochlear nerve action potential-AP (*first and second trace*). Their sum, shown in the bottom trace, (or using alternating polarity clicks) results in the resolution of the summating potential (SP), preceding the AP.

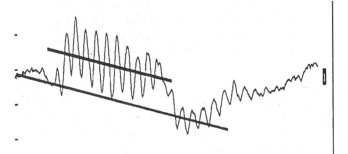

Figure 23–4. Cochlear microphonic recorded using a tympanic membrane electrode superimposed on prominent summating potential. The amplitude of the summating potential amplitude is defined by the two parallel lines.

the ECochG occur within an approximately 3 ms poststimulus time window at stimulus intensities ranging from 80 to 95 dB nHL. The latency of the summating potential (SP) for click stimuli ranges from less than 1 to no more than 1.5 ms. This value refers to the peak and not the onset of the SP. The onset is approximately 0.5 ms poststimulus. The latency of the AP ranges from about 1.5 to 2.5 ms depending upon hearing status. It is possible to also record the later components of the ABR, such as waves III and V. If this is of interest, a recording epoch of 10 ms is sufficient, as the latency of Wave V is between 5.5 and 6.5 ms. A 10-ms window provides sufficient resolution to the early components of interest such as the SP and AP, and also allows the resolution of waves III and V. Another important aspect of the recording protocol is to have a 1- to 2-ms prestimulus baseline. This is necessary as it serves as the reference point for measuring the amplitudes of the SP and the AP. It is highly desirable for this prestimulus baseline to be as electrically neutral as possible, so that it appears as a reasonably flat line. Since the prestimulus baseline occurs prior to the delivery of the stimulus, in theory it is not affected by auditory system activation. In reality, depending on the repetition rate, this prestimulus segment may be somewhat affected by auditory pathway activation. The recommended stimulus rate for ECochG is typically lower than the recommended rate for auditory brainstem response testing, and we recommend a rate ranging from approximately 9 to 11 per second. The lower the rate the less the prestimulus baseline is affected by auditory pathway activation and is likely to remain more neutral. At times movement or muscle artifact may affect the prestimulus baseline to the point that averaging is not sufficient to eliminate the artifact within the time period. If that is the case, my recommendation is to delete the response and begin a new average closely monitoring the status of the baseline. This is very important for the accuracy of the components of interest. Some individuals have a tendency to measure the SP and AP amplitudes from the lowest "valley" preceding the SP which is actually the onset of the SP, and thus not electrically neutral. This mode of amplitude measurement is likely to introduce inaccuracies as it is not an electrically neutral reference point as is the prestimulus baseline. Figure 23–6 illustrates an ECochG recorded as outlined above. The baseline,

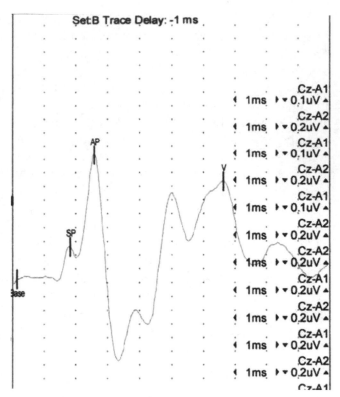

Figure 23–6. Typical ECochG recorded with a tympanic membrane surface electrode. A prestimulus baseline is necessary to serve as the reference for the SP and AP amplitudes.

which is reasonably flat, serves as the common reference point for the measurement of the SP and AP amplitudes. This then results in an accurate SP-to-AP ratio.

RATIONALE AND PRINCIPLE OF ELECTROCOCHLEOGRAPHY AND SUMMATING POTENTIAL TO ACTION POTENTIAL RATIO (SP/AP RATIO)

The principles of the SP and AP recording, and diagnostic applications are based on extensive experimental animal studies where these components were recorded either directly from scala tympani or scala vestibuli or from an electrode in direct contact of the round window. Early work by Davis and associates in the 1950s defined the summating potential and demonstrated that static pressure to the scala tympani could change the amplitude of the summating potential and change its polarity. Eggermont (1976) summarized the effects of specific recording site, stimulus frequency, and stimulus intensity on the polarity of the SP relative to the AP. He expressed the opinion that the polarity of the SP reflects an anatomical difference relative the specific site of the electrode. In the majority of the cases recorded from human subjects and patients, he observed the SP with the same polarity as the AP. Eggermont concluded that while the polarity may be subject to recording site relative to scala tympani or scala vestibuli since the promontory SP probably reflects responses from both scalae, the sign of the SP is not a reflection of cochlear pathology. However, the magnitude of the SP may be associated with "some form of cochlear disorder." Eggermont evaluated input/output functions for the SP, and the AP at various frequencies for normal hearing controls, Ménière's patients and patients with cochlear hearing loss without hearing loss and without Ménière's. He also evaluated SP/AP ratio for different frequencies and at different intensities and found that the mean value, or overall value, was slightly higher than in normal ears, and in normal ears, the ratio was stimulus intensity dependent increasing from low to high intensity. In Ménière's patients there was no correlation between stimulus intensity and SP/AP ratio, that is, the ratio which was overall higher than in normal ears was the same at low and high intensities. The SP/AP ratio difference was highest between Ménière's ears and ears with non- Ménière's sensory hearing loss.

There has been extensive literature regarding the utility of ECochG in the diagnosis of Ménière's disease and in monitoring the effects of treatment. The SP/AP amplitude ratio has been reported to exceed a specificity of 90% (Ferraro, Best, & Arenberg, 1983; Murphy & Gates, 1999). In terms of sensitivity most reports agree that approximately 60% to 65% of patients with Ménière's disease present with an increased SP/AP amplitude ratio. In an attempt to improve the sensitivity, Ferraro and his colleagues (Al-Momani, Ferraro, Gajewski, & Ator, 2009) recommended to augment the measurement of the SP/AP amplitude ratio with the SP and AP area under the curve. This addition substantially increased the sensitivity of ECochG for Ménière's disease to 92% based on this study.

It is clear from experimental animal studies and human clinical studies that the position of the basi-

lar membrane that would be displaced in the presence of endolymphatic hydrops, does have an effect on the amplitude of the summating potential. It is thought that in the presence endolymphatic hydrops, the basilar membrane is statically displaced toward the scala tympani. While it is thought that under normal conditions the SP is generated by the inner hair cells, when the basilar membrane is displaced toward scala tympani, there is a larger contribution from the outer hair cells due to a change in their electrical properties influenced by the abnormal position of the basilar membrane, thus increasing the magnitude of the summating potential.

DIAGNOSTIC APPLICATIONS OF ELECTROCOCHLEOGRAPHY

ECochG in Ménière's Disease

It stands to reason that the diagnostic applications of ECochG will pertain to conditions that alter the mechanics of the cochlea which in turn would contribute to the change in the magnitude or nature of cochlear potentials, such as the summating potential. Ménière's disease continues to represent a diagnostic challenge for the clinician. Given that effective treatment depends on accurate diagnosis, clinicians continue to make every effort to improve diagnostic accuracy in Ménière's disease.

Histopathologic studies of temporal bones with classic Ménière's disease signs and symptoms, have demonstrated the presence of distortion and dilation of the endolymphatic spaces in the membranous labyrinth. This phenomenon is typically referred to as endolymphatic hydrops, which is considered to be the pathologic basis of Ménière's disease. It is of note, however, that these pathologic changes do not always correspond to clinical manifestations. Some studies have shown a complete match of pathologic and clinical findings (Rauch, Merchant, & Thedinger, 1989). Others did not find such close correspondence (Minor, Schessel, & Carey, 2004). The American Academy of Otolaryngology-Head and Neck Surgery (AAO-HNS) has provided criteria for the diagnosis of Ménière's disease based on the nature of the recurrent spontaneous vertigo, hearing loss, aural fullness, tinnitus, as well as audiological documentation of hearing loss (Committee on Hearing and Equilibrium Guidelines, 1995). Signs and symptoms, including hearing loss, tend to fluctuate, and physical findings in general are lacking in this condition. Appropriately summarized are the questions confronting the clinicians relative to the diagnosis of Ménière's disease. The questions outlined included whether the patient had Ménière's disease and this can be based on audiologic and vestibular evaluations as well as on the AAO-HNS criteria; which ear is causing the symptoms? This question may be answered by results of audiologic and vestibular tests, especially if vestibular and auditory results coincide, such as low-frequency, fluctuating sensorineural hearing loss and vestibular weakness in the same ear. The next important question is whether there is bilateral disease, as this will significantly impact the treatment plan. Finally, we need to ask whether the treatment that has been initiated for a given patient is effective. ECochG can be used to address the questions posed in the diagnosis of Ménière's disease. One of the main clinical advantages of ECochG is that the results are ear specific and therefore the question of which ear is responsible for the symptoms and whether the patient presents with bilateral disease may be answered by the results of this test. The typical expected result in an ear positive for Ménière's disease is an increase in the summating potential amplitude relative to the action potential amplitude—that is, an increase in the SP/AP ratio (Coats, 1981; Dauman et al., 1988). As mentioned elsewhere in this chapter, it is believed that the presence of hydrops affects the resting position of the basilar membrane, displacing it toward the scala tympani which in turn results in changes in the electro-anatomy of the hair cells, increasing the magnitude of the summating potential. Instead of measuring and reporting the absolute amplitude of the summating potential, the SP/AP amplitude ratio is used, in order to avoid individual variability. Most investigators have used a value range for the SP/AP ratio, 0.3 to 0.5 as the outer limits of the normal range. Using these values approximately two-thirds of Ménière's patients presented with abnormally elevated SP/AP ratios (Aso, Watanabe, & Mizukoshi, 1991). Due in part to differences in measurement, there is some variation in the literature in terms of normal values of SP/AP ratio in subjects without Ménière's disease. In order to eliminate this vari-

ability, Margolis, Rieks, Fournier, and Levine (1995) published a study on normative ECochG data from 53 subjects. They used tympanic surface electrodes and found that the SP/AP ratios were dependent on stimulus level, ranging from 0.22 at 78 db nHL to 0.29 at 68 db nHL. The 95th percentile for the SP/AP ratio ranged from 0.40 to 0.49. Based on these data they considered 0.35 or less to be a normal value and 0.5 or above to be a definitely abnormal result. Based on our own normative data and the Margolis publication, the definition of the upper limit normal range in our clinic is 0.40. Values above 0.40 are considered to be elevated. The following case study illustrates our diagnostic protocol including the interpretation of the ECochG.

The patient was a 38-year-old woman with a 2-year history of episodic vertigo lasting 10 to 15 min, accompanied by nausea and occasional emesis. These episodes had been occurring every 2 weeks and their severity varied. Each one of these episodes left the patient fatigued and incapacitated for a few hours. In between attacks, she was functioning quite well with the exception of some disequilibrium she experienced for a few days after the attacks. She also reported right-sided aural fullness and a mid-frequency tinnitus that was essentially constant, but at times it would become more noticeable. She was unclear whether the tinnitus increase coincided with the onset the vertiginous episodes. She also noticed hearing loss in her right ear, but she felt that her hearing in her right ear was at times better. Her left ear was completely symptom-free. There was no family history of hearing loss or diagnosed Ménière's disease. She was otherwise in good health with no history of hypertension or diabetes.

An audiogram obtained in our clinic showed normal hearing in the left ear across the frequency range with a word discrimination score of 100% and an SRT of 5 dB. In the right ear, she presented with an up-sloping, moderate, low-frequency sensorineural hearing loss with normal thresholds, but in the 3000- to 4000-Hz range. The SRT in the right ear was 30 dB and the word recognition score was 92% when obtained at 70 dBHL. On the day she had her audiogram, she indicated that this was a day when her hearing was subjectively relatively good in the right ear. We carried out an ECochG evaluation using a tympanic surface electrode as described elsewhere in this chapter. We used both clicks and tone-bursts as stimuli in an attempt to determine the presence or absence of an elevated summating potential in the right ear to support the diagnosis of Ménière's disease. With left ear stimulation using clicks, the summating potential to action potential ratio was within normal limits based on our criteria, with a value of 0.3. With right ear stimulation, the summating potential to action potential ratio was elevated with a value of 0.6, as illustrated in Figure 23–7.

Both the summating potential and the action potential amplitudes were measured referenced to a prestimulus baseline, which was quite flat, and

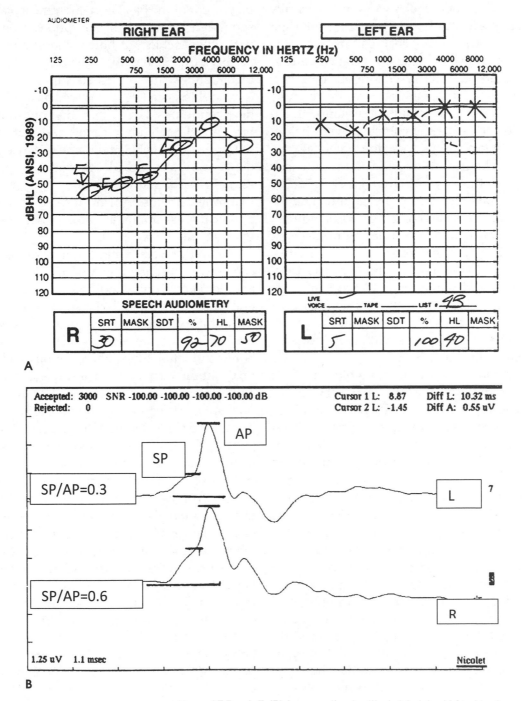

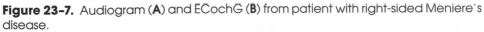

Figure 23–7. Audiogram (**A**) and ECochG (**B**) from patient with right-sided Ménière's disease.

as such it was an ideal reference for the respective amplitudes of the two potentials of interest. Measurements were also carried out using a 1000-Hz tone-burst used to elicit a cochlear microphonic and to further evaluate the presence or absence of an elevated summating potential. With left ear stimulation, the summating potential was difficult to identify as the cochlear microphonic cycles were symmetrically displaced relative to baseline. In contrast, with right ear stimulation, the entire cochlear microphonic wave form appeared elevated above the baseline as though displaced on a ramp. This ramp represents the summating potential which was much more prominent with right ear stimulation than with left ear stimulation. This finding coincides with the elevated summating potential to action potential ratio obtained with click stimulation in the right ear. It is of note that in this case, vestibular testing identified some left-beating positional nystagmus, and the caloric test results consisted of increased slow-phase velocity with warm water stimulation in the right ear. This of course may be interpreted as an irritative lesion at this time in the right ear; however, the presence of an increased summating potential amplitude in the right ear, coinciding with the low-frequency sensorineural hearing loss made a significant contribution to a definitive diagnosis of Ménière's disease in this patient's right ear.

Note the following about possible effects of hearing loss on the clinical utility of ECochG: Hearing loss exceeding 40 to 50 dB HL in mid and high frequencies is considered by some to be a contraindication for ECochG due to poor resolution of the SP and the AP, and the possibility of an altered amplitude relationship between those two components (Mori, Asai, & Sakagami, 1993; Ferraro, 2010). The latter could result in inaccurate SP/AP ratios thus decreasing the measure's clinical utility. In this author's experience, reliable SP, AP, and SP/AP ratios can be obtained up to 60 to 70 dB HL hearing loss across the frequency range with tympanic membrane recording. Very likely as a consequence of recruitment, in my practice I have experienced highly resolved SP and AP components elicited by 95 dB nHL clicks in patients with 70 dB HL flat or high-frequency , sloping pure tone thresholds. Therefore, I consider patients with up to 70 dB cochlear hearing loss as appropriate candidates for ECochG.

Electrocochleography in Superior Semicircular Canal Dehiscence

It is important to note that changes in the magnitude of the summating potential and the elevation of the SP/AP ratio are not specific to Ménière's disease. Given that other conditions can result in a static displacement of the basilar membrane, it stands to reason that an elevated SP/AP ratio can be associated with other cochleo-vestibular conditions. Recently, it has been established that the SP/AP ratio is elevated in patients with confirmed superior semicircular canal dehiscence (SSCD) as well as other third window conditions. Given that this condition has been recognized relatively recently, and that much of the literature on ECochG and Ménière's disease precede the recognition and identification of the superior semicircular canal dehiscence, it is quite possible that some patients with an elevated SP/AP ratio and a clinical presentation atypical for Ménière's disease may actually have SSCD.

Superior semicircular canal dehiscence syndrome was described by Minor, Solomon, Zinreigh, and Zee (1998). This condition is associated with several auditory and vestibular signs and symptoms. In the auditory domain, these include hypersensitive bone conduction thresholds, meaning a subzero dB bone conduction threshold resulting in what appears on the audiogram to be an air-bone gap, overall sensitivity to sounds including one's own footstep and one's own voice (autophony), audible eye movements, and some degree of hyperacusis. The air-bone gap appearing on the audiogram coexists with typically normal, type A tympanogram and intact acoustic reflexes. Among vestibular symptoms, patients complain of overall disequilibrium, hypersensitivity to stimulation, sound- and pressure-evoked vertigo or imbalance, and sensation of a bouncing horizon when walking, but no evidence of oscillopsia.

Several years ago (Arts, Adams, Telian, El-Kashlan, & Kileny, 2008), we made the initial observation in a few patients with confirmed superior canal dehiscence, that they all presented with elevated summating potential to action potential ratio values. Subsequently, we evaluated the ECochG results of 11 patients, seven with unilateral SSCD and four with bilateral SSCD (15 ears with SSCD). In all these patients we included ECochG in the preoperative evaluation. Additionally, all these patients underwent an audiologic evaluation as well as vestibular-evoked myogenic potential (VEMP) testing and high-resolution temporal bone computed tomography, reformatted to optimally view the semicircular canal. In this series, 14 of the 15 ears with confirmed SSCD on computed tomography were found to have an elevated SP/AP ratio (exceeding 0.40). Four of these patients underwent surgery to repair the dehiscence and in all, the SP/AP ratio normalized postoperatively. In one of these four patients, we continuously monitored ECochG during the dehiscence repair and were able to document an immediate intraoperative resolution of the abnormalities. Subsequently, we began monitoring intraoperatively all SSCD repair procedures. We concluded following this initial study that the SP/AP ratio was highly sensitive to SSCD and that it was advisable to include ECochG in the diagnostic evaluation of patients suspected of SSCD.

The following cases illustrate ECochG findings in SSCD. This is the case of a 38-year-old female patient with a 1- to 2-year history of autophony localized to her right ear, right-sided pulsatile tinnitus and fullness sensation, sensitivity to loud sounds, and a sense of disequilibrium, in particular when walking along the aisle of a store flanked by large shelves on either side. Figure 23–8A shows her audiogram which demonstrates normal hearing and no air-bone gap in the left ear, and an apparent low-frequency mild conductive hearing loss in the right ear with air-bone gaps from 250 to 1000 Hz and sub-zero dB bone conduction thresholds for those same frequencies. Mid-frequency and high-frequency hearing is in the normal limits with absent air-bone gap in the right ear. Tympanic ECochG was carried out in this patient as described elsewhere in this chapter. An elevated SP/AP ratio, 0.53 was obtained with right ear stimulation, while the SP/AP value for left ear stimulation was within normal limits with a value of 0.34, as shown in Figure 23–8B. Auditory brainstem response interpeak latencies were also evaluated and these were normal and symmetrical bilaterally. VEMP measurements were also carried out in this patient resulting in a 65-dB threshold for the right ear, a 75-dB threshold for the left ear, and overall larger VEMP amplitudes for right ear responses. The patient was referred for CT imaging for a study of the temporal bones with reformatting

to bring the superior canal in the viewing plane. As illustrated in Figure 23–8C, there is a clear dehiscence on the right side while the left superior canal was covered with bone, albeit somewhat thin.

The second case is that of a 45-year-old woman presenting with left ear symptoms consistent with SSCD. These included autophony localized to the left ear, left-sided fullness sensation, and an overall sense of disequilibrium exacerbated when exercising. This patient also reported two to three episodes when loud sounds elicited a sense of disequilibrium. Her audiogram was normal for her right ear and was characterized by bone conduction hypersensitivity in the left ear for frequencies ranging from 250 to 1000 kHz. Her bone conduction thresholds ranged from −5 to −10 dB. This was not the case for the right ear.

ECochG resulted in an SP/AP ratio of 0.78 for the left, symptomatic ear and a normal SP/AP ratio of 0.36 for the asymptomatic right ear, as illustrated in Figure 23–9A. Figures 23–9B and 23–9C illustrate CT imaging studies clearly demonstrating a dehiscent left-sided superior canal and a right-sided canal that was covered by bone. This patient underwent repair of her left-sided superior canal dehiscence and her SP/AP ratio diminished intraoperatively from 0.78 to 0.34. This was subsequently confirmed 2 months postoperatively with an SP/AP ratio of 0.3 for the left ear. The right ear continued to have a normal SP/AP ratio.

We subsequently reviewed ECochG findings for 45 affected ears. The mean SP/AP ratio for these 45 ears was 0.62 with a standard deviation of 0.21. We also evaluated SP/AP ratios in 21 unaffected ears of the same patients resulting in a mean SP/AP ratio of 0.29 with a standard deviation of 0.17. A statistical analysis indicated that the difference in SP/AP ratio between the affected and unaffected ears was significant with a P value of 0.0001.

What is the pathophysiological phenomenon underlying the elevated SP in SSCD? Rosowski et al. (2004) offered the following explanation: As a result of the dehiscence, impedance may be higher on the scala vestibuli side of the cochlea than on the scala tympani side. This may be more prominent at certain stimulus frequencies. If this is the case, it may result in a basilar membrane bias toward scala tympani, and a resultant increase in the summating potential (SP)

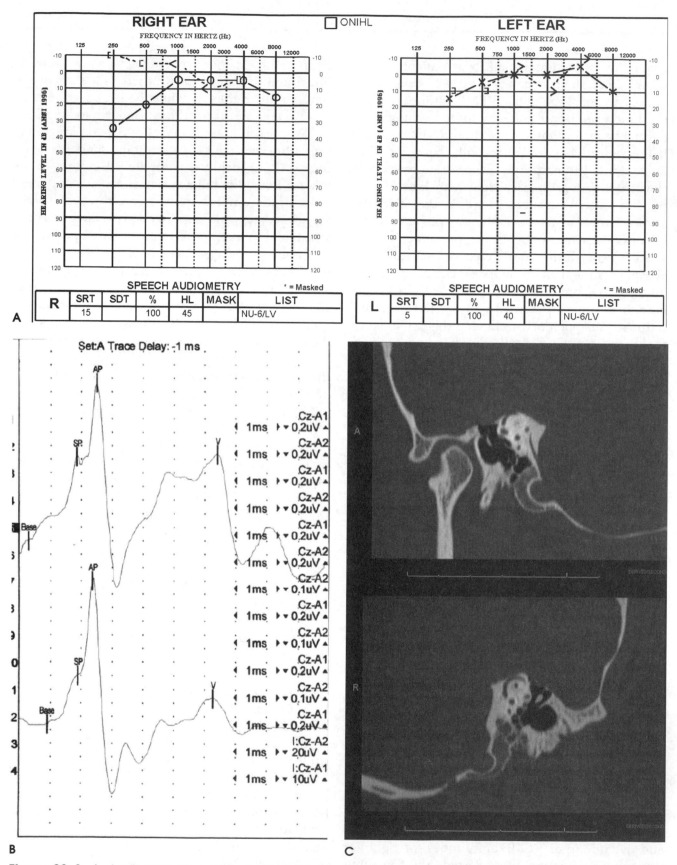

Figure 23-8. A. Audiogram from patient with right-sided SSCD. **B.** ECochG from patient with right-sided SSCD. **C.** CT scans from patient with right-sided SSCD (*top, left side; bottom, right side*). The absence of bone over the right superior canal is evident.

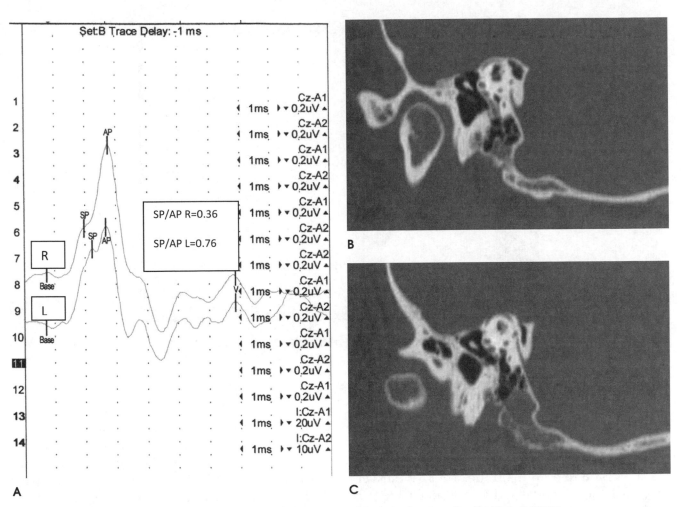

Figure 23–9. **A.** ECochG from patient with left SSCD. **B–C.** CT scans from patient with left SSCD.

It is possible that the presence of a third window contributes to the alteration of hydrodynamic forces within the cochlea, resulting in the aforementioned basilar membrane bias.

The following example serves as a proof of principle for an elevated SP in the presence of a third window. We monitored ECochG continuously during a canal occlusion procedure of the right posterior semicircular canal for benign paroxysmal positional vertigo. Preoperatively, in the absence of endolymphatic hydrops or a third window, this patient presented with a normal SP/AP ratio. Canal occlusion involved an initial exposure of the membranous canal by drilling an opening of the bony posterior semicircular canal, thus creating an artificial third window. As shown in Figure 23–10, as soon as the membranous labyrinth was exposed, the summating potential increased. When the canal occlusion

was complete and the bony defect was restored, the SP returned to its normal, preoperative value. This example does not explain the mechanism of SP elevation any further, but it does confirm that the presence of a third window exposing the membranous labyrinth, contributes to an elevation of the summating potential, and that this phenomenon is reversible when closing the third window.

INTRAOPERATIVE APPLICATIONS OF ELECTROCOCHLEOGRAPHY IN SUPERIOR SEMICIRCULAR CANAL DEHISCENCE REPAIR

Soon after recognizing that superior canal dehiscence was characterized by an SP/AP elevation, we began systematically and consistently monitoring

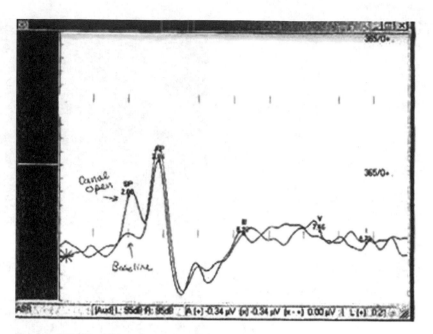
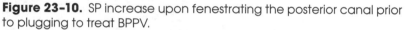

Figure 23–10. SP increase upon fenestrating the posterior canal prior to plugging to treat BPPV.

the ECochG intraoperatively during SSCD repair. In our first four cases we were able to document intraoperative reductions of the SP/AP ratio with the completion of the repair from an abnormally elevated ratio to a normal ratio. Thus, in our very first case, the ratio was reduced from 0.62 to 0.25, the second case from 0.56 to 0.32, the third from 0.84 to 0.36, and the fourth case with a larger SP than AP, the ratio declined from 1.48 to 0.10. Of the next 29 consecutive cases (24 repaired via a middle-fossa approach, and 5 via a transmastoid approach), in 23 cases we documented an intraoperative normalization of the SP/AP ratio which was maintained until the end of the case. In three cases operated via the transmastoid approach, fluid in the middle ear during surgery affected the accuracy of the ECochG; therefore, ECochG was not useful intraoperatively. In three additional cases, the SP/AP ratio initially decreased, and then inexplicably increased gradually following repair. The surgeon inspected the site to ascertain a complete occlusion of the dehiscence, which was confirmed. Therefore, it is not clear what created that late increase in the SP/AP ratio. However, all six cases where the SP/AP ratio was unreliable due to fluid in the middle ear, or those that the SP/AP increased again following repair, the

ratio was normal postoperatively when follow-up ECochG was carried out in the outpatient clinic.

Figure 23–11 illustrates an intraoperative sequence of ECochG during the repair of a superior canal dehiscence. Initial values prior to occlusion for the SP/AP ratio range from 0.86 to 0.68, all considered to be abnormal. At the conclusion of the repair, the ratio normalized to a value ranging from 0.2 to 0.32. This normal value was maintained until the end of the case and confirmed again postoperatively when the ECochG was repeated in the outpatient clinic. It is also of note that following the repair this patient was symptom free.

SUMMARY

ECochG is a useful and effective clinical tool in the evaluation, treatment planning, and treatment effectiveness confirmation in patients with balance disorders. In particular, ECochG is useful in the management of patients suspected of endolymphatic hydrops/Ménière's disease and third window conditions. One of the important properties of ECochG is that it provides ear-specific information, and the

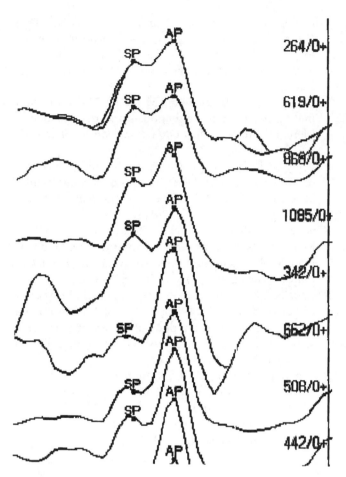

Figure 23-11. ECochG intraoperative monitoring sequence in SSCD repair.

not reaching the tympanic membrane, especially in narrow and in extremely curved ear canals. If the electrode makes contact with the ear canal only, it is no more effective than the ineffective tip-trode. Health-care providers such as audiologists can be effectively trained to carry out this test in an optimal manner; however, this type of training may have to take place postgraduation, as such experience cannot be obtained in most typical audiology training programs. It is important to note that operator skill can greatly influence the quality of the measurement and the efficacy of this diagnostic test.

REFERENCES

Al-Momani, M. O., Ferraro, J. A., Gajewski, B. J., & Ator, G. (2009). Improved sensitivity of electrocochleography in the diagnosis of Meniere's disease. *International Journal of Audiology, 48*(11), 811–819. doi:10.3109/14992020903019338.

American Academy of Otolaryngology-Head and Neck Surgery (AAO-HNS) Committee on Hearing and Equilibrium. (1995). Guidelines for the diagnosis and evaluation of therapy in Meniere's disease. *Otolaryngology-Head and Neck Surgery, 113*, 181–185.

Arts, H. A., Adams, M. E., Telian, S. A., El-Kashlan, H., & Kileny, P. R. (2008). Reversible electrocochleographic abnormalities in superior canal dehiscence. *Otology & Neurotology, 30*(1), 79–86.

Aso, S., Watanabe, Y., & Mizukoshi, K. (1991). A clinical study of electrocochleography in Menière's disease. *Acta Oto-Laryngologica, 111*(1), 44–52.

Coats, A. C. (1981). Summating potential amplitude in Meniere and non-Meniere ears. *Archives of Otolaryngology, 107*(4), 199–208.

Dallos, P. (1976). Cochlear receptor potentials. In R. Ruben (Ed.), *Electrocochleography* (pp. 5–21). Baltimore, MD: University Park Press.

Dauman, R., Aran, J. M., Charlet de Sauvage, R., & Portmann, M. (1988). Clinical significance of the summating potential in Meniere's disease. *American Journal of Otology, 9*(1), 31–38

Davis, H., Deatherage, B. H., Eldredge, D. H., & Smith, C. A. (1958). Summating potentials of the cochlea. *American Journal of Physiology, 195*(2), 251–261.

Eggermont, J. J. (1976). Summating potentials in electrocochleography: Return to hearing disorders. In R. Ruben (Ed.), *Electrocochleography* (pp. 67–89). Baltimore, MD: University Park Press.

results are not affected by the condition of the contralateral ear. As such, ECochG can be useful in determining which side may cause the symptoms related by the patient, in those situations where vestibular testing provides equivocal information regarding the laterality of the lesion. Tympanic ECochG is well suited to both outpatient and intraoperative applications. It is well accepted by patients as it is not uncomfortable, invasive, or traumatic. There is a certain level of technical skill necessary involving manual dexterity, in addition to a good working knowledge of clinical auditory neurophysiology. It is imperative that the tympanic electrode be introduced via microscopic visualization of the ear canal and tympanic membrane. It is unadvisable to introduce the electrode "blindly" into the ear canal: this could result in patient discomfort, and the electrode

Ferraro, J. A. (2010). Electrocochleography: A review of recording approaches, clinical applications and new findings in adults and children. *Journal of the American Academy of Audiology, 21*(3), 145–152.

Ferraro, J., Best, L. G., & Arenberg, I. K. (1983). The use of electrocochleography in the diagnosis, assessment, and monitoring of endolymphatic hydrops. *Otolaryngology Clinics of North America, 16*(1), 69–82.

Guttman, J., & Barrera, S. E. (1934). Persistence of cochlear electrical disturbance on auditory stimulation in the presence of cochlear ganglion degeneration. *American Journal of Physiology, 109*, 704–708.

Jewett, D. L., & Williston, J. S. (1971). Auditory-evoked far fields averaged from the scalp of humans. *Brain, 94*(4), 681–696.

Lempert, J., Wever, E. G., & Lawrence, M. (1947). The cochleogram and its clinical application: A preliminary report. *Archives of Otolaryngology-Head and Neck Surgery, 45*, 61–67.

Margolis, R. H., Rieks, D., Fournier, E. M., & Levine, S. E. (1995). Tympanic electrocochleography for diagnosis of Menière's disease. *Archives of Otolaryngology-Head and Neck Surgery, 121*(1), 44–55.

Merchant, S. N., Rosowski, J. J., & McKenna, M. J. (2007). Superior semicircular canal dehiscence mimicking otosclerotic hearing loss. *Advances in Oto-Rhino-Laryngology, 65*, 137–145.

Minor, L. B., Schessel, D. A., & Carey, J. P. (2004). Ménière's disease [Review]. *Current Opinion in Neurology, 17*(1), 9–16.

Minor, L. B., Solomon, D., Zinreich, J. S., & Zee, D. S. (1998). Sound- and/or pressure-induced vertigo due to bone dehiscence of the superior semicircular canal. *Archives of Otolaryngology-Head & Neck Surgery, 24*(3), 249–258.

Mori, N., Asai, H., & Sakagami, M. (1993). The role of summating potential in the diagnosis and management of Meniere's disease. *Acta Oto-Laryngologica (Stockholm), 501*(Suppl.), 51–53.

Murphy, M. P., & Gates, G. A. (1999). Measuring the effects of Meniere's disease: Results of the Patient-Oriented Severity Index (MD POSI) version 1. *Annals of Otology, Rhinology and Laryngology, 108*(4), 331–337.

Rauch, S. D., Merchant, S. N., & Thedinger, B. A. (1989). Meniere's syndrome and endolymphatic hydrops. Double-blind temporal bone study. *Annals of Otology, Rhinology and Laryngology, 98*(11), 873–883.

Rosowski, J. J., Songer, J. E., Nakajima, H. H., Brinsko, K. M., & Merchant, S. N. (2004). Clinical, experimental and theoretical investigations of the effect of superior semicircular canal dehiscence on hearing mechanisms. *Otology & Neurotology, 25*, 323–332.

Ruben, R. J., Elberling, C., & Salomon, G. (1976). *Electrocochleography.* Baltimore, MD: University Park Press.

Terkildsen, K., Osterhammel, P., & Huis in't Veld, F. (1973). Far field electrocochleography, electrode positions. *Scandinavian Audiology, 2*, 141–148.

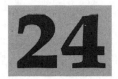

Topological Localization of Vestibular System Impairment[1]

Gary P. Jacobson, Devin L. McCaslin, Erin G. Piker, Jill M. Gruenwald, Sarah L. Grantham, and Lauren L. English

INTRODUCTION

The physiological origins of the common vestibular function measures provide the clinician with a unique opportunity to, in many cases, make statements about (1) if an impairment exists, (2) if one exists, whether the impairment affects the peripheral or central vestibular system, (3) if it is a peripheral impairment, which of the end-organ structures are impaired, (4) if the peripheral impairment is unilateral or bilateral, (5) the degree of impairment, and (6) whether static and/or dynamic compensation has occurred in the wake of the injury.

VESTIBULAR FUNCTION TESTS AND THE STRUCTURES THEY ASSESS

Caloric Test

The electronystagmography/videonystagmography (ENG/VNG) examination culminates in either the monothermal warm or bithermal caloric tests. The caloric test provides a means to assess the physiological integrity of the horizontal semicircular canals and superior vestibular nerves. It should be noted that attempts have been made (Aoki et al., 2009) to extract additional information from the caloric test by tilting the patient's head from midline toward the examiner 45 deg (which activates the posterior semicircular canal following warm caloric irrigation and results in an up-beating nystagmus) and then 45 deg away from midline (which activates the anterior semicircular canal following warm caloric irrigation and results in a down-beating nystagmus). We have had little success with this technique.

cVEMP

It is now well-accepted that the saccule and inferior vestibular nerve represent the peripheral origins of the cervical vestibular-evoked myogenic potential (cVEMP) recorded from the sternocleidomastoid muscle (SCM) in response to high-intensity air-conducted tone-bursts or mechanical stimulation

[1]Portions of this text have been reproduced with permission from the American Academy of Audiology from Jacobson, G. P., McCaslin, D. L., Piker, E. G., Gruenwald, J., Grantham, S. L., and Tegel, L. (2011). Patterns of abnormality in cVEMP, oVEMP, and caloric tests may provide topological information about vestibular impairment. *Journal of the American Academy of Audiology, 22,* 1–11.

(i.e., either vibratory stimulation of the head or skull taps). The cVEMP consists of two primary components that are referred to by their mean latencies of P13 and N23, or, as P1 and N1. The response is present ipsilaterally and represents the electrophysiological manifestation of the vestibulo-collic reflex. This reflex begins in the saccule with afferent connections through the inferior vestibular nerve up to the vestibular nucleus and with efferent connections down through the vestibulospinal tract to the spinal accessory nucleus of cranial nerve XI and finally to the motor neurons of the SCM.

oVEMP

In addition to the cVEMP, it is possible to record a biphasic response from the infraorbital region following stimulation types identical to those used to record the cVEMP. The oVEMP is present bilaterally (i.e., through the vestibulo-ocular reflex [VOR]) but is largest recorded from beneath the contralateral eye when gaze is directed upward (Chihara, Iwasaki, Ushio, & Murofushi, 2007; Iwasaki et al., 2007; Todd, Rosengren, Aw, & Colebatch, 2007). The biphasic response is referred to by its mean latencies of N10 and P15, or, as N1 and P1. Following bone conduction stimulation, the contralateral response is believed to emanate from the inferior oblique muscle following activation of the utricle (Iwasaki et al., 2007; Todd et al., 2007; Welgampola, Migliaccio, Myrie, Minor, & Carey, 2009). The origin of the oVEMP evoked by air-conducted stimuli has been attributed to either saccular afferents only or a combination of saccular and utricular afferents. However, (the following) evidence has suggested that the oVEMP to air conduction stimulation derives its peripheral origins predominately from the utricle and superior vestibular nerve.

1. Saccule receptors are not the only vestibular receptors activated by air conduction. Murofushi and Curthoys (1997) recorded responses from irregular otolith afferents in both the inferior and superior vestibular nerves of guinea pigs in response to air conduction clicks (Murofushi & Curthoys, 1997). Curthoys and Vulovic (2010) presented evidence of neurons sensitive to both air-conduction and bone-conduction stimuli that originated from both the utricular and saccular maculae (Curthoys & Vulovic, 2010). Accordingly, air-conduction stimulation does not selectively activate saccular receptors, as some utricular afferents coursing through the superior vestibular nerve also respond to an air-conducted stimulus.

2. The placement of electrodes below an averted contralateral eye places the inferior oblique muscle in an advantageous position for recording (i.e., superficial to the noninverting electrode). Following peripheral transduction, the utricle routes electrical output to the ipsilateral inferior rectus and contralateral inferior oblique muscles via the VOR. Conversely, the saccule has relatively weak projections to the ocular muscles (Curthoys, 2010). Thus, strategic placement of recording electrodes in the environment of muscles innervated by nerves receiving the electrical output from the utricle predominately is a method of limiting the peripheral sources contributing to the oVEMP response.

3. Perhaps most compelling has been empirical evidence demonstrating that the cVEMP and oVEMP may vary independent of one another in patients with peripheral vestibular system impairments (e.g. Govender et al. 2011). For example, Manzari, Burgess, and Curthoys (2010) presented a case report of a patient with left-sided *inferior* vestibular neuritis. The authors reported that regardless of mode of stimulation (i.e., air- or bone-conducted stimuli), the cVEMP was absent on the ipsilesioned side, whereas the oVEMP response was present and normal bilaterally (Manzari, Burgess, & Curthoys, 2010). Manzari, Tedesco, Burgess, and Curthoys (2010a) then reported a series of patients with *superior* vestibular neuritis who demonstrated an abnormal contralesional oVEMP and bilaterally normal cVEMPs (Manzari et al., 2010a). The patients with a unilaterally abnormal oVEMP (and normal cVEMP) also had a unilateral caloric weakness on the same side. The caloric exam assesses the function of the horizontal semicircular canal (SCC) and the superior vestibular nerve. Accordingly, these results are consistent with the oVEMP response measuring a part of

the peripheral vestibular system akin to what the caloric evaluates (i.e., superior vestibular nerve) and different from what the cVEMP measures (i.e., inferior vestibular nerve). Evidence from patients with Ménière's disease (MD) also lends support to the argument that the cVEMP and oVEMP evaluate independent parts of the peripheral vestibular system. Manzari, Tedesco, Burgess, and Curthoys (2010b) have reported that while the cVEMP is not altered in the early stages of endolymphatic hydrops, the contralesional oVEMP is enhanced (i.e., larger amplitude) (Manzari et al., 2010b).

INNERVATION AND PERFUSION PATTERNS OF THE VESTIBULAR (AND AUDITORY) END ORGAN

Innervation Patterns

The bipolar ganglion cells of the vestibular branch of the CN VIII divide in the internal auditory canal to form the inferior and superior branches (Figure 24–1). The superior vestibular nerve (SNV) sends

the anterior ampullary nerve to innervate the anterior/superior semicircular canal. The superior vestibular nerve (SVN) also sends the horizontal ampullary nerve to innervate the horizontal/lateral semicircular canal. Finally, the SVN sends the utricular nerve to innervate the utricle.

The inferior branch of the vestibular nerve, the inferior vestibular nerve (IVN), sends a saccular nerve to innervate the saccule. Additionally, the IVN innervates the posterior semicircular canal with the posterior ampullary nerve.

Given these innervation patterns, it is possible but not probable to have a discrete injury affecting one or more of the ampullary nerves and/or nerves innervating the otolith end organs. It is far more likely for injury to affect one or both of the branches of the vestibular nerve. For example, an injury affecting the SVN would produce an impairment in nerve conduction from the anterior and horizontal semicircular canals, and the utricle. This would be reflected in abnormal test results for the ipsilesional caloric and oVEMP tests and normal cVEMP test results. Alternately, a lesion affecting the IVN would be expected to produce an abnormal cVEMP test but normal caloric and oVEMP tests.

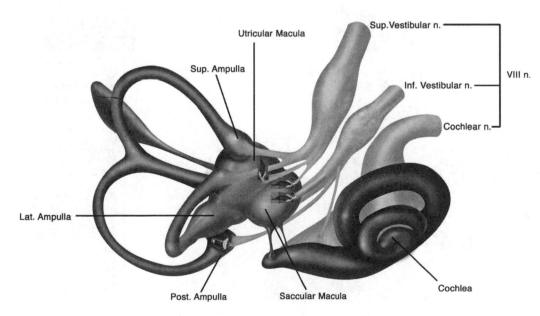

Figure 24–1. Innervation of the peripheral vestibular system. *Sup.* = superior, *Inf.* = inferior, *Lat.* = lateral, *n* = nerve.

Vascular Perfusion Patterns

Perfusion of the labyrinth begins with the major feeder, the basilar artery that sends a branch called the anterior inferior cerebellar artery (AICA) (Figure 24–2). The AICA sends out a branch called the labyrinthine artery and that artery splits to form the common cochlear and anterior vestibular arteries. The common cochlear artery sends out a branch called the vestibulocochlear artery and that splits to form main cochlear and modiolar arteries and the posterior vestibular artery. The main cochlear and modiolar arteries supply blood to the cochlea. The posterior vestibular artery carries blood to the poste-

rior semicircular canal and the saccule. The anterior vestibular artery perfuses the utricle, a small part of the saccule, and the horizontal and anterior semicircular canals.

A loss of blood supply from the AICA or the labyrinthine artery will produce a devastating injury affecting the function of the ipsilesioned membranous labyrinth.

A loss of blood supply from either the common cochlear artery or vestibulocochlear artery will produce a lesion affecting the cochlea, the posterior semicircular canal, and the saccule. This means the patient will show significant sensorineural hearing loss and an abnormal/absent cVEMP on the ipsile-

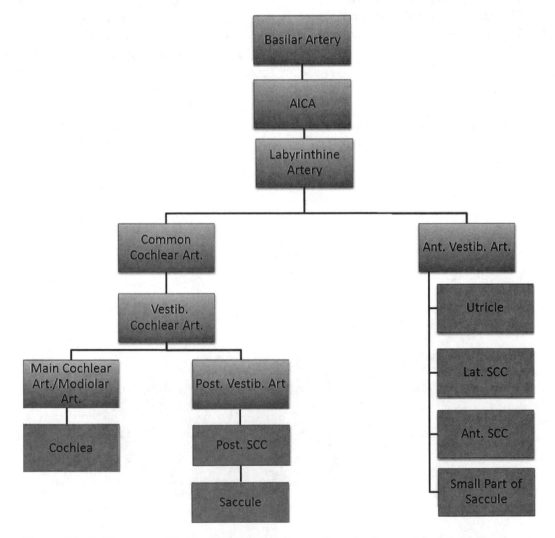

Figure 24–2. Diagram of the vascular perfusion pattern for the peripheral vestibular system. *Art.* = artery, *Lat* = lateral, *Post.* = posterior, *Ant.* = anterior, *SCC* = semicircular canal.

sional side and will be expected to show both normal caloric and oVEMP tests on the ipsilesioned side.

A loss of blood supply from the anterior vestibular artery will produce an injury affecting the ipsilesional utricle and lateral and anterior semicircular canals. Accordingly, this patient would be expected to show unaffected ipsilesional hearing and cVEMP tests and abnormal/absent caloric and oVEMP tests.

A loss of blood flow from the main cochlear artery would produce sudden deafness on the affected side. An isolated injury to the posterior vestibular artery would have no effect on auditory function or the caloric and oVEMP tests but would have an effect on the cVEMP test on the ipsilesioned side.

CASE REPORTS DEMONSTRATING REPRODUCIBLE PATTERNS THAT OCCUR IN CLINICAL DATA

Case 1

For purposes of comparison, Case 1 (Figure 24–3) shows caloric, cVEMP, and oVEMP test results obtained from a patient with bilaterally normal peripheral and central vestibular system function. Figure 24–4 is a summary indicating the absence of peripheral vestibular system impairment.

Case 2

The patient is a 43-year-old male with a previous diagnosis of Ménière's disease on the left side in 1993. In 1995 he underwent a left vestibular nerve section as a definitive procedure. The patient reported vertigo following the nerve section. The patient also reported a history of tinnitus and hearing loss on the left side. He reported that his hearing has become poorer on the left side. Over the past 6 months the patient felt slightly off-balance but denied vertigo, nausea, or vomiting. His medical history was significant for anxiety, ulcerative colitis, and gastroesophageal reflex disease (GERD). His physical examination was unremarkable. A brain MRI was interpreted as normal. Immittance testing showed the patient to have bilaterally normal tympanometry and normal ipsilateral and contralateral acoustic reflex thresholds. An audiometric examination (Figure 24–5) showed the patient to have essentially normal pure tone thresholds on the right side and a mild, flat sensorineural hearing loss on the left side (i.e., the ipsilesional side).

Quantitative vestibular testing (Figure 24–6) showed the patient to have an absent caloric response, absent cVEMP, and an absent oVEMP on the left side (i.e., the side of the vestibular nerve section). The results were consistent with a deafferentation of the superior and inferior vestibular nerves (Figure 24–7).

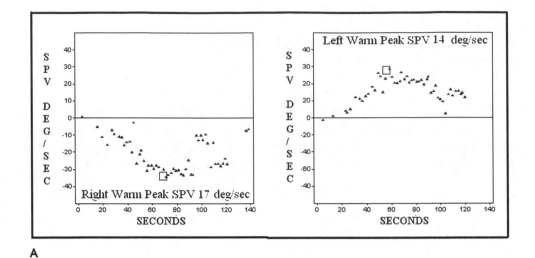

A

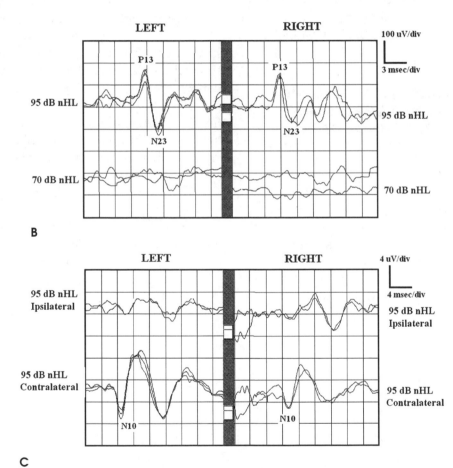

B

C

Figure 24-3. Case 1. **A.** Summary of caloric examination from a patient with bilaterally normal peripheral vestibular system function. The caloric asymmetry was 10% (laboratory upper limit for asymmetry for the monothermal warm caloric test is 25%). **B.** A bilaterally symmetrical cVEMP examination (Right P13 latency 15 ms; Left P13 latency 15 ms; Right P1–N1 amplitude 358.58 µV; Left P1–N1amplitude 224.85 µV). The P1–N1 interaural amplitude asymmetry is 23% (the laboratory normal upper limit is 43%). **C.** A bilaterally symmetrical oVEMP examination (Right N1 latency 10 ms; Left N1 latency 12 ms; Right N1–P1 amplitude 11 µV; Left N1–P1amplitude 8.8 µV). The N1–P1 interaural amplitude asymmetry is 12% (the laboratory normal upper limit is 33%).

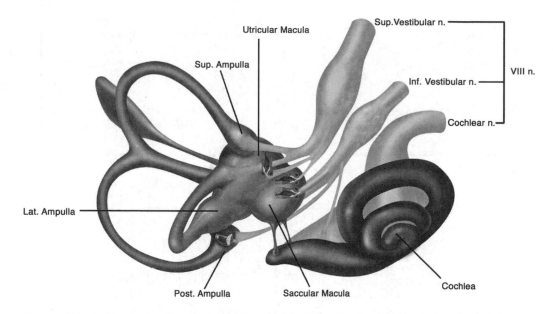

Figure 24-4. Summary figure indicating normal functioning of the lateral semicircular canals, utricle, saccule, and both the inferior and superior vestibular nerves.

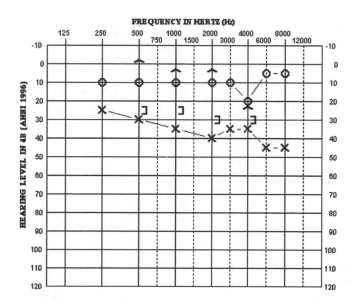

Figure 24-5. Audiometric test results for Case 2.

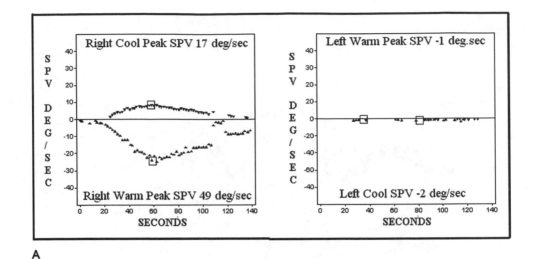

A

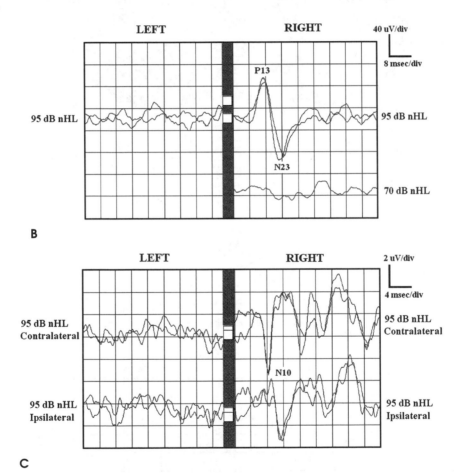

B

C

Figure 24-6. A. Summary of caloric examination from Case 2 who has had a left vestibular neurectomy for intractable vertigo. The caloric asymmetry was 100% on the left side (laboratory upper limit for Alternate Binaural Bithermal Caloric Test asymmetry is 22%). **B.** An abnormal cVEMP examination (Right P1 latency 15 ms; Left P1 latency—absent response; Right P1–N1 amplitude 142 μV; Left P1–N1 amplitude—absent response). The P1 interaural amplitude asymmetry is 100% (the laboratory normal upper limit is 43%). That is, the cVEMP is absent on the left side. **C.** An abnormal oVEMP examination (Right N1 latency 11 ms; Left N1 latency—absent; Right N1–P1 amplitude 7 μV; Left N1–P1—absent). The N1–P1 interaural amplitude asymmetry is 100% (the laboratory normal upper limit is 33%).

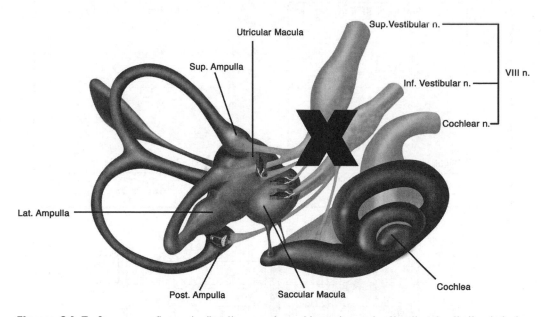

Figure 24-7. Summary figure indicating profound impairment affecting both the inferior and superior vestibular nerves, and/or the entire vestibular membranous labyrinth on the left side.

Case 3

The patient is a 50-year-old female with a 6-week history of persistent true vertigo. The patient stated that the vertigo increased in severity with changes in her head position. The patient also reported a headache history although she did not report a temporal relationship between the headaches and the vertigo. Her medical history was significant only for deep vein thrombosis in the left lower extremity and right upper extremity deep vein thrombosis. Immittance testing showed the patient to have normal tympanometry and ipsilateral and contralateral stapedial reflex thresholds bilaterally. Pure tone audiometry (Figure 24–8) was bilaterally normal with the exception of a notched mild hearing loss at 2000 Hz and 4000 Hz on the left side.

Quantitative vestibular system testing showed the patient to have a significant left-sided caloric asymmetry (43%; Figure 24–9A), a bilaterally symmetrical cVEMP examination (5%; Figure 24–9B) and a significant left-sided oVEMP asymmetry (36%;

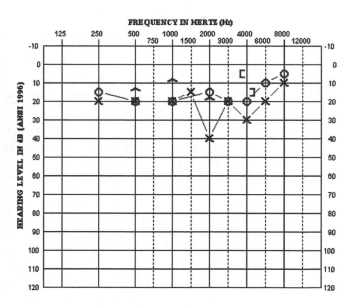

Figure 24-8. Audiometric test results for Case 3.

Figure 24–9C). Collectively the findings suggest a left-sided peripheral vestibular system impairment affecting the superior vestibular nerve (Figure 24–10).

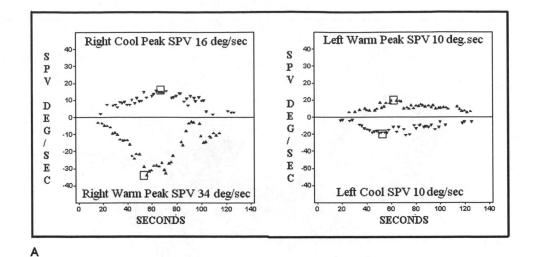

A

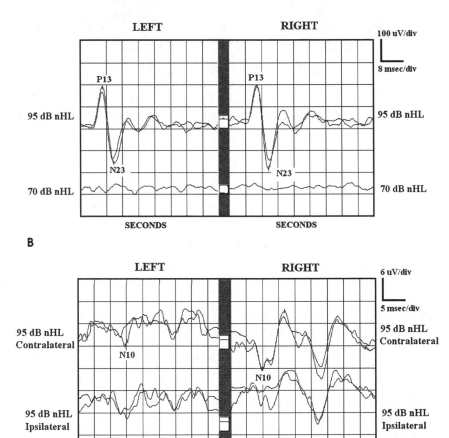

B

C

Figure 24-9. A. Summary of caloric examination from Case 3 who was a patient with a left-sided vestibular peripheral vestibular system impairment affecting the utricle and horizontal semicircular canal, or more likely, the superior vestibular nerve. The caloric asymmetry was 43% on the left side (laboratory upper limit for asymmetry is 22%). **B.** A bilaterally symmetrical cVEMP examination (Right P1 latency 15 ms; Left P1 latency 14 ms; Right P1–N1 amplitude 370 μV; Left P1–N1 amplitude 335 μV). The P1–N1 interaural amplitude asymmetry is 5% (the laboratory normal upper limit is 43%). **C.** An abnormal oVEMP examination on the left side (Right N1 latency 11 ms; Left N1 latency 10; Right N1–P1 amplitude 7 μV; Left N1–P1 3.3 μV). The N1–P1 interaural amplitude asymmetry is 36% (the laboratory normal upper limit is 33%).

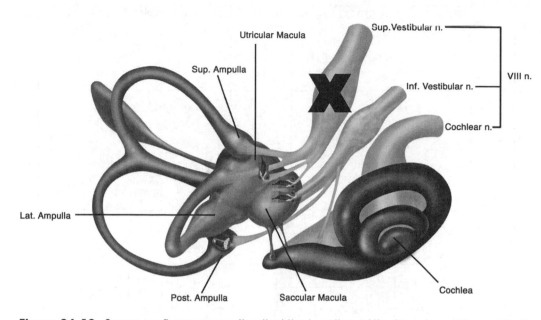

Figure 24–10. Summary figure suggesting that the location of the impairment is most likely at the left superior vestibular nerve.

Case 4

The patient is a 46-year-old female with a diagnosis of left Ménière's disease. She received this diagnosis in 2000. The Ménière's disease began with fluctuant vertigo and hearing loss, fullness, and tinnitus in her left ear. Over the past 10 years she has had spells of vertigo, hearing loss, and tinnitus occurring approximately every 3 months. In the more recent past the spells have occurred one to two times per week. She has been managed conservatively with a low-salt diet, oral vestibular suppressants (diazepam), and transtympanic dexamethasone. The patient reported having had an MRI that was interpreted as normal. An audiometric examination (Figure 24–11) showed the patient to have an asymmetrical sensorineural hearing loss. The impairment affected the high frequencies on the right side and was moderate in degree. On the left side the hearing loss was flat and moderate in degree. The patient demonstrated normal tympanometry and normal ipsilateral and contralateral acoustic reflex thresholds bilaterally.

Quantitative vestibular system testing showed the patient to have symmetrical caloric responses (16%), an abnormally small cVEMP on the left side

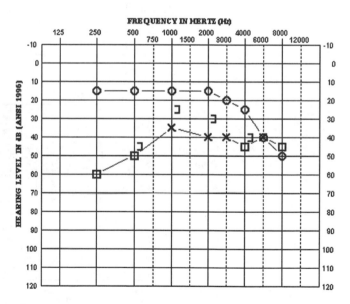

Figure 24–11. Audiometric test results for Case 4.

(50%), and bilaterally symmetrical oVEMPs (8%; Figure 24–12). Collectively the findings suggested a left-sided peripheral vestibular system impairment affecting the saccule and/or the inferior vestibular nerve (Figure 24–13).

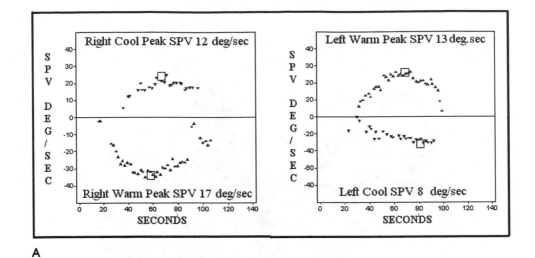

A

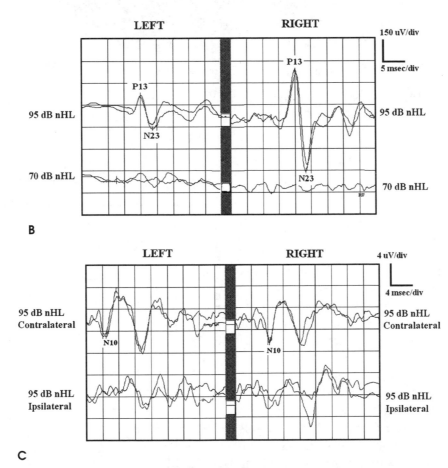

B

C

Figure 24–12. A. Summary of caloric examination from Case 4 who had a peripheral vestibular system impairment affecting the saccule and/or inferior vestibular nerve. The patient demonstrated a bilaterally symmetrical caloric examination. The caloric asymmetry was 16% (laboratory upper limit for asymmetry is 22%). **B.** An abnormal cVEMP examination (Right P1 latency 15 ms; Left P1 latency 17 ms; Right P1–N1 amplitude 725 µV; Left P1–N1 amplitude 240 µV). The P1–N1 interaural amplitude asymmetry is 50% (the laboratory normal upper limit is 43%). That is, the cVEMP was reduced in amplitude on the left side. **C.** A bilaterally symmetrical oVEMP examination (Right N1 latency 11 ms; Left N1 latency 9 ms; Right N1–P1 amplitude 8 µV; Left N1–P1 amplitude 6.8 µV). The N1–P1 interaural amplitude asymmetry was 8% (the laboratory normal upper limit is 33%).

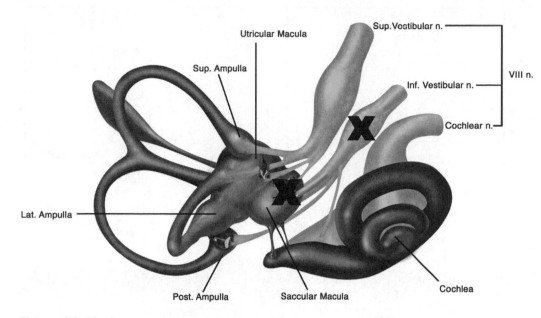

Figure 24-13. Summary figure suggesting the presence of an impairment affecting the inferior vestibular nerve and/or the saccule.

OTHER DIAGNOSTIC PATTERNS THAT HAVE BEEN DESCRIBED

Case 5

This patient demonstrates a 68% right unilateral weakness (Figure 24–14A). However, the cVEMP examination is bilaterally normal (Figure 24–14B) as is the oVEMP examination (Figure 24–14C). Taken together the results suggest that the saccule and inferior vestibular nerve are functioning normally. Additionally, the superior vestibular nerves are functioning normally (i.e., the oVEMPs are normal). The sole aberration is the asymmetric caloric responses suggesting an impairment affecting the right horizontal semicircular canal (Figure 24–15).

Case 6

This patient shows a symmetrical (i.e., a 5% asymmetry) monothermal warm caloric examination (Figure 24–16A). Additionally, the patient's cVEMP test is bilaterally normal (e.g., there is a 2% amplitude asymmetry; Figure 24–16B). Last, the oVEMP examination reveals a 47% amplitude asymmetry which is abnormal (Figure 24–16C). In total, the normal cVEMP suggests that both saccule and inferior vestibular nerve function are bilaterally normal. The normal caloric test tells us that the horizontal semicircular canal cristae are functioning normally as is the superior division of the vestibular nerve. In this example the abnormal right oVEMP examination suggests a selective impairment of the right utricle (Figure 24–17).

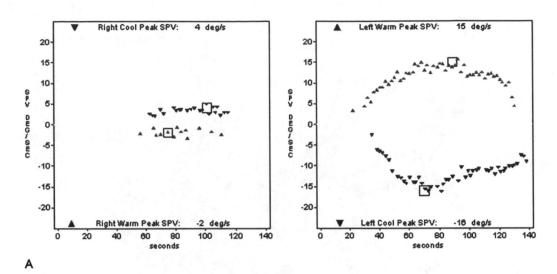

A

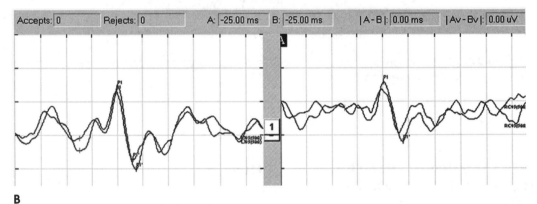

B

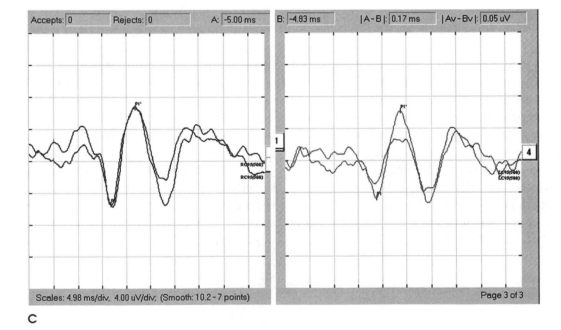

C

Figure 24-14. A. Caloric examination summary figure for Case 5 showing a 68% right unilateral weakness. **B.** Symmetrical cVEMP and **C.** oVEMP latencies and amplitudes.

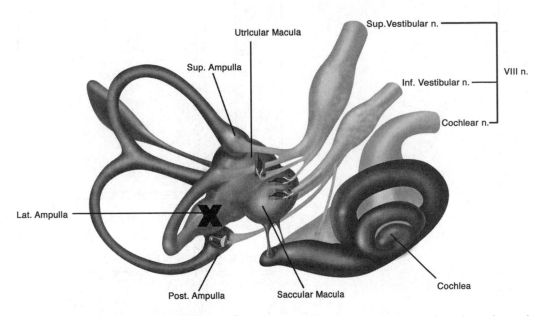

Figure 24-15. Summary figure for Case 5 suggesting the presence of an impairment affecting the right lateral semicircular canal in isolation.

SUMMARY

The six patterns discussed herein that have been summarized in Table 24–1, are those that are encountered most commonly and illustrate the test results observed for the largest number of peripheral impairments. There is one final pattern that we have identified that occurs infrequently. That is, an absent cVEMP in a patient with a normal caloric test and a normal oVEMP but who has a posterior semicircular canal canalithiasis on the same side as the absent

cVEMP might suggest an isolated injury to the saccule since a patient with an inferior vestibular nerve impairment should not be capable of demonstrating BPPV affecting the posterior semicircular canal.

As of the time of this writing there is cautious optimism that the video head impulse test (i.e., vHIT) will add additional power to our ability to localize the site or sites of injury to the peripheral vestibular system (see Chapter 16). This technique should give us the ability to identify patients with lesions affecting individual canals and otolith end organs when combined with caloric and VEMP tests.

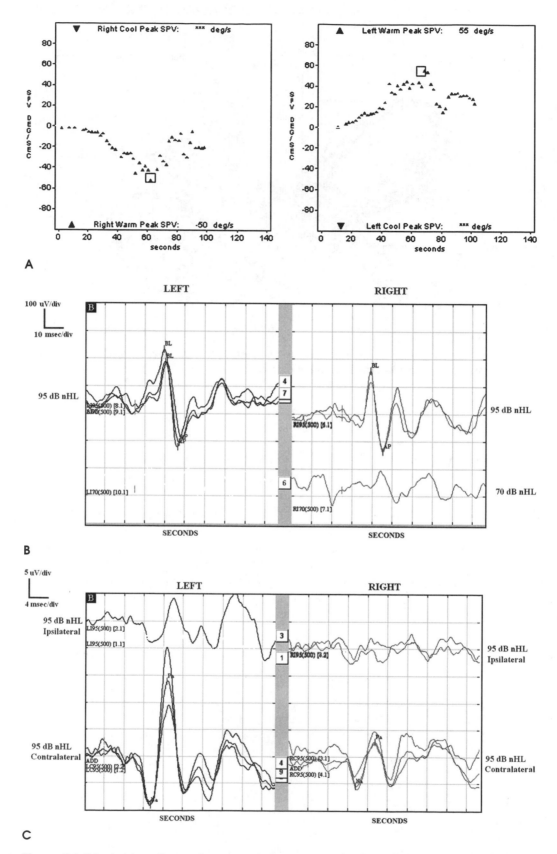

Figure 24–16. **A.** Monothermal warm caloric summary for Case 6 showing a normal result (i.e., 5% asymmetry). **B.** Normal cVEMP test. **C.** The 47% right asymmetry on oVEMP testing.

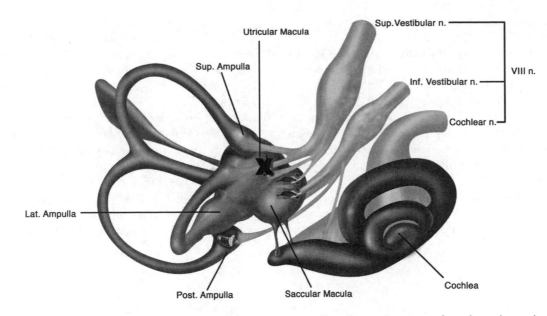

Figure 24–17. Summary figure for Case 6 suggesting the presence of an impairment affecting the right utricle.

Table 24–1. Summary of the Patterns of Abnormality (and Clinical Significance of the Patterns) That Are Most Frequently Observed in a Tertiary Care Otology/Neurotology Clinic

Type	Caloric	cVEMP	oVEMP	Impairment
1	Normal	Normal	Normal	None
2	Abnormal	Abnormal	Abnormal	Entire end organ, or superior and inferior vestibular nerve
3	Normal	Abnormal	Normal	Saccule or inferior vestibular nerve
4	Abnormal	Normal	Abnormal	Superior vestibular nerve and/or lateral semicircular canal and utricle
5	Abnormal	Normal	Normal	Lateral semicircular canal
6	Normal	Normal	Abnormal	Utricle

REFERENCES

Aoki, S., Arai, Y., Yoda, K., & Nishida S. (2009). A head-tilt caloric test for evaluating the vertical semicircular canal function. *Acta Oto-laryngologica, 129*(11), 1226–1231.

Chihara, Y., Iwasaki, S., Ushio, M., & Murofushi, T. (2007). Vestibular-evoked extraocular potentials by air-conducted sound: Another clinical test for vestibular function. *Clinical Neurophysiology, 118*(12), 2745–2751.

Curthoys, I. S. (2010). A critical review of the neurophysiological evidence underlying clinical vestibular testing using sound, vibration and galvanic stimuli. *Clinical Neurophysiology, 121*(2), 132–144.

Curthoys, I. S., & Vulovic, V. (2010). Vestibular primary afferent responses to sound and vibration in the guinea pig. *Experimental Brain Research, 210*(3–4), 347–352.

Govender, S., Rosengren, S. M., & Colebatch, J. G. (2011). Vestibular neuritis has selective effects on air- and bone-conducted cervical and ocular vestibular evoked myogenic potentials. *Clinical Neurophysiology. 122*(6), 1246–1255.

Iwasaki, S., McGarvie, L. A., Halmagyi, G. M., Burgess, A. M., Kim, J., Colebatch, J. G., & Curthoys, I. S. (2007).

Head taps evoke a crossed vestibulo-ocular reflex. *Neurology, 68*(15), 1227–1229.

Manzari, L., Burgess, A. M., & Curthoys, I. S. (2010). Dissociation between cVEMP and oVEMP responses: Different vestibular origins of each VEMP? *European Archives of Oto-Rhino-Laryngology, 267*(9), 1487–1489.

Manzari, L., Tedesco, A., Burgess, A. M., & Curthoys, I. S. (2010a). Ocular vestibular-evoked myogenic potentials to bone-conducted vibration in superior vestibular neuritis show utricular function. *Otolaryngology-Head and Neck Surgery, 143*(2), 274–280.

Manzari, L., Tedesco, A. R., Burgess, A. M., & Curthoys, I. S. (2010b). Ocular and cervical vestibular-evoked myogenic potentials to bone conducted vibration in Meniere's disease during quiescence vs. during acute attacks. *Clinical Neurophysiology, 121*(7), 1092–1101.

Murofushi, T., & Curthoys, I. S. (1997). Physiological and anatomical study of click-sensitive primary vestibular afferents in the guinea pig. *Acta Oto-Laryngologica, 117*(1), 66–72.

Todd, N. P., Rosengren, S. M., Aw, S. T., & Colebatch, J. G. (2007). Ocular vestibular evoked myogenic potentials (OVEMPs) produced by air- and bone-conducted sound. *Clinical Neurophysiology, 118*(2), 381–390.

Welgampola, M. S., Migliaccio, A. A., Myrie, O. A., Minor, L. B., & Carey, J. P. (2009). The human sound-evoked vestibulo-ocular reflex and its electromyographic correlate. *Clinical Neurophysiology, 120*(1), 158–166.

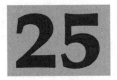

Pediatric Vestibular Testing

Kristen Janky and Neil T. Shepard

INTRODUCTION

Presented in this chapter are techniques and interpretation of the results for assessing children with problems of dizziness and balance dysfunction. First, there is a need to define what is meant by a child —when are the testing and interpretations of vestibular and balance function assessment for the adult appropriately applicable to "a child"? This question could be addressed by age alone, but it seems logical that the approach should be by the maturational status of the underlying peripheral sensory end organs and the neurological substrate that needs to respond to the inputs from the sensory end organs. Using this premise we would define the need for an alternative approach for testing and alternative normative data at different ages for the child.

The peripheral vestibular system is anatomically fully developed at birth. Physiologically the vestibulo-ocular reflex (VOR) functions at a level similar to the adult, but there is evidence to suggest that there is a maturational effect of the VOR and may require age-appropriate normative ranges (see the discussion below on use of Rotary Chair in the laboratory testing section). This is, however, not the case for the visual system's ability to capture small targets via saccades or track targets in a smooth manner. The performance of these tasks is not well developed for smooth pursuit or saccades until upward of 4 to 6 months (Jacobs, Harris, Shawkat, & Taylor, 1997; Von Hofsten & Rosander, 1997) with the ability to attend to large moving targets in repeated tracking manner (optokinetic nystagmus) seen by 2 to 4 months (Valmaggia et al., 2004). However, all of these tasks are estimated to not have full adult development until much later—OKN about 4 years (Valmaggia et al., 2004) and smooth pursuit up to preadolescence (Katsanis, Iacono, & Harris, 1998; Tajik-Parvinchi, Lillakas, Irving, & Steinbach, 2003). Therefore, saccade tasks and smooth pursuit tracking tasks with typical small targets are not acceptable for use in the child under age 6 months with the use of adult normative ranges; age-specific normative ranges are needed (Mezzalira, Neves, Maudonnet, Bilecki, & de Avila, 2005; Valmaggia et al., 2004). Optokinetic (OKN) stimuli can be used for the very young child with a sinusoidal protocol as a substitute for smooth pursuit (see discussion in Chapters 9 and 10 on OKN and its dominance by smooth pursuit), yet the normative data range does not match that of the adult until after age 4 (Valmaggia et al., 2004). The ability of the child to maintain quiet stance in an adult-like manner is fully developed between 7 and 10 years of age (Forssberg & Nashner, 1982; Woollacott, Debu, & Mowatt, 1987). Therefore, adult normative data for postural control and gait tasks are not applicable to the child until pre-teen to mid-teen years.

Interestingly, even though the peripheral vestibular system and the visual systems are fully functional at the adult level early in development (< age 24 months), the change in the strategy for use of these cues from a child set of rules to the adult integrated set of internal rules occurs slowly between

3 and 6 years of age and is not considered complete until age 7.5 to 8 (Frossberg & Nashner, 1982). These changes in the use of visual, proprioceptive/somatosensory and vestibular cues for maintaining upright stance are parallel with the changes in linguistic and syntactic child rules to the adult rules over the same ages. Therefore, although the VOR can be evaluated at birth by rotary chair and caloric tests and saccade and smooth pursuit tasks by age 4 years, all with expected adult normative ranges, the complexity for evaluating integrated postural control assessment by the adult normative ranges needs to wait until age 15. Yet, the same tools for this task such as dynamic posturography and other developmental assessments specific to balance and ambulation are applicable to children from age 3, but this normative range specific to the age of the child is different from that of the adult (Christy, Payne, Azuero, & Formby, 2014; Rine, 2007). For all of the assessment tools for the peripheral and central vestibular system, and those for postural control, modifications in the testing protocol are needed to make the tests of interest to young child (<7) similar to the modifications used for the evaluation of hearing for this same age group. For the young child one must remember that the next test that you acquire may well be the last test you are going to get. Therefore, not only is the test used of importance but so is selecting what evaluations are going to be used which must be given some thought for each child seen. The concept of planning the evaluation of the child will be discussed in more detail below.

We now turn our attention to the estimates of incidence of vestibular and balance and gait abnormalities in children 15 years of age and younger. Because of the inescapable anatomical and physiological relationship between the auditory and peripheral vestibular systems, and the better-documented information on hearing loss, we use hearing loss in children 15 and under as an index for discussion of the incidence of problems with balance and dizziness.

Incidence of Vestibular and Balance Problems in Children

As a reference point the incidence of hearing loss in children 6 to 19 years of age is estimated through the third National Health and Nutrition examination survey. This survey from the years of 1988 to 1994 gives an incidence of 14.9% of children who have a slight or greater loss of hearing defined as 16 dB HL or greater loss. The majority of the loss was determined to be unilateral (Niskar et al., 1998). In contrast there is not a nationwide estimate of the incidence of vestibular and balance problems in children partly because it is felt to be uncommon and because of the difficulty of verifying the issue of a vestibular deficit in children under age 3 without extensive evaluations and expensive equipment. There are, however, isolated studies that have tried to provide estimates of dizziness in specific groups of children (e.g., in 10-year-olds, suggesting a prevalence of 5.7%) (Humphriss & Hall, 2011). In an extensive retrospective study of a pediatric health system over a 4-year interval (O'Reilly et al., 2010), records were searched for encounters related to ICD-9 codes related to balance disorders. This resulted in over 550,000 individual entries. These were then searched for chief complaints related to balance and other otologic/neuro-otologic diagnoses. Out of the total patients, 1.03% had primary complaint related to balance issues. Out of this group 35.8% were diagnosed with a vestibular disorder; 38% with peripheral, and 21% with central vestibular disorders. They went on to calculate the odds ratio of syncope and found that to be 21 times higher in the patients with unspecified dizziness than in the general pediatric population. Also the odds ratio was 43 times higher for simultaneous presence of sensorineural hearing loss in those with peripheral vestibular disorders than in the general pediatric group. In the group with central vestibular disorders, the odds ratio of headache complaints was 16 times higher than in the general pediatric group.

In a recent systematic review with meta-analysis, the prevalence and diagnosis of vestibular disorders in children were reviewed (Gioacchini, Alicandri-Ciufelli, Kaleci, & Re, 2014). Of the 10 articles they identified for the review, the total number of children was 724. Of the overall group the most common forms of dizziness were vestibular migraine (27.82%), benign paroxysmal vertigo of childhood (15.68%), and vestibular neuritis (9.81%) with head trauma as the third most common cause of vertigo at 14%.

From these studies it is clear that there is a common association with hearing loss and headaches in children with dizziness. These figures also suggest that the general occurrence of dizziness in children is approximately that of adults, but there is a difference in the frequency of presentation of the various forms of dizziness (Agrawal, Carey, Della Santina, Schubert, & Monor, 2009; Kerber, Meurer, West, & Fendrick, 2008).

DEVELOPMENT OF THE VESTIBULAR AND BALANCE SYSTEMS— A GUIDE TO EVALUATION

Anatomically, the vestibular system is fully developed at birth; however, maturation of our overall ability to maintain "balance" is thought to continue until the age of 12 to 15 years. Balance function is attained with information from the visual, vestibular, and proprioceptive (awareness and perception of our body in space) systems. Each of these three systems has an important role in the maintenance of overall balance. Therefore, the maturation process includes integration of information from these three systems and is reflected in the attainment of gross motor milestones (i.e., the ability to sit, stand, walk, crawl, run, and jump) as well as the integration of this information for everyday ambulation and postural control. Pediatric assessments differ from those for adults because these systems are at various stages of development in children. Understanding this maturation process can be helpful in interpreting tests of vestibular function as well as the normal variation in gross motor milestone development and postural control. As discussed below, when vestibular loss occurs, it can cause a significant disruption in the timeliness of this maturation process.

The vestibular system is responsible for initiating three important reflexes in the maintenance of overall balance: the vestibulo-ocular reflex (VOR), the vestibulo-colic reflex (VCR), and the vestibulospinal reflex (VSR). These reflexes are responsible for stabilizing the eyes during head movement, the head during body movement, and the body for postural control. Each of these reflexes is explained below as well as the specific clinical tests that are used to assess these reflex pathways.

Vestibulo-Ocular Reflex (VOR)

The primary goal of the vestibular system is to maintain steady vision during head movement. The mechanism by which the vestibular system maintains this goal is the VOR. With the VOR, the vestibular system detects velocity of head movement and initiates an equal and opposite movement of the eyes. Specifically, the semicircular canals (horizontal, anterior, and posterior) are responsible for detecting angular accelerations (i.e., moving the head "yes" or "no"), while the otolith organs (utricle and saccule) detect linear accelerations (i.e., accelerating in a car or airplane). In response to these types of movements, the VOR is responsible for keeping visual targets on the fovea of the retina, where the sensitivity of the eye is the greatest.

The VOR is typically responsible for maintaining clear vision in response to head movements that exceed approximately 100 deg/s. When head movements are slower than that, or when the head is still, the visual, or ocular motor system, helps maintain images on the fovea of the retina. The three primary reflexive eye movements that help achieve this goal are smooth pursuit, saccade, and optokinetic eye movements. For example, the smooth pursuit system is responsible for maintaining clear vision during head movements and is able to track visual targets moving up to approximately 100 deg/s, after which the VOR takes over. Studies involving the VOR suggest that this pathway reaches maturity in the first 6 to 12 months of life, while the ocular motor system matures at a slower pace. Examinations of the VOR include the video head impulse test (vHIT), rotary chair, ocular vestibular-evoked myogenic potential (VEMP), and caloric test, while the ocular motor exam is used to assess the visual system.

Vestibulo-Colic Reflex (VCR)

The primary goal of the vestibulo-colic reflex is to stabilize the head during body movement. Information from the vestibular system is utilized to relax and contract muscles in the neck to keep the head upright. Evidence of the vestibular system's role in stabilizing head is that children with significant vestibular loss are delayed in the age they gain head control (Inoue et al., 2013). Examinations of the VCR include the cervical VEMP. The cervical VEMP utilizes this pathway in that when stimulating the saccule with an acoustic stimulus, we measure a release from the contracted sternocleidomastoid (SCM) muscle in the neck.

Vestibulo-Spinal Reflex (VSR)— General Postural Control

The primary goal of the vestibulo-spinal reflex (VSR) is to stabilize the body for postural control. This system is somewhat more complex as it involves a larger number of connections to muscles throughout the body (i.e., the arms, hands, legs, feet, etc.). There are three primary tracts that make up the VSR: lateral vestibulospinal, medial vestibulospinal, and reticulospinal. Given the strategy changes discussed below, this system is not considered mature until ages 12 to 15 years. Examinations of the VSR include assessments of postural control, such as the Sensory Organization Test (SOT) or tests of gross motor development.

Gross Motor Developmental Norms and Their Predictability of Peripheral/Central Vestibular Loss

Gross motor developmental delay has been observed in children with hearing loss. In infancy, the presence of vestibular loss has been shown to significantly affect the attainment of gross motor milestones (Abadie et al., 2000; Inoue et al., 2013; Kaga, 1999; Kaga, Shinjo, Jin, & Takegoshi, 2008), meaning children with vestibular loss have been documented to hold their head upright, then sit, stand, walk, and crawl later than their age-matched, normal developing peers. This delay is even greater when coupled with cognitive impairment (Kaga, 1999). Although typically developing children sit, stand, walk, and crawl at 6 to 8 months, 10 to 11 months, and 10 to 12 months, respectively, children with vestibular loss can sit as late 8 to 18 months, stand by 9 to 20 months, and walk independently at 12 to 33 months (Kaga,1999).

Few studies exist examining the relationship between degree of vestibular loss and degree of gross motor delay, but there does appear to be a relationship. Abadie et al. (2000) reported that in 17 children diagnosed with coloboma-heart-atresia-genital-ear (CHARGE) syndrome, all children had some degree of vestibular loss and achieved their motor milestones later than normal developing peers (mean age): holding head steady (6.8 months), stable sitting (14 months), standing supported (19.8 months), standing unsupported (23.9 months),

and walking indoors (29.8 months). When ranked according to degree of vestibular loss, children with greater vestibular loss achieved motor milestones later than those with less severe vestibular loss (Abadie et al., 2000). In a retrospective chart review (unpublished data), parents were more likely to report gross motor developmental delay in children with documented bilateral vestibular loss on rotary chair than in children with normal rotary chair findings. Although sensitivity and specificity values do not exist for the predictability of gross motor delay and vestibular loss, these preliminary data suggest that some degree of a relationship exists; however, additional data are needed from children with varying etiologies and degrees of vestibular and hearing loss. The presence of this relationship would suggest that parents be questioned on the attainment of gross motor milestones, and vestibular loss should be suspected if gross motor delay exists, particularly when coupled with hearing loss.

Evidence is emerging regarding the relative contribution of the otolith organs in the development of postural control. In typically developing infants, preliminary evidence suggests that the otoliths undergo changes during development, which correlate with walking (Wiener-Vacher, Toupet, & Narcy, 1996). With the ability to assess otolith function via vestibular-evoked myogenic potentials (VEMP, described below), infants with absent VEMP responses have been reported to walk later than those with present VEMP (Inoue et al., 2013). Likewise, older children with residual otolith function (present cervical VEMP) are reported to have better static balance than those without otolith function (absent cervical VEMP) (De Kegel, Maes, Baetens, Dhooge, & Van, 2012; Jafari & Asad, 2011; Shall, 2009). It should be noted, however, that this relationship has not always been consistently observed (Cushing, Papsin, Rutka, James, & Gordon, 2008b). These findings are preliminary, and other factors, such as overall degree of vestibular system loss, should also be considered.

Although children with vestibular loss do eventually meet their motor milestones, developmental delays can persist as the child gets older. Some speculate that gross motor developmental delay as a result of vestibular loss can be naturally overcome in children due to the large degree of plasticity in the developing brain (Kaga et al., 2008); however, in some children gross motor delay has been found to be persistent or even progressive, suggesting that plasticity is not enough (Rine et al., 2000, 2004). In older children, gross motor developmental delays have been documented on standardized tests of motor proficiency, such as the Bruininks-Oseretsky Test of Motor Proficiency II (BOT-2), and balance dysfunction has been documented on the Sensory Organization Test (SOT). Abnormalities on these tests have been found to be a positive predictor for the presence of vestibular loss (Brookhouser, Cyr, & Beauchaine, 1982; Cushing et al., 2008a, 2008b, 2009; De Kegel et al., 2012). Poor motor performance has been documented in children with both unilateral and bilateral vestibular loss (DeKegel et al., 2012).

Strategy Changes With Development

Visual, vestibular, and proprioceptive information must be adequately integrated in order to maintain balance and postural control. During development, the *effective use* of each of these systems changes as children transition to adult-like strategies. Children tend to be more dominant on their visual system in the early years. Utilizing the SOT, which is described in more detail below, children have demonstrated adequate use of somatosensory information between 4 and 6 years of age; however, they are not able to adequately use vision or vestibular information for postural control (Charpiot, Tringali, Ionescu, Vital-Durand, & Ferber-Viart, 2010; Hirabayashi & Iwasaki, 1995; Rine, Rubish, & Feeney, 1998). Hirabayashi and Iwasaki (1995) report that by age 14 to 15, utilization of visual information is adult-like; however, the effective use of vestibular information is still continuing to mature. There is some disagreement on the exact time frame children are able mimic adult-like strategies, but this transition is thought to occur by age 12 to 15 years (Peterka & Black, 1990; Peterson, Christou, & Rosengren, 2006). Regardless of the exact time frames, these findings collectively suggest that there is continued maturation of sensory integration (Casselbrant et al., 2010; Charpiot et al., 2010; Hirabayashi & Iwasaki, 1995; Rine et al., 1998). It can take up to ages 10 to 15 for final refinement, but the basics of use of the adult strategies for using the three inputs and an adult-weighted manner emerge around ages 7 to 8 (Forssberg & Nashner, 1982).

VESTIBULAR EVALUATION OF THE CHILD

As stated above, planning the evaluation can be more important in the young child under age 5 than the older child or adult. Where we would have a similar routine with the older child and adult that we would proceed through, this is not the case with the younger child. One needs to remember that the evaluation may be more than a 1-day process, especially for the very young child under 2 years of age or the infant. For this very young age group, the next result you obtain may well be the last one you are going to get on that day. Since it is possible that the child may have to return the next day for completion of testing or would need to return in 6 to 12 months as they are older and can participate in more evaluative studies, you do not want to leave a memory in the child of a bad experience. Therefore, if the child becomes fussy and clearly does not wish to continue to participate, then it is time to stop. As with hearing evaluations in very young children, the tasks performed need to keep the child's attention and be made age appropriate for the child—made fun if possible. Whereas with older children and adults we will repeat some of the testing multiple times for best performance, this is not possible with the young child. You typically get a single opportunity for obtaining data from a test being performed. Therefore, if the dominant complaints from the parents/child by observation are related to gait difficulties and unsteadiness, we would start the evaluation with a very brief review of possible bilateral peripheral vestibular hypofunction via head thrust test. If negative, then move onto evaluations of gait and postural control and then come back to further evaluation of the VOR system. If a quick screen for unilateral or bilateral peripheral involvement or the primary complaint is interpreted to imply episodic events of vertigo, move first to the evaluation of the VOR and then on to gait and balance evaluation.

The child with persistent verbal or action complaints related to balance or the possible onset of vertigo event as witnessed by abnormal eye movement or the child suddenly stopping playing and sitting quietly are felt to be in need of a formal office and laboratory evaluation. The child who has short duration symptoms that are not repeated over time may do well with the direct office evaluation and the interview of the child and parents for determination of what had occurred.

History and Clinical Presentation

The following information is needed to assist in the determination of the possible etiology of the balance or vestibular disorder:

- Are the symptoms episodic or of a more persistent nature?
- Do the symptoms seem to represent a sensation of movement of the child's environment or of the child within the environment?
- If the symptoms are episodic, how frequently do they occur?
- If episodic how long do the symptom last for a given episode or given exacerbation in constant background symptoms?
- Is there a history of childhood diseases since birth, disorders of the mother during pregnancy, or any problems during or shortly after the birth process?
- Are there any known or suspected hearing loss issues?

The above information for the nonverbal child will clearly need to be obtained from the parent. The details of the sensations, whether in spells, duration of the spells, and frequency, may be difficult to obtain. However, it is worth the investment in time as many times asking questions about the child's general behavior, playing activities, and child's avoidances (such as heights) can come together in a picture of what may be happening as the parents reflect on what they have observed. This also gives the child time to play in your presence to start to become familiar with you and the surroundings.

As the child starts to be able to verbalize, engaging the child in helping to better define the above information, especially that of the sensation the child feels can be very useful. Be careful not to lead the child as to what you are looking for in an answer. Then find several ways to get the same information to see if the responses are consistent. As the child gets up to 2 to 4 years of age, some can be very specific as to what it is they are experiencing. As you

can engage the child, it is helpful in the interview so the child is not left out of the discussion and the discussion is not just about and around the child but includes the child. As the child is older the questions can start to be focused to give information that would be more specific to the disorders that could be occurring based on what causes for dizziness are the most common (discussed below).

Direct Office Examination

The office examination can be useful for the child of any age. The older the child, the more aspects of the examination can be used, and the more reliable are the findings. Very little in the way of equipment is needed for the basic office examination, but having a clown nose, stickers, or other child toys can be quite useful to attract and hold the child's attention during the task at hand.

Infant Through Start of Independent Walking

The following elements would be included in the typical office examination:

- Head thrust test—the infant/child on the parent's lap facing the clinician. This is where having a sticker on the forehead or nose of the clinician can be very helpful.
- Pursuit tracking—using a large sticker, see if the child will follow the movement. This ability may not be developed if the child is under 4 months of age.
- Saccade testing— using two large and different stickers or finger puppets, have one pop up to the left and then as it disappears have the other pop up to the right. If the child's head is free you would need to watch for the eye movement first and then the head. If the child will tolerate a gentle hold of the chin by the parent, then watch for the eye saccade movement. Again at ages under 2 to 3 months, the child may be involved in a searching behavior with the eyes before capturing the target.
- Optokinetic nystagmus—for the child under 4 months who may not be able to perform pursuit, this could be an alternative to dem-

onstrate pursuit ability (see discussion in the introduction). For this have a strip of cloth with repeating stickers that can be drawn slowly across the child's visual field, and if the nystagmus can be generated this would be a good indicator of gross ability of smooth pursuit. If no nystagmus can be generated, nothing can be decided from a negative result.

- Rotational chair—for this the child needs to sit on the examiner's lap facing the examiner. The examiner is in a swivel office chair. Without any visually attracting target, just the examiner's face, the chair is oscillated back and forth looking for nystagmus. It is important that the child's eyes be on the examiner and not looking elsewhere to avoid optokinetic stimulation. At the young ages in this group the visual fixation suppression system is not well developed so you can typically see nystagmus unless they have significant bilateral hypofunction.

Child Walking Independently

For this age grouping typically about 18 months or over, the same elements in the direct examination given for the younger child above would still be included. The variations would be that smaller objects could be used for pursuit, and saccade testing and the rotary chair evaluation would now not be used in office format. For the child at 6 years of age or older, then the same activities would be used as in the adult but several other office examination activities can be added that have reasonable predictability for what would occur in the formal laboratory tests discussed below—the interested reader is referred to the recent work by Christy et al. (2014).

For the child 18 months or over, we would vary the head thrust test by having the child sit by himself or herself in a chair or again on a parent's lap and get the child to watch the examiner's nose as we do in an adult (Figure 25–1). Since the child can walk independently, motor milestones can be used to look at normal motor gait activity (Rine, 2007). Also, we can now start to perform the Modified Clinical Test for Sensory Interaction on Balance (Shumway-Cook & Horak, 1986). The modification is that the test is performed with only four conditions: standing on firm surface with and without vision, then

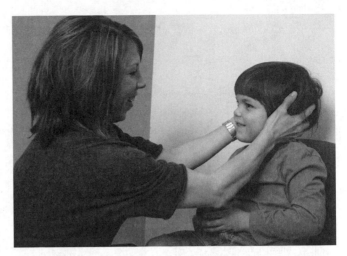

Figure 25–1. Example of a child and examiner in preparation for a head thrust test.

standing on a compliant surface with and without vision. For the young child who will not keep his or her eyes closed on command, the examiner and child are together and a third person (typically the parent) would take care of switching the lights on or off in the room. Have the child hold loosely to the examiner's little finger so the examiner knows when the lights are shut off if the child is swaying. Figure 25–2 illustrates this setup with the child on a foam cushion.

Laboratory Testing— What Studies at What Ages

In children, vestibular loss can be congenital or acquired, can occur with or without hearing loss, and can differentially affect the vestibular sensory structures (otoliths versus semicircular canals). Therefore, the purpose of vestibular assessment may be for determination of (1) the pathophysiology of dizziness complaints, (2) the etiology of hearing loss, or (3) the underlying cause of gross motor developmental delay. Although we have the capability to assess each of the vestibular sensory structures independently with a combination of tests: VEMP (assessing both utricle and the saccule), the video head impulse test (vHIT, assessing each semicircular canal), as well as caloric and rotary chair testing (assessing the horizontal canal), it is important to understand which assessments are appropriate for

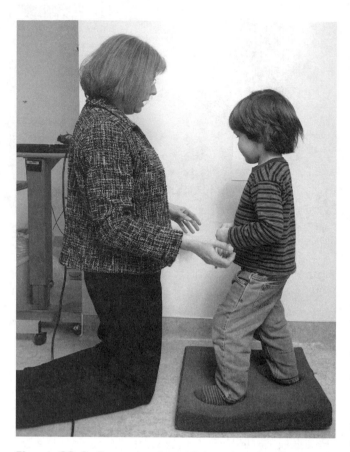

Figure 25–2. Example of a child performing the modified CTSIB standing on foam with visual fixation present.

children and at which age. Following is a description of common vestibular assessments and normative data across ages.

Recording Technique: Video Versus Electrodes

Some method of recording eye movements must be utilized for a variety of the outcomes listed below (i.e., pursuit tracking, random saccade, caloric testing, etc.). There are a variety of techniques for eye movement recording; however, the two main techniques for recording eye movements during vestibular assessment are video goggles (video-oculography), which use infrared to track pupil direction, or electrodes (electro-oculography), which record the corneo-retinal potential. While video goggles are preferred for vestibular testing in adults due to their increased resolution and ability to enable patients to keep their eyes open during

tasks without fixation, they are not always ideal for use with children. Video goggles are expensive, are often too big, or are not tolerated by small children, in which case, electrodes must be used. It would be the recommendation of the authors to utilize video goggles whenever possible and defer to electrodes when video is not an option.

Rotational Chair

Rotary chair, using traditional paradigms, is an assessment of the horizontal semicircular canals. One downfall of rotary chair is that it does not provide ear-specific information but is an overall indicator of vestibular responsiveness across a range of frequencies (0.01 to 0.64 Hz); therefore, rotary chair cannot be used to localize unilateral peripheral vestibular system involvement but is an excellent assessment for diagnosing bilateral vestibular loss. The two main rotary chair paradigms utilized with children are the sinusoidal harmonic acceleration (SHA) test and the step test (refer to Chapters 14 and 15 for additional information on these paradigms). One advantage of rotary chair is that unlike caloric testing, middle-ear abnormalities (i.e., PE tubes, atresia, etc.) do not preclude testing.

Rotary chair testing is tolerated by most children. Children can sit in the chair independently or can be seated on a parent's lap. For children younger than 5 years, SHA testing is preferred because of its gentle nature. Electrodes are used for eye movement recording and a chair-mounted camera is used to monitor the child during rotation. The chair-mounted camera is used to ensure that the child is awake and alert. On occasion, children will not tolerate the use of electrode placement on the face, in which case the chair-mounted camera can be used to subjectively observe nystagmus during rotation (Figure 25–3). When testing infants, the infant is seated on the parent's lap and the parent is asked to place a hand over the child's head, attempting to keep the head still. For children greater than 5 years, either step or SHA can be completed and eye movements are recorded with video goggles. Similar to adults, some degree of mental tasking is recommended during rotation as rotary chair gain can decrease with decreased alertness. Older children are generally engaged in conversation or simple cognitive tasks such as counting

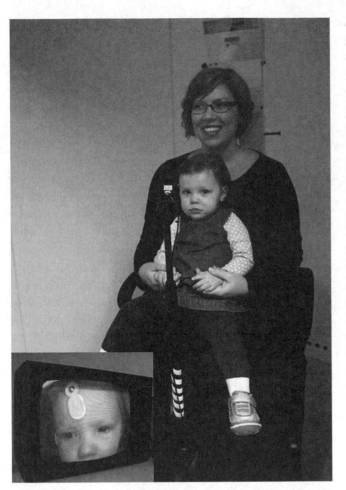

Figure 25-3. Example of child seated on parent's lap during rotary chair. The child's eyes can be subjectively observed on an external monitor via an infrared chair-mounted camera (*Inset*).

or spelling, and younger children are kept alert by singing nursery rhymes or children's songs. Difficulty lies in alerting children with significant hearing loss. In this instance, children are encouraged to wear their hearing aids. If the child is seated on the parent's lap the parents are encouraged to talk or sing to the child for maintaining alertness.

Outcome parameters with rotary chair are gain, phase (time constant), and symmetry. In children, rotary chair outcomes are similar to those of adults. Figure 25–4 demonstrates abnormal rotary chair SHA gain in a 12 year-old child with history of meningitis. In children with normal vestibular function, higher rotary chair gains have consistently been reported compared to adults (Charpiot et al., 2010; Maes, De Kegel, Van, & Dhooge, 2014; Valente, 2007), with the exception of Casselbrant et al. (2010) who found a linear increase in rotary chair gain in children ages 3 to 9 years. Because of these findings, high gain in young children is not considered a pathologic finding unless coupled with other indications for central pathology. However, some data suggest significant differences in phase between adults and normal children. In infants, phase has been found to be more variable and have a tendency to exhibit a phase lag. This variability and lag both improve with age. The variability in phase is attributed to lack of steady head position during testing (Staller, Goin, & Hildebrandt, 1986). In older children, larger phase values have been found compared to adults (Valente, 2007). Because larger phase values (i.e., phase leads)

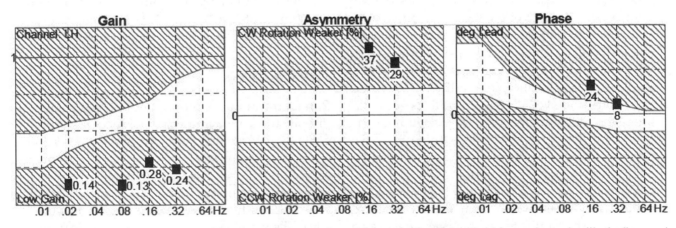

Figure 25-4. Example of abnormal rotary chair gain in a 12-year-old child with history of meningitis. Left panel shows low gain for all frequencies assessed (0.02, 0.08, 0.16, and 0.32 Hz), middle panel shows asymmetry, and right panel shows phase. This child also had low vHIT gains, as shown in Figure 25–5.

can be indicative of peripheral vestibular system involvement, age-appropriate normative data are needed to determine appropriate clinical cutoffs. Collectively, these findings suggest that the VOR undergoes maturation from childhood to adulthood and that age-appropriate normative data are needed when assessing children.

Rotary chair can be completed on children of any age; however, it is typically completed on children older than 4 months due to development of the VOR (Staller et al., 1986). A relationship between nystagmus amplitude and weight has been reported with higher amplitude nystagmus being associated with heavier babies (Eviatar & Eviatar, 1979). Staller et al. (1986) report 10% of infants less than 60 days old do not generate measurable nystagmus in response to rotation. It has been recommended that if children less than 6 months of age do not elicit nystagmus to rotation, that testing should be repeated once they are older than 6 months to rule out maturational effects (Eviatar & Eviatar, 1979).

Postural Control Assessment

The Sensory Organization Test (SOT) is a routine assessment of balance function for both adults and children. The SOT evaluates use of visual, vestibular, and proprioceptive sensory inputs in the maintenance of balance. During SOT, postural sway is measured over three trials for each of the following six conditions: (1) eyes open, stable platform; (2) eyes closed, stable platform; (3) eyes open, sway surround; (4) eyes open, sway platform; (5) eyes closed, sway platform; and (6) eyes open, sway surround, sway platform. In each of these conditions, some facet of the visual, vestibular, and/or proprioceptive system is disrupted; providing a functional assessment of overall balance. For example, condition 5 is primarily assessing how well the subject utilizes vestibular inputs for maintaining balance; in this condition, the subject has his or her eyes closed, eliminating use of the visual system, and the platform sways, eliminating effective use of proprioception.

Outcome parameters for the SOT include an equilibrium score for each trial and an overall composite score. The equilibrium score is a percentage of degree of sway, from 0 to 100, and assumes an anterior posterior postural sway envelope of 12.5°, so a score of 0 means the child swayed maximally 12.5°

(or more), and a score of 100 means the child was perfectly still. Children must weigh at least 30 lbs to put enough weight on the platform to record postural sway. Normative data for the SOT exist in children down to age 3 (Hirabayashi & Iwasaki, 1995; Rine et al., 1998). Overall composite scores improve with age, meaning that younger children demonstrate greater degrees of sway than older children and adults (Casselbrant et al., 2010; Peterson et al., 2006; Rine et al., 1998; Valente, 2007). As reviewed above, children make appropriate use of somatosensory information by age 6; however, use of visual and vestibular information is still undergoing maturation. This provides evidence that age-appropriate normative data are necessary for SOT and a framework for normal expectations. In younger children, where use of somatosensory information is mature, performance on conditions 1 to 3 can be expected to mimic that of adults; however, in the remaining conditions where visual and vestibular information are predominantly utilized, greater degrees of sway can be expected for younger children. By age 12 to 15 years, children can be expected to perform adult-like under all SOT conditions (Peterka & Black, 1990; Peterson et al., 2006).

The purpose of the SOT in children is to detect balance dysfunction, but it can also be used to monitor various disorders known to affect the postural control pathway (Hirabayashi & Iwasaki, 1995). Children often require extensive coaching, reinforcement, and encouragement. Some children have fear of closing their eyes during testing. In this instance, fun glasses can be used to eliminate clear vision, or the room lights can be dimmed or turned off for brief periods in order to eliminate visual cues.

Pursuit Tracking

Pursuit tracking, or smooth pursuit, is the ability to visually track a moving visual target. The purpose of evaluating pursuit tracking is to assess the vestibulo-cerebellum and, more generally, the brainstem and cerebellum. During pursuit tracking, patients view a computer-generated visual target, which oscillates back and forth at frequencies ranging from 0.2 to 1 Hz. The main outcome parameter is gain, which is calculated by dividing eye velocity by target velocity. In adults, it has been well described that the ability to perform pursuit tracking declines with age.

Children have the ability to perform smooth pursuit eye movements as young as 2 months of age (Jacobs et al., 1997); however, smooth pursuit gains are significantly lower and more variable when compared to adults and continue to mature with age (Accardo, Pensiero, Da, & Perissutti, 1995). Children should be able to achieve normal smooth pursuit by age 5 (Levens,1988). Pursuit tracking is significantly affected by level of attentiveness; therefore, children should be coached throughout testing. For all ocular motor testing, use of fun, colorful targets can be helpful in the assessment of children. Some manufacturers allow the programming of cartoon characters as visual targets.

Random Saccade

A saccade is a rapid eye movement from one point of fixation to another. There are a variety of paradigms to assess saccade performance; however, the most widely used is the random saccade test. With the random saccade test the main outcome parameters are latency, velocity, and accuracy. Saccade latency is calculated as the time from target onset to the initiation of eye movement; velocity is the speed of the eye movement as it moves to the target; and accuracy is precision with which the eyes meet the target. These outcome parameters are all analyzed via commercial systems. In general, saccade accuracy is thought to arise from the posterior vermis region with velocity and latency originating by the parapontine reticular formation. Because these outcome parameters are engendered by different substrates, abnormalities of saccade latency, velocity, and accuracy can help to further determine site of lesion. In children, saccade latency decreases with age while saccade velocity is stable during childhood. Maturation of saccades is thought to be complete by age 12 (Bucci & Seassau, 2012).

OKN Up to Age 7

The optokinetic response is a reflexive eye movement, optokinetic nystagmus (OKN), in response to moving objects in the visual field. When visual targets are moving to the right, left-beat OKN occurs and vice versa for visual targets moving to the left. A true test of the OKN system requires that at minimum, the target (stripes, dots, etc.) takes up 90% of the visual field. OKN is thought to reach maturation by age 7 (D'Agostino, Melagrana, Pasquale, & Taborelli, 1997). For children less than 7 years of age, gain values decrease with the younger age and do require age-specific normative ranges. As with the adult OKN is dominated with smooth pursuit tracking even though saccades are also involved. As in the discussion in the introduction this can be taken advantage of to get an estimate of smooth pursuit by using OKN (Mezzalira et al., 2005; Valmaggia et al., 2004). Like other tests of ocular motor function, cartoon characters can be substituted for standard visual targets. Children generally do not require any special instructions as OKN is a reflexive eye movement; however, they can be asked to simply watch or attempt to count the visual stimuli.

Hallpike and Roll Tests

The Dix-Hallpike and roll tests are bedside assessments for the presence of benign paroxysmal positional vertigo (BPPV) in the vertical and horizontal canals, respectively. As described below, BPPV is rare in children; however, it should not be disregarded in the pediatric population, particularly in the event of head trauma or if the child complains of positional dizziness. There are no specific modifications in the way the Dix-Hallpike or roll maneuvers are completed in children. Outcome parameters with the Dix-Hallpike and roll maneuver are the subjective assessment of nystagmus consistent with BPPV, which is not different than nystagmus observed in adults. BPPV has been reported in children as young as 3 years (Saka et al., 2013). Treatment of BPPV in the pediatric population utilizing canalith repositioning maneuvers is the same as with adults. However, issues with both assessment and treatment of BPPV in children are fear of being dizzy and keeping their eyes open during these provoking maneuvers. Reassurance and use of fun visual targets, stickers, or finger puppets, can be helpful.

Gaze Testing and Positional Testing

The purpose of gaze testing is to assess for the presence of spontaneous and/or gaze-evoked nystagmus. During gaze testing, the presence of nystagmus is evaluated while patients view a visual target directly in front of them (center position), eccentrically 30–40° to the right, left, up and down and then in these same eye positions with fixation removed. Gaze-evoked nystagmus can originate from either the peripheral or the central vestibular system with differences in clinical presentation between the two (see Chapter 10 for details). Nystagmus that is peripheral in origin will generally have a linear slow component, be direction fixed, and enhance with fixation removed. Nystagmus is considered to be of central origin if it has a rounded (versus linear) slow component velocity, if it evidences rebound (where the fast component of the nystagmus changes with the direction of the last eye movement), or it enhances or does not change in intensity with fixation. In children, at minimum a subjective assessment of spontaneous nystagmus should be completed. Like adults, gaze testing can uncover evidence of an acute peripheral vestibular disorder or provide evidence for central vestibular system involvement.

The purpose of static positional testing is to examine the effect of gravity on positional changes of the head. During static positional testing, eye movements are recorded with fixation removed in the sitting, supine, body-right, body-left, and precaloric positions. Additionally, positional testing can be completed with the head turned right and left in the sitting, supine, and head-hanging positions to examine the influence of cervical head movement. The interpretation of positional nystagmus in children is similar to that of adults. Positional nystagmus is classified as either direction fixed (e.g., right-beating in all positions) or direction changing (e.g., right-beating in some positions and left-beating in others). Direction-changing nystagmus may be further categorized as geotropic (nystagmus beating toward the earth) or ageotropic (nystagmus beating away from the earth).

The clinical significance of positional nystagmus is determined by its intensity, frequency, and direction. In terms of intensity, positional nystagmus is considered clinically significant if it meets the following criteria: (1) the slow phase velocity is greater than 5 degrees per second in any given position, or (2) the slow phase velocity is less than 6 degrees per second, however, is present in more than 50% of positions (minimum two out of four positions). Significant positional nystagmus is localized as peripheral, central, or nonlocalizing based on the

direction and pattern of nystagmus. Direction-fixed positional nystagmus is typically localized to the peripheral vestibular system, specifically when there are no other indications of central vestibular system involvement on either direct exam or case history. Direction-changing nystagmus, within any given position, is localized to the central vestibular system, while direction-changing nystagmus between positions can localize to either the periphery or central system or be considered nonlocalizing.

VEMPs: Cervical and Ocular

VEMPs are used to assess otolith function by measuring muscle potential changes in response to acoustic stimulation. There are two types of VEMP responses: cervical and ocular. Cervical VEMPs measure muscle potential changes in the sternocleidomastoid muscle and provide information regarding the saccule and the inferior vestibular nerve (Colebatch, Halmagyi, & Skuse, 1994), while ocular VEMPs measure muscle potential changes in the inferior oblique eye muscle and are speculated to provide information regarding the utricle and superior portion of the vestibular nerve (Rosengren, McAngus, & Colebatch, 2005). Both the cervical and ocular VEMP are recorded in response to acoustic stimulation, either air conduction or bone conduction. The cVEMP is an ipsilateral, inhibiting response, meaning acoustic sound delivered to the ear causes the ipsilateral contracted sternocleidomastoid muscle to relax. The oVEMP is a contralateral, excitatory response, wherein acoustic sound delivered to the ear causes the contralateral inferior oblique muscle to contract. VEMPs have been shown to be purely vestibular in nature as they are preserved in patients with sensorineural hearing loss (Colebatch et al., 1994).

Outcome parameters in cervical VEMP are the p13 and n23 latencies and the p13/n23 peak-to-peak amplitude. Cervical VEMP have been measured in children as young as 1 to 4 weeks in response to 95 to 100 nHL, 500-Hz tone-bursts (Erbek et al., 2007; Sheykholeslami, Megerian, Arnold, & Kaga, 2005). Cervical VEMP responses in children are similar in morphology to those of adults with the exception that both the p13 and n23 latencies are shorter in children and prolong with age; there is also greater variability in the p13/n23 peak-to-peak amplitude in children (Chang, Yang, Wang, & Young, 2007;

Kelsch, Schaefer, & Esquivel, 2006; Sheykholeslami et al., 2005; Valente, 2007). Prolongation of the p13 latencies with age has been attributed to neck length in children (Chang et al., 2007). The presence of cervical VEMP responses at birth provide evidence for their early development.

The outcome parameters in ocular VEMP are the n10 and p16 latencies and the n10/p16 peak-to-peak amplitude. Wang, Hsieh, and Young (2013) report that oVEMP are not present in children until 12 months and do not report reliable response rates in children until 4 years. These responses are difficult to obtain in infants as sustained up-gaze is necessary for measuring ocular VEMP. However, ocular VEMPs have also been recorded when children gently close their eyes, taking advantage of Bell's phenomenon, which can be attempted in young children (Huang, Yang, & Young, 2012; Wang et al., 2013). No significant differences in ocular VEMP latency or amplitude have been reported compared to adults; however, few studies to date have documented ocular VEMP in children.

VEMPs are fairly quick to administer and are especially helpful in the pediatric population as they provide information about unilateral vestibular function without inducing symptoms of dizziness. Difficulties in obtaining these responses in the pediatric population are that children must sustain contraction of the SCM muscle (background tonic EMG) for cervical VEMPs and sustain up-gaze for ocular VEMPs. Kelsch et al. (2006) report less SCM fatigue when children are allowed to prop up on their elbows. We have found toys and computer animations as well as continued verbal reinforcement to be helpful for maintaining head turn and contraction with cervical VEMP. For ocular VEMP, stickers placed on the ceiling have been helpful for maintaining up-gaze. For either type of VEMP one final concern is the high stimulus level required to record these responses. In adults, stimulus levels of 120 to 125 dB SPL are typically used. Although these stimulus levels are considered safe in adult-sized ears, there is concern for high sound pressure levels in small ear canals.

Caloric Irrigations

Bithermal caloric testing is currently regarded as the gold standard in assessment of the horizontal canal and, subsequently, the superior branch of the VIII cranial nerve. The main benefit of caloric testing is that it yields ear-specific information. Caloric testing can be completed with either air or water stimuli. With either method, a cool (inhibitory) or a warm (excitatory) stimulus is delivered to each ear. While air is a more convenient stimulus type, water has been shown to result in higher slow phase velocities, specifically in response to warm water (Maes et al., 2007; Zangemeister & Bock, 1980; Zapala, Olsholt, & Lundy, 2008). Water calorics have been deemed the stimulus of choice with air stimulation recommended when water is contraindicated.

Interpretation of caloric responses in children is identical to that of adults. Interpretation is completed two ways: (1) the magnitude of slow component velocities are first identified as being reduced, normal, or hypermetric, and (2) comparisons between right and left irrigations are made inserting the peak of the response using Jongkees formula (Jongkees, Maas, & Philipszoon, 1962). Comparisons between right and left are not routinely completed when caloric responses are reduced bilaterally. A wide range of accepted normal caloric responses have been reported. Caloric responses are considered hypermetric when slow phase velocities exceed 60 to 70°/s and are considered bilaterally reduced when either the sum of all responses is less than 20°/s or the peak response is less than 10°/s for warm irrigations and less than 15°/s for ice water irrigations. When comparing right and left responses, individual labs should determine their own cutoff criteria; however, caloric asymmetries and directional preponderances greater than 25% to 30% are traditionally considered significant. Sensitivity and specificity of the caloric test in response to air has been reported as 0.82 and 0.82, respectively, and in response to water as 0.84 and 0.84, respectively (Zapala et al., 2008).

Caloric responses have been reported in children as young as 2 months of age with complete maturation by 6 to 12 months (Eviatar & Eviatar, 1979); however, appropriate calibration is a concern in these small children. The slow phase velocity of nystagmus in response to caloric stimulation has been found to decrease with age, similar to that noted during rotary chair testing (Andrieu-Guitrancourt, Peron, & Aubet, 1981). Children may be fearful of completing caloric testing because it causes symptoms of dizziness, fixation is removed during testing, and they temporarily cannot hear out of the ear receiving the irrigation. If reinforcement and reassurance are not enough, the duration of the stimulus can be decreased to lessen the effect or two irrigations can be performed instead of four.

Video Head Impulse Test (vHIT)

The video head impulse test (vHIT) is a new assessment of semicircular canal function. With vHIT, patients wear lightweight goggles, which simultaneously measure both eye and head velocity (100 to 250°/s). During vHIT, patients are asked to fixate on a visual target approximately 1 m in front of them while head impulses are delivered in the plane of each semicircular canal.

The main outcome parameter in vHIT is gain, which is a ratio of eye and head velocity. Generally, gains above about 0.8 are consistent with normal VOR function, indicating that the eye and head are moving in an equal and opposite direction during the head thrust. An additional outcome is the presence of refixation saccades, either overt (occurring after the head thrust) or covert (occurring during the head impulse). There are currently no reports of vHIT in children with the exception of a case report in a 4-year-old child (Manzari, Burgess, MacDougall, & Curthoys, 2012). Experience within our clinic at Boys Town suggests that vHIT is a reliable test of semicircular canal function and can be completed in children down to age 6. Preliminary data in our

lab suggest there is no significant difference in vHIT gains between children and adults. Figure 25–5 demonstrates abnormal vHIT gain in a 12-year-old child with history of meningitis. Overt saccades, refixation saccades that occur *after* the head impulse, can be seen in response to head impulses to the left and covert saccades, refixation saccades that occur *during* the head impulse, can be seen in response to head impulses to the right.

The advantage of vHIT is that it not only provides information regarding unilateral peripheral vestibular system function, but provides canal specific information without inducing symptoms of dizziness. Difficulties in obtaining these responses in the pediatric population are that children must sustain gaze on a visual target while delivering head impulses. We have found the use of child-appropriate stickers to be engaging enough for young children and yet small enough to serve as a fixation point. Sustained gaze on this fixed target is reinforced by asking the child questions about the character on the sticker.

Regardless of whether the focus is for determination of pathophysiology of symptoms, etiology of hearing loss, or to determine the underlying cause of gross motor developmental delay, we have found that all children are able to complete an assessment of canal function and an assessment of otolith function. For children greater than 5 years of age, both ocular and cervical VEMP testing are feasible as well as any assessment of canal function (rotary

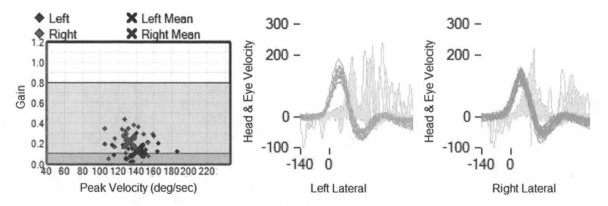

Figure 25–5. Example of abnormal vHIT gain in a 12-year-old child with history of meningitis. Left panel shows mean gain for left and right horizontal (lateral) canals with the large Xs. Right-side panels show raw head velocity in the smooth trace for the labeled left and right lateral canals, with the eye velocities in the nonsmooth trace to the right of the head velocities in each of the graphs labeled left and right lateral canals. This finding was confirmed by low rotary chair gains, as shown above.

chair, calorics, or vHIT). For children younger than 5, the first tier assessment is rotary chair and cervical VEMP with an attempt at bedside head impulse and questions regarding the child's attainment of gross motor milestones. With regard to other assessments, the SOT can be completed on children greater than 3 years who weigh at least 30 pounds, while ocular motor testing can be attempted on children of any age.

Correlation of Test Outcomes to Gross Motor Function

Does the presence of vestibular loss necessarily indicate that children will have abnormal gross motor function? Early studies demonstrated that performance on the tandem Romberg was predictive of vestibular loss in children (Brookhouser et al., 1982). Later studies have shown that rotary chair and caloric testing are both predictive of performance on functional balance outcomes, where children with low rotary chair gain or low caloric slow phase velocities will have poorer balance function (Cushing et al., 2008b; De Kegel et al., 2012).

DISORDERS THAT CAUSE VESTIBULAR AND BALANCE PROBLEMS

All of the disorders that can cause dizziness and balance disorders in adults have been reported in children; however, the frequency of the occurrence in children differs from that of the adult. A brief discussion of the disorders that are typically associated with dizziness and balance disorders of a peripheral and central origin in adults is presented first. Following that, presentation of diseases and syndromes that are more specific to childhood will be presented.

Disorders of Dizziness and Balance Typically Associated With Adults—Occurrence in Children

In consideration of disorders that cause primary symptoms of vertigo, dizziness (light-headedness), and/or unsteadiness in adults seen in tertiary care facilities and national health surveys, the order by typical incidence (most common to least) would be as follows:

1. Benign paroxysmal positional vertigo
2. Vestibular migraine (Lempert & Neuhauser, 2009)
3. Persistent postural-perceptual dizziness (formerly chronic subjective dizziness syndrome) (Chapter 30)
4. Vestibular neuronitis
5. Labyrinthitis
6. Herpes zoster oticus
7. Ménière's disease
8. Tumors of the cerebellar pontine angle; vascular causes; central nervous system degenerative disorders; B12 deficiency, collectively

In children, the few studies that have performed general reviews of the incidence of the more common disorders (Balatsouras et al., 2007; Gioacchini et al., 2014) consistently list the top three causes of dizziness in children:

1. Vestibular migraine
2. Benign paroxysmal vertigo of childhood
3. Viral insults to include otitis media
4. Head trauma
5. Benign paroxysmal positional vertigo (in older children) (rare)
6. Ménière's disease (rare)
7. Tumors and vascular insults (rare)

Those listed as one and two made up 65% of the cases reviewed by Balatsouras et al. (2007). The systematic review by Gioacchini et al. (2014) showed vestibular migraine at a rate of 27.82% and benign paroxysmal vertigo of childhood to be 15.68%, while Ménière's is mentioned far less than its incidence in adults which in a busy neurotologic clinic with a dedicated balance center <5% and <1% in estimates of the general population (Kerber et al., 2008).

The disorder of benign paroxysmal vertigo of childhood is considered a migraine precursor and is listed in the International Classification of Headache Disorders, 3rd edition (beta version) and listed in the first and second editions as well, as an episodic disorder associated with migraine headaches. Therefore, by far the most common disorder to cause dizziness in children would be developed or developing migraine headaches.

Childhood Diseases and Syndromes

Vestibular loss can occur in varying degrees (unilateral, mild bilateral, or severe bilateral), can differentially affect the different sensory structures (semicircular canal versus otolith), and can affect different nerve portions (superior versus inferior nerve involvement). Similarly, the time course of vestibular loss can vary, occurring either in utero or acquired after birth. The presence of vestibular loss is highly associated with the presence of hearing loss (O'Reilly et al., 2010). In fact, the likelihood of vestibular loss has been shown to increase with greater degrees of hearing loss (Brookhouser et al., 1982; Tribukait, Brantberg, & Bergenius, 2004). Hearing loss worse than 90 dB has shown a greater tendency to be associated with vestibular loss (Tribukait et al., 2004). As described below, vestibular loss is also associated with specific childhood diseases and syndromes. However, the presence of vestibular loss in children can be difficult to detect by observation as children do not typically complain of dizziness. Below is a brief description of childhood diseases/syndromes, their prevalence/incidence, and the estimated degree of vestibular loss associated with each. When a child has been diagnosed with any of these conditions, vestibular loss should be suspected.

In Utero

Cytomegalovirus. Congenital cytomegalovirus (CMV) infection is the leading cause of hearing loss in children, resulting in progressive and fluctuating sensorineural hearing loss. CMV is estimated to occur in approximately 40,000 children each year in the United States (Cannon & Davis, 2005). Vestibular loss is commonly associated with CMV, with severity ranging from unilateral to bilateral and affecting both the saccule and horizontal semicircular canals. In infants with congenital CMV abnormalities on rotary chair, the caloric test and cervical VEMP have been reported (Inoue et al., 2013; Zagolski, 2008b). Inoue et al. (2013) report 60% of children with CMV to have abnormal caloric responses and 33% to have absent cervical VEMP responses.

Rubella. The rubella virus (commonly known as the German measles) is seen less frequently due to vaccination. Degree of vestibular loss is variable. With rubella, the degree of vestibular loss has been documented to be higher as the degree of hearing loss increases (Zagolski, 2009); however, this relationship has not been found by all (Nishida, 1983). Both canal and saccule loss has been documented, with canal loss (via caloric responses) reported between 30–43% of cases and saccule loss (via cervical VEMP) in approximately 43% of ears (Nishida, Ueda, & Fung, 1983; Zagolski, 2009).

Usher Syndrome. Usher syndrome is an autosomal recessive genetic condition. Usher syndrome is characterized by sensorineural hearing loss and retinitis pigmentosa (RP). There are three classifications of Usher syndrome: Type I is characterized by congenital, profound sensorineural hearing loss, RP, and bilateral vestibular hypofunction. In children with Type I Usher syndrome, vestibular function is generally absent, and subsequently these children acquire motor milestones later. The average age for independent walking in children with Usher has been reported at 21.9 months (range 12 to 30 months) (Jatana et al., 2013). Type II has moderate-to-severe sensorineural hearing loss, progressive RP beginning in the second decade of life, and normal vestibular function. Last, Type III has progressive RP and progressive hearing and vestibular loss.

Waardenburg. Waardenburg syndrome is a genetic condition that is commonly associated with congenital hearing loss, heterochromia iridum (different-colored eyes) and a white forelock, among other features. It is estimated to affect 1 in 40,000 (Genetics Home Reference, 2012). The presentation of Waardenburg syndrome can be variable and similarly the occurrence of vestibular loss can be variable. As many as 77% have been reported to demonstrate some abnormality on vestibular function testing (Black, Pesznecker, Allen, & Gianna, 2001).

Auditory Neuropathy. Auditory neuropathy, or dyssynchrony, occurs when hearing in the inner ear is normal, but there is a breakdown in transmitting that information to the brain. In addition to the auditory nerve, the vestibular nerve can also be affected. In cases of auditory neuropathy, vestibular testing shows variable abnormality of the superior and inferior vestibular nerves. Few studies have documented vestibular function in a large group with auditory neuropathy. Cervical VEMP responses have been shown to be absent in the majority of cases (Akdogan, Selcuk, Ozcan, & Dere, 2008; Sazgar, Yazdani, Rezazadeh, & Yazdi, 2010). Similarly, abnormal caloric responses have also been noted (Fujikawa & Starr, 2000; Sheykholeslami, Kaga, Murofushi, & Hughes, 2000). Vestibular function has been reported to decline with age in individuals with auditory neuropathy (Fujikawa & Starr, 2000; Masuda & Kaga, 2011), which helps explain the variability in reported findings. For example, in one cohort of children (*n* = 3), caloric responses were reported to be normal in all cases (Akdogan et al., 2008). Some individuals with auditory neuropathy affecting the vestibular nerve are reportedly asymptomatic in spite of documented vestibular involvement (Sinha, Barman, Singh, Rajeshwari, & Sharanya, 2013).

GJB2 (Connexin 26 Mutations). GJB2 (Connexin 26 mutations) is the most common cause of nonsyndromic deafness. In children with GJB2, variable vestibular function has been reported ranging from normal, to unilateral, to bilateral vestibular hypofunction. Likewise, a range in incidence of vestibular involvement has been reported. In 25 children diagnosed with homozygous connexin 26 mutations, 10 children exhibited a unilateral weakness in response to caloric stimulation and 1 child exhibited bilateral vestibular loss (Cushing, Gordon, Rutka, James, & Papsin, 2013). Cervical VEMP was completed in 24 of those children, and VEMP responses were absent bilaterally in 6 and unilaterally in 10 (Cushing et al., 2013). In other reports, 5/7 children with GJB2 had at least one abnormality on vestibular function tests (VEMP and caloric) (Kasai et al., 2010). However, in other reports normal canal function has been found in all cases (*n* = 13) with isolated absent VEMP responses in one child (Inoue et al., 2013).

Large Vestibular Aqueduct Syndrome. Within the vestibular aqueduct is the endolymphatic duct and sac. The criterion used to determine whether the vestibular aqueduct is considered enlarged can vary, but commonly LVAS is diagnosed when the diameter of the vestibular aqueduct is greater than 1.5 mm or when its diameter is twice the size of the posterior canal, as seen on computed tomography (CT) (Valvassori & Clemis, 1978; Wilson, Hodgson, & Talbot, 1997). LVAS is considered one type of third window disorder (similar to superior canal dehiscence syndrome) and therefore demonstrates the same pattern of findings on audiometric and VEMP testing, that is, conductive hearing loss not of middle-ear origin and large ocular and cervical VEMP amplitudes with significantly lower thresholds (Merchant et al., 2007; Merchant & Rosowski, 2008; Sheykholeslami, Schmerber, Habiby, & Kaga, 2004; Taylor et al., 2012; Zhou & Gopen, 2011; Zhou, Gopen, & Kenna, 2008). However, individuals with LVAS can also have complaints of dizziness and imbalance and in addition to showing an enhancement on VEMP testing, evidence vestibular loss on caloric testing (Yetiser, Kertmen, & Ozkaptan, 1999). An estimated 30% of individuals with LVAS report some type of vestibular-related symptom (Jackler & De La Cruz, 1989; Yetiser et al., 1999). A relationship between LVAS and BPPV in patients (children and adults) has also been reported (Manzari, 2008; Song, Hong, Kim, & Koo, 2012).

LVAS can be associated with both syndromic and nonsyndromic hearing loss. LVAS is a characteristic feature in branchio-oto-renal (BOR), Pendred syndrome, and Mondini malformation. BOR is characterized by malformations in the outer, middle, and inner ear (LVAS among other malformations) and the kidneys. Pendred syndrome, a type of syndromic hearing loss, consists of hearing loss, LVAS, and goiter (enlargement of the thyroid). Last, while Mondini malformation can occur in isolation, coupled with LVAS, it can also be found in the constellation of Pendred syndrome. In unselected children with inner-ear malformation, dysfunction on at least one vestibular test (rotary chair, calorics, or VEMP) has been noted in greater than 50% of cases (Cushing et al., 2013; Inoue et al., 2013).

Neurofibromatosis Type 2. Neurofibromatosis Type 2 (NF2) is a genetic condition that facilitates the growth of noncancerous tumors. The most common tumor growth associated with NF2 is that of vestibular schwannomas. The incidence of NF2 is 1 in 33,000 (Genetics Home Reference, 2013). Symptoms associated with NF2 usually present during adolescence; however, isolated cases have been reported of NF2 in the first year of life (Ruggieri et al., 2013). NF2 is presumed to affect the superior branch of the vestibular nerve more often than the inferior branch as caloric abnormalities are more common than absent or reduced VEMP responses (Wang, Hsu, & Young, 2005).

Vestibular loss has also been reported variably in the following conditions: fetal alcohol syndrome and other inner-ear congenital malformations, such as CHARGE syndrome and Scheibe dysplasia.

Acquired

Meningitis. In the majority of children with meningitis some degree of semicircular canal involvement is exhibited, either complete loss of function or reduced function; however, a subset can have normal function or preserved otolith function (Arnvig, 1955; Cushing et al., 2013; Wiener-Vacher, Obeid, & Abou-Elew, 2012). Cushing et al. (2013) report bilateral areflexia in 9/10 and bilateral hypofunction in 1/10 children with meningitis and preserved saccule function (as diagnosed by cervical VEMP) in 14/22 ears. Meningitis has been shown to delay the acquisition of motor milestones (Wiener-Vacher et al., 2012) and in some cases can cause a regression in gross motor function. Balance has also been found to be poorer in older children with history meningitis (Cushing et al., 2009).

Ototoxic Drug Use. Medications proven to be vestibulo-toxic include aminoglycosides such as gentamicin and streptomycin, among others. Not all individuals with exposure to aminoglycosides will experience vestibular loss; however, when vestibular loss does occur it can be widespread throughout the vestibular periphery affecting both the otolith organs and the semicircular canals (Zagolski, 2008a). Toxicity has been reported to be dose dependent in some medications, with greater dosage over a longer course of days increasing susceptibility (Chen, Bach, Shoup, & Winick, 2013). However, gentamicin is the exception as it can be vestibulotoxic regardless of the dose or duration (Ahmed, Hannigan, MacDougall, Chan, & Halmagyi, 2012). When assessing residual otolith function in patients with known bilateral canal loss, individuals with history of ototoxicity were noted to have the least amount of residual vestibular function (Agrawal, Bremova, Kremmyda, & Strupp, 2013).

Measles and Mumps. Vestibular loss has also been reported variably in the following conditions: measles (a respiratory virus resulting in fever, runny nose, coughing, and rash) and mumps (a virus resulting in fever, headache, malaise, and swollen glands); however, both the measles and mumps are not frequently encountered due to vaccination. Mumps has its association with a prior common cause of unilateral hearing loss that as an adult has been indicated as a cause for delayed endolymphatic hydrops, a condition that can present like that of Ménière's disease but without the auditory symptoms since the person already has the severe hearing loss (Schuknecht, Suzuka, & Zimmerman, 1990).

While none of the above-mentioned diseases/syndromes show an exclusive relationship with vestibular loss, vestibular testing in children should be considered when hearing loss of any of the above etiologies has been diagnosed. Techniques for determining the etiology of hearing loss are improving; however, in many instances the etiology of hearing loss is unknown. Vestibular loss in these cases should be suspected with greater degrees of hearing loss and when coupled with significant gross motor delay; although again, this relationship is not mutually exclusive.

REFERENCES

Abadie, V., Wiener-Vacher, S., Morisseau-Durand, M. P., Poree, C., Amiel, J., Amanou, L., Peigne, C., Lyonnet, S., & Manac'h, Y. (2000). Vestibular anomalies in CHARGE syndrome: Investigations on and consequences for postural development. *European Journal of Pediatrics, 159*, 569–574.

Accardo, A. P., Pensiero, S., Da, P. S., & Perissutti, P. (1995). Characteristics of horizontal smooth pursuit eye movements to sinusoidal stimulation in children of primary school age. *Vision Research, 35*, 539–548.

Agrawal, Y., Bremova, T., Kremmyda, O., & Strupp, M. (2013). Semicircular canal, saccular and utricular function in patients with bilateral vestibulopathy: Analysis based on etiology. *Journal of Neurology, 260*, 876–883.

Agrawal, Y., Carey, J. P., Della Santina, C. C., Schubert, M. C., & Minor, L. B. (2009). Disorder of balance and vestibular function in the US adults: Data from the National Health and Nutrition Examination Survey, 2001–2004. *Archives of Internal Medicine, 169*(10), 938–944.

Ahmed, R. M., Hannigan, I. P., MacDougall, H. G., Chan, R. C., & Halmagyi, G. M. (2012). Gentamicin ototoxicity: A 23-year selected case series of 103 patients. *Medical Journal of Australia, 196,* 701–704.

Akdogan, O., Selcuk, A., Ozcan, I., & Dere, H. (2008). Vestibular nerve functions in children with auditory neuropathy. *International Journal of Pediatric Otorhinolaryngology, 72,* 415–419.

Andrieu-Guitrancourt, J., Peron, J. M. D. D., & Aubet, J. C. P. (1981). Normal vestibular responses to air caloric tests in children. *International Journal of Pediatric Otorhinolaryngology, 3*(3), 245–250.

Arnvig, J. (1955). Vestibular function in deafness and severe hardness of hearing. *Acta Oto-Laryngologica, 45,* 283–288.

Balatsouras, D. G., Kaberos, A., Assimakopoulos, D., Katotomichelakis, M., Economou, N. C., & Korres, S. G. (2007). Etiology of vertigo in children. *International Journal of Pediatric Otorhinolaryngology, 71,* 487–494.

Black, F. O., Pesznecker, S. C., Allen, K., & Gianna, C. (2001). A vestibular phenotype for Waardenburg syndrome? *Otology and Neurotology, 22,* 188–194.

Brookhouser, P. E., Cyr, D. G., & Beauchaine, K. A. (1982). Vestibular findings in the deaf and hard of hearing. *Otolaryngology-Head and Neck Surgery, 90,* 773–777.

Bucci, M. P., & Seassau, M. (2012). Saccadic eye movements in children: A developmental study. *Experimental Brain Research, 222,* 21–30.

Cannon, M. J., & Davis, K. F. (2005). Washing our hands of the congenital cytomegalovirus disease epidemic. *BMC, Public Health, 5,* 70.

Casselbrant, M. L., Mandel, E. M., Sparto, P. J., Perera, S., Redfern, M. S., Fall, P. A., & Furman, J. M. (2010). Longitudinal posturography and rotational testing in children three to nine years of age: Normative data. *Otolaryngology-Head and Neck Surgery, 142,* 708–714.

Chang, C. H., Yang, T. L., Wang, C. T., & Young, Y. H. (2007). Measuring neck structures in relation to vestibular evoked myogenic potentials. *Clinical Neurophysiology, 118,* 1105–1109.

Charpiot, A., Tringali, S., Ionescu, E., Vital-Durand, F., & Ferber-Viart, C. (2010). Vestibulo-ocular reflex and balance maturation in healthy children aged from six to twelve years. *Audiology and Neurotology, 15,* 203–210.

Chen, K. S., Bach, A., Shoup, A., & Winick, N. J. (2013). Hearing loss and vestibular dysfunction among children with cancer after receiving aminoglycosides. *Pediatric Blood and Cancer, 60,* 1772–1777.

Christy, J. B., Payne, J., Azuero, A., & Formby, C. (2014). Reliability and diagnostic accuracy of clinical tests of vestibular function for children. *Pediatric Physical Therapy, 26,* 180–190.

Colebatch, J. G., Halmagyi, G. M., & Skuse, N. F. (1994). Myogenic potentials generated by a click-evoked vestibulocollic reflex. *Journal of Neurology, Neurosurgery, and Psychiatry, 57,* 190–197.

Cushing, S. L., Chia, R., James, A. L., Papsin, B. C., & Gordon, K. A. (2008a). A test of static and dynamic balance function in children with cochlear implants: The vestibular olympics. *Archives of Otolaryngology-Head and Neck Surgery, 134,* 34–38.

Cushing, S. L., Gordon, K. A., Rutka, J. A., James, A. L., & Papsin, B. C. (2013). Vestibular end-organ dysfunction in children with sensorineural hearing loss and cochlear implants: An expanded cohort and etiologic assessment. *Otology and Neurotology, 34,* 422–428.

Cushing, S. L., Papsin, B. C., Rutka, J. A., James, A. L., Blaser, S. L., & Gordon, K. A. (2009). Vestibular end-organ and balance deficits after meningitis and cochlear implantation in children correlate poorly with functional outcome. *Otology and Neurotology, 30,* 488–495.

Cushing, S. L., Papsin, B. C., Rutka, J. A., James, A. L., & Gordon, K. A. (2008b). Evidence of vestibular and balance dysfunction in children with profound sensorineural hearing loss using cochlear implants. *Laryngoscope, 118,* 1814–1823.

D'Agostino, R., Melagrana, A., Pasquale, G., & Taborelli, G. (1997). The study of optokinetic "look" nystagmus in children: Our experience. *International Journal of Pediatric Otorhinolaryngology, 40,* 141–146.

De Kegel, A., Maes, L., Baetens, T., Dhooge, I., & Van, W. H. (2012). The influence of a vestibular dysfunction on the motor development of hearing-impaired children. *Laryngoscope, 122,* 2837–2843.

Erbek, S., Erbek, S. S., Gokmen, Z., Ozkiraz, S., Tarcan, A., & Ozluoglu, L. N. (2007). Clinical application of vestibular evoked myogenic potentials in healthy newborns. *International Journal of Pediatric Otorhinolaryngology, 71,* 1181–1185.

Eviatar, L., & Eviatar, A. (1979). The normal nystagmic response of infants to caloric and perrotatory stimulation. *Laryngoscope, 89,* 1036–1045.

Forssberg, H., & Nashner, L. M. (1982). Ontogenetic development of postural control in man: Adaptation to altered support and visual conditions during stance. *Journal of Neuroscience, 2,* 545–552.

Fujikawa, S., & Starr, A. (2000). Vestibular neuropathy accompanying auditory and peripheral neuropathies. *Archives of Otolaryngology-Head and Neck Surgery, 126,* 1453–1456.

Genetics Home Reference. (2012). *Waardenburg syndrome.* Retrieved from http://ghr.nlm.nih.gov/condition/waardenburg-syndrome

Genetics Home Reference. (2013). *Neurofibromatosis type 2.* Retrived from http://ghr.nlm.nih.gov/condition/neurofibromatosis-type-2

Gioacchini, F. M., Alicandri-Ciufelli, M., Kaleci, S., & Re, M. (2014). Prevalence and diagnosis of vestibular disorders in children: A review. *International Journal of Pediatric Otorhinolaryngology, 78,* 718–724.

Headache Classification Committee of the International Headache Society (IHS). (2013). The International Classification of Headache Disorders, 3rd edition (Beta version). *Cephalalgia, 33,* 629–808.

Hirabayashi, S., & Iwasaki, Y. (1995). Developmental perspective of sensory organization on postural control. *Brain and Development, 17,* 111–113.

Huang, Y. C., Yang, T. L., & Young, Y. H. (2012). Feasibility of ocular vestibular-evoked myogenic potentials (oVEMPs) recorded with eyes closed. *Clinical Neurophysiology, 123,* 376–381.

Humphriss, R. L., & Hall, A. J. (2011). Dizziness in 10 year old children: An epidemiological study. *International Journal of Pediatric Otorhinolaryngology, 75,* 395–400.

Inoue, A., Iwasaki, S., Ushio, M., Chihara, Y., Fujimoto, C., Egami, N., & Yamasoba, T. (2013). Effect of vestibular dysfunction on the development of gross motor function in children with profound hearing loss. *Audiology and Neurotology, 18,* 143–151.

Jackler, R. K., & De La Cruz, A. (1989). The large vestibular aqueduct syndrome. *Laryngoscope, 99,* 1238–1242.

Jacobs, M., Harris, C. M., Shawkat, F., & Taylor, D. (1997). Smooth pursuit development in infants. *Australian and New Zealand Journal of Ophthalmology, 25,* 199–206.

Jafari, Z., & Asad, M. S. (2011). The effect of saccular function on static balance ability of profound hearing-impaired children. *International Journal of Pediatric Otorhinolaryngology, 75,* 919–924.

Jatana, K. R., Thomas, D., Weber, L., Mets, M. B., Silverman, J. B., & Young, N. M. (2013). Usher syndrome: Characteristics and outcomes of pediatric cochlear implant recipients. *Otology and Neurotology, 34,* 484–489.

Jongkees, L. B., Maas, J. P., & Philipszoon, A. J. (1962). Clinical nystagmography. A detailed study of electronystagmography in 341 patients with vertigo. *Practica Otorhinolaryngologica (Basel), 24,* 65–93.

Kaga, K. (1999). Vestibular compensation in infants and children with congenital and acquired vestibular loss in both ears. *International Journal of Pediatric Otorhinolaryngology, 49,* 215–224.

Kaga, K., Shinjo, Y., Jin, Y., & Takegoshi, H. (2008). Vestibular failure in children with congenital deafness. *International Journal of Audiology, 47,* 590–599.

Kasai, M., Hayashi, C., Iizuka, T., Inoshita, A., Kamiya, K., Okada, H., . . . Ikeda, K. (2010). Vestibular function of patients with profound deafness related to GJB2 mutation. *Acta Oto-Laryngologica, 130,* 990–995.

Katsanis, J., Iacono, W., & Harris, M. (1998). Development of ocular functioning in preadolescence, adolescence, and adulthood. *Psychophysiology, 35,* 64–72.

Kelsch, T. A., Schaefer, L. A., & Esquivel, C. R. (2006). Vestibular evoked myogenic potentials in young children: Test parameters and normative data. *Laryngoscope, 116,* 895–900.

Kerber, K. A., Meurer, W. J., West, B. T., & Fendrick, A. M. (2008). Dizziness presentations in U.S. emergency departments, 1995–2004. *Academic Emergency Medicine, 15,* 744–750.

Lempert, T., & Neuhauser, H. (2009). Epidemiology of vertigo, migraine and vestibular migraine. *Journal of Neurology, 256,* 333–338.

Levens, S. L. (1988). Electronystagmography in normal children. *British Journal of Audiology, 22,* 51–56.

Maes, L., De Kegel, A., Van, W. H., & Dhooge, I. (2014). Rotatory and colic vestibular evoked myogenic potential testing in normal-hearing and hearing-impaired children. *Ear and Hearing, 35*(2), e21–32. doi:10.1097/ AUD.0b013e3182a6ca91

Maes, L., Dhooge, I., De, V. E., D'haenens, W., Bockstael, A., & Vinck, B. M. (2007). Water irrigation versus air insufflation: A comparison of two caloric test protocols. *International Journal of Audiology, 46,* 263–269.

Manzari, L. (2008). Enlarged vestibular aqueduct (EVA) related with recurrent benign paroxysmal positional vertigo (BPPV). *Medical Hypotheses, 70,* 61–65.

Manzari, L., Burgess, A. M., MacDougall, H. G., & Curthoys, I. S. (2012). Objective measures of vestibular function during an acute vertigo attack in a very young child. *European Archives of Otorhinolaryngology, 269,* 2589–2592.

Masuda, T., & Kaga, K. (2011). Influence of aging over 10 years on auditory and vestibular functions in three patients with auditory neuropathy. *Acta Oto-Laryngologica, 131,* 562–568.

Merchant, S. N., Nakajima, H. H., Halpin, C., Nadol, J. B., Jr., Lee, D. J., Innis, W. P., . . . Rosowski, J. J. (2007). Clinical investigation and mechanism of air-bone gaps in large vestibular aqueduct syndrome. *Annals of Otology, Rhinology, and Laryngology, 116,* 532–541.

Merchant, S. N., & Rosowski, J. J. (2008). Conductive hearing loss caused by third-window lesions of the inner ear. *Otology and Neurotology, 29,* 282–289.

Mezzalira, R., Neves, L. C., Maudonnet, O. A. Q., Bilecki, M. M. D. C., & de Avila, F. G. (2005). Oculomotricity in childhood: Is the normal range the same as in adults? *Brazilian Journal of Otorhinolaryngology, 71,* 680–685.

Nishida, Y., Ueda, K., & Fung, K. C. (1983). Congenital rubella syndrome: Function of equilibrium of 80 cases with deafness. *Laryngoscope, 93,* 938–940.

Niskar, A. S., Kieszak, S. M., Holmes, A., Esteban, E., Rubin, C., & Brody, D. J. (1998). Prevalence of hearing loss among children 6 to 19 years of age—The Third

National Health and Nutrition Examination Survey. *JAMA, 279,* 1071–1075.

O'Reilly, R. C., Morlet, T., Nicholas, B. D., Josephson, G., Horlbeck, D., Lundy, L., & Mercado, A. (2010). Prevalence of vestibular and balance disorders in children. *Otology and Neurotology, 31,* 1441–1444.

Peterka, R. J., & Black, F. O. (1990). Age-related changes in human posture control: Sensory organization tests. *Journal of Vestibular Research, 1,* 73–85.

Peterson, M. L., Christou, E., & Rosengren, K. S. (2006). Children achieve adult-like sensory integration during stance at 12-years-old. *Gait and Posture, 23,* 455–463.

Rine, R. M. (2007). Management of the pediatric patient with vestibular hypofunction. In S. J. Herdman (Ed.), *Vestibular rehabilitation* (3rd ed.). Philadelphia, PA: F. A. Davis, 360–374.

Rine, R. M., Braswell, J., Fisher, D., Joyce, K., Kalar, K., & Shaffer, M. (2004). Improvement of motor development and postural control following intervention in children with sensorineural hearing loss and vestibular impairment. *International Journal of Pediatric Otorhinolaryngology, 68,* 1141–1148.

Rine, R. M., Cornwall, G., Gan, K., LoCascio, C., O'Hare, T., Robinson, E., & Rice, M. (2000). Evidence of progressive delay of motor development in children with sensorineural hearing loss and concurrent vestibular dysfunction. *Perceptual and Motor Skills, 90,* 1101–1112.

Rine, R. M., Rubish, K., & Feeney, C. (1998). Measurement of sensory system effectiveness and maturational changes in postural control in young children. *Pediatric Physical Therapy, 10,* 16–20.

Rosengren, S. M., McAngus Todd, N. P., & Colebatch, J. G. (2005). Vestibular-evoked extraocular potentials produced by stimulation with bone-conducted sound. *Clinical Neurophysiology, 116,* 1938–1948.

Ruggieri, M., Gabriele, A. L., Polizzi, A., Salpietro, V., Nicita, F., Pavone, P., . . . Quattrone, A. (2013). Natural history of neurofibromatosis type 2 with onset before the age of 1 year. *Neurogenetics, 14,* 89–98.

Saka, N., Imai, T., Seo, T., Ohta, S., Fujimori, K., Masumura, C., . . . Sakagami, M. (2013). Analysis of benign paroxysmal positional nystagmus in children. *International Journal of Pediatric Otorhinolaryngology, 77,* 233–236.

Sazgar, A. A., Yazdani, N., Rezazadeh, N., & Yazdi, A. K. (2010). Vestibular evoked myogenic potential (VEMP) in patients with auditory neuropathy: Auditory neuropathy or audiovestibular neuropathy? *Acta Oto-Laryngologica, 130,* 1130–1134.

Schuknecht, H. F., Suzuka, Y., & Zimmerman, C. (1990) Delayed endolymphatic hydrops and its relationship to Meniere's disease. *Annals of Otology, Rhinology, and Laryngology, 99,* 843.

Shall, M. S. (2009). The importance of saccular function to motor development in children with hearing impairments. *International Journal of Otolaryngology, 2009,* Article ID: 972565. doi:10.1155/2009/972565

Sheykholeslami, K., Kaga, K., Murofushi, T., & Hughes, D. W. (2000). Vestibular function in auditory neuropathy. *Acta Oto-Laryngologica, 120,* 849–854.

Sheykholeslami, K., Megerian, C. A., Arnold, J. E., & Kaga, K. (2005). Vestibular-evoked myogenic potentials in infancy and early childhood. *Laryngoscope, 115,* 1440–1444.

Sheykholeslami, K., Schmerber, S., Habiby, K. M., & Kaga, K. (2004). Vestibular-evoked myogenic potentials in three patients with large vestibular aqueduct. *Hearing Research, 190,* 161–168.

Shumway-Cook, A., & Horak, F. B. (1986). Assessing the influence of sensory interaction on balance. *Physical Therapy, 66,* 1548–1550.

Sinha, S. K., Barman, A., Singh, N. K., Rajeshwari, G., & Sharanya, R. (2013). Involvement of peripheral vestibular nerve in individuals with auditory neuropathy. *European Archives of Otorhinolaryngology, 270,* 2207–2214.

Song, J. J., Hong, S. K., Kim, J. S., & Koo, J. W. (2012). Enlarged vestibular aqueduct may precipitate benign paroxysmal positional vertigo in children. *Acta Oto-Laryngologica, 132*(Suppl. 1), S109–S117.

Staller, S. J., Goin, D. W., & Hildebrandt, M. (1986). Pediatric vestibular evaluation with harmonic acceleration. *Otolaryngology-Head and Neck Surgery, 95,* 471–476.

Tajik-Parvinchi, D. J., Lillakas, L., Irving, E., & Steinbach, M. J. (2003). Children's pursuit eye movements: A developmental study. *Vision Research, 43,* 77–84.

Taylor, R. L., Bradshaw, A. P., Magnussen, J. S., Gibson, W. P., Halmagyi, G. M., & Welgampola, M. S. (2012). Augmented ocular vestibular evoked myogenic potentials to air-conducted sound in large vestibular aqueduct syndrome. *Ear and Hearing, 33,* 768–771.

Tribukait, A., Brantberg, K., & Bergenius, J. (2004). Function of semicircular canals, utricles and saccules in deaf children. *Acta Oto-Laryngologica, 124,* 41–48.

Valente, M. (2007). Maturational effects of the vestibular system: A study of rotary chair, computerized dynamic posturography, and vestibular evoked myogenic potentials with children. *Journal of the American Academy of Audiology, 18,* 461–481.

Valmaggia, C., Rutsche, A., Baumann, A., Pieh, C., Shavit, Y. B., Proudlock, F., & Gottlob, I. (2004). Age related change of optokinetic nystgmus in healthy subjects: A study from infancy to senescence. *British Journal of Ophthalmology, 88,* 1577–1581.

Valvassori, G. E., & Clemis, J. D. (1978). The large vestibular aqueduct syndrome. *Laryngoscope, 88,* 723–728.

Von Hofsten, C., & Rosander, K. (1997). Development of smooth pursuit tracking in young infants. *Vision Research, 37*(13), 1799–1810.

Wang, C. P., Hsu, W. C., & Young, Y. H. (2005). Vestibular evoked myogenic potentials in neurofibromatosis 2. *Annals of Otology, Rhinology, and Laryngology, 114,* 69–73.

Wang, S. J., Hsieh, W. S., & Young, Y. H. (2013). Development of ocular vestibular-evoked myogenic potentials in small children. *Laryngoscope, 123,* 512–517.

Wiener-Vacher, S. R., Obeid, R., & Abou-Elew, M. (2012). Vestibular impairment after bacterial meningitis delays infant posturomotor development. *Journal of Pediatrics, 161,* 246–251.

Wiener-Vacher, S. R., Toupet, F., & Narcy, P. (1996). Canal and otolith vestibulo-ocular reflexes to vertical and off vertical axis rotations in children learning to walk. *Acta Oto-Laryngologica, 116,* 657–665.

Wilson, D. F., Hodgson, R. S., & Talbot, J. M. (1997). Endolymphatic sac obliteration for large vestibular aqueduct syndrome. *American Journal of Otology, 18,* 101–106.

Woollacott, M., Debu, B., & Mowatt, M. (1987). Neuromuscular control of posture in the infant and child. *Journal of Motor Behavior, 19,* 167–186.

Yetiser, S., Kertmen, M., & Ozkaptan, Y. (1999). Vestibular disturbance in patients with large vestibular aqueduct syndrome (LVAS). *Acta Oto-Laryngologica, 119,* 641–646.

Zagolski-, O. (2008a). Vestibular system in infants after systemic therapy with amikacin. *Journal of Otolaryngology-Head and Neck Surgery, 37,* 534–539.

Zagolski, O. (2008b). Vestibular-evoked myogenic potentials and caloric stimulation in infants with congenital cytomegalovirus infection. *Journal of Laryngology and Otology, 122,* 574–579.

Zagolski, O. (2009). Vestibular-evoked myogenic potentials and caloric tests in infants with congenital rubella. *B-ENT, 5,* 7–12.

Zangemeister, W. H., & Bock, O. (1980). Air versus water caloric test. *Clinical Otolaryngology and Allied Sciences, 5,* 379–387.

Zapala, D. A., Olsholt, K. F., & Lundy, L. B. (2008). A comparison of water and air caloric responses and their ability to distinguish between patients with normal and impaired ears. *Ear and Hearing, 29,* 585–600.

Zhou, G., & Gopen, Q. (2011). Characteristics of vestibular evoked myogenic potentials in children with enlarged vestibular aqueduct. *Laryngoscope, 121,* 220–225.

Zhou, G., Gopen, Q., & Kenna, M. A. (2008). Delineating the hearing loss in children with enlarged vestibular aqueduct. *Laryngoscope, 118,* 2062–2066.

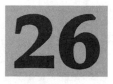

26

Nonmedical Management of Positional Vertigo

Richard A. Clendaniel

INTRODUCTION

Benign paroxysmal positional vertigo (BPPV) is one of the most common causes of dizziness, in some studies (Kroenke, Hoffman, & Einstadter, 2000) accounting for 16% of all cases of dizziness. In clinics specializing in the treatment of individuals with dizziness, BPPV is diagnosed in close to 30% of the individuals (Neuhauser, Leopold, von Brevern, Arnold, & Lempert, 2001). Estimates of the 1-year incidence of BPPV range from 0.01% to 2.4%, with a lifetime prevalence of 2.4% (Froehling et al., 1991; Mizukoshi, Watanabe, Shojaku, Okubo, & Watanabe, 1988; von Brevern et al., 2007). Fortunately, BPPV is easily diagnosed with relatively simple clinical tests and is, generally, effectively treated with various treatment maneuvers. In this chapter, we will review the signs and symptoms associated with BPPV, the presumed pathophysiology behind BPPV, and the treatment techniques for BPPV.

The first detailed description of positional vertigo was supplied by Bárány in 1921 (in Lanska & Remler, 1997), in which he noted several of the key characteristics of BPPV: mixed vertical and torsional nystagmus, the brief duration of the nystagmus and vertigo, as well as the decreased response, or fatigability, of the nystagmus and vertigo with repetitive provocations. In 1931 and 1950 Nylén (1931,

1950) described a series of test positions used for the assessment of positional nystagmus. While Nylén included many positions in his tests, none of which were analogous to the currently accepted provocative test for BPPV, he did make a clinically important, marked distinction between positional nystagmus and positioning nystagmus. The positional tests are performed slowly, taking 5 s to move the patient 90 degrees, and the resulting nystagmus is thought to be due to the position of the head in space, as compared to the positioning tests, which are performed rapidly, and the resulting nystagmus is due to the *movement* of the head into a specific position. Based on this distinction, BPPV is technically benign paroxysmal *positioning* vertigo (Brandt, 1990).

It wasn't until 1952 that Dix and Hallpike (1952) described the technique that we know as the Dix-Hallpike test. In addition, Dix and Hallpike confirmed the key characteristics of BPPV described earlier by Bárány and identified two other key characteristics of BPPV: (1) the latency to the onset of the nystagmus and vertigo, and (2) the reversal of the nystagmus when the patient sits up. They labeled this "positional vertigo of the benign paroxysmal type" and felt that it was caused by an irritative lesion of the peripheral vestibular system. Dix and Hallpike further postulated that it was irritation of the utricle that was responsible for the signs and symptoms of BPPV.

The utricular origin of BPPV was a matter of debate for several years. In the early 1960s, Schuknecht (1962) proposed that it was actually a gravity-dependent movement of loose otoconia that caused stimulation of the posterior semicircular canal (SCC) ampulla, producing the nystagmus and vertigo observed in BPPV. This model accounted for the latency, duration, and fatigability of the signs and symptoms associated with BPPV. However, the model was anatomically incorrect and did not fit with the known physiology of the hair cells within the posterior SSC. This hypothesis was subsequently revised based in part on the finding of deposits attached to the cupula, primarily of the posterior SCC, and to fit with the known anatomy and physiology of the vestibular system. The revised hypothesis (Schuknecht & Ruby, 1973), cupulolithiasis, proposed that the otoconia were attached to the cupula of the posterior SSC making the cupula gravity dependent, which would cause the cupula to deflect in a direction that excites the hair cells in the posterior SSC during the provocative tests. This hypothesis, while explaining the direction and latency of the observed nystagmus in BPPV, does not explain the typical short duration of the nystagmus.

Hall, Ruby, and McClure (1979) proposed an alternative mechanism behind BPPV, *canalolithiasis* (commonly called *canalithiasis*), in which the displaced otoconia, or canaliths, are freely mobile within the semicircular canal. This model accounts for all the characteristic of typical BPPV: latency, duration, direction of the nystagmus, reversal of the nystagmus, and fatigability. They also recognized a second form of BPPV where the canaliths are attached to the cupula, giving rise to nystagmus of prolonged duration.

There is some physical evidence to support these hypotheses. Schuknecht and Ruby (1973) did observe granular deposits adherent to the cupula of the posterior SCC in temporal bone studies of individuals who had a history of BPPV. Others (Parnes & McClure, 1992) have observed mobile particulate matter within the endolymph of the posterior SCC during canal plugging surgical procedures for BPPV, lending some anatomical support for canalithiasis. In addition, one study (Welling et al., 1997) evaluated the particulate matter removed from one posterior SCC under electron microscopy and reported that the material appeared consistent with degenerating otoconia. There are, however, studies that raise some questions about canalithiasis and cupulolithiasis. Kveton and Kashgarian (1994) reported finding particulate matter in posterior SCC of individuals who had no symptoms of BPPV. Moriarty and colleagues (Moriarty, Rutka, & Hawke, 1992) conducted temporal bone studies and measured the frequency and size of deposits on the cupulae of over 1,000 semicircular canals. They found deposits on close to 22% of the cupulae. The clinical histories were available for most of the patients, and there was no history of BPPV. Based on these findings, the significance of the deposits and particulate matter is unclear.

ETIOLOGY

There are few large series studies assessing the cause of BPPV. In the two studies (Baloh, Honrubia, & Jacobson, 1987; Katsarkas & Kirkham, 1978) that each looked at over 200 patients with BPPV, the most common etiology was idiopathic, accounting for 49% and 66% of the cases. BPPV secondary to head trauma was the next most common cause, accounting for 18% of the patients in both studies. BPPV was seen secondary to viral neurolabyrinthitis in 2% and 15% of the patients, and secondary to vertebrobasilar insufficiency in 1% and 5% of the cases. Miscellaneous disorders, including Ménière's, migraine, otosclerosis, and other ear disorders, were associated with BPPV in 12.5% and 13% of the patients in the two studies. Baloh and colleagues (1987) found that across all diagnostic groups the ratio of females to males was 1.6:1. While BPPV can be seen across all age ranges, it is unusual to see BPPV in children, and the idiopathic form of BPPV most frequently occurs to individuals in their 60s (Baloh et al., 1987).

Even though the earlier studies proposed that BPPV was due to stimulation of the posterior SCC, BPPV can be seen in the anterior and horizontal SCCs as well. Several studies (Herdman, Tusa, & Clendaniel, 1994; Korres et al., 2002; Prokopakis et al., 2005) have documented the occurrence rate of BPPV affecting the different semicircular canals. All three studies found that the posterior SCC was the most commonly affected canal, accounting for 83%

to 91% of the identified cases. The study by Korres and colleagues (2002) as well as the study by Prokopakis and colleagues (2005) found that horizontal SCC BPPV accounted for 8% and 10% of the cases, and that anterior SCC BPPV accounted for only 1% and 2% of the cases. In the study by Herdman and colleagues (1994), the prevalence of anterior SCC BPPV, 15%, was greater than horizontal SCC BPPV, 2%. In this study, there were a substantial number of individuals with BPPV who were not included in the analysis because the pattern of nystagmus, and the affected semicircular canal, could not be ascertained secondary to either eye closure during the nystagmus, or a vertical component that could not be determined. This may have affected the observed distribution of the affected semicircular canals.

CLINICAL PRESENTATION

Individuals suffering from BPPV experience brief but often intense symptoms of vertigo associated with changes in head position, or orientation, relative to gravity. These individuals commonly complain of vertigo associated with lying down, rolling over in bed, and sitting up from a reclined position. They will often note symptoms of vertigo with bending over and looking up for objects on a high shelf, prompting the name "top-shelf vertigo" (Squires, Weidman, Hain, & Stone, 2004). In addition to the symptoms of vertigo, individuals with BPPV typically also experience symptoms of nonspecific dizziness, lightheadedness, imbalance, and nausea (Baloh et al., 1987; Blatt, Georgakakis, Herdman, Clendaniel, & Tusa, 2000; Bloom & Katsarkas, 1989; von Brevern et al., 2007).

Before describing the clinical tests for BPPV, it is important to keep two facts in mind. One, what is critical in the testing (and treatment) of BPPV is the position of the head in space, not the position of the head relative to the patient's body. The tests that we will describe can be modified to accommodate individuals who have restricted cervical and trunk mobility. Two, the pattern and duration of the elicited nystagmus will indicate which of the semicircular canals is affected and whether it is a case of canalithiasis or cupulolithiasis. For both the canali-

thiasis and cupulolithiasis models of posterior semicircular canal BPPV, the provoking test will cause excitation of the posterior SCC hair cells, which will result in a mixed up-beating and torsional nystagmus, with the torsional nystagmus beating toward the affected ear. In cases of anterior SCC BPPV, the provoking test will cause excitation of the anterior SCC hair cells, leading to a mixed down-beating and torsional nystagmus, again with the torsional nystagmus beating toward the affected ear. BPPV affecting the horizontal SCC will produce a horizontal nystagmus. For horizontal SCC canalithiasis, when the displaced otoconia are located in the posterior aspect of one horizontal SCC, the provoking test will evoke nystagmus beating to the right when the head is turned to the right, and to the left when the head is turned to the left. In both cases, the nystagmus will beat toward the ground and is referred to as geotropic nystagmus. In cases of horizontal SCC cupulolithiasis, as well as canalithiasis where the displaced otoconia are located in the anterior arm of the horizontal SCC, the provoking test will cause the opposite pattern of stimulation to the hair cells, and produce left-beating nystagmus when the head is turned to the right and right-beating nystagmus when the head is turned to the left. In both cases, the nystagmus will beat away from the ground and is referred to as ageotropic, or apogeotropic, nystagmus. The elicited pattern of nystagmus in the provocative tests is summarized in Table 26–1.

The classic test for BPPV is the Dix-Hallpike test, originally described in 1952 (Dix & Hallpike, 1952). To perform this test the patient starts sitting on a treatment table with his or her neck rotated 45 degrees to one side (Figure 26–1A). This neck rotation places the ipsilateral posterior SCC in the sagittal plane, which will be the plane of the movement during the test. This will also place the ipsilateral posterior SCC in a gravity dependent position when the patient is supine, which should maximize the effect of gravity on the displaced otoconia within the semicircular canal. The clinician can stand either facing the patient (as shown) or behind the patient. The clinician will guide and assist the patient into lying supine with neck now in 20 to 30 degrees of extension (Figure 26–1B). The position change from sitting to supine should be performed relatively quickly, over the course of a couple of seconds. This

Table 26-1. Elicited Nystgmus in BPPV by Semicircular Canal Involvement

Affected Semicircular Canal	Right	Left
Posterior	Up-beating Right torsion	Up-beating Left torsion
Anterior	Down-beating Right torsion	Down-beating Left torsion
Horizontal		
Canalithiasis	Geotropic[a]	Geotropic[a]
Cupulolithiasis and anterior arm canalithiasis	Ageotropic[a]	Ageotropic[a]

[a]BPPV on one side will produce nystagmus with provocative test to both sides.

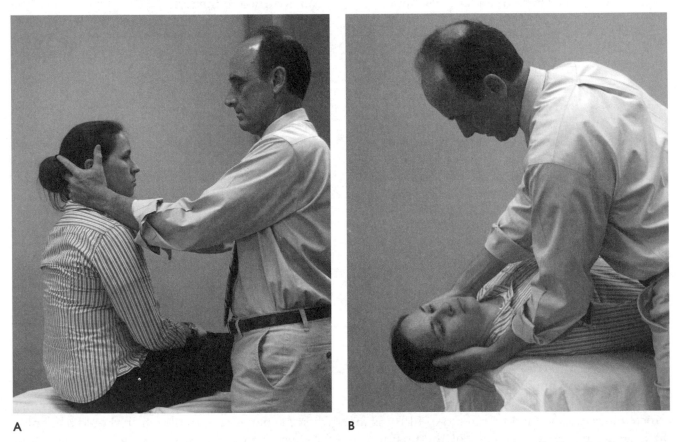

A   B

Figure 26-1. The Dix-Hallpike test on the right. **A.** Patient sits lengthwise on the treatment table. The clinician rotates the patient's neck 45 degrees to the right. **B.** The patient lies down quickly, assisted by the clinician, and extends the neck approximately 30 degrees. The undermost ear, in this case the right ear, should be below the level of the patient's shoulder. The clinician monitors the patient's symptoms and eye movements. *continues*

position is maintained and the clinician monitors the patient's symptoms and eye movements, looking for nystagmus. The test can be performed in room light or with vision blocked using Frenzel goggles (either optical or video). Patients typically cannot suppress the nystagmus associated with BPPV, so

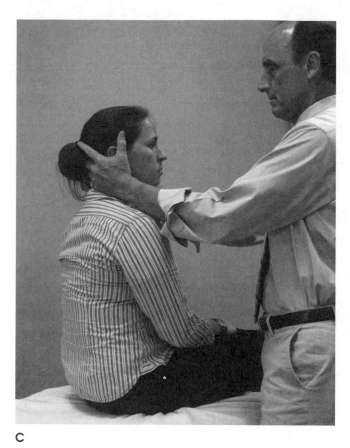

C

Figure 26–1. *continued* **C.** The clinician maintains the 45 degrees of neck rotation and assists the patient back into a sitting position, again monitoring for symptoms and nystagmus.

Frenzel goggles are not required; however, the Frenzel goggles will make it easier to observe the nystagmus. There is typically a short latency to the onset of the nystagmus and vertigo once the patient is in the supine position, but in some cases the latency can be prolonged, so when performing the Dix-Hallpike test, it is recommended that the patient be kept in the supine position for 30 s. Once the nystagmus and symptoms have stopped, or after the 30 s in the test position. The patient is assisted to a seated position (Figure 26–1C). Again, the clinician will monitor the patient for symptoms and nystagmus. Patients who have BPPV will often develop symptoms and nystagmus on coming back to a seated position, so it is critical that the clinician maintains contact and guards the patient after the patient sits up. The test is then repeated with the neck rotated 45 degrees to the other side. If the patient has limited cervical exten-

sion, the test can be modified by having the patient lie on an inclined table, with the head of the table lower than the foot of the table.

Another test is the side-lying test, described by Cohen (2004) as an alternative to the traditional Dix-Hallpike test for individuals with limited mobility, especially cervical extension. To perform this test, the patient starts sitting on the treatment table with his or her neck rotated 45 degrees away from the side to be tested. The clinician will assist and guide the patient into a side-lying position on the side to be tested (Figure 26–2). Like the Dix-Hallpike test, this movement is performed rapidly, and then the clinician monitors the patient for provocation of symptoms and nystagmus. The clinician will then assist the patient back to a seated position, maintaining the cervical rotation during the movement. Once upright, the patient rotates his or her neck to neutral and the clinician monitors the patient for nystagmus and symptoms. The test is then repeated to the opposite side with the neck rotated in the opposite direction. Rotating the patient's neck 45 degrees to one side will place the contralateral posterior semicircular canal in the frontal plane, which will be the plane of the movement during the test. This again places the posterior SCC in a gravity dependent position when the patient is side-lying and should maximize the effect of gravity on the displaced otoconia within the semicircular canal. Cohen (2004) found no statistical difference between the side-lying and Dix-Hallpike tests in the initial study.

Although the Dix-Hallpike test is thought to primarily test the posterior and anterior semicircular canals, patients with horizontal semicircular canal BPPV may have a positive Dix-Hallpike test. The roll test is a positioning test designed to specifically assess for horizontal canal BPPV. The basis of this test was discussed briefly by McClure (1985) and then formally described by Pagnini, Nuti, and Vannucchi (1989). To perform this test, the patient starts sitting on the treatment table with his or her neck in neutral. The patient then lies supine, with the head elevated approximately 30 degrees, which places the horizontal SCC in an earth vertical orientation. The clinician will then assist the patient in rotating his or her neck 90 degrees to one side (Figure 26–3A–B). Like the Dix-Hallpike test, this movement is performed rapidly through the available range of cervical rotation. If the patient has

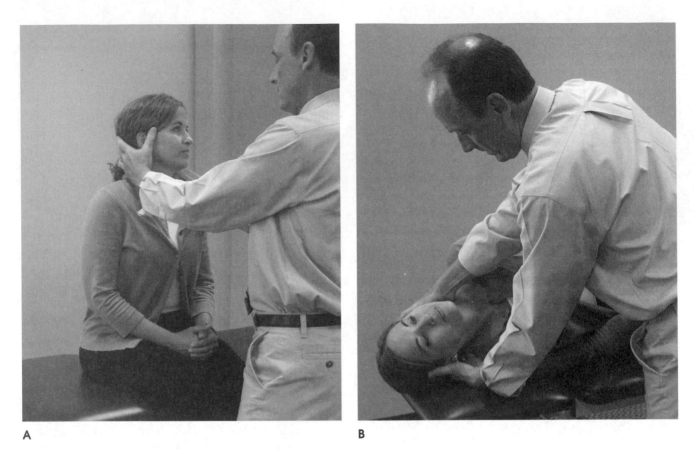

A   B

Figure 26-2. The side-lying test for the right. **A.** Patient sits on the treatment table. The clinician rotates the patient's neck 45 degrees to the left. **B.** The patient lies down quickly on the right side, assisted by the clinician, and side bends the neck to bring the head to the table. The clinician monitors the patient's symptoms and eye movements. The clinician will then assist the patient back up to a seated position, again monitoring the patient's symptoms and nystagmus.

limited cervical rotation, then the patient can simply roll to one side. The clinician monitors the patient for provocation of symptoms and nystagmus. The patient will then rotate the neck to a neutral position. This process will then be repeated to the other side (Figure 26–3C).

What constitutes a positive, or abnormal, positioning test? One can make the diagnosis of BPPV when the positioning test induces vertigo and nystagmus that meet the following criteria:

1. Vertigo and nystagmus that are consistent with stimulation of the posterior SCC (mixed up-beating and torsion), the anterior SCC (mixed down-beating and torsion), or horizontal SCC (horizontal nystagmus, geotropic or ageotropic, when testing both sides);

2. A latency (generally less than 5 s) to the onset of the symptoms and nystagmus once the patient is in the testing position;

3. Paroxysmal vertigo and nystagmus (duration less than 1 min, displaying an increase and then decrease in intensity); and

4. Fatigability of the nystagmus and vertigo with repeated testing (Bhattacharyya et al., 2008; Furman & Cass, 1999).

From a clinical perspective, the fatigability of the nystagmus and symptoms are often not tested, as the patients will typically be treated following the diagnosis of BPPV. The duration of the nystagmus shows some variability. The nystagmus associated with horizontal SCC canalithiasis may last longer than 1 min secondary to the velocity storage system.

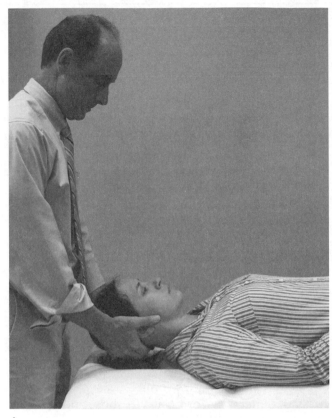

A

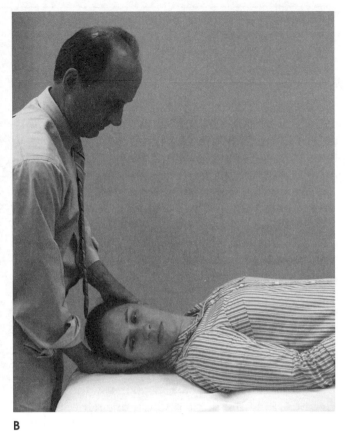

B

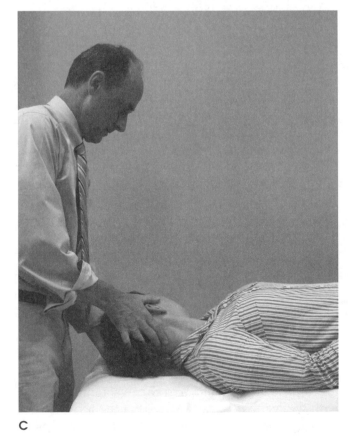

C

Figure 26-3. Roll test for horizontal SCC BPPV. **A.** The patient starts in supine with the neck flexed approximately 30 degrees. **B.** The clinician assists the patient in rotating the neck 90 degrees to the right. The clinician monitors the patient's symptoms and nystagmus. Then the patient will return the neck to neutral rotation. **C.** The clinician assists the patient in rotating the neck 90 degrees to the left, again monitoring the patient's symptoms and nystagmus. Then the patient will return the neck to neutral rotation.

In cases of cupulolithiasis affecting any of the semicircular canals, the nystagmus may persist as long as the individual remains in the provoking position.

The elicited pattern of nystagmus is critical for determining the affected semicircular canal. For the posterior SCC, the diagnosis is usually straightforward, as the Dix-Hallpike test on the affected side will generate the expected pattern of nystagmus, and the Dix-Hallpike test on the healthy side will be negative (no nystagmus or vertigo). The clinical presentation of anterior SCC BPPV is not as clear. There are reports in the literature that for anterior SCC BPPV, the Dix-Hallpike test will be positive when the neck is rotated away from the affected ear (Y. K. Kim, Shin, & Chung, 2005), toward the affected ear (Bertholon, Bronstein, Davies, Rudge, & Thilo, 2002; Crevits, 2004), and with cervical rotation in both directions (Bertholon et al., 2002). The variability of the provocative test is due to the orientation of the anterior SCC during the testing. For example, when performing the right Dix-Hallpike test, the left anterior SCC is in the plane of the movement and ends up in an earth vertical orientation. Canaliths within that canal could then fall away from the ampulla, leading to excitation of the hair cells with a resultant down-beating, left torsional nystagmus. If one were to perform the left Dix-Hallpike in this same patient, the left anterior SCC would not be aligned with the movement or end up in an earth vertical orientation. However, due to the cervical extension in the Dix-Hallpike, the left anterior SCC will tilt below horizontal. Again, canaliths within the canal could then fall away from the ampulla, leading to excitation of the hair cells, again with a resultant down-beating, left torsional nystagmus. The clinician must base the determination of the affected anterior SCC on the direction of the torsional nystagmus, not on the side of the provocative Dix-Hallpike test.

The horizontal SCC poses additional diagnostic challenges. Due to the orientation of the horizontal SCCs during the provoking tests, one horizontal SCC will be stimulated with tests to both sides. The elicited nystagmus will either be geotropic, or ageotropic with positioning tests to both sides. Geotropic nystagmus is attributed to canalithiasis of the horizontal SCC (Baloh, Jacobson, & Honrubia, 1993; McClure, 1985). Ageotropic nystagmus may be caused by either cupulolithiasis of the horizontal

SCC, or by a variant of canalithiasis where the canaliths are located in the anterior arm of the horizontal SCC near the cupula (Baloh, Yue, Jacobson, & Honrubia, 1995; Fife, 1998; Nuti, Vannucchi, & Pagnini, 1996; Steddin & Brandt, 1996). Determination of the affected ear may be made based on the intensity of the elicited nystagmus and symptoms. For horizontal SCC canalithiasis, it is hypothesized (McClure, 1985; Pagnini et al., 1989) that the direction of the head rotation that elicits the greatest nystagmus and symptoms is the affected side. This is based in part on Ewald's second law (Baloh, Honrubia, & Konrad, 1977) whereby an excitatory stimulus generates a greater response than an inhibitory stimulus of equal magnitude. The observed response asymmetry may also be due to the distance between the canaliths and the cupula, as well as the diminished effect as the canaliths move out of the canal into the utricular space (Baloh et al., 1993). For horizontal SCC cupulolithiasis and the anterior arm variant of canalithiasis, the positioning tests will generate cupular deflections opposite to those induced by typical horizontal SCC canalithiasis. Thus, a positioning test to the involved side will lead to inhibition of the hair cells of that canal, and a decreased response as compared to the response elicited by the positioning test to the unaffected side (Baloh et al., 1977; Steddin & Brandt, 1996).

Another test to determine the affected horizontal SCC is the bow and lean test described by Choung, Shin, Kahng, Park, and Choi (2006). Once the direction of the nystagmus, geotropic or ageotropic, has been determined, the bow and lean test can be performed. The patient starts seated upright. To perform the "bow," the patient will flex his or her cervical and upper thoracic spine to bow the head 90 degrees. Once in this position, the clinician will determine the direction of the elicited nystagmus. After the patient returns to an upright, seated position, the "lean" component of the test is performed by having the patient extend the neck and trunk to lean the head back 45 degrees. Again, the clinician will determine the direction of the elicited nystagmus. For patients with horizontal SCC canalithiasis, the nystagmus elicited with the bow will beat toward the affected ear, and the nystagmus elicited with the lean will beat away from the affected ear. For example, consider right-sided, horizontal SCC canalithiasis. The "bow" will cause the canaliths to fall toward the ampulla, ampullopetal stimulation, leading to excitation of the hair cells in the right horizontal SCC, which will elicit nystagmus beating to the right (toward the affected ear). The "lean" will cause the canaliths to fall away from the ampulla, ampullofugal stimulation, leading to inhibition of the hair cells in the right horizontal SCC, which will elicit nystagmus beating to the left (away from the affected ear). For patients with horizontal SCC cupulolithiasis, the opposite pattern is seen; the nystagmus elicited by the bow will beat away from the affected ear, and that elicited by the lean will beat toward the affected ear. As an example, now consider right-sided, horizontal SCC cupulolithiasis. The "bow" will cause the canaliths to fall away from the ampulla, ampullofugal stimulation, leading to inhibition of the hair cells in the right horizontal SCC, which will elicit nystagmus beating to the left (away from the affected ear). The "lean" will cause the canaliths to fall toward the ampulla, ampullopetal stimulation, leading to excitation of the hair cells in the right horizontal SCC, which will elicit nystagmus beating to the right (toward the affected ear). In the initial study (Choung et al., 2006) of 26 patients with horizontal SCC BPPV, there was agreement between the bow and lean test and the intensity of the nystagmus in determination of the affected side in 50% of the cases. There were three patients where the investigators could not determine an intensity difference but there were clear findings with the bow and lean test. Likewise, there were three patients who had no nystagmus in the bow and lean test. There was disagreement between the two testing methods in seven patients. In all seven, treatment based on the results of the bow and lean test was successful.

TREATMENT

Posterior Semicircular Canal BPPV

Brandt-Daroff Exercise

Thomas Brandt and Robert Daroff (Brandt & Daroff, 1980) were the first to describe a treatment for BPPV.

The treatment, now commonly called the Brandt-Daroff exercise, is a series of position changes carried out by the patient, multiple times during the day. To perform this exercise, the patient sits on the edge of a bed, rotates the neck 45 degrees away from the affected ear, and then, with eyes closed, lies down on the affected side (Figure 26–4A–B). The patient remains in this position until the vertiginous symptoms stop. Then, keeping the neck rotated, the patient sits up. Once back in a seated position, the patient rotates the head back to neutral. After waiting 30 s, longer if needed for any vertiginous symptoms to pass, the patient rotates the neck 45 degrees toward the affected ear, and then rapidly lies down on the unaffected side (Figure 26–4C–D). After 30 s, or longer if needed for any vertiginous symptoms to pass, the patient sits back up and rotates the neck back to neutral. In the original study, this sequence of position changes was repeated within one exercise session until the vertigo was not provoked with the position changes. The patients performed the exercises every 3 hr while awake, and the exercises were continued until they were free of symptoms for two consecutive days. In current clinical practice, patients are commonly asked to perform 10 to 15 sequences in a row, three times a day. Brandt and Daroff reported that 66 of the 67 patients had a resolution of their signs and symptoms within 3 to 14 days. While the Brandt-Daroff exercise has often been referred to as a habituation exercise, Brandt and Daroff argued that the observed changes were too rapid for habituation and were most likely due to a mechanical displacement of the canaliths.

Whereas the study by Brandt and Daroff was uncontrolled, a more recent study (Amor-Dorado et al., 2012) compared the Brandt-Daroff exercise (five cycles per session, three sessions per day) to the particle, or canalith, repositioning maneuver, PRM. There was a statistically significant difference in the remission rate 1 week after the treatment, with 80.5% of the patients in the CRM group having negative Dix-Hallpike tests as compared to only 25% of the patients performing the Brandt-Daroff exercises. This statistically significant difference was present at 1 month as well. Based on these studies, there is some evidence that supports the use of the Brandt-Daroff exercise; however, other treatments may be more effective.

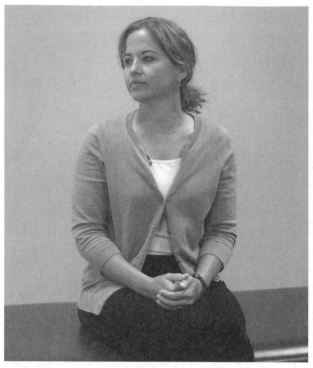

A

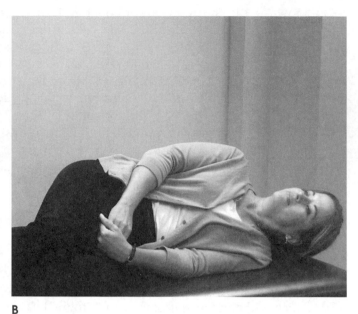

B

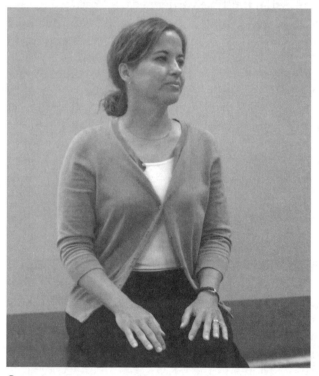

C

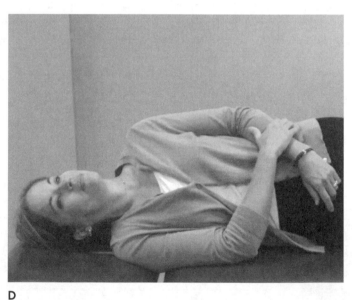

D

Figure 26-4. The Brandt-Daroff exercise for left posterior SCC BPPV. **A.** Patient starts sitting on a bed with the neck rotated 45 degrees to the right (to the unaffected side). **B.** Patient lies down quickly onto the left side (the affected side), maintaining the neck rotation. Once the vertigo and nystagmus have stopped the patient sits up still maintaining the neck rotation. The patient again waits until the vertigo and nystagmus have stopped, or 30 s if he or she has no symptoms. **C.** Patient rotates the neck 45 degrees to the left. **D.** Patient lies down quickly onto the right side, maintaining the neck rotation. The patient again waits until the vertigo and nystagmus have stopped, or 30 s if he or she has no symptoms, and then the patient sits up. This sequence is repeated 10 to 15 times in a row, or until the patient is asymptomatic with the position changes.

Particle Repositioning Maneuvers

The particle repositioning maneuvers (PRMs) are a set of prescribed head movements and head positions designed to move the canaliths through the involved canal and into the utricular space. These movements are often called the canalith repositioning procedure, CRP, (or canalith repositioning maneuver, or treatment). The term *canalith repositioning procedure* was used by Epley (1992) to describe treatment of posterior SCC BPPV, and we reserve the use of CRP for that particular treatment and use PRM as a more general term. As with testing for BPPV, the position of the head in space is the critical factor during the PRMs. The treatments described in the following sections may be modified to accommodate the patient and their physical limitations. For example, an individual with thoracic kyphosis and limited cervical extension may not be able to extend the neck sufficiently during the CRP. The treatment can be modified by placing the patient on a tilt table with the head of the bed lower than the foot. This positioning will allow the patient's head to tilt beyond horizontal, the critical position of the head, while accommodating the patient's kyphotic posture and limited cervical range of motion.

Canalith Repositioning Procedure. John Epley (1992) described the canalith repositioning procedure for treatment of posterior SCC canalithiasis. The treatment was based on the idea that the displaced otoconia, the canaliths, were freely mobile in the semicircular canal and that one could use gravity and a series of head positions to pull the canaliths away from the ampulla and into the utricular space. To perform the treatment, the patient starts sitting lengthwise on a treatment table, with the neck rotated 45 degrees to the affected side (Figure 26–5A). The clinician, maintaining the cervical rotation, then assists and guides the patient into a supine position with the neck extended 30 degrees off the edge of the treatment table, essentially repeating the Dix-Hallpike test (Figure 26–5B). The patient is kept in this position until the nystagmus stops. The clinician will guide the patient's head as the patient rotates the neck so that it is rotated 45 degrees to the other side (Figure 26–5C). The patient is again kept in this position until the nystagmus stops. If no nystagmus is observed with the change in head position, then the patient maintains this position for a time equal to the duration of the nystagmus observed in the Dix-Hallpike test. The patient will then roll onto the unaffected side (Figure 26–5D). During this movement,

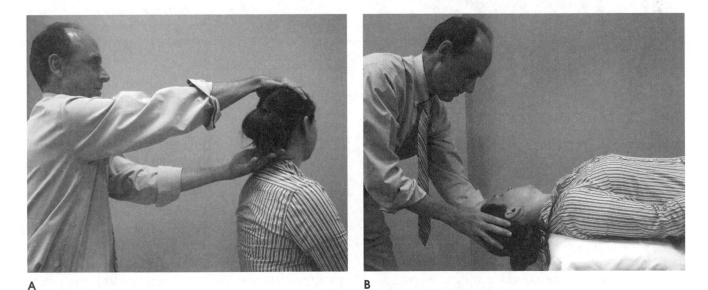

A   B

Figure 26-5. The canalith repositioning procedure (CRP) for treating left-sided posterior (or anterior) SCC canalithiasis. **A.** The patient starts sitting lengthwise on the treatment table, with the neck rotated 45 degrees to the affected side. **B.** The clinician assists and guides the patient into supine, extending the patient's neck off the edge of the treatment table approximately 30 degrees below horizontal. The patient stays in this position at least until the nystagmus stops, if not 15 to 30 s longer. *continues*

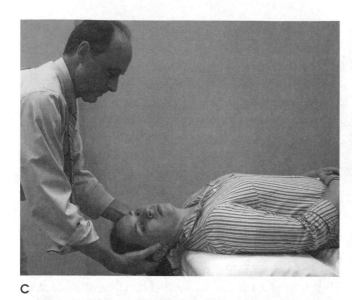

C

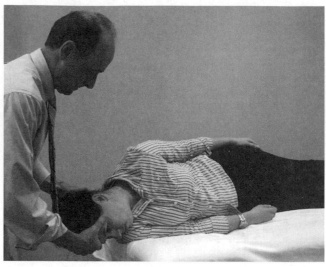

D

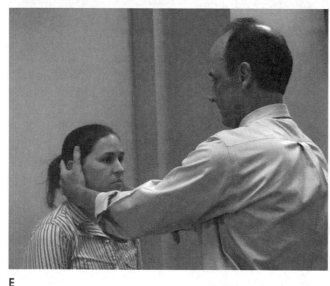

E

Figure 26–5. *continued* **C.** The clinician will then rotate the patient's neck 90 degrees, so the patient ends up in 45 degrees rotation to the right, maintaining the neck extension throughout the movement. The patient will remain in this position until the nystagmus stops, or as long as he or she remained in the previous position. **D.** The clinician will then assist and guide the patient into right side lying. The patient maintains the 45 degrees of neck rotation, but as the patient rolls to the side, the clinician will guide the patient's neck from extension to side bending to the right, bringing the patient's chin toward the right shoulder. The patient will remain in this position until the nystagmus stops, or as long as the patient remained in the first supine position. **E.** The clinician assists the patient into a seated position, maintaining the cervical rotation and side bending as the patient sits up. Once upright, the patient's neck can be brought to an upright and straight-ahead position.

the 45 degrees of cervical rotation is maintained, and as the patient rolls onto the side, the neck is brought out of extension and into lateral flexion, side bending, toward the treatment table. The patient will end up in a side-lying position with the chin tucked down near the undermost shoulder. Care should be taken during this position change to avoid bringing the patient's head above horizontal. The side lying position is again maintained until the nystagmus stops, or if no nystagmus is observed, the patient maintains this position for a time equal to the duration of the nystagmus observed in the Dix-Hallpike test. Maintaining the head position relative to the body, the clinician will assist the patient back to sitting, at which point the patient can rotate the neck

back to neutral and come out of the flexed position (Figure 26–5E). Since the patient can develop nystagmus and vertigo once he or she sits upright, the clinician should hold onto the patient and observe the eyes upon completion of the treatment.

Clinicians have modified some aspects of the original CRP. Epley (1992) recommended the use of medications (transdermal scopolamine or diazepam) to reduce nausea and prevent vomiting during the test and treatment. There is no mention of the use of medication for these symptoms in the current clinical practice guidelines (Bhattacharyya et al., 2008; Fife et al., 2008). However, for patients with a history of vomiting with the BPPV, antiemetic medications such as Phenergan and Compazine may be useful. Epley also recommended the use of mastoid vibration during treatment to help move the canaliths through the canal. Studies (Hain, Helminski, Reis, & Uddin, 2000; Ruckenstein & Shepard, 2007) to date have shown that vibration does not improve the efficacy of the treatment. In addition, a Cochrane Review (Hunt, Zimmermann, & Hilton, 2012) concluded that there was no evidence that vibration added to the treatment outcomes. Last, Epley recommended that patients avoid lying down for 48 hr after the treatment. Massoud and Ireland (1996) demonstrated no difference in outcomes between those who received the posttreatment restrictions and those who did not. Similar findings were seen in another study (Nuti, Nati, & Passali, 2000), and the Cochrane Review (Hunt et al., 2012) concluded that there was no clinical benefit to the posttreatment restrictions.

Semont Maneuver. Another PRM was described by Semont, Freyss, and Vitte (1988), which is often referred to as the Semont maneuver, Liberatory maneuver, or Brisk maneuver. In the original paper, they suggested that this treatment would work for either canalithiasis or cupulolithiasis by moving the particles through the posterior SCC, or off of the cupula. To perform the treatment as originally described, the patient starts sitting on a treatment table. The clinician assists and guides the patient into a side-lying position on the affected side, letting the neck side bend to bring the head to the table. If there is no nystagmus, then the clinician rotates the patient's neck 45 degrees, facing away from the table (Figure 26–6A–B). The patient will remain in this position for 2 to 3 min after the nystagmus has stopped. Maintaining the 45 degrees of cervical rotation, the patient is quickly moved into the opposite side-lying position, with a sudden deceleration of the head in the clinician's hands (Figure 26–6C). If there is no nystagmus, the clinician slowly rotates the patient's neck 90 degrees, and then rapidly rotates back down to the original 45 degrees, nose-down position (Figure 26–6D–E) to induce the nystagmus and vertigo. The patient remains in this position for at least 5 min and is then slowly brought back to the seated position. Others have modified the timing of the treatment such that the patient remains in the initial side-lying position for 2 min and the final side-lying position for 3 min (Levrat, van Melle, Monnier, & Maire, 2003), or 4 min in each position (Herdman, Tusa, Zee, Proctor, & Mattox, 1993). Others (Cohen & Kimball, 2005) actually modified the movements such that from the initial side-lying position, the patient's neck was rotated to a 45 degree nose-down position, rather than moving into side lying on the opposite side.

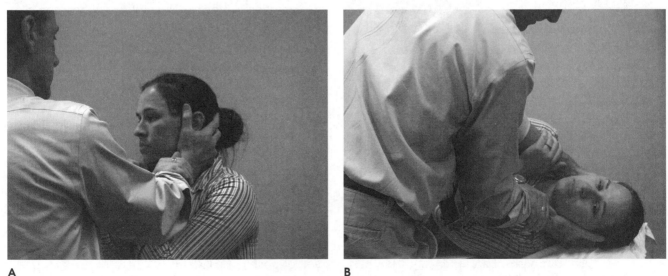

A   B

Figure 26–6. The Semont maneuver for left-sided posterior SCC canalithiasis or cupulolithiasis. **A.** The patient starts sitting on the treatment table with the neck rotated 45 degrees to the right, which places the affected posterior SCC in the plane of the movement. The patient may want to cross the arms and grasp the clinician's forearms for extra support. **B.** The patient is brought rapidly into left side lying, maintaining the 45 degrees of cervical rotation. The neck can then side bend to the left, bringing the head down to the table. The patient remains in this position for 1 to 2 min after the nystagmus has stopped. *continues*

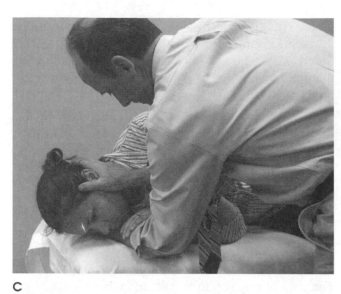

C

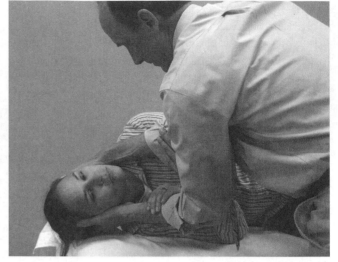

D

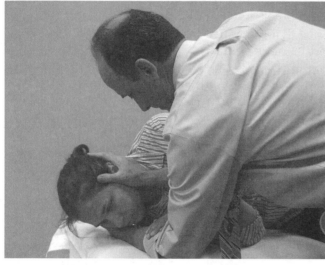

E

Figure 26–6. *continued* **C.** The clinician, along with assistance from the patient, rapidly moves the patient from left side lying to right side lying, maintaining the rightward neck rotation throughout the movement. There is a sudden deceleration of the patient's head in the clinician's hands as the patient's shoulder and the clinician's forearm hit the treatment table. The patient should experience vertigo at this point. If not, the clinician can rotate the patient's neck 90 degrees to the left (**D**) and then rapidly back down toward the treatment table (**E**). The original description of the treatment called for the patient to remain in this position for 5 min after the cessation of the vertigo and nystagmus. In clinical practice today, the patient typically remains in this position for 2 min after the vertigo and nystagmus stop. The clinician will then guide the patient back to a seated position, maintaining the cervical rotation until the patient is upright. Note that this treatment may be performed with the clinician standing behind the patient.

Outcomes

There is strong evidence to support the use of the PRMs in the treatment of posterior SCC BPPV. There are numerous randomized controlled trials demonstrating the effectiveness of the CRP for the treatment of posterior SCC BPPV (Cohen & Kimball, 2005; Froehling et al., 2000; Lynn, Pool, Rose, Brey, & Suman, 1995; Simhadri, Panda, & Raghunathan, 2003; von Brevern et al., 2006; Yimtae, Srirompotong, Srirompotong, & Sae-Seaw, 2003). These studies reported success rates of 41% to 95% in the treatment groups as compared to 4% to 35% in the control groups. Some of the variability in these numbers is due to the timing of the posttreatment assessments,

which ranged from 24 hr to 4 weeks. In addition to the RCTs, there have been Cochrane reviews (Hilton & Pinder, 2004; Hunt et al., 2012) and meta-analyses (White, Savvides, Cherian, & Oas, 2005; Woodworth, Gillespie, & Lambert, 2004), which all support the use of the CRP. The two published clinical practice guidelines (Bhattacharyya et al., 2008; Fife et al., 2008) both recommend the use of the CRP for treatment of posterior SCC BPPV.

Even though there have not been as many investigations of the Semont maneuver, numerous studies have demonstrated the effectiveness of this treatment approach. Semont and colleagues (1988) reported an 84% success rate with one maneuver and a 93% success rate with two maneuvers. Herdman and colleagues (1993) reported a 70% success rate with one treatment; while Levrat and colleagues (2003) reported a 63% success rate after one treatment and an 84% success rate with two treatments. In a controlled study, where the sham treatment was the Semont maneuver to the unaffected side, Mandalà and colleagues (2012) reported an 87% success rate in the treatment arm at 24 hr, as compared to a 0% success rate in the sham arm. Cohen and Kimball (2005) showed a similar decrease in vertigo frequency and intensity in patients treated with either the CRP or their modified Semont maneuver. The vertigo frequency and intensity in both of these groups were markedly less than that observed in the sham treatment group. Published clinical practice guidelines (Bhattacharyya et al., 2008; Fife et al., 2008) support the use of the Semont maneuver for the treatment of posterior SCC BPPV, but due to the paucity of studies comparing the Semont maneuver to the CRP, the practice guidelines did not make recommendations regarding the comparative effectiveness of two PRMs.

Treatment Considerations

Since the posttreatment restrictions are not required, clinicians may retest and repeat treatment as needed within one treatment session. There is marked variability in the literature in terms of the number of maneuvers performed in a treatment session, from one per session (Lynn et al., 1995) to repeated maneuvers (maximum of five) until there is resolution of the nystagmus in the Dix-Hallpike test (Froehling et al., 2000). Due to this variability, the clinical practice guideline (Bhattacharyya et al., 2008) makes no recommendations as to the number of maneuvers performed in a treatment session. Based on the literature, repeat testing and treatment within a given session are not contraindicated. The clinician, however, should be mindful of the patient's overall symptoms, as repeated provocation can lead to nausea and emesis.

Complications from the PMRs are rare and mild. No serious complications were reported in the RCTs. Mild complications of nausea, vomiting, fainting, and canal conversions were present in 6% to 12% of the patients (Herdman & Tusa, 1996; Yimtae et al., 2003). Herdman and Tusa (1996) reported that of 85 patients treated with the CRP for posterior SCC BPPV, 6% presented with a canal conversion on reassessment. Three individuals developed horizontal SCC BPPV, and two individuals developed anterior SCC BPPV. Yimtae and colleagues (2003) reported that two of 22 patients treated for posterior SCC BPPV with the CRP developed canal conversions, and in both cases it was the horizontal SCC that was affected. Canal conversions are infrequent and, based on the above studies, are more likely to occur in the horizontal SCC. A modeling study of BPPV (Rajguru, Ifediba, & Rabbitt, 2004) suggests that during the CRP, as the patient is lying on his or her side, the neck should be laterally flexed away from the table to decrease the conversion of posterior to anterior SCC BPPV. As canal conversions to the anterior SCC are rare, and as this is a modeling study with no clinical data to support it, the recommended modification to the CRP seems premature at this time.

Anterior Semicircular Canal BPPV

There are numerous treatments that have been proposed for the treatment of anterior SCC BPPV; unfortunately, all the studies are purely descriptive in nature. Initially, the "reverse Epley" maneuver was suggested as a treatment for anterior SSC canalithiasis (Epley, 2001; Honrubia, Baloh, Harris, & Jacobson, 1999); this maneuver is simply the CRP performed as if treating the contralateral posterior SCC. The data supporting this treatment are meager at best, with less than five patients in each of the studies and unclear outcomes (Honrubia et al., 1999; Korres, Riga, Balatsouras, & Sandris, 2008; Seok, Lee, Yoo, & Lee, 2008). Also, from an anatomical perspective, this series of head positions would not appear to be effective in clearing the particles from the anterior SCC. We describe here the three treatment approaches that have moderate evidence to support their use.

Particle Repositioning Maneuvers

The CRP, as described in the previous section for posterior SCC BPPV, has been used successfully for the treatment of anterior SCC canalithiasis (Jackson, Morgan, Fletcher, & Krueger, 2007; Lopez-Escamez, Molina, & Gamiz, 2006). Lopez-Escamez and colleagues (2006) reported that 11 of 14 individuals with anterior SCC canalithiasis had resolution of their signs and symptoms after one CRP. Similarly, Jackson et al. (2007) reported that 40 patients with anterior SCC canalithiasis required an average of 1.34 maneuvers to clear their signs and symptoms of BPPV. Note that if, for example, it is the *right* anterior SCC that is involved, the patients start the treatment with their neck rotated 45 degrees to the *right*, just as if they were treating the *right* posterior SCC BPPV.

Y. K. Kim and colleagues (2005) proposed a different treatment for anterior SCC BPPV. For this treatment, the patient starts by sitting on a treatment table and rotates the neck 45 degrees to the unaffected side (Figure 26–7A). Maintaining the cervical rotation, the clinician will assist and guide the patient in to a supine position, with the neck extended 30 to 45 degrees off the end of the table (Figure 26–7B); note that there is this discrepancy in the original article about the degree of neck extension. The patient remains in this position for 2 min. The clinician then brings the patient's neck back to 0 degrees of extension (Figure 26–7C), and the patient remains in this position for 1 min. The clinician will

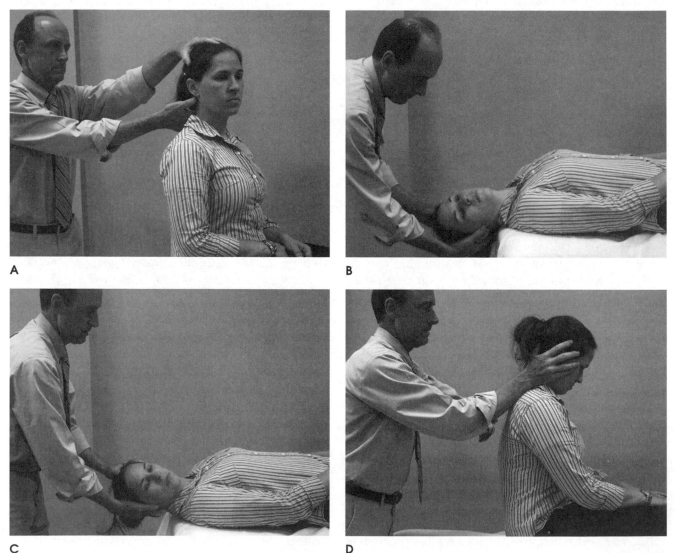

A

B

C

D

Figure 26-7. Treatment of left anterior SCC canalithiasis as described by Y. K. Kim et al. (2005). **A.** The patient starts sitting lengthwise on the treatment table, with the neck rotated 45 degrees to the right, which places the affected anterior SCC in the sagittal plane. **B.** The clinician guides the patient into supine and extends the neck 45 degrees below horizontal, maintaining the cervical rotation. The patient remains in this position for 2 min. **C.** The clinician will then raise the patient's head so that there is no neck extension. The patient stays in this position for 1 min. **D.** The clinician then assists the patient into sitting, and guides the patient's neck into flexion (chin to chest) and into neutral rotation. The patient remains in this position for 30 to 60 s.

then assist and guide the patient to a seated position, with the neck in 0 degrees of rotation and 30 degrees of flexion (Figure 26–7D). In a study of 60 patients with anterior SCC canalithiasis, Kim and colleagues (2005) found resolution of signs and symptoms in 46.7% following one treatment, and 80% after two treatments. Six patients required more than two treatments, and 96.7% of the patients ultimately had resolution of the signs and symptoms.

A different PRM was described by Yacovino, Hain, and Gualtieri (2009). For this treatment, the

patient starts by sitting lengthwise on a treatment table with no neck rotation (Figure 26–8A). The clinician will assist and guide the patient into a supine position, with the neck extended 30 degrees off the end of the table (Figure 26–8B). The patient remains in this position for 30 s. The clinician then quickly flexes the patient's neck to a chin to chest position (Figure 26–8C), and the patient remains in this position for 30 s. The clinician will then assist and guide the patient to a seated position, maintaining the neck in the flexed position (Figure 26–8D). After 30 s in

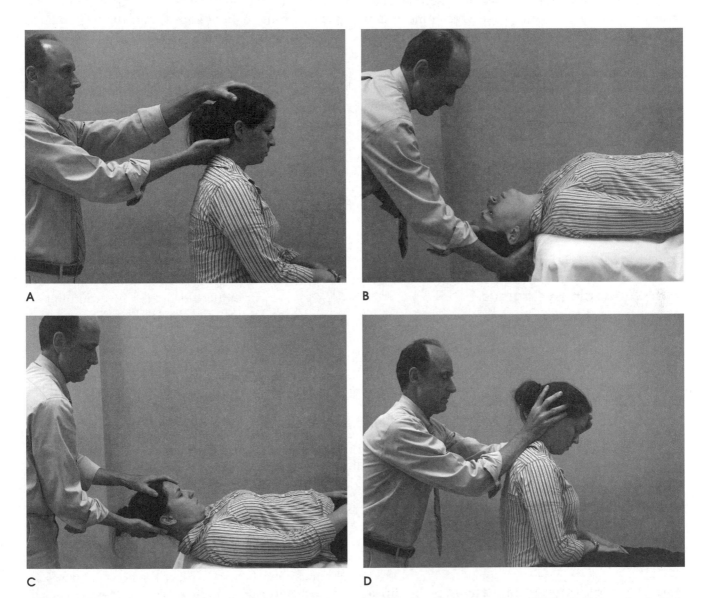

Figure 26–8. Treatment of anterior SCC canalithiasis as described by Yacovino et al. (2009). **A.** The patient starts sitting lengthwise on the treatment table, with the neck in neutral. **B.** The clinician guides the patient into supine and extends the neck 30 degrees below horizontal, with no cervical rotation. The patient remains in this position for 30 s. **C.** The clinician will then quickly flex the patient's neck, bringing the chin to the chest. The patient stays in this position for 30 s. **D.** The clinician then assists the patient into sitting, maintaining the neck flexion for another 30 s.

this position, the patient can lift the chin off of the chest. In the initial study of 13 individuals with anterior SCC canalithiasis, Yacovino et al. (2009) found that 84.6% of the patients had resolution of their signs and symptoms following one treatment, and 100% had resolution of their signs and symptoms after two treatments.

The CRP and the procedures described by Kim et al. (2005) and Yacovino et al (2009) were all assessed as a case series without a control group for comparison. Without a control group or comparison studies, one cannot determine if the treatments are truly effective, nor can one make a recommendation for one of these treatments over another.

Anterior SCC cupulolithiasis is a rare entity and is not often described in the literature. As such there is no evidence to support any given treatment. Jackson and colleagues (2007) reported that in their sample of 55 patients with anterior SCC BPPV, 15 had cupulolithiasis based on the duration of the nystagmus elicited in the Dix-Hallpike test. These patients were treated with either the CRP with applied mastoid vibration, or the Semont maneuver followed by the CRP. There was no indication in their study if either of these treatment regimens were beneficial.

Horizontal Semicircular Canal BPPV with Geotropic Nystagmus

As discussed previously, the finding of bilateral geotropic nystagmus during the positioning tests is consistent with horizontal SCC canalithiasis, with the canaliths located in the posterior arm of the horizontal SCC. There are several treatment procedures that have been proposed for treatment of this condition: (1) the particle repositioning maneuver incorporating a 270 degree to 360 degree roll; (2) the Appiani maneuver, sometimes referred to as the Gufoni maneuver; and (3) forced prolonged positioning. These treatments are described and supporting studies are reviewed.

Particle Repositioning Maneuvers

Barbecue Roll/Lempert Maneuver. A modification of the CRP for the posterior canal was suggested to treat horizontal SCC canalithiasis (Lempert & Tiel-Wilck, 1996). The treatment consisted of a series

of rapid 90 degree rotations away from the affected ear, with the patient starting in a supine position. The total rotation encompassed 270 degrees, so the patient would end up lying on the affected side. Others (Honrubia et al., 1999; J. S. Kim et al., 2012a; Tirelli & Russolo, 2004) have performed the treatment starting with the patient supine with the neck rotated 90 degrees to the affected side, and then performed a series of 90 degree rotations, completing the treatment with the patient either prone (270 degree rotation) or side lying on the affected side (360 degree rotation). In theory, starting the treatment with the patient supine and the neck rotated to the affected side would allow canaliths in the anterior aspect of the horizontal SCC to migrate to a more posterolateral position in the canal. There have been no studies comparing the efficacy of the two ending positions (prone or side lying), so that decision will rest with the clinician based in part on the mobility and physical capabilities of the patient. To perform the treatment the patient starts lying supine with the neck rotated 90 degrees to the affected ear (Figure 26–9A). The patient will remain in this position for 30 to 60 s until the nystagmus stops. Note that if the patient has limited cervical rotation, he or she will simply start in side-lying position on the affected side. From this initial position, the clinician will guide the patient as he or she rotates the neck 90 degrees away from the affected ear, incorporating 20 to 30 degrees of neck flexion to place the horizontal SCC in an earth vertical orientation (Figure 26–9B). Again, the patient will remain in this position for 30 to 60 s until the nystagmus stops. From this position, the patient will rotate the neck another 90 degrees to the right. Given the subsequent position changes, it is often easier to simply have the patient rotate the entire body 90 degrees so that he or she is lying on the unaffected side, without the cervical rotation (Figure 26–9C). Again, the patient will remain in this position for 30 to 60 s until the nystagmus stops. From this position, clinician will guide and assist the patient as he or she rotates the entire body to assume a prone on elbows position. The patient's neck remains in neutral relative to rotation but assumes some flexion to place the horizontal SCC in an earth vertical orientation (Figure 26–9D). The clinician should take care in the placement of his or her hands to ensure appropriate support of the patient's head. One hand will typically be supporting the

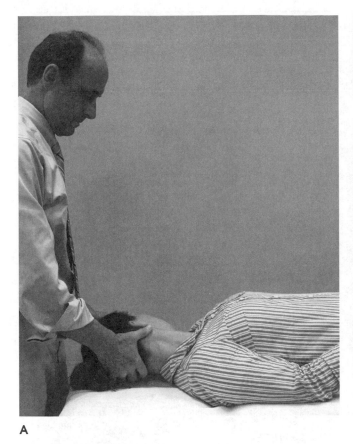

A

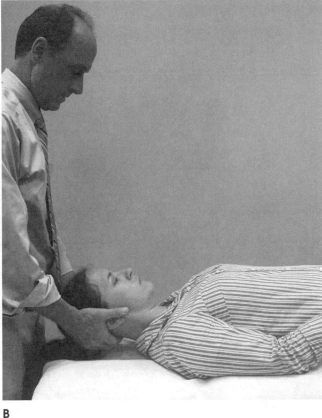

B

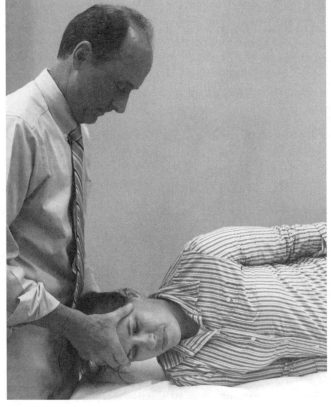

C

Figure 26-9. The Barbecue Roll, or Lempert maneuver, for left-sided, horizontal SCC canalithiasis. **A.** Patient starts in supine with the neck rotated 90 degrees to the left. The clinician will support the patient's head. The patient remains in this position for 30 to 60 s, or until the nystagmus stops. **B.** The clinician guides the patient's head to neutral rotation, and holds the head in 30 degrees of flexion to place the horizontal SCC in an earth vertical orientation. The patient remains in this position for 30 to 60 s, or until the nystagmus stops. **C.** The clinician then assists and guides the patient into right side lying, keeping the neck in 0 degrees of rotation. The patient remains in this position for 30 to 60 s, or until the nystagmus stops. Note, the treatment can be performed by simply rotating the neck 90 degrees, which makes the subsequent position change a bit more involved. *continues*

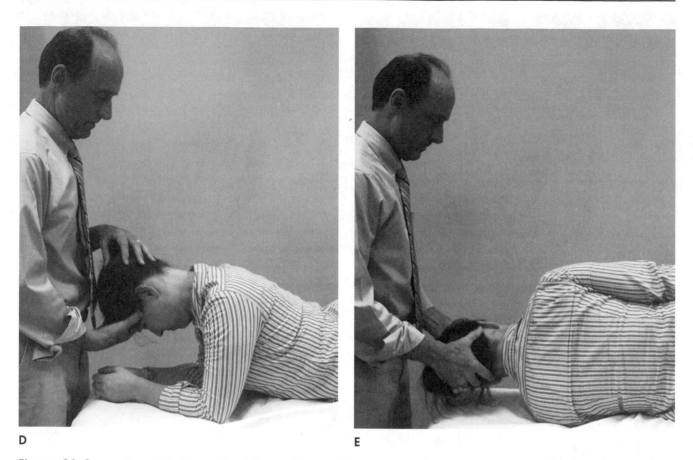

D   E

Figure 26–9. *continued* **D.** The patient then rolls over into prone and props up on the elbows. The clinician will support the patient's head in some flexion to place the horizontal SCC in an earth vertical orientation. The patient again remains in this position for 30 to 60 s, or until the nystagmus stops. **E.** The patient can get up from this position, or can roll another 90 degrees onto the left side and sit up from a side-lying position.

patient's forehead, while the other hand is placed on the patient's occiput. Again, the patient will remain in this position for 30 to 60 s until the nystagmus stops. At this point the patient has completed 270 degrees of rotation, and the canaliths should have exited the horizontal SCC. If the patient is able, he or she can get up from this position. There are several methods that can be used: (1) the patient can rise up on hands and knees, and then rock back so he or she is sitting on the heels; (2) the patient can rise up on the hands and knees, rotate the lower trunk to one side and drop the pelvis to the treatment table, and then sit up from that position; or (3) if the patient is very mobile, from the prone on elbows position, the patient can rotate the lower trunk so the pelvis and legs are in essentially a side-lying position, and then push up from the prone on elbows position. The other, and often simpler, alternative is to have the patient rotate the entire body another 90 degrees

into the side-lying position (so that the patient has completed 360 degrees of rotation, Figure 26–9E), and then sit up from that position.

Regardless of the method used to get the patient into a seated position, the provider should maintain contact with the patient once sitting, just in case the patient develops vertigo with the final position change. Also, as with the CRP for the posterior SCC, the provider is simply guiding the patient's head through the movements.

Liberatory Maneuver for Horizontal SCC Canalithiasis (Appiani or Gufoni Maneuver). This treatment was first published in English in a 2001 manuscript written by Appiani and colleagues (Appiani, Catania, & Gagliardi, 2001). In this article the authors credit the technique to Gufoni in a 1999 Italian manuscript written by Asprella, Libonati, and Gufoni. Hence, there is some confusion in the literature regarding the naming of the technique, and it may be called either the Appiani or the Gufoni. The premise of this technique is similar to other treatments of canalithiasis, which is the use of gravity to move the canaliths through the affected horizontal SCC.

To perform the treatment, the patient starts in sitting on a treatment table. The clinician faces the patient, and assists and guides the patient into a side-lying position on the unaffected side (Figure 26–10A–B). The patient remains in this position for 2 min. In this position, gravity should cause the canaliths to migrate posteriorly in the HSC. After the 2 min, the clinician rotates the patient's neck 45 degrees, bringing the nose down toward the treatment table (Figure 26–10C), which should cause the canaliths to migrate out of the horizontal SCC and into the utricular space. The patient remains in this position for an additional 2 min and is then brought back to a seated position. Once the patient is upright, the neck is brought back to a neutral position (Figure 26–10D).

Forced Prolonged Positioning (FPP)

This treatment was described by Vannuchi, Giannoni, and Pagnini (1997) as an alternative treatment for horizontal SCC canalithiasis. This is a treatment that the patient will perform on his or her own at home. The patient starts by lying on the affected side for 30 to 60 s until the vertiginous symptoms stop, during which the canaliths should migrate to the most lateral aspect of the horizontal SCC. The patient then slowly rolls through supine, onto the unaffected side and remains in this position for 12 hr. The patient can get up to eat, and so forth, but then returns to the bed to continue the treatment.

Outcomes

There is evidence to support the use of the PRMs in the treatment of horizontal SCC canalithiasis that generates geotropic nystagmus in the positioning tests. Nuti et al. (1996) found that 71% of the 36 patients treated with the barbecue roll had resolution of their signs and symptoms of horizontal SCC canalithiasis. Likewise, Kim and colleagues (2012a) found a statistically significant difference in the resolution of signs and symptoms following the barbecue roll as compared to a sham treatment.

In the same study, they also reported a similar statistically significant difference in the resolution of signs and symptoms following the Appiani maneuver (referred to as the Gufoni in the study) as compared to a sham treatment. They found no difference between the resolution rates for the barbecue roll and Appiani treatments. Mandalà and colleagues (2013) also found a statistically significant difference between the Appiani (88.9%) as compared to a sham treatment (8.6%). Results of the FPP treatment appear to be beneficial as well. In the original study, 22 of 29 patients with horizontal SCC canalithiasis had resolution of their signs and symptoms following one treatment session (Vannucchi et al., 1997). Nuti and colleagues (1996) reported a 76.2% success rate (n = 63) with the FPP treatment. A recent meta-analysis (Buzzell, Frank, Williams, Goode, & Clendaniel, 2014) showed the barbecue roll, Appiani, and FPP all to be effective methods of treating horizontal SCC BPPV with geotropic nystagmus.

Horizontal Semicircular Canal BPPV with Ageotropic Nystagmus

As discussed previously, the finding of bilateral ageotropic nystagmus during the positioning tests is consistent with either horizontal SCC cupulolithiasis, or canalithiasis with the canaliths located in the anterior arm of the horizontal SCC. There are different treatment procedures that have been proposed for each of these conditions. One of the difficulties in treating this condition is differentiating between horizontal SCC cupulolithiasis and anterior arm canalithiasis. In theory, the elicited nystagmus will be persistent in cupulolithiasis and of a shorter duration in the anterior arm canalithiasis.

Modified Semont Maneuver for Horizontal SCC Cupulolithiasis

This treatment was described by Casani, Vannucci, Fattori, and Berrettini (2002) as a method of treating horizontal SCC cupulolithiasis. While the treatment is often called the Casani maneuver, in the article the authors reference the technique to an Italian publication by Gufoni and colleagues in 1998. So elsewhere in the literature, this same technique is called the Gufoni maneuver. To perform the treatment, the patient will start sitting on the treatment

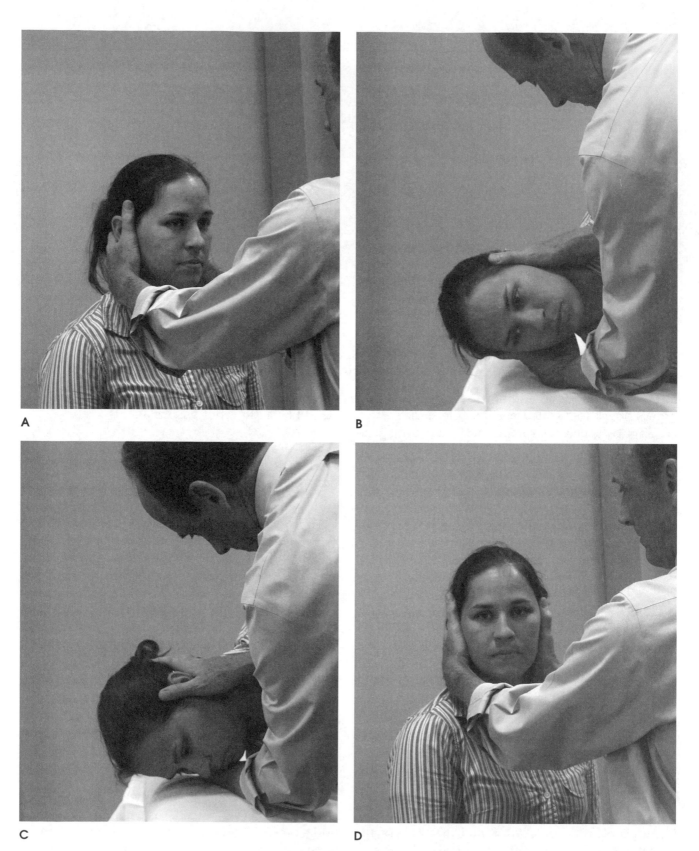

A

B

C

D

Figure 26-10. The Liberatory maneuver for left horizontal SCC canalithiasis (Appiani or Gufoni maneuver). **A.** The patient starts sitting on the treatment table, with the neck in neutral. **B.** The patient lies down quickly on the right side. The clinician maintains the neutral neck position. The patient remains in this position for 2 min. **C.** The patient rotates the neck 45 degrees to the right (nose-down position) and remains in this position for 2 min. **D.** Maintaining the neck rotation, the patient sits back up. Once upright the patient can bring the neck back to a neutral position.

table with the neck in neutral. The clinician will hold onto the patient's head and rapidly guide the patient into a side-lying position toward the affected ear (Figure 26–11). As soon as the patient is in the side-lying position, the clinician will rapidly rotate the patient's neck 45 degrees nose down toward the table. The patient remains in this position for 2 to 3 min and then sits upright.

Gufoni Maneuver for Horizontal SCC Canalithiasis of the Anterior Arm

This Gufoni maneuver, as it is commonly called, was described by Appiani and colleagues (Ciniglio Appiani, Catania, Gagliardi, & Cuiuli, 2005) as a method to transform anterior arm horizontal SCC canalithiasis into the typical posterior arm horizontal SCC canalithiasis. To perform the treatment, the patient starts in sitting. The clinician faces the patient and rapidly assists and guides the patient into a side-lying position on the affected side (Figure 26–12A–B). The patient remains in this position for 1 min following the cessation of the nystagmus. In this position, gravity should cause the canaliths to migrate posteriorly in the HSC. The clinician quickly rotates the patient's neck 45 degrees, bringing the nose up away from the treatment table (Figure 26–12C), which should cause the canaliths to migrate posteriorly in the horizontal SCC. The patient remains in this position for an additional 2 min and is then brought back to a seated position. Once the patient is upright, the neck is brought back to a neutral position (Figure 26–12D). If the treatment was successful, on retesting the clinician will observe geotropic nystagmus, which will be treated with the barbecue roll, the Appiani maneuver, or FPP.

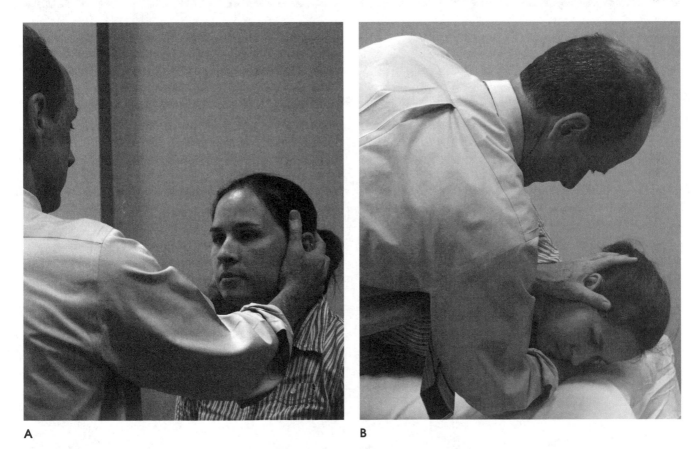

A

B

Figure 26–11. Modified Semont maneuver for left horizontal SCC cupulolithiasis (Casani maneuver). **A.** The patient starts sitting on the treatment table, with the neck in neutral. **B.** The patient lies down quickly on the left side. As soon as the patient is side lying, the clinician rapidly rotates the patient's neck 45 degrees to the left (nose-down position). The patient remains in this position for 2 to 3 min and then sits back up. Once upright the patient can bring the neck back to a neutral position.

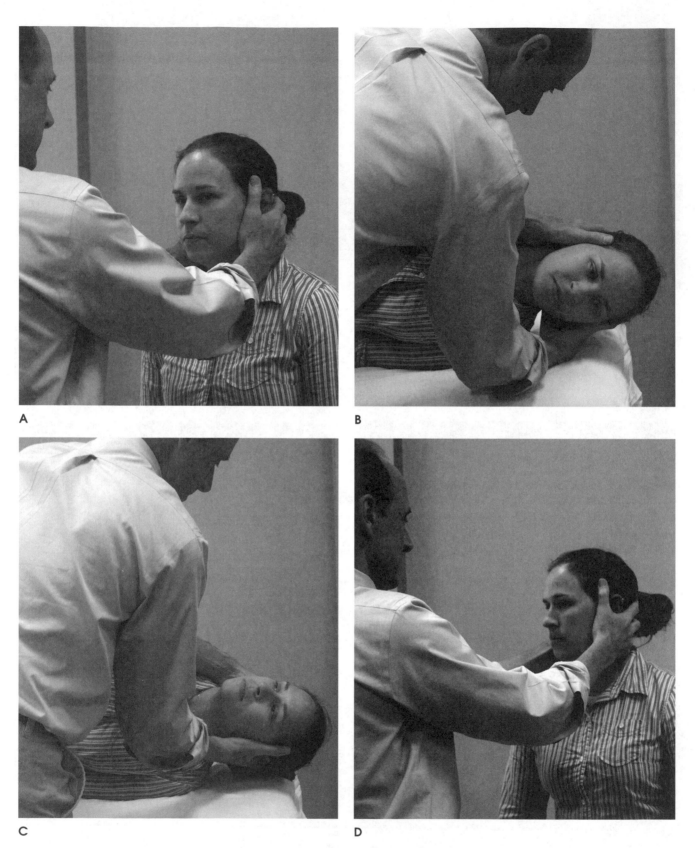

Figure 26–12. Gufoni maneuver for left anterior arm horizontal SCC canalithiasis. **A.** The patient starts sitting on the treatment table, with the neck in neutral. **B.** Assisted by the clinician, the patient lies down quickly on the left side. The patient remains in this position for 1 min after the nystagmus stops. **C.** The clinician then rotates the patient's neck 45 degrees to the right (nose up). The patient remains in this position for 2 min. **D.** The patient then sits back up. Once upright the patient can bring the neck back to a neutral position.

Outcomes

There is limited evidence to support the use of the modified Semont maneuver for horizontal SCC cupulolithiasis. Casani and colleagues (2002) reported that six of nine patients (66.7%) with presumed horizontal SCC cupulolithiasis had resolution of their signs and symptoms following one or two treatments. A similar study (Oh et al., 2009) demonstrated less impressive results, 17 out of 84 individuals (20.2%) had resolution of the signs and symptoms following one treatment. The use of the Gufoni maneuver for treatment of anterior arm horizontal SCC canalithiasis has stronger support in the literature. Ciniglio Appiani et al. (2005) reported on 16 patients with this form of horizontal SCC BPPV. All 16 showed a transition from ageotropic to geotropic nystagmus in the provoking tests following treatment. A recent RCT (J. S. Kim et al., 2012b) demonstrated that the Gufoni maneuver was more successful than a sham treatment, 45/52 (86.5%) as compared to 22/49 (44.9%), respectively, for the treatment of anterior arm horizontal SCC canalithiasis. Other treatments, such as head shaking, and FPP lying on the affected side have been suggested as treatments for horizontal SCC BPPV with ageotropic nystagmus. There are insufficient data to support these treatments at this time.

CENTRAL POSITIONAL NYSTAGMUS AND CENTRAL POSITIONAL VERTIGO

While benign paroxysmal positioning vertigo (BPPV) is a common finding that is relatively easy to diagnose and treat, there are causes of positional nystagmus and positional vertigo that are due to either abnormalities within the central nervous system, or other peripheral vestibular conditions. These conditions do not respond to the interventions described for the treatment of BPPV. The goal of this section is to help the clinician identify the signs and symptoms of positional nystagmus and positional vertigo that are not consistent with BPPV and are suggestive of other disorders.

Central Positional Nystagmus

Two types of central positional nystagmus have been identified, central positional nystagmus without vertigo (CPN) and central positional nystagmus with vertigo (CPV) (Harrison & Ozsahinoglu, 1972; Sakata, Ohtsu, Shimura, & Sakai, 1987). Central positional nystagmus without vertigo is characterized by nystagmus that persists as long as the head is held in the provoking position (Harrison & Ozsahinoglu, 1972). The nystagmus is typically in one direction (vertical, horizontal, or torsional), unlike the mixed vertical torsional nystagmus seen in posterior and anterior semicircular canal BPPV. Central positional nystagmus may be seen in elderly patients when they are supine. The elicited nystagmus is typically vertical. In the absence of other findings on the examination, the CPN is thought to be benign. In other individuals the CPN may be seen in conjunction with either up-beating or down-beating spontaneous nystagmus while the patient is seated. The CPN in these cases is typically greater than the spontaneous nystagmus observed in sitting.

The down-beating spontaneous nystagmus and CPN have been associated with a variety of central disorders including Chiari malformation, multiple sclerosis, olivopontocerebellar atrophy, and brainstem infarction (Baloh & Spooner, 1981). These patients had other oculomotor signs such as impaired smooth pursuit and impaired VOR cancellation. The actual pathophysiology causing the down-beating nystagmus is not well understood at this point, but it is thought that the down-beating nystagmus results from an imbalance between the anterior and posterior semicircular canal pathways. Recall that the semicircular canal inputs are separated at the level of the vestibular nuclei into vertical (pitch), horizontal (yaw), and roll pathways. A lesion that causes either an increase in the central anterior semicircular canal pathways or a decrease in the central posterior semicircular canal pathways would lead to down-beating nystagmus.

The up-beating spontaneous nystagmus and CPN have been associated with central disorders such as tumor, stroke, and multiple sclerosis affecting brachium conjunctivum or the ventral tegmental tract (Fisher, Gresty, Chambers, & Rudge, 1983). Many of these patients also had findings of abnormal smooth pursuit. The presumed pathophysiology for the up-beating nystagmus is thought to be the opposite of that for the down-beating nystagmus. The up-beating nystagmus is due to a higher level of neural activity in the central posterior semicircular canal pathways relative to the central anterior semicircular canal pathways.

Given the lack of symptoms of vertigo with the positional tests, the unidirectionality of the positional nystagmus, and the other oculomotor findings, it should not be difficult for the clinician to differentiate between CPN and BPPV.

Central positional nystagmus with vertigo can present with persistent positional-induced nystagmus and vertigo. In this type of CPV, the nystagmus is down-beating without a torsional component, the nystagmus and vertigo persist as the long as the head is in the provoking position, the nystagmus and vertigo do not fatigue, and they do not habituate with repeated testing. This pattern of CPV has been attributed to cerebellar tumors, or to hemorrhage dorsolateral to the fourth ventricle (Brandt, 1990; Harrison & Ozsahinoglu, 1975).

Unlike CPN, CPV may present in a manner remarkably similar to BPPV. Central positioning nystagmus with vertigo is often characterized by brief episodes of positioning vertigo and nystagmus, which has been called pseudo-BPPN (Buttner, Helmchen, & Brandt, 1999; Sakata et al., 1987). Based on clinical and experimental studies, there is a large degree of overlap in the signs and symptoms associated with BPPV and CPV. For example, the latency to the onset of nystagmus in cases of CPV has been reported to be between 0 and 5 s (Gregorius, Crandall, & Baloh, 1976; Jacobson, Butcher, Newman, & Monsell, 1995; Watson, Barber, Deck, & Terbrugge, 1981). The pattern of nystagmus in CPV can take a variety of forms. Findings from clinical studies have reported pure vertical (down-beating or up-beating), pure torsional, pure horizontal, and mixed vertical and horizontal patterns of nystagmus (Barber, 1984; Gregorius et al., 1976; Kattah, Kolsky, & Luessenhop, 1984; H. A. Kim, Yi, & Lee, 2012; Sakata et al., 1987). The duration of the elicited nystagmus and symptoms is typically relatively brief (5 to 60 s) and mimics that seen in BPPV (Barber, 1984; Gregorius et al., 1976). Fatigability of the response to repeated testing within a short time frame, although not always tested in the clinic, is a hallmark of BPPV and may also be seen in individuals with CPV (Gregorius et al., 1976; Kattah et al., 1984). However, fatigability of the response is not seen in all patients with CPV (Gregorius et al., 1976; Sakata et al., 1987). As can be seen from these studies, in terms of latency,

duration, and fatigability, there are marked similarities between BPPV and CPV. There do appear to be differences in the patterns of elicited nystagmus; however, down-beating torsional nystagmus could be due to anterior semicircular canal BPPV or CPV, and horizontal nystagmus could be due to horizontal semicircular canal BPPV or CPV. While the other patterns of nystagmus seen in CPV do not fit with the classical descriptions of the nystagmus seen in BPPV, the nystagmus seen in individuals with BPPV may not appear to fit the pattern of mixed vertical and torsional nystagmus seen in posterior and anterior semicircular canal BPPV. For example, the lateral position of the eye in the orbit will accentuate either the vertical or torsional component of the nystagmus, which may make it difficult to determine if the nystagmus is mixed vertical and torsional, pure vertical, or pure torsional. Also, lid closure or rapid blinking, may make it difficult to assess the pattern of nystagmus. Either scenario would increase the difficulty in making an accurate diagnosis.

The presence of other neurologic findings and symptoms would not be expected in cases of BPPV. Associated symptoms, such as sudden hearing loss, tinnitus, fainting sensations, progressive imbalance, and vomiting have been reported in individuals with paroxysmal, positioning vertigo of central origin (CPV) (Dunniway & Welling, 1998; Shoman & Longridge, 2007). An abnormal oculomotor exam is often seen in individuals with CPV (Buttner et al., 1999). The presence of other neurologic signs and symptoms, however, is not a requirement for CPV. There are numerous reports of individuals with CPV and no other signs or symptoms (Barber, 1984; Gregorius et al., 1976; H. A. Kim et al., 2012; Watson et al., 1981). The similarities and differences between BBPV, CPV, and CPN are summarized in Table 26–2.

Various causes of CPV have been reported in the literature, including cerebellopontine angle tumors, lesions affecting the cerebellar vermis or the fourth ventricle, and an infarction of the cerebellar nodulus (Dunniway & Welling, 1998; H. A. Kim et al., 2012; Shoman & Longridge, 2007). A more common form of CPV is migrainous vertigo and positional nystagmus. Spontaneous, positional, or a combination of spontaneous and positional nystagmus can be seen during an acute migraine with associated symptoms of dizziness (von Brevern, Zeise, Neuhauser, Clarke, & Lempert, 2005). In these cases the nystagmus can

Table 26–2. Common Features of Peripheral and Central Positional Vertigo and Nystagmus

Features	BPPV	CPV	CPN
Latency	1–15	0–5	0
Duration	5–60 s (longer in horizontal canal and in cupulolithiasis)	5–60 s	Persistent as long as the head is in the provoking position
Direction of nystagmus	In the plane of the stimulated canal. Most commonly mixed up-beating and torsion, may be down-beating and torsion, or horizontal	Pure vertical, pure torsional, or horizontal	Typically pure down-beating, may be pure up-beating or horizontal
Symptoms	Vertigo	Vertigo	No vertigo
Fatigability	Typical	Possible	No
Nausea and vomiting	Unusual with a single test; may develop with repeat testing	More frequently seen with a single test	No
Associated neurological signs and symptoms	None	None, cerebellar signs, or oculomotor signs	None, spontaneous nystagmus, or oculomotor abnormalities

be vertical, horizontal, or torsional and may change with different positional tests. In patients with a history of migrainous vertigo who were assessed when they were asymptomatic, 12% to 28% (depending on the time of assessment) demonstrated significant positional nystagmus (Radtke, von Brevern, Neuhauser, Hottenrott, & Lempert, 2012).

Other Causes of Positional Nystagmus/Vertigo

Vertebrobasilar insufficiency (VBI) has been reported to produce episodic bouts of vertigo and nystagmus (Grad & Baloh, 1989; Strupp et al., 2000). These findings have been seen in both positional testing as well as in sitting with cervical rotation. Symptoms associated with VBI would be dependent on the position of the head on the trunk (neck position), rather than the position of the head in space (positional testing). Consequently, nystagmus and vertigo seen in the Dix-Hallpike test should be reproducible in sitting with cervical extension and rotation, if the cause of the signs and symptoms were due to VBI. Vertigi-

nous symptoms are common in cases of VBI, but isolated episodes of vertigo in VBI is controversial, with conflicting reports as to the incidence of this finding (Gomez, Cruz-Flores, Malkoff, Sauer, & Burch, 1996; Wityk et al., 1998).

Perilymphatic fistula and superior canal dehiscence can make the membranous labyrinth susceptible to pressure changes such as Valsalva maneuvers, or the Dix-Hallpike test, where the head is hanging below the horizontal plane. These conditions are typically accompanied by hearing loss. The production of nystagmus and symptoms are not dependent on the position of the head in space and can often be reproduced in an upright (seated) position with the Valsalva maneuver.

Last, positional nystagmus may be seen following a unilateral vestibular loss. The nystagmus is horizontal (geotropic or ageotropic), and the pattern of nystagmus will remain constant (geotropic or ageotropic) in each Dix-Hallpike, or roll test. Thus the nystagmus may appear similar to horizontal semicircular canal BPPV (canalithiasis or cupulolithiasis). Whereas individuals with horizontal semicircular canal BPPV are very symptomatic, individuals with positional nystagmus as a result of unilateral vestibular loss are either asymptomatic or have mild symptoms.

Summary

There are causes of positional vertigo and nystagmus that are not due to BPPV. The challenge to the clinician is to identify the cause of the positional vertigo, such that appropriate treatment can be initiated. There are differences in the clinical presentation of the various causes of positional vertigo, but at times it may be difficult to determine whether the positional vertigo is due to BPPV or another cause, such as CPV. The latency, duration, and symptoms may be similar in cases of BPPV and CPV. There are generally differences in the pattern of elicited nystagmus in BPPV and CPV. The one consistent difference between BPPV and CPV is that BPPV will respond to maneuvers such as the canalith repositioning maneuver or Semont maneuver, while CPV will not respond to these treatments. If the presumed BPPV is not responding to the therapeutic maneuvers, the clinician should be suspicious of possible CPV.

REFERENCES

Amor-Dorado, J. C., Barreira-Fernandez, M. P., Aran-Gonzalez, I., Casariego-Vales, E., Llorca, J., & Gonzalez-Gay, M. A. (2012). Particle repositioning maneuver versus Brandt-Daroff exercise for treatment of unilateral idiopathic BPPV of the posterior semicircular canal: A randomized prospective clinical trial with short- and long-term outcome. *Otology and Neurotology, 33*(8), 1401–1407.

Appiani, G. C., Catania, G., & Gagliardi, M. (2001). A liberatory maneuver for the treatment of horizontal canal paroxysmal positional vertigo. *Otology and Neurotology, 22*(1), 66–69.

Baloh, R. W., Honrubia, V., & Jacobson, K. (1987). Benign positional vertigo: Clinical and oculographic features in 240 cases. *Neurology, 37*(3), 371–378.

Baloh, R. W., Honrubia, V., & Konrad, H. R. (1977). Ewald's second law re-evaluated. *Acta Oto-Laryngologica, 83*(5–6), 475–479.

Baloh, R. W., Jacobson, K., & Honrubia, V. (1993). Horizontal semicircular canal variant of benign positional vertigo. *Neurology, 43*(12), 2542–2549.

Baloh, R. W., & Spooner, J. W. (1981). Downbeat nystagmus: A type of central vestibular nystagmus. *Neurology, 31*(3), 304–310.

Baloh, R. W., Yue, Q., Jacobson, K. M., & Honrubia, V. (1995). Persistent direction-changing positional nystagmus: Another variant of benign positional nystagmus? *Neurology, 45*(7), 1297–1301.

Barber, H. O. (1984). Positional nystagmus. *Otolaryngology-Head and Neck Surgery, 92*(6), 649–655.

Bertholon, P., Bronstein, A. M., Davies, R. A., Rudge, P., & Thilo, K. V. (2002). Positional down beating nystagmus in 50 patients: Cerebellar disorders and possible anterior semicircular canalithiasis. *Journal of Neurology, Neurosurgery, and Psychiatry, 72*(3), 366–372.

Bhattacharyya, N., Baugh, R. F., Orvidas, L., Barrs, D., Bronston, L. J., Cass, S., . . . Haidari, J. (2008). Clinical practice guideline: Benign paroxysmal positional vertigo. *Otolaryngology-Head and Neck Surgery, 139*(5 Suppl. 4), S47–S81.

Blatt, P. J., Georgakakis, G. A., Herdman, S. J., Clendaniel, R. A., & Tusa, R. J. (2000). The effect of the canalith repositioning maneuver on resolving postural instability in patients with benign paroxysmal positional vertigo. *American Journal of Otology, 21*(3), 356–363.

Bloom, J., & Katsarkas, A. (1989). Paroxysmal positional vertigo in the elderly. *Journal of Otolaryngology, 18*(3), 96–98.

Brandt, T. (1990). Positional and positioning vertigo and nystagmus. *Journal of the Neurological Sciences, 95*(1), 3–28.

Brandt, T., & Daroff, R. B. (1980). Physical therapy for benign paroxysmal positional vertigo. *Archives of Otolaryngology, 106*(8), 484–485.

Buttner, U., Helmchen, C., & Brandt, T. (1999). Diagnostic criteria for central versus peripheral positioning nystagmus and vertigo: A review. *Acta Oto-Laryngologica, 119*(1), 1–5.

Buzzell, B., Frank, K., Williams, A., Goode, A., & Clendaniel, R. (2014). *Treatment of horizontal canal benign paroxysmal positional vertigo: A systematic review and meta-analysis.* Paper presented at the Combined Sections Meeting, Las Vegas, NV.

Casani, A. P., Vannucci, G., Fattori, B., & Berrettini, S. (2002). The treatment of horizontal canal positional vertigo: Our experience in 66 cases. *Laryngoscope, 112*(1), 172–178.

Choung, Y. H., Shin, Y. R., Kahng, H., Park, K., & Choi, S. J. (2006). "Bow and lean test" to determine the affected ear of horizontal canal benign paroxysmal positional vertigo. *Laryngoscope, 116*(10), 1776–1781.

Ciniglio Appiani, G., Catania, G., Gagliardi, M., & Cuiuli, G. (2005). Repositioning maneuver for the treatment of the apogeotropic variant of horizontal canal benign paroxysmal positional vertigo. *Otology and Neurotology,* 26(2), 257–260.

Cohen, H. S. (2004). Side-lying as an alternative to the Dix-Hallpike test of the posterior canal. *Otology and Neurotology,* 25(2), 130–134.

Cohen, H. S., & Kimball, K. T. (2005). Effectiveness of treatments for benign paroxysmal positional vertigo of the posterior canal. *Otology and Neurotology,* 26(5), 1034–1040.

Crevits, L. (2004). Treatment of anterior canal benign paroxysmal positional vertigo by a prolonged forced position procedure. *Journal of Neurology, Neurosurgery, and Psychiatry,* 75(5), 779–781.

Dix, M., & Hallpike, C. (1952). The pathology, symptomatology and diagnosis of certain common disorders of the vestibular systems. *Annals of Otology, Rhinology and Laryngology,* 61, 987.

Dunniway, H. M., & Welling, D. B. (1998). Intracranial tumors mimicking benign paroxysmal positional vertigo. *Otolaryngology-Head and Neck Surgery,* 118(4), 429–436.

Epley, J. M. (1992). The canalith repositioning procedure: For treatment of benign paroxysmal positional vertigo. *Otolaryngology-Head and Neck Surgery,* 107(3), 399–404.

Epley, J. M. (2001). Human experience with canalith repositioning maneuvers. *Annals of the New York Academy of Sciences,* 942, 179–191.

Fife, T. D. (1998). Recognition and management of horizontal canal benign positional vertigo. *American Journal of Otology,* 19(3), 345–351.

Fife, T. D., Iverson, D. J., Lempert, T., Furman, J. M., Baloh, R. W., Tusa, R. J., . . . Quality Standards Subcommittee, A. A. o. N. (2008). Practice parameter: Therapies for benign paroxysmal positional vertigo (an evidence-based review): Report of the Quality Standards Subcommittee of the American Academy of Neurology. *Neurology,* 70(22), 2067–2074.

Fisher, A., Gresty, M., Chambers, B., & Rudge, P. (1983). Primary position upbeating nystagmus. A variety of central positional nystagmus. *Brain,* 106(Pt. 4), 949–964.

Froehling, D. A., Bowen, J. M., Mohr, D. N., Brey, R. H., Beatty, C. W., Wollan, P. C., & Silverstein, M. D. (2000). The canalith repositioning procedure for the treatment of benign paroxysmal positional vertigo: A randomized controlled trial. *Mayo Clinic Proceedings,* 75(7), 695–700.

Froehling, D. A., Silverstein, M. D., Mohr, D. N., Beatty, C. W., Offord, K. P., & Ballard, D. J. (1991). Benign positional vertigo: Incidence and prognosis in a population-based study in Olmsted County, Minnesota. *Mayo Clinic Proceedings,* 66(6), 596–601.

Furman, J. M., & Cass, S. P. (1999). Benign paroxysmal positional vertigo. *New England Journal of Medicine,* 341(21), 1590–1596.

Gomez, C. R., Cruz-Flores, S., Malkoff, M. D., Sauer, C. M., & Burch, C. M. (1996). Isolated vertigo as a manifestation of vertebrobasilar ischemia. *Neurology,* 47(1), 94–97.

Grad, A., & Baloh, R. W. (1989). Vertigo of vascular origin: Clinical and ENG features in 84 cases. *Archives of Neurology,* 46, 281.

Gregorius, F. K., Crandall, P. H., & Baloh, R. W. (1976). Positional vertigo with cerebellar astrocytoma. *Surgical Neurology,* 6(5), 283–286.

Hain, T. C., Helminski, J. O., Reis, I. L., & Uddin, M. K. (2000). Vibration does not improve results of the canalith repositioning procedure. *Archives of Otolaryngology-Head and Neck Surgery,* 126(5), 617–622.

Hall, S. F., Ruby, R. R., & McClure, J. A. (1979). The mechanics of benign paroxysmal vertigo. *Journal of Otolaryngology,* 8(2), 151–158.

Harrison, M. S., & Ozsahinoglu, C. (1972). Positional vertigo: Aetiology and clinical significance. *Brain,* 95(2), 369–372.

Harrison, M. S., & Ozsahinoglu, C. (1975). Positional vertigo. *Archives of Otolaryngology,* 101(11), 675–678.

Herdman, S. J., & Tusa, R. J. (1996). Complications of the canalith repositioning procedure. *Archives of Otolaryngology-Head and Neck Surgery,* 122(3), 281–286.

Herdman, S. J., Tusa, R. J., & Clendaniel, R. A. (1994). Eye movement signs in verical canal benign paroxysmal positional vertigo. In A. F. Fuchs, T. Brandt, U. Buttner, & D. S. Zee (Eds.), *Contemporary ocular motor and vestibular research: A tribute to David A. Robinson* (pp. 385–387). New York, NY: Thieme Medical.

Herdman, S. J., Tusa, R. J., Zee, D. S., Proctor, L. R., & Mattox, D. E. (1993). Single treatment approaches to benign paroxysmal positional vertigo. *Archives of Otolaryngology-Head and Neck Surgery,* 119(4), 450–454.

Hilton, M. P., & Pinder, D. K. (2004). The Epley (canalith repositioning) manoeuvre for benign paroxysmal positional vertigo. *Cochrane Database of Systematic Reviews,* (2). Retrieved from http://onlinelibrary.wiley.com/doi/10.1002/14651858.CD003162.pub2/abstract

Honrubia, V., Baloh, R. W., Harris, M. R., & Jacobson, K. M. (1999). Paroxysmal positional vertigo syndrome. *American Journal of Otology,* 20(4), 465–470.

Hunt, W. T., Zimmermann, E. F., & Hilton, M. P. (2012). Modifications of the Epley (canalith repositioning) manoeuvre for posterior canal benign paroxysmal positional vertigo (BPPV). *Cochrane Database of Systematic Reviews,* (4). Retrieved from http://onlinelibrary.wiley.com/doi/10.1002/14651858.CD008675.pub2/abstract

Jackson, L. E., Morgan, B., Fletcher, J. C., Jr., & Krueger, W. W. (2007). Anterior canal benign paroxysmal positional vertigo: An underappreciated entity. *Otology and Neurotology,* 28(2), 218–222.

Jacobson, G. P., Butcher, J. A., Newman, C. W., & Monsell, E. M. (1995). When paroxysmal positioning vertigo isn't benign. *Journal of the American Academy of Audiology, 6*(4), 346–349.

Katsarkas, A., & Kirkham, T. H. (1978). Paroxysmal positional vertigo—a study of 255 cases. *Journal of Otolaryngology, 7*(4), 320–330.

Kattah, J. C., Kolsky, M. P., & Luessenhop, A. J. (1984). Positional vertigo and the cerebellar vermis. *Neurology, 34*(4), 527–529.

Kim, H. A., Yi, H. A., & Lee, H. (2012). Apogeotropic central positional nystagmus as a sole sign of nodular infarction. *Neurological Sciences, 33*(5), 1189–1191.

Kim, J. S., Oh, S. Y., Lee, S. H., Kang, J. H., Kim, D. U., Jeong, S. H., . . . Kim, H. J. (2012a). Randomized clinical trial for geotropic horizontal canal benign paroxysmal positional vertigo. *Neurology, 79*(7), 700–707.

Kim, J. S., Oh, S. Y., Lee, S. H., Kang, J. H., Kim, D. U., Jeong, S. H., . . . Kim, H. J. (2012b). Randomized clinical trial for apogeotropic horizontal canal benign paroxysmal positional vertigo. *Neurology, 78*(3), 159–166.

Kim, Y. K., Shin, J. E., & Chung, J. W. (2005). The effect of canalith repositioning for anterior semicircular canal canalithiasis. *ORL Journal for Oto-Rhino-Laryngology and Its Related Specialties, 67*(1), 56–60.

Korres, S., Balatsouras, D. G., Kaberos, A., Economou, C., Kandiloros, D., & Ferekidis, E. (2002). Occurrence of semicircular canal involvement in benign paroxysmal positional vertigo. *Otology and Neurotology, 23*(6), 926–932.

Korres, S., Riga, M., Balatsouras, D., & Sandris, V. (2008). Benign paroxysmal positional vertigo of the anterior semicircular canal: Atypical clinical findings and possible underlying mechanisms. *International Journal of Audiology, 47*(5), 276–282.

Kroenke, K., Hoffman, R. M., & Einstadter, D. (2000). How common are various causes of dizziness? A critical review. *Southern Medical Journal, 93*(2), 160–167.

Kveton, J. F., & Kashgarian, M. (1994). Particulate matter within the membranous labyrinth: Pathologic or normal? *American Journal of Otology, 15*(2), 173–176.

Lanska, D. J., & Remler, B. (1997). Benign paroxysmal positioning vertigo: Classic descriptions, origins of the provocative positioning technique, and conceptual developments. *Neurology, 48*(5), 1167–1177.

Lempert, T., & Tiel-Wilck, K. (1996). A positional maneuver for treatment of horizontal-canal benign positional Vertigo. *Laryngoscope, 106,* 476–478.

Levrat, E., van Melle, G., Monnier, P., & Maire, R. (2003). Efficacy of the Semont maneuver in benign paroxysmal positional vertigo. *Archives of Otolaryngology-Head and Neck Surgery, 129*(6), 629–633.

Lopez-Escamez, J. A., Molina, M. I., & Gamiz, M. J. (2006). Anterior semicircular canal benign paroxysmal positional vertigo and positional downbeating nystagmus. *American Journal of Otolaryngology, 27*(3), 173–178.

Lynn, S., Pool, A., Rose, D., Brey, R., & Suman, V. (1995). Randomized trial of the canalith repositioning procedure. *Otolaryngology-Head and Neck Surgery, 113*(6), 712–720.

Mandalà, M., Pepponi, E., Santoro, G. P., Cambi, J., Casani, A., Faralli, M., . . . Nuti, D. (2013). Double-blind randomized trial on the efficacy of the Gufoni maneuver for treatment of lateral canal BPPV. *Laryngoscope, 123*(7), 1782–1786.

Mandalà, M., Santoro, G. P., Asprella Libonati, G., Casani, A. P., Faralli, M., Giannoni, B., . . . Nuti, D. (2012). Double-blind randomized trial on short-term efficacy of the Semont maneuver for the treatment of posterior canal benign paroxysmal positional vertigo. *Journal of Neurology, 259*(5), 882–885.

Massoud, E. A., & Ireland, D. J. (1996). Post-treatment instructions in the nonsurgical management of benign paroxysmal positional vertigo. *Journal of Otolaryngology, 25*(2), 121–125.

McClure, J. A. (1985). Horizontal canal BPV. *Journal of Otolaryngology, 14*(1), 30–35.

Mizukoshi, K., Watanabe, Y., Shojaku, H., Okubo, J., & Watanabe, I. (1988). Epidemiological studies on benign paroxysmal positional vertigo in Japan. *Acta Oto-Laryngologica Supplementum, 447,* 67–72.

Moriarty, B., Rutka, J., & Hawke, M. (1992). The incidence and distribution of cupular deposits in the labyrinth. *Laryngoscope, 102*(1), 56–59.

Neuhauser, H., Leopold, M., von Brevern, M., Arnold, G., & Lempert, T. (2001). The interrelations of migraine, vertigo, and migrainous vertigo. *Neurology, 56*(4), 436–441.

Nuti, D., Nati, C., & Passali, D. (2000). Treatment of benign paroxysmal positional vertigo: No need for postmaneuver restrictions. *Otolaryngology-Head and Neck Surgery, 122*(3), 440–444.

Nuti, D., Vannucchi, P., & Pagnini, P. (1996). Benign paroxysmal positional vertigo of the horizontal canal: A form of canalolithiasis with variable clinical features. *Journal of Vestibular Research, 6*(3), 173–184.

Nylén, C. O. (1931). Clinical study on positional nystagmus in cases of brain tumor. *Acta Oto-Laryngologica, supplementum, 15,* 1–111.

Nylén, C. O. (1950). Positional nystagmus; a review and future prospects. *Journal of Laryngology and Otology, 64*(6), 295–318.

Oh, S. Y., Kim, J. S., Jeong, S. H., Oh, Y. M., Choi, K. D., Kim, B. K., . . . Lee, J. J. (2009). Treatment of apogeotropic benign positional vertigo: Comparison of therapeutic head-shaking and modified Semont maneuver. *Journal of Neurology, 256*(8), 1330–1336.

Pagnini, P., Nuti, D., & Vannucchi, P. (1989). Benign paroxysmal vertigo of the horizontal canal. *ORL Journal for Oto-Rhino-Laryngology and Its Related Specialties, 51*(3), 161–170.

Parnes, L. S., & McClure, J. A. (1992). Free-floating endolymph particles: A new operative finding during posterior semicircular canal occlusion. *Laryngoscope, 102*(9), 988–992.

Prokopakis, E. P., Chimona, T., Tsagournisakis, M., Christodoulou, P., Hirsch, B. E., Lachanas, V. A., . . . Velegrakis, G. A. (2005). Benign paroxysmal positional vertigo: 10-year experience in treating 592 patients with canalith repositioning procedure. *Laryngoscope., 115*(9), 1667–1671.

Radtke, A., von Brevern, M., Neuhauser, H., Hottenrott, T., & Lempert, T. (2012). Vestibular migraine: Long-term follow-up of clinical symptoms and vestibulo-cochlear findings. *Neurology, 79*(15), 1607–1614.

Rajguru, S. M., Ifediba, M. A., & Rabbitt, R. D. (2004). Three-dimensional biomechanical model of benign paroxysmal positional vertigo. *Annals of Biomedical Engineering, 32*(6), 831–846.

Ruckenstein, M. J., & Shepard, N. T. (2007). The canalith repositioning procedure with and without mastoid oscillation for the treatment of benign paroxysmal positional vertigo. *ORL Journal for Oto-Rhino-Laryngology and Its Related Specialties, 69*(5), 295–298.

Sakata, E., Ohtsu, K., Shimura, H., & Sakai, S. (1987). Positional nystagmus of benign paroxysmal type (BPPN) due to cerebellar vermis lesions. Pseudo-BPPN. *Auris Nasus Larynx, 14*(1), 17–21.

Schuknecht, H. F. (1962). Positional vertigo: Clinical and experimental observations. *Transactions of the American Academy of Ophthalmology and Otolaryngology, 66,* 319–332.

Schuknecht, H. F., & Ruby, R. R. (1973). Cupulolithiasis. *Advances in Otorhinolaryngology, 20,* 434–443.

Semont, A., Freyss, G., & Vitte, E. (1988). Curing the BPPV with a liberatory maneuver. *Advances in Otorhinolaryngology, 42,* 290–293.

Seok, J. I., Lee, H. M., Yoo, J. H., & Lee, D. K. (2008). Residual dizziness after successful repositioning treatment in patients with benign paroxysmal positional vertigo. *Journal of Clinical Neurology, 4*(3), 107–110.

Shoman, N., & Longridge, N. (2007). Cerebellar vermis lesions and tumours of the fourth ventricle in patients with positional and positioning vertigo and nystagmus. *Journal of Laryngology and Otology, 121*(2), 166–169.

Simhadri, S., Panda, N., & Raghunathan, M. (2003). Efficacy of particle repositioning maneuver in BPPV: A prospective study. *American Journal of Otolaryngology, 24*(6), 355–360.

Squires, T. M., Weidman, M. S., Hain, T. C., & Stone, H. A. (2004). A mathematical model for top-shelf vertigo: The role of sedimenting otoconia in BPPV. *Journal of Biomechanics, 37*(8), 1137–1146.

Steddin, S., & Brandt, T. (1996). Horizontal canal benign paroxysmal positioning vertigo (h-BPPV): Transition of canalolithiasis to cupulolithiasis. *Annals of Neurology, 40,* 918–922.

Strupp, M., Planck, J. H., Arbusow, V., Steiger, H. J., Bruckmann, H., & Brandt, T. (2000). Rotational vertebral artery occlusion syndrome with vertigo due to "labyrinthine excitation." *Neurology, 54*(6), 1376–1379.

Tirelli, G., & Russolo, M. (2004). 360-Degree canalith repositioning procedure for the horizontal canal. *Otolaryngology-Head and Neck Surgery, 131*(5), 740–746.

Vannucchi, P., Giannoni, B., & Pagnini, P. (1997). Treatment of horizontal semicircular canal Benign Paroxysmal Positional Vertigo. *Journal of Vestibular Research, 7*(1), 1–6.

von Brevern, M., Radtke, A., Lezius, F., Feldmann, M., Ziese, T., Lempert, T., & Neuhauser, H. (2007). Epidemiology of benign paroxysmal positional vertigo: A population based study. *Journal of Neurology, Neurosurgery, and Psychiatry, 78*(7), 710–715.

von Brevern, M., Seelig, T., Radtke, A., Tiel-Wilck, K., Neuhauser, H., & Lempert, T. (2006). Short-term efficacy of Epley's manoeuvre: A double-blind randomised trial. *Journal of Neurology, Neurosurgery, and Psychiatry, 77*(8), 980–982.

von Brevern, M., Zeise, D., Neuhauser, H., Clarke, A. H., & Lempert, T. (2005). Acute migrainous vertigo: Clinical and oculographic findings. *Brain, 128*(Pt. 2), 365–374.

Watson, P., Barber, H. O., Deck, J., & Terbrugge, K. (1981). Positional vertigo and nystagmus of central origin. *Canadian Journal of Neurological Sciences, 8*(2), 133–137.

Welling, D. B., Parnes, L. S., Obrien, B., Bakaletz, L., Brackmann, D. E., & Hinojosa, R. (1997). Particulate matter in the posterior semicircular canal. *Laryngoscope, 107*(1), 90–94.

White, J., Savvides, P., Cherian, N., & Oas, J. (2005). Canalith repositioning for benign paroxysmal positional vertigo. *Otology and Neurotology, 26*(4), 704–710.

Wityk, R. J., Chang, H. M., Rosengart, A., Han, W. C., Dewitt, L. D., Pessin, M. S., & Caplan, L. R. (1998). Proximal extracranial vertebral artery disease in the New England Medical Center Posterior Circulation Registry. *Archives of Neurology, 55*(4), 470–478.

Woodworth, B. A., Gillespie, M. B., & Lambert, P. R. (2004). The canalith repositioning procedure for benign positional vertigo: A meta-analysis. *Laryngoscope, 114*(7), 1143–1146.

Yacovino, D. A., Hain, T. C., & Gualtieri, F. (2009). New therapeutic maneuver for anterior canal benign paroxysmal positional vertigo. *Journal of Neurology, 256*(11), 1851–1855.

Yimtae, K., Srirompotong, S., Srirompotong, S., & Sae-Seaw, P. (2003). A randomized trial of the canalith repositioning procedure. *Laryngoscope, 113*(5), 828–832.

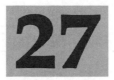

Medical Management of Vertigo That Is Otologic in Origin

Brian Neff and R. Mark Wiet

INTRODUCTION

Once the peripheral vestibular system has been isolated as the cause of a patient's vertigo, an appropriate course of management is chosen. Depending on the etiology of the symptoms, conservative management options include observation, physical therapy, and medical management. In contemporary medicine, surgical management of the vertigo that is otologic in origin is also occasionally appropriate in carefully selected patients. However, even in most busy neurotologic practices, operations for vertigo are infrequent.

Pharmacologic treatment typically used to treat peripheral vestibular disorders is nonspecific. Often, medication is used only to relieve a symptom (such as vertigo) and not its cause. Generally, medications fall into two basic categories: those used for general vestibular suppression, and those used for treatment or prophylaxis of specific vertiginous conditions such as Ménière's disease or vestibular migraine.

VESTIBULAR SUPPRESSION

A multitude of medicines can be considered to help the patient with vertigo or motion sickness. These include benzodiazepines, antihistamines, anticho-

linergics, neuroleptics, calcium channel antagonists, tricyclic antidepressants, and serotonergics (Tables 27–1 and 27–2) (Wackym & Schumacher-Monfre, 2005; Zajonc & Roland, 2006). The more commonly prescribed medications including benzodiazepines, antihistamines, and anticholinergic agents are reviewed here. These medications will not prevent vertigo from occurring but usually reduce the intensity of the spell and associated nausea. Their major side effect is central sedation. In the setting of an uncompensated, fixed peripheral vestibular lesion, active head and eye movements produce sensory error signals, triggering the central nervous system to generate compensation mechanisms via the mechanism of adaptive plasticity. It is thought that persisting use of vestibular suppressants for dizziness inhibits the brain's ability to properly apprehend visual, proprioceptive, and remaining vestibular input, thus hampering the central process of compensation (Peppard, 1986). Thus, for an uncompensated, fixed unilateral lesion, vestibular suppressants are effective and appropriate in the acute setting but should not be used on a chronic basis. Occasionally, patients will present with chronic motion provoked vestibular symptoms or dysequilibrium. However, they only improve with vestibular therapy after being weaned from these medications in order to allow compensation to occur. These same patients should also be considered for the possible diagnosis of chronic subjective dizziness (CSD) if they meet

Table 27–1. Selected Medications Approved in the United States for Vertigo and Motion Sickness

Medication	MS	AV	CD	Action	Precaution
Benzodiazepines					
Diazepam (Valium)	+	+	+	GABA-A mediated inhibition in the vestibular nuclei	Sedation; avoid in patients with pulmonary insufficiency, sleep apnea, liver or kidney disease; addiction is possible
Lorazepam (Ativan)	+	+		Same as diazepam	Same as diazepam
Clonazepam	+	+		Same as diazepam	Same as diazepam
Antihistamines					
Diphenhydramine	+		+	H1 blockade; anticholinergic effects	Sedation
Dimenhydrinate	+		+	Same as diphenhydramine	Sedation
Meclizine	+		+	Same as diphenhydramine	Sedation
Cyclizine	+		+	Same as diphenhydramine	Sedation; may aggravate severe heart failure
Promethazine	++			H1 blockade; very strong anticholinergic effects	Sedation; use with caution in patients with renal failure
Anticholinergics					
Scopolamine	+		+	M1, M2, and M3 blockade; M3 blockade is likely the most important	Sedation, dry mouth, blurred vision, acute angle closure glaucoma, contact dermatitis, possible withdrawal symptoms; rare psychosis reported
Scopolamine/ ephedrine	++			Same as scopolamine alone; plus adrenergic and dopaminergic effects	Same as scopolamine; hypertension, anxiety, arrhythmia; use with caution in patients with hyperthyroidism, diabetes, or glaucoma
Scopolamine/ d-amphetamine	++			Same as scopolamine/ ephedrine	Same as scopolamine/ ephedrine
Neuroleptics					
Droperidol/fentanyl		+	?	Antiadrenergic and antidopaminergic effects; analgesia with fentanyl	Hypotension, respiratory depression; use with caution in patients with liver or kidney disease

Note. Both adrenergics are effective as monotherapy. *MS* = motion sickness; *AV* = acute vertigo; *CD* = chronic dizziness.

the clinical criteria (see Chapter 30). In the management of patients with bilateral vestibular paresis, one should also attempt to eliminate vestibular suppressant medications, as these will often make symptoms worse. Medications that have central anticholinergic side effects should also be avoided in these patients because of their vestibular suppressant effects (Hain & Yacovino, 2005). Benign paroxysmal positional vertigo (BPPV) is best treated with canalith repositioning procedures (CRPs) since

Table 27–2. Selected Medications Used for Vestibular Symptoms but Not Approved for Use in the United States

Medication	MS	Vertigo	Suspected Drug Action
Anticholinergics			
Idaverine	+		M1 and M2 receptor blockade
Zamifenacin	+		M3 and M5 receptor blockade
Calcium antagonists			
Flunarizine	+	+	Labyrinth suppression; possibly at the level of the vestibular hair cells
Cinnarizine	+	+	Same as flunarizine
Serotonergics			
8-OH-DPAT	++		5-HT1A agonist effects; probably in the vestibular nuclei
DOI			5-HT2 agonist effects
Other			
Betahistine		+	Weak H1 agonist; moderate H3 antagonist; used primarily for Ménière's disease

Note. MS = motion sickness; 8-OH-DPAT = 8-hydroxy-2-(di-n-propylamino) tetralin; DOI = l-(2,5-dimethoxy-4-iodophenyl)-2-aminopropane.

this treatment is highly effective and vestibular suppressants should only be used sparingly in the most severe symptomatic cases.

Benzodiazepines

Diazepam (Valium), clonazepam (Klonopin), lorazepam (Ativan), and alprazolam (Xanax) are benzodiazepines that are commonly prescribed for vertigo and prophylaxis of motion sickness. They potentiate the effects of γ-aminobutyric acid (GABA), an inhibitory neurotransmitter, at GABA-A receptors in the vestibular nuclei, thus causing vestibular suppression (Hain & Yacovino, 2005; Sekitani, McCabe, & Ryu, 1971). This is the most effective class of medications for the suppression of severe vertigo. The senior author has had good results with both lorazepam and diazepam in the management of acute vertigo in Ménière's patients. Diazepam has a longer duration of action, whereas lorazepam has a shorter half-life and is more suitable for attacks lasting less

than 4 hr. Due to diazepam's long half-life, lower dosages should be administered to elderly patients to avoid excessive and prolonged sedation or altered consciousness. The nongeneric form of lorazepam (Ativan) will dissolve if administered sublingually and is a wise choice when vertigo with associated vomiting makes oral medication use problematic. Of note, alprazolam is effective in controlling acute dizziness associated with panic disorder, and clonazepam may provide specific benefit in patients with vestibular migraine. However, medications less likely to cause dependence are generally preferred in the chronic treatment of both disorders.

In the acute care setting such as an emergency room, diazepam can be administered intravenously in incremental doses of 1 to 2 mg until the patient is comfortable. Resolution of nystagmus may provide a good measure of a proper therapeutic effect. After the majority of the symptoms subside, the patient may be discharged and use the oral form of the drug as needed. However, both diazepam and lorazepam can be prescribed as rectal suppositories for use during times of severe vomiting. Benzodiazepines seem to assist in the early phases of compensation, perhaps by allowing for earlier ambulation and facilitating the head movements required to initiate vestibular compensation (Martin, Gilchrist, Smith, & Darlington, 1996). To prevent physiologic addiction and to facilitate central compensation, the patient must be weaned from these medications once the acute symptoms are resolving.

Antihistamines

Milder vestibular suppressants, such as meclizine (Antivert), dimenhydrinate (Dramamine), diphenhydramine (Benadryl), and promethazine (Phenergan) are the most commonly prescribed antihistamines for vertigo and motion sickness. They are known to function as histamine-1 receptor (H_1) antagonists. The precise mechanism for their effect on central vestibular processing is unclear but is probably due to their significant central anticholinergic effects. Any antihistamine that crosses the blood-brain barrier can be expected to provide some relief of vertigo and motion sickness. In particular, meclizine enjoys considerable popularity. It is a safe, well-tolerated medication and is frequently adequate for the symptomatic management of milder vertigo associated with Ménière's spells. The newer second-generation antihistamines do not cross the blood-brain barrier and are not appropriate to treat vertigo (Hain & Yacovino, 2005).

Some patients, particularly those with nonspecific dizziness syndromes associated with seasonal allergy symptoms, note considerable benefit from the regular use of oral antihistamines. Otherwise, these medications are best reserved for use only when vertigo spells occur. Most clinicians recommend the use of meclizine or Phenergan at the first sign of a Ménière's attack, particularly when the patient has a predictable interval between the onset of hearing symptoms and the episode of vertigo. Meclizine has the disadvantage of slow onset with peak effect up to 9 hr after dosing. The dose for meclizine ranges from 12.5 to 50 mg, three times daily. However, if no benefit is seen from 25 mg, it is unlikely to be effective at higher doses. Side effects are not common with all these medications but include dry mouth, sedation, fatigue, and blurry vision. Tachyphylaxis

is common with these medications, which provides further rationale for avoiding indiscriminate long-term use.

Anticholinergics

One medication in this class that is used in the management of dizziness is transdermal scopolamine (Transderm Scop). It is a nonspecific muscarinic receptor antagonist. Among the side effects listed in Table 27–1, blurred vision and dry mouth are the most common. Because this preparation may cause confusion or other more disturbing mental status changes, it should be used cautiously in elderly individuals. Like other vestibular suppressants, it is thought to slow the rate of vestibular compensation. Conventional practice is to avoid its use in the management of chronic vertigo (Hain & Yacovino, 2005). It is most effective in the prophylaxis of motion sickness associated with car, plane, or boat travel.

Transdermal scopolamine is absorbed transcutaneously into the circulation and therefore can be placed anywhere on the skin. Although bypassing the gastrointestinal tract in patients with nausea or emesis is a great advantage, local dermatologic sensitivity can develop. In this case, the patient merely needs to move the patch to an alternative hairless location. If a more dramatic diffuse dermatologic sensitivity reaction occurs, the patient must discontinue use of this product promptly, and should wash the skin thoroughly where the patch had been applied to remove any residual drug. Occasionally, topical or systemic corticosteroids are required to control the skin reaction. Both scopolamine and meclizine should be used with care in patients with asthma, prostate hypertrophy, narrow angle glaucoma, and pulmonary edema due to their stronger anticholinergic effects.

TREATMENT OF THE ACUTE VESTIBULAR CRISIS

It is appropriate to select one of the above vestibular suppressants when treating a patient with a recent onset of severe vertigo due to presumed labyrinthitis or vestibular neuritis. In addition, oral corticosteroid therapy has been demonstrated to reduce symptom intensity and abbreviate the time required to resolve the disabling vertigo symptoms in a double-blind, prospective, placebo-controlled crossover study (Ariyasu, Byl, Sprague, & Adour, 1990). Other data support these findings and add that antivirals do not seem to provide incremental benefit in the management of vestibular neuritis (Strupp et al., 2004).

Vestibular symptoms associated with labyrinthitis or vestibular neuritis usually last in the range of days to weeks. After the acute symptoms subside, patients may experience chronic imbalance or motion-provoked symptoms. Depending on the patient's age and functional status, these residual symptoms may have a protracted time course. In that case, provided the correct diagnosis has been made and the lesion is stable, vestibular rehabilitation therapy should be of benefit.

TREATMENT OF MÉNIÈRE'S DISEASE

Clinical history is of the utmost importance in the diagnosis of Ménière's disease. The suspected diagnosis is confirmed by appropriate diagnostic testing to rule out other disorders, as discussed elsewhere in this text. The management of Ménière's disease involves several unique dietary, medical, and operative treatments that are inappropriate for other vestibular disorders. Most otologists continue to believe that the combination of salt restriction and diuretics represents the best medical therapy for Ménière's disease (Jackson, Glasscock, Davis, Hughes, & Sismanis, 1981). Once control of vertigo has been achieved, stabilization of hearing and decreased tinnitus and aural fullness may follow. If medical therapy fails to control the vertigo, surgical options may be appropriate and the procedure selected will depend upon the level of residual hearing in the involved ear. These options are discussed in detail in Chapter 28.

Dietary Modification

Each day, the average American consumes over 4 g of sodium. Dietary salt reduction is the most widely used initial therapy for treatment of Ménière's disease. The level of restriction is not widely agreed

upon and varies per treating physician between 1000 and 2000 mg of sodium per day. It is also felt to be helpful to divide the total daily salt intake, as equally as possible, by the number of daily meals in order to avoid sodium loading. Frequently, weeks of carefully restricting salt intake will pass before there is improvement in the vertiginous symptoms. Pitfalls occur when patients eat outside the home and when they consume prepared foods that are high in sodium. Dieticians can help patients establish and strictly monitor low-salt intake. The mechanism of action is frequently explained as lowering total body and inner ear fluid levels. Studies have shown that dietary sodium restriction does not alter serum or endolymph sodium concentration. It has also been hypothesized that sodium restriction may alter serum osmolality via vasopressin; however, the definitive mechanism of dietary sodium reduction is truly not known (Coelho & Lalwani, 2008). Some patients note that caffeine ingestion, nicotine use, or certain specific foods may exacerbate their symptoms. This situation may be a result of the high prevalence of migraine conditions associated with Ménière's syndrome (Radtke et al., 2002).

Diuretics

If sodium restriction fails, the concomitant or sequential addition of thiazide diuretics (such as hydrochlorothiazide with or without triamterene) may help reduce the frequency of Ménière's attacks. Thiazide diuretics function by inhibiting sodium and chloride transport in the cortical thick ascending limb and early distal tubule of the nephron. They have a milder diuretic action than the loop diuretics, and they are not known to be ototoxic. Triamterene, a potassium-sparing diuretic, is frequently added to avoid the hypokalemia that can accompany the use of thiazide diuretics. The compound formulation of triamterene and hydrochlorothiazide (Dyazide) is frequently used as a first-line treatment in patients with Ménière's disease. It should be avoided in patients who are allergic to sulfa medications or who have kidney disease. The mechanism of action within the inner ear is widely hypothesized, but it is not really known. The use of thiazide diuretics has been shown to control vertigo in 58% of patients and stabilize hearing in 60% of patients (Klockhoff

& Lindblom, 1967). Another study conducted with Dyazide showed a significant effect on vertigo but failed to demonstrate any effect on hearing (van Deelen & Huizing, 1986). A Cochrane review of the literature up to April 2009 found that there were no diuretic treatment trials for Ménière's disease that even met review criteria, and thus, a best practice standard is currently not possible (Burgess & Kunda, 2010). If patients are unable to tolerate Dyazide, acetazolamide (Diamox), a carbonic anhydrase inhibitor, can be used as an alternative (Hain & Yacovino, 2005). Both hydrochlorothiazide and acetazolamide are sulfonamide derivatives and should be avoided in patients with severe sulfa allergies.

Oral Steroids

The use of oral steroids during flares of Ménière's disease vertigo or hearing fluctuations is extrapolated from experience with sudden sensorineural hearing loss (SNHL) and autoimmune hearing loss treatment. At times, it is initially difficult to distinguish Ménière's disease from a sudden SNHL. Additionally, there is circumstantial evidence that some cases of Ménière's disease might have an autoimmune character. This is especially the case when considering simultaneous presenting bilateral Ménière's disease. The effectiveness of oral steroids in Ménière's disease is largely anecdotal with no universal recommendation. One prospective randomized study of 16 patients looked at the effects of 18 weeks of low-dose oral prednisone and found a 50% reduction in the frequency, and 30% reduction in the duration of vertiginous symptoms. There remained a significant advantage in the treated group 12 months later (Morales-Luckie, Cornejo-Suarez, Zaragoza-Contreras, & Gonzlez-Perez, 2005). Like many Ménière's disease studies, design flaws and a lack of corroborative results have limited the usefulness of this study. Most treating physicians do not see a role for oral steroids in stereotypically presenting unilateral Ménière's disease for either the vertiginous or aural complaints. There is also no definitive evidence that oral steroids impact the long-term hearing outcomes in patients with Ménière's disease. Occasionally, patients will note a strong association between activity of Ménière's disease and allergic symptoms. Quality studies evaluating anti-allergy treatments in the control of Ménière's disease symptoms are lacking. Given the lack of beneficial medical Ménière's disease treatments, a trial of antihistamine therapy during the peak seasons of allergy sensitivity can be tried in this subgroup of patients. Allergic desensitization therapy should not be routinely recommended until effectiveness is better established in outcome studies.

Vasodilators (Betahistine Hydrochloride, Serc, Betaserc)

Betahistine is a structural homolog of histamine and is a weak histamine H_1-receptor agonist and a strong H_3-receptor antagonist. Clinical trials suggest betahistine might reduce the frequency of vertigo attacks in Ménière's disease patients. Betahistine is not currently available by subscription in the United States. Betahistine has significant first-pass metabolism when delivered orally, and caution or avoidance of medication usage should be followed in patients with severe liver failure. Dosages used in trials include 16 mg TID, 24 mg TID, and 48 mg TID. The 48 mg was the most effective. There are some retrospective trials suggesting more benefit up to 160 mg TID. Betahistine, at clinically effective human doses, caused an increase in cochlea stria vascularis capillary blood flow in a dose-dependent manner in guinea pigs (Bertlich et al., 2014). Betahistine also seems to inhibit the vestibular nuclei, independent of blood flow changes (Coelho & Lalwani, 2008). As of a November 2010 Cochrane Review, a review of seven prospective trials did not find enough unbiased evidence to determine whether betahistine was effective at vertigo control. None of the trials showed any effect on hearing loss, and only one quality trial looked at tinnitus and showed no effect (James & Burton, 2011). A further PubMed search for betahistine studies since the Cochrane Review date of November 25, 2010, utilizing the Cochrane search method found no further studies that would meet their review criteria or lend any further clarity to betahistine effectiveness in Ménière's disease (Gürkov et al., 2013; James & Burton, 2011; Lezius, Adrion, Mansmann, Jahn, & Strupp, 2011; Monzani et al., 2012).

Calcium Channel Blockers

Nimodipine has been shown to cross the blood-brain barrier and the blood-perilymph barrier and may act to mitigate calcium ion disturbances in the inner ear of Ménière's disease patients. It is also possible that this is not correct, and it may, in fact, act centrally on vestibular inputs or act to mitigate migraine-induced vestibular abnormalities. The true mechanism, like Ménière's disease pathophysiology, is not well understood. Judgment of clinical effectiveness also suffers from a lack of high-quality clinical trials. In a retrospective U.S. review of 12 patients, nimodipine 30 mg BID was found to control vertigo in 67% (8/12) and stabilize or improve hearing in 58% (7/12). Side effects are rare and include hypotension, constipation, anemia, and hepatitis (Lassen, Hirsch, & Kamerer, 1996).

Meniett Device

The Meniett device is an option that may be a useful adjunct for the management of Ménière's disease in some patients. The basis for this device's development centers on the observation that changes in ambient pressure improved Ménière's symptoms (Densert & Densert, 1982). Densert et al. reported reduced symptoms and improved electrocochleographic findings in a randomized, blinded study using intermittent overpressures from a portable, low-intensity, alternating-pressure generator (Densert, Sass, & Arlinger, 1995). The U.S. Food and Drug Administration cleared the commercially available Meniett device (Medtronic, Minneapolis, Minnesota) for use in the United States in 1999. After a tympanostomy tube is surgically placed in the affected ear, the Meniett device is used to apply repetitive low-pressure pulses through the tympanostomy tube, three times daily. Although its mechanism of action is not fully understood, one theory is that the pressure pulses on the inner ear fluid system via the round window, combined with physiologic reactions in the ear, reduce excess endolymphatic fluid and restore the inner ear's homeostatic balance. This theory is based on the concept that endolymphatic hydrops has a cause-and-effect relationship with symptoms. However, recent evidence suggests

that the overproduction of endolymph may well be an epiphenomenon of whatever is the primary cause for the Ménière's disease; therefore, a change in the endolymphatic hydropic state may simply serve as an indication of improvement in the underlying cause (Merchant, Adams, & Nadol, 2005). The pressure may also have a direct effect on labyrinthine hydrodynamics by stimulating increased flow of endolymph through the utriculoendolymphatic valve, a primary site of pathology in Ménière's disease. As additional endolymph is continually produced and released into the scala media, the patient must use the Meniett on a continuous basis for control of symptoms. It is recommended that patients use the Meniett three times a day, and the tympanostomy tube should be checked frequently for patency.

A multi-institution Meniett study documented a significant reduction of severe vertigo attacks within 4 months, compared with a control group using a placebo device (Gates, Green, Tucci, & Telian, 2004). The 2-year follow-up data regarding the study participants were subsequently published (Gates, Verrall, Green, Tucci, & Telian, 2006). All patients enrolled in the study were surgical candidates. Of the 43 participants who entered the 2-year follow-up study with active Ménière's disease, 20 went into remission. On average, participants achieved remission in approximately 3 months. The probability of achieving remission was more likely in the first 5 months (72%). Of the 23 participants who did not reach remission, 13 dropped out and sought alternative options including labyrinthectomy, endolymphatic sac surgery, and gentamicin injections. The conditions of eight improved, and the conditions of two worsened or the participants saw no improvement yet continued to participate in the 2-year follow-up. Although the U.S. study did not replicate the favorable European data on hearing improvement, it did corroborate their finding that the Meniett device can be very effective for vertigo control. It has been particularly helpful in highly anxious patients, patients with bilateral Ménière's disease, and others who are poor surgical candidates. The main drawback to this treatment is that it is expensive, and oftentimes, is not paid for by insurance. The effectiveness of Meniett treatment is similar to historic placebo results for Ménière's disease treatments, and some would argue that studies of this device could show false benefit due to inadequate blinding in long-term studies or limitations in the placebo arm design (Shen & Ruckenstein, 2010).

More recently, the P-100 (Enttex GmbH, Hannover, Germany) device has offered a less expensive alternative to the Meniett device. It is a small handheld device that delivers positive low-pressure therapy to the ear via a manual hand pump. A safety valve limits the amount of pressure that can be generated. To date, P-100 efficacy studies compared to the Meniett device are insufficient due to limited patient sample sizes (Franz & Van der Laan, 2005).

Intratympanic Steroid Therapy

Intratympanic steroid injections have been gaining popularity in the treatment of Ménière's disease. Advocates of this treatment tout advantages such as avoidance of the systemic effects of steroids, potential avoidance of surgery, ease of administration, the treatment is nonablative and can be utilized in bilateral disease, and low risk of iatrogenic hearing loss and imbalance. Published rates of vertigo control using this treatment range from 47% to 82% (Barrs, 2004; Barrs, Keyser, Stallworth, & McElveen, 2001; Morales-Luckie et al., 2005; Doyle et al., 2004). A Cochrane Review through January 2011 found only one small prospective, randomized, blinded, placebo controlled trial that had an acceptable risk of bias. In this study, 22 patients were randomized and the treatment group received five injections of 4 mg/mL dexamethasone in 5 days (once per day). The authors demonstrated a significant reduction in vertigo at 24 months in the treatment group as measured by American Academy of Otolaryngology Head and Neck Surgery (AAO-HNS) functional level, vertigo class (AAO-HNS definition), Dizziness Handicap Inventory (DHI) score, and subjective vertigo improvement (Garduno-Anaya, Couthino De Toledo, Hinojosa, Pane, & Rios Castenada, 2005; Phillips, & Westerberg, 2011). Since that time, an additional prospective, randomized, blinded, placebo-controlled trial found vertigo reduction with a single 12 mg injection of OTO-104. OTO-104 is a dexamethasone suspension in a thermoreversible glycol polymer that allows prolonged delivery of the drug to the inner ear (Lambert et al., 2012). Both of these studies show promise that intratympanic steroids truly relieve Ménière's disease vertigo, but larger studies are still needed. It is still true that reliable evidence of intratympanic steroids in relieving Ménière's disease-related hearing loss, tinnitus, and aural fullness is missing. Additionally, optimum dosage, vehicle (sustained release), and administration schedule are not known (Alles, der Gaag, & Stokroos, 2006).

Intratympanic Aminoglycoside Therapy

Since the middle of the 20th century, systemic and intratympanic aminoglycosides have been used to treat Ménière's disease. Streptomycin, widely used during the 1950s for the management of tuberculosis, was found to have ototoxic side effects. Initially, this was exploited to produce complete vestibular ablation through the intramuscular injections of streptomycin (Schuknecht, 1956). Although this was frequently complicated by oscillopsia, most patients reported improved functional capacity compared to their pretreatment level. In later years, subtotal ablation of vestibular function was preferentially used to avoid this potentially disabling oscillopsia (Graham & Kemink, 1984). A typical subtotal ablation treatment schedule is 1 g intramuscularly twice daily, 5 days per week, while carefully monitoring audiometric and electronystagmographic data. Typical effective total doses range from 10 to 30 g, but some patients required up to 50 g to control symptoms. Serial rotational chair VOR gain measurements can be used to monitor the response to therapy. When low-frequency gain values begin to decrease, or after 20 g have been administered, treatment is discontinued and the patient is observed. Persistent symptoms can be treated with additional doses of streptomycin, as the therapeutic effect appears to be cumulative.

Direct intratympanic application of ototoxic aminoglycoside antibiotics into the middle ear has gained widespread popularity for the management of Ménière's disease that is refractory to more conservative measures. Also introduced by Schuknecht, its main advantage is avoidance of an ablative surgical procedure (Schuknecht, 1956). Gentamicin is currently the aminoglycoside of choice due to its relatively selective vestibulotoxicity. Streptomycin may even be a better choice for this use due to its limited cochleotoxicity. Unfortunately, this drug is rather complex to obtain due to FDA restrictions related to its importance in the treatment of multi-drug-resistant tuberculosis.

A variety of intratympanic gentamicin treatment protocols have been studied, but no protocol predictably produces a complete "chemical labyrinthectomy" and a low incidence of hearing loss. A recent meta-analysis evaluated different techniques (Chia, Grant, Anderson, & Harris, 2004). The highest rate of complete vertigo control (81.7%) was found with the "titration" method. In six articles that reported using the titration method, the frequency of the gentamicin injections varied, but administration was terminated with the onset of signs or symptoms of inner ear disturbance. Hearing loss observed with the titration method was 24%. Among the various techniques reported, the rates of hearing loss were between 13% and 35%. The lowest rate of hearing loss was paradoxically seen in studies using the "weekly" technique. This involves giving patients a single dose of gentamicin once a week for a total of four predetermined treatments, without regard to observed treatment effects.

Intratympanic gentamicin adds an effective ablative treatment option for patients with both serviceable and nonserviceable hearing, where in the distant past, only ablative surgical procedures existed. As of a June 2011 Cochrane Review, there were two prospective, double-blind, placebo-controlled, randomized clinical trials evaluating intratympanic gentamicin effects on vertigo control in Ménière's disease patients. Both showed a significant reduction of vertigo in the gentamicin treated group (Pullens & van Benthem, 2011). There are no prospective or unbiased comparison studies on the hearing outcomes and vertigo control rates between gentamicin and vestibular nerve section in Ménière's disease patients with serviceable hearing. Even if one adopted a conservative attitude, both likely have vertigo control rates >80% and significant hearing losses occurring immediately or in a delayed fashion in ≤20% (Colletti, Carner, & Colletti, 2007; Huon, Fang, & Wang, 2012; Teufert & Doherty, 2010). Choosing which treatment is best for a patient will require some common sense as well as largely being directed by patient risk assessment and treatment goals. The role that surgery plays in the management of this disease is outlined further in Chapter 28. Figure 27–1 depicts one potential algorithm,

among many, for use of the available management options in Ménière's disease.

Treatment of Vestibular Migraine

Vestibular migraine is also known as migraine-related vertigo or migrainous vertigo. Vestibular migraine is thought to be the second most common cause of recurrent vertigo after benign paroxysmal positional vertigo (Neuhauser, 2007). Neuhauser et al. have proposed diagnostic criteria (Neuhauser, Leopold, von Brevern, Arnold, & Lempert, 2001). Treatment methods include modification of diet and lifestyle, as well as potential use of medications. In general, prophylactic medications are prescribed, although abortive medications may be useful in rare cases.

A retrospective review of a systematic regimen of therapy for vestibular migraine has been published (Reploeg, & Goebel, 2002). Patients in their study were initially treated with dietary manipulation that included avoidance of foods such as caffeine, chocolate, cheese, processed meats, and red wines. If the patient's symptoms continued, they were prescribed a low dose of the tricyclic antidepressant, nortriptyline (Pamelor). This was started at 10 or 25 mg and slowly titrated to a maximum of 50 mg based on the patient's symptoms. If titration was unsuccessful, atenolol (Tenormin), a beta-blocker, was prescribed to be taken alone or in combination with the nortriptyline. Vestibular suppressants and abortive migraine medications were not used in the study. One to 2 months passed before doses were changed or treatment failure was considered. If these medications showed no efficacy, the patient was referred to a neurologist for consultation. The neurologist prescribed various medications including selective serotonin reuptake inhibitors, valproic acid, carbamazepine (Tegretol), and gabapentin (Neurontin). Overall, 72% of their patients (58/81 patients) experienced greater than 75% reduction in symptom frequency. Only 16% of patients (13/81 patients) were able to achieve this level of relief with dietary modification alone. The next 30% (24/81 patients) achieved significant reduction of symptoms with the addition of nortriptyline. An additional 26% (21/81 patients) had significant reduction of symptoms when atenolol or a calcium-channel blocker was added. More recently a prospective observational

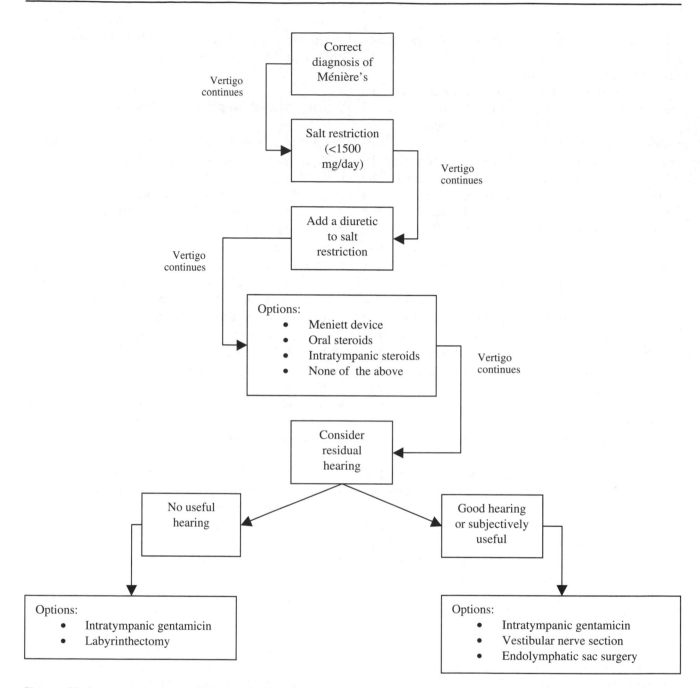

Figure 27-1. Management of Ménière's disease.

study has shown a similar rate of satisfactory control (69%) in patients using prophylactic medications in vestibular migraine. However, that study utilized a wider range of medications, including a calcium channel blocker (Flunarizine) not available in the United States (Maione, 2006).

In 1998, Johnson published a detailed retrospective study on the medical management of vestibular migraine (Johnson, 1998). His technique combined the use of dietary changes, lifestyle adaptation, medication, physical therapy, and acupuncture. Dietary modifications included elimination of aspartame (NutraSweet), reduction or elimination of chocolate, caffeine, and alcohol. Lifestyle adaptations included stress reduction, sleep modification, and initiation of regular exercise. Pharmacologic treatment was chosen based on the patient's age, general health issues, history of drug reactions, and coincident factors such as anxiety disorder, panic attacks, or depression. A total of 10 different medications were used either alone or in combination, including benzodiazepines, calcium-channel blockers, beta-blockers, tricyclic antidepressants, and selective serotonin reuptake inhibitors. Overall, he reported complete or substantial control of vestibular symptoms in 92% of patients. In addition to the discussed classes of vestibular migraine prophylactic medications, topiramate (Topamax) and venlafaxine (Effexor) have also shown benefit in vestibular migraine vertigo and headache reduction in nonrandomized, non-placebo-controlled treatment trials and anecdotal reports, respectively (Gode et al., 2010; Walker, 2006). It has been the author's experience that vestibular migraine patients have a significant rate of medication intolerance to all medication classes that requires low starting doses, slow medication titra-

tion, and extended patient counseling in an effort to improve patient compliance. Table 27–3 lists the migraine prophylactic medications most used at the author's institution.

Comorbid Ménière's Disease and Vestibular Migraine

There are not any clinical studies to evaluate best practice treatment approaches for comorbid Ménière's disease and vestibular migraine. Only recently have epidemiology studies looked at their coexistence and clinical presentation overlap. Ménière's disease and vestibular migraine seem to coexist in 28% of Ménière's disease patients with large clinical overlap in vertigo and associated aural symptom presentation (Neff et al., 2012). The most distinguishing clinical characteristics for Ménière's disease were the pure tone average (PTA) and audiometry standards

Table 27–3. Prophylactic Medications for the Treatment of Vestibular Migraine With or Without Concomitant Ménière's Disease

Medication	Drug Class	Starting Dose	Goal Dose	Maximum Dose	Titration	Common Side Effects
Verapamil (Verelan)	Calcium channel blocker	120 mg QD	240 mg QD	240 mg BID; caution arrhythmia	Increase by 60 mg every week	Constipation, palpitations, peripheral edema, hypotension, fatigue
Venlafaxine XR (Effexor XR)	Serotonin-norepinephrine reuptake inhibitor (SNRI)	37.5 mg QD	75–150 mg QD	225 mg QD	Increase by 37.5 mg every 2 weeks	Drug withdrawal, headache exacerbation, increased blood pressure, perioral or extremity tingling, vivid dreams, sexual dysfunction, suicidal ideation
Gabapentin (Neurontin)	Anticonvulsant	300 mg QD	600 mg TID	1200 mg TID	Increase by 300 mg per day every 7 days	Drowsiness, dizziness, unsteadiness, weight gain, fatigue, extremity fluid retention, blurred vision
Nortriptyline (Pamelor)	Tricyclic antidepressant	10 mg QHS	50–70 mg QHS	150 mg QHS	Increase by 10 mg every 7 days	Dry mouth, constipation, weight gain, somnolence
Topiramate (Topamax)	Anticonvulsant	25 mg QD	50 mg BID	200 mg BID	Increase by 25 mg every 7 days	Word-finding difficulty, trouble concentrating, mental fogginess, weight loss, tingling in extremities

set forth by the 1995 AAO-HNS Ménière's disease criteria (Committee on Hearing and Equilibrium, 1995). The most distinguishing characteristics of vestibular migraine were moderate to severe headache and photophobia during vestibular symptoms (Neff et al., 2012).

There are two reasonable approaches to treating concomitant Ménière's disease and vestibular migraine (MDVM). The author's preferred approach is to treat the vestibular migraine component first with dietary modification and prophylactic migraine medications. This is for several reasons. First, treatment risk is really limited to medication side effects, and these are nearly always self-limited with reduction or termination of medical therapy. There are not the permanent risks of hearing loss and worsened dysequilibrium associated with Ménière's disease treatments, to varying degrees. Second, as previously mentioned, some migraine prophylactics may have beneficial treatment effects for Ménière's disease, for example, calcium channel blockers. Last, many of these patients have comorbid chronic subjective dizziness and health anxiety issues that make them less than ideal candidates for procedural or surgical interventions until these issues are addressed and improved.

Another reasonable treatment algorithm is to first treat Ménière's disease or vestibular migraine based on the predominance of symptom support for either diagnoses. In cases where Ménière's disease is felt to be playing a primary role in vertigo persistence, the author favors nonablative Ménière's disease treatments as a first-line therapy, such as intratympanic steroid injections, Meniett device use, or endolymphatic sac surgery. This is because many of these patients have bilateral ear symptomology, bilateral vestibular test abnormalities, and may be at higher risk to develop contralateral Ménière's disease even if they are currently presenting with unilateral disease complaints. In these cases that have failed vertigo control with nonablative Ménière's disease treatments, the author prefers to treat with at least two different classes of vestibular migraine prophylactic medications prior to moving on to ablative Ménière's disease treatments, if the migraine medication trials are unsuccessful. It should be noted that not tolerating a medication is not deemed a failed medication trial, and every effort should be made to try to find a medication class that is tolerable to the patient.

With either approach, a few combined MDVM patients will be treatment resistant to initial therapies. In cases where MDVM patients continue to have spontaneous vertigo of >20 min duration and have failed migraine prophylactic medications and nonablative Ménière's disease treatments, then the author favors intratympanic gentamicin given via a titration method. This approach often leads to vertigo control without completely ablating the vestibular system. This may be important if the contralateral ear develops Ménière's disease in the future. Titrated intratympanic gentamicin can be used after failed medical and nonablative treatments in the second ear due to the residual, yet reduced, vestibular function that was maintained in the initial ear after previous intratympanic gentamicin. Although very effective for vertigo control, vestibular nerve section and labyrinthectomy both lead to complete vestibular ablation in the initially treated ear and cannot be done in both ears without disabling oscillopsia. Although not definitively proven, the author's anecdotal experience is that this MDVM group has a much higher rate of initial and eventual bilateral Ménière's disease development. The author favors using IM streptomycin primarily in cases of bilateral simultaneous Ménière's disease or MDVM (bilateral involvement) not responsive to initial therapy. Last, the author has also done a few sequential (right ear then 6 weeks later left ear, or vice versa) bilateral intratympanic gentamicin injections followed by vestibular rehabilitation on patients with treatment-resistant MDVM (bilateral simultaneous involvement) or bilateral Ménière's disease with some success. Simultaneous (both ears at same visit) intratympanic gentamicin in bilateral Ménière's disease cases has not been tried, to date, by the author or reported in the literature.

SUMMARY

Management of the patient with vestibular disorder can be very challenging. Careful and thorough evaluation of the patient, followed by comprehensive counseling about the nature of vestibular dysfunction is essential. Proper counseling will allay many of the patient's fears and helps produce an understanding of the patient's disease that will allow them to participate meaningfully in management decisions. Using this strategy, along with the judicious selection of medical, surgical, and/or rehabilitative measures, should result in substantial improvement in many cases of peripheral vestibular dysfunction, even if the symptoms cannot be entirely eliminated.

REFERENCES

Alles, M. J. R. C., der Gaag, M. A., & Stokroos, R. J. (2006). Intratympanic steroid therapy for inner ear diseases: A review of the literature. *European Archives of Oto-Rhino-Laryngology, 263*(9), 791–797.

Ariyasu, L., Byl, F. M., Sprague, M. S., & Adour, K. K. (1990). The beneficial effect of methylprednisolone in acute vestibular vertigo. *Archives of Otolaryngology-Head and Neck Surgery, 116*(6), 700–703.

Barrs, D. M. (2004). Intratympanic injections of dexamethasone for long-term control of vertigo. *Laryngoscope, 114*(11), 1910–1914.

Barrs, D. M., Keyser, J. S., Stallworth, C., & McElveen, Jr., J. T. (2001). Intratympanic steroid injections for intractable Meniere's disease. *Laryngoscope, 111*(12), 2100–2104.

Bertlich, M., Ihler, F., Sharaf, K., Weiss, B. G., Strupp, M., & Canis, M. (2014). Betahistine metabolites, Aminoethylpyridine, and hydroxyethylpyridine increase cochlear blood flow in guinea pigs in vivo. *International Journal of Audiology, 53*(10), 753–759.

Burgess, A., & Kundu, S. (2010). Diuretics for Ménière's disease or syndrome (review). *Cochrane Database of Systematic Reviews* 2006, Issue 3, Art. No.: CD003599. Updated 2010, Issue 4.

Chia, S. H., Grant, A. C., Anderson, J. P., & Harris, J. P. (2004). Intratympanic gentamicin therapy for Meniere's disease: A meta-analysis. *Otology and Neurotology, 25*(4), 554–552.

Coelho, D. H., & Lalwani, A. K. (2008). Medical management of Meniere's disease. *Laryngoscope, 118*, 1099–1108.

Colletti, V., Carner, M., & Colletti, L. (2007). Auditory results after vestibular nerve section and intratympanic gentamicin for Meniere's disease. *Otology and Neurotology, 28*(2), 145–151.

Committee on Hearing and Equilibrium guidelines for the diagnosis and evaluation of therapy in Meniere's disease. (1995). *Otolaryngology-Head and Neck Surgery, 113*(3), 181–185.

Densert, B., & Densert, O. (1982). Overpressure in the treatment of Meniere's disease. *Laryngoscope, 92*(11), 1285–1292.

Densert, B., Sass, K., & Arlinger, S. (1995). Short-term effects of induced middle ear pressure changes on the electrocochleogram in Meniere's disease. *Acta Oto-Laryngologica, 115*(6), 732–737.

Doyle, K. J., Bauch, C., Battista, R., Beatty, C. W., Hughes, G. B., Mason, J., . . . Musiek, F. L. (2004). Intratympanic steroid treatment: A review. *Otology and Neurotology, 25*(6), 1034–1039.

Franz, B., & Van der Laan, F. (2005). P-100 in the treatment of Meniere's disease: A clinical study. *International Tinnitus Journal, 11*(2), 146–149.

Garduno-Anaya, M. A., Couthino De Toledo, H., Hinojosa, G. R., Pane, P. C., & Rios Castenada, L. C. (2005). Dexamethasone inner ear perfusion by intratympanic injection in unilateral Meniere's disease: A two-year prospective, placebo-controlled, double-blind, randomized trial. *Otolaryngology-Head and Neck Surgery, 133*(2), 285–294.

Gates, G. A., Green, J. D. Jr., Tucci, D. L., & Telian, S. A. (2004). The effects of transtympanic micropressure treatment in people with unilateral Meniere's disease. *Archives of Otolaryngology-Head and Neck Surgery, 130*(6), 718–725.

Gates, G. A., Verrall, A., Green, J. D. Jr., Tucci, D. L., & Telian, S. A. (2006). Meniett clinical trial: Long-term follow-up. *Archives of Otolaryngology-Head and Neck Surgery, 132*(12), 1311–1316.

Gode, S., Celebisoy, N., Kirazli, T., Akyuz, A., Bilgen, C., Karapolat, H., . . . Gokcay, F. (2010). Clinical assessment of topiramate therapy in patients with migrainous vertigo. *Headache, 50*(1), 77–84.

Graham, M. D., & Kemink, J. L. (1984). Titration streptomycin therapy for bilateral Meniere's disease. *American Journal of Otology, 5*(6), 534–535.

Gürkov, R., Flatz, W., Keeser, D., Strupp, M., Ertl-Wagner, B., & Krause, E. (2013). Effect of standard-dose Betahistine on endolymphatic hydrops: An MRI pilot study. *European Archives of Otorhinolaryngology, 270*(4), 1231–1235.

Hain, T. C., & Yacovino, D. (2005). Pharmacologic treatment of persons with dizziness. *Neurology Clinics, 23*(3), 831–853, vii.

Huon, L. K., Fang, T. Y., & Wang, P. C. (2012). Outcomes of intratympanic gentamicin injection to treat Meniere's disease. *Otology and Neurotology, 33*(5), 706–714.

Jackson, C. G., Glasscock, M. E., Davis, W. E., Hughes, G. B., & Sismanis, A. (1981). Medical management of Meniere's disease. *Annals of Otology, Rhinology, and Laryngology, 90*(2, Pt.1), 142–147.

James, A., & Burton, M. J. (2011). Betahistine for Ménière's disease or syndrome (review). *Cochrane Database of Systematic Reviews* 2001, Issue 1. Art. No.: CD001873. Updated 2011, Issue 3.

Johnson, G. D. (1998). Medical management of migraine-related dizziness and vertigo. *Laryngoscope, 108*(1, Pt.2), 1–28.

Klockhoff, I., & Lindblom, U. (1967). Meniere's disease and hydrochlorothiazide (Dichlotride)—a critical analysis of symptoms and therapeutic effects. *Acta Oto-Laryngologica, 63*(4), 347–365.

Lambert, P. R., Nguyen, S., Maxwell, K. S., Tucci, D. L., Lustig, L. R., Fletcher, M., . . . Lebel, C. (2012). A randomized, double-blind, placebo-controlled clinical study to assess the safety and clinical activity of OTO-104 given as a single intratympanic injection in patients with unilateral Meniere's disease. *Otology and Neurotology, 33*(7), 1257–1265.

Lassen, L. F., Hirsch, B. E., & Kamerer, D. B. (1996). Use of nimodipine in the medical treatment of Meneire's disease: Clinical experience. *American Journal of Otology, 17*, 577–580.

Lezius, F., Adrion, C., Mansmann, U., Jahn, K., & Strupp, M. (2011). High-dosage betahistine dihydrochloride between 288 and 480 mg/day in patients with severe Meniere's disease: A case series. *European Archives of Otorhinolaryngology, 268*(8), 1237–1240.

Maione, A. (2006). Migraine-related vertigo: Diagnostic criteria and prophylactic treatment. *Laryngoscope, 116*(10), 1782–1786.

Martin, J., Gilchrist, D. P., Smith, P. F., & Darlington, C. L. (1996). Early diazepam treatment following unilateral labyrinthectomy does not impair vestibular compensation of spontaneous nystagmus in guinea pig. *Journal of Vestibular Research, 6*(2), 135–139.

Merchant, S. M., Adams, J. C., & Nadol, J. B. Jr. (2005). Pathophysiology of Meniere's syndrome: Are symptoms caused by endolymphatic hydrops? *Otology and Neurotology, 26*(1), 74–81.

Monzani, D., Barillari, M. R., Alicandri Ciufelli, M., Aggazzotti Cavazza, E., Neri, V., Presutti, L., & Genovese, E. (2012). Effect of a fixed combination of nimodipine and betahistine versus betahistine as monotherapy in the long-term treatment of Meniere's disease: A 10-year experience. *Acta Otorhinolaryngologica Italica, 32*(6), 393–403.

Morales-Luckie, E., Cornejo-Suarez, A., Zaragoza-Contreres, M. A., & Gonzalez-Perez, O. (2005). Oral administration of prednisone to control refractory vertigo in Meniere's disease: A pilot study. *Otology and Neurotology, 26*(5), 1022–1026.

Neff, B. A., Staab, J. P., Eggers, S. D., Carlson, M. L., Schmitt, W. R., Van Abel, K. M., . . . Shepard, N. T. (2012). Auditory and vestibular symptoms and chronic subjective dizziness in patients with Ménière's disease, vestibular migraine, and Ménière's disease with concomitant vestibular migraine. *Otology and Neurotology, 33*(7), 1235–1244.

Neuhauser, H. K. (2007). Epidemiology of vertigo. *Current Opinion in Neurology, 20*(1), 40–46.

Neuhauser, H. K., Leopold, M., von Brevern, M., Arnold, G., & Lempert, T. (2001). The interrelations between migraine, vertigo, and migrainous vertigo. *Neurology, 56*(4), 436–441.

Peppard, S. B. (1986). Effect of drug therapy on compensation from vestibular injury. *Laryngoscope, 96*(8), 878–898.

Phillips, J. S., & Westerberg, B. (2011). Intratympanic steroids for Meniere's disease or syndrome. *Cochrane Database of Systemic Reviews*, Issue 7. Article No.: CD008514.

Pullens, B., & van Benthem, P. P. (2011). Intratympanic gentamicin for Ménière's disease or syndrome. *Cochrane Database of Systematic Reviews*, Issue 3. Art. No.: CD008234.

Radtke, A., Lempert, T., & Gresty, M. A., Brookes, G. B., Bronstein, A. M., & Neuhauser, H. (2002). Migraine and Meniere's disease: Is there a link? *Neurology, 59*, 1700–1704.

Reploeg, M. D., & Goebel, J. A. (2002). Migraine-associated dizziness: Patient characteristics and management options. *Otology and Neurotology, 23*(3), 364–371.

Schuknecht, H. F. (1956). Ablation therapy for the relief of Meniere's disease. *Laryngoscope, 66*(7), 859–870.

Sekitani, T., McCabe, B. F., & Ryu, J. H. (1971). Drug effects on the medial vestibular nucleus. *Archives of Otolaryngology, 93*(6), 581–589.

Shen, J., & Ruckenstein, M. J. (2010). Medical treatment of Meniere's disease. In M. J. Ruckenstein (Ed.), *Meniere's disease: Evidence and outcomes* (pp. 97–104). San Diego, CA: Plural.

Strupp, M., Zingler, V. C., Arbusow, V., Niklas, D., Maag, K. P., Dieterich, M., . . . Brandt, T. (2004). Methylprednisolone, valacyclovir, or the combination for vestibular neuritis. *New England Journal of Medicine, 351*(4), 354–361.

Teufert, K. B., & Doherty, J. (2010). Endolymphatic sac shunt, labyrinthectomy, and vestibular nerve section in Meniere's Disease. *Otolaryngologic Clinics of North America, 43*(5), 1091–1111.

Van Deelen, G. W., & Huizing, E. H. (1986). Use of a diuretic (Dyazide) in the treatment of Meniere's disease. A double-blind cross-over placebo-controlled study. *ORL Journal of Otorhinolaryngology and Its Related Specialties, 48*(5), 287–292.

Wackym, P. A., & Schumacher-Monfre, T. S. (2005). Pharmacotherapy for vestibular dysfunction. In R. K. Jackler (Ed.), *Neurotology* (2nd ed., pp. 659–672). Philadelphia, PA: Elsevier Mosby.

Walker, M. F. (2006). Vertigo and dysequilibrium. In R. Tidball Johnson (Ed.), *Current therapy in neurologic diseases* (p. 6). Philadelphia, PA: Mosby Elsevier.

Zajonc, T. P., & Roland, P. S. (2006). Vertigo and motion sickness. Part II: Pharmacologic treatment. *Ear, Nose, and Throat Journal, 85*(1), 25–35.

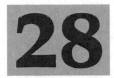

Surgical Management of Vertigo That Is Otologic in Origin

Steven A. Telian and R. Mark Wiet

INTRODUCTION

In balance disorder patients, surgical management is usually the last treatment offered but can offer dramatic benefit when appropriately indicated. By the time an operation is considered, vertiginous patients have often sought consultation from multiple physicians and tried many potential remedies without success. As such, they are often eager for relief, making them vulnerable to even more intense disappointment from poor postoperative outcomes. This chapter aims to provide the reader with a framework for understanding the surgical treatment options in the management of vertigo, and a deeper understanding of appropriate surgical patient selection for these procedures. It is beyond the scope of this text to discuss detailed technical aspects of the surgical procedures that are used for the management of vertigo. More comprehensive details are available elsewhere (Telian, 2010). However, a general description of it is provided to help the reader understand the nature and potential limitations of each procedure.

RATIONALE FOR SURGERY

The ideal operative candidate with vestibular disease is one with a fluctuating or progressive unilateral peripheral lesion, who has previously failed appropriate medical management. Vestibular system surgery is most likely to succeed when it is undertaken to stabilize an unstable inner ear disorder, either by correcting a defect that underlies the condition or by ablating any residual function in the pathologic ear. It is unlikely to be successful when a fixed labyrinthine lesion is present but the patient has been unable to compensate centrally. For example, patients with vestibular neuritis initially have intense symptoms that gradually subside. In most cases, central vestibular compensation will relieve dizziness by adjusting to the altered, but stable, sensory inputs from the periphery. If the patient continues to be symptomatic, it is usually because of inability to compensate centrally. Thus, the patient would be more appropriately treated with vestibular rehabilitation methods.

Certain surgical procedures are only appropriate for particular diagnoses. Examples include posterior semicircular canal occlusion for intractable benign paroxysmal positional vertigo (BPPV), repair of superior semicircular canal dehiscence, or repair of a perilymphatic fistula. Success in these settings hinges on making the exact etiologic diagnosis, and choosing the correct procedure to reverse the pathologic process. In these cases, it is possible to preserve or restore inner ear function.

The quintessential example of a fluctuating peripheral lesion is Ménière's disease. The peripheral lesion in this condition is unstable by definition and often is progressive in nature. The disease is characterized by fluctuation between normal labyrinthine function and dramatic cochleovestibular pathology. Central compensation is not possible, or really a primary consideration, until the ear can be stabilized by effective medical or surgical management. Specific procedures designed to relieve Ménière's disease that have been advocated to achieve peripheral stabilization are discussed later in the chapter. The ablative vestibular operations can be grouped into two general categories: labyrinthectomy or vestibular neurectomy. Either of these may be applied successfully in the management of Ménière's disease or any other unstable peripheral vestibular disorder. For the latter category, the exact etiologic diagnosis is not as critical. Instead, the physician simply needs to be certain that the problem is attributable to unstable unilateral peripheral vestibular dysfunction and that the pathologic ear has been correctly identified.

PROCEDURES FOR BENIGN PAROXYSMAL POSITIONAL VERTIGO (BPPV)

BPPV is generally believed to be the most common human vestibular disorder. Cupulolithiasis was the original pathogenic hypothesis proposed for BPPV. It was believed that otoconial debris became lodged within the ampulla of the posterior semicircular canal, rendering it sensitive to gravity. As early as the 1970s, objections to this theory arose since a disorder in the biomechanics of cupular function could not produce the nystagmus pattern most frequently observed in patients with BPPV (McCabe & Ryu, 1979). In the 1990s, evidence accumulated to support the concept of otoconia floating freely in the endolymphatic space of the membranous semicircular canals. This theory is known as canalithiasis (Epley, 2001; Parnes & McClure, 1991; Welling et al., 1997). BPPV generally affects the posterior semicircular canal, but canalithiasis in particular can involve any of the three canals. Diagnosis is based on a history of brief vertigo associated with rapid changes in head position, such as rolling over in bed, along with a positive Hallpike maneuver on examination. With canalithiasis, the clinician should observe a brief latent period, followed by rotary nystagmus developing with a fast component that beats toward the dependent ear. There is a crescendo-decrescendo

pattern, after which the nystagmus passes and the vertigo subsides within 20 to 30 s. If the maneuver is repeated, the response fatigues. Assuming BPPV has been correctly diagnosed, treatment options include observation, nonsurgical procedures performed by the physician or trained vestibular physical therapist, or surgery for intractable BPPV. It has been estimated that less than 1% of patients with posterior canal BPPV will require surgical intervention (Shaia et al., 2006).

Singular Neurectomy for BPPV

The singular nerve, also known as the posterior ampullary nerve, is a branch of the inferior vestibular nerve that selectively innervates the posterior semicircular canal ampulla. An operation promoted by Gacek known as the singular neurectomy involves sectioning the singular nerve via a transcanal approach (Gacek & Gacek, 1994). The singular nerve is accessed by drilling posteroinferiorly to the posterior margin of the round window. The posterior canal ampulla and the bony vestibule are at high risk during the procedure, and injury to either one can result in severe vertigo and sensorineural hearing loss. Control of vertigo from BPPV can be achieved in 95% of patients. The estimated risk of sensorineural hearing loss in expert hands is 3%. Anatomic studies in human cadaveric temporal bones have shown variable results in regard to the feasibility of this operation. Some authors believe the singular nerve is approachable via the external auditory canal in 98% of temporal bones (Kos et al., 2006), whereas other authors are not as optimistic and quote numbers as low as 20% (Leuwer & Westhofen, 1996). Experience dictates that this is a technically challenging operation that should not be undertaken unless it has first been mastered in the temporal bone laboratory. Although this procedure is safe and highly reliable in experienced hands, it has largely been supplanted by the technically simpler posterior semicircular canal occlusion procedure.

Posterior Canal Occlusion for BPPV

Posterior semicircular canal occlusion for relief of BBPV was introduced in 1991 by Parnes and McClure. Success of this procedure requires that the canalithiasis variant of BPPV has been properly diagnosed. Following a complete mastoidectomy, the surgeon identifies the dense bone of the posterior semicircular canal between the facial nerve and the posterior fossa dural plate. The bony lumen of the posterior semicircular canal is opened carefully with a diamond drill. Periosteum is used to occlude the membranous canal, and the lumen is obliterated (Figure 28–1). The temporal bone CT shown in Figure 28–2 depicts the postoperative appearance on imaging. Retrospective studies have shown that nearly 100% of BPPV patients treated with this procedure receive control of their vertigo. In addition, hearing loss is uncommon when the operation is properly performed (Shaia et al., 2006).

REPAIR OF PERILYMPHATIC FISTULA

Perilymphatic fistula (PLF) should be considered in any patient with vertigo after head trauma, barotrauma, or previous stapedectomy but rarely occurs spontaneously (Shea, 1992). The disturbance to the vestibular system in this disorder is due to a leak of perilymph from the inner ear into the middle ear through the oval window, round window, or other natural fissures in the bony labyrinth (Goodhill, 1981). For the most part, traumatic perilymphatic fistulae are thought to heal spontaneously. Typically when this diagnosis is entertained in acute cases, a 3-day period of bed rest with oral corticosteroid therapy will be recommended. Patients with persistent vertigo after penetrating middle ear trauma should undergo immediate exploration and repair. In chronic cases, where this diagnosis is considered but uncertain, a trial of vestibular rehabilitation is appropriate prior to any surgical intervention provided that the hearing is stable (Shepard et al., 1992).

Surgical exploration for PLF is warranted when conservative measures have failed and a high clinical suspicion remains. Appropriate exposure involves elevation of a tympanomeatal flap and bone removal from the posterior superior quadrant of the medial external auditory canal. The main areas of interest are the round window and oval window niches. In

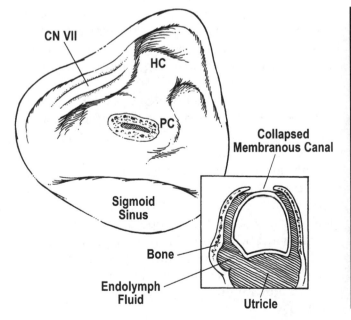

Figure 28-1. Surgical view of posterior semicircular canal procedure in a left temporal bone. Inset shows a cross section of the posterior canal after the bone has been drilled away and the membranous canal has collapsed. From Chapter 144, Surgery for vestibular disorders, by Steven A. Telian. In C. W. Cummings (Ed.), *Otolaryngology head and neck surgery*, 4th ed., p. 3292. Copyright 2005, Elsevier. Reproduced with permission.

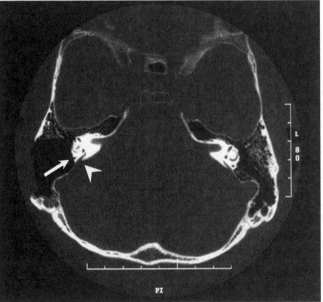

Figure 28-2. Axial CT scan without contrast of the temporal bones at the level of the horizontal semicircular canals in a patient who has undergone a right posterior semicircular canal occlusion. There is a mastoidectomy defect and the bone lateral to the posterior semicircular canal has been removed (*arrow*). The vestibular aqueduct is marked also (*arrowhead*).

addition, particular attention should be paid to the areas anterior to the oval window and inferior to the round window for abnormally patent fissures. Obvious defects should be repaired by patching with fascia or perichondrium. Suspicious areas are typically treated in the same manner. In negative explorations, routine patching of the round window niche is appropriate. Packing of the oval window when the footplate and annular ligament are normal should be avoided or performed very judiciously to prevent an additional conductive component to the hearing loss.

Controversy exists around the diagnosis of perilymphatic fistula due to the difficulty associated with identifying a microfistula at the time of surgery and uncertainty regarding the clinical diagnostic criteria (Shepard et al., 1992). A molecule known for its utility in confirmation of cerebrospinal fluid leaks, β-2 transferrin, has also been identified in perilymph. Attempts have been made to use this as a marker for PLF as well. However, results have been conflicting with this technique (Levenson, Desloge, & Parisier, 1996; Skedros, Cass, Hirsch, & Kelly, 1993). Small sample sizes and variability in sensitivity of the assays are the likely sources of these discrepant results.

REPAIR OF SUPERIOR SEMICIRCULAR CANAL DEHISCENCE

Minor and his colleagues have described and characterized superior semicircular canal dehiscence (SSCD) as an important and previously overlooked cause of vertigo (Minor, 2005). In this condition, an acquired defect violating the bony lumen of the superior canal develops, resulting in direct contact between the perilymph and the dura of the middle cranial fossa. This creates a "third window phenomenon" resulting in a reduction in the transmission of auditory energy by motion of the stapes footplate as well as potential disturbances of the micromechanics within the vestibular labyrinth. The symptoms that often lead to the identification of this syndrome are vertigo and eye movements induced by loud sound or pressure (coughing, sneezing, straining, or the Valsalva maneuver). These symptoms are associated with evoked torsional eye movements in a pattern consistent with the innervation of the dehiscent superior canal. This complex is known as the Tullio phenomenon when sound is the provocative factor and Hennebert's sign when the stimulus is pressure in the external auditory canal. These patients may complain of autophony and hyperacusis for bone-conducted sounds. It has also been recognized that patients with SSCD often have a low-frequency conductive hearing loss, perhaps without the vestibular signs and symptoms mentioned above. The air-bone gap in these patients is partly due to inefficient transmission of stapedial vibration to the basilar membrane due to the third window phenomenon, but there is also an increased sensitivity to bone-conducted sound. This leads to supranormal thresholds for bone conduction testing, especially in the low frequencies. If the audiologist suspects this disorder and remembers to test for bone conduction thresholds below 0 dB, the patient may have responses as low as −15 dB. Since the tympanic membrane is intact and the middle ear appears healthy, patients may be wrongly diagnosed with otosclerosis, particularly when there is no history of vertigo. The ear surgeon should not hesitate to close the ear and evaluate for SSCD if the stapes appears normally mobile upon inspection. The critical feature for distinguishing between these two diagnoses is the routine presence of intact acoustic reflexes in SSCD. Thus, patients with a conductive loss should ideally undergo acoustic reflex testing before stapedectomy surgery is undertaken.

Vestibular-evoked myogenic potentials (VEMP) have been shown to be present at reduced thresholds in ears with SSCD. In addition, electrocochleography (ECoG) in these ears will almost always demonstrate an increased summating potential to action potential ratio, which will return to normal after surgical correction (Adams et al., 2011). The diagnosis also requires a CT scan of the temporal bones that is consistent with SSCD. The scan must be performed with high-resolution scanning and reconstructions in the parasagittal plane containing the superior canal.

To illustrate this diagnosis, we present a case of SSCD:

A 51-year-old registered nurse presented with right hearing loss, intermittent right tinnitus, mild episodic vertigo, and a sense of disequilibrium for several months. Physical exam showed normal ears, and the fistula test was a negative in the right ear. With a 512-Hz tuning fork, the Weber test lateralized to the right ear, and air conduction was greater than bone conduction bilaterally. With a 256-Hz tuning fork, bone conduction was greater than air conduction in the right ear, and unchanged in the left. Audiologic testing showed only a slight high-frequency hearing loss the left ear. In the right ear (Figure 28–3), she had a mild-to-moderate low-frequency conductive component to her hearing loss. Speech recognition scores and tympanometry were normal bilaterally. Acoustic reflexes were also present bilaterally, indicating an absence of middle ear pathology. ECoG showed a summating potential to action potential ratio of 0.82 (Figure 28–4). The history, physical exam findings, and audiologic results prompted further evaluation. She underwent a cervical VEMP study (Figure 28–5) and a CT

scan of the temporal bones (Figure 28–6). The results of both tests were consistent with a diagnosis of right superior semicircular canal dehiscence. Given that she had very intermittent vertigo and only a mild low-frequency hearing loss, we recommended continued observation, and consideration for audiometric amplification. Her condition did not progress over the ensuing 5 years. If her hearing loss had worsened, or if she had developed worsening vestibular symptoms, we would have considered surgical repair by a middle fossa approach.

Conservative management of SSCD includes avoidance of the evoking stimulus. For those who are debilitated by the vestibular manifestations of SSCD, surgery is an option. This classically involves a middle cranial fossa approach, and plugging of the superior canal similar to that described for

Frequency in Hertz

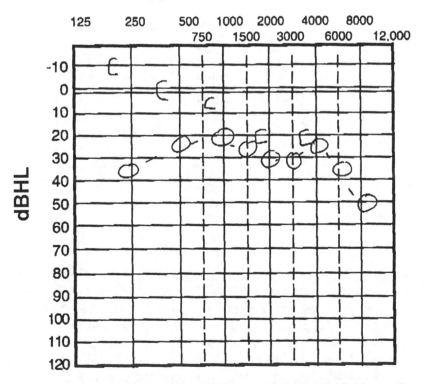

Figure 28–3. Right ear audiogram from a patient with right superior semicircular canal dehiscence. In addition to a bilateral high-frequency moderate sensorineural hearing loss, this patient has a superimposed low-frequency air-bone gap, as can be seen in patients with superior canal dehiscence.

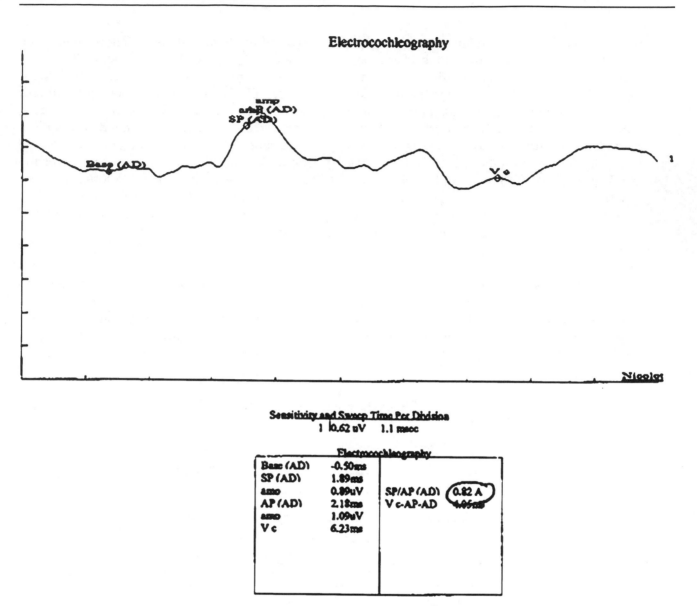

Figure 28–4. Electrocochleography (ECoG) for the right ear was carried out utilizing a tympanic membrane surface electrode. Responses were elicited by click stimuli, and the summating potential to action potential ratio was abnormally elevated to a value of 0.82.

posterior canal occlusion, and/or resurfacing of the dehiscence with bone cement. In Minor's 2005 landmark initial report of surgery for SSCD, eight of nine patients who underwent plugging, but only 7 of 11 who underwent resurfacing, had complete resolution of their symptoms. Thus, the current recommendation is to perform canal plugging rather than resurfacing. This recommendation was reinforced when two patients had delayed postoperative moderate to severe sensorineural hearing loss after a revision procedure for SSCD after failure with

resurfacing (Limb, Carey, Srireddy, & Minor, 2006). Hillman, Kertesz, Hadley, and Shelton reported a series of 30 patients, 13 of whom were operated on with a 93% success rate (Hillman et al., 2006) One of their patients had a decrease in sensorineural hearing function of 10 dB following surgery. Interestingly, the postoperative improvement in the conductive hearing loss is frequently modest. One study of 43 patients with SSCD repaired via the middle fossa approach documented that the mean air-bone gap decreased from 16 to 8 dB after surgery, with a

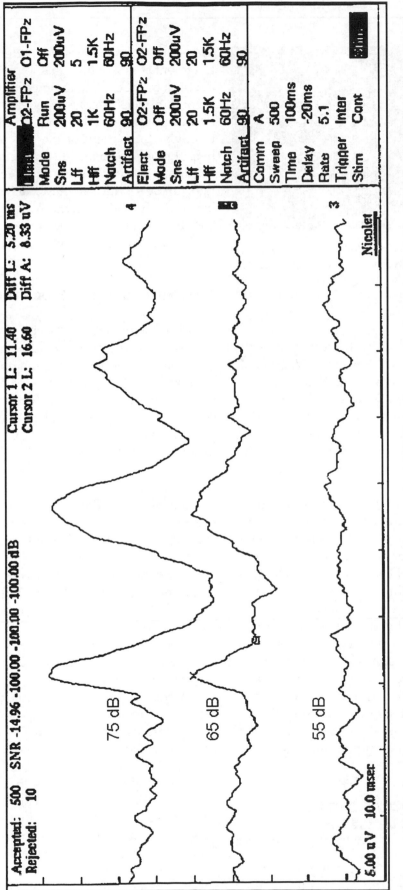

Figure 28–5. Right ear cervical vestibular-evoked myogenic potential (cVEMP) testing was carried out with right ear stimulation. Responses with rather large amplitudes were obtained at 75 and 65 dB. A small amplitude response could still be identified at 55 dB. Left ear stimulation in the range of 75 to 90 dB produced no discernible response (*not shown*). Thus, the VEMP was considered to be positive for a right SSCD.

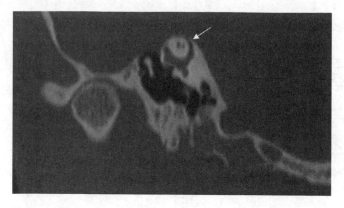

Figure 28-6. CT scan showing a widely dehiscent right superior semicircular canal (*arrow*). This image was reformatted in a plane parallel to the right superior semicircular canal (*Poschl view*) from an axial CT without contrast.

decreased air-conducted pure tone average offset by increased bone conduction thresholds (Ward et al., 2012). In addition, 25% of patients had a new sustained mild high-frequency sensory hearing loss, but there were no changes in speech discrimination. Thus, surgery is not generally recommended unless vestibular symptoms or troublesome auditory phenomena such as autophony or Tullio's phenomenon are also present.

In recent years, a transmastoid approach for repair of SSCD has been advocated as an alternative (Beyea, Agrawal, & Parnes, 2012). This approach is less risky to the patient, because it does not require a middle fossa craniotomy. However, because the repair is generally performed through a second surgically created fenestration in the semicircular canal lumen, it may prove to be more risky to the inner ear function. In general, this approach is preferred for patients who suffer from chronic migraine, TMJ disorders, intracranial hypertension, or other headache syndromes. It is also very suitable for dehiscences that could be difficult to expose from above, such as those that are located medial to the dome of the canal or those that are in contact with the superior petrosal sinus.

SPECIFIC OPERATIONS FOR MÉNIÈRE'S DISEASE

Recurrent episodic vertigo, fluctuating sensorineural hearing loss, tinnitus, and aural fullness are a complex of symptoms that signify the presence of Ménière's disease. Typically after a 4 to 6 month treatment course with suitable medical therapy, the decision may be made to proceed with further treatment if intractable episodic spells of vertigo persist. At this point, it is the responsibility of the surgeon to advise the patient of the treatment options and help the patient to decide on the appropriate intervention. Ablative operations will reliably relieve vertigo, but do sacrifice any residual vestibular function in the involved ear. Alternatively, operations such as endolymphatic sac procedures are designed to preserve function while stabilizing the inner ear.

Endolymphatic Sac Procedures

There is histopathologic evidence that Ménière's disease is associated with endolymphatic hydrops, producing distention of the membranous labyrinth (Schuknecht, 1993). As first described by Portmann, the endolymphatic sac (ELS) can be approached surgically through a complete mastoidectomy and opened, ostensibly to drain endolymph into the mastoid cavity (Portmann, 1927). Variations to this operation were subsequently proposed by Shambaugh, House, and Shea (House, 1965; Shambaugh, 1975; Shea, 1966). These include wide bony decompression, endolymphatic-subarachnoid shunt, and endolymphatic-mastoid shunt, respectively. Somewhat later, insertion of a pressure-sensitive valve into the endolymphatic duct was proposed (Arenberg, Zoller, & Wan de Water, 1983). Regardless of the method used, there is very little evidence-based literature to support the efficacy of endolymphatic sac operations. As such, the use of these operations has been continually debated, and their popularity has waxed and waned.

A creative randomized clinical study was performed in Denmark that compared endolymphatic sac decompression with a control group having cortical mastoidectomy only using double-blind design (Bretlau, Thomsen, Tos, & Johnsen, 1989). Both groups demonstrated improvements that were not found to be statistically different. The authors thus concluded that improvements in vertigo after ELS surgery could be attributed to a "placebo effect." Proponents of sac surgery argue that the sample size was too small to detect clinically important differences. Furthermore, they point out that both groups improved, arguing in favor of the operation even if the effect was nonspecific. The same group subsequently performed another small controlled study comparing endolymphatic sac decompression and insertion of a tympanostomy tube, again with similar results (Thomsen, Bonding, Becker, Stage, & Tos, 1998). Because neither study included a nonsurgical control group, any influence of the favorable natural history of Ménière's disease on the reported efficacy could not be assessed. A reanalysis of the data from the first Danish study was completed years later using more sophisticated nonparametric statistical methods (Welling & Nagaraja, 2000). This analysis demonstrated that the active sac surgery group did have statistically significant improvements in postoperative vertigo, nausea, vomiting, and tinnitus compared with the mastoidectomy alone group.

Traditionally, advocates of these procedures report a 50% to 80% success rate and believe that this operation is preferable to initial use of an ablative procedure given the natural history of this disease (Convert, Franco-Vidal, Bebear, & Darrouzet, 2006). Graham and Kemink (1984) were able to show that wide bony decompression without shunting compares favorably to operations that include shunt procedures. One uncontrolled observational study claimed that vertigo and vestibular disability could be largely corrected in 85% of patients 2 years after wide bony decompression of the sac and sigmoid sinus (Gianoli, Larouere, Kartush, & Wayman, 1998).

An argument against the use of ELS surgery may be justified, given the following considerations. Schucknecht argued convincingly that the endolymphatic hydrops observed in Ménière's disease is due to malfunction at the level of the utriculoendolymphatic valve, rather than in the ELS itself (Schucknecht, 1993). If this is indeed true, then any apparent benefit obtained from surgical manipulation of the ELS or endolymphatic duct must be a nonspecific or indirect effect of the surgery. Furthermore, when sac surgery is performed, any foreign material placed within the sac for shunting purposes will usually become encapsulated with fibrous tissue, blocking any potential outflow of endolymph. With these considerations in mind, Gates documented in a prospective observational trial that Innovar (a potent neuroleptic analgesic) provided lasting relief of vertigo for most patients who failed medical management (Gates, 1999). Thus, at least some of the reported benefit of ELS surgery may be attributable to the general anesthesia rather than the

surgical intervention. Each practitioner must come to a conclusion whether endolymphatic sac surgery is sufficiently reliable to routinely recommend its use to patients seeking relief of Ménière's disease symptoms.

Cochlear Endolymphatic Shunt

The cochlear endolymphatic shunt procedure (often called cochleosacculotomy) involves an attempt to create a permanent communication between the perilymphatic space and the endolymphatic compartment (Schuknecht, 1991a; Schuknecht & Bartley, 1985). Using a transcanal tympanotomy approach, the round window is exposed. A right-angled hook is inserted through the round window membrane and directed toward the oval window niche, hugging the lateral wall of the inner ear (Figure 28–7). Ideally, the osseous spiral lamina is penetrated, leading to permanent internal fistulization of the endolymphatic system into perilymph of the scala tympani. By creating this small fistula, the surgeon hopes to allow the ear to equilibrate pressure between the perilymphatic and endolymphatic compartments. It has been reported that 70% of patients who undergo

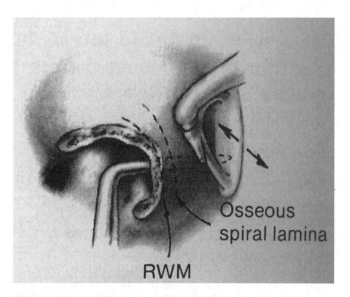

Figure 28–7. Left ear transcanal view of a cochleosacculotomy procedure depicts a right angle hook in the round window niche, piercing the round window membrane and the osseous spiral lamina. From Chapter 144, Surgery for vestibular disorders, by Steven A. Telian. In C. W. Cummings (Ed.), *Otolaryngology head and neck surgery*, 4th ed., p. 3294. Copyright 2005, Elsevier. Reproduced with permission.

this operation achieve long-term relief of their vertigo. However, the operation is associated with a 25% incidence of high-frequency sensorineural hearing loss, and a 10% incidence of profound deafness (Schuknecht, 1991a). Thus, it has had very limited application, though it is viewed by some authors as a safe alternative to labyrinthectomy in elderly patients (Kinney, Nalepa, Hughes, & Kinney, 1995).

ABLATIVE VESTIBULAR SURGERY

When patients with balance disorder are refractory to maximal medical therapy and conservative surgical measures, the final option would be to perform an ablative vestibular procedure. A labyrinthectomy is appropriate if the hearing is quite poor, while vestibular nerve section may be advised if the hearing remains useful in the involved ear. These procedures are designed to ablate residual function in the diseased ear, eliminating the spontaneous episodes of vertigo that result from fluctuation of labyrinthine input to the central nervous system. They are most often applied to patients with Ménière's disease but can also be used in the treatment of any unstable peripheral vestibular disorder where the offending labyrinth has been correctly identified (Benecke, 1994; Kemink, Telian, El-Kashlan, & Langman, 1991).

Patient Selection: Poor Compensation Versus Unstable Labyrinthine Disease

A surgical ablation procedure in a patient who lacks the ability to compensate centrally for the new deficit is likely to be fruitless. This may seem inherently obvious, but prior to the advent of vestibular rehabilitation therapy in the late 1980s, this principle was poorly appreciated. Such procedures were offered somewhat indiscriminately to any patient who had a localized peripheral lesion documented with ongoing symptoms of any kind. It was demonstrated at the University of Michigan that vestibular rehabilitation was superior to vestibular nerve section for treating symptoms caused by uncompensated vestibular neuritis (Table 28–1). Therefore, high priority should be placed on distinguishing patients with poor compensation from those with unstable ves-

Table 28–1. University of Michigan Treatment Results in Uncompensated Vestibular Neuritis

	Vestibular Nerve Section (*n* = 16)	Vestibular Rehabilitation (*n* = 59)
Complete improvement	0%	25%
Dramatic improvement	25%	47%
Mild improvement	45%	13%
No improvement	25%	15%
Worse	5%	0%

tibular lesions. To accomplish this goal, the clinician needs to pay close attention to the clinical history as well as the vestibular testing results. It is also wise to undertake a therapeutic trial of vestibular rehabilitation prior to considering surgical treatment when this distinction is unclear.

Clinical History

Incomplete compensation despite a stable vestibular lesion, as may be the case after severe vestibular neuritis or labyrinthitis, is signified by a history of an index event of a severe vertiginous crisis, then followed by continuous unsteadiness and/or mild motion-provoked vertigo. Such patients are best treated with vestibular rehabilitation. An unstable vestibular lesion is suggested by recurrent episodic spells that are at least equal in severity to the initial insult. Documentation of a progressive or fluctuating sensorineural hearing loss also provides a strong indication of an unstable ear.

Balance Function Testing

Three major goals of balance function testing may inform the physician regarding the suitability of surgical treatment:

- site-of-lesion localization of the offending vestibular periphery,
- assessment of the level of vestibular compensation, and

■ assessment of integrated use of available sensory systems.

Peripheral localization may be accomplished by video- or electronystamography (VNG/ENG), particularly by measuring the response to caloric irrigations in each ear. In addition, VNG can assist with assessment of vestibular compensation. Incomplete compensation is suggested by clinically significant spontaneous nystagmus, positional nystagmus, or a directional preponderance.

Rotational chair testing may inform the clinician whether the location of the lesion is central or peripheral. Gain reduction generally signifies the presence of a bilateral peripheral vestibulopathy, but false-positive results occur due to sedation of the patient or conscious suppression of the response due to efforts to suppress nausea. Abnormalities in the timing relationship (phase) of the vestibulo-ocular reflex (VOR) or a reduction in the time constant provide evidence for peripheral vestibular dysfunction but do not inform the clinician regarding site of lesion or level of compensation.

However, a persistent asymmetry in the slow phase eye velocity responses to clockwise versus counter-clockwise rotation strongly suggests that the lesion is uncompensated.

Posturography may demonstrate that there is a functional impairment in the balance system despite normal physiologic responses as measured on VNG or rotational chair testing. A patient unable to integrate input from the visual, vestibular, and somatosensory systems to maintain stable stance may have incomplete compensation for a vestibular lesion. Also, sensory preference abnormalities may be defined in which unreliable sensory signals are inappropriately selected, destabilizing the patient. This information may be useful when counseling the patient or designing a vestibular rehabilitation program (Table 28–2).

Therapeutic Trial of Vestibular Rehabilitation Therapy

A trial of supervised vestibular therapy is justified whenever there is diagnostic uncertainty. An

Table 28–2. Clinical Usefulness of Vestibular Test Results

Evidence for peripheral labyrinthine dysfunction	Unilateral caloric weakness
	Spontaneous or positional nystagmus with normal oculomotor findings
	Classical nystagmus after Hallpike maneuver
	Rotational chair phase or asymmetry
Evidence for uncompensated status	Persistent spontaneous or positional nystagmus
	Rotational chair asymmetry
	Abnormalities on sensory organization posturography test
Explanations for poor compensation caused by central nervous system pathology	Vertical or perverted nystagmus
	Oculomotor test abnormalities on electronystagmogram battery
	Failure of visual suppression of nystagmus
	Failure of visual enhancement of nystagmus
	Abnormalities on motor coordination test without musculoskeletal disorder
Evidence for improved compensation status after treatment	Resolution of nystagmus
	Resolution of rotational chair asymmetry
	Improved performance on posturography

example would be a patient with a head injury who has evidence of both central and peripheral vestibular dysfunction, along with comorbid symptoms such as chronic headache, cognitive impairment, and depression. After therapy, there may be improvement in the balance symptoms, validating the previous notion that there was incomplete compensation. On the contrary, if the patient fails to make progress after several weeks of therapy, it becomes more likely that the patient has an unstable lesion.

Identifying the Offending Labyrinth

The best indicator of the offending labyrinth is an asymmetric hearing loss, especially if there is a fluctuating or progressive sensorineural hearing loss in one ear (Shone, Kemink, & Telian, 1991). Another reliable lateralizing feature is a consistently reproducible unilateral reduction of responsiveness to caloric irrigations, assuming that the patient does not report new auditory symptoms in the better hearing ear. Less reliable features include aural fullness, tinnitus, the direction of spontaneous or positional nystagmus, and rotary chair testing asymmetries. It is important to consider the entire clinical picture. For example, if a patient complains of roaring tinnitus and hearing fluctuation in the ear with better caloric responses, then it is likely that the second ear has become involved. In this case, surgery directed toward the weaker ear should be avoided.

Identification of Intracranial Pathology

Vestibular test findings suggesting central pathology include vertical or perverted nystagmus, failure of fixation suppression, and oculomotor control abnormalities. Increased saccade latencies, decreased saccade velocities, and pursuit tracking worse than expected for the patient's age are central oculomotor findings that the clinician needs to evaluate prior to considering vestibular surgery. Ultimately, most vestibular patients should undergo magnetic resonance imaging of the brain focused on the posterior fossa (Figure 28–8). Gadolinium enhancement should always be administered. This study provides a reliable means of detecting tumors, demyelinating disease, and subtle lesions of the brainstem. Classical

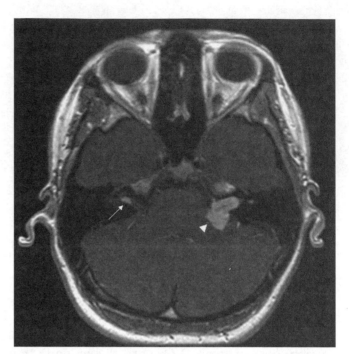

Figure 28–8. T1 Axial MRI with gadolinium-NF2 patient with a right internal auditory canal lesion (*white arrow*), and a left cerebellopontine angle lesion with extension into left internal auditory canal (*white arrowhead*).

vertigo syndromes can be mimicked by intracranial lesions, especially vestibular schwannomas (Disher, Telian, & Kemink, 1991).

Preservation of Residual Hearing

There is mounting evidence that hearing preserved by conservation surgery will usually continue to deteriorate, especially in Ménière's disease. In this case, the riskier intracranial procedure required for a vestibular neurectomy may provide no incremental benefit to the patient (Eisenman, Speers, & Telian, 2001; Tewary, Riley, & Kerr, 1998). This realization, coupled with the increased use of intratympanic gentamicin treatment, has led to a dramatic reduction of intracranial procedures for vertigo. Regardless, the patient's perception of useful hearing is the most important factor when determining whether or not to sacrifice residual hearing. Some patients claim subjective benefit from amplification of hearing ordinarily considered useless by audiologic standards. On the other hand, there are patients who have clinically measurable hearing that should be useful, but report no benefit from amplification and/or refuse to use a hearing aid. Thus, no specific hearing threshold or speech discrimination score should be used as a strict criterion to clarify this decision, and each case must be considered on an individual basis.

Labyrinthectomy

Labyrinthectomy procedures are reserved for patients who have minimal, if any, residual hearing. When the contralateral ear is stable and the patient is convinced that the involved ear is functionally useless, one may recommend a labyrinthectomy. This can be accomplished chemically with intratympanic aminoglycosides (discussed elsewhere in this volume) or surgically using a transcanal or transmastoid labyrinthectomy.

Also known as the oval window labyrinthectomy, the transcanal labyrinthectomy procedure is performed through the external auditory canal (Pulec, 1974; Schuknecht, 1991b). A tympanomeatal flap is elevated and the stapes is removed from the oval window, giving the surgeon access to the labyrinth. Some surgeons remove bone between the oval window and the round window to improve visualization of the vestibule. The saccule and the utricle are then removed. Removal of the horizontal and superior canal ampullae is not possible with this approach, but the surgeon may choose to section the singular nerve or remove the posterior canal ampulla. Control of vertigo may be augmented by placing absorbable packing material soaked with an aminoglycoside antibiotic into the vestibule. This procedure reliably eliminates episodic vertigo, even though removal of the sensory neuroepithelium in its entirety is not achieved. A threefold increase in postoperative disequilibrium compared to the transmastoid approach (63 versus 23%, respectively) has been documented (Langman & Lindeman, 1998).

The transmastoid labyrinthectomy, considered by the senior author to be the "gold standard" for surgical relief of vertigo, is accomplished though a postauricular incision. A complete mastoidectomy is performed and the surgeon identifies the horizontal semicircular canal in the mastoid antrum. When the labyrinthine bone has been drilled away appropriately, the surgeon will be able to visualize and remove all three ampullae and both otolithic maculae (Figure 28–9). The wound is then irrigated and closed. As one would expect, this procedure results in highly

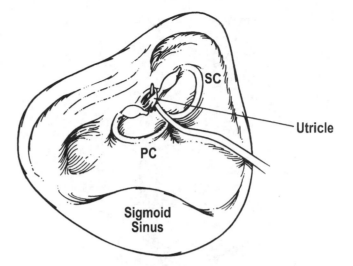

Figure 28–9. Surgical view of left temporal bone following transmastoid labyrinthectomy. Semicircular canals and vestibule are open. From Chapter 144, Surgery for vestibular disorders, by Steven A. Telian. In C. W. Cummings (Ed.), *Otolaryngology head and neck surgery*, 4th ed., p. 3301. Copyright 2005, Elsevier. Reproduced with permission.

reliable relief of vertigo (Kemink, Telian, Graham, & Joynt,1989; Schwaber, Pensak, & Reiber, 1995).

Vestibular Neurectomy

If a decision has been made to ablate vestibular function but hearing preservation is desired, a vestibular nerve section may be performed. This operation is more risky and slightly less reliable than labyrinthectomy procedures, but it does offer relief from episodic vertigo in the vast majority of cases. Reported rates of vertigo control range from 80% to 95%. The three most widely used approaches are the retrolabyrinthine approach, the retrosigmoid approach, and the middle fossa approach.

The retrolabyrinthine approach involves a complete mastoidectomy, with decompression of the posterior fossa dura and the sigmoid sinus. The bone anterior to the sinus is removed until the labyrinth is outlined and the endolymphatic sac is exposed. The dura and the endolymphatic sac are incised anterior to the sigmoid sinus, opening the cerebellopontine angle. The eighth nerve complex is identified and the vestibular portion of the eighth cranial nerve is divided, taking care to avoid injury to the facial nerve, the auditory fibers, or the nervus intermedius (Figure 28–10). The major disadvantage

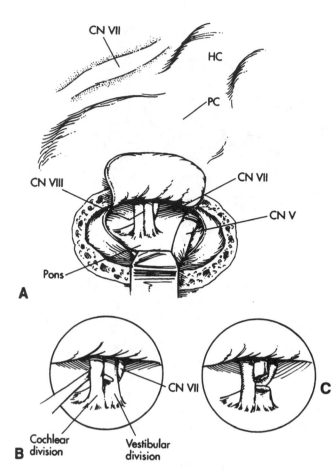

Figure 28-10. Left retrolabyrinthine vestibular nerve section. **A.** Depiction of the surgeon's view into the cerebellopontine angle through the craniotomy. **B.** Higher power magnification showing the separation of the cochlear and vestibular portions of the eighth cranial nerve. Under the same magnification, **C.** depicts the separation of the sectioned vestibular nerve. From Chapter 144, Surgery for vestibular disorders, by Steven A. Telian. In C. W. Cummings (Ed.), *Otolaryngology head and neck surgery*, 4th ed., p. 3305. Copyright 2005, Elsevier. Reproduced with permission.

of this approach is the uncertainty about the plane of dissection between the cochlear and vestibular nerve bundles. This may result in an incomplete transection of the vestibular nerve fibers or inadvertent sectioning of some fraction of the auditory fibers. This is a reliable approach with a low incidence of hearing loss and facial nerve injury (J. W. House, Hitselberger, McElveen, & Brackmann, 1984; Kemink & Hoff, 1986; Silverstein & Norrell, 1980).

The retrosigmoid approach may allow for more selective sectioning of the vestibular nerve than the retrolabyrinthine approach. Because this procedure involves less temporal bone dissection, thus improving the speed of the procedure, it is the preferred approach by many neurotologists today. However, patient positioning and the surgeon's proximity to the nerve are less favorable than with the retrolabyrinthine approach. There is also an increased need for retraction of the cerebellum. This operation is also known to produce a higher incidence of postoperative headaches, especially if intradural drilling is performed to achieve more lateral exposure of the eighth nerve within the internal auditory canal (Colletti, Camer, & Colletti, 2007; McKenna, Nadol, Ojemann, & Halpin, 1996; Silverstein, Norrell, & Smouha, 1987).

The middle fossa approach was popularized in the 1970s by Fisch and Glasscock (Fisch, 1974; Glasscock & Miller, 1977). It is the most technically demanding approach used for vestibular neurectomy. However, it permits the most definitive section of the vestibular fibers, in that the surgeon can specifically identify the superior and inferior vestibular nerves within the lateral portion of the internal auditory canal (Figure 28–11). In this location, the auditory fibers are clearly separated from the vestibular nerves. Unfortunately, this procedure places the cochlear blood supply at higher risk, and is known to carry the highest rate of injury to the facial nerve among conventional approaches to vestibular neurectomy, with temporary paresis rates as high as 33% (Gacek & Gacek, 1996; Garcia-Ibanez & Garcia-Ibanez, 1980).

Translabyrinthine vestibular neurectomy and transcochlear cochleovestibular neurectomy are two rarely employed approaches for vestibular nerve section that involve sacrifice of hearing (Jones, Silverstein, & Smouha, 1989; Pulec, 1968). Translabyrinthine vestibular neurectomy involves completing a transmastoid labyrinthectomy and then proceeding to transect the superior and inferior vestibular nerves medial to Scarpa's ganglion. The addition of a vestibular neurectomy should be unnecessary given the high success rates using transmastoid labyrinthectomy alone (Langman & Lindeman, 1993). Transcochlear cochleovestibular neurectomy extends a transcanal labyrinthectomy to open the cochlea and the distal end of the internal auditory canal. Ostensibly, this is performed to allow sectioning of the cochlear nerve along with the vestibular

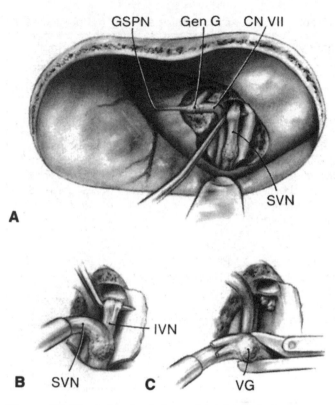

Figure 28–11. **A.** Surgical view of right middle fossa vestibular nerve section procedure. The brain is retracted medially. Note locations of facial nerve (CN VII) and superior vestibular nerve (SVN). **B.** Increased magnification of the lateral internal auditory canal. The SVN has been cut and is retracted anteriorly. The surgeon has isolated the inferior vestibular nerve (IVN) beneath the SVN. **C.** Shows the surgeon preparing to cut proximal to the vestibular ganglion (VG). *Gen G,* geniculate ganglion. From Chapter 144, Surgery for vestibular disorders, by Steven A. Telian. In C. W. Cummings, (Ed.), *Otolaryngology head and neck surgery,* 4th ed., p. 3304. Copyright 2005, Elsevier. Reproduced with permission.

nerve, in hopes of decreasing tinnitus. However, most reports of cochlear nerve section for tinnitus have shown a dismal success rate.

The overall complication rate for vestibular neurectomy is low, although facial nerve paralysis, hearing loss, meningitis, stroke, subdural hematoma, and wound infections have all been reported. Facial nerve paralysis is rare, especially when using the retrosigmoid or retrolabyrinthine approach. Hearing loss occurs following <10% of procedures. Most patients are capable of returning to normal activities approximately 2 to 4 months following the nerve section. The period of postoperative vestibular com-

pensation may be more prolonged than that which is encountered following labyrinthectomy (Gacek & Gacek, 1996). Each of the above-mentioned ablative procedures for the treatment of vertigo is summarized in Table 28–3.

Postoperative Course

Failures have been reported following ablative surgery. Reasons that symptoms persist after surgery may include an incorrect diagnosis, incomplete removal of the neuroepithelium during a labyrinthectomy, incomplete division of the vestibular fibers in vestibular neurectomy, or inadequate vestibular compensation. Late relapses following ablative surgery may result from central decompensation (Katsarkas & Segal, 1988). Whenever incomplete compensation or decompensation is a possibility, a trial of vestibular rehabilitation is appropriate before considering revision surgery.

Patient satisfaction with ablative procedures is variable because the process of vestibular compensation is also variable. Although some patients compensate fully following ablative surgery, up to 30% may be left with considerable chronic disequilibrium or motion-provoked vertigo. One study showed that even though most labyrinthectomy patients are relieved of vertigo, only 50% of them returned to work (Pereira & Kerr, 1996). But, vestibular neurectomy has been shown to cause a longer delay before returning to work (Gacek & Gacek, 1996). Eisenman compared long-term postoperative compensation measured 3 to 10 years after vestibular neurectomy or labyrinthectomy. There were no differences noted in self-assessment of balance abilities, functional balance performance, or hearing handicap (Eisenman et al., 2001). The majority in both groups showed physiologic evidence of incomplete compensation, even though all were free of episodic vertigo. Vestibular exercises should be prescribed for all patients who undergo vestibular ablation, and customized programs are appropriate for those who have poor initial progress or show evidence of incomplete vestibular compensation later in the postoperative course. Patients who are at particular risk for incomplete recovery include those with additional sensory deficits or central neurologic conditions, those taking sedating medications, and patients with poor psychological motivation for recovery.

Table 28–3. Ablative Procedures for Control of Vertigo

	Procedure	Hearing Result	Control of Vertigo	Advantages	Disadvantages	References
Labyrinthectomy (Procedures That Destroy Hearing)	Transcanal labyrinthectomy	Complete ipsilateral loss of hearing	86% (J. L. Pulec, 1974)	Less invasive, quicker operation	Threefold increase in postoperative disequilibrium in the elderly population in comparison to the transmastoid approach	Langman & Lindeman, 1998; Pulec, 1974
	Transmastoid labyrinthectomy	Complete ipsilateral loss of hearing	97%	*Most reliable ablative procedure;* Less postoperative imbalance than transcanal.	Hearing loss	Kemink, Telian, Graham, & Joynt, 1989
	Translabyrinthine vestibular neurectomy	Complete ipsilateral loss of hearing		Division of vestibular nerve medial to Scarpa's ganglion	Risk of CSF leak and meningitis	Pulec, 1968
	Transcochlear cochleovestibular neurectomy	Complete ipsilateral loss of hearing	89%	Small possibility of tinnitus relief	Risk of CSF leak and meningitis	Jones, Silverstein, & Smouha, 1989
Vestibular Nerve Section (Procedures That Preserve Hearing)	Retrolabyrinthine approach for vestibular neurectomy	86%–100% Hearing preservation	85%	Lower incidence of hearing loss and facial nerve injury; technically simpler than the MCF approach	The eighth cranial nerve is exposed only in the cerebellopontine angle where it is difficult to separate auditory nerve fibers from vestibular fibers; risk of CSF leak and meningitis	House et al., 1984; Kemink & Hoff, 1986
	Retrosigmoid approach for vestibular neurectomy	75% Hearing preservation	90%–100%	No temporal bone dissection is required to expose the eighth cranial nerve which improves the speed of the procedure	Poorer proximity to the nerve from the wound, increased retraction of the cerebellum, increase in postoperative headaches; risk of CSF leak and meningitis	Colletti et al., 2007; McKenna et al., 1996; Silverstein et al., 1987
	Middle cranial fossa approach for vestibular neurectomy	76%–83% Hearing preservation	94%–99%	Permits the most definitive sectioning of the vestibular nerve fibers	Technically demanding, highest rate of injury to the facial nerve, endangers the cochlear blood supply; risk of CSF leak and meningitis	Fisch, 1974; Garcia-Ibanez & Garcia-Ibanez, 1980; Glasscock & Miller, 1977

REFERENCES

Adams, M. E., Kileny, P. R., Telian, S. A., El-Kashlan, H. K., Heidenreich, K. D., Mannarelli, G. R., & Arts, H. A. (2011). Electrocochleography as a diagnostic and intraoperative adjunct in superior semicircular canal dehiscence. *Otology and Neurotology, 32*, 1506–1512.

Arenberg, I. K., Zoller, S. A., & Van de Water, S. M. (1983). The results of the first 300 consecutive endolymphatic system-mastoid shunts with valve implants for hydrops. *Otolaryngology Clinics of North America, 16*(1), 153–174.

Benecke, J. E. (1994). Surgery for non-Meniere's vertigo. *Acta Oto-Laryngologica Supplementum, 513*, 37–39.

Beyea, J. A., Agrawal, S. K., & Parnes, L. S. (2012). Transmastoid semicircular canal occlusion: A safe and highly effective treatment for BPPV and SSCD. *Laryngoscope, 122*, 1862–1866.

Bretlau, P., Thomsen, J., Tos, M., & Johnsen, N. J. (1989). Placebo effect in surgery for Meniere's disease: Nine-year follow-up. *American Journal of Otology, 10*(4), 259–261.

Colletti, V., Carner, M., & Colletti, L. (2007). Auditory results after vestibular nerve section and intratympanic gentamicin for Meniere's disease. *Otology and Neurotology, 28*(2), 145–151.

Convert, C., Franco-Vidal, V., Bebear, J. P., & Darrouzet, V. (2006). Outcome-based assessment of endolymphatic sac decompression for Meniere's disease using the Meniere's disease outcome questionnaire: A review of 90 patients. *Otology and Neurotology, 27*(5), 687–696.

Disher, M. J., Telian, S. A., & Kemink, J. L. (1991). Evaluation of acute vertigo: Unusual lesions imitating vestibular neuritis. *American Journal of Otology, 12*(3), 227–231.

Eisenman, D. J., Speers, R., & Telian, S. A. (2001). Labyrinthectomy versus vestibular neurectomy: Long-term physiologic and clinical outcomes. *Otology and Neurotology, 22*(4), 539–548.

Epley, J. M. (2001). Human experience with canalith repositioning maneuvers. *Annals of the New York Academy of Sciences, 942*, 179–191.

Fisch, U. (1974). Vestibular and cochlear neurectomy. *Transactions of the American Academy of Ophthalmology and Otolaryngology, 78*(4), 252–255.

Gacek, R. R., & Gacek, M. R. (1994). Singular neurectomy in the management of paroxysmal positional vertigo. *Otolaryngologic Clinics of North America, 27*(2), 363–379.

Gacek, R. R., & Gacek, M. R. (1996). Comparison of labyrinthectomy and vestibular neurectomy in the control of vertigo. *Laryngoscope, 106*(2, Pt. 1), 225–230.

Garcia-Ibanez, E., & Garcia-Ibanez, J. L. (1980). Middle fossa vestibular neurectomy: A report of 373 cases. *Otolaryngology-Head and Neck Surgery, 88*(4), 486–490.

Gates, G. A. (1999). Innovar treatment for Meniere's disease. *Acta Oto-laryngologica, 119*(2), 189–193.

Gianoli, G. J., Larouere, M. J., Kartush, J. M., & Wayman, J. (1998). Sac-vein decompression for intractable Meniere's disease: Two-year treatment results. *Otolaryngology-Head and Neck Surgery, 118*(1), 22–29.

Glasscock, M. E., 3rd, & Miller, G. W. (1977). Middle fossa vestibular nerve section in the management of Meniere's disease. *Laryngoscope, 87*(4, Pt. 1), 529–541.

Goodhill, V. (1981). Ben H. Senturia lecture. Leaking labyrinth lesions, deafness, tinnitus and dizziness. *Annals of Otology, Rhinology, and Laryngology, 90*(2, Pt. 1), 99–106.

Graham, M. D., & Kemink, J. L. (1984). Surgical management of Meniere's disease with endolymphatic sac decompression by wide bony decompression of the posterior fossa dura: Technique and results. *Laryngoscope, 94*(5 Pt. 1), 680–683.

Hillman, T. A., Kertesz, T. R., Hadley, K., & Shelton, C. (2006). Reversible peripheral vestibulopathy: The treatment of superior canal dehiscence. *Otolaryngology-Head and Neck Surgery, 134*(3), 431–436.

House, J. W., Hitselberger, W. E., McElveen, J., & Brackmann, D. E. (1984). Retrolabyrinthine section of the vestibular nerve. *Otolaryngology-Head and Neck Surgery, 92*(2), 212–215.

House, W. F. (1965). Subarachnoid shunt for drainage of hydrops. A report of 146 cases. *Laryngoscope, 75*(10), 1547–1551.

Jones, R., Silverstein, H., & Smouha, E. (1989). Long-term results of transmeatal cochleovestibular neurectomy: An analysis of 100 cases. *Otolaryngology-Head and Neck Surgery, 100*(1), 22–29.

Katsarkas, A., & Segal, B. N. (1988). Unilateral loss of peripheral vestibular function in patients: Degree of compensation and factors causing decompensation. *Otolaryngology-Head and Neck Surgery, 98*(1), 45–47.

Kemink, J. L., & Hoff, J. T. (1986). Retrolabyrinthine vestibular nerve section: Analysis of results. *Laryngoscope, 96*(1), 33–36.

Kemink, J. L., Telian, S. A., El-Kashlan, H. K., & Langman, A. W. (1991). Retrolabyrinthine vestibular nerve section: Efficacy in disorders other than Meniere's disease. *Laryngoscope, 101*(5), 523–528.

Kemink, J. L., Telian, S. A., Graham, M. D., & Joynt, L. (1989). Transmastoid labyrinthectomy: Reliable surgical management of vertigo. *Otolaryngology-Head and Neck Surgery, 101*(1), 5–10.

Kinney, W. C., Nalepa, N., Hughes, G. B., & Kinney, S. E. (1995). Cochleosacculotomy for the treatment of Meniere's disease in the elderly patient. *Laryngoscope, 105*(9, Pt. 1), 934–937.

Kos, M. I., Feigl, G., Anderhuber, F., Wall, C., Fasel, J. H.,& Guyot, J. P. (2006). Transcanal approach to the singular nerve. *Otology and Neurotology, 27*(4), 542–546.

Langman, A. W., & Lindeman, R. C. (1993). Surgery for vertigo in the nonserviceable hearing ear: Transmastoid labyrinthectomy or translabyrinthine vestibular nerve section. *Laryngoscope, 103*(12), 1321–1325.

Langman, A. W., & Lindeman, R. C. (1998). Surgical labyrinthectomy in the older patient. *Otolaryngology-Head and Neck Surgery, 118*(6), 739–742.

Leuwer, R. M., & Westhofen, M. (1996). Surgical anatomy of the singular nerve. *Acta Oto-Laryngologica, 116*(4), 576–580.

Levenson, M. J., Desloge, R. B., & Parisier, S. C. (1996). Beta-2 transferrin: Limitations of use as a clinical marker for perilymph. *Laryngoscope, 106*(2, Pt. 1), 159–161.

Limb, C. J., Carey, J. P., Srireddy, S., & Minor, L. B. (2006). Auditory function in patients with surgically treated superior semicircular canal dehiscence. *Otology and Neurotology, 27*(7), 969–980.

McCabe, B. F., & Ryu, J. H. (1979). Vestibular physiology in understanding the dizzy patient. *Continuing education manual; American Academy of Otolaryngology.* Alexandria, VA: American Academy of Otolaryngology.

McKenna, M. J., Nadol, J. B., Jr., Ojemann, R. G., & Halpin, C. (1996). Vestibular neurectomy: Retrosigmoid-intracanalicular versus retrolabyrinthine approach. *American Journal of Otology, 17*(2), 253–258.

Minor, L. B. (2005). Clinical manifestations of superior semicircular canal dehiscence. *Laryngoscope, 115*(10), 1717–1727.

Parnes, L. S., & McClure, J. A. (1991). Posterior semicircular canal occlusion in the normal hearing ear. *Otolaryngology-Head and Neck Surgery, 104*(1), 52–57.

Pereira, K. D., & Kerr, A. G. (1996). Disability after labyrinthectomy. *Journal of Laryngology and Otology, 110*(3), 216–218.

Portmann, G. (1927). Vertigo: Surgical treatment by opening of the saccus endolymphaticus. *Archives of Otolaryngology, 6,* 301–319.

Pulec, J. L. (1968). Translabyrinthine section of the VIIIth cranial nerve in Meniere's disease. In J. Pulec (Ed.), *Meniere's disease.* Philadelphia, PA: W. B. Saunders.

Pulec, J. L. (1974). Labyrinthectomy: Indications, technique and results. *Laryngoscope, 84*(9), 1552–1573.

Schuknecht, H. F. (1991a). Cochleosacculotomy for Meniere's disease: Internal endolymphatic shunt. *Operative Techniques in Otolaryngology-Head and Neck Surgery, 2,* 35.

Schuknecht, H. F. (1991b). Transcanal labyrinthectomy. *Operative Techniques in Otolaryngology-Head and Neck Surgery, 2,* 17.

Schuknecht, H. F. (1993). Disorders of unknown causes: A. Endolymphatic hydrops. In H. F. Schuknecht (Ed.), *Pathology of the ear* (2nd ed., pp. 499–524). Philadelphia, PA: Lea & Febiger.

Schuknecht, H. F., & Bartley, M. (1985). Cochlear endolymphatic shunt for Meniere's disease. *American Journal of Otology, Nov*(Suppl.), 20–22.

Schwaber, M. K., Pensak, M. L., & Reiber, M. E. (1995). Transmastoid labyrinthectomy in older patients. *Laryngoscope, 105*(11), 1152–1154.

Shaia, W. T., Zappia, J. J., Bojrab, D. I., LaRouere, M. L., Sargent, E. W., & Diaz, R. C. (2006). Success of posterior semicircular canal occlusion and application of the dizziness handicap inventory. *Otolaryngology-Head and Neck Surgery, 134*(3), 424–430.

Shambaugh, G. E., Jr. (1975). Effect of endolymphatic sac decompression on fluctuant hearing loss. *Otolaryngological Clinics of North America, 8*(2), 537–540.

Shea, J. J. (1966). Teflon film drainage of the endolymphatic sac. *Archives of Otolaryngology-Head and Neck Surgery, 83*(4), 316–319.

Shea, J. J. (1992). The myth of spontaneous perilymph fistula. *Otolaryngology-Head and Neck Surgery, 107*(5), 613–616.

Shepard, N. T., Telian, S. A., Niparko, J. K., Kemink, J. L., & Fujita, S. (1992). Platform pressure test in identification of perilymphatic fistula. *American Journal of Otology, 13*(1), 49–54.

Shone, G., Kemink, J. L., & Telian, S. A. (1991). Prognostic significance of hearing loss as a lateralizing indicator in the surgical treatment of vertigo. *Journal of Laryngology and Otology, 105*(8), 618–620.

Silverstein, H., & Norrell, H. (1980). Retrolabyrinthine surgery: A direct approach to the cerebellopontine angle. *Otolaryngology-Head and Neck Surgery, 88*(4), 462–469.

Silverstein, H., Norrell, H., & Smouha, E. E. (1987). Retrosigmoid-internal auditory canal approach vs. retrolabyrinthine approach for vestibular neurectomy. *Otolaryngology-Head and Neck Surgery, 97*(3), 300–307.

Skedros, D. G., Cass, S. P., Hirsch, B. E., & Kelly, R. H. (1993). Sources of error in use of beta-2 transferrin analysis for diagnosing perilymphatic and cerebral spinal fluid leaks. *Otolaryngology-Head and Neck Surgery, 109*(5), 861–864.

Telian, S. A. (2010). Surgery for vestibular disorders. *Cummings otolaryngology head and neck surgery* (5th ed., Vol. 3, pp. 2359–2371). Philadelphia, PA: Elsevier.

Tewary, A. K., Riley, N., & Kerr, A. G. (1998). Long-term results of vestibular nerve section. *Journal of Laryngology and Otology, 112*(12), 1150–1153.

Thomsen, J., Bonding, P., Becker, B., Stage, J., & Tos, M. (1998). The non-specific effect of endolymphatic sac surgery in treatment of Meniere's disease: A prospective, randomized controlled study comparing "classic" endolymphatic sac surgery with the insertion of a ventilating tube in the tympanic membrane. *Acta Oto-Laryngologica, 118*(6), 769–773.

Ward, B. K., Agrawal, Y., Nguyen, E., Della Santina, C. C., Limb, C. J., Francis, H. W., . . . Carey, J. P. (2012). Hearing outcomes after plugging of the superior semicircular canal by a middle crania fossa approach. *Otology and Neurotology, 33,* 1386–1391.

Welling, D. B., & Nagaraja, H. N. (2000). Endolymphatic mastoid shunt: A re-evaluation of efficacy. *Otolaryngology-Head and Neck Surgery, 122*(3), 340–345.

Welling, D. B., Parnes, L. S., O'Brien, B., Bakaletz, L. O., Brackmann, D. E., & Hinojosa, R. (1997). Particulate matter in the posterior semicircular canal. *Laryngoscope, 107*(1), 90–94.

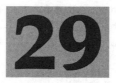

Neurologic Origins of Dizziness and Vertigo

Joseph M. Furman and Susan L. Whitney

INTRODUCTION

Dizziness and vertigo can be caused by both peripheral (i.e., inner ear) and central (i.e., neurological) vestibular abnormalities. In some patients there is involvement of both central and peripheral vestibular structures. It is important clinically to distinguish among these localizations in order to make an accurate diagnosis and develop an efficacious treatment plan. Arriving at a correct localization and etiologic diagnosis depends upon obtaining an accurate history, performing an appropriate physical examination, and obtaining relevant laboratory testing and imaging. In some patients, successful treatment can provide additional information regarding the accuracy of diagnosis.

Differentiating between peripheral and central vestibular disorders can be challenging without sophisticated laboratory testing and imaging. However, there are several clinical clues that can be used to make this distinction. In general, because unilateral peripheral vestibular abnormalities and central vestibular abnormalities lead to dizziness and possibly vertigo, distinguishing between central and peripheral vestibular abnormalities usually requires the recognition of other signs and symptoms referable to either the inner ear or the central nervous system. Table 29–1 indicates clinical features that can aid in determining whether or not the patient has a peripheral or central abnormality. Nausea and vomiting are typically severe in peripheral vestibular disorders and less common and less severe in central disorders. Imbalance is typically mild in peripheral vestibular abnormalities, whereas imbalance is usually severe in central disorders. In the emergency department environment, the ability of the patient to ambulate can be extremely helpful in enabling the clinician to ascribe the patient symptoms to a peripheral cause. As expected, hearing loss is much more common in peripheral vestibular abnormalities as compared to central vestibular abnormalities.

Table 29–1. Differentiation Between Peripheral (End Organ and Nerve) and Central Causes of Vertigo

	Nausea and Vomiting	Imbalance	Hearing Loss	Oscillopsia	Neurologic Symptoms	Compensation
Peripheral	Severe	Mild	Common	Mild	Rare	Rapid
Central	Moderate	Severe	Rare	Severe	Common	Slow

A notable exception is the anterior inferior artery syndrome, which is typically associated with unilateral hearing impairment. Oscillopsia (i.e., jumbling of the visual surround) is most commonly seen in bilateral vestibular loss. Oscillopsia can also be seen in central disorders and less likely in unilateral peripheral vestibular disorders. As noted earlier, neurologic symptoms, for example, diplopia, facial numbness or weakness, dysarthria, or dysphagia, are more commonly seen with central abnormalities. Patients with peripheral vestibular abnormalities may complain of blurred vision likely resulting from vestibular nystagmus. Central nervous system compensation for a unilateral peripheral vestibular abnormality usually leads to a reduction of signs and symptoms of vestibulopathy. Compensation is usually slower in patients with neurologic abnormalities that are either a cause of their dizziness and disequilibrium or are present in addition to a peripheral vestibular abnormality.

Vestibular compensation is a jargon term that refers to the ability of the central nervous system to use information from a single functional labyrinth to overcome the loss of sensory information from an impaired labyrinth. Acutely following a unilateral peripheral vestibular deficit, patients develop nystagmus secondary to involvement of the vestibulo-ocular system, postural instability secondary to involvement of the vestibulo-spinal system, spatial disorientation secondary to involvement of the vestibular projections to the cerebrum, and nausea and vomiting secondary to involvement of the vestibulo-autonomic system. In some patients, vestibular compensation does not progress normally. These patients often come to the attention of their doctors because of prolonged symptoms. When encountering a patient with delayed or impaired compensation, it is appropriate to consider several possibilities. These are rated in Table 29–2. In patients with fluctuating vestibular function, such as patients with a stuttering course of vestibular neuritis or in patients with endolymphatic hydrops, the central nervous system is challenged by encountering different vestibular function at different times. The central nervous system for these patients has difficulty compensating because of variability in vestibular function. Abnormal peripheral vestibular function rather than loss of peripheral vestibular function may provide the central nervous system with a vestibular signal that cannot be interpreted. In this case, there may be dif-

Table 29–2. Failure to Compensate

Fluctuating vestibular function
Abnormal peripheral vestibular input
Central nervous system abnormality
Sedentary lifestyle
Multisensory loss
Somatosensory disorders
Visual disorders
Cervical or spine disorders
Medication
Immobility
Aging

ficulty ignoring the abnormal peripheral vestibular signals. This may impair compensation. Abnormalities of the central nervous system such as vascular disease, neurodegenerative disease, and demyelinating disease may impair the ability of the central nervous system to undergo the compensation process, which involves rebalancing vestibular nucleus activity and altering sensory integration, which are complex neural processes. Another factor that can interfere with compensation is a lack of physical activity by the patient, which is necessarily associated with diminished coordinated sensorimotor activity. A lack of physical activity can be a result of a sedentary lifestyle or a physical ailment, for example, a musculoskeletal abnormality of the hips or knees. Presumably, adequate sensory input is required for the central nervous system to accomplish the compensation process. Thus, comparable to inadequate motor activity, sensory loss such as that seen with peripheral neuropathy, or visual abnormalities can impair compensation. Multisensory loss such as that seen in patients with diabetes secondary to combined peripheral neuropathy and retinopathy, can be especially problematic. Of particular recent interest, fall risk can increase with progressive corrective lenses in older persons (Lord, Dayhew, & Howland, 2002). Cervical and spinal vertebral abnormalities can adversely affect compensation. The reason for this interference with compensation is uncertain. Medications, especially vestibular suppressant medications, are notorious for their ability to interfere with the compensation process. Common medications such as meclizine should be discontinued or limited as much as possible in patients who have evidence for impaired compensation.

For older patients who manifest inadequate compensation, age alone can be a negative factor in the compensation process. However, prior to ascribing impaired compensation to advanced age, all other factors should be considered as advanced age alone generally does not lead to an inability to compensate centrally for a peripheral vestibular deficit.

MAJOR DIAGNOSTIC CATEGORIES

Neurologic causes of dizziness and vertigo can be categorized based upon etiology and pathophysiology. Table 29–3 lists eight disease categories that are discussed individually and several of which are highlighted by case vignettes. Vestibular migraine is clearly the most common of these disorders even though until recently a diagnosis of vestibular migraine was relatively unknown or dismissed as a diagnostic entity. Concussion as a cause of dizziness and vertigo has recently received much attention largely as a result of professional sports, although actually, sport concussion is largely a condition seen in school-age children and young adults.

Vestibular Migraine

Vestibular migraine is a now widely recognized condition thought to occur in approximately 1% of the population with a female-to-male predominance

Table 29–3. Major Diagnostic Categories

Vestibular migraine
Cerebrovascular disease
Head trauma
Neurodegenerative disease
Chiari malformation
Acoustic neuroma (vestibular schwannoma)
Demyelinating disease
Mal de Debarquement syndrome

of about 5:1 (Furman, Marcus, & Balaban, 2013). Historically, vestibular migraine had been called migraine-related dizziness, migraine-associated dizziness, migraine-vestibulopathy, and migrainous vertigo. Vestibular migraine should be considered a migraine equivalent. That is, vestibular migraine is a migrainous disorder that may cause neurologic symptoms other than headache. Benign recurrent vertigo of childhood, which has been recognized for many years, is likely a childhood form of vestibular migraine (Basser, 1964). A related condition, basilar-type migraine, which is a migrainous disorder associated with loss of consciousness, is being phased out of the International Headache Society nomenclature. The recognition of vestibular migraine as a distinct clinical entity began with a landmark study by Kayan and Hood (1984) with the recognition that patients with migraine headache were much more likely to complain of vestibular symptoms than patients with tension headache. Current diagnostic practice for vestibular migraine dates to 2001 when Neuhauser, Leopold, von Brevern, Arnold, and Lempert published a study of 200 patients with dizziness 38% of whom had migraine. The most recent diagnostic criteria, largely based on the original Neuhauser et al. criteria, have been developed by a working group of the Bárány Society (Lempert et al., 2012). These criteria are illustrated in Figure 29–1. The key features of these diagnostic criteria include a diagnosis of migraine, a currently active migrainous disorder, episodic vertigo or imbalance, and a temporal association between vestibular symptoms and migrainous symptoms. These criteria should be considered specific rather than sensitive. That is, if a patient meets the criteria, the patient is highly likely to be suffering from vestibular migraine, whereas if a patient does not meet these criteria, the patient may actually be suffering from this disorder. Also, dizziness may not be clearly temporarily associated with migraine headache or other migrainous phenomena. The mean age of onset of vestibular migraine is about 38 years for women and 42 years for men. Overall, migraine headache predates the onset of dizziness by about 8 years. Symptoms of vestibular migraine are quite varied and can include all types of dizziness such as light-headedness, swimming sensation, a rocking or swimming sensation, and motion sickness. Vestibular migraine usually occurs in attacks that can last for seconds, minutes, or hours. In some patients, symptoms can

Flow chart for the Diagnosis of Vestibular Migraine

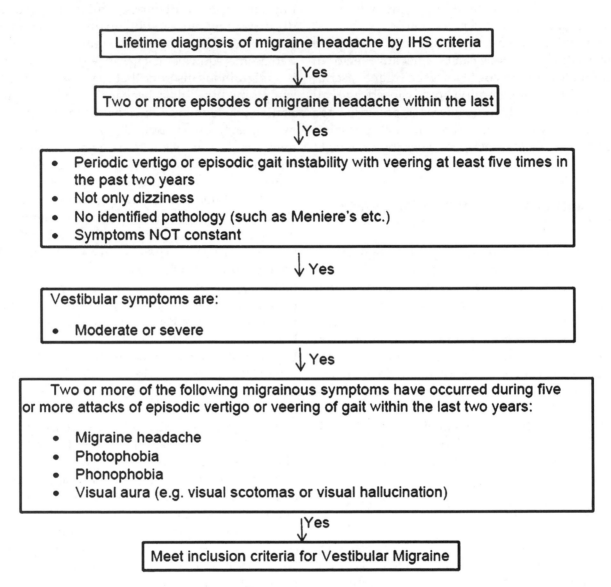

Figure 29–1. Flow chart for the diagnosis of vestibular migraine.

last for days or be nearly constant. Physical examination is usually normal except during an acute vestibular migraine attack at which time nystagmus can be seen indicative of either a peripheral vestibular abnormality, a central vestibular abnormality, or a combined central and peripheral vestibular abnormality (von Brevern, Zeise, Neuhauser, Clarke, & Lempert, 2005). Vestibular laboratory testing in vestibular migraine may be normal but often includes a directional preponderance on rotational testing.

Other abnormalities include a unilateral peripheral vestibular reduction based on either caloric testing or vestibular-evoked myogenic potentials in about one-fourth of the patients. The pathophysiology of vestibular migraine is uncertain but has recently been discussed in an article by Furman et al. (2013) and is illustrated in Figure 29–2. The treatment for vestibular migraine is similar to the treatment for migraine headache and should always begin with the identification of triggers, especially food triggers.

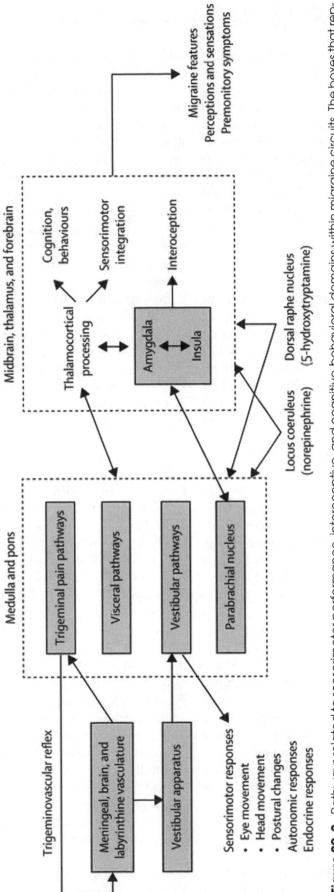
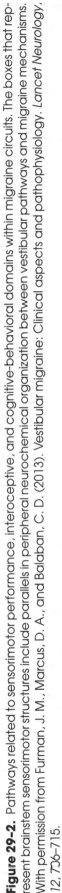

Figure 29–2. Pathways related to sensorimotor performance, interoceptive, and cognitive-behavioral domains within migraine circuits. The boxes that represent brainstem sensorimotor structures include parallels in peripheral neurochemical organization between vestibular pathways and migraine mechanisms. With permission from Furman, J. M., Marcus, D. A., and Balaban, C. D. (2013). Vestibular migraine: Clinical aspects and pathophysiology. *Lancet Neurology, 12,* 706–715.

Otherwise, as for migraine headache, treatment options can be categorized into preventative, abortive, and symptomatic. Preventative pharmacotherapy for vestibular migraine is similar to that for migraine headache. Few studies have addressed abortive treatments, but triptans are a therapeutic option. Symptomatic treatments include vestibular suppressant medications and antinausea agents. Also, vestibular rehabilitation should be considered for patients with vestibular migraine who manifest ongoing vestibulo-ocular or postural abnormalities.

Case Vignette 1

A 48-year-old woman presented with a complaint of dizziness that had been worsening for the past 6 months. The patient had a history of migraine headache as a teenager and as a young adult but headache had largely resolved following the birth of her second child in her early 30s. The patient had not had a migraine headache for several years. The patient's dizziness was characterized by a sense of light-headedness and disequilibrium in association with photophobia and phonophobia and nausea without headache. When questioned, the patient related that aside from the absence of headache and the presence of dizziness, the patient's associated symptoms were comparable to those experienced with migraine headache. Physical examination was normal. Vestibular laboratory testing revealed a borderline abnormal caloric reduction and a directional preponderance on rotational testing. Magnetic resonance imaging (MRI) of the brain, which had been ordered by the patient's primary care physician, revealed mild periventricular white matter changes consistent with either microvascular disease or migraine. A diagnosis of vestibular migraine was reached and the patient was advised to decrease her dietary intake of foods that might be provoking migraine and prescribed a vestibular suppressant medication to be used on an as-needed basis. A follow-up appointment was scheduled at which time migraine prophylaxis treatment would be considered.

Cerebrovascular Disease

Infrequently, cerebrovascular disease can involve the posterior fossa and lead to dizziness or vertigo as a result of ischemia of central vestibular structures with or without involvement of peripheral vestibular structures. The vascular supply of the posterior fossa includes the vertebral arteries combining to form the basilar artery and then branching into the posterior cerebral arteries. Major arteries in the posterior fossa also include the posterior inferior cerebellar arteries, which arise from the vertebral arteries, the anterior inferior cerebellar artery which arises from the basilar artery and gives rise to the internal auditory artery, and the superior cerebellar artery. Also, multiple perforating arteries arise from the vertebral and basilar arteries to supply the brainstem. The blood supply to the labyrinth and cochlea arises from the anterior inferior cerebellar artery and includes the common cochlear artery and the vestibular artery. The blood supply to the vestibular labyrinth is considered end-arterial (i.e., without collateral circulation). Historically, a diagnosis of vertebrobasilar insufficiency was commonly given to patients who had episodic signs and symptoms referable to the brainstem. However, vertebrobasilar insufficiency is not a common diagnosis at this time since noninvasive angiography has led to the recognition that few patients actually have significant posterior fossa arterial disease. The two most common posterior fossa ischemic conditions include the posterior inferior cerebellar artery syndrome, commonly known as Wallenberg syndrome, and the anterior inferior cerebellar artery syndrome. Both of these vascular syndromes include vestibular symptoms. The posterior inferior cerebellar artery syndrome is also known as the lateral medullary syndrome because of the location of the infarction. Involvement of the vestibular nuclei leads to dizziness, vertigo, and disequilibrium. Other signs and symptoms of the lateral medullary syndrome often include saccadic lateropulsion, asymmetrically impaired ocular pursuit, spontaneous vestibular nystagmus, gaze-evoked nystagmus when looking toward the side of the lesion, diminished facial sensation, ipsilateral limb dysmetria, a dissociated sensory loss contralateral to the lesion, and gait instability. The diagnosis of lateral medullary infarction is confirmed by MRI. The anterior inferior cerebellar artery syndrome also leads to dizziness, vertigo, facial numbness, disequilibrium, and incoordination but in addition can lead to tinnitus, hearing loss, and facial weakness as a result of damage to the labyrinth and seventh and eighth cranial nerves. The management of posterior fossa ischemia and infarction is beyond the scope of this chapter but is comparable to management of strokes elsewhere in the central nervous system.

The rotational vertebral artery syndrome, though quite rare, is worth mentioning because of its propensity to cause dizziness and vertigo. The condition results from a combination of a dominant vertebral artery and structural anatomy that causes the dominant vertebral artery to become compressed with head turning. The diagnosis of this condition is confirmed only with conventional angiography wherein vascular compromise is seen with the head turned. Endovascular or surgical treatment may be indicated.

Head Trauma

Head trauma can cause dizziness and vertigo. The pathophysiology for traumatic dizziness and vertigo includes damage to the central nervous system, vestibular labyrinth, the neck, or some combination thereof. Mild traumatic brain injury, also known as concussion, can involve structures important for dizziness, vertigo, and disequilibrium such as the brainstem and cerebellum. The precise mechanism for brain concussion is unknown but may include a cascade of metabolic and neurochemical changes that lead to abnormal brain function. The symptoms of concussion can include impaired cognition, somatic symptoms such as dizziness and vertigo, mood and behavioral alterations, and abnormalities of sleep. Head trauma also can damage inner ear structures via labyrinthine or cochlear concussion. The precise mechanism of labyrinthine concussion is uncertain but may include other supporting cells or hair cells leading to labyrinthine dysfunction. The role of the neck in traumatic head injury is uncertain. However, proprioceptors from the neck are clearly important for normal balance and spatial orientation. Thus, when evaluating a patient suffering from dizziness or vertigo in association with concussion, it is essential to consider all three localizations including the central nervous system, the labyrinth, and the neck. Physical examination is often normal although some patients with dizziness or vertigo following head trauma may manifest typical benign paroxysmal positional nystagmus and vertigo. Vestibular laboratory testing and audiometry can be particularly helpful in identifying an inner ear component. Diagnosing a cervicogenic component may be challenging and often relies on the patient's history of

worsening of dizziness in association with exacerbation of neck pain. Management of patients with concussion generally requires the combined resources of neuropsychologists, physiatrists, neurologists, and physical therapists. Appropriate treatment depends on the localization of the patient's abnormalities.

Case Vignette 2

A 50-year-old male was seen for a complaint of dizziness following a motor vehicle accident. The patient was involved in a rear-end collision in which his vehicle was struck from behind. The patient was not wearing a seat belt and struck his head against the steering wheel. It is uncertain whether he had a loss of consciousness. The patient believes that he suffered from a whiplash, flexion-extension neck injury. The patient was prescribed meclizine but continued to experience dizziness and neck pain. Despite physical therapy for neck discomfort, the patient's symptoms persisted. The patient's physical examination revealed that head thrust testing could not be performed because of limited range of motion at the neck. Examination was otherwise normal. Dix-Hallpike maneuvers were negative. Vestibular laboratory testing revealed a low-amplitude left-beating spontaneous vestibular nystagmus, no positional nystagmus, and an absent response to bithermal caloric stimulation of the right ear with a minimal response to ice water irrigation of the right ear. Rotational testing showed a moderately severe left directional preponderance. Platform posturography indicated excessive sway on SOT conditions 5 and 6. A CT scan of the head performed on the day of the patient's motor vehicle accident was negative. The patient's most likely diagnosis was thought to be a right peripheral vestibulopathy based on labyrinthine concussion in combination with cervicogenic dizziness. The patient was treated with a combination of vestibular rehabilitation therapy and very low dose diazepam on an as-needed basis. Meclizine was discontinued. Physical therapy for the patient's neck discomfort was continued.

Neurodegenerative Disease

Neurodegenerative disorders can present with dizziness and disequilibrium. This group of diseases is quite diverse. Disorders such as cerebellar degeneration and progressive supranuclear palsy primarily involve the balance system. Alzheimer's disease and other dementias and Parkinson's disease and their variants can also present with dizziness and disequilibrium. Cerebellar degeneration, often called spinocerebellar atrophy, spinocerebellar degeneration, or spinocerebellar ataxia, can involve solely the cerebellum or can involve both the cerebellum and brainstem. The cerebellar degeneration syndromes are now categorized based on the genetic abnormalities underlying these disorders. More than 30 different types of spinocerebellar ataxia have been identified. However, despite genetic differences, there is much phenotypic overlap. Also, there are numerous sporadic forms of spinocerebellar ataxia that have not been categorized genetically. There is a large degree of phenotypic variability among these disorders in terms of age of onset, rate of progression, severity, the presence of episodic features, and the presence of dizziness. Physical examination always includes ataxia and may include various degrees of ocular motor abnormalities including abnormal saccadic function especially saccadic dysmetria. A family history of ataxia suggests a diagnosis of familial spinocerebellar ataxia, but only about two-thirds of patients with spinocerebellar ataxia can establish a diagnosis using genetic analysis. Vestibular findings in spinocerebellar ataxia usually include ocular motor abnormalities with preservation of peripheral vestibular function. Visual-vestibular interaction testing is generally abnormal. In some forms of spinocerebellar ataxia, there may be peripheral vestibular reduction, for example, in Friedreich's ataxia. There is no specific treatment for spinocerebellar ataxia.

Progressive supranuclear palsy is a degenerative disorder sometimes confused with Parkinson's disease. The hallmark feature of progressive supranuclear palsy is a limitation of volitional vertical gaze, particularly downward gaze with preservation of reflexive vertical eye movement. Patients are usually in their 50s and present with gait instability and falls. Physical examination reveals extrapyramidal findings such as increased tone and bradykinesia. Other clinical features include impaired cognition and square wave jerks. Vestibular laboratory testing is usually not necessary to make a diagnosis and, because of abnormal eye movements, caloric testing may be abnormal artifactually. Treatment with antiparkinsonian agents is generally not helpful.

Another condition to be considered in a discussion of neurodegenerative disorders is orthostatic tremor, a disorder of uncertain etiology presumed related to action tremors. Patients with orthostatic tremor often complain of a sense of imbalance when standing rather than when walking. Physical examination reveals a palpable lower extremity tremor that usually does not develop until the patient has been standing for more than 1 or 2 min and worsens with prolonged standing. Vestibular testing is normal in orthostatic tremor. Treatment with gabapentin may be helpful.

Chiari Malformation

Chiari malformation refers to a malformation of the brain in which cerebellar tissue extends below the foramen magnum. A related malformation, named the Arnold-Chiari malformation, has an associated syrinx of the spinal cord. Patients with Chiari malformation often present with dizziness and disequilibrium. Physical examination usually reveals down-beating nystagmus, which may be seen only with oblique lateral-down gaze. Although down-beat nystagmus may be seen with other abnormalities of the craniocervical junction, Chiari malformation is the most common. Other ocular motor abnormalities seen with Chiari malformation include gaze-evoked nystagmus and abnormal ocular pursuit. Vestibular laboratory testing is generally not required for establishing a diagnosis. MRI of the brain with sagittal images is essential for confirming a diagnosis of Chiari malformation. Treatment options for Chiari malformation include a suboccipital craniectomy and decompression.

Case Vignette 3

An 18-year-old woman complained of nearly constant dizziness and imbalance that had been present for several years and seemed to be getting gradually worse. The patient did not complain of vertigo but noted that certain head positions, particularly looking up, increased a sense of disequilibrium. Physical examination revealed gaze-evoked nystagmus and down-beating nystagmus on oblique down-lateral gaze. Gait was normal and Romberg was negative but the patient had difficulty standing on a compliant foam pad with eyes closed. MRI of the brain revealed that the cerebellar tonsils extended into the spinal canal by approximately 6 mm. A diagnosis of Chiari malformation was made and a neurosurgical opinion was sought.

Acoustic Neuroma (Vestibular Schwannoma)

Acoustic neuroma, which is actually a schwannoma usually on the vestibular rather than the auditory portion of the eighth cranial nerve, infrequently presents with dizziness. However, some patients with acoustic neuroma may present with disequilibrium or mild disorientation. The typical presenting symptoms acoustic neuroma are unilateral hearing loss and tinnitus. Physical examination is usually normal with the exception of a unilateral hearing loss unless the patient has a large cerebellar pontine angle tumor. With large cerebellar pontine angle tumors, there may be distortion of the brainstem and cerebellum leading to nystagmus and vestibular findings. In particular, Brun's nystagmus may be seen, which is a combination of a gaze-evoked nystagmus when looking toward the side of the lesion and a vestibular nystagmus when looking contralateral to the side of the lesion. Additionally, gait instability and a positive Romberg may be seen. Laboratory testing usually indicates a unilateral sensorineural hearing loss often with impaired word recognition. Vestibular laboratory testing generally reveals a unilateral vestibular reduction and may additionally show a directional preponderance. A diagnosis of acoustic neuromas is established via MRI. Treatment options for acoustic neuroma include watchful waiting, resection, and radiation. The appropriate choice of therapy depends on numerous factors including the patient's age and health status and the size and location of the tumor.

Demyelinating Disease

Dizziness and disequilibrium can be the presenting symptoms in demyelinating disease (i.e., multiple sclerosis) in about 5% of patients. Alternatively, dizziness and disequilibrium can complicate the presentation of someone who has an established diagnosis of demyelinating disease. The basis for the vestibular and balance symptoms in demyelinating disease in some patients relates to lesions at the eighth nerve root entry zone. In some patients with demyelinating disease, no root entry zone lesion is visible. In these patients, dizziness and disequilibrium may be related to a root entry zone lesion that is not seen, to involvement of other brainstem or higher centers, or to a disorder unrelated to demyelinating disease. A combination of physical examination, vestibular laboratory testing, and MRI is required to establish an etiology, either of demyelinating disease or of some other disorder that is exacerbating the patient's current complaints. Typical findings referable to the ocular motor system in patients with demyelinating disease include internuclear ophthalmoplegia and gaze-evoked nystagmus. Patients with demyelinating disease thus may present with a mixture of peripheral and central signs and symptoms. Treatment options for patients with demyelinating disease are numerous and should be coordinated with an expert in this disorder. Vestibular rehabilitation is often considered in conjunction with pharmacotherapy.

Mal de Debarquement Syndrome

A diagnosis of mal de debarquement syndrome should be reserved for patients who have experienced a long-duration exposure to a motion environment such as an oceangoing cruise, or a long distance air flight. Typically, patients with mal de debarquement syndrome experience prolonged symptoms of dizziness and disequilibrium. Symptoms may last for weeks or even months following exposure to the motion environment. Patients often feel less symptomatic when in moving environments such as automobile as compared to when they are stationary. Physical examination, laboratory testing, and imaging are usually normal. Treatment options include vestibular suppressant medications, antidepressants, and the carbonic anhydrase inhibitor acetazolamide.

Case Vignette 4

A 40-year-old woman complained of persistent dizziness that began approximately 1 week after disembarking from a Caribbean cruise. The patient had been symptomatic for approximately 1 month when she was evaluated. Symptoms included a sense of dizziness and disequilibrium and a persistent rocking sensation as if she were still on a cruise. There were no complaints of difficulty with hearing or balance when walking. The patient's physical examination was normal as was vestibular laboratory testing. The patient's primary care physician had obtained MRI, which was negative. This patient was given a diagnosis of mal debarquement syndrome. The patient was treated with low-dose clonazepam. When seen in follow-up in 3 months, the patient noted reduced but not absent symptoms. A subsequent follow-up 6 months following the initial evaluation found that the patient was essentially asymptomatic. The patient was advised to avoid oceangoing vessels and was also advised to use a vestibular suppressant medication on long-duration air flights.

SUMMARY

Neurological origins for dizziness and vertigo include disorders of various types. Proper management of patients with neurologic causes of dizziness and vertigo requires an accurate diagnosis and recognition of both localization and etiology.

REFERENCES

Basser, L. (1964). Benign paroxysmal vertigo of childhood. *Brain, 87*, 141–152.

Furman, J. M., Marcus, D. A., & Balaban, C. D. (2013). Vestibular migraine: Clinical aspects and pathophysiology. *Lancet Neurology, 12*, 706–715.

Kayan, A., & Hood, J. D. (1984). Neuro-otological manifestations of migraine. *Brain, 107*(Pt 4), 1123–1142.

Lempert, T., Olesen, J., Furman, J., Waterston, J., Seemungal, B., Carey, J., . . . Newman-Toker, D. (2012). Vestibular migraine: Diagnostic criteria. *Journal of Vestibular Research, 22*, 167–172.

Lord, S. R., Dayhew, J., & Howland, A. (2002). Multifocal glasses impair edge-contrast sensitivity and depth perception and increase the risk of falls in older people. *Journal of the American Geriatric Society, 50*, 1760–1766.

Neuhauser, H., Leopold, M., von Brevern, M., Arnold, G., & Lempert, T. (2001). The interrelations of migraine, vertigo, and migrainous vertigo. *Neurology, 56*, 436–441.

von Brevern, M., Zeise, D., Neuhauser, H., Clarke, A. H., & Lempert, T. (2005). Acute migrainous vertigo: Clinical and oculographic findings. *Brain, 128*, 365–374.

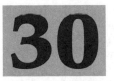

Behavioral Factors in Dizziness and Vertigo

Jeffrey P. Staab

Patients want an explanation for their suffering, but do not want to be laughed at, or worse, considered to be insane.
—Carl Westphal, 1871

INTRODUCTION

In classic medical texts, dizziness was considered to be an illness of the head and a symptom of trouble below the diaphragm (i.e., in the hypochondria) (Balaban & Jacob, 2001). These observations foretold the modern differential diagnosis of vestibular symptoms, which extends beyond neurotologic illnesses. Medical writings from the 1870s gave the first recognizable indication that vestibular symptoms could have psychiatric as well as physical causes. Table 30–1 paraphrases three 19th century descriptions of conditions that caused dizziness, visual motion sensitivity, and anxiety as patients approached the open space of town squares (Balaban & Jacob, 2001; Kuch & Swinson, 1992). Moriz Benedikt maintained that his syndrome of Platzschwindel was a neuro-ophthalmologic disorder and that any fear or anxiety reported by patients was a normal reaction to their neurologic illness. Carl Westphal and Emil Cordes focused more on anxiety as a principal component of patients' symptoms. Westphal coined the term *agoraphobia* (literally fear of open squares or fear of the marketplace), and Cordes wrote one of the earliest, most unmistakable descriptions of panic attacks found anywhere in the medical literature. The debate among these three German physicians as to the cause(s) of their patients' distress was never resolved. A few years later, several French physicians recorded additional observations about vestibular symptoms, anxiety, and predisposing psychological factors. As reviewed by Balaban and Jacob (2001), Legrande du Saulle described "fear of fear," a core concept in modern cognitive and behavioral theories of anxiety disorders. Lannois and Tournier noted that agoraphobia occurred in individuals with preexisting psychic anxiety, and was elicited by otologic diseases that produced vertigo, observations confirmed in recent years. Perroud espoused treatment by self-exposure to seemingly impassable plazas, a forerunner of behavioral therapy. In the early 20th century, the founders of clinical neurotology (e.g., Bárány, Hallpike) and clinical psychiatry (Freud and other psychoanalysts) diverged from their predecessors as they developed the procedures of the neurotologic examination and psychoanalysis, respectively. Vertigo was clearly identified with deficits in vestibular function, while anxiety and psychosomatic symptoms, including psychogenic dizziness, were considered manifestations of unconscious conflicts.

Table 30-1. Late 19th Century Descriptions of Dizziness and Anxiety

Platzschwindel (vertigo in open spaces)	Benedikt (1870)	Persons feel well in their rooms or on narrow streets; however, as soon as they arrive at a wider street or especially an open square, they become overcome by vertigo, such that they either fear they might tumble or develop such a fear that they do not dare to pass by such a place.[a]
Die Agoraphobie (agoraphobia, fear of open squares, fear of marketplace)	Westphal (1871)	Patients find it impossible to cross open squares and to walk along certain streets. Fear restricts their mobility, (but) they insist that they are not aware of any reasons for their anxiety. It seems to arise as an alien force as soon as a square is crossed or approached. With the anxiety, as part of one process, occurs the thought of not being able to cross and an image or perception of an enormous expanse of space.[b]
Platzangst, Platzfurcht (fear of open spaces, dread of open spaces)	Cordes (1872)	This fear now escalates, partially via a cognitive-intellectual path and partially via a somatic path, such that one fearsome image gives birth to the next. To this are added severe, escalating heart palpitations, an unspeakable precordial anxiety, chest oppression and fighting for breath, and alternating sensations of hot, cold, and shivering. These sensations go chaotically through one another and elicit sequences of most poorly defined thoughts.[a]

[a]Abstracted from a translation by Balaban and Jacob (2001).
[b]Abstracted from a translation by Kuch and Swinson (1992).

More than a century after panic attacks and agoraphobia were first described, they reemerged as independent disorders in the official psychiatric nomenclature with the publication of the third edition of the *Diagnostic and Statistical Manual of Mental Disorders* (*DSM-III*) in 1980 and its revision (*DSM-III-R*) in 1987 (American Psychiatric Association, 1980, 1987). This prompted a series of studies that reexamined the links between vestibular symptoms and anxiety using late 20th century knowledge about vestibular dysfunction and anxiety disorders (Hoffman, O'Leary & Munjack, 1994; Jacob, Furman, Durrant, & Turner, 1996, 1997; Sklare, Stein, Pikus, & Uhde, 1990; Stein, Asmundson, Ireland, & Walker, 1994; Swinson, Cox, Rutka, Mai, Kerr, & Kuch, 1993; Tecer, Tukel, Erdamar, & Sunay, 2004). These studies, reviewed in more detail below, suggested that patients with panic disorder had higher than expected rates of vestibular deficits and that patients with vestibular dysfunction had higher than expected rates of panic disorder (i.e., that the relationship between dizziness and anxiety was bidirectional—psychosomatic and somatopsychic) (Furman & Jacob, 2001). Investigators in three countries described syndromes of nonvertiginous dizziness in an effort to advance clinical diagnosis and scientific understanding of persistent vestibular symptoms (Table 30–2). In Germany, Brandt and Dieterich (1986) described phobic postural vertigo (PPV) as a common, clearly identifiable condition manifested by subjective dizziness and illusory perturbations of the body. Brandt and Dieterich asserted that PPV was a neurotologic condition distinct from panic or other anxiety disorders, though their definition included anxiety symptoms and follow-up studies revealed that 75% of PPV patients had clinically significant anxiety and depression (Huppert, Strupp, Rettinger, Hecht, & Brandt, 2005; Kapfhammer et al., 1997). Similarly, Jacob et al. (1993) in the United States and Bronstein (1995) in the United Kingdom defined syndromes of uneasiness in complex motion environments and hypersensitivity to visual motion cues, which they termed space-motion discomfort (SMD) and visual vertigo (now visually-induced dizziness [VID]), respectively. Initially, SMD and VID were described in patients with neurotologic dysfunction, but they were subsequently identified in individuals with primary anxiety disorders (Bronstein, 2004). Therefore, despite 100 years of scientific advances in neurotology and psychiatry, the 20th century came to a close much like the century before, with an unresolved conundrum about the relationship between vestibular symptoms and anxiety. Limited data were available to guide treatment.

Table 30-2. Late 20th Century Syndromes of Persistent Vestibular Symptoms

Phobic postural vertigo (PPV)	Brandt & Dieterich (1986)	• Dizziness or subjective imbalance with normal exam • Fluctuating unsteadiness or illusory body perturbations • Anxiety and autonomic arousal • Obsessive-compulsive personality, mild depression • Provocative stimuli—bridge, street, crowds • Onset after stress, medical illness, or vestibular disorder
Space motion discomfort (SMD)	Jacob et al. (1993)	• Uneasiness about balance or spatial orientation • Feelings of swaying or rocking when still • Heightened awareness of normal movement • Provocative stimuli—environments with inexact or potentially conflicting visual and somatosensory cues (e.g., heights, bridges, open spaces)
Visual vertigo (VV)	Bronstein (1995)	• Dizziness in environments with complex visual stimuli (e.g., grocery stores, crowded places, complex décor) • Sensitivity to destabilizing effects of visual stimuli (e.g., tilted frame, rotating pinwheel)

The early years of the 21st century have yielded a number of promising developments. Several investigators (Adkin, Frank & Carpenter, 2002; Brown, Gage, Polych, Sleik, & Winder, 2002; Carpenter, Frank, Adkin, Paton, & Allum, 2004; Ohno, Wada, Saitoh, Sunaga, & Nagai, 2004) demonstrated the effects that perceived threat and anxiety have on normal balance function, providing a better framework for understanding links between the brain's threat/anxiety and balance systems in normal individuals and patients with vestibular symptoms. Huppert and colleagues (2005) showed that PPV was a stable clinical entity that could be distinguished reliably from active neurotologic illnesses. Redfern, Furman, and Jacob (Furman, Redfern, & Jacob, 2006; Redfern, Furman, & Jacob, 2007) clarified the relationships between SMD, vestibular deficits, panic symptoms, and agoraphobia. Staab and Ruckenstein (2003, 2007; Staab, 2006a, 2006b, 2012) reformulated PPV, SMD, and VID into the concept of chronic subjective dizziness (CSD), which just evolved further into the diagnosis of persistent postural-perceptual dizziness (PPPD), recently added to the beta (draft) version of the 11th edition of the International Classification of Diseases (ICD-11 beta) by the World Health Organization (2014) (Table 30–3). Godemann and colleagues (Godemann, Koffroth, Neu, & Heuser, 2004; Godemann et al., 2005; Godemann

Schabowska, Naetebusch, Heinz, & Strohle, 2006), Heinrichs, Edler, Eskens, Mielczarek, and Moschner (2007), and Cousins and colleagues (2014) published prospective studies of medical and behavioral outcomes in patients following acute vestibular neuritis and benign paroxysmal positional vertigo (BPPV) illuminating the longitudinal interactions of medical and psychological factors that determine the clinical course of persistent vestibular symptoms, observations that support the key features of PPPD. Finally, and most importantly for patients, the 21st century brought the first studies of successful therapies for vestibular symptoms and anxiety, including treatment with serotonin reuptake inhibitors (Horii et al., 2004, 2007, 2008; Simon et al., 2005; Staab, 2011a; Staab, Ruckenstein, & Amsterdam, 2004; Staab, Ruckenstein, Solomon, & Shepard, 2002), vestibular and balance rehabilitation therapy (VBRT) (Jacob, Whitney, Detweiler-Shostak & Furman, 2001; Pavlou, Lingeswaran, Davies, Gresty, & Bronstein, 2004; Yardley, Beech, & Weinman, 2001), and cognitive behavior therapy (CBT) (Edelman, Mahoney, & Cremer, 2012; Holmberg, Karlberg, Harlacher, Rivano-Fischer, & Magnusson, 2006; Holmberg, Karlberg, Harlacher, & Magnusson, 2007; Johansson, Akerlund, Larsen, & Andersson, 2001; Mahoney, Edelman, & Cremer, 2013). This chapter reviews these advances. It is hoped that they will replace dated concepts such

Table 30-3. Persistent Postural-Perceptual Dizziness (PPPD)

Definition	Explanatory Notes
Persistent nonvertiginous dizziness, unsteadiness, or both lasting 3 months or more.	Symptoms must be present for more than 15 of every 30 days, though most patients experience daily symptoms.
Symptoms are present most days, often increasing throughout the day, but may wax and wane. Momentary flares may occur spontaneously or with sudden movement.	Symptoms need not be continuous but must be present for prolonged (hours-long) periods throughout the day. Momentary symptoms alone do not fulfill this criterion.
Affected individuals feel worst when upright, exposed to moving or complex visual stimuli, and during active or passive head motion. These situations may not be equally provocative.	These situations may be troublesome for individuals with other neuro-otologic disorders during active phases of illness (e.g., flares of Ménière's disease), but they cause persistent difficulty for patients with PPPD.
Typically, the disorder follows occurrences of acute or episodic vestibular or balance-related problems (e.g., peripheral or central vestibular disorders, migraine, concussion, orthostatic intolerance, panic attacks with dizziness). Symptoms may begin intermittently, and then consolidate. Gradual onset is uncommon.	It may not be possible to identify a specific trigger in all cases, but a slow, insidious onset is unusual. PPPD commonly coexists with other diseases or disorders. Evidence of other active illnesses does not necessarily exclude PPPD but may indicate comorbid condition(s).

Source: Expanded from World Health Organization (2014).

as recurrent vestibulopathy and psychogenic dizziness in the minds and practices of physicians and other medical professionals, allowing patients with vestibular symptoms to benefit from developments that are deciphering a centuries-old enigma.

PSYCHOLOGICAL INFLUENCES ON BALANCE FUNCTION IN NORMAL INDIVIDUALS

Table 30–4 lists several investigations of the effect of perceived threat on balance function in normal individuals (i.e., subjects with no neurotologic or psychiatric diagnoses). Healthy subjects rose to tiptoes from a flat-footed stance more slowly when standing on a high compared to low platform and when near compared to away from the edge of the platform (Adkin et al., 2002). Adults of all ages reduced gait speed and stride length when walking on narrow as opposed to wide and high as opposed to low walkways. Older adults were most conservative in this regard (Brown et al., 2002). The added demands of a cognitive task increased the effects of

perceived threat on gait speed (Gage et al., 2003). When subjects were asked to respond to auditory cues while walking on walkways, gait speeds and reaction times were slower on high versus low and narrow versus wide pathways. In making these gait and posture adjustments, subjects reported anxiety about falling, reduced confidence in balance, and greater sensations of instability (Adkin et al., 2002).

Investigators also measured state and trait anxiety in various studies of postural control. State anxiety is the amount of anxiety that an individual has at a specific point in time. A person with high level of state anxiety may not necessarily have an anxiety disorder, but may simply be worried about a specific circumstance. Trait anxiety is the tendency to be anxious and worried. An individual with a high level of trait anxiety is frequently known as a worrywart. On a posture platform, individuals with high state anxiety swayed more than those with low state anxiety with eyes open, but not eyes closed (Ohno et al., 2004). The frequency content of postural sway suggested that state anxiety influenced the processing of visual cues more than vestibular or somatosensory stimuli (Wada, Sunaga, & Nagai, 2001). State anxiety also affected postural control. When given rotational

Table 30-4. Effects of Perceived Threat, State, and Trait Anxiety on Normal Balance Function

Balance Challenge	Effect
• Rise to toes from a normal stance (Adkin et al., 2002)	• Time to complete task was slower on a high versus low platform, slowest at edge of high platform.
• Walk on a walkway (Brown et al., 2002)	• Gait speed was slower on a high versus low walkway, slowest on a high narrow walkway. • Stride length was shorter on a high versus low walkway, shortest on a high narrow walkway.
• Dual task—respond to auditory cues while walking on a walkway (Gage, Sleik, Polych, McKenzie, & Brown, 2003)	• Gait and response times to auditory cues were slower on higher and narrower walkways.
• Maintain stance on a stationary posture platform (Ohno et al., 2004)	• Postural sway was greater for subjects with high versus low state anxiety in the eyes-open condition. • No differences in the eyes-closed condition.
• Maintain stance during rotary perturbations to posture platform (Carpenter et al., 2004)	• Subjects with high versus low state anxiety had shorter response latencies to platform perturbations and made more postural corrections.
• Maintain stance on posture platform with eyes closed (Hainaut, Caillet, Lestienne, & Bolmont, 2011)	• Subjects with high versus low trait anxiety exhibited stiffer postural control with reduced sway after performing a demanding mental task.
• Visual adaptation in a virtual reality environment (Viaud-Delmon, Ivanenko, Berthoz, & Jouvent, 2000a)	• Subjects with high versus low trait anxiety were more strongly affected by erroneous visual stimuli.

perturbations on a posture platform, individuals with higher state anxiety employed stiffer postural control strategies with shorter response latencies and more postural corrections than less anxious subjects (Carpenter et al., 2004). State anxiety also seemed to exacerbate the age-related degeneration of balance reflexes in older adults (Carpenter, Adkin, Brawley, & Frank, 2006).

Subjects with high trait anxiety reduced their body sway whereas individuals with low trait anxiety swayed more while standing with eyes closed after performing a demanding mental task (Hainault et al., 2011). Normal individuals utilize this type of stiffened postural control under threatening circumstances (e.g., when standing at heights) (Adkin, Frank, Carpenter & Peysar, 2000). Trait anxiety also may influence the processing of visual stimuli. In a virtual reality environment, subjects with high trait anxiety had greater adaptation to erroneous visual feedback gains than individuals with low trait anxiety, even when accurate vestibular and somatosensory stimuli were available (Viaud-Delmon et al., 2000). In other words, subjects with high trait anxiety relied more on visual cues, even when they were misleading. The effect of state and trait anxiety on clinical balance function tests is not as clear, though state, but not trait, anxiety may increase canal-ocular reflex gain (Viaud-Delmon et al., 2000; Yardley et al., 1995b).

BALANCE FUNCTION IN PATIENTS WITH ANXIETY DISORDERS

During the last two decades, several research groups have investigated vestibular function in patients with panic and other anxiety disorders (Hoffman et al., 1994; Jacob et al., 1996, 1997; Sklare, et al., 1990; Swinson et al., 1993; Tecer et al., 2004). Most found that patients with panic disorder were more likely than normal control subjects to have at least one abnormality on caloric, optokinetic, or autorotation tests (i.e., one parameter outside of the normal range). However, the findings varied from one subject to another, both within and between investigations, revealing no consistent pattern of diagnosable vestibular deficits. In the most detailed studies to date, Jacob et al. (1997) found that persistent hypersensitivity to motion stimuli and agoraphobic avoidance (i.e., widespread avoidance of situations related to dizziness) were associated with compensated peripheral vestibular deficits on balance function tests. Furman and colleagues (Furman et al., 2006; Jacob, Redfern, & Furman, 2009) found that patients with anxiety disorders had slightly higher gains and shorter time constants of the canal-ocular reflex as well as slightly higher gains of the otolith-ocular reflex than nonanxious control subjects, a pattern that is not consistent with either central or peripheral vestibular deficits. In total, these data suggest that patients with anxiety disorders are quite likely to demonstrate nonspecific, nondiagnostic abnormalities on tests of semicircular canal function (e.g., caloric stimulation, rotary chair, or autorotation), but the cause of these abnormalities is not clear. Most investigators concluded that they reflect subtle vestibular deficits (Hoffman et al., 1994; Jacob et al., 1996; Sklare et al., 1990; Swinson et al., 1993; Tecer et al., 2004), but the absence of clinical correlates to support this conjecture requires that other possibilities, such as the effects of heightened anxiety on otherwise normal balance reflexes, must be considered (Yardley, Watson, Britton, Lear, & Bird, 1995b). The findings of Furman, Jacob, and colleagues (Furman et al., 2006; Jacob et al., 1997; Jacob, Redfern, & Furman, 2009) are best understood in the light of longitudinal studies of vestibular systems and anxiety (Cousins et al., 2014; Godemann et al., 2004, 2005, 2006; Staab & Ruckenstein, 2003), which show an evolution from acute vestibular insults to chronic motion sensitivity and persistent visual dependence in patients with comorbid anxiety.

Investigations using static and dynamic posturography have given a clearer picture of the effects of anxiety disorders on balance function than studies using tests of canal- and otolith-ocular reflexes. Patients with panic disorder had more body sway on static posturography than nonanxious control subjects (Perna et al., 2001) and were more likely to be destabilized by disorienting perceptual cues during dynamic posturography (Yardley, Britton, Lear, Bird,

& Luxon, 1995a). The extent of postural instability correlated strongly with the severity of agoraphobic behaviors (Perna et al., 2001; Yardley et al., 1995a) and anticipatory anxiety (i.e., trepidation in advance of situations related to dizziness) (Perna et al., 2001). Jacob and colleagues (Jacob et al., 1997; presented/unpublished), using the sensory organization test (SOT), found that patients with anxiety disorders were more vision or surface dependent than normal control subjects. That is, anxious patients relied more heavily on visual or somatosensory information than vestibular inputs for balance control. Subjects with anxiety disorders plus heightened sensitivity to motion cues performed particularly poorly on Conditions 3 (stable platform, sway referenced surround) and 4 (sway referenced platform, stable surround), where visual or somatosensory information is misleading. Querner, Krafczyk, Dieterich, & Brandt (2000) and Yardley et al. (1995a) described comparable performance difficulties in patients with nonvertiginous dizziness and anxiety.

Redfern et al. (2007) compared the postural stability of patients with anxiety disorders and normal controls exposed to an optic flow stimulus (i.e., a projected visual pattern that streamed past them) while standing on a static posture platform. Subjects with anxiety disorders had greater postural sway than normal individuals during optic flow, even though they had adequate vestibular and somatosensory data to control their posture. The degree of postural instability was mediated by the severity of motion sensitivity (SMD). Taken together, these posturographic studies suggest that patients with anxiety disorders, especially those with strong motion sensitivity, rely mostly on vision, somewhat less on somatosensory cues, and least on vestibular inputs for balance control (i.e., they appear to be visually dependent). In a study of 15 patients with panic disorder, treatment with the anxiolytic SSRI, paroxetine, countered this effect (Perna et al., 2003).

These physiologic investigations provide an explanation for the SOT patterns observed in a study by Cevette, Puetz, Marion, Wertz, and Muenter (1995) who compared SOT performance in patients with vestibular deficits, patients with dizziness due to psychiatric disorders, and normal control subjects. The three groups had distinctly different test results as shown in Figure 30–1. Normal subjects had gradually decreasing scores from Conditions

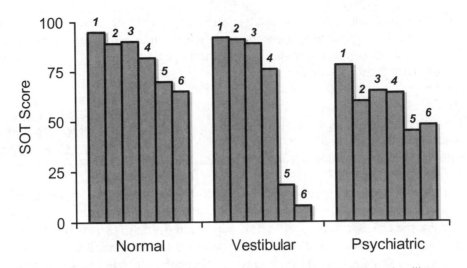

Figure 30–1. SOT performance by normal subjects and individuals with vestibular or psychiatric disorders. Cevette et al., "Aphysiologic Performance on Dynamic Posturography" (*Otolaryngology-Head and Neck Surgery* Vol. 112 #6) p. 13, Copyright © 1995 by SAGE Publications. Reprinted by Permission of SAGE Publications.

1 to 6, consistent with the increasing difficulty of balance challenges in successive SOT conditions. Subjects with central or peripheral vestibular deficits performed poorly on Conditions 5 and 6, which test patients' abilities to use vestibular information in the presence of misleading visual and somatosensory stimuli. Patients with anxiety, depressive, or somatic symptom disorders had lower than normal scores across all conditions. In some cases, patients with psychiatric disorders had their lowest scores on Conditions 3 and 4 and did better on Conditions 5 and 6. The authors called this an "aphysiologic" pattern, an unfortunate misnomer that has been incorrectly equated with malingering (Gianoli, McWilliams, Soileau, & Balafsky, 2000; Goebel et al., 1997; Morgan, Beck. & Dobie, 2002). In actuality, this pattern represents the physiologic effects of anxiety on balance function (Jacob et al., 1997; Querner et al., 2000; Yardley et al., 1995a). Therefore, the SOT cannot be used to identify malingering.

PSYCHIATRIC CAUSES OF DIZZINESS AND VERTIGO

Since the time of Westphal and Cordes, the medical literature has described patients with dizziness and imbalance caused by panic disorder with or without agoraphobia. Panic attacks may cause dizziness, unsteadiness, and mild vertigo, but not ataxia (Staab, 2006a, 2006b). In some cases, patients with dizziness due to panic disorder report unmistakable, classic panic attacks with sudden, overwhelming fear accompanied by palpitations, chest pain, dyspnea, tremulousness, and diaphoresis. However, patients whose primary panic symptom is dizziness are more likely to report light-headedness, nonspecific swirling sensations, or fogginess in the head with autonomic symptoms reminiscent of motion sickness. When they acknowledge anxiety, patients often attribute it to worry about being dizzy, downplaying the fear as a primary symptom. This presentation of panic disorder may obscure the diagnosis, but there are very few other causes of episodic, nonvertiginous dizziness with autonomic symptoms that peak in 2 to 5 min, and then decrease spontaneously over 15 to 60 min, sometimes lingering for a few hours at a low level. The other common cause of this clinical presentation, vestibular migraine, often coexists with anxiety disorders (Staab & Ruckenstein, 2007). On physical examination, patients with panic disorder may experience increased dizziness during provocative procedures, such as the Dix-Hallpike test, but they will not show objective signs of vestibular dysfunction such as pathological nystagmus. In fact, the observation of nystagmus or ataxia in patients with panic disorder suggests co-occurring neurotologic illness (Shepard, Solomon, Ruckenstein, & Staab, 2003). In tertiary care centers, a primary diagnosis of panic disorder was identified in one-third of patients with chronic, nonvertiginous dizziness or 8% to 10% of all patients referred for evaluation of dizziness or imbalance (Eckhardt et al., 1996; Eckhardt-Henn, Breuer, Thomalske, Hoffmann, & Hopf, 2003; Staab & Ruckenstein, 2003, 2007).

In contrast to the noteworthy prevalence of anxiety disorders as causes of dizziness, unsteadiness, and mild vertigo, psychiatric causes of severe vertigo and ataxia are less common. Functional neurologic disorders (aka conversion or dissociative sensorimotor disorders) and factitious disorders may cause these signs and symptoms, but the unusual spinning sensations and gait abnormalities that they produce reveal their psychological origins (Staab, 2006a, 2006b; Honaker, Gilbert, & Staab, 2010). Only 2 of 345 (0.6%) tertiary care patients in a large study of individuals with chronic, nonvertiginous dizziness were diagnosed with functional disorders and none with factitious disorder (Staab & Ruckenstein, 2007). Patients with functional disorders may report symptoms that superficially suggest structural disorders, but their physical signs are not consistent with structural peripheral or central vestibular deficits (Honaker, Gilbert, & Staab, 2010). In some cases, functional disorders can lead to physical injury, such as a patient who developed degenerative arthritis in both hips after years of walking with the unusual wide-based gait of a functional gait disorder. Patients with factitious disorder (aka Munchhausen's syndrome) intentionally produce physical or psychological symptoms, but do so for unconscious reasons such as a pathological need for attention. Depending on their methods, patients with factitious disorders may produce bona fide medical impairments (e.g., dizziness and orthostasis from surreptitious use of a diuretic). For this reason, factitious disorder is difficult to diagnose but should be suspected when patients fail to improve, worsen, or develop new symptoms despite adequate diagnosis and treatment. Patients with functional and factitious disorders are not malingerers. Illness behaviors in both disorders are driven by serious psychological distress that may require considerable effort to identify or treat. Malingerers, on the other hand,

are fully aware of their deceit and the reasons that they are lying. Fortunately, true malingering is rare among patients with balance disorders.

PSYCHOLOGICAL PREDISPOSING, PRECIPITATING, PROVOKING, AND PERPETUATING FACTORS

A full accounting of psychological mechanisms in patients with vestibular symptoms requires an understanding of factors that trigger, exacerbate, and sustain illness (Staab, 2006a). These concepts provide a portrait of medical-psychiatric interactions that can inform effective diagnostic evaluations, patient education, and treatment plans. Table 30–5 lists psychological predisposing, precipitating, provoking, and perpetuating factors. Two predisposing factors have been identified. The first is the anxiety-related personality traits of neuroticism and introversion. Patients with neuroticism are dysphoric worrywarts who have persistent low levels of anxiety and depression that tend to increase under stress, accompanied by psychosomatic symptoms (e.g., headache, dyspepsia). Patients with introversion tend to be shy, reserved, unassertive, and disinclined to be thrillseekers. Neuroticism has been linked to generalized anxiety disorder and depression following stressful life events, whereas introversion has been linked to panic and social anxiety disorders (Fox, Henderson, Marshall, Nichols, & Ghera, 2005; Kalin, 2004). These personality traits may influence the development of persistent symptoms after acute vestibular syndromes. Staab, Rohe, Eggers, and Shepard (2014) found that individuals with neurotic, introverted personality traits were significantly overrepresented among patients with CSD compared to other neurotologic conditions producing similar levels of vestibular symptoms, anxiety, and depression. Tschan and colleagues (2011) found that individuals with higher levels of resilience, self-confidence, and optimism (essentially the opposite of neuroticism and introversion) were less likely to develop chronic symptoms after acute vestibular events. Indovina and colleagues (2014) may have identified the neural correlates underlying these findings. In a functional magnetic resonance imaging study, they found that neuroticism was associated with increased central

Table 30–5. Behavioral Factors and Their Relationship to Vestibular Symptoms

Factor	Role	Effect
Neurotic, introverted temperament (trait anxiety)	Predisposing	Anxiety-related personality traits may increase the reactivity of vestibular and anxiety systems in the brain to vestibular stimulation and may increase the risk of developing PPPD after a precipitating event.
Preexisting anxiety disorder	Predisposing	Anxiety disorders that predate the occurrence of an acute vestibular syndrome appear to increase the likelihood of developing chronic dizziness as a sequela.
Panic attacks	Precipitating	Panic attacks are the most common psychiatric cause of episodic vestibular symptoms.
Elevated state anxiety	Provoking	Events that increase state anxiety (e.g., illness, life stress) may exacerbate vestibular disorders.
Cognitive processes	Perpetuating	Several cognitive symptoms maintain behavioral morbidity in patients with vestibular symptoms.
Catastrophic thinking		Catastrophic thoughts about vestibular symptoms and their potential adverse consequences maintain a high level of dizziness-related worry and anxiety.
Anticipatory anxiety and phobic avoidance		Patients may develop high levels of anxiety in advance of circumstances that they associate with vestibular symptoms. This often leads to excessive avoidance of activities inside and outside the home.

vestibular system activity and increased connectivity between vestibular and anxiety pathways in the brain in response to vestibular stimulation and that introversion was associated with increased anxiety system responses to the same stimuli. Perhaps the vulnerabilities inherent in neurotic, introverted personality traits may explain the observations that stressful life events seem to provoke recurrences of Ménière's disease, vestibular migraine, panic disorder, and depression, at least in vulnerable individuals (Brantberg, Trees, & Baloh, 2005; Fox et al., 2005; Furman, Balaban, Jacob, & Marcus, 2005; Kalin, 2004; Takahashi, Ishida, Iida, Yamashita, & Sugawara, 2001). The second predisposing factor is a history of anxiety disorders pre-dating the onset of vestibular symptoms. Retrospective (Staab & Ruckenstein, 2005) and prospective (Best et al., 2006; Godemann et al., 2006) data suggest that patients with preexisting anxiety disorders may be more likely to develop chronic dizziness in the aftermath of acute vestibular syndromes. These predisposing factors may also affect treatment response. Staab and Ruckenstein

(2005) found that patients with CSD and an anxiety diathesis experienced a less robust response to treatment with serotonin reuptake inhibitors than patients without anxiety-related risk factors. Thus, the long-term medical and psychological outcomes of patients who experience acute vestibular syndromes may be determined, in part, by their personality traits and preexisting psychopathological state.

Psychological events may precipitate dizziness even in the absence of medical problems (Horii et al., 2007; Jacob et al., 1996; Staab & Ruckenstein, 2003, 2007). Dizziness and light-headedness are common symptoms of panic attacks, second in frequency only to chest pain and dyspnea. Panic attacks occur as part of panic disorder and also in social and specific phobias (including fear of falling), posttraumatic stress disorder, obsessive-compulsive disorder, and several medical conditions. Psychological conflicts that trigger functional or factitious disorders also fall into the category of psychological precipitants of vestibular and balance symptoms, but they require assessment on a case-by-case basis because of their relative infrequency.

Cognitive processes, including catastrophic thinking about the consequences of being dizzy (e.g., "I'll crash the car.") and anxious ruminations about chronic symptoms (e.g., "I'll never get better.") maintain a conscious focus on vestibular symptoms and promote disability over daily functioning (Yardley, Verschuur, Masson, Luxon, & Haacke, 1992; Yardley, Luxon, & Haake, 1994; Yardley et al., 2001). Anticipatory anxiety and phobic avoidance add considerable morbidity as they greatly restrict participation in work, social, and home activities.

Clinicians who identify their patients' psychological predisposing, precipitating, provoking, and perpetuating factors during the medical evaluation of dizziness are in a position to help their patients develop a clearer understanding of their clinical state and have a firmer foundation for successful interventions (Best et al., 2006; Staab, 2006a, 2006b; Yardley et al., 2001). Clinical experience shows that patients understand these processes and appreciate attention to them as part of a multimodality treatment plan.

A 21ST CENTURY INTERACTIVE MODEL OF BEHAVIORAL FACTORS AND VESTIBULAR SYMPTOMS

The concepts of space-motion discomfort (Jacob et al., 1993) and visual-induced dizziness (Bronstein, 1995, 2004) codified the phenomenon of hypersensitivity to motion stimuli in modern terminology (see Table 30–2). Both were originally described in patients with vestibular deficits, but were later identified in patients with psychiatric causes of dizziness as well. This suggests that they share a common pathophysiologic mechanism that is related to the experience of being dizzy, regardless of the underlying trigger.

Jacob and colleagues extensively studied the relationships among SMD, anxiety, and vestibular deficits (Furman et al., 2006; Jacob et al., 1993, 1996, 1997; Redfern et al., 2007). They found partial overlaps between SMD, panic disorder, and height phobia and linked SMD to compensated peripheral vestibular deficits and agoraphobic behaviors. They also discovered that SMD predicted sensitivity to destabilizing motion stimuli (e.g., optic flow on a posture platform) better than neurotologic or psychiatric diagnoses (Redfern et al., 2007). This led Furman and Jacob (2001) to suggest that SMD provides the link between vestibular dysfunction and psychiatric morbidity in patients with chronic dizziness.

Patients with chronic dizziness also experience VID (Bronstein, 1995, 2004). Guerraz et al. (2001) measured the susceptibility of patients with VID to the destabilizing influences of static (tilted frame) and dynamic (rotating pinwheel) visual stimuli. Patients with VID had more postural sway than patients with unilateral peripheral vestibular losses or normal individuals. The severity of anxiety was similar in the VID and peripheral deficit groups and higher than in normal controls. This suggests that VID, like SMD, is a manifestation of links between dizziness and anxiety.

From PPV to CSD and Now to PPPD

The introduction of phobic postural vertigo in 1986 by Brandt and Dieterich provided a neurotologic diagnosis for patients with persistent dizziness and motion sensitivity in the absence of active vestibular deficits (see Table 30–2) (see Brandt, 1996, for review). Subsequent studies found PPV to be a reliably identifiable clinical entity (Huppert et al., 2005; Kapfhammer et al., 1997) with a natural course of waxing and waning, typically improving, dizziness and imbalance. In contrast to this benign physical picture, two-thirds of patients developed clinically significant anxiety or depression, which is not explained by the anxiety symptoms that are part of the definition of PPV. In laboratory studies, patients with PPV used postural control strategies (e.g., co-contraction of postural muscles, especially at the ankles) that normal individuals typically employ only in challenging balance situations (Krafczyk, Schlamp, Dieterich, Haberhauer, & Brandt, 1999). As a result, they showed greater postural instability than normal controls during low demand balance tasks. In more challenging situations, where high demand strategies are adaptive, patients with PPV and normal individuals had similar postural stability (Querner et al., 2000). These findings are consistent with Brandt's hypothesis that patients with PPV become sensitized to their own postural control movements through classical conditioning and misinterpret normal body sway as a need for greater attention to postural mechanisms.

The diagnosis of PPV moved the field of neurotology beyond the vague concept of psychogenic dizziness, which was defined as dizziness without an identifiable medical cause. This was a crucial advance, but the definition of PPV did not fully elaborate its physical symptoms, and the inclusion of psychological elements confounded comorbid symptoms (anxiety and depression) and predisposing factors (personality traits) with core elements of the syndrome. Furthermore, this grouping of physical, psychiatric, and personality criteria did not easily guide clinicians to effective treatments (Staab, 2006a, 2006b). To address these concerns, Staab and Ruckenstein (2005, 2007) introduced the syndrome of chronic subjective dizziness (CSD), which streamlined the definition of PPV, influenced by the concepts of SMD and VID. Subsequent research clarified the differential diagnosis of CSD and its medical and psychiatric comorbidities, and prompted treatment studies (Staab, 2012). In 2010, the Bárány Society commissioned a subcommittee of its vestibular disorders classification project to define the most important behavioral neurotologic disorders and reconcile the definitions of PPV and CSD. That was completed in May 2014. A single syndrome encompassing knowledge gained from a quarter century of research and clinical experience with PPV and CSD was defined and renamed persistent postural-perceptual dizziness (PPPD) in recognition of its core features—persistent nonvertiginous dizziness that is exacerbated by upright postural and spatial perception stimuli. PPPD has been added to the draft version of the ICD-11 (World Health Organization, 2014). Its definition and explanatory notes are contained in Table 30–3.

The primary physical symptoms of PPPD are persistent nonvertiginous dizziness or unsteadiness that are present most of the time for 3 months or more. Patients often describe feelings of rocking or swaying when upright, but they do not report falls or ataxia. These perceptual symptoms were adapted from descriptions not only of PPV and CSD, but also SMD and VID. Patients with PPPD may have histories of past vestibular deficits, but their active symptoms should be those described in Table 30–3. PPPD may coexist with other neurotologic conditions (e.g., vestibular migraine, Ménière's disease) that produce episodic exacerbations of vestibular symptoms, superimposed on its persistent daily dizziness and unsteadiness. This is a change from the original concepts of PPV and CSD, which excluded other active neurotologic conditions, a restriction found to be incorrect in studies of the differential diagnosis of the disorder (Staab, 2012). One distinction between patients with other neurotologic disorders and those with PPPD is that patients with other neurotologic illnesses can usually minimize their symptoms by holding their heads still, while most patients with PPPD are symptomatic even when stationary. Neurotologic examination may provoke dizziness in patients with PPPD, but PPPD alone does not produce evidence of active vestibular dysfunction (e.g., pathological nystagmus). Vestibular laboratory tests are usually normal, but sometimes show nondiagnostic abnormalities, evidence of previous vestibular deficits (e.g., compensated peripheral loss from prior vestibular neuritis), or active deficits from coexisting illnesses (e.g., unilateral hearing and vestibular deficits from Ménière's disease).

Anxiety and depressive disorders commonly coexist with PPPD, but research studies in patient cohorts with PPV and CSD showed that 25% of individuals had no psychiatric disorders (Brandt, 1996; Staab & Ruckenstein, 2007; Staab, Eggers, Neff, & Shepard, 2010). Therefore, the symptoms of anxiety and depression that were part of the definition of PPV were not included in PPPD, though clinicians should maintain an appreciation for this frequent psychiatric comorbidity. Similarly, the obsessive-compulsive personality traits included in PPV were more precisely identified in subsequent studies to be elements of neuroticism and introversion (Staab et al., 2014) and better considered to be predisposing factors than core criteria for PPPD. A detailed review of the evolution of PPV to CSD to PPPD can be found in Staab (2012).

Psychiatric Complications of Neurotologic Illnesses

The prevalence of anxiety and depressive disorders is higher in patients with neurotologic illnesses (Clark, Hirsch, Smith, Furman & Jacob, 1994; Eckhardt et al., 1996; Eckhardt-Henn, Breuer, Thomalske, Hoffmann, & Hopf, 2003; Grunfeld, Gresty,

Bronstein & Jahanshahi, 2003; Persoons, Luyckx, Desloovere, Vandenberghe, & Fischler, 2003; Ruckenstein & Staab, 2001) than in general medical outpatients (Evans et al., 1999). Moreover, anxiety and depression may be stronger predictors of long-term functional impairment than neurotologic status. In two studies that investigated clinical outcomes 3 to 6 years after patients suffered acute vestibular losses, rates of anxiety and depression (Eagger, Luxon, Davies, Coelho, & Ron, 1992) and persistent dizziness (Kammerlind, Ledin, Skargren, & Odkvist, 2005) were both about 50%. In both studies, psychiatric morbidity, not neurotologic function, determined symptomatic outcomes. In a prospective study of 101 patients with dizziness, Yardley et al. (1994) found that the severity of anxiety at study entry was the single best predictor of functional impairment after 7 months. Therefore, improving the prognosis of patients with dizziness depends on adequate recognition and treatment of coexisting anxiety and depression (Best et al., 2006; Eagger et al., 1992; Eckhardt et al., 1996; Staab, 2006a, 2006b).

Vestibular Neuronitis and BPPV

In retrospective, cross-sectional, and prospective studies, several investigators have shown that anxiety adversely affects the clinical course and recovery of patients with vestibular neuronitis (VN) and BPPV. Patients with generalized anxiety disorder coexisting with labyrinthine defects due to VN had more postural instability than patients with VN alone (Monzani et al., 2004). Individuals who employed rigid postural control strategies to compensate for their balance deficits, a hallmark of anxiety, were less likely to recover without residual symptoms (Alessandrini, D'Erme, Bruno, Napolitano, & Magrini, 2003). Godemann et al. (2004, 2005) followed 75 patients prospectively for 1 year after hospitalization for acute VN. Twenty-two subjects (29%) had persistent dizziness at 1 year, but only two had uncompensated vestibular deficits at that time. The other 20 demonstrated full vestibular recovery, despite their ongoing symptoms. Seventeen of those 20 (85%) experienced high levels of anxiety during the acute period of their illnesses. In a second study (Godemann et al., 2006), the investigators followed an expanded sample of 93 subjects for 2 years.

Excluding individuals with preexisting psychiatric disorders, seven patients (7.5%) had new onset panic disorder and five others (5.4%) developed persistent dizziness despite neurotologic recovery. Logistical regression found that fear of vertigo, levels of anxiety 10 days after vertigo onset, and catastrophic thoughts about dizziness were the strongest predictors of psychiatric outcomes at 2 years. Persistence of these symptoms at 6 months was an even stronger predictor of incidence of psychiatric illness. Heinrichs and colleagues (2007) found strikingly similar results in a 3-month study of patients recruited after acute VN or new onset BPPV. In summary, high levels of anxiety during acute vestibular syndromes and catastrophic thoughts about being dizzy predicted persistent physical symptoms and poor psychiatric outcomes despite neurotologic recovery. Emerging evidence suggests that early anti-anxiety interventions may reduce long-term morbidity (see psychotherapy below).

Meniérè's Disease

Several studies have found that Meniérè's disease is associated with high rates of depression (Coker, Coker, Jenkins, & Vincent, 1989), anxiety (Celestino, Rosini, Carucci, Marconi, & Vercillo, 2003; Takahashi et al., 2001), and poor quality of life (Söderman et al., 2002). Depression is most common during active phases of illness, when up to 70% of patients have clinically significantly depressive symptoms (Coker et al., 1989). Even during quiescent periods, significantly more patients with Ménière's disease are depressed (32%) (Coker et al., 1989) than general medical outpatients (9%) (Evans et al., 1999). Rates of depression and anxiety tend to increase with the duration of illness and number of episodes, but not with measures of neurotologic function (Celestino et al., 2003; Savastano, Maron, Mangialaio, Longhi, & Rizzardo, 1996). Ménière's patients with high levels of neuroticism had more psychological distress, rated their physical symptoms as more severe, and focused more on being ill than patients who had few neurotic traits (Savastano et al., 1996). In two studies, Takahashi and colleagues (Onuki, Takahashi, Odagiri, Wada, & Sato, 2005; Takahashi et al., 2001) found that individuals with anxious personality traits had greater progression of low-frequency hearing loss than less anxious individuals. External life events, rural versus urban living, and preferred styles of relaxation did not affect the course of illness.

Anxiety may adversely affect the outcomes of medical-surgical treatment of Meniérè's disease. In one prospective study of 103 patients treated with transtympanic gentamicin, anxiety-related, pretreatment functional impairment predicted the persistence of chronic nonvertiginous dizziness 5 years after transtympanic gentamicin treatment, despite good control of episodic vertigo attacks (Boleas-Aguirre, Sánchez-Ferrandiz, Guillén-Grima, & Perez, 2007).

Migraine

Vestibular migraine is the most common cause of episodic vestibular symptoms without hearing loss. Approximately 60% to 80% of patients who have recurrent vertigo without hearing loss suffer from migraine (Brantberg et al., 2005; Furman et al., 2005). Chronic, nonvertiginous dizziness also has been associated with vestibular migraine, though this may represent coexisting PPPD. Patients with migraine and episodic or chronic vestibular symptoms frequently have comorbid anxiety (Staab & Ruckenstein, 2007). Anxiety and headache may be so intertwined that it is nearly impossible to separate their effects on the patients' morbidity (Furman et al., 2005). In such cases, clinical experience suggests that treatment of both anxiety and migraine are required to reduce patients' vestibular symptoms.

DIAGNOSIS AND TREATMENT OF PSYCHIATRIC MORBIDITY IN PATIENTS WITH DIZZINESS

The Clinical History, Examination, and Laboratory Findings

Medical and psychiatric diagnoses often coexist in patients with dizziness, but the severity of one does not predict the severity of the other (Best et al., 2006; Jacobson & McCaslin, 2003; Nagarkar, Gupta, & Mann, 2000; Yardley et al., 1992). Therefore, physical and psychiatric symptoms must be evaluated simultaneously, but independently (Best et al., 2006;

Eckhardt et al., 1996; Yardley et al., 1992). Otorhinolaryngologists, neurologists, primary care clinicians, physical therapists, and audiologists bear the primary responsibility for detecting psychiatric morbidity in patients with dizziness because dizzy patients rarely consult psychiatrists or psychologists for their symptoms (Best et al., 2006; Staab, 2006a, 2006b). Fortunately, simple methods exist to help these clinicians detect psychiatric morbidity. These methods can be incorporated into routine office practice with little effort and no formal training.

The clinical history is the best guide to both medical and psychiatric causes of dizziness (Ruckenstein & Staab, 2001; Shepard et al., 2003). When taking a history, three mental notes may help clinicians identify patients with psychiatric illness (Staab, 2006c):

1. Does the patient have an *active* neurotologic condition?
2. Does the neurotologic condition explain *all* of the patient's symptoms?
3. Does the patient have behavioral symptoms indicative of psychiatric morbidity?

The first question helps to separate past and present illnesses, which is especially important in light of research that has revealed the common evolution of acute vertigo into chronic dizziness (e.g., development of PPPD). The second question focuses on comorbidity, which is important for choosing treatment interventions. (Does the patient with Ménière's disease and chronic, nonvertiginous dizziness require gentamicin for Ménière's or sertraline for coexisting PPPD?) The third question helps to identify behavioral symptoms in patients who may not appear to be overtly anxious or depressed. It calls the clinician's attention to anticipatory anxiety, phobic avoidance behaviors, and alterations in activities that may be out of proportion to identifiable vestibular deficits. A compassionate discussion about these symptoms may help patients understand the need for psychiatric interventions.

The physical examination is more likely be positive in patients with acute rather than chronic vestibular symptoms and in those with complaints of vertigo, ataxia, diplopia, or oscillopsia than dizziness, unsteadiness, or vague visual complaints (Guidetti, Monzani, & Civiero, 2002). Therefore, many patients with dizziness-related psychiatric symptoms will have unremarkable neurotologic examinations, except for patients with functional or factitious disorders who may show dramatic findings incompatible with medical illnesses.

Laboratory tests must be interpreted in concert with the clinical history and physical examination findings. For cases in which the history suggests a past or present vestibular insult, evidence of a vestibular lesion (compensated or not) would be expected on balance function tests and the extent of compensation may be a useful guide for therapeutic interventions. If there is no historical evidence of neurotologic illness, then nonspecific test abnormalities should not be overcalled (Best et al., 2006; Shepard et al., 2003; Staab, 2006a, 2006b). Anxiety, migraine, and mild traumatic brain injuries may cause nondiagnostic abnormalities on balance function tests (Staab & Ruckenstein, 2007). Dynamic posturography, including the SOT, is a test of integrated balance function (Furman, 1994). As discussed above, the pattern of low scores across the board suggests the influence of anxiety (Cevette et al., 1995). However, the SOT cannot be used as the basis for diagnosing psychiatric comorbidity. Table 30–6 gives a general guide to the differential diagnosis for PPPD.

Psychiatric Screening Tools

A simple and effective means of detecting psychiatric problems is to have patients with dizziness complete validated questionnaires at home or in the waiting room prior to consultation. Table 30–7 lists several self-report scales that have proven utility in neurotologic settings. The Dizziness Handicap Inventory (DHI) is a widely used self-report for patients with dizziness (Jacobson & Newman, 1990). It contains 25 questions about physical symptoms (P), functional impairment (F), and emotional symptoms (E). Most of the questions on the E subscale are about depression. Some of the problems on the F subscale may be caused by anxiety. These subscales cannot be used to make psychiatric diagnoses, and the total DHI score may be more valid than subscales scores. In our experience, patients may be more likely to acknowledge behavioral problems on the DHI (through total scores >25) than on dedicated anxiety or depression scales, though we employ both in daily practice.

The Hospital Anxiety and Depression Scale (HADS) has seven questions for anxiety and seven for depression (Zigmond & Snaith, 1983). It is self-explanatory, easy to score, and correlates well with formal psychiatric assessments. The HADS has been used in patients with dizziness to screen for anxiety and depression (Grunfeld et al., 2003) and track the progress of medication treatment (Horii et al., 2007). The original Patient Health Questionnaire (PHQ) contained modules that screen for five types of psychiatric disorders (Spitzer, Kroenke, & Williams, 1999). Persoons et al. (2003) validated the anxiety and depression modules in 268 adults with vestibular symptoms. The depression module (PHQ-9) has nine questions. It is easy to score and correlates well with formal psychiatric evaluations. The anxiety module has been supplanted by the Generalized Anxiety Disorder Scale (GAD-7), which is an effective screening tool for anxiety disorders overall, not just generalized anxiety. The PHQ-9 and GAD-7 have become the most common depression and anxiety screeners in primary care, but the HADS remains a fine alternative. It is perfectly reasonable to choose either the combination of the PHQ-9/GAD-7 or the HADS to screen for anxiety and depression in neurotologic, audiologic, and physical therapy practices.

TREATMENT OPTIONS

To date, there have been no large-scale, randomized, controlled trials of medications or other treatments for behavioral morbidity in patients with vestibular symptoms. Researchers continue to examine the benefits of medication, vestibular rehabilitation, and psychotherapy. Table 30–8 lists published trials of each of these interventions, demonstrating the considerable promise of these treatments. In clinical practice, these three therapies may be combined depending on the needs of individual patients, though there no studies of combined treatments.

Medications

Six uncontrolled studies (two case series and four open-label prospective trials) involving 200 patients in the United States and Japan support the use of

Table 30–6. Differential Diagnosis of PPPD With Associated Psychiatric Disorders

	%	Neurotologic and Other Medical Conditions	Anxiety and Depressive Disorders
Primary and secondary anxiety disorders	59.7		
• Primary anxiety disorder	34.2	None	1. Panic/phobic anxiety 2. Generalized anxiety 3. Minor anxiety 4. Major depression
• Secondary anxiety disorder triggered by a precipitating vestibular/balance event	10.1	1. Peripheral vestibular disorders 2. Central vestibular disorders	1. Minor anxiety 2. Panic/phobic anxiety 3. Generalized anxiety 4. Major depression
• Preexisting anxiety disorder exacerbated by a precipitating vestibular/balance event	15.4	1. Peripheral vestibular disorders 2. Central vestibular disorders	1. Generalized anxiety 2. Panic/phobic anxiety 3. Minor anxiety 4. Major depression
CNS illnesses	38.6		
• Migraine	16.5	Vestibular migraine	1. Panic/phobic anxiety 2. Generalized anxiety 3. Minor anxiety 4. No psychiatric diagnosis 5. Major depression
• Traumatic brain injury (TBI)	15.1	1. Mild TBI 2. Moderate TBI	1. Postconcussional syndrome 2. Posttraumatic stress disorder 3. Panic/phobic anxiety 4. Major depression 5. No psychiatric diagnosis
• Dysautonomia	7.0	1. Postural orthostatic tachycardia syndrome (POTS) 2. Neurally mediated reflex (vasovagal) syncope	1. No psychiatric diagnosis 2. Panic/phobic anxiety 3. Generalized anxiety 4. Minor anxiety 5. Major depression
Other medical conditions	1.7		
• Dysrhythmia	1.7	1. Atrial dysrhythmias 2. Ventricular dysrhythmias	1. Panic/phobic anxiety 2. Generalized anxiety 3. No psychiatric diagnosis 4. Major depression
• Adverse drug reaction		1. Side effect of dizziness 2. Allergic reaction with dizziness	
• Debilitating medical illness with serious physical deconditioning		Medical or surgical condition with extended convalescence	

Source: Adapted from Staab and Ruckenstein (2007).

Table 30–7. Questionnaires for Detecting Behavioral Morbidity in Patients With Vestibular Symptoms

Tool	Description	Advantages and Disadvantages
Dizziness Handicap Inventory (DHI)	• 25-item self-report of physical, functional, and emotional symptoms of dizziness • Functional and emotional scales capture behavioral symptoms • Versions in several languages	• Widely employed in dizziness research • Quantitative, can be used to track progress • Total score is more useful than subscales. • Limited correlation with balance function tests
Vertigo Symptom Scale (VSS)	• 36-item self-report with two subscales, a vertigo scale for vestibular symptoms and an autonomic/anxiety scale for anxiety • Versions in several European languages	• Not used as widely as the DHI, but has better psychometric properties. • Subscales correlate with objective measures of vestibular symptoms and standard ratings of psychological symptoms.
Activities-specific Balance Confidence Scale (ABC)	• Self-rated confidence in doing 16 activities of daily living involving movement	• Developed and validated for use in the elderly • Correlates reasonably well with the Dizziness Handicap Inventory and Dynamic Gait Index
Patient Health Questionnaire (PHQ-9)	• Nine-item self-report of depressive symptoms • Validated in many languages	• Identifies significant depressive symptoms • Quantitative, can be used to track progress • *Download free of charge at:* http://www.phqscreeners.com
Generalized Anxiety Disorder Questionnaire (GAD-7)	• Seven-item self-report of various anxiety symptoms, not just generalized anxiety • Validated in many languages	• Identifies significant anxiety symptoms • Quantitative, can be used to track progress • *Download free of charge at:* http://www.phqscreeners.com
Hospital Anxiety and Depression Scale (HADS)	• 14-item self-report of anxiety and depressive symptoms • Validated in many languages	• Identifies clinically significant symptoms • Quantitative, can be used to track progress • *Request permission for use at:* permissions@gl-assessment.co.uk

Source: Reprinted from Staab (2013). Used with permission.

selective serotonin reuptake inhibitors (SSRIs) to treat chronic dizziness and unsteadiness (Horii et al., 2004, 2007; Simon et al., 2005; Goto et al., 2014; Staab et al., 2002, 2004). A synthesis of the findings is that SSRIs are safe and well tolerated by patients with persistent vestibular symptoms, despite dizziness being listed as a common side effect for this class of medications. SSRIs reduced chronic dizziness in patients with CSD (now PPPD) regardless of the severity of coexisting psychiatric illness (Simon et al., 2005; Staab et al., 2002, 2004). Sertraline improved daily dizziness that persisted in three patients after medical-surgical treatment for Ménière's disease (Goto et al., 2014). However, SSRIs were not

Table 30–8. Treatment Studies for Persistent Vestibular Symptoms

Medications		
Selective serotonin reuptake inhibitors (SSRIs)	Staab et al. (2002)	Retrospective case series of 60 patients with chronic dizziness ± anxiety/depression treated with various SSRIs
	Horii et al. (2004)	Prospective open trial of 47 patients with chronic dizziness ± anxiety/depression treated with paroxetine
	Staab et al. (2004)	Prospective open trial of 20 patients with chronic dizziness ± anxiety/depression treated with sertraline
	Simon et al. (2005)	Prospective open trial of five patients with chronic dizziness ± anxiety/depression treated with fluoxetine
	Horii et al. (2007)	Prospective open trial of 60 patients with chronic dizziness ± anxiety/depression treated with fluvoxamine
	Goto, Tsutsumi, & Ogawa (2014)	Case series of three patients with persistent dizziness after treatment for Ménière's disease treated with sertraline
Serotonin-norepinephrine reuptake inhibitors (SSRIs)	Horii et al. (2008)	Prospective open trial of 40 patients with chronic dizziness ± anxiety/depression treated with milnacipran.
	Staab (2011a)	Retrospective case series of 32 patients with CSD (now PPPD) and vestibular migraine ± anxiety disorders treated with venlafaxine

Physical Therapy		
Vestibular and balance rehabilitation therapy (VBRT)	Jacob et al. (2001)	Pilot study of nine patients with persistent dizziness treated with 2 weeks of self-exposure exercises, then 8 to 12 of therapist-directed VBRT
	Yardley et al. (2001)	Randomized study comparing 33 patients with persistent dizziness treated with self-exposure exercises to 43 untreated control subjects with similar symptoms
	Cohen & Kimball (2003)	Comparison of three home-based rehabilitation programs in 53 patients with chronic vestibular symptoms
	Pavlou et al. (2004)	Parallel group study comparing 20 patients with persistent visually induced dizziness treated with VBRT to 20 similar patients treated with VBRT plus desensitization exercises using a visual motion simulator
	Yardley et al. (2004)	Randomized trial of 83 patients with persistent dizziness treated with home-based VBRT directed by primary care nurses versus 87 patients treated with usual primary care
	Meli, Zimatore, Badaracco, De Angelis, & Tufarelli (2007)	Randomized study of 40 patients with chronic vestibular symptoms treated with VBRT versus 40 untreated controls

Psychotherapy		
Cognitive behavioral therapy (CBT)	Johansson et al. (2001)	Study of nine elderly patients with persistent dizziness treated with CBT elements added to VBRT versus 10 patients on a waiting list
	Holmberg et al. (2006)	Parallel group study of 31 patients with PPV (now PPPD) comparing 16 treated with CBT to 15 treated with self-exposure exercises
	Holmberg et al. (2007)	One-year follow-up of the authors' 2006 study
	Edelman et al. (2012)	Single arm trial of 44 patients with evolving CSD (essentially early onset PPPD) treated with CBT
	Mahoney et al. (2013)	Six-month follow-up of the authors' 2012 study

effective for patients with other chronic vestibular symptoms and low levels of anxiety and depression (Horii et al., 2004, 2007; Simon et al., 2005). Studies using serotonin-norepinephrine reuptake inhibitors (SNRIs) yielded similar results (Horii et al., 2008; Staab, 2011a), with the possibility that SNRIs might also benefit patients with vestibular migraine (Staab, 2011a). These findings await conformation by adequately powered, randomized controlled trials.

Vestibular Rehabilitation

Vestibular and balance rehabilitation therapy (VBRT) is now commonly used to improve compensation in patients who have sustained acute vestibular losses, but it was first developed to treat patients with long-standing chronic dizziness, including many who now would be diagnosed with PPPD (Staab, 2011b). Randomized, comparative studies involving more than 400 patients have established VBRT as an effective treatment for chronic vestibular symptoms (see Table 30–8), though the mechanism is likely to be habituation (i.e., systematic desensitization), not compensation. In fact, VBRT was initially called vestibular habituation (Staab, 2011b). When used to habituate chronic vestibular symptoms, VBRT must be started more gently and advanced more slowly than is commonly done to enhance compensation after acute vestibular syndromes. In this manner, VBRT is also effective in reducing comorbid anxiety and depression (Meli et al., 2007).

Psychotherapy

Two sets of studies have investigated the efficacy of a type of psychotherapy called cognitive behavior therapy (CBT) for patients with PPV and CSD (now PPPD). Originally, CBT was developed to treat major depression, but variations on the core techniques have expanded its indications to anxiety, traumatic stress, and somatic symptom disorders as well as several functional conditions. Holmberg et al. (2006) showed that CBT reduced physical symptoms and related functional impairments in patients with chronic PPV, but its benefits did not persist at one year of follow-up (Holmberg et al., 2007). Edelman and colleagues (Edelman et al., 2012; Mahoney et al., 2013) were more successful. They captured patients at about 8 weeks following acute vestibular syndromes, essentially as CSD (now PPPD) was evolving, but not fully established, and showed that a short course of CBT produced rapid benefits (Edelman et al., 2012) that were sustained 6 months later (Mahoney et al., 2013). This suggests that CBT may have prophylactic benefits for patients who demonstrate evidence of emerging PPPD, offering secondary prevention of this chronic condition before it develops completely.

CBT and VBRT are complementary treatments that can be used together clinically. The hope is that CBT will address cognitive patterns that reinforce vestibular symptoms (e.g., "I'll crash the car.") (Yardley et al., 2001), while VBRT will extinguish motion hypersensitivity and improve balance confidence. Pilot studies support this notion (Jacob et al., 2001; Johansson et al., 2001; Pavlou et al., 2004).

CONCLUSIONS

Perceived threats and anxiety have profound effects on balance function in completely normal individuals and patients with vestibular symptoms caused by neurotologic or psychiatric conditions. The threat/anxiety system changes the speed and intensity of postural control movements in response to perceived threats. Anxiety disorders may cause vestibular symptoms in the absence of neurotologic illnesses, while neurotologic illnesses may trigger new anxiety disorders or exacerbate preexisting ones. Patients with temperamental predispositions (neuroticism and introversion) seem to suffer greater physical and psychiatric morbidity in the aftermath of medical or psychiatric triggers of vestibular symptoms than patients without a significant anxiety diathesis. A syndrome of persistent postural-perceptual dizziness (PPPD) may sustain chronic morbidity long after the inciting events have resolved.

The principal barriers to detecting behavioral morbidity in patients with vertigo, unsteadiness, and dizziness are a single-minded focus on the vestibular system as the source of these symptoms and misconceptions about the role of psychological mechanisms in sustaining vestibular complaints. Patients and practitioners frequently share this single-mindedness. With epidemiologic research showing that 30% to 50% of balance patients have psychiatric comorbidity, authors in Asia (Horii et al., 2007), Europe (Best et al., 2006), and the United States (Staab, 2006a, 2006b) have recommended that psychiatric screening become an integral part of neurotologic evaluations for patients presenting with acute or chronic vestibular symptoms. Simple and effective psychiatric screening tools are available for this purpose. Recent data suggest that serotonergic antidepressants, vestibular rehabilitation, and cognitive behavior therapy may alleviate physical and psychiatric morbidity in patients with chronic vestibular symptoms.

REFERENCES

Adkin, A. L., Frank, J. S., & Carpenter, M. G. (2002). Fear of falling modifies anticipatory postural control. *Experimental Brain Research, 143,* 160–170.

Adkin, A. L., Frank, J. S., Carpenter, M. G., & Peysar, G. W. (2000). Postural control is scaled to level of postural threat. *Gait and Posture, 12,* 87–93.

Alessandrini, M., D'Erme, G., Bruno, E., Napolitano, B., & Magrini, A. (2003). Vestibular compensation: Analysis of postural re-arrangement as a control index for unilateral vestibular deficit. *NeuroReport, 14,* 1075–1079.

American Psychiatric Association. (1980). *Diagnostic and statistical manual of mental disorders* (3rd ed.). Washington, DC: Author.

American Psychiatric Association. (1987). *Diagnostic and statistical manual of mental disorders* (3rd ed., Rev.). Washington, DC: Author.

Balaban, C. D., & Jacob, R. G. (2001). Background and history of the interface between anxiety and vertigo. *Journal of Anxiety Disorders, 15,* 27–51.

Best, C., Eckhardt-Henn, A., Diener, G., Bense, S., Breuer, P., & Dieterich, M. (2006). Interaction of somatoform and vestibular disorders. *Journal of Neurology, Neurosurgery, and Psychiatry, 77,* 658–664.

Boleas-Aguirre, M. S., Sánchez-Ferrandiz, N., Guillén-Grima, F., & Perez, N. (2007). Long-term disability of class A patients with Ménière's disease after treatment with intratympanic gentamicin. *Laryngoscope, 117,* 1474–1481.

Brandt, T. (1996). Phobic postural vertigo. *Neurology, 46,* 1515–1519.

Brandt, T., & Dieterich, M. (1986). Phobischer Attacken-Schwank-schwindel, ein neues Syndrom? *Munch Med Wschr, 28,* 247–250.

Brantberg, K., Trees, N., & Baloh, R. W. (2005). Migraine-associated vertigo. *Acta Oto-Laryngologica, 125,* 276–279.

Bronstein, A. M. (1995). Visual vertigo syndrome: Clinical and posturography findings. *Journal of Neurology, Neurosurgery, and Psychiatry, 59,* 472–476.

Bronstein, A. M. (2004). Vision and vertigo: Some visual aspects of vestibular disorders. *Journal of Neurology, 251,* 381–387.

Brown, L. A., Gage, W. H., Polych, M. A., Sleik, R. J., & Winder, T. R. (2002). Central set influences on gait. Age-dependent effects of postural threat. *Experimental Brain Research, 145,* 286–296.

Carpenter, M. G., Adkin, A. L., Brawley, L. R., & Frank, J. S. (2006). Postural, physiological and psychological reactions to challenging balance: Does age make a difference? *Age and Ageing, 35,* 298–303.

Carpenter, M. G., Frank, J. S., Adkin, A. L., Paton, A., & Allum, J. H. (2004). Influence of postural anxiety on postural reactions to multi-directional surface rotations. *Journal of Neurophysiology, 92,* 3255–3265.

Celestino, D., Rosini, E., Carucci, M. L., Marconi, P. L., & Vercillo, E. (2003). Meniere's disease and anxiety disorders. *Acta Otorhinolaryngologica Italica, 23,* 421–427.

Cevette, M. J., Puetz, B., Marion, M. S., Wertz, M. L., & Muenter, M. D. (1995). Aphysiologic performance on dynamic posturography. *Otolaryngology-Head and Neck Surgery, 112,* 676–688.

Clark, D. B., Hirsch, B. E., Smith, M. G., Furman, J. M., & Jacob, R. G. (1994). Panic in otolaryngology patients presenting with dizziness or hearing loss. *American Journal of Psychiatry, 151,* 1223–1225.

Cohen, H. S., & Kimball, K. T. (2003). Increased independence and decreased vertigo after vestibular rehabilitation. *Otolaryngology-Head and Neck Surgery, 128,* 60–70.

Coker, N. J., Coker, R. R., Jenkins, H. A., & Vincent, K. R. (1989). Psychological profile of patients with Meniere's disease. *Archives of Otolaryngology-Head and Neck Surgery, 115,* 1355–1357.

Cousins, S., Cutfield, N. J., Kaski, D., Palla, A., Seemungal, B. M., Golding, J. F., . . . Bronstein, A. M. (2014). Visual dependency and dizziness after vestibular neuritis. *PLoS One, 9*(9), e105426. doi:10.1371/journal.pone.0105426

Eagger, S., Luxon, L. M., Davies, R. A., Coelho, A., & Ron, M. A. (1992). Psychiatric morbidity in patients with peripheral vestibular disorder: A clinical and neuro-otological study. *Journal of Neurology, Neurosurgery, and Psychiatry, 55,* 383–387.

Eckhardt, A., Tettenborn, B., Krauthauser, H., Thomalske, C., Hartmann, O., Hoffmann, S. O., & Hopf, H. C. (1996). Vertigo and anxiety disorders—Results of interdisciplinary evaluation. *Laryngorhinootologie, 75,* 517–522.

Eckhardt-Henn, A., Breuer, P., Thomalske, C., Hoffmann, S. O., & Hopf, H. C. (2003). Anxiety disorders and other psychiatric subgroups in patients complaining of dizziness. *Journal of Anxiety Disorders, 17,* 369–388.

Edelman, S., Mahoney, A. E., & Cremer, P. D. (2012). Cognitive behavior therapy for chronic subjective dizziness: A randomized, controlled trial. *American Journal of Otolaryngology, 33*(4), 395–401.

Evans, D. L., Staab, J. P., Petitto, J. M., Morrison, M. F., Szuba, M. P., Ward, H. E., . . . O'Reardon, J. P. (1999). Depression in the medical setting: Biopsychological interactions and treatment considerations. *Journal of Clinical Psychiatry, 60*(Suppl. 4), 40–55.

Fox, N. A., Henderson, H. A., Marshall, P. J., Nichols, K. E., & Ghera, M. M. (2005). Behavioral inhibition: Linking biology and behavior within a developmental framework. *Annual Review of Psychology, 56,* 235–262.

Furman, J. M. (1994). Posturography: Uses and limitations. *Baillieres Clinical Neurology, 3,* 501–513.

Furman, J. M., Balaban, C. D., Jacob, R. G., & Marcus, D. A. (2005). Migraine-anxiety related dizziness (MARD): A new disorder? *Journal of Neurology, Neurosurgery, and Psychiatry, 76,* 1–8.

Furman, J. M., & Jacob, R. G. (2001). A clinical taxonomy of dizziness and anxiety in the otoneurological setting. *Journal of Anxiety Disorders, 15,* 9–26.

Furman, J. M., Redfern, M. S., & Jacob, R. G. (2006). Vestibulo-ocular function in anxiety disorders. *Journal of Vestibular Research, 16,* 209–215.

Gage, W. H., Sleik, R. J., Polych, M. A., McKenzie, N. C., & Brown, L. A. (2003). The allocation of attention during locomotion is altered by anxiety. *Experimental Brain Research, 150,* 385–394.

Gianoli, G., McWilliams, S., Soileau, J., & Belafsky, P. (2000). Posturographic performance in patients with the potential for secondary gain. *Otolaryngology-Head and Neck Surgery, 122,* 11–18.

Godemann, F., Koffroth, C., Neu, P., & Heuser, I. (2004). Why does vertigo become chronic after neuropathia vestibularis? *Psychosomatic Medicine, 66,* 783–787.

Godemann, F., Schabowska, A., Naetebusch, B., Heinz, A., & Strohle, A. (2006). The impact of cognitions on the development of panic and somatoform disorders: A prospective study in patients with vestibular neuritis. *Psychological Medicine, 36,* 99–108.

Godemann, F., Siefert, K., Hantschke-Bruggemann, M., Neu, P., Seidl, R., & Strohle, A. (2005). What accounts for vertigo one year after neuritis vestibularis—Anxiety or a dysfunctional vestibular organ? *Journal of Psychiatric Research, 39,* 529–534.

Goebel, J. A., Sataloff, R. T., Hanson, J. M., Nashner, L. M., Hirshout, D. S., & Sokolow, C. C. (1997). Posturographic evidence of nonorganic sway patterns in normal subjects, patients, and suspected malingerers. *Otolaryngology-Head and Neck Surgery, 117,* 293–302.

Goto, F., Tsutsumi, T., & Ogawa, K. (2014). Successful treatment of relapsed Ménière's disease using selective serotonin reuptake inhibitors: A report of three cases. *Experimental and Therapeutic Medicine, 7*(2), 488–490.

Grunfeld, E. A., Gresty, M. A., Bronstein, A. M., & Jahanshahi, M. (2003). Screening for depression among neuro-otology patients with and without identifiable vestibular lesions. *International Journal of Audiology, 42,* 161–165.

Guerraz, M., Yardley, L., Bertholon, P., Pollak, L., Rudge, P., Gresty, M. A., & Bronstein, A. M. (2001). Visual vertigo: Symptom assessment, spatial orientation and postural control. *Brain. 124*(Pt. 8), 1646–1656.

Guidetti, G., Monzani, D., & Civiero, N. (2002). Head-shaking nystagmus in the follow-up of patients with vestibular diseases. *Clinical Otolaryngology, 27,* 124–128.

Hainaut, J. P., Caillet, G., Lestienne, F. G., & Bolmont, B. (2011). The role of trait anxiety on static balance performance in control and anxiogenic situations. *Gait and Posture. 33*(4), 604–608.

Heinrichs, N., Edler, C., Eskens, S., Mielczarek, M. M., & Moschner, C. (2007). Predicting continued dizziness after an acute peripheral vestibular disorder. *Psychosomatic Medicine, 69,* 700–707.

Hoffman, D. L., O'Leary, D. P., & Munjack, D. J. (1994). Autorotation test abnormalities of the horizontal and vertical vestibulo-ocular reflexes in panic disorder. *Otolaryngology-Head and Neck Surgery, 110,* 259–269.

Holmberg, J., Karlberg, M., Harlacher, U., & Magnusson, M. (2007). One-year follow-up of cognitive behavioral therapy for phobic postural vertigo. *Journal of Neurology. 254,* 1189–1192.

Holmberg, J., Karlberg, M., Harlacher, U., Rivano-Fischer, M., & Magnusson, M. (2006). Treatment of phobic postural vertigo: A controlled study of cognitive-behavioral therapy and self-controlled desensitization. *Journal of Neurology, 253,* 500–506.

Honaker, J. A., Gilbert, J. M., & Staab, J. P. (2010). Chronic subjective dizziness versus conversion disorder: Discussion of clinical findings and rehabilitation. *American Journal of Audiology, 19,* 3–8.

Horii, A., Kitahara, T., Masumura, C., Kizawa, K., Maekawa, C., & Kubo, T. (2008). *Effects of milnacipran, a serotonin noradrenaline reuptake inhibitor (SNRI) on subjective handicaps and posturography in dizzy patients.* Abstracts from the XXVth Congress of the Bárány Society, Kyoto, Japan. Retrieved July 9, 2011, from http://www.acplan.jp/barany2008

Horii, A., Mitani, K., Kitahara, T., Uno, A., Takeda, N., & Kubo, T. (2004). Paroxetine, a selective serotonin reuptake inhibitor, reduces depressive symptoms and subjective handicaps in patients with dizziness. *Otology and Neurotology, 25,* 536–543.

Horii, A., Uno, A., Kitahara, T., Mitani, K., Masumura, C., Kizawa, K. & Kubo, T. (2007). Effects of fluvoxamine on anxiety, depression, and subjective handicaps of chronic dizziness patients with or without neuro-otologic diseases. *Journal of Vestibular Research, 17,* 1–8.

Huppert, D., Strupp, M., Rettinger, N., Hecht, J., & Brandt, T. (2005). Phobic postural vertigo—A long-term follow-up (5 to 15 years) of 106 patients. *Journal of Neurology, 252,* 564–569.

Indovina, I., Riccelli, R., Staab, J. P., Lacquaniti, F., & Passamonti, L. (2014). Personality traits modulate subcortical and cortical vestibular and anxiety responses to sound-evoked otolithic receptor stimulation. *Journal of Psychosomatic Research.* doi:10.1016/j.jpsychores.2014.09.005

Jacob, R. G., Furman, J. M., Durrant, J. D., & Turner, S. M. (1996). Panic, agoraphobia, and vestibular dysfunction. *American Journal of Psychiatry, 153,* 503–512.

Jacob, R. G., Furman, J. M., Durrant, J. D., & Turner, S. M. (1997). Surface dependence: A balance control strategy in panic disorder with agoraphobia. *Psychosomatic Medicine, 59,* 323–330.

Jacob, R. G., Redfern, M. S., & Furman, J. M. (2009). Space and motion discomfort and abnormal balance control in patients with anxiety disorders. *Journal of Neurology, Neurosurgery, and Psychiatry, 80*(1), 74–78.

Jacob, R. G., Whitney, S. L., Detweiler-Shostak, G., & Furman, J. M. (2001). Vestibular rehabilitation for patients with agoraphobia and vestibular dysfunction: A pilot study. *Journal of Anxiety Disorders, 15,* 131–146.

Jacob, R. G., Woody, S. R., Clark, D. B., Lilienfeld, S. O., Hirsch, B. E., Kucera, G. D., . . . Durrant, J. D. (1993). Discomfort with space and motion: A possible marker of vestibular dysfunction assessed by the Situational Characteristics Questionnaire. *Journal of Psychopathology and Behavioral Assessment, 15,* 299–324.

Jacobson, G. P., & McCaslin, D. L. (2003). Agreement between functional and electrophysiologic measures in patients with unilateral peripheral vestibular system impairment. *Journal of the American Academy of Audiology, 14,* 231–238.

Jacobson, G. P., & Newman, C. W. (1990). The development of the Dizziness Handicap Inventory. *Archives of Otolaryngology-Head and Neck Surgery, 116,* 424–427.

Johansson, M., Akerlund, D., Larsen, H. C., & Andersson, G. (2001). Randomized controlled trial of vestibular rehabilitation combined with cognitive-behavioral therapy for dizziness in older people. *Otolaryngology-Head and Neck Surgery, 125,* 151–156.

Kalin NH. (2004). Studying non-human primates: A gateway to understanding anxiety disorders. *Psychopharmacology Bulletin, 38,* 8–13.

Kammerlind, A. S., Ledin, T. E., Skargren, E. I., & Odkvist, L. M. (2005). Long-term follow-up after acute unilateral vestibular loss and comparison between subjects with and without remaining symptoms. *Acta Oto-Laryngologica (Stockholm), 125,* 946–953.

Kapfhammer, H. P., Mayer, C., Hock, U., Huppert, D., Dieterich, M., & Brandt, T. (1997). Course of illness in phobic postural vertigo. *Acta Neurologica Scandinavica, 95,* 23–28.

Krafczyk, S., Schlamp, V., Dieterich, M., Haberhauer, P., & Brandt, T. (1999). Increased body sway at 3.5–8 Hz in patients with phobic postural vertigo. *Neuroscience Letters, 259,* 149–152.

Kuch, K., & Swinson, R. P. (1992). Agoraphobia: What Westphal really said. *Canadian Journal of Psychiatry, 37,* 133–136.

Mahoney, A. E. J., Edelman, S., & Cremer, P. D. (2013). Cognitive behavior therapy for chronic subjective dizziness: Longer-term gains and predictors of disability. *American Journal of Otolaryngology, 34*(2), 115–120.

Meli, A., Zimatore, G., Badaracco, C., De Angelis, E., & Tufarelli, D. (2007). Effects of vestibular rehabilitation therapy on emotional aspects in chronic vestibular patients. *Journal of Psychosomatic Research, 63,* 185–190.

Monzani, D., Marchioni, D., Bonetti, S., Pellacani, P., Casolari, L., Rigatelli, M., & Presutti, L. (2004). Anxiety affects vestibulospinal function of labyrinthine-defective patients during horizontal optokinetic stimulation. *Acta Otorhinolaryngologica Italica, 24,* 117–124.

Morgan, S. S., Beck, W. G., & Dobie, R. A. (2002). Can posturography identify informed malingerers? *Otology and Neurotology, 23,* 214–217.

Nagarkar, A. N., Gupta, A. K., & Mann, S. B. (2000). Psychological findings in benign paroxysmal positional vertigo and psychogenic vertigo. *Journal of Otolaryngology, 29,* 154–158.

Ohno, H., Wada, M., Saitoh, J., Sunaga, N., & Nagai, M. (2004). The effect of anxiety on postural control in humans depends on visual information processing. *Neuroscience Letters, 364,* 37–39.

Onuki, J., Takahashi, M., Odagiri, K., Wada, R., & Sato, R. (2005). Comprative study of the daily lifestyle of patients with Meniere's disease and controls. *Annals of Otology, Rhinology, and Laryngology, 114,* 927–933.

Pavlou, M., Lingeswaran, A., Davies, R. A., Gresty, M. A., & Bronstein, A. M. (2004). Simulator based rehabilitation in refractory dizziness. *Journal of Neurology, 251,* 983–995.

Perna, G., Dario, A., Caldirola, D., Stefania, B., Cesarani, A., & Bellodi, L. (2001). Panic disorder: The role of the balance system. *Journal of Psychiatric Research, 35,* 279–286.

Perna, G., Alpini, D., Caldirola, D., Raponi, G., Cesarani, A., & Bellodi, L. (2003). Serotonergic modulation of the balance system in panic disorder: An open study. *Depression and Anxiety, 17*, 101–106.

Persoons, P., Luyckx, K., Desloovere, C., Vandenberghe, J., & Fischler, B. (2003). Anxiety and mood disorders in otorhinolaryngology outpatients presenting with dizziness: Validation of the self-administered PRIME-MD Patient Health Questionnaire and epidemiology. *General Hospital Psychiatry, 25*, 316–323.

Querner, V., Krafczyk, S., Dieterich, M., & Brandt, T. (2000). Patients with somatoform phobic postural vertigo: The more difficult the balance task, the better the balance performance. *Neuroscience Letters, 285*, 21–24.

Redfern, M. S., Furman, J. M., & Jacob, R. G. (2007). Visually induced postural sway in anxiety disorders. *Journal of Anxiety Disorders, 21*(5), 704–716.

Ruckenstein, M. J., & Staab, J. P. (2001). The Basic Symptom Inventory-53 and its use in the management of patients with psychogenic dizziness. *Otolaryngology-Head and Neck Surgery, 125*, 533–556.

Savastano, M., Maron, M. B., Mangialaio, M., Longhi, P., & Rizzardo, R. (1996). Illness behaviour, personality traits, anxiety, and depression in patients with Meniere's disease. *Journal of Otolaryngology. 25*, 329–333.

Shepard, N. T., Solomon, D., Ruckenstein, M., & Staab, J. (2003). Evaluation of the vestibular (balance) system. In J. B. Snow & J. J. Ballenger (Eds.), *Ballenger's otorhinolaryngology head and neck surgery* (16th ed., pp. 161–194). Hamilton, Ontario, Canada: B. C. Decker.

Simon, N. M., Parker, S. W., Wernick-Robinson, M., Oppenheimer, J. E., Hoge, E. A., Worthington, J. J., . . . Pollack, M. H. (2005). Fluoxetine for vestibular dysfunction and anxiety: A prospective pilot study. *Psychosomatics. 46*, 334–339.

Sklare, D. A., Stein, M. B., Pikus, A. M., & Uhde, T. W. (1990). Dysequilibrium and audiovestibular function in panic disorder: Symptom profiles and test findings. *American Journal of Otology, 11*, 338–341.

Söderman, A. C., Bagger-Sjöbäck, D., Bergenius, J., & Langius, A. (2002). Factors influencing quality of life in patients with Ménière's disease, identified by a multidimensional approach. *Otology & Neurotology, 23*(6), 941–948.

Spitzer, R. L., Kroenke, K., & Williams, J. B. (1999). Validation and utility of a self-report version of PRIME-MD: The PHQ Primary Care Study. *JAMA, 282*, 1737–1744.

Staab, J. P. (2006a). Chronic dizziness: The interface between psychiatry and neuro-otology. *Current Opinion in Neurology, 19*, 41–48.

Staab, J. P. (2006b). Assessment and management of psychological problems in the dizzy patient. *Continuum: Lifelong Learning in Neurology, 12*, 189–213.

Staab, J. P. (2006c). Anxiety and depression in older patients with otorhinolaryngologic illnesses. In K. Calhoun, D.

E. Eibling, M. K. Wax, & K. Kost (Eds.), *Geriatric otolaryngology* (pp. 633–646). New York, NY: Marcel Dekker.

Staab, J. P. (2011a). Clinical clues to a dizzying headache. *Journal of Vestibular Research, 21*(6), 331–340.

Staab, J. P. (2011b). Behavioral aspects of vestibular rehabilitation. *NeuroRehabilitation, 29*(2), 179–183.

Staab, J. P. (2012). Chronic subjective dizziness. *Continuum (Minneapolis, Minnesota), 18*(5 Neuro-otology), 1118–1141.

Staab, J. P. (2013). Behavioural neuro-otology. In A. M. Bronstein (Ed.), *Oxford textbook of vertigo and imbalance* (pp. 333–346). New York, NY: Oxford University Press.

Staab, J., Eggers, S., Neff, B., & Shepard, N. (2010). Validation of a clinical syndrome of persistent dizziness and unsteadiness. Abstracts from the XXVI Bárány Society Meeting, Reykjavik, Iceland, August 18–21, 2010. *Journal of Vestibular Research, 20*(3–4), 172–173.

Staab, J. P., Rohe, D. E., Eggers, S. D., & Shepard, N. T. (2014). Anxious, introverted personality traits in patients with chronic subjective dizziness. *Journal of Psychosomatic Research, 76*(1), 80–83.

Staab, J. P., & Ruckenstein, M. J. (2003). Which comes first? Psychogenic dizziness versus otogenic anxiety. *Laryngoscope, 113*, 1714–1718.

Staab, J. P., & Ruckenstein, M. J. (2005). Chronic dizziness and anxiety: Effect of course of illness on treatment outcome. *Archives of Otolaryngology-Head and Neck Surgery, 131*, 675–679.

Staab, J. P., & Ruckenstein, M. J. (2007). Expanding the differential diagnosis of dizziness. *Archives of Otolaryngology-Head and Neck Surgery, 13*, 170–176.

Staab, J. P., Ruckenstein, M. J., & Amsterdam, J. D. (2004). A prospective trial of sertraline for chronic subjective dizziness. *Laryngoscope, 114*, 1637–1641.

Staab, J. P., Ruckenstein, M. J., Solomon, D., & Shepard, N. T. (2002). Serotonin reuptake inhibitors for dizziness with psychiatric symptoms. *Archives of Otolaryngology-Head and Neck Surgery, 128*, 554–560.

Stein, M. B., Asmundson, G. J. G., Ireland, D., & Walker, J. R. (1994). Panic disorder in patients attending a clinic for vestibular disorders. *American Journal of Psychiatry, 151*, 1697–1700.

Swinson, R. P., Cox, B. J., Rutka, J., Mai, M., Kerr, S., & Kuch, K. (1993). Otoneurological functioning in panic disorder patients with prominent dizziness. *Comprehensive Psychiatry, 34*, 127–129.

Takahashi, M., Ishida, K., Iida, M., Yamashita, H., & Sugawara, K. (2001). Analysis of lifestyle and behavioral characteristics in Meniere's disease patients and a control population. *Acta Oto-Laryngologica (Stockholm), 121*, 254–256.

Tecer, A., Tukel, R., Erdamar, B., & Sunay, T. (2004). Audiovestibular functioning in patients with panic disorder. *Journal of Psychosomatic Research, 57*, 177–182.

Tschan, R., Best, C., Beutel, M. E., Knebel, A., Wiltink, J., Dieterich, M., & Eckhardt-Henn, A. (2011). Patients' psychological well-being and resilient coping protect from secondary somatoform vertigo and dizziness (SVD) 1 year after vestibular disease. *Journal of Neurology, 258*, 104–112.

Viaud-Delmon, I., Ivanenko, Y. P., Berthoz, A., & Jouvent, R. (2000a). Adaptation as a sensorial profile in trait anxiety: A study with virtual reality. *Journal of Anxiety Disorders, 14*, 583–601.

Viaud-Delmon, I., Siegler, I., Israel, I., Jouvent, R., & Berthoz, A. (2000b). Eye deviation during rotation in darkness in trait anxiety: An early expression of perceptual avoidance? *Biological Psychiatry, 47*, 112–118.

Wada, M., Sunaga, N., & Nagai, M. (2001). Anxiety affects the postural sway of the antero-posterior axis in college students. *Neuroscience Letters, 302*, 157–159.

World Health Organization. (2014). *International classification of diseases* (11th ed., ICD-11 Beta draft). Retrieved August 22, 2014 from apps.who.int/classifications/icd11/browse/f/en

Yardley, L., Beech, S., & Weinman, J. (2001). Influence of beliefs about the consequences of dizziness on handicap in people with dizziness, and the effect of therapy on beliefs. *Journal of Psychosomatic Research, 50*, 1–6.

Yardley, I.., Britton, J., Lear, S., Bird, J., & Luxon, L. M. (1995a). Relationship between balance system function and agoraphobic avoidance. *Behavior Research and Therapy, 33*, 435–439.

Yardley, L., Donovan-Hall, M., Smith, H. E., Walsh, B. M., Mullee, M., & Bronstein, A. M. (2004). Effectiveness of primary care-based vestibular rehabilitation for chronic dizziness. *Annals of Internal Medicine, 141*, 598–605.

Yardley, L., Luxon, L. M., & Haacke, N. P. (1994). A longitudinal study of symptoms, anxiety and subjective well-being in patients with vertigo. *Clinical Otolaryngology and Allied Sciences, 19*, 109–116.

Yardley, L., Verschuur, C., Masson, E., Luxon, L., & Haacke, N. (1992). Somatic and psychological factors contributing to handicap in people with vertigo. *British Journal of Audiology, 26*, 283–290.

Yardley, L., Watson, S., Britton, J., Lear, S., & Bird, J. (1995b). Effects of anxiety arousal and mental stress on the vestibulo-ocular reflex. *Acta Oto-Laryngologica, 115*, 597–602.

Zigmond, A. S., & Snaith, R. P. (1983). The Hospital Anxiety and Depression Scale. *Acta Psychiatrica Scandinavica, 67*, 361–370.

Vestibular Rehabilitation

Susan L. Whitney and Joseph M. Furman

OVERVIEW

Vestibular rehabilitation is increasingly becoming an indispensable treatment modality for patients with dizziness and/or balance problems. Vestibular rehabilitation has taken on many forms over the years, from a group exercise class in the 1940s (Cawthorne, 1944; Cooksey, 1946) to its present form where people receive a customized exercise program (Herdman, 2000; Pavlou, Lingeswaran, Davies, Gresty, & Bronstein, 2004; Shepard & Telian, 1995). This chapter provides an overview of the history of vestibular rehabilitation, what types of patients might be aided with a rehabilitation program, some basic principles of vestibular rehabilitation, and the typical outcomes from vestibular rehabilitation including the positive and negative predictors of success.

Vestibular rehabilitation was first described in the 1940s by Cooksey and Cawthorne (Cawthorne, 1944; Cooksey, 1946), who developed and published their description of a group exercise program that was designed to decrease dizziness in persons with vestibular dysfunction from head injuries (postconcussion disorder and other cases of "giddiness") (Cawthorne, 1944). Cawthorne (1944) noted that their exercise program was effective following postconcussion and with unilateral peripheral vestibular hypofunction.

Cawthorne (1944) suggested that vestibular disorders can cause people to limit their activities of daily living and also cause people to restrict their activities outside the home (e.g., work activities).

Cawthorne's (1944) group exercise program incorporated eye-head exercises designed to stimulate the semicircular canals and the otolith organs. Exercise was started early after onset of symptoms (i.e., as soon as it was deemed "safe"). Exercises were prescribed that gradually became faster and more difficult as the person improved. Patients participated in the Cawthorne group exercise program between 10 days up to a month with the exercise program encompassing the "entire day" (Cawthorne, 1944).

Ironically, parts of the Cawthorne-Cooksey exercise program today would be considered dangerous (Table 31–1). The original group exercise program had advanced patients walking up and down steps and ladders with eyes closed (Cawthorne, 1944; Cooksey, 1946).

Cawthorne (1944) and Dix (1976) advocated that persons had better outcomes if seen early after vestibular insult, a thought supported by recent findings (Bamiou, Davies, McKee, & Luxon, 2000). Both Cawthorne (1944) and Cooksey (1946) suggested a gradually more difficult program of mental exercise and physical and occupational therapy in their program that occupied their entire day. Exercises generally started in supine position and progressed to walking with eyes open and closed. Mental exercises were incorporated 1 hr a day, and in occupational therapy, patients were advised to progress to perform their exercises in crowded or noisy circumstances. "Mental exercises" are not generally used today but all patients are encouraged to progress their exercise program in more visually challenging environments, such as crowded or visually stimulating

Table 31–1. Cawthorne-Cooksey Exercises as Adapted by Dix

(A) In bed	(1) Eye movements—at first slow, then quick,
	   (a) up and down,
	   (b) from side to side, and
	   (c) focusing on finger movement from 3 feet to 1 foot away from face.
	
	 (2) Head movements at first slow, then quick; later with eyes closed,
	   (a) bending forward and backward, and
	   (b) turning from side to side.

(B) Sitting (in class)	(1) and (2) as in (A) (3) Shoulder shrugging and circling (4) Bending forward and picking up objects from the ground
(C) Standing (in class)	(1) Exercises (1) and (2) in (A), and (3) in (B) (2) Changing from sitting to standing position with EO and EC (3) Throwing a small ball from hand to hand (above eye level) (4) Throwing a ball from hand to hand under knee (5) Change from sitting to standing and turning round in between
(D) Moving about (in class)	(1) Circle round center person who will throw a large ball and return it (2) Walk across the room with EO and EC (3) Walk up and down slope with EO and EC (4) Walk up and down steps with EO and EC (5) Any game involving stooping or stretching and aiming such as skittles, bowls, or basketball

Note. EO = eyes open; EC = eyes closed.
Source: Reproduced from Dix, M. R. The physiological basis and practical value of head exercises in the treatment of vertigo. *Practitioner* 1976;(217):919–924. Reprinted with permission from Practitioner Medical Publishing Ltd.

situations as they improve. Dual-tasking is commonly incorporated into exercise programs of persons who are at less risk for falling (Lei-Rivera, Sutera, Galatioto, Hujsak, & Gurley, 2013). Cawthorne (1944) also advocated performing the exercises preoperatively so that patients were familiar with the exercises prior to surgery (Cawthorne, 1944), which has recently been supported in the literature prior to inner ear surgery (Magnusson et al., 2009; Magnusson, Karlberg, & Tjernstrom, 2011).

Cooksey suggested that the exercise programs were both physical and psychological (Cooksey, 1946). Recently, there have been links established between anxiety and vestibular disorders (Balaban & Thayer, 2001; Beidel & Horak, 2001; Eagger, Luxon, Davies, Coelho, & Ron, 1992; Guerraz et al., 2001; Gurr & Moffat, 2001; Holmberg, Karlberg, Harlacher, Rivano-Fischer, & Magnusson, 2006; R. G.

Jacob & Furman, 2001; R. G. Jacob, Whitney, Detweiler-Shostak, & Furman, 2001; Nagaratnam, Ip, & Bou-Haidar, 2005; Nagarkar, Gupta, & Mann, 2000; Pollak, Klein, Rafael, Vera, & Rabey, 2003; Sklare, Konrad, Maser, & Jacob, 2001; Yardley, 1994; Yardley, Luxon, & Haacke, 1994; Yardley & Putman, 1992; Yardley & Redfern, 2001). Studies also support the connections between the vestibular system and the autonomic nervous system (Balaban, 1999; Balaban & Porter, 1998; Balaban & Thayer, 2001), suggesting that there is an anatomic link between the vestibular apparatus and the regulation of blood pressure and breathing (Yates, 1996; Yates, Billig, Cotter, Mori, & Card, 2002; Yates & Bronstein, 2005).

Most of the original ideas of Cooksey and Cawthorne are in use today in some form, although walking up slopes and stair climbing with eyes closed is not done in the United States. Group exercises are not typically performed because it is very difficult to organize groups of persons with similar complaints. Due to safety considerations, walking with eyes closed on any surface is performed with extreme caution and only with highly advanced patients. Eye/head exercises are performed with almost every person with vestibular dysfunction, as suggested by Cooksey and Cawthorne and their general principles of gradually increasing the difficulty and the speed of the activity appear to have been incorporated into all exercise programs used to address vestibular dysfunction.

Dix (1976) suggested that people with head injuries, drug intoxication, and those with psychogenic dizziness were good candidates for rehabilitation. Dix (1976) was the first to describe the typical "stiff" gait that patients with vestibular disorders display, especially the difficulty with turning their trunk during gait. Fatigue was also described by Dix (1976), which is a common complication of vestibular disorders. Fatigue, especially at the end of the day for the patient, can complicate their rehabilitation progress. The original exercises that Dix (1976) suggested for a home exercise program were performed for 5 min, three times a day for up to 1 to 3 months until the symptoms resolved (Dix, 1976).

Today, it is commonly thought that exercise may need to be "dosed" in smaller quantities for the patient to be compliant with the exercise program. If exercises are done all at one time, the patient may feel worse, which is a negative factor related to exercise compliance.

Norré and DeWeerdt (1981) suggested that habituation therapy might help to provoke dizziness and remediate dizziness symptoms in persons with vestibular disorders. Patients were asked to move into the dizziness provocative positions to decrease the intensity of the response. Differences in their program compared to the Cooksey-Cawthorne program were that their program was individualized and only patients with motion provoked symptoms were included. Thirty-four different positions were tested and the number of provocative positions decreased by over 50% within a 2-month period (Norre & DeWeerdt, 1981). Fifty-three percent of the patients were symptom-free with 92% reporting at least partial improvement in symptoms.

The Brandt-Daroff exercise was also developed in the 1980s to treat patients with motion-provoked

dizziness (Brandt & Daroff, 1980). Brandt and Daroff suggested that people perform the exercise two times each day for at least 10 repetitions while they were hospitalized for up to 14 days. A 99% positive response rate was reported from the exercise with complete resolution of the patient's BPPV.

Norré and Beckers later suggested that vestibular exercises needed to be customized based on their findings after developing a measure to record symptoms in 19 provocative positions (Norré & Beckers, 1988). Patients selectively had symptoms only in some of the positions tested, and Norré and Beckers suggested that the exercise program needed to be customized to meet the patient's needs (Norre & Beckers, 1988). Norré and Beckers recorded the intensity and duration of symptoms after passive head movements and treated patients based on the specific deficits that they identified in their provocative movement testing. Active exercise was performed at home five times daily. Norre (1987) later reported that his individualized exercise program of habituation exercises was more effective in the reduction of symptoms than a general exercise program. (Norre, 1987)

McCabe (1970) suggested that patients with unstable vestibular disorders are not good candidates for rehabilitation, which is still true 44 years later. He reported on 15 years of experience with vestibular rehabilitation and stated the following patient diagnoses benefited from exercises: central and peripheral postural vertigo, the "irritable labyrinth" with motion intolerance, labyrinthitis, temporal bone fracture, traumatic vertigo, destructive labyrinthectomy, and Wallenberg's syndrome (McCabe, 1970). He reported that drugs used to mask symptoms appeared to prevent or slow the recovery process.

Horak, Jones-Rycewicz, Black, and Shumway-Cook (1992) subsequently attempted to determine if medication to suppress dizziness, a general conditioning program, or a vestibular rehabilitation program would be more effective in decreasing symptoms and enhancing postural control in persons with chronic vestibular hypofunction. Patients were treated twice a week for 6 weeks and there were improvements in dizziness in all groups. The only group that demonstrated changes in balance was the vestibular rehabilitation group (Horak et al., 1992). Most studies have demonstrated changes in postural control after vestibular rehabilitation (Asai, Watanabe, & Shimizu, 1997; Bamiou et al., 2000; Brown, Whitney, Wrisley, & Furman, 2001; Cass, Borello-France, & Furman, 1996; Clendaniel & Tucci, 1997; Cohen & Kimball, 2004b; Cowand, Wrisley, Walker, Strasnick, & Jacobson, 1998; Di Fabio, 1995; el Kashlan, Shepard, Asher, Smith-Wheelock, & Telian, 1998; Gill-Body & Krebs, 1994; Gottshall, Hoffer, Moore, & Balough, 2005; Gurr & Moffat, 2001; Jacob et al., 2001; Konrad et al., 1992; Krebs, Gillbody, Riley, & Parker, 1993; Medeiros et al., 2005; Meli, Zimatore, Badaracco, De Angelis, & Tufarelli, 2006; Pavlou et al., 2004; Shepard & Telian, 1995; Smith-Wheelock, Shepard, & Telian, 1991; Suarez et al., 2003; Telian, Shepard, Smith-Wheelock, & Hoberg, 1991; Viirre & Sitarz, 2002).

More recent studies have supported the use of vestibular rehabilitation in persons with both peripheral and central vestibular disorders. There is much more evidence for the use of vestibular rehabilitation in persons with peripheral vestibular hypofunction than any other vestibular condition, primarily because they are the easiest group to study and also because it is a common diagnostic category (Hillier & McDonnell, 2011). There is much more heterogeneity in central vestibular disorders, making it more difficult to study this group (Furman & Whitney, 2000).

THEORETICAL CONSIDERATIONS

Vestibular Compensation and Recovery

Patients with vestibular disorders often experience dizziness, vertigo, motion sickness, nausea, vomiting, difficulty with their vision, and difficulty with walking especially with head movements. It is not understood why some patients have all of the above symptoms and others only have a few.

Time to recovery of function can vary from person to person, suggesting that there are many factors that affect recovery of function. Patients seem to recover from (i.e., compensate for) unilateral vestibular loss through movement, possibly via the brain's ability to suppress the aberrant signal from the involved ear and the uncontrolled excitation from the intact ear. Central nervous system plasticity

seems the most likely basis of recovery. For example, with a unilateral vestibular abnormality, VOR gain partially recovers over time, though never reaches its prelesion function, especially at high velocities of head movement (Curthoys & Halmagyi, 1995). A study by Bowman supports the concept of only partial recovery in persons with vestibular disorders; persons who have compensated well for a unilateral vestibular disorder continued to have functional deficits when queried (Bowman, 2004).

Disorders of the cerebellum affect recovery. An intact cerebellar flocculus is important for vestibular adaptation to occur (Courjon, Flandrin, Jeannerod, & Schmid, 1982; Furman, Balaban, & Pollack, 1997).

Vestibular adaptation is thought to be context specific (Zee, 2000); hence, exercise is often performed in various positions and in different environmental contexts and velocities. Smooth pursuit most likely stabilizes gaze at slower speeds. An error signal induces vestibular adaptation via slipping of the image on the retina during head movement (Zee, 2000).

Visual stimulation appears to be critical for adapting the dynamic VOR. Zee (2000) reports that there is no increase in VOR gain if the person is not exposed to light. Beyond light exposure and movement, there is some emerging evidence of neural "rewiring" within the CNS after insult. The concept of neural sprouting (a form of plasticity) as a result of the sensory experiences from movement after a vestibular insult has been postulated as a mechanism for recovery (Dieringer, 1995).

Sensory substitution is used to aid in the rehabilitation process. Patients are taught to use vision, somatosensation, and the signals remaining from the intact labyrinth to aid in the recovery process. Patients are instructed to use predictive saccades and the visual pursuit system to compensate for bilateral vestibular loss. Through practice, patients can learn to increase smooth pursuit gain (Herdman, 1998) or to generate saccades to decrease the visual blurring that occurs with fast head movements (Berthoz, 1988; Schubert & Zee, 2010).

The cervico-ocular reflex (COR)—that is, eye movements elicited by changes in the position of the head on the torso—is sometimes utilized to attempt to substitute for the loss of VOR function, even though it appears that not all people may be able to utilize this reflex response (Schubert, Das, Tusa, & Herdman, 2004; Schubert & Minor, 2004). Schubert et al. (2004) have suggested that the COR may be adaptable with exercise training in some people with vestibular dysfunction.

Age and gender do not appear to affect vestibular compensation (Herdman, Schubert, Das, & Tusa, 2003; Topuz et al., 2004; S. L. Whitney, Wrisley, Marchetti, & Furman, 2002). Length of symptoms also does not appear to affect the ultimate outcome in persons with unilateral vestibular hypofunction (Herdman et al., 2003). Generally, it is thought that people with peripheral vestibular disorders will have a better outcome than those with central vestibular disorders, especially disorders of the cerebellum, which is critical for VOR function (Brown, Whitney, Marchetti, Wrisley, & Furman, 2006; Furman & Whitney, 2000).

Factors that appear to affect compensation abilities resulting in a negative outcome include a history of migraine (Wrisley, Whitney, & Furman, 2002), a history of anxiety and/or depression (Bowman, 2004), being younger (Bowman, 2004; Herdman, Blatt, Schubert, & Tusa, 2000; S. L. Whitney, Hudak, & Marchetti, 2000; S. L. Whitney et al., 2002), cerebellar dysfunction (Brown et al., 2006), visual impairments (Herdman, 2000; Luxon, 2003), decreased distal sensation (Herdman, 2000; S. L. Whitney & Rossi, 2000), head injury (Davies & Luxon, 1995; Kentala, Viikki, Pyykko, & Juhola, 2000; Rubin, Woolley, Dailey, & Goebel, 1995; Shepard, Telian, Smith-Wheelock, & Raj, 1993; S. Whitney & Unico, 2001), intermittent symptoms (Clendaniel & Tucci, 1997; Herdman, 2000; S. L. Whitney & Rossi, 2000), progressive vestibular dysfunction (S. L. Whitney & Rossi, 2000), medical comorbidities (Shepard & Telian, 1995; S. A. Telian & Shepard, 1996; S. Whitney & Unico, 2001), vestibular suppressant medication (Bamiou et al., 2000; Herdman, 2000; Peppard, 1986), and physical restriction of daily activities (Fetter & Zee, 1988; Gustave et al., 1998; Lacour, Roll, & Appaix, 1976; Luxon, 2003). Table 31–2 presents additional reasons for negative outcomes. Youth as a negative predictive factor appears to be counterintuitive. It has been suggested that persons who are younger and seen in a vestibular clinic are more impaired than their older counterparts (S. L. Whitney, Hudak, et al., 2000) and that they may have higher expectations for recovery (Bowman, 2004).

VOR gain can be significantly impaired after a vestibular disorder. Vertical VOR gain has been

Table 31-2. Negative Predictive Factors Related to Rehabilitation Outcomes

- A history of a ocular motor tropia or phoria
- A history of migraine (even a remote history)
- Ankylosing spondylitis
- Charcot-Marie Tooth disease
- Coexisting neurologic dysfunction (visual field loss, ptosis, cognitive impairment, spasticity)
- Convergence insufficiency
- Convergence spasm
- Involvement of the contralateral labyrinth
- Diabetes
- Externally restricted cervical range of motion (four-poster collar)
- Fluctuating vestibular functioning
- Glaucoma
- Macular degeneration
- Medication (certain CNS depressants)
- Myopathy that results in loss of distal muscle strength
- Parkinson disease
- Peripheral neuropathy
- Inactive lifestyle
- Visual aids (progressive or trifocal lenses, monocular contact lenses)

reported to be decreased by as much as 66%, whereas horizontal VOR gain was reduced by 50% toward the involved side and 25% toward the noninvolved side of the vestibular dysfunction (Allum, Yamane, & Pfaltz, 1988). Even after rehabilitation, dynamic gain deficits remain (Curthoys & Halmagyi, 1995). Bowman (2004) suggests that people who are well compensated continue to have some remaining functional limitations that adversely affect their lives.

Evidence That Exercise Can Help Persons With Peripheral and Central Vestibular Disorders

The evidence appears clear that function improves following vestibular rehabilitation for persons with unilateral hypofunction (Clendaniel & Tucci,

1997; B. Cohen, John, Yakushin, Buettner-Ennever, & Raphan, 2002; H. Cohen, 1992, 1994; H. Cohen, Ewell, & Jenkins, 1995; H. Cohen, Kanewineland, Miller, & Hatfield, 1995; H. S. Cohen & Kimball, 2003, 2004a, 2004b; Corna et al., 2003; Cowand et al., 1998; Gill-Body, Krebs, Parker, & Riley, 1994; Herdman, 1990; Herdman, Blatt, & Schubert, 2000; Herdman, Clendaniel, Mattox, Holliday, & Niparko, 1995; Herdman et al., 2003; Horak et al., 1992; Krebs et al., 1993; Mruzek, Barin, Nichols, Burnett, & Welling, 1995; Norre, 1984; Norre & Beckers, 1988; Pavlou et al., 2004; Shepard & Telian, 1995; Shepard, Telian, & Smith-Wheelock, 1990; Shepard et al., 1993; Strupp, Arbusow, Maag, Gall, & Brandt, 1998; Szturm, Ireland, & Lessing-Turner, 1994; Telian & Shepard, 1996; Topuz et al., 2004; S. L. Whitney & Rossi, 2000; Yardley, Beech, Zander, Evans, & Weinman, 1998; Yardley, Burgneay, Andersson, et al., 1998; Yardley, Burgneay, Nazareth, & Luxon, 1998; Yardley et al., 2004). Persons with vestibular hypofunction are the best studied group, because they are more homogeneous than persons with central vestibular disorders.

There is no consensus in the literature as to what is the best way to treat vestibular hypofunction. Treatment lengths vary from 4 to 12 weeks. The longer treatment times are primarily for persons with bilateral vestibular hypofunction or for persons with significant comorbid medical disorders, space and motion symptoms, or psychiatric symptoms associated with their dizziness.

There is little evidence that persons with central vestibular disorders can be aided with vestibular rehabilitation (Furman & Whitney, 2000). A recent pilot randomized trial suggests that rehabilitation is effective with older adults with central vestibular disorders (Marioni et al., 2013) and with persons poststroke in the vertebro-basilar circulation (Balci, Akdal, Yaka, & Angin, 2013). Studies of persons with head trauma, cervical dizziness, cerebellar disorders, AICA and PICA stroke, and migraine have reported beneficial results following vestibular rehabilitation (K. E. Brown et al., 2006; H. Cohen, 1992; H. Cohen, Kanewineland, Miller, & Hatfield, 1995; Cowand et al., 1998; Gill-Body, Popat, Parker, & Krebs, 1997; Karlberg, Magnusson, Malmstrom, Melander, & Moritz, 1996; Rubin et al., 1995; Shepard & Telian, 1995; Suarez et al., 2003; S. Whitney & Unico, 2001; S. Whitney, Wrisley, et al., 2000; Wrisley, Sparto,

Whitney, & Furman, 2000; Wrisley et al., 2002). Treatment lengths vary for persons with central vestibular disorders, but generally these patients are more difficult to treat and require more time for optimal rehabilitation outcomes. Those with central vestibular disorders have a better prognosis than those with combined peripheral and central vestibular disorders. Persons with cervical dizziness are often co-treated with physical therapy specifically for the neck as it is not uncommon for a person's dizziness to persist until their neck pain resolves. However, there is no strong evidence that manual therapy and vestibular rehabilitation in combination is superior to either intervention alone (Lystad, Bell, Bonnevie-Svendsen, & Carter, 2011).

When considering an exercise program, patient safety is of optimal importance. Encouragement is essential as patients do not like to make themselves dizzy. Experience in treating patients with vestibular disorders may make a difference in a patient's outcome, as it is sometimes difficult to know how much exercise is excessive. Our general rule is that patients should not have symptoms for longer than 20 min after they complete their exercise program. Patients are strongly encouraged to bring on their symptoms during the exercises, although for some patients this is very difficult. Fear of dizziness can become a problem with persons with chronic symptoms, as patients begin to avoid activities or situations that provoke their symptoms.

Computerized dynamic posturography, dizziness, fear of falling, balance confidence, self-efficacy, quality of life, anxiety, static postural measures, number of falls, gait measures, dynamic visual acuity, VOR gain, and the ability to perform transitional movements have all been shown to improve following rehabilitation (I. Brown, Renwick, & Raphael, 1995; K. E. Brown et al., 2001, 2006; H. Cohen, Heaton, Congdon, & Jenkins, 1996; H. Cohen, Kanewineland, et al., 1995; H. S. Cohen & Kimball, 2003, 2004b, 2005; H. S. Cohen, Kimball, & Stewart, 2004; K.M. Gill-Body & Krebs, 1994; K.M. Gill-Body et al., 1994, 1997; Gill et al., 2002; S. J. Herdman, 1990, 1997; S. J. Herdman et al., 2000; S. J. Herdman et al., 1995, 2003; Shepard & Telian, 1995; Shepard et al., 1990, 1993; Szturm et al., 1994; Vitte, Semont, & Berthoz, 1994; S. Whitney et al., 2000; S. L. Whitney & Rossi, 2000; S. L. Whitney, Sparto, et al., 2006).

THE VESTIBULAR EVALUATION

History

The most important aspect of the vestibular evaluation is the patient history. The patient usually can provide enough information by the end of the history to positively identify what the diagnosis is if the correct questions are asked. In order to standardize the questions, forms are used to assist the clinician in gaining a better understanding of the patient's medical comorbidities and additional factors that may affect the dizziness. The data from the forms can speed up history taking and allow for more probing questions based on the already completed intake forms. The questions that are answered can guide additional queries by the clinician that can assist in determining patient diagnosis.

In addition to the health intake forms, it is very important to ask specific questions about whether headache is related to the patient's dizziness symptoms. Migraine is highly prevalent and is much more common in women than men. Most studies suggest that the vestibular population is approximately 60% to 65% women, suggesting that migraine may be a contributing factor in the high proportion of persons with vestibular disorders. It is not uncommon for persons with migraine headache to present with dizziness, vertigo, and space and motion symptoms as presenting complaints to an otology clinic (Cass et al., 1997; Neuhauser, Leopold, von Brevern, Arnold, & Lempert, 2001; S. Whitney et al., 2000).

Migraine has been shown to be a negative predictor of recovery after vestibular rehabilitation, even with a remote history of migraine (Wrisley et al., 2002). Marcus and Furman have developed a screening questionnaire for both migraine (Appendix 31–A) (Marcus, Kapelewski, Jacob, Rudy, & Furman, 2004) and for vestibular migraine (Appendix 31–B) (Marcus, Kapelewski, Rudy, Jacob, & Furman, 2004). The questionnaires help the clinician to determine if a patient has migraine, which is often either not previously diagnosed or is considered sinus disease by the patient. Patients often report that they get sinus headaches or head pressure, without ever having had the diagnosis of migraine prior to attending a vestibular clinic. Once it is clear that a patient has migraines, a more specific questionnaire

based on Neuhauser et al.'s (2001) work can be used to determine if the patient has migraine-related dizziness.

A history of the person's falls is very important. Persons with vestibular disorders fall more frequently than others in the community (Agrawal, Carey, Della Santina, Schubert, & Minor, 2009; Herdman et al., 2000; Kristinsdottir, Jarnlo, & Magnusson, 2000; Murray, Hill, Phillips, & Waterston, 2005; S. L. Whitney, Hudak, et al., 2000; S. L. Whitney, Marchetti, Schade, & Wrisley, 2004; S. L. Whitney, Marchetti, & Schade, 2006). Determining the cause and circumstances surrounding the fall and also whether there was any injury is an important part of the history. Some causes of falls may require immediate medical notification, such as syncope, which is clearly not associated with a vestibular disorder. The area of assessment of falls risk is addressed in Chapter 33.

Physical Examination

Strength, range of motion, and sensation are assessed to determine if they are negative factors that will affect recovery. Lower extremity weakness will affect the person's ability to move, which is very important for vestibular compensation. In addition, it is very important to have adequate neck and foot range of motion. Neck range of motion will affect the ability of the person to compensate and foot range of motion will affect the ability of the lower extremities to assist with compensation through increased weighting of somatosensation for postural control. Persons who have poor sensation distally fall frequently (Hughes, Duncan, Rose, Chandler, & Studenski, 1996; S. R. Lord & Clark, 1996; Maki, Perry, Norrie, & McIlroy, 1999; Marchetti & Whitney, 2005; Richardson & Ashton-Miller, 1996; Richardson, Ashton Miller, Lee, & Jacobs, 1996), only adding to the dysfunction associated with inadequate vestibular function.

The typical oculomotor examination includes assessing motor performance of cranial nerves III, IV, and VI and an assessment of spontaneous nystagmus. In addition, gaze-evoked nystagmus is assessed. Typically, smooth pursuit and saccades are assessed visually for any major disruption in function. Patients are asked to follow a moving target and also to quickly move their eyes from one target to another. In addition, vergence is assessed by asking the patient to follow a target moved toward the nose. Vergence is more difficult for older adults, but they should be able to follow the finger for at least part of the motion.

With infrared (IR) goggles, the therapist will determine if the patient has a positive Dix-Hallpike test and also determine if there is any nystagmus at rest without fixation. If the patient can fixate with no nystagmus in room light but has spontaneous nystagmus with IR goggles in place, it suggests a peripheral vestibular disorder. An inability to suppress nystagmus while fixating on a target with eyes open could indicate either an acute peripheral vestibular disorder or a central vestibular disorder.

Head-shaking nystagmus is also assessed whereby the head is rotated in about 20 to 30 degrees of flexion (Hain, Fetter, & Zee, 1987). The head is rotated quickly to the right and left with IR goggles in place and after approximately 20 head shakes, the movement is stopped and the examiner visualizes any nystagmus and describes it. A normal response is no nystagmus when the motion is stopped by the examiner.

The head impulse test is performed without goggles in order to assess the semicircular canals (Halmagyi & Curthoys, 1988). The person's head is moved quickly either toward neutral (nose straight ahead) or away from neutral approximately 10 to 20 degrees while the patient focuses on an object in front of him or her. If the eyes are unable to maintain on the fixation point and one or more saccades are visualized, a peripheral vestibular disorder is suspected (Halmagyi & Curthoys, 1988; Kattah, Talkad, Wang, Hsieh, & Newman-Toker, 2009).

Dynamic visual acuity is assessed while viewing an eye chart (Herdman et al., 2003; Herdman, Schubert, & Tusa, 2001; Rine & Braswell, 2003). The therapist first determines the patient's static visual acuity. Then, the patient's head is moved at approximately 2 Hz to the right and left while the patient is asked to read the letters on the chart. A drop of more than two lines often indicates a vestibular disorder. Improvement in dynamic visual acuity has been recorded after rehabilitation (Herdman et al., 2003).

At the end of the oculomotor examination, the Dix-Hallpike maneuver is performed to determine if the patient has BPPV. Extremes of neck extension or rotation are avoided. Tests are also performed to determine if the patient has horizontal canal BPPV (see Chapter 26 for specifics about testing and treatment). Baseline data for the above are recorded and used for comparison at discharge. In addition, balance and gait data are collected to determine if there is any change over time.

THE VESTIBULAR EXERCISE PROGRAM

Exercises are incorporated that attempt to enhance remaining vestibular, somatosensory, or visual functioning in persons with vestibular disorders. The most common diagnostic categories seen in physical therapy that have demonstrated positive change after vestibular rehabilitation are shown in Table 31–3.

The most commonly provided vestibular exercise is VOR × 1 for people with vestibular dysfunc-

Table 31–3. Diagnostic Groups That Have Improved After Vestibular Rehabilitation

- AICA and PICA stroke
- Anxiety-related dizziness
- Benign paroxysmal positional vertigo
- Bilateral hypofunction
- Cerebellar disorders
- Cervical vertigo
- Head trauma
- Labyrinthitis
- Mal de Debarquement
- Ménière's disease
- Migraine dizziness
- Multiple sclerosis
- Multisensory disequilibrium
- Neuronitis
- Panic disorder with agoraphobia and dizziness
- Postacoustic schwannoma
- Posttraumatic dizziness (postconcussion disorders
- Unilateral hypofunction

tion, whereby the person is asked to focus on a target while moving the head in either the pitch or yaw plane. The VOR × 1 exercise is advanced by changing the backgrounds, the speed of the movement of the head, and also the position of the patient. It is very important the patient always have the target in focus as he or she performs the exercise.

Once VOR × 1 is mastered, the patient is often asked to perform VOR × 2, which is more difficult than VOR × 1. The head always goes in the opposite direction as the target is held at arm's length, while the eyes remain focused on the target. The exercise requires a fair amount of coordination and intellect, so some patients are never able to perform the exercise.

More recently, equipment such as disco balls and virtual reality (Figure 31–1) have been used to

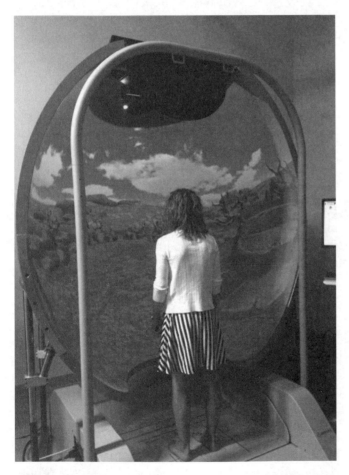

Figure 31–1. The person is viewing the virtual scene while standing on a platform that can be manipulated with a keystroke on the computer. Picture courtesy of Dr. Lewis Nashner, Bertec Corporation, Columbus, OH.

improve dizziness and function in persons with head trauma and those with uncompensated peripheral vestibular disorders (Garcia et al., 2013; Gottshall, Sessoms, & Bartlett, 2012; Llorens, Colomer-Font, Alcaniz, & Noe-Sebastian, 2013; Meldrum et al., 2012; Pavlou et al., 2012; Sparto, Furman, Whitney, Hodges, & Redfern, 2004; Sparto, Whitney, Hodges, Furman, & Redfern, 2004; Viirre, 1996; Whitney, Sparto, et al., 2006; Whitney, Sparto, Brown, et al., 2001). The equipment seems to be particularly useful in persons who are sensitive to motion in their environment, such as the person who cannot tolerate grocery shopping or going to a shopping mall. Gradual exposure seems to be a key factor in recovery.

Typically, exercises are started in the sitting position and then advanced to standing, then standing in more difficult positions, and finally during gait on flat surfaces progressing to gait on more unstable support surfaces. There is always a risk of the patient falling, so the therapist must be careful to avoid injury to the patient. Exercises should be written down and demonstrated to the patient. Pictures are ideal, as most patients forget what was said to them in the clinic and come back after practicing doing "novel" exercises, as they may not have fully understood the instructions.

Exercises are provided to patients to attempt to enhance their somatosensation. Novel somatosensory devices are being employed to attempt to substitute for vestibular loss including a vibrotactile vest (Honegger, Hillebrandt, van den Elzen, Tang, & Allum, 2013; Peterka, Wall, & Kentala, 2006; Sienko, Balkwill, Oddsson, & Wall, 2013; Wall, Oddsson, Horak, Wrisley, & Dozza, 2004) and vibrating insoles (Galica et al., 2009; Priplata, Niemi, Harry, Lipsitz, & Collins, 2003; Priplata et al., 2006). Exercises are performed in sitting and standing positions with the goal of having the person reweigh somatosensory inputs for enhanced postural control. Standing weight shifts with emphasis on "feeling" the feet with eyes open and closed is emphasized. Patients are asked to roll balls under their feet in sitting with eyes closed to better "feel" where the ball is and to increase intrinsic toe strength. Rocking back and forth on the feet is also encouraged in sitting and standing.

Lower extremity strengthening is always encouraged. Patients are asked to perform strengthening exercises in standing as much as possible, as most patients have difficulty with their balance in standing or walking rather than sitting.

It is always important to ask the patient to increase his or her activity level, especially with walking. A walking program is encouraged for all patients in safe environments progressing to more difficult circumstances. One should avoid uneven terrain if the patient falls on the modified test of sensory integration and balance (mCTSIB) eyes open on a foam surface (see the detailed description of this assessment later in this chapter). If the patient is very impaired, walking in the house with a finger against the wall may help to provide additional proprioceptive input and steady the person's gait pattern (Jeka, 1997). Obviously, the patient will be weaned from the wall as soon as possible and will be progressed to more difficult circumstances and environments. Walking in a grocery store is one of the most difficult activities for persons with vestibular disorders (S. L. Whitney et al., 2001).

Standing on uneven surfaces, mini-tramps, or on a piece of foam with eyes open are all methods used to enhance the use of vision. By disturbing proprioceptive inputs, one must use vision to assist with postural control if vestibular inputs are disrupted. Visual inputs are very important for postural control, and when removed make balance much more difficult.

Standing with eyes closed on a flat surface usually will cause the somatosensory system to be used extensively, yet when you have the person stand on a foam pad, the patient may have to reweigh sensory inputs and rely more on vestibular inputs. If there is severe vestibular damage, the person may not be able to maintain the position. Thus, all three senses are used in daily activities, and when the vestibular system is disrupted, there is a shift in responsibilities with the other sensors having to work optimally to maintain postural control.

Exercises are progressed in an incremental manner and as quickly as possible in order to improve function and return the person to work or play activities. Most people with vestibular disorders are older adults, yet some younger people experience vestibular dysfunction and are often disabled by their symptoms (Luxon, 2003). In addition to exercise, there is some evidence that behavioral therapy, relaxation/breathing exercises, and environmental modifications can be helpful with persons with ves-

tibular disorders (Herdman, 2000; Johansson, Akerlund, Larsen, & Andersson, 2001; Monahan, Sharpe, Drury, Ertl, & Ray, 2002; Schmid, Henningsen, Dieterich, Sattel, & Lahmann, 2011; Siniaia & Miller, 1996; S. L. Whitney & Rossi, 2000; Yates, 1996).

Patients are treated differently based on their presenting diagnoses and lab findings. Patients who have no remaining VOR, at least as well as we are able to test, are less likely to benefit from VOR exercises. Sensory substitution exercises are advised, especially for persons with bilateral vestibular hypofunction (Gillespie & Minor, 1999; S. A. Telian et al., 1991; S. L. Whitney & Rossi, 2000). It is very important to know not only the diagnosis, but also the laboratory findings in order to develop a customized exercise program. In one tertiary vestibular clinic, 22% of all the patients seen had a diagnosis of BPPV (S. L. Whitney, Marchetti, & Morris, 2005). Benign paroxysmal positional vertigo is often seen in addition to peripheral or central vestibular disorders, and should always be considered as a possibility either as the primary or as a secondary concern. The Dix-Hallpike maneuver should be performed on all patients presenting to the therapist.

SELECTED CASES

Patients with various vestibular pathologies require targeted physical therapy interventions. A few cases follow to attempt to illustrate how patients are treated differently based on their diagnosis, presenting symptoms, and comorbidities. To better understand the cases, basic rules about the measurement tools are provided. Generally, DHI scores of 0 to 30 are considered mild, 31 to 60 are moderate, and >60 indicate severe dizziness (S. L. Whitney & Wrisley, 2004). Activities-Specific Balance Confidence scores range from 0 to 100, with scores <67 indicating a high risk for falling (Myers, Fletcher, Myers, & Sherk, 1998). Dynamic Gait Index scores of <20 indicate fall risk (S. L. Whitney, Hudak, et al., 2000). Scores of >15 on the FTSST indicate that a patient is one standard deviation slower than the mean and the score represents the average of 80-year-old people (Lord, Murray, Chapman, Munro, & Tiedemann, 2002). Slower gait speeds indicate higher risk for falling, with a decrease of 0.1 m/s over a 6-month period considered clinically significant (Perera, Mody, Woodman, & Studenski, 2006).

Case 1

A 35-year-old female accountant presented to physical therapy with a chief complaint of vertigo that started 12 days ago. She initially complained of nausea and vertigo that lasted for several hours. Following the episode, she complained of disequilibrium, gait instability, and poor vision for 2 days. Her primary care physician referred her to physical therapy with a diagnosis of "vertigo." The patient had no complaint of hearing loss, tinnitus, or aural fullness. After questioning the patient, she reported that she had had a flu episode 2 weeks prior to experiencing the vertigo episode.

Prior to the physical therapy examination, the patient had completed the DHI and the ABC. Her score on the DHI was 40 and her score on the ABC was 65. She stated that she felt off balance and was having difficulty walking outside on the grass and was having some difficulty walking at home at night in the dark. She reported that she continued to experience dizziness with walking, especially in grocery stores and malls and had symptoms with fast movements on the television screen. She had no difficulty with reading but was having difficulty playing tennis. Normally, she played tennis twice a week. She has no significant past medical history other than occasional shoulder pain after playing tennis.

Her strength, coordination, and sensation were normal with no complaints of weakness or numbness. The patient's DGI score was 19 out of 24 with significant instability with walking with head turns and up/down movements and some reported dizziness. She also felt that she needed to hold onto the rail while going up and down steps. Her gait speed was 1.0 m/s and her TUG score was 14 s. Her five times sit to stand test (FTSST) was 9 s. She was unable to stand on high-density T-foam without falling with eyes closed. She could stand on the foam with eyes open. She also had a negative Romberg test.

During her eye examination with IR Frenzel goggles, she had a left-beating nystagmus. In room light, no nystagmus could be visualized. She had a

positive head thrust test to the right and lost three lines during dynamic visual acuity testing. She also experienced moderate symptoms when asked to perform the VOR × 1 exercise (focus on a target that is stationary, then move the head to the right/left or up/down while keeping the target in focus). No vestibular laboratory testing had been performed.

Based on the positive head thrust test, no reported changes in hearing, a normal neurologic exam, and the spontaneous nystagmus that resolved in room light, the patient's most likely diagnosis is vestibular neuritis.

The patient was seen in physical therapy once per week for 6 weeks in six 1-hr sessions with the following goals: to decrease the DHI score from 40 to 20, improve ABC from 65 to 80, return to tennis, increase the DGI score from 19 to 23, increase gait speed from 1.0 m/s to 1.3 m/s, and decrease the TUG score from 14 to 9 s.

The patient was asked to perform VOR × 1 while standing with a blank background at her first session and to work on walking slowly with head movements. In addition, she was asked to bounce a tennis ball on her racquet 20 times and to try to increase the number of times that she could watch the ball and bounce it over the next week as part of her home exercise program. Her goal was to keep the ball in focus as she did the ball bounce. In addition, she was asked to walk outside for at least 10 min a day.

Over the next 5 weeks, she worked on the following activities and exercises, including walking with head turns, standing and walking on and over compliant surfaces, walking faster on level surfaces, progressing in tennis, VOR × 1 with a busy background in standing to walking while performing VOR × 1, progressing to VOR × 2 in standing with various backgrounds (while focused on a target that was moving to the left as the head moved to the right with the eyes always in focus on the target).

At the end of the sixth session, the patient was discharged from physical therapy. She had met or exceeded all of her goals. She was back to playing tennis and stated that she felt much better. She continued to have some symptoms in grocery stores but otherwise felt fine. She was able to stand on foam with her eyes closed and all of her scores significantly improved. The patient was told to continue to play tennis and to do things that she enjoyed. She was told to call if she had any future problems and was discharged from care.

Case 2

A 22-year-old woman was referred to physical therapy with a chief complaint of fullness in her head, feeling off balance, and headaches. Six years prior she had a Chiari malformation decompression. Since the surgery she has complained of bilateral tinnitus. She states that she has had several episodes of vertigo that feel like the caloric testing that she has previously undergone. The patient reports that she veers to the left while ambulating. Symptoms are worse with sit to stand, bending, looking up, with fatigue, exertion, and stress. She also complains of getting dizzy with stairs, escalators, and elevators. She complains of weakness and clumsiness in the arms and legs, greatest in the left lower extremity. She has had migraines since childhood. Balance symptoms are worse with headaches. The patient has photophobia and phonophobia with her headaches and had difficulty with her concentration when she is experiencing a headache.

She complains of pressure in her head and tingling around her cheeks and eyes with the headaches. She has occasional numbness in her hands and a history of panic attacks (none recently) and depression. Patient had been prescribed Depakote for her headaches but had not taken the medicine.

The physician had reported that her cranial nerves were intact and strength and range of motion were normal. Sensation was normal as well as her deep tendon reflexes (DTRs). During Romberg testing, she fell to the left with a dropping of her left hip. All vestibular testing (calorics, ocular motor, positional, rotational chair) and audiometry were normal. The physician's differential diagnosis included migraine-related dizziness, possible endolymphatic hydrops, status post-Chiari malformation surgery, and astasia abasia. Recommended treatment included clonazepam and physical therapy.

During the physical therapy examination, the patient reported that she worked as a receptionist and expressed that she disliked her job. She was living with her family after dropping out of college. She was complaining of blurred vision, headaches, and that her vision "zig-zags" when she has headaches.

The patient's ABC score was 19 and her DHI score was 80. She has not been driving because she felt that she was not safe. She reported that quick head movements increased her symptoms. She reported two falls in the last 4 weeks and six falls in the last 6 months. Upon questioning, she stated that the falls were related to her dizzy spells.

Her baseline dizziness was rated as 10 out of 100 with 100 indicating the worst dizziness one could experience. She was unsteady in the Romberg position and she had excessive arm movement while trying to maintain her balance in tandem Romberg eyes open. She fell in tandem Romberg eyes closed, again to the left. Her DGI score was 13/24 and her FTSST was 11.8 s. Her TUG score was 8.5 s, and her gait speed was 1.36 m/s. She did not complain of any symptoms with any eye/head coordination activities. The following goals were identified for this patient: to increase her DGI score from 13 to 19/24, decrease her DHI score from 80 to 60, and increase her ABC score from 19 to 30.

The patient was provided with exercises to perform at home that included standing on a pillow in a corner with eyes closed, walking with head movements in the pitch and yaw planes, and walking at different speeds.

Upon return to physical therapy 1 week later, she reported that her dizziness and balance were improving. At the beginning of the second therapy session she rated her symptoms as 0 out of 100 and she had decreased the clonazepam dose. She stated that the pillow exercise was very difficult for her to perform as it made her dizzy and she lost her balance. During the SOT of computerized dynamic posturography, she had a tendency to lean to the left. Her ABC score had increased to 46, her DHI had decreased to 58, her DGI had increased to 22, her FTSST had decreased to 8.5 s, and her gait speed was unchanged. Her composite SOT score was 52 (Figure 31–2A). Her new exercises included shifting weight with emphasis on the right foot in the anterior/posterior and medial/lateral planes.

At her third visit, her dizziness and balance were "better." Baseline dizziness was 0. She reported that

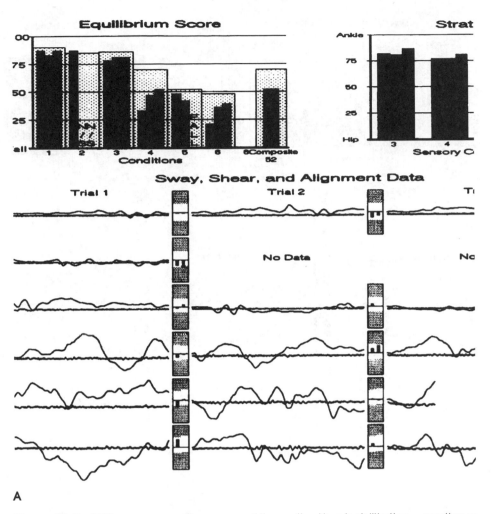

Figure 31–2. SOT scores over the course of the patient's rehabilitation. *continues*

leaning to the right was difficult and that her ability to shift weight had improved. The patient reported that walking up hills and going up escalators were the only times that she noticed symptoms now. She had no dizziness with head movements and had a negative Romberg. No lateral hip movement was noted during gait. The ABC was now 95%, DHI–16, DGI–22, and her FTSST remained at 8.5 s. Her TUG score decreased to 7 s and gait speed increased to 1.52 m/s. Her SOT had improved from 52 to 63 (Figure 31–2B). She had met all three of her goals and was discharged from physical therapy care.

In this case it is not clear what her diagnosis was, yet the patient improved. Her balance significantly improved as did her subjective complaints.

Case 3

Mrs. J is a 65-year-old woman who presents with a chief complaint of dizziness, difficulty with her vision, and difficulty walking in the dark. Mrs. J. recently bought a cane at the local pharmacy to help her walk outside the house. She states that she is having difficulty walking on her gravel driveway and reading grocery labels while pushing the cart at the grocery store. Mrs. J has no complaints of dizziness when she is seated or lying down unless she moves her head quickly. She also complains of having difficulty as a passenger in the car. She was previously provided meclizine, which the patient reports has not helped her. The patient had no

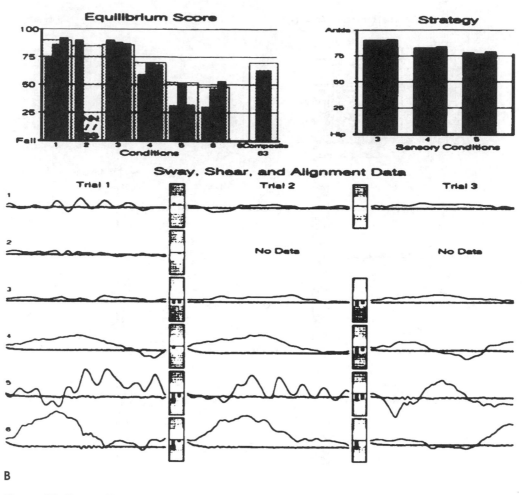

Figure 31–2. *continued*

complaints of double vision, weakness, loss or changes of sensation, or changes in her coordination.

Mrs. J was referred to physical therapy with a diagnosis of vertigo/instability of gait 4 weeks after first developing her symptoms. She has been referred by her primary care physician. On additional questioning, she stated that she had recently been hospitalized with a complicated cholecystitis 6 weeks ago. She had been treated with 2 weeks of IV gentamicin.

The patient had a DHI score of 60 and an ABC of 45. She stated that she was not leaving the house without holding onto her husband. She used furniture to ambulate around the house by holding onto it as she feels unstable.

On physical examination, she had a DGI score of 14, a TUG score of 22 s, gait speed was 0.8 m/s with

unsteadiness, a positive Romberg, a FTSST score of 17 s, and she fell while standing on foam with eyes open. She lost four lines with the Dynamic Visual Acuity test and had a positive head thrust test to the right and the left. Based on the findings, it appeared that the patient had bilateral vestibular hypofunction. Her trouble with reading in the grocery store is most likely related to oscillopsia, and she demonstrated some ataxia while walking. Her vestibular suppressant had been discontinued by her physician and she was provided exercises to improve her stability. No vestibular testing was available to confirm the physical therapy diagnosis.

Mrs. J's goals included decreasing her DHI score from 60 to 40, increasing her ABC score from 45 to 60, increasing her DGI score from 14 to 17, decreasing her TUG score from 22 to 19, increasing her gait speed to 1.0 m/s, decreasing her FTSST score from 17 to 14, and being able to stand on foam with eyes open for 5 s.

Mrs. J was treated in physical therapy for eight visits over a period of 9 weeks. She was provided with home safety instructions that emphasized adequate light wherever she went. Motion detector lights were suggested for outside her home and within the house. She was advised to carry a small flashlight with her at all times in case the lights went out so as to prevent a fall. Thick rugs in her home were discouraged, and it was suggested that she consider the installation of a grab bar in the shower and a rubber mat in the shower for increased grip under her feet.

For this patient, it is unclear if she has any remaining vestibular function. Therefore, it was decided to have her attempt VOR × 1 while standing in a corner with a chair in front of her, feet apart, starting slowly moving her head in the pitch and yaw planes while keeping the target in focus that was on the wall at eye level in front of her. In addition, exercises to enhance her proprioceptive abilities were attempted including shifting weight anterior/posterior and medial/lateral. She was encouraged to think about the slow weight shifting under her feet as she performed the exercises.

Her exercises were progressed by performing VOR × 1 in more difficult standing postures, and she was encouraged to walk as much as possible. She was instructed in proper cane use and the height of the cane was adjusted. Mrs. J also was told to hold two targets in front of her at arm's length, then to move her eyes to one target, followed by head movement to line up both her head and eyes up with the target, then repeating the same movement in the opposite direction. It has been suggested that saccadic eye movements may help to compensate for bilateral vestibular loss (Herdman et al., 2001; Schubert & Zee, 2010). In addition, she was instructed to focus on a target and remember where the target was in the distance. Then she moved her head to the right or left (up or down) while trying to keep her eyes on the target with her eyes closed. She then opened her eyes with the goal of her eyes being lined up with the "remembered" target.

More advanced balance exercises were provided and the patient met the above goals. She continued to be impaired and had difficulty walking, especially on uneven surfaces. Patients with bilateral loss do improve but remain impaired. She could not stand or walk on uneven surfaces in dim light and could not walk in the dark. Her risk of falling remained high and most likely will continue to remain high because of the loss of vestibular function. As she gets older, it is likely that her balance will get worse. She was strongly encouraged at discharge to continue with her more active lifestyle of daily walks to maintain her physical therapy gains. Her balance would get worse if she developed a distal sensory or motor neuropathy. Maintaining good visual health was also emphasized so that her two remaining balance sensors (somatosensory and visual) were optimized.

Case 4

A 75-year-old woman was referred to the balance and vestibular clinic with a diagnosis of instability of gait. She reported that her chief complaint was that she is afraid of falling. Mrs. M reported that she has fallen four times in the last 6 months and two of those falls were within the last month. She stated that she trips over things: twice over a rug, once over a curb after getting out of her car, and once over furniture in her daughter's house. She does not remember how she fell the other two times. Three months ago she fractured her distal radius and ulna when trying to break one of the falls. From the Colles fracture, she has resultant ulnar deviation at the wrist and decreased grip strength in her right hand.

Mrs. M lives alone and does not use an assistive device. She had previously used a walker and a cane after her total knee replacements, the most recent 2 years ago. She drives her car and wants to continue her active lifestyle, although she is unable to get on the floor and clean after the second total knee replacement. Her daughter helps her with grocery shopping and heavy cleaning. Otherwise, she is back to managing independently after the upper extremity fractures. She did require more assistance from her daughter when her arm was in a cast for 7 weeks. Mrs. M is now taking five different medications for her hypertension, diabetes, cholesterol, the beginnings of macular degeneration, and has some early distal sensory changes in her lower extremities.

Mrs. M is bright and energetic. She is motivated to maintain her lifestyle, which is very positive for her prognosis. Her score on the ABC scale was 45 and on the DHI her score was 0, as she had no reports of dizziness.

Mrs. M's TUG score was 18 s, Berg Balance Scale (BBS) score was 47, gait speed was 0.9 m/s, FTSST score was 22 s, and DGI score was 16. She was unable to stand on foam with eyes open without falling. Overall, Mrs. M was at significant risk for a future fall. Her four previous falls in the past 6 months is significant for future fall risk. In addition, she is taking more than four medications, has hypertension, has visual problems, and has fear of falling. She is walking more slowly than normal for her age and her BBS score and reports of previous falls indicated that within the next 6 months she has a 78% chance of falling (Shumway-Cook, Baldwin, Polissar, & Gruber, 1997). Also, she is most likely developing distal sensory loss from the diabetes. All of the above factors suggest that Mrs. M should undergo physical therapy intervention to attempt to decrease her fall risk. She agreed to participate after discussing what her risk factors were and the importance of improving her function to attain her goal of staying independent in her home.

Goals were developed with Mrs. M that included decreasing her number of falls over the next month to 0, increasing her ABC score from 45 to 65, decreasing her TUG score from 18 to 14 s, increasing her BBS from 47 to 52, increasing her DGI score from 16 to 19, decreasing her FTSST score from 22 to 18 s, and increasing her gait speed to 1.1 m/s.

Mrs. M was seen in physical therapy one to two times each week for 10 weeks. According to the American Geriatrics Association's Guidelines (American Geriatrics & American Association for Geriatric, 2003), in older adults it often requires a minimum of 10 weeks to achieve changes in balance. Mrs. M was advised about home modifications during her first visit that included a printed home safety checklist, information about fall hazards outside the home, and adequate lighting because of her macular degeneration. In addition, foot safety was discussed that included regular foot inspection, proper shoe fit, and regular visits to the doctor for toenail trimming.

Mrs. M states that she does not know why she falls, except that she feels that she may not be picking up her feet when she walks. It was noted that the patient had a tendency to drag her feet during swing-through rather than dorsiflex normally at heel strike.

On physical therapy examination, Mrs. M's blood pressure was 145/90 at rest and her pulse was 82. Her standing BP was 135/88 immediately after rising to standing after lying flat for 5 min, suggesting that postural hypotension was not a factor related to her frequent falls. It was hoped that through a regular walking program, her hypertension might be reduced.

Mrs. M started on a walking program. She was instructed to go to the grocery store and walk with a cart in order to increase her endurance. Mrs. M was also told to buy a few groceries each trip to the store to avoid fatigue when taking them up the flight of stairs at home to her kitchen. There was a railing on the right side as she ascends the steps. Hand and right upper extremity strengthening was initiated to increase the strength in her right upper extremity. She worked on standing in a corner in the Romberg position with eyes open and then began to stand on uneven surfaces so that she would be able to walk and stand on compliant surfaces such as thick carpets and gravel in a driveway. She also began a lower extremity strengthening program including sit to stand with no use of the upper extremities, standing mini-squats, marching in place, single leg stance, lifting one foot at a time to tap a low stool, increasing the speed of the activity as she improved, and moving her trunk while standing. In addition, over the 10 weeks, she ambulated faster on level surfaces, at different speeds, and with head movements in a safe environment. She used her cane throughout in order to provide her some additional somatosensory input as she ambulated.

The patient met all of the above goals except for decreasing her FTSST score to 18 s. She did decrease her time to 20 s but complained of knee soreness in performing the sit to stand exercise at home. Mrs. M was happy with her functional gains and was instructed to continue to exercise daily to maintain the gains achieved by her efforts. Each session, she was provided with exercises to perform at home in a safe manner. Mrs. M also began a community-based senior exercise program two to three times a week to maintain her level of fitness to address her multisensory disequilibrium.

ASSESSING PROGRESS IN VESTIBULAR REHABILITATION

Subjective Assessments

There are several subjective measures that are commonly used to assess change in persons with vestibular disorders including the Dizziness Handicap Inventory (DHI) (Jacobson & Newman, 1990), the Activities-Specific Balance Confidence (ABC) scale (Powell & Myers, 1995), the Vestibular Activities of Daily Living Scale (H. S. Cohen & Kimball, 2000; H. S. Cohen, Kimball, & Adams, 2000), the Short Form Medical Outcomes-36 items quality of life measure (Ware & Sherbourne, 1992), visual and verbal analog scales (Hall & Herdman, 2006; S. Whitney et al., 2000; S. L. Whitney & Rossi, 2000; Wrisley et al., 2002), and the Vertigo Symptom Scale (VSS) (Yardley, Masson, Verschuur, Haacke, & Luxon, 1992). Each is discussed below.

Dizziness Handicap Inventory

The DHI is the most commonly used subjective scale in vestibular clinics (Jacobson & Newman, 1990). It has been translated into several languages and is the most studied measure of perceived dizziness to date (Nyabenda, Briart, Deggouj, & Gersdorff, 2004; Vereeck, Truijen, Wuyts, & Van de Heyning, 2006). There are two American versions: the original and a short version of the DHI (G. P. Jacobson & Calder, 1998; G. P. Jacobson & Newman, 1990; Tesio, Alpini, Cesarani, & Perucca, 1999).

The original DHI consists of 25 items in three categories: functional (36 points), physical (28 points), and emotional (36 points). The DHI can provide four scores: the total DHI and a score for each of the three subcategories. Patients read each item and determine if the motion or activity bothers them all of the time, some of the time, or never. If the respondent answers "yes" to the question they receive a score of "4" for that item, "sometimes" a "2", and "no" a "0." The worst score possible is "100" and the best is "0." Jacobson and Newman developed the DHI to attempt to objectify the handicapping effects of dizziness that can occur from vestibular disease

(Jacobson & Newman, 1990). The tool helps to provide information about the handicapping effects of dizziness on a person's well-being. It has been used to determine if patients are improving after intervention (Ekvall Hansson, Mansson, Ringsberg, & Hakansson, 2006).

Scores above 60 on the DHI have been related to recurrent falls and have been designated as severe dizziness (S. L. Whitney, Wrisley, Brown, & Furman, 2004). Scores between 0 and 30 are related to mild dizziness and 31 to 60 to moderate dizziness (Whitney, Wrisley, Brown, & Furman, 2004). A decrease on the DHI of 18 is considered a clinically significant improvement (Jacobson & Newman, 1990). The DHI is often used to assess change in patients with vestibular loss.

The DHI has recently been used to assist in the diagnosis of benign paroxysmal positional vertigo (BPPV) (S. L. Whitney, Marchetti, et al., 2005). BPPV has been reported in 22% of patients treated at a tertiary vestibular clinic (S. L. Whitney, Marchetti, et al., 2005). The DHI was tested to determine if answers to the DHI could assist the clinician in making the diagnosis of BPPV. The five-item DHI was a significant predictor of the likelihood of having BPPV. The five items included dizziness with looking up, getting out of bed, quick head movements, rolling in bed, and bending.

The two-item BPPV subscale suggested that if a person "always" had symptoms with supine to sit and rolling in bed, they were 4.3 times more likely to have a positive Dix-Hallpike than those people who scored 0 on the 8-point scale (S. L. Whitney, Marchetti, et al., 2005). The response of "always" indicated that patients consistently became dizzy during supine to sit and rolling in bed.

Data from the two- or five-item DHI are is particularly important because not all patients who have BPPV have a positive Dix-Hallpike test (Nunez, Cass, & Furman, 2000; Viirre, Purcell, & Baloh, 2005). The Dix-Hallpike has been documented to be affected by the speed of the movement (Nunez et al., 2000) and may need to be repeated in order for it to be positive (Viirre et al., 2005). Haynes et al. (2002) have suggested that persons may have "subjective" BPPV, whereby they complain of vertigo in the Dix-Hallpike position, but no torsional nystagmus is visualized. After repositioning, persons had resolution of their BPPV (86% resolution for those with "subjective" BPPV versus 91% in those with a positive Dix-Hallpike test) (Haynes et al., 2002).

The DHI provides another check in the system to help guide the clinician in determining if the patient has BPPV. It is not uncommon, even with a negative Dix-Hallpike, to see torsional nystagmus in the second stage of the Epley maneuver, validating that the person does have BPPV. The DHI can assist in making the diagnosis of BPPV, especially in people who have a negative Dix-Hallpike maneuver.

In older adults, making the diagnosis of BPPV may be especially important. Oghalai et al. (Oghalai, Manolidis, Barth, Stewart, & Jenkins, 2000) reported that older adults with BPPV were more likely to have reported a fall, had lower ADL scores, and also reported greater levels of depression. They reported that 9 out of 100 older adults seen in the clinic had undiagnosed BPPV (Oghalai et al., 2000). Using the DHI may speed the diagnosis of BPPV and reduce the risk of a fall event in older adults.

Activities-Specific Balance Confidence Scale (ABC)

The ABC was developed by Powell and Myers to assess balance confidence while performing common activities both in the home and in the community (Myers et al., 1998; Powell & Myers, 1995). The ABC tool is very easy to administer and is often given to patients to complete prior to examination. The ABC consists of a leading phrase that states "How confident are you that you will not lose your balance or become unsteady when" with 16 various stems such as "reaching for an object off a shelf at eye level or walking outside on icy sidewalks." The 16 items vary from easy to difficult.

Each respondent checks a response between 0% indicating no confidence to 100% indicating complete confidence in completing the task. Responses to the 16 items are averaged and a total ABC score is reported. The tool was validated and compared to other balance tools (Myers et al., 1998; Powell & Myers, 1995) and also the DHI (S. L. Whitney, Hudak, & Marchetti, 1999). A moderately strong negative correlation ($r = -0.64$) was reported between the DHI and the ABC in persons with a vestibular disorder (S. L. Whitney et al., 1999).

Scores on the ABC of less than 67% have been related to increased fall risk in community-living older adults with a sensitivity of 84% and a specificity of 88% (Lajoie & Gallagher, 2004). Scores below 50 on the ABC have indicated that the people are more likely to be homebound or have low physical functioning, those between 50 and 80 have moderate functional limitations, and those 80 and above on the ABC are likely to be active community-living older adults (Myers et al., 1998). The ABC provides some insight with a simple paper and pencil test as to how impaired the person perceives that they are. The ABC has been compared to the Berg Balance Scale, and scores on the ABC are significantly lower for people who report falls as compared to nonfallers (Lajoie & Gallagher, 2004). Older adults who scored low on computerized dynamic posturography also reported low ABC scores (Myers et al., 1998; Powell & Myers, 1995).

The ABC score validates the clinician's clinical impression. If a person presents to the clinic with an ABC score of 95, one would not expect that person to have severely impaired postural control during CDP or when walking. A high ABC score coupled with poor performance on CDP would be highly unlikely, suggesting that further investigation is warranted. The ABC score can be used as a means to check that the person's perceived balance confidence matches what the clinician visualizes.

Yardley et al. (1994) have suggested that persons with vestibular disorders restrict their activities to avoid dizziness or embarrassment from their vestibular condition. The ABC can help to identify restriction of activities and lack of confidence in performing functional activities in persons living with vestibular dysfunction (S. L. Whitney et al., 1999). The ABC has been used to document change over time (K. E. Brown et al., 2001; 2006; S. L. Whitney & Rossi, 2000; S. L. Whitney, Wrisley, Brown, & Furman, 2000; Wrisley et al., 2002). Scores on the ABC allow the clinician to determine if the patient's balance confidence has changed over the course of rehabilitation.

Vestibular Disorders Activities of Daily Living (VADL) Scale

Cohen and Kimball developed the VADL to objectify change in ADL performance over time in persons with vestibular disorders (H. S. Cohen & Kimball, 2000; H. S. Cohen et al., 2000). The VADL scale has three subscales: functional, instrumental, and ambulation. Test-retest reliably was 0.87 and the VADL had an internal consistency of 0.90 (H. S. Cohen & Kimball, 2000). The tool consists of 38 items, whereby the patient rates the tasks from a range of "independence" to "no longer can perform, too difficult" on a 10-point scale. The tool has been used to document change over time and provides information about higher-level activities that patients may have difficulty accomplishing such as driving a car or getting into or out of a shower or tub (H. S. Cohen & Kimball, 2003, 2004a, 2004b).

Visual Analog Scales

Hall and Herdman (2006) have reported an interclass correlation coefficient CC of 0.48 with the head movement visual analog scale when tested twice within the same therapy session. Subjects were asked to mark on a vertical line how they felt before and after moving their heads for 1 min. This was repeated at the end of the session for comparison. Others have used either a verbal or visual analog scale to report symptoms (K. E. Brown et al., 2001; Horak et al., 1992; S. Whitney et al., 2000; Wrisley et al., 2002).

Vertigo Symptom Scale (VSS)

The VSS was developed by Yardley et al. (1992) to help quantify frequently observed symptoms in persons with vestibular disorders. Patients are asked to rate symptom frequency over the past year from "0" indicating "never" to "5" indicating "very often": on average more than once a week (Yardley et al., 1992). After statistical analysis, the test loads on three main factors: (1) items related to autonomic nervous system function or anxiety; (2) perceived disorientation and imbalance, nausea, and vomiting; and (3) dizziness and short duration unsteadiness (Yardley et al., 1992). Test-retest reliability of the subscales of the VSS ranged from 0.89 to 0.96 (Yardley et al., 1992). The tool has been used as an outcome of vestibular rehabilitation intervention (H. S. Cohen & Kimball, 2003; H. S. Cohen et al., 2004; Holmberg et al., 2006).

The Medical Outcomes Survey: 36-Item Short Form (MOS-SF36)

The MOS-SF36 has been used to assess quality of life in persons with vestibular disorders (Enloe & Shields, 1997; Fielder, Denholm, Lyons, & Fielder, 1996; Gamiz & Lopez-Escamez, 2004; Kinney, Sandridge, & Newman, 1997; Solomon, Skobieranda, & Genzen, 1995). The tool consists of eight subscales and requires about 5 to 10 min to complete. It can be cumbersome for older adults with visual problems. Gamiz demonstrated good internal consistency with persons with BPPV (Cronbach's alpha >0.7) (Gamiz & Lopez-Escamez, 2004).

STANDING MEASURES OF BALANCE

Romberg, Tandem Romberg, Single Leg Stance, and Functional Reach

Several simple measures are often employed to determine change over time. One of the easiest is to ask the patient to stand in the Romberg position. Patients stand with their feet together with eyes open and then later, if successful, with eyes closed. Time that the person can maintain the position is recorded with a stopwatch while the patient is carefully guarded to prevent a fall. Most clinicians time the standing position for 30 s. The patient should not use the arms for balance during the test and the feet should not move on the floor. The test is used frequently to assess change over time (Herdman, 2000). Tandem Romberg is often tested if the person is able to maintain the feet-together Romberg position without falling. The patient is asked to stand with the feet in a straight line with the heel touching the toes of the other foot. Again, time to maintain the position is recorded with a stopwatch.

Single leg standing is another simple test that is used to record change over time (F.B. Horak et al., 1992; Mann, Whitney, Redfern, Borello-France, & Furman, 1996; Messier et al., 2000). The patient is asked to stand on one leg with the other leg not touching the weight-bearing limb. The person's weight-bearing limb should not move on the floor, nor should the arms move from the start position. Time to maintain the position is recorded, and changes are noted over the course of rehabilitation. It is important to attempt to test under the same conditions so that comparisons can be made between therapy visits. Movement in the periphery could affect postural control in persons with vestibular disorders adversely, causing them to place their foot on the floor prematurely.

Mann et al. (1996) reported that persons with high DHI scores (worse perceived dizziness) had lower functional reach scores than those persons with lower DHI scores. Functional reach has been used to assess fall risk in older adults and persons with vestibular dysfunction (Duncan, Studenski, Chandler, & Prescott, 1992; S. L. Whitney & Rossi, 2000). The further the person can reach horizontally, the less risk there is of falling (Duncan, Weiner, Chandler, & Studenski, 1990). Generally, it has been reported that functional reach scores of 6 inches or less are highly related to an increase in falling within the next 6 months. Scores of between 6 and 10" indicate moderate risk, and functional reach scores of >10" indicate less risk (Duncan et al., 1992).

One always has some risk of falling, as accidents happen frequently, but it does appear that some fall risk behavior can be predicted. Wernick-Robinson, Krebs, and Giorgetti (1999) have suggested that functional reach scores were similar in older healthy adults and persons with vestibular hypofunction. They suggest that the functional reach test is not a good measure of dynamic balance, yet it did demonstrate moderate correlations with AP sway. The ability to reach safely for an object is a component of balance but may not relate strongly to dynamic postural control in gait.

Foam Posturography

Brandt and colleagues were the first to suggest that standing on foam with eyes open and closed could be used as a form of rehabilitative exercise and also as a measurement tool (Brandt, Krafczyk, & Malsbenden, 1981). They demonstrated improvements in postural sway in control subjects after standing on foam eyes open and closed with neck extension over a period of 5 days. They suggested that it could be used for rehabilitation. Different types of foam pads may yield different results, so care should be

utilized to test the patient on the same type of foam (Figure 31–3).

The Clinical Test of Sensory Integration and Balance (CTSIB) was later developed based on Brandt et al.'s work (Shumway-Cook & Horak, 1986b) and the work of Nashner (Forssberg & Nashner, 1982; Horak & Nashner, 1986; Nashner, 1982; Nashner, Shumway-Cook, & Marin, 1983). The CTSIB consists of six conditions, that is, standing on a flat firm surface and on a compliant foam surface under three different visual circumstances: eyes open, eyes closed, and while wearing a sensory conflict dome with feet together and shoes removed (Shumway-

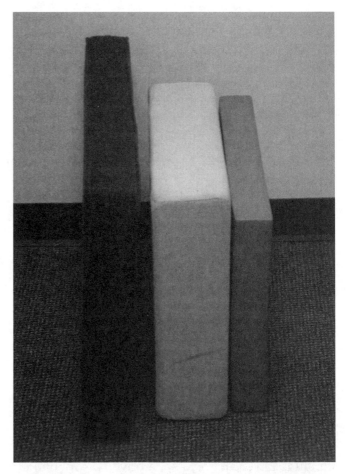

Figure 31–3. When testing or treating patients with vestibular disorders, the thickness of the foam may affect patient performance. High-density foam versus very compliant foam will change patient behavior. All patients should be carefully watched when getting onto the foam, while standing on it, and while getting off the foam pad.

Cook & Horak, 1986a). The CTSIB can also be performed with feet comfortably apart (normal stance width) and with shoes on without a difference in score compared to standing with feet together, shoes removed (S. L. Whitney & Wrisley, 2004; Wrisley & Whitney, 2004).

The CTSIB is easy to perform but the patient must be closely guarded to ensure that the patient does not fall. The foam pad must be secure on a firm surface so that it does not slip. Patients have been known to fall getting onto or off the foam pad, so care should be exercised not just during standing. The CTSIB was designed to assess reliance on visual, vestibular, and proprioceptive sensors for postural control. Time to maintain the position (30 s in the original paper) (Shumway-Cook & Horak, 1986b), amount of sway (as assessed with a sway grid) (Shumway-Cook & Horak, 1986b), fall or no fall (Cass et al., 1996), and sway angles (also assessed with a sway grid) (Shumway-Cook & Horak, 1986b) have been used as objective measures of CTSIB performance. The test has been widely used for patients with vestibular disorders (H. Cohen, Blatchly, & Gombash, 1993; H. Cohen et al., 1996; el Kashlan et al., 1998; S. L. Whitney & Wrisley, 2004; Wrisley & Whitney, 2004). Test-retest reliability of the CTSIB is high with an r equal to or greater than 0.75 in older, community-living adults (Anacker & Di Fabio, 1992) and an r equal to 0.99 for inter-rater reliability and test-retest reliability in young adults (H. Cohen et al., 1993). Weber and Cass (1993) have reported a 90% agreement between the CTSIB and the Sensory Organization Test (SOT) (Figure 31–4) of computerized dynamic posturography (CDP) and a 90% sensitivity and 95% specificity in adults with vestibular dysfunction using the foam pad in their office, yet there was no correlation between caloric or rotational chair findings and CTSIB findings (Weber & Cass, 1993). The CTSIB measures something different than what other vestibular findings provide.

Performance on the CTSIB has been used to assess fall risk in persons with vestibular disorders (H. Cohen et al., 1993; el Kashlan et al., 1998; Weber & Cass, 1993), older adults (Baloh, Corona, Jacobson, Enrietto, & Bell, 1998; R. P. Di Fabio & Seay, 1997; Sherrington & Lord, 1998), and also persons with peripheral neuropathies (Dickstein, Shupert, & Horak, 2001). The CTSIB was able to identify 63%

of older adults who were at risk for falling (R. P. Di Fabio & Seay, 1997).

The CTSIB is used clinically to help the therapist design an appropriate exercise program based on the deficits identified during test performance (Shumway-Cook & Horak, 1986b). Generally, it is thought that all persons without disease should be able to stand with their eyes open, feet together. If a patient cannot stand under these circumstances, one might suspect a central nervous system disorder. For example, many patients with multiple sclerosis (MS) cannot stand with eyes open, feet together. Patients with MS often have dorsal column dysfunction, resulting in a loss of distal sensation causing them to fall in the Romberg position, eye open. Persons with acute peripheral vestibular disorders may have difficulty standing on a firm surface with eyes open, that is, Condition 1 of the CTSIB, but it is unlikely.

Condition 2, standing in the Romberg position with eyes closed removes vision as an aid to postural control, yet if the somatosensory and vestibular pathways are intact, the person will remain standing. Persons with severe central nervous system disorders or peripheral neuropathies may fall on Condition 2. Standing near a wall during testing so that you can use the wall to help you guard a large patient may serve your best interests and that of the patient to protect them from falling. Having the patient wear a gait belt around the waist to grab hold of if needed can be very beneficial. Touching the patient during testing will most likely affect the performance and should be avoided (Jeka, 1997). Being vigilant is very important during testing so that the examiner and the patient remain safe.

Condition 3 consists of having the patient stand with his or her eyes open while wearing a visual conflict dome. The dome moves as the person's head and body move in the same direction and has been called a visual conflict dome. If a patient relies almost exclusively on vision for postural control, he or she will be very unstable or may even fall during testing.

Older adults are often prone to falling during Condition 3. Most people have felt something similar to Condition 3 while watching a train move past you. It can be difficult to determine if you are moving or if the train is moving, as the optic flow influences the person's visual system into believing that they may be moving also. The dome is not used as

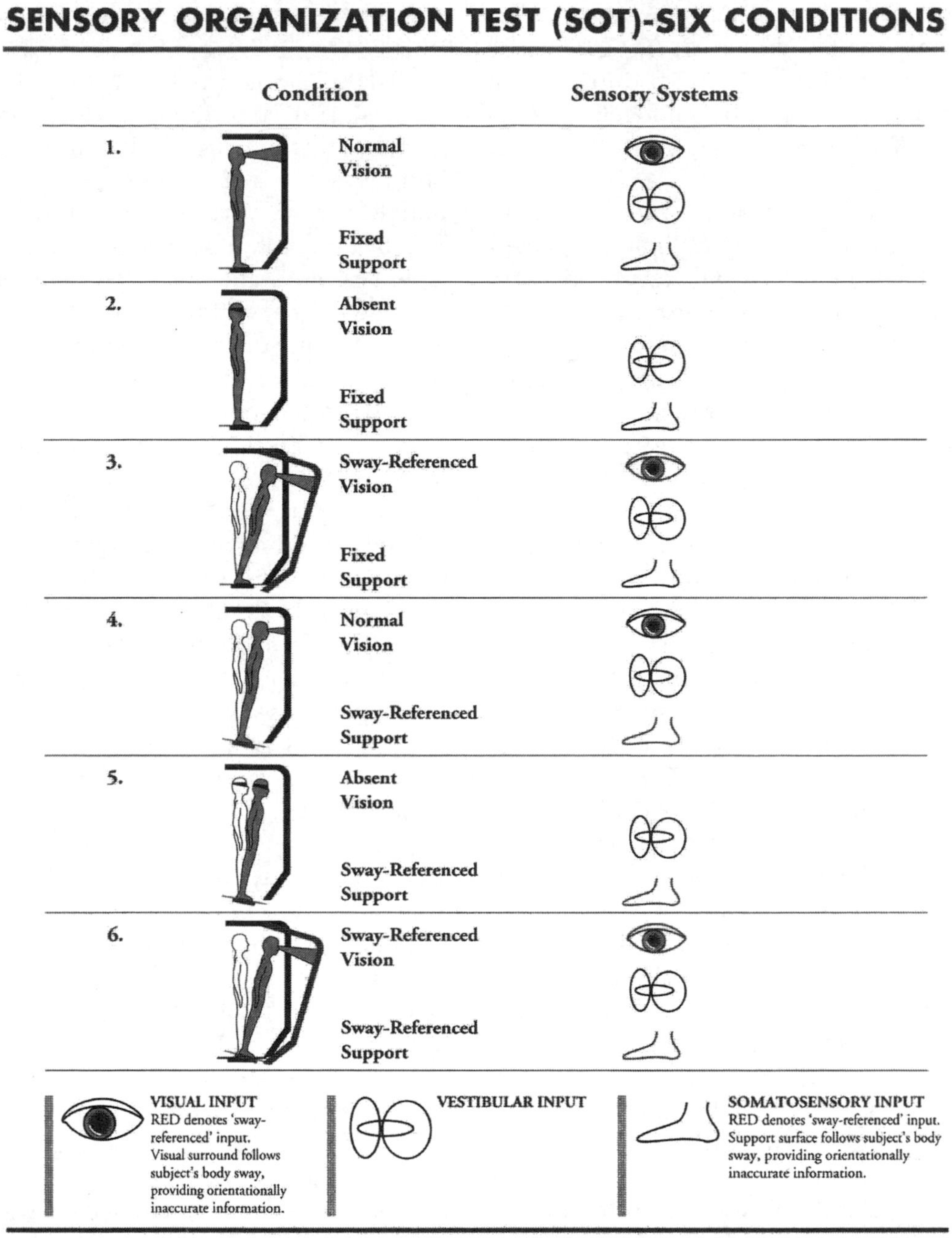

SENSORY ORGANIZATION TEST (SOT)-SIX CONDITIONS

	Condition	Sensory Systems
1.	Normal Vision / Fixed Support	
2.	Absent Vision / Fixed Support	
3.	Sway-Referenced Vision / Fixed Support	
4.	Normal Vision / Sway-Referenced Support	
5.	Absent Vision / Sway-Referenced Support	
6.	Sway-Referenced Vision / Sway-Referenced Support	

VISUAL INPUT RED denotes 'sway-referenced' input. Visual surround follows subject's body sway, providing orientationally inaccurate information.

VESTIBULAR INPUT

SOMATOSENSORY INPUT RED denotes 'sway-referenced' input. Support surface follows subject's body sway, providing orientationally inaccurate information.

Figure 31-4. SOT results can help determine how to treat the patient. Most patients with vestibular disorders fall on Conditions 5 and 6. Patients who fall under Conditions 4 through 6 have a surface-dependent pattern. With exercise and movement, SOT scores can be improved. The use of SOT can be used to quantify change over time in persons with vestibular disorders. From NeuroCom International, Inc.

much clinically as when the test was first devised. Wrisley and Whitney (2004) suggested a version of the test called the modified CTSIB (mCTSIB, Figure 31–5), where the dome is not used. The mCTSIB omits Conditions 3 and 6. It was reported by Cohen et al. (H. Cohen et al., 1993) that there were no differences between Conditions 2 and 3 and between Conditions 5 and 6.

Condition 1

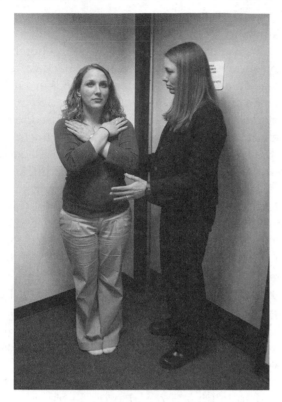

Condition 2

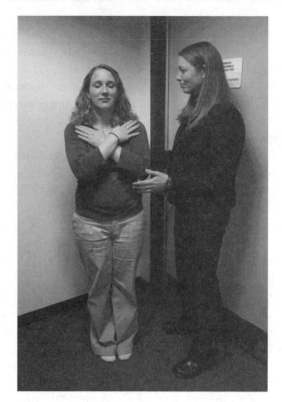

Condition 4

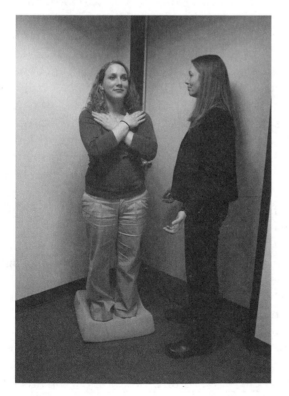

Condition 5

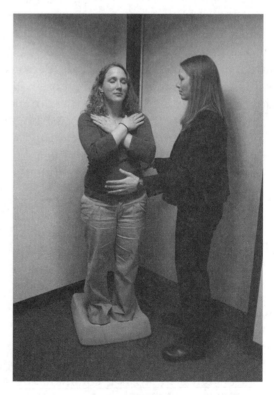

Figure 31-5. The modified Clinical Test of Sensory Integration and Balance (mCTSIB) consists of four tests: standing on a solid surface eyes open and closed, and standing on a compliant surface eyes open and closed.

Patients who cannot stand on foam with eyes open (Condition 4) are not able to walk safely on uneven surfaces, such as sand or gravel. Those who cannot stand on foam with eyes closed should not walk in the dark, especially on uneven surfaces. Having difficulty with Condition 4 is very common in older adults.

Patients are asked to stand with eyes closed on the foam pad during Condition 5. Generally, persons with peripheral vestibular hypofunction fall on Conditions 5 and 6, although not always, if they are well compensated (Herdman, 2000). Even persons with decreased bilateral hypofunction may be able to stand during Condition 5 if they are well compensated (K. E. Brown et al., 2001; Telian et al., 1991).

Condition 6 is the most difficult task, as they are ranked in hierarchical order with Condition 1 the easiest and Condition 6 the hardest to accomplish. The test involves standing with the visual dome in place while standing on the foam with eyes open. Sway is usually the greatest during Condition 6, although Cohen et al. found little difference in CTSIB 5 and 6 scores when tested with young and older adults, and persons with vestibular dysfunction (H. Cohen et al., 1993). Typically, persons with unilateral vestibular hypofunction fall on both Conditions 5 and 6.

Biomechanical constraints can affect the performance of the patient (Horak, 1987). Persons who have limited ankle range of motion, those with pain, or those with decreased strength or endurance will have their scores on the CTSIB affected because of physiologic constraints that are not related to their visual, vestibular, or proprioceptive systems. Careful examination of additional factors that might affect CTSIB performance should be made before one can be assured that there is dysfunction from one of the sensory pathways. Ankle dorsiflexion weakness could result in a fall on compliant surfaces, resulting in an erroneous conclusion as to why the patient is unstable.

Computerized Dynamic Posturography (CDP)

The Sensory Organization Test (SOT) of the Equi-Test™ (see Figure 31–4), is a commercially available device available to quantify postural control.

In addition to the SOT, the EquiTest device also includes a motor control test (MCT), whereby the floor is moved quickly forward or backward, and pitches up and down at different speeds around the patient's ankle joint while load sensors detect forces exerted by the feet. The SOT cannot be used to make a definitive diagnosis of vestibular dysfunction nor can the CTSIB, although the SOT is often used to corroborate other physical examination findings.

Scores on the CTSIB have been shown to moderately correlate with the SOT of CDP (el Kashlan et al., 1998; Weber & Cass, 1993). The six conditions are virtually the same, but instead of a visual conflict dome, the SOT incorporates a three-sided visual surround. During the SOT, there are combinations of the floor being sway-referenced and the walls being sway-referenced, providing a strong stimulus. The CDP attempts to isolate various aspects of postural controls, that is, reliance on visual, somatosensory, or vestibular information. Scores on the SOT can help to plan the treatment intervention, have been related to fall history, and provide objective data that can be used to assess change over time (Black, Angel, Pesznecker, & Gianna, 2000; S. L. Whitney, Marchetti, et al., 2006). O'Neill, Gill-Body, and Krebs (1998) reported improvements in the SOT score over time with patients with vestibular hypofunction undergoing vestibular rehabilitation, yet there was not a correlation between changes in functional performance and the SOT change scores.

The relationship between the SOT of CDP and falls risk is somewhat controversial (Girardi, Konrad, Amin, & Hughes, 2001; S. L. Whitney, Marchetti, et al., 2006). Girardi et al. (2001) and Whitney et al. (S. L. Whitney, Marchetti, et al., 2006) report that the SOT is helpful in identifying persons who are at risk for falling. Improvements in SOT scores and fewer falls during the SOT have been reported by Black et al. at the end of an episode of care consisting of an individualized vestibular rehabilitation program (Black et al., 2000). Recurrent fallers had significantly lower SOT scores than those who were one-time fallers or those who did not report a fall (Whitney, Marchetti, & Schade, 2006). Those patients who scored less than 38 on the SOT composite were 4.1 times more likely to be a recurrent faller (S. L. Whitney, Marchetti, et al., 2006). Tinetti and Williams (1997) have suggested that community-living older adults who fall are more likely to be admitted to long-term care facilities. As a result, some older adults may not be completely honest when they report their frequency of falling and objective testing may be helpful.

The SOT has been used to assist in identifying malingerers (Goebel et al., 1997; Krempl & Dobie, 1998; Mallinson & Longridge, 2005). Certain patterns of sway or unusual findings on CDP (both the SOT and MCT) suggest that the person may not be making his or her best effort or that he or she may have a psychiatric/psychologic condition. Mallinson and Longridge (2005) developed nine criteria that may reflect aphysiologic behavior in persons tested on CDP (Table 31–4). Computerized dynamic posturography helps to identify inconsistencies of postural performance, although one should also be concerned about mislabeling conversion disorder as malingering. Keim (1993) has reported that there was a higher prevalence of abnormal SOT scores in persons with central vestibular dysfunction, suggesting that brain disorders may be identified more easily than peripheral vestibular disorders by the SOT. Jacobson et al. (G.P. Jacobson, Newman, Hunter, & Blazer, 1991) stated that studying the vestibulo-ocular reflex does not provide a complete picture of the patients' functional performance. Computerized dynamic posturography or the CTSIB provides additional data to assist in making a diagnosis and in treatment planning.

GAIT ASSESSMENT

Gait Speed

The most acceptable measure of gait performance is gait speed (Guralnik et al., 2000; Perera et al., 2006; Studenski et al., 2011). Changes in older adults of 0.1 m/s are considered clinically significant (Perera et al., 2006). The slower an older adult ambulates, the greater his or her risk of falling (Guralnik et al., 2000). Using a value of 0.56 m/s as a lower limit of normal, Van Swearingen and colleagues identified a sensitivity of 72% and a specificity of 74% in frail older adults for recurrent falls (Van Swearingen, Paschal, Bonino, & Chen, 1998).

Normal walking speed to cross a signaled intersection is 1.27 m/s in young adults (Hoxie &

Table 31–4. Criteria Established To Determine Malingering in Persons Tested With Computerized Dynamic Posturography

Criterion	Description
1	Better performance on Conditions 1 and 2 when unaware
2	Conditions 1 and 2 markedly below normal
3	Conditions 5 and 6 relatively better than Conditions 1 and 2
4	Circular sway (i.e., lateral and anteroposterior together) without any falls
5	High intertrial variability on all SOT trials
6	Repeated suspiciously consistent sway patterns throughout the SOT trials
7	Exaggerated MCT responses
8	Inconsistent MCT responses
9	"Gut feeling" (i.e., clinical judgment)

Note. Scores of less than three do not indicate aphysiologic behavior; scores three and four are suspicious of aphysiologic behavior; scores of five or more suggest aphysiologic behavior. *SOT* = Sensory Organization Test; *MCT* = Motor Control Test. *Source*: Mallinson and Longridge (2005). Adapted and used with permission.

Rubenstein, 1994). The speed of older adults crossing an intersection was reported at 0.86 m/s, with 27% of the older adults not reaching the other side of the road before the light changed at the intersection (Hoxie & Rubenstein, 1994). Vestibular disorders generally slow gait speed, making functional mobility in the community even more difficult for older persons.

When observing a patient arrive for testing or treatment, it is very important to assess the patient's gait. Gait speed can easily be recorded by timing ambulation with a stopwatch over a specified distance. Patients who look unstable need to be guarded closely, but care should be taken to avoid touching the patient as it will change their gait performance (Jeka, 1997). Recent evidence suggests that gait speed, age, and gender are strong predictors of life expectancy (Studenski et al., 2011).

Gait speed can be recorded with any assistive device, including canes or walkers. Generally, patients are asked to walk over a 5-m walkway. If a patient cannot walk 5 m (approximately 20 feet), the walkway can be shortened as long as the patient can attain his or her normal gait speed before the clinician starts recording the timed gait.

It is best to have the patient walking at his or her normal gait speed before starting the stopwatch. The patient should walk past both lines on the floor or wall rather than stopping and starting at the lines, as you will be recording their acceleration and deceleration rather than ambulation at a constant velocity. Thus, the gait speed recorded will not reflect the patient's normal gait velocity. Distance divided by time equals velocity in feet/s. Most clinicians then convert the feet/s to m/s by multiplying by 0.3048.

Patients with vestibular disorders are often asked to walk at different speeds to determine if they can accelerate or decelerate upon command. Patients with vestibular dysfunction have a tendency to walk with little trunk or head rotation, especially during turning. This "stiff gait" is classic of persons with vestibular disorders.

One of the goals of rehabilitation is to incorporate eye/head rotation during functional activities as part of the exercise program. Without encouragement, some patients rarely walk because of their fear of becoming vertiginous or dizzy, and some develop a fear of falling (S. L. Whitney et al., 1999). Walking quickly may be more difficult than walking slowly for persons with vestibular disorders. Record-ing a person's self-selected and fast gait speed can enhance the therapist's understanding of gait performance since gait performance can vary depending on the speed at which the patient walks.

Walking in busy environments around many people and in environments where there is high visual contrast (stripes, checkered floors) will make ambulation much more difficult for persons with vestibular disorders (Bowman, 2004; Bronstein, 2004). In fact, some patients may completely avoid such environments. Patients with significant space and motion symptoms may become ill in the above circumstances (Bowman, 2004; R. Jacob, Furman, & Balaban, 1996; R. Jacob, Furman, & Perel, 1996; R. Jacob et al., 1993). After one or two exposures, some patients will avoid going out to stores and large social events to avoid feeling ill (Bowman, 2004). This avoidance behavior can lead to significant functional deficits (Bowman, 2004).

Timed "Up and Go" Test (TUG)

Another commonly used tool to assess progress over time is the TUG (Podsiadlo & Richardson, 1991). The tool was developed for use with frail older adults and it is one of the best validated tests used to assess balance during gait. The examiner asks the patient to rise from a chair, walk 3 m, turn around, and come back and sit down in a chair. They can use the armrests to rise from the chair and are also permitted to use an assistive device.

The TUG has been used to assess change over time in persons with vestibular disorders (Gill-Body, Beninato, & Krebs, 2000; S. Whitney et al., 2000; S. L. Whitney, Marchetti, et al., 2004; S. L. Whitney & Rossi, 2000; S. L. Whitney, Sparto, et al., 2006; S. L. Whitney, Wrisley, et al., 2000, 2004, 2005) and is often used to assess fall risk (Bischoff et al., 2003; H. S. Cohen & Kimball, 2004b; R. P. Di Fabio & Seay, 1997; Dite & Temple, 2002; Newton, 1997; Rockwood, Awalt, Carver, & MacKnight, 2000; Shumway-Cook, Brauer, & Woollacott, 2000). It has also been reported to be related to difficulty performing activities of daily living (Podsiadlo & Richardson, 1991).

The test-retest reliability of the TUG test has been reported as $r = 0.99$ in community-dwelling older adults with multiple comorbidities (Podsiadlo & Richardson, 1991). With increasing age,

TUG scores increase (Medley & Thompson, 1997) and increase by the use of a walking aid (Medley & Thompson, 1997; Shumway-Cook et al., 2000). The height of the chair used will also affect TUG performance (Siggeirsdottir, Jonsson, Jonsson, & Iwarsson, 2002), with lower chairs making it more difficult for persons to perform the test, resulting in increased (worse) TUG scores.

Standardization of procedures is very important for consistent results with the TUG. One should use the same chair each time and be consistent with the instructions. The voice command is important. Podsiadlo and Richardson (1991) suggested that the test be performed at the person's comfortable speed. If the examiner speaks loudly, the person is more likely to ambulate as quickly as possible, making comparisons between visits more difficult.

In older adults, scores of ≥13.5 s on the TUG test have been related to fall risk (Shumway-Cook et al., 2000). In persons with vestibular disorders, people who scored >13.5 s to perform the TUG were 3.7 times more likely to have reported falling within the last 6 months (S. L. Whitney, Marchetti, et al., 2004). Patients with scores >11.1 s were five times more likely to have reported a fall in the last 6 months (S. L. Whitney, Marchetti, et al., 2004), suggesting that the TUG is a very useful tool to assess fall risk in persons with vestibular disorders.

Whitney et al. have reported that the TUG scores of persons with vestibular disorders were similar to healthy people in their 80s (Steffen, Hacker, & Mollinger, 2002; S. L. Whitney, Marchetti, et al., 2004). Healthy men and women in their 70s often score between 8.5 and 9 s on the TUG (Podsiadlo & Richardson, 1991), suggesting that patients with vestibular disorders have significant gait impairment as the mean TUG score of a cohort of persons with vestibular disorders was 12 s (S. L. Whitney, Marchetti, et al., 2004).

Dynamic Gait Index (DGI)

The Dynamic Gait Index (DGI) was developed to record dynamic gait performance (Shumway-Cook & Woollacott, 1995). Shumway-Cook and Woollacott first published the tool in their textbook (Shumway-Cook & Woollacott, 1995). It has been used in persons with vestibular disorders to record change over time in their dynamic gait (K. E. Brown et al., 2006; K. E. Brown et al., 2001; Hall, Schubert, & Herdman, 2004; S. L. Whitney, Wrisley, et al., 2000). The DGI consists of eight walking tasks including: (1) walking; (2) walking at different speeds; (3) walking with yaw head movements; (4) walking with pitch head movements; (5) walking over objects; (6) walking around objects; (7) walking, turning, and stopping quickly on command; and (8) walking up and down steps. Each item is scored on a 0 to 3 scale, where 0 indicates that they could not perform the gait task or had to stop, and 3 indicates normal performance. Scores on the tool range from 0 to 24. Reliability of the DGI has been reported to range between .64 and .88 in persons with vestibular disorders (Hall & Herdman, 2006; Wrisley, Walker, Echternach, & Strasnick, 2003).

The DGI takes about 5 to 10 min to complete and provides the clinician with information about fall risk. Scores of ≤19 on the DGI have been related to fall risk in persons with vestibular disorders (Hall et al., 2004; S. L. Whitney, Hudak, et al., 2000; S. L. Whitney, Marchetti, et al., 2004). The functional gait assessment (FGA) has recently been reported to be more sensitive to change than the original DGI (Marchetti & Whitney, 2006; Marchetti, Lin, Alghdir, & Whitney, 2014). Marchetti and Whitney developed a four-item DGI that appears to provide similar data to the eight-item DGI, but takes half of the time (Marchetti & Whitney, 2006). The four-item DGI consists of the following items: walking on a level surface, walking with changes of speed, and walking with head movements in the pitch and yaw planes. The DGI-4 had slightly higher sensitivity and specificity than the eight-item DGI for identifying persons who had reported one fall (Marchetti & Whitney, 2006). Recently, Woollacott et al. (2013) modified the original DGI to try to expand the capabilities of the test (Shumway-Cook, Taylor, Matsuda, Studer, & Whetten, 2013).

SUMMARY

Graded balance and eye/head exercises help patients with vestibular disorders recover from the vestibular insult. Movement is key to functional recovery. Recovery most likely occurs as a result of plasticity within the nervous system. Patients must be encouraged to move after a vestibular disorder. There is clear evidence that balance function in people with peripheral vestibular disorders can be enhanced by rehabilitation. There is less evidence available about functional changes in persons with central vestibular disorders. The central vestibular group is much more difficult to study as they are a very heterogeneous group. There is emerging evidence to support vestibular rehabilitation for persons with central vestibular disorders.

REFERENCES

Agrawal, Y., Carey, J. P., Della Santina, C. C., Schubert, M. C., & Minor, L. B. (2009). Disorders of balance and vestibular function in US adults: Data from the National Health and Nutrition Examination Survey, 2001–2004. *Archives of Internal Medicine, 169*(10), 938–944. doi:10.1001/archinternmed.2009.66

Allum, J. H., Yamane, M., & Pfaltz, C. R. (1988). Long-term modifications of vertical and horizontal vestibulo-ocular reflex dynamics in man. I. After acute unilateral peripheral vestibular paralysis. *Acta Oto-Laryngologica, 105*(3–4), 328–337.

American Geriatrics Society & American Association for Geriatric Psychiatry. (2003). The American Geriatrics Society and American Association for Geriatric Psychiatry recommendations for policies in support of quality mental health care in U.S. nursing homes. *Journal of the American Geriatric Society, 51*(9), 1299–1304.

Anacker, S., & Di Fabio, R. (1992). Influence of sensory inputs on standing balance in community-dwelling elders with a recent history. *Physical Therapy, 72,* 575–583.

Asai, M., Watanabe, Y., & Shimizu, K. (1997). Effects of vestibular rehabilitation on postural control. *Acta Oto-Laryngologica Supplementum, 528,* 116–120.

Balaban, C. D. (1999). Vestibular autonomic regulation (including motion sickness and the mechanism of vomiting). *Current Opinion in Neurology, 12*(1), 29–33.

Balaban, C. D., & Porter, J. D. (1998). Neuroanatomic substrates for vestibulo-autonomic interactions. *Journal of Vestibular Research, 8*(1), 7–16.

Balaban, C. D., & Thayer, J. F. (2001). Neurological bases for balance-anxiety links. *Journal of Anxiety Disorders, 15*(1–2), 53–79.

Balci, B. D., Akdal, G., Yaka, E., & Angin, S. (2013). Vestibular rehabilitation in acute central vestibulopathy: A randomized controlled trial. *Journal of Vestibular Research, 23*(4–5), 259–267. doi:10.3233/VES-130491

Baloh, R. W., Corona, S., Jacobson, K. M., Enrietto, J. A., & Bell, T. (1998). A prospective study of posturography in normal older people. *Journal of the American Geriatric Society, 46*(4), 438–443.

Bamiou, D. E., Davies, R. A., McKee, M., & Luxon, L. M. (2000). Symptoms, disability and handicap in unilateral peripheral vestibular disorders. Effects of early presentation and initiation of balance exercises. *Scandinavian Audiology, 29*(4), 238–244.

Beidel, D. C., & Horak, F. B. (2001). Behavior therapy for vestibular rehabilitation. *Journal of Anxiety Disorders, 15*(1–2), 121–130.

Berthoz, A. (1988). The role of gaze in compensation of vestibular disfunction: The gaze substitution hypothesis. *Progress in Brain Research, 76,* 411–420.

Bischoff, H. A., Stahelin, H. B., Monsch, A. U., Iversen, M. D., Weyh, A., von Dechend, M., . . . Theiler, R. (2003). Identifying a cut-off point for normal mobility: A comparison of the timed "up and go" test in community-dwelling and institutionalised elderly women. *Age and Ageing, 32*(3), 315–320.

Black, F. O., Angel, C. R., Pesznecker, S. C., & Gianna, C. (2000). Outcome analysis of individualized vestibular rehabilitation protocols. *American Journal of Otology, 21*(4), 543–551.

Bowman, A. (2004). *Psychological and visual-perceptual explanations of poor compensation following unilateral vestibular loss.* (Doctor of Philosophy), The University of Sydney, Sydney, Australia.

Brandt, T., & Daroff, R. B. (1980). Physical therapy for benign paroxysmal positional vertigo. *Archives of Otolaryngology, 106*(8), 484–485.

Brandt, T., Krafczyk, S., & Malsbenden, I. (1981). Postural imbalance with head extension: Improvement by training as a model for ataxia therapy. *Annals of the New York Academy of Sciences, 374,* 636–649.

Bronstein, A. M. (2004). Vision and vertigo: Some visual aspects of vestibular disorders. *Journal of Neurology, 251*(4), 381–387.

Brown, I., Renwick, R., & Raphael, D. (1995). Frailty: Constructing a common meaning, definition, and conceptual framework. *18*(2), 93–102.

Brown, K. E., Whitney, S. L., Marchetti, G. F., Wrisley, D. M., & Furman, J. M. (2006). Physical therapy for central vestibular dysfunction. *Archives of Physical Medicine and Rehabilitation, 87*(1), 76–81.

Brown, K. E., Whitney, S. L., Wrisley, D. M., & Furman, J. M. (2001). Physical therapy outcomes for persons with bilateral vestibular loss. *Laryngoscope, 111*(10), 1812–1817.

Cass, S. P., BorelloFrance, D., & Furman, J. M. (1996). Functional outcome of vestibular rehabilitation in patients with abnormal sensory-organization testing. *American Journal of Otology, 17*(4), 581–594.

Cass, S. P., Furman, J. M., Ankerstjerne, J. K. P., Balaban, C., Yetiser, S., & Aydogan, B. (1997). Migraine-related vestibulopathy. *Annals of Otology, Rhinology, and Laryngology, 106*(3), 182–189.

Cawthorne, T. (1944). The physiological basis for head exercises. *Journal of the Chartered Society of Physiotherapy, 3,* 106–107.

Clendaniel, R. A., & Tucci, D. L. (1997). Vestibular rehabilitation strategies in Meniere's disease. *Otolaryngologic Clinics of North America, 30*(6), 1145–1158.

Cohen, B., John, P., Yakushin, S. B., Buettner-Ennever, J., & Raphan, T. (2002). The nodulus and uvula: Source of cerebellar control of spatial orientation of the angular vestibulo-ocular reflex. *Annals of the New York Academy of Sciences, 978,* 28–45.

Cohen, H. (1992). Vestibular rehabilitation reduces functional disability. *Otolaryngology-Head and Neck Surgery, 107*(5), 638–643.

Cohen, H. (1994). Vestibular rehabilitation improves daily life function. *American Journal of Occupational Therapy, 48*(10), 919–925.

Cohen, H., Blatchly, C. A., & Gombash, L. L. (1993). A study of the clinical test of sensory interaction and balance. *Physical Therapy, 73*(6), 346–351.

Cohen, H., Ewell, L. R., & Jenkins, H. A. (1995). Disability in Menieres disease. *Archives of Otolaryngology-Head and Neck Surgery, 121*(1), 29–33.

Cohen, H., Heaton, L. G., Congdon, S. L., & Jenkins, H. A. (1996). Changes in sensory organization test scores with age. *Age and Ageing, 25*(1), 39–44.

Cohen, H., Kanewineland, M., Miller, L. V., & Hatfield, C. L. (1995). Occupation and visual-vestibular interaction in vestibular rehabilitation. *Otolaryngology-Head and Neck Surgery, 112*(4), 526–532.

Cohen, H. S., & Kimball, K. T. (2000). Development of the Vestibular Disorders Activities of Daily Living Scale. *Archives of Otolaryngology-Head and Neck Surgery, 126*(7), 881–887.

Cohen, H. S., & Kimball, K. T. (2003). Increased independence and decreased vertigo after vestibular rehabilitation. *Otolaryngology-Head and Neck Surgery, 128*(1), 60–70.

Cohen, H. S., & Kimball, K. T. (2004a). Changes in a repetitive head movement task after vestibular rehabilitation. *Clinical Rehabilitation, 18*(2), 125–131.

Cohen, H. S., & Kimball, K. T. (2004b). Decreased ataxia and improved balance after vestibular rehabilitation. *Otolaryngology-Head and Neck Surgery, 130*(4), 418–425.

Cohen, H. S., & Kimball, K. T. (2005). Effectiveness of treatments for benign paroxysmal positional vertigo of the posterior canal. *Otology and Neurotology, 26*(5), 1034–1040.

Cohen, H. S., Kimball, K. T., & Adams, A. S. (2000). Application of the Vestibular Disorders Activities of Daily Living Scale. *Laryngoscope, 110*(7), 1204–1209.

Cohen, H. S., Kimball, K. T., & Stewart, M. G. (2004). Benign paroxysmal positional vertigo and comorbid conditions. *ORL Journal of Otorhinolaryngology and Its Related Specialties, 66*(1), 11–15.

Corna, S., Nardone, A., Prestinari, A., Galante, M., Grasso, M., & Schieppati, M. (2003). Comparison of Cawthorne-Cooksey exercises and sinusoidal support surface translations to improve balance in patients with unilateral vestibular deficit. *Archives of Physical Medicine and Rehabilitation, 84*(8), 1173–1184.

Cooksey, F. S. (1946). Rehabilitation in vestibular injuries. *Proceedings of the Royal Society of Medicine, 39,* 273–278.

Courjon, J. H., Flandrin, J. M., Jeannerod, M., & Schmid, R. (1982). The role of the flocculus in vestibular compensation after hemilabyrinthectomy. *Brain Research, 239*(1), 251–257.

Cowand, J. L., Wrisley, D. M., Walker, M., Strasnick, B., & Jacobson, J. T. (1998). Efficacy of vestibular rehabilitation. *Otolaryngology-Head and Neck Surgery, 118*(1), 49–54.

Curthoys, I. S., & Halmagyi, G. M. (1995). Vestibular compensation: A review of the oculomotor, neural, and clinical consequences of unilateral vestibular loss. *Journal of Vestibular Research, 5*(2), 67–107.

Davies, R. A., & Luxon, L. M. (1995). Dizziness following head injury: A neuro-otological study. *Journal of Neurology, 242*(4), 222–230.

Di Fabio, R. (1995). Sensitivity and specificity of platform posturography for identifying patients with vestibular dysfunction. *Physical Therapy, 75*(4), 46–61.

Di Fabio, R. P., & Seay, R. (1997). Use of the "fast evaluation of mobility, balance, and fear" in elderly community dwellers: Validity and reliability. *Physical Therapy, 77*(9), 904–917.

Dickstein, R., Shupert, C. L., & Horak, F. B. (2001). Fingertip touch improves postural stability in patients with peripheral neuropathy. *Gait and Posture., 14*(3), 238–247.

Dieringer, N. (1995). "Vestibular compensation": Neural plasticity and its relations to functional recovery after labyrinthine lesions in frogs and other vertebrates. *Progress in Neurobiology, 46*(2–3), 97–129.

Dite, W., & Temple, V. A. (2002). A clinical test of stepping and change of direction to identify multiple falling older adults. *Archives of Physical Medicine and Rehabilitation, 83*(11), 1566–1571.

Dix, M. R. (1976). The physiological basis and practical value of head exercises in the treatment of vertigo. *The Practitioner, 217*, 919–925.

Duncan, P. W., Studenski, S., Chandler, J., & Prescott, B. (1992). Functional reach-predictive-validity in a sample of elderly male veterans. *Journals of Gerontology, 47*(3), M93–M98.

Duncan, P. W., Weiner, D. K., Chandler, J., & Studenski, S. (1990). Functional reach: A new clinical measure of balance. *Journals of Gerontology, 45*(6), M192–M197.

Eagger, S., Luxon, L. M., Davies, R. A., Coelho, A., & Ron, M. A. (1992). Psychiatric morbidity in patients with peripheral vestibular disorder: A clinical and neuro-otological study. *Journal of Neurology, Neurosurgery, and Psychiatry, 55*(5), 383–387.

Ekvall Hansson, E., Mansson, N. O., Ringsberg, K. A., & Hakansson, A. (2006). Dizziness among patients with whiplash-associated disorder: A randomized controlled trial. *Journal of Rehabilitation Medicine, 38*(6), 387–390.

el Kashlan, H. K., Shepard, N. T., Asher, A. M., Smith-Wheelock, M., & Telian, S. A. (1998). Evaluation of clinical measures of equilibrium. *Laryngoscope, 108*(3), 311–319.

Enloe, L. J., & Shields, R. K. (1997). Evaluation of health-related quality of life in individuals with vestibular disease using disease-specific and general outcome measures. *Physical Therapy, 77*(9), 890–903.

Fetter, M., & Zee, D. S. (1988). Recovery from unilateral labyrinthectomy in rhesus monkey. *Journal of Neurophysiology, 59*(2), 370–393.

Fielder, H., Denholm, S. W., Lyons, R. A., & Fielder, C. P. (1996). Measurement of health status in patients with vertigo. *Clinical Otolaryngology, 21*(2), 124–126.

Forssberg, H., & Nashner, L. M. (1982). Ontogenetic development of postural control in man: Adaptation to altered support and visual conditions during stance. *Journal of Neuroscience, 2*(5), 545–552.

Furman, J. M., Balaban, C. D., & Pollack, I. F. (1997). Vestibular compensation in a patient with a cerebellar infarction. *Neurology, 48*(4), 916–920.

Furman, J. M., & Whitney, S. L. (2000). Central causes of dizziness. *Physical Therapy, 80*(2), 179–187.

Galica, A. M., Kang, H. G., Priplata, A. A., D'Andrea, S. E., Starobinets, O. V., Sorond, F. A., . . . Lipsitz, L. A. (2009). Subsensory vibrations to the feet reduce gait variability in elderly fallers. *Gait and Posture, 30*(3), 383–387. doi:10.1016/j.gaitpost.2009.07.005

Gamiz, M. J., & Lopez-Escamez, J. A. (2004). Health-related quality of life in patients over sixty years old with benign paroxysmal positional vertigo. *Gerontology, 50*(2), 82–86.

Garcia, A. P., Gananca, M. M., Cusin, F. S., Tomaz, A., Gananca, F. F., & Caovilla, H. H. (2013). Vestibular rehabilitation with virtual reality in Meniere's disease. *Brazilian Journal of Otorhinolaryngology, 79*(3), 366–374. doi:10.5935/1808-8694.20130064

Gill, T. M., Baker, D. I., Gottschalk, M., Peduzzi, P. N., Allore, H., & Byers, A. (2002). A program to prevent functional decline in physically frail, elderly persons who live at home. *New England Journal of Medicine, 347*(14), 1068–1074.

Gill-Body, K. M., Beninato, M., & Krebs, D. E. (2000). Relationship among balance impairments, functional performance, and disability in people with peripheral vestibular hypofunction. *Physical Therapy, 80*(8), 748–758.

Gill-Body, K. M., & Krebs, D. E. (1994). Locomotor stability problems associated with vestibulopathy: Assessment and treatment. *Physical Therapy Practice, 3*(4), 232–245.

Gill-Body, K. M., Krebs, D. E., Parker, S. W., & Riley, P. O. (1994). Physical therapy management of peripheral vestibular dysfunction: Two clinical case reports. *Physical Therapy, 74*(2), 129–142.

Gill-Body, K. M., Popat, R. A., Parker, S. W., & Krebs, D. E. (1997). Rehabilitation of balance in two patients with cerebellar dysfunction. *Physical Therapy, 77*(5), 534–552.

Gillespie, M. B., & Minor, L. B. (1999). Prognosis in bilateral vestibular hypofunction. *Laryngoscope, 109*(1), 35–41.

Girardi, M., Konrad, H. R., Amin, M., & Hughes, L. F. (2001). Predicting fall risks in an elderly population: Computer dynamic posturography versus electronystagmography test results. *Laryngoscope, 111*(9), 1528–1532.

Goebel, J. A., Sataloff, R. T., Hanson, J. M., Nashner, L. M., Hirshout, D. S., & Sokolow, C. C. (1997). Posturographic evidence of nonorganic sway patterns in normal subjects, patients, and suspected malingerers. *Otolaryngology-Head and Neck Surgery, 117*(4), 293–302.

Gottshall, K. R., Hoffer, M. E., Moore, R. J., & Balough, B. J. (2005). The role of vestibular rehabilitation in the treatment of Meniere's disease. *Otolaryngology-Head and Neck Surgery, 133*(3), 326–328.

Gottshall, K. R., Sessoms, P. H., & Bartlett, J. L. (2012). Vestibular physical therapy intervention: Utilizing a computer assisted rehabilitation environment in lieu of traditional physical therapy. *Conference Proceedings-IEEE Engineering in Medicine and Biology Society, 2012*, 6141–6144. doi:10.1109/EMBC.2012.6347395

Guerraz, M., Yardley, L., Bertholon, P., Pollak, L., Rudge, P., Gresty, M. A., & Bronstein, A. M. (2001). Visual vertigo: Symptom assessment, spatial orientation and postural control. *Brain, 124*(Pt. 8), 1646–1656.

Guralnik, J. M., Ferrucci, L., Pieper, C. F., Leveille, S. G., Markides, K. S., Ostir, G. V., . . . Wallace, R. B. (2000). Lower extremity function and subsequent disability:

Consistency across studies, predictive models, and value of gait speed alone compared with the short physical performance battery. *Journals of Gerontology, Series A: Biological Sciences and Medical Sciences, 55*(4), M221–M231.

Gurr, B., & Moffat, N. (2001). Psychological consequences of vertigo and the effectiveness of vestibular rehabilitation for brain injury patients. *Brain Injury, 15*(5), 387–400.

Gustave, D., Duflo, S., Borel, L., Harlay, F., Leonard, J., & Lacour, M. (1998). Short-term changes in neck muscle and eye movement responses following unilateral vestibular neurectomy in the cat. *Experimental Brain Research, 120*(4), 439–449.

Hain, T. C., Fetter, M., & Zee, D. S. (1987). Head-shaking nystagmus in patients with unilateral peripheral vestibular lesions. *American Journal of Otolaryngology, 8*(1), 36–47.

Hall, C. D., & Herdman, S. J. (2006). Reliability of clinical measures used to assess patients with peripheral vestibular disorders. *Journal of Neurologic Physical Therapy, 30*(2), 74–81.

Hall, C. D., Schubert, M. C., & Herdman, S. J. (2004). Prediction of fall risk reduction as measured by dynamic gait index in individuals with unilateral vestibular hypofunction. *Otology and Neurotology, 25*(5), 746–751.

Halmagyi, G. M., & Curthoys, I. S. (1988). A clinical sign of canal paresis. *Archives of Neurology, 45*(7), 737–739.

Haynes, D. S., Resser, J. R., Labadie, R. F., Girasole, C. R., Kovach, B. T., Scheker, L. E., & Walker, D. C. (2002). Treatment of benign positional vertigo using the semont maneuver: Efficacy in patients presenting without nystagmus. *Laryngoscope, 112*(5), 796–801.

Herdman, S. J. (1990). Treatment of vestibular disorders in traumatically brain-injured patients. *Journal of Head Trauma Rehabilitation, 5*(4), 63–76.

Herdman, S. J. (1997). Advances in the treatment of vestibular disorders. *Physical Therapy, 77*(6), 602–618.

Herdman, S. J. (1998). Role of vestibular adaptation in vestibular rehabilitation. *Otolaryngology-Head and Neck Surgery, 119*(1), 49–54.

Herdman, S. J. (2000). *Vestibular rehabilitation* (2nd ed.). Philadelphia, PA: F. A. Davis.

Herdman, S. J., Blatt, P. J., & Schubert, M. C. (2000). Vestibular rehabilitation of patients with vestibular hypofunction or with benign paroxysmal positional vertigo. *Current Opinion in Neurology, 13*(1), 39–43.

Herdman, S. J., Blatt, P., Schubert, M. C., & Tusa, R. J. (2000). Falls in patients with vestibular deficits. *American Journal of Otology, 21*(6), 847–851.

Herdman, S. J., Clendaniel, R. A., Mattox, D. E., Holliday, M. J., & Niparko, J. K. (1995). Vestibular adaptation exercises and recovery: Acute stage after acoustic neu-roma resection. *Otolaryngology-Head and Neck Surgery, 113*(1), 77–87.

Herdman, S. J., Schubert, M. C., Das, V. E., & Tusa, R. J. (2003). Recovery of dynamic visual acuity in unilateral vestibular hypofunction. *Archives of Otolaryngology-Head and Neck Surgery, 129*(8), 819–824.

Herdman, S. J., Schubert, M. C., & Tusa, R. J. (2001). Role of central preprogramming in dynamic visual acuity with vestibular loss. *Archives of Otolaryngology-Head and Neck Surgery, 127*(10), 1205–1210.

Hillier, S. L., & McDonnell, M. (2011). Vestibular rehabilitation for unilateral peripheral vestibular dysfunction. *Clinical Otolaryngology, 36*(3), 248–249.

Holmberg, J., Karlberg, M., Harlacher, U., Rivano-Fischer, M., & Magnusson, M. (2006). Treatment of phobic postural vertigo. A controlled study of cognitive-behavioral therapy and self-controlled desensitization. *Journal of Neurology, 253*(4), 500–506.

Honegger, F., Hillebrandt, I. M., van den Elzen, N. G., Tang, K. S., & Allum, J. H. (2013). The effect of prosthetic feedback on the strategies and synergies used by vestibular loss subjects to control stance. *Journal of Neuroengineering and Rehabilitation, 10*, 115. doi:10.1186/1743-0003-10-115

Horak, F. B. (1987). Clinical measurement of postural control in adults. *Physical Therapy, 67*(12), 1881–1885.

Horak, F. B., Jones-Rycewicz, C., Black, F. O., & Shumway-Cook, A. (1992). Effects of vestibular rehabilitation on dizziness and imbalance. *Otolaryngology-Head and Neck Surgery, 106*(2), 175–180.

Horak, F. B., & Nashner, L. M. (1986). Central programming of postural movements: Adaptation to altered support-surface configurations. *Journal of Neurophysiology, 55*(6), 1369–1381.

Hoxie, R. E., & Rubenstein, L. Z. (1994). Are older pedestrians allowed enough time to cross intersections safely? *Journal of the American Geriatric Society, 42*(3), 241–244.

Hughes, M. A., Duncan, P. W., Rose, D. K., Chandler, J. M., & Studenski, S. A. (1996). The relationship of postural sway to sensorimotor function, functional performance, and disability in the elderly. *Archives of Physical Medicine and Rehabilitation, 77*(6), 567–572.

Jacob, R., Furman, J., & Balaban, C. (1996). Psychiatric aspects of vestibular disorders. In R. W. Baloh & G. M. Halmagyi (Eds.), *Disorders of the vestibular system* (pp. 509–528). New York, NY: Oxford University Press.

Jacob, R., Furman, J., & Perel, J. (1996). Panic, phobia, and vestibular dysfunction. In B. Yates & A. Miller (Eds.), *Vestibular autonomic regulation* (pp. 197–227). New York, NY: CRC Press.

Jacob, R., Woody, S. R., Clark, D. B., Lilienfeld, S. O., Hirsch, B. E., Kucera, G. D., . . . Durrant, J. D. (1993). Discomfort with space and motion: A possible marker of vestibular dysfunction assessed by the Situational

Characteristics Questionnaire. *Journal of Psychopathology and Behavioral Assessment, 15*(4), 299–324.

Jacob, R. G., & Furman, J. M. (2001). Psychiatric consequences of vestibular dysfunction. *Current Opinion in Neurology, 14*(1), 41–46.

Jacob, R. G., Whitney, S. L., Detweiler-Shostak, G., & Furman, J. M. (2001). Vestibular rehabilitation for patients with agoraphobia and vestibular dysfunction: A pilot study. *Journal of Anxiety Disorders, 15*(1–2), 131–146.

Jacobson, G. P., & Calder, J. H. (1998). A screening version of the Dizziness Handicap Inventory (DHI-S). *American Journal of Otology, 19*(6), 804–808.

Jacobson, G. P., & Newman, C. W. (1990). The development of the Dizziness Handicap Inventory. *Archives of Otolaryngology-Head and Neck Surgery, 116*(4), 424–427.

Jacobson, G. P., Newman, C. W., Hunter, L., & Blazer, G. K. (1991). Balance Function Test correlates of the Dizziness Handicap Inventory. *Journal of the American Academy of Audiology, 2,* 253–260.

Jeka, J. J. (1997). Light touch contact as a balance aid. *Physical Therapy, 77*(5), 476–487.

Johansson, M., Akerlund, D., Larsen, H. C., & Andersson, G. (2001). Randomized controlled trial of vestibular rehabilitation combined with cognitive-behavioral therapy for dizziness in older people. *Otolaryngology-Head and Neck Surgery, 125*(3), 151–156.

Karlberg, M., Magnusson, M., Malmstrom, E. M., Melander, A., & Moritz, U. (1996). Postural and symptomatic improvement after physiotherapy in patients with dizziness of suspected cervical origin. *Archives of Physical Medicine and Rehabilitation, 77*(9), 874–882.

Kattah, J. C., Talkad, A. V., Wang, D. Z., Hsieh, Y. H., & Newman-Toker, D. E. (2009). HINTS to diagnose stroke in the acute vestibular syndrome: Three-step bedside oculomotor examination more sensitive than early MRI diffusion-weighted imaging. *Stroke, 40*(11), 3504–3510. doi:10.1161/STROKEAHA.109.551234

Keim, R. J. (1993). Clinical comparisons of posturography and electronystagmography. *Laryngoscope, 103*(7), 713–716.

Kentala, E., Viikki, K., Pyykko, I., & Juhola, M. (2000). Production of diagnostic rules from a neurotologic database with decision trees. *Annals of Otology Rhinology and Laryngology, 109*(2), 170–176.

Kinney, S. E., Sandridge, S. A., & Newman, C. W. (1997). Long-term effects of Meniere's disease on hearing and quality of life. *American Journal of Otology, 18*(1), 67–73.

Konrad, H. R., Tomlinson, D., Stockwell, C. W., Norre, M., Horak, F. B., Shepard, N. T., & Herdman, S. J. (1992). Rehabilitation therapy for patients with disequilibrium and balance disorders. *Otolaryngology-Head and Neck Surgery, 107*(1), 105–108.

Krebs, D. E., Gillbody, K. M., Riley, P. O., & Parker, S. W. (1993). Double-blind, placebo-controlled trial of rehabilitation for bilateral vestibular hypofunction—Preliminary report. *Otolaryngology-Head and Neck Surgery, 109*(4), 735–741.

Krempl, G. A., & Dobie, R. A. (1998). Evaluation of posturography in the detection of malingering subjects. *American Journal of Otology, 19*(5), 619–627.

Kristinsdottir, E. K., Jarnlo, G. B., & Magnusson, M. (2000). Asymmetric vestibular function in the elderly might be a significant contributor to hip fractures. *Scandinavian Journal of Rehabilitation Medicine, 32*(2), 56–60.

Lacour, M., Roll, J. P., & Appaix, M. (1976). Modifications and development of spinal reflexes in the alert baboon (*Papio papio*) following an unilateral vestibular neurotomy. *Brain Research, 113*(2), 255–269.

Lajoie, Y., & Gallagher, S. P. (2004). Predicting falls within the elderly community: Comparison of postural sway, reaction time, the Berg balance scale and the Activities-specific Balance Confidence (ABC) scale for comparing fallers and non-fallers. *Archives of Gerontology and Geriatrics, 38*(1), 11–26.

Lei-Rivera, L., Sutera, J., Galatioto, J. A., Hujsak, B. D., & Gurley, J. M. (2013). Special tools for the assessment of balance and dizziness in individuals with mild traumatic brain injury. *Neurorehabilitation, 32*(3), 463–472.

Llorens, R., Colomer-Font, C., Alcaniz, M., & Noe-Sebastian, E. (2013). BioTrak virtual reality system: Effectiveness and satisfaction analysis for balance rehabilitation in patients with brain injury. *Neurologia, 28*(5), 268–275. doi:10.1016/j.nrl.2012.04.016

Lord, S. R., & Clark, R. D. (1996). Simple physiological and clinical tests for the accurate prediction of falling in older people. *Gerontology, 42*(4), 199–203.

Lord, S. R., Murray, S. M., Chapman, K., Munro, B., & Tiedemann, A. (2002). Sit-to-stand performance depends on sensation, speed, balance, and psychological status in addition to strength in older people. *Journals of Gerontology, Series A: Biological Sciences and Medical Sciences, 57*(8), M539–M543.

Luxon, L. L. (2003). *Textbook of audiological medicine clinical aspects of hearing and balance.* London, UK: Martin Dunitz.

Lystad, R. P., Bell, G., Bonnevie-Svendsen, M., & Carter, C. V. (2011). Manual therapy with and without vestibular rehabilitation for cervicogenic dizziness: A systematic review. *Chiropractic and Manual Therapies, 19*(1), 21. doi:10.1186/2045-709X-19-21

Magnusson, M., Kahlon, B., Karlberg, M., Lindberg, S., Siesjo, P., & Tjernstrom, F. (2009). Vestibular "PREHAB". *Annals of the New York Academy of Sciences, 1164,* 257–262.

Magnusson, M., Karlberg, M., & Tjernstrom, F. (2011). "PREHAB": Vestibular prehabilitation to ameliorate the effect of a sudden vestibular loss. *Neurorehabilitation, 29*(2), 153–156.

Maki, B. E., Perry, S. D., Norrie, R. G., & McIlroy, W. E. (1999). Effect of facilitation of sensation from plantar foot-surface boundaries on postural stabilization in young and older adults. *Journals of Gerontology, Series A: Biological Sciences and Medical Sciences, 54*(6), M281–M287.

Mallinson, A. I., & Longridge, N. S. (2005). A new set of criteria for evaluating malingering in work-related vestibular injury. *Otology and Neurotology, 26*(4), 686–690.

Mann, G. C., Whitney, S. L., Redfern, M. S., Borello-France, D. F., & Furman, J. M. (1996). Functional reach and single leg stance in patients with peripheral vestibular disorders. *Journal of Vestibular Research, 6*(5), 343–353.

Marchetti, G. F., Lin, C. C., Alghadir, A., & Whitney, S. L. (2014). Responsiveness and minimal detectable change of the Dynamic Gait Index and Functional Gait Index in persons with balance and vestibular disorders. *Journal of Neurologic Physical Therapy, 38*(2), 119–124.

Marchetti, G. F., & Whitney, S. L. (2005). Older adults and balance dysfunction. *Neurologic Clinics, 23*(3), 785–805, vii.

Marchetti, G. F., & Whitney, S. L. (2006). Construction and validation of the 4-item Dynamic Gait Index. *Physical Therapy, 86*(12), 1651–1660. doi:10.2522/ptj.20050402

Marcus, D. A., Kapelewski, C., Jacob, R. G., Rudy, T. E., & Furman, J. M. (2004). Validation of a brief nurse-administered migraine assessment tool. *Headache, 44*(4), 328–332. doi:10.1111/j.1526-4610.2004.04076.x

Marcus, D. A., Kapelewski, C., Rudy, T. E., Jacob, R. G., & Furman, J. M. (2004). Diagnosis of migrainous vertigo: Validity of a structured interview. *Medical Science Monitor, 10*(5), CR197–CR201.

Marioni, G., Fermo, S., Lionello, M., Fasanaro, E., Giacomelli, L., Zanon, S., . . . Staffieri, A. (2013). Vestibular rehabilitation in elderly patients with central vestibular dysfunction: A prospective, randomized pilot study. *Age (Dordrecht, the Netherlands), 35*(6), 2315–2327. doi:10.1007/s11357-012-9494-7

McCabe, B. F. (1970). Labyrinthine exercises in the treatment of diseases characterized by vertigo: Their physiologic basis and methodology. *Laryngoscope, 80*(9), 1429–1433.

Medeiros, I. R., Bittar, R. S., Pedalini, M. E., Lorenzi, M. C., Formigoni, L. G., & Bento, R. F. (2005). Vestibular rehabilitation therapy in children. *Otology and Neurotology, 26*(4), 699–703.

Medley, A., & Thompson, M. (1997). The effect of assistive devices on the performance of community dwelling elderly on the timed up and go test. *Issues on Aging, 20*, 3–7.

Meldrum, D., Herdman, S., Moloney, R., Murray, D., Duffy, D., Malone, K., . . . McConn-Walsh, R. (2012). Effectiveness of conventional versus virtual reality based vestibular rehabilitation in the treatment of dizziness, gait and balance impairment in adults with unilateral peripheral vestibular loss: A randomised controlled trial. *BMC Ear, Nose, and Throat Disorders, 12*, 3. doi:10.1186/1472-6815-12-3

Meli, A., Zimatore, G., Badaracco, C., De Angelis, E., & Tufarelli, D. (2006). Vestibular rehabilitation and 6-month follow-up using objective and subjective measures. *Acta Oto-Laryngologica, 126*(3), 259–266.

Messier, S. P., Royer, T. D., Craven, T. E., O'Toole, M. L., Burns, R., & Ettinger, W. H. (2000). Long-term exercise and its effect on balance in older, osteoarthritic adults: Results from the fitness, arthritis, and seniors trial (FAST). *Journal of the American Geriatric Society, 48*(2), 131–138.

Monahan, K. D., Sharpe, M. K., Drury, D., Ertl, A. C., & Ray, C. A. (2002). Influence of vestibular activation on respiration in humans. *American Journal of Physiology—Regulatory, Integrative and Comparative Physiology, 282*(3), R689–R694.

Mruzek, M., Barin, K., Nichols, D. S., Burnett, C. N., & Welling, D. B. (1995). Effects of vestibular rehabilitation and social reinforcement on recovery following ablative vestibular surgery. *Laryngoscope, 105*(7 Pt. 1), 686–692.

Murray, K. J., Hill, K., Phillips, B., & Waterston, J. (2005). A pilot study of falls risk and vestibular dysfunction in older fallers presenting to hospital emergency departments. *Disability and Rehabilitation, 27*(9), 499–506.

Myers, A. M., Fletcher, P. C., Myers, A. H., & Sherk, W. (1998). Discriminative and evaluative properties of the activities-specific balance confidence (ABC) scale. *Journals of Gerontology, Series A: Biological Sciences and Medical Sciences, 53*(4), M287–M294.

Nagaratnam, N., Ip, J., & Bou-Haidar, P. (2005). The vestibular dysfunction and anxiety disorder interface: A descriptive study with special reference to the elderly. *Archives of Gerontology and Geriatrics, 40*(3), 253–264.

Nagarkar, A. N., Gupta, A. K., & Mann, S. B. (2000). Psychological findings in benign paroxysmal positional vertigo and psychogenic vertigo. *Journal of Otolaryngology, 29*(3), 154–158.

Nashner, L. M. (1982). Adaptation of human movement to altered enviroments. *Trends in Neurosciences, 5*, 358–361.

Nashner, L. M., Shumway-Cook, A., & Marin, O. (1983). Stance posture control in select groups of children with cerebral palsy: Deficits in sensory organization and muscular coordination. *Experimental Brain Research, 49*(3), 393–409.

Neuhauser, H., Leopold, M., von Brevern, M., Arnold, G., & Lempert, T. (2001). The interrelations of migraine, vertigo, and migrainous vertigo. *Neurology, 56*(4), 436–441.

Newton, R. A. (1997). Balance screening of an inner city older adult population. *Archives of Physical Medicine and Rehabilitation, 78*(6), 587–591.

Norre, M. E. (1984). Treatment of unilateral vestibular hypofunction. In W. Oosterveld (Ed.), *Otoneurology* (pp. 23–39). Hoboken, NJ: Wiley.

Norre, M. E. (1987). Rationale of rehabilitation treatment for vertigo. *American Journal of Otolaryngology, 8*(1), 31–35.

Norre, M. E., & Beckers, A. M. (1988). Vestibular habituation training. Specificity of adequate exercise. *Archives of Otolaryngology-Head and Neck Surgery, 114*(8), 883–886.

Norre, M. E., & DeWeerdt, W. (1981). Positional (provoked) vertigo treated by postural training vestibular habituation training. *Agressologie, 22*(B), 37–44.

Nunez, R. A., Cass, S. P., & Furman, J. M. (2000). Short- and long-term outcomes of canalith repositioning for benign paroxysmal positional vertigo. *Otolaryngology-Head and Neck Surgery, 122*(5), 647–652.

Nyabenda, A., Briart, C., Deggouj, N., & Gersdorff, M. (2004). [Normative study and reliability of French version of the dizziness handicap inventory]. *Annales de Readaptation et de Medecine Physique, 47*(3), 105–113.

Oghalai, J. S., Manolidis, S., Barth, J. L., Stewart, M. G., & Jenkins, M. A. (2000). Unrecognized benign paroxysmal positional vertigo in elderly patients. *Otolaryngology-Head and Neck Surgery, 122*(5), 630–634.

O'Neill, D. E., Gill-Body, K. M., & Krebs, D. E. (1998). Posturography changes do not predict functional performance changes. *American Journal of Otology, 19*(6), 797–803.

Pavlou, M., Kanegaonkar, R. G., Swapp, D., Bamiou, D. E., Slater, M., & Luxon, L. M. (2012). The effect of virtual reality on visual vertigo symptoms in patients with peripheral vestibular dysfunction: A pilot study. *Journal of Vestibular Research, 22*(5–6), 273–281. doi:10.3233/VES-120462

Pavlou, M., Lingeswaran, A., Davies, R. A., Gresty, M. A., & Bronstein, A. M. (2004). Simulator based rehabilitation in refractory dizziness. *Journal of Neurology, 251*(8), 983–995.

Peppard, S. B. (1986). Effect of drug therapy on compensation from vestibular injury. *Laryngoscope, 96*(8), 878–898.

Perera, S., Mody, S. H., Woodman, R. C., & Studenski, S. A. (2006). Meaningful change and responsiveness in common physical performance measures in older adults. *Journal of the American Geriatric Society, 54*(5), 743–749.

Peterka, R. J., Wall, C., 3rd, & Kentala, E. (2006). Determining the effectiveness of a vibrotactile balance prosthesis. *Journal of Vestibular Research, 16*(1–2), 45–56.

Podsiadlo, D., & Richardson, S. (1991). The timed "Up & Go": A test of basic functional mobility for frail elderly persons. *Journal of the American Geriatric Society, 39*(2), 142–148.

Pollak, L., Klein, C., Rafael, S., Vera, K., & Rabey, J. M. (2003). Anxiety in the first attack of vertigo. *Otolaryngology-Head and Neck Surgery., 128*(6), 829–834.

Powell, L. E., & Myers, A. M. (1995). The Activities-specific Balance Confidence (ABC) Scale. *Journals of Gerontology, Series A: Biological Sciences and Medical Sciences, 50A*(1), M28–M34.

Priplata, A. A., Niemi, J. B., Harry, J. D., Lipsitz, L. A., & Collins, J. J. (2003). Vibrating insoles and balance control in elderly people. *Lancet, 362*(9390), 1123–1124.

Priplata, A. A., Patritti, B. L., Niemi, J. B., Hughes, R., Gravelle, D. C., Lipsitz, L. A., . . . Collins, J. J. (2006). Noise-enhanced balance control in patients with diabetes and patients with stroke. *Annals of Neurology, 59*(1), 4–12.

Richardson, J. K., & Ashton-Miller, J. A. (1996). Peripheral neuropathy: An often-overlooked cause of falls in the elderly. *Postgraduate Medicine, 99*(6), 161–172.

Richardson, J. K., Ashton-Miller, J. A., Lee, S. G., & Jacobs, K. (1996). Moderate peripheral neuropathy impairs weight transfer and unipedal balance in the elderly. *Archives of Physical Medicine and Rehabilitation, 77*(11), 1152–1156.

Rine, R. M., & Braswell, J. (2003). A clinical test of dynamic visual acuity for children. *International Journal of Pediatric Otorhinolaryngology, 67*(11), 1195–1201.

Rockwood, K., Awalt, E., Carver, D., & MacKnight, C. (2000). Feasibility and measurement properties of the functional reach and the timed up and go tests in the Canadian study of health and aging. *Journals of Gerontology, Series A: Biological Sciences and Medical Sciences, 55*(2), M70–M73

Rubin, A. M., Woolley, S. M., Dailey, V. M., & Goebel, J. A. (1995). Postural stability following mild head or whiplash injuries. *American Journal of Otology, 16*(2), 216–221.

Schmid, G., Henningsen, P., Dieterich, M., Sattel, H., & Lahmann, C. (2011). Psychotherapy in dizziness: A systematic review. *Journal of Neurology, Neurosurgery, and Psychiatry, 82*(6), 601–606. doi:10.1136/jnnp.2010.237388

Schubert, M. C., Das, V., Tusa, R. J., & Herdman, S. J. (2004). Cervico-ocular reflex in normal subjects and patients with unilateral vestibular hypofunction. *Otology and Neurotology, 25*(1), 65–71.

Schubert, M. C., & Minor, L. B. (2004). Vestibulo-ocular physiology underlying vestibular hypofunction. *Physical Therapy, 84*(4), 373–385.

Schubert, M. C., & Zee, D. S. (2010). Saccade and vestibular ocular motor adaptation. *Restorative Neurology and Neuroscience, 28*(1), 9–18.

Shepard, N. T., & Telian, S. A. (1995). Programmatic vestibular rehabilitation. *Otolaryngology-Head and Neck Surgery, 112*(1), 173–182.

Shepard, N. T., Telian, S. A., & Smith-Wheelock, M. (1990). Habituation and balance retraining therapy. A retrospective review. *Neurologic Clinics, 8*(2), 459–475.

Shepard, N. T., Telian, S. A., Smith-Wheelock, M., & Raj, A. (1993). Vestibular and balance rehabilitation therapy. *Annals of Otology, Rhinology, and Laryngology, 102*(3 Pt. 1), 198–205.

Sherrington, C., & Lord, S. R. (1998). Increased prevalence of fall risk factors in older people following hip fracture. *Gerontology, 44*(6), 340–344.

Shumway-Cook, A., Baldwin, M., Polissar, N. L., & Gruber, W. (1997). Predicting the probability for falls in community-dwelling older adults. *Physical Therapy, 77*(8), 812–819.

Shumway-Cook, A., Brauer, S., & Woollacott, M. (2000). Predicting the probability for falls in community-dwelling older adults using the Timed Up & Go Test. *Physical Therapy, 80*(9), 896–903.

Shumway-Cook, A., & Horak, F. (1986a). Assessing the influence of sensory interaction on balance. *Physical Therapy, 66*(10), 1548–1550.

Shumway-Cook, A., & Horak, F. B. (1986b). Assessing the influence of sensory interaction of balance. Suggestion from the field. *Physical Therapy, 66*(10), 1548–1550.

Shumway-Cook, A., Taylor, C. S., Matsuda, P. N., Studer, M. T., & Whetten, B. K. (2013). Expanding the scoring system for the Dynamic Gait Index. *Physical Therapy, 93*(11), 1493–1506. doi:10.2522/ptj.20130035

Shumway-Cook, A., & Woollacott, M. (1995). *Motor control: Theory and practical applications.* Baltimore, MD: Williams & Wilkins.

Sienko, K. H., Balkwill, M. D., Oddsson, L. I., & Wall, C., 3rd. (2013). The effect of vibrotactile feedback on postural sway during locomotor activities. *Journal of Neuroengineering and Rehabilitation, 10*, 93. doi:10.1186/1743-0003-10-93

Siggeirsdottir, K., Jonsson, B. Y., Jonsson, H., Jr., & Iwarsson, S. (2002). The timed "Up & Go" is dependent on chair type. *Clinical Rehabilitation, 16*(6), 609–616.

Siniaia, M. S., & Miller, A. D. (1996). Vestibular effects on upper airway musculature. *Brain Research, 736*(1–2), 160–164.

Sklare, D. A., Konrad, H. R., Maser, J. D., & Jacob, R. G. (2001). Special issue on the interface of balance disorders and anxiety: An introduction and overview. *Journal of Anxiety Disorders, 15*(1–2), 1–7.

Smith-Wheelock, M., Shepard, N. T., & Telian, S. A. (1991). Physical therapy program for vestibular rehabilitation. *American Journal of Otology, 12*(3), 218–225.

Solomon, G. D., Skobieranda, F. G., & Genzen, J. R. (1995). Quality of life assessment among migraine patients treated with sumatriptan. *Headache, 35*(8), 449–454.

Sparto, P. J., Furman, J. M., Whitney, S. L., Hodges, L. F., & Redfern, M. S. (2004). Vestibular rehabilitation using a wide field of view virtual environment. *Conference Proceedings-IEEE Engineering in Medicine and Biology Society, 7*, 4836–4839. doi:10.1109/IEMBS.2004.1404338

Sparto, P. J., Whitney, S. L., Hodges, L. F., Furman, J. M., & Redfern, M. S. (2004). Simulator sickness when performing gaze shifts within a wide field of view optic flow environment: Preliminary evidence for using virtual reality in vestibular rehabilitation. *Journal of Neuroengineering and Rehabilitation, 1*(1), 14. doi:10.1186/1743-0003-1-14

Steffen, T. M., Hacker, T. A., & Mollinger, L. (2002). Age- and gender-related test performance in community-dwelling elderly people: Six-Minute Walk Test, Berg Balance Scale, Timed Up & Go Test, and gait speeds. *Physical Therapy, 82*(2), 128–137.

Strupp, M., Arbusow, V., Maag, K. P., Gall, C., & Brandt, T. (1998). Vestibular exercises improve central vestibulospinal compensation after vestibular neuritis. *Neurology, 51*(3), 838–844.

Studenski, S., Perera, S., Patel, K., Rosano, C., Faulkner, K., Inzitari, M., . . . Guralnik, J. (2011). Gait speed and survival in older adults. *JAMA, 305*(1), 50–58. doi:10.1001/jama.2010.1923

Suarez, H., Arocena, M., Suarez, A., De Artagaveytia, T. A., Muse, P., & Gil, J. (2003). Changes in postural control parameters after vestibular rehabilitation in patients with central vestibular disorders. *Acta Oto-Laryngologica, 123*(2), 143–147.

Szturm, T., Ireland, D. J., & Lessing-Turner, M. (1994). Comparison of different exercise programs in the rehabilitation of patients with chronic peripheral vestibular dysfunction. *Journal of Vestibular Research, 4*(6), 461–479.

Telian, S. A., & Shepard, N. T. (1996). Update on vestibular rehabilitation therapy. *Otolaryngologic Clinics of North America, 29*(2), 359–371.

Telian, S. A., Shepard, N. T., Smith-Wheelock, M., & Hoberg, M. (1991). Bilateral vestibular paresis: Diagnosis and treatment. *Otolaryngology-Head and Neck Surgery, 104*(1), 67–71.

Tesio, L., Alpini, D., Cesarani, A., & Perucca, L. (1999). Short form of the Dizziness Handicap Inventory: Construction and validation through Rasch analysis. *American Journal of Physical Medicine and Rehabilitation, 78*(3), 233–241.

Tinetti, M. E., & Williams, C. S. (1997). Falls, injuries due to falls, and the risk of admission to a nursing home. *The New England Journal of Medicine, 337*(18), 1279–1284.

Topuz, O., Topuz, B., Ardic, F. N., Sarhus, M., Ogmen, G., & Ardic, F. (2004). Efficacy of vestibular rehabilitation on chronic unilateral vestibular dysfunction. *Clinical Rehabilitation, 18*(1), 76–83.

Van Swearingen, J. M., Paschal, K. A., Bonino, P., & Chen, T. W. (1998). Assessing recurrent fall risk of community-dwelling, frail older veterans using specific tests of mobility and the physical performance test of function. *The Journals of Gerontology Series A: Biological Sciences and Meidcal Sciences, 53*(6), M457–M464.

Vereeck, L., Truijen, S., Wuyts, F., & Van de Heyning, P. H. (2006). Test-retest reliability of the Dutch version of the Dizziness Handicap Inventory. *B-ENT, 2*(2), 75–80.

Viirre, E. (1996). Vestibular telemedicine and rehabilitation. Applications for virtual reality. *Studies in Health Technology and Informatics, 29,* 299–305.

Viirre, E., Purcell, I., & Baloh, R. W. (2005). The Dix-Hallpike test and the canalith repositioning maneuver. *Laryngoscope, 115*(1), 184–187.

Viirre, E., & Sitarz, R. (2002). Vestibular rehabilitation using visual displays: Preliminary study. *Laryngoscope, 112*(3), 500–503.

Vitte, E., Semont, A., & Berthoz, A. (1994). Repeated optokinetic stimulation in conditions of active standing facilitates recovery from vestibular deficits. *Experimental Brain Research, 102*(1), 141–148.

Wall, C., 3rd, Oddsson, L. E., Horak, F. B., Wrisley, D. W., & Dozza, M. (2004). Applications of vibrotactile display of body tilt for rehabilitation. *Conference Proceedings-IEEE Engineering in Medicine and Biology Society, 7,* 4763–4765. doi:10.1109/IEMBS.2004.1404318

Ware, J. E., Jr., & Sherbourne, C. D. (1992). The MOS 36-item short-form health survey (SF-36). I. Conceptual framework and item selection. *Medical Care, 30*(6), 473–483.

Weber, P. C., & Cass, S. P. (1993). Clinical-assessment of postural stability. *American Journal of Otology, 14*(6), 566–569.

Wernick-Robinson, M., Krebs, D. E., & Giorgetti, M. M. (1999). Functional reach: Does it really measure dynamic balance? *Archives of Physical Medicine and Rehabilitation, 80*(3), 262–269.

Whitney, S., & Unico, J. (2001). Vestibular disorders in mild head injury. *Athletic Therapy Today, 6*(1), 33–39.

Whitney, S., Wrisley, D. M., Brown, K. E., & Furman, J. M. (2000). Physical therapy for migraine-related vestibulopathy and vestibular dysfuction with history of migraine. *Laryngoscope, 110,* 1528–1534.

Whitney, S. L., Hudak, M. T., & Marchetti, G. F. (1999). The activities-specific balance confidence scale and the dizziness handicap inventory: A comparison. *Journal of Vestibular Research, 9*(4), 253–259.

Whitney, S. L., Hudak, M. T., & Marchetti, G. F. (2000). The dynamic gait index relates to self-reported fall history in individuals with vestibular dysfunction. *Journal of Vestibular Research-Equilibrium and Orientation, 10*(2), 99–105.

Whitney, S. L., Marchetti, G. F., & Morris, L. O. (2005). Usefulness of the dizziness handicap inventory in the screening for benign paroxysmal positional vertigo. *Otology and Neurotology, 26*(5), 1027–1033.

Whitney, S. L., Marchetti, G. F., & Schade, A. I. (2006). The relationship between falls history and computerized dynamic posturography in persons with balance and vestibular disorders. *Archives of Physical Medicine and Rehabilitation, 87*(3), 402–407.

Whitney, S. L., Marchetti, G. F., Schade, A., & Wrisley, D. M. (2004). The sensitivity and specificity of the Timed "Up & Go" and the Dynamic Gait Index for self-reported falls in persons with vestibular disorders. *Journal of Vestibular Research, 14*(5), 397–409.

Whitney, S. L., & Rossi, M. M. (2000). Efficacy of vestibular rehabilitation. *Otolaryngology Clinics of North America, 33*(3), 659–672.

Whitney, S. L., Sparto, P. J., Brown, K. E., Furman, J. M., Redfern, M. S., & Jacobson, J. (2001). The potential use of virtual reality in persons with vestibular disorders. Preliminary findings with the BNAVE. *Neurology Report, 26*(2), 72–78.

Whitney, S. L., Sparto, P. J., Hodges, L. F., Babu, S. V., Furman, J. M., & Redfern, M. S. (2006). Responses to a virtual reality grocery store in persons with and without vestibular dysfunction. *Cyberpsychology and Behavior, 9*(2), 152–156. doi:10.1089/cpb.2006.9.152

Whitney, S. L., & Wrisley, D. M. (2004). The influence of footwear on timed balance scores of the modified clinical test of sensory interaction and balance. *Archives of Physical Medicine and Rehabilitation, 85*(3), 439–443.

Whitney, S. L., Wrisley, D. M., Brown, K. E., & Furman, J. M. (2000). Physical therapy for migraine-related vestibulopathy and vestibular dysfunction with history of migraine. *Laryngoscope, 110*(9), 1528–1534.

Whitney, S. L., Wrisley, D. M., Brown, K. E., & Furman, J. M. (2004). Is perception of handicap related to functional performance in persons with vestibular dysfunction? *Otology and Neurotology, 25*(2), 139–143.

Whitney, S. L., Wrisley, D. M., Marchetti, G. F., & Furman, J. M. (2002). The effect of age on vestibular rehabilitation outcomes. *Laryngoscope, 112*(10), 1785–1790.

Whitney, S. L., Wrisley, D. M., Marchetti, G. F., Gee, M. A., Redfern, M. S., & Furman, J. M. (2005). Clinical measurement of sit-to-stand performance in people with balance disorders: Validity of data for the

Five-Times-Sit-to-Stand Test. *Physical Therapy, 85*(10), 1034–1045.

Wrisley, D. M., Sparto, P. J., Whitney, S. L., & Furman, J. M. (2000). Cervicogenic dizziness: A review of diagnosis and treatment. *Journal of Orthopaedic and Sports Physical Therapy, 30*(12), 755–766.

Wrisley, D. M., Walker, M. L., Echternach, J. L., & Strasnick, B. (2003). Reliability of the dynamic gait index in people with vestibular disorders. *Archives of Physical Medicine and Rehabilitation, 84*(10), 1528–1533.

Wrisley, D. M., & Whitney, S. L. (2004). The effect of foot position on the modified clinical test of sensory interaction and balance. *Archives of Physical Medicine and Rehabilitation, 85*(2), 335–338.

Wrisley, D. M., Whitney, S. L., & Furman, J. M. (2002). Vestibular rehabilitation outcomes in patients with a history of migraine. *Laryngoscope, 23*(4), 483–487.

Yardley, L. (1994). Contribution of symptoms and beliefs to handicap in people with vertigo—A longitudinal study. *British Journal of Clinical Psychology, 33*, 101–113.

Yardley, L., Beech, S., Zander, L., Evans, T., & Weinman, J. (1998). A randomized controlled trial of exercise therapy for dizziness and vertigo in primary care. *British Journal of General Practice, 48*(429), 1136–1140.

Yardley, L., Burgneay, J., Andersson, G., Owen, N., Nazareth, I., & Luxon, L. (1998). Feasibility and effectiveness of providing vestibular rehabilitation for dizzy patients in the community. *Clinical Otolaryngology and Allied Sciences, 23*(5), 442–448.

Yardley, L., Burgneay, J., Nazareth, I., & Luxon, L. (1998). Neuro-otological and psychiatric abnormalities in a community sample of people with dizziness: A blind, controlled investigation. *Journal of Neurology, Neurosurgery, and Psychiatry, 65*(5), 679–684.

Yardley, L., Donovan-Hall, M., Smith, H. E., Walsh, B. M., Mullee, M., & Bronstein, A. M. (2004). Effectiveness of primary care-based vestibular rehabilitation for chronic dizziness. *Annals of Internal Medicine, 141*(8), 598–605.

Yardley, L., Luxon, L. M., & Haacke, N. P. (1994). A longitudinal study of symptoms, anxiety and subjective well-being in patients with vertigo. *Clinical Otolaryngology, 19*(2), 109–116.

Yardley, L., Masson, E., Verschuur, C., Haacke, N., & Luxon, L. (1992). Symptoms, anxiety and handicap in dizzy patients: Development of the Vertigo Symptom Scale. *Journal of Psychosomatic Research, 36*(8), 731–741.

Yardley, L., & Putman, J. (1992). Quantitative analysis of factors contributing to handicap and distress in vertiginous patients: A questionnaire study. *Clinical Otolaryngology and Allied Sciences, 17*(3), 231–236.

Yardley, L., & Redfern, M. S. (2001). Psychological factors influencing recovery from balance disorders. *Journal of Anxiety Disorders, 15*(1–2), 107–119.

Yates, B. J. (1996). Vestibular influences on the autonomic nervous system. *Annals of the New York Academy of Sciences, 781*, 458–473.

Yates, B. J., Billig, I., Cotter, L. A., Mori, R. L., & Card, J. P. (2002). Role of the vestibular system in regulating respiratory muscle activity during movement. *Clinical and Experimental Pharmacology and Physiology, 29*(1–2), 112–117.

Yates, B. J., & Bronstein, A. M. (2005). The effects of vestibular system lesions on autonomic regulation: Observations, mechanisms, and clinical implications. *Journal of Vestibular Research, 15*(3), 119–129.

Zee, D. S. (2000). Vestibular adaptation. In S. J. Herdman (Ed.), *Vestibular rehabilitation* (2nd ed., pp. 77–87). Philadelphia, PA: F. A. Davis.

Headache Diagnostic Interview for Determination of Migraine

Subject name: _____ Date: _____ Examiner: _____

1. Did the headaches start within 2 weeks of a head injury, trauma, or medical illness?

    YES   NO (If no, proceed to next question.)

2. Do you have any brain abnormality, like tumors or hydrocephalus?

    YES   NO (If no, proceed to next question.)

3. Do you have a headache every day or take over-the-counter or prescription pain or headache medications (e.g., Excedrin) more than 4 days per week?

    YES   NO (If no, proceed to next question.)

4. Do you have an intermittent or constant headache?

    Constant   Intermittent (If intermittent, proceed to the next question.)

5. How long does each individual headache episode last?

    <2 hr   ≥2 hr (If ≥2 hr, proceed to next question.)

6. Do you have **any** of the following neurological symptoms immediately before or during your headache episodes?

    _____ Visual scotoma

    _____ Visual hallucination (zig-zag or wavy lines, colored lights or balls, shimmering patterns)

    _____ Weakness or numbness on one side of your body

    If YES, diagnose MIGRAINE. No further questions needed.

    If NO, proceed with question #7.

7. Do you have at least **two** of the following symptoms with your headache?

    _____ Pain is on one side of the head during a headache episode

    _____ Pain feels like throbbing or pulsing sensation

    _____ Pain limits, restricts, or interferes with routine activities

    _____ Pain is made worse by performing routine activities, such as stair climbing

    NO (STOP! No diagnosis of migraine   YES (If yes, proceed to next question.)

8. Do you have at least **one** of the following symptoms with your headache?

    _____ Nausea or vomiting

    _____ Markedly increased sensitivity to **BOTH** normal room lighting **AND** conversational speech (The person should report a need to turn down or off lights, close curtains or blinds, turn down or off radio or television, or need to retreat to dark, quiet room.)

    If YES, then diagnose MIGRAINE. If NO, no diagnosis of migraine.

Diagnostic Interview for Determination of Vestibular Migraine

Note that STOP during the interview means that the patient does not have typical vestibular migraine symptoms and may require additional evaluations for the etiology of vertigo.

Patient name: _____ Date: _____

1. Does the patient have a lifetime diagnosis of migraine according to the IHS criteria?

    NO (STOP)   YES (Proceed to next question.)

2. Have any of the following symptoms been experienced within the last 2 years at least twice (not necessarily related to a headache episode)?
    - ☐ Vertigo (i.e., a sensation of spinning)
    - ☐ A feeling of abnormal motion
        - ○ Like walking on the deck of a boat
        - ○ Objects in the room seem to spin or turn around the patient
        - ○ Feeling like spinning or turning when stationary
    - ☐ Sense of imbalance or nausea when moving the head
    - ☐ Tendency to veer to the side when trying to walk straight
    - ☐ None of the above (STOP)

3. Do vestibular symptoms persist all the time (i.e., for more than 1 to 2 weeks) or do they come and go? If balance symptoms persist all the time, does the severity fluctuate?
    a. Intermittent or fluctuating in severity
    b. Constant AND nonfluctuating (STOP)

4. Has one of the following symptoms occurred at least twice at the same time as either episodic imbalance attacks or experiencing increased severity of fluctuating balance symptoms?
    - ☐ Migraine headache
    - ☐ Markedly increased sensitivity to either normal room lighting or conversational speech (The person should report a need to turn down or turn off lights, close curtains or blinds, turn down or turn off radio or television, or need to retreat to a dark, quiet room.)
    - ☐ Migrainous aura (e.g., visual scotoma, visual hallucination, weakness or numbness on one side of the body. DO NOT score positive if the "aura" symptom is dizziness)
    - ☐ None of the above (STOP)

5. To what degree do the balance symptoms just discussed affect the patient? That is, if not experiencing any headaches, how much would he or she still be affected by the balance symptoms?
    - ☐ Balance symptoms usually *interfere* with daily activities or are endured with distress (Rate as moderate)
    - ☐ Balance symptoms usually *prohibit* daily activities or are endured with *extreme* distress (Rate as severe)
    - ☐ Balance symptoms do not usually interfere with daily activities and are endured with minimal distress (STOP)

continues

If symptoms are either moderate or severe, diagnose patient with vestibular migraine.

[Note that additional pathology may be responsible, in part, for the patient's vertigo.]

Proceed to the next question.

6. Is hearing loss or ringing in the ears temporally related to the balance problem?

> YES: A detailed evaluation may be required to determine whether the patient has a nonmigrainous comorbid otologic disorder.

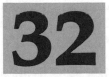

The Aging Vestibular System: Implications for Rehabilitation

Courtney D. Hall and Dara Meldrum

INTRODUCTION

It is well documented that there is an increase in falls incidence and fall-related injury with increased age. Approximately one-third of community-dwelling individuals 65 years and older fall in a given year (Tromp et al., 2001) with that rate increasing to approximately 42% in individuals 75 years and older (Downton & Andrews, 1991). Overall the rate of fall-related injury is low with approximately 10% of all falls resulting in injury; however, the rate of fall-related injuries rises dramatically with age: the annualized rate in adults 65 to 74 years of age is 55 per 1,000 and in adults 75 years and older is 115 per 1,000 with the injury rate of women being twice that of men (Adams, Martinez, Vickerie, & Kirzinger, 2011; Peel, Kassulke, & McClure, 2002). Of concern is that fewer than half of older fallers report a fall to their physicians; thus, it is incumbent on health-care providers to direct the case history to identify falls incidence and fall risk in their older patients (Stevens et al., 2012).

There are many contributors to falls including, but not limited to, gait and balance impairments, lower extremity weakness, and dizziness and vertigo. A recent systematic review revealed that dizziness/vertigo is a major risk factor for falls and increases the risk of falling twofold (Deandrea et al., 2010). In fact, dizziness is among the most preva-

lent complaints for which people seek medical help and the incidence increases with advancing age (Colledge, Wilson, Macintyre, & MacLennan, 1994). Individuals with vestibular deficits demonstrate a greater incidence of falls than their age-matched healthy counterparts, and the degree of deficit appears to impact the incidence of falling: individuals with bilateral versus unilateral vestibular hypofunction have a greater incidence of falls (Herdman, Blatt, Schubert & Tusa, 2000). Dizziness is often related to vestibular dysfunction which is treated effectively with vestibular exercises.

Most of our knowledge about the role of the vestibular system in postural control is derived from studies of individuals with loss of vestibular function and animal studies. Vestibular pathology, although more severe than age-related changes in vestibular function, provides insight into the contribution of age-related decrements in vestibular function to postural instability. However, two caveats need to be taken into account. Interpretation of information garnered from studies involving vestibular loss is confounded by the fact that the findings reflect both the loss of vestibular function and the compensation for that loss. Additionally, until recently vestibular loss was defined by measuring the function of the horizontal semicircular canals only. Thus, studies of people with vestibular loss may be muddled because of remaining otolith or even vertical canal function in some but not all subjects. We are now able to measure the function of the vertical semicircular canals, the saccule, and the utricle using such methods such as video head impulse testing, off-axis rotational testing, vestibular evoked myogenic responses, and measurement of subjective visual vertical. However, little is known about differences in postural control in people with loss of horizontal semicircular canal versus otolith organs function and even less about the interaction of vestibular loss and aging.

This chapter provides a general review of the effect of aging on the sensory systems contributing to postural stability, the functional impact of VOR functioning on postural control, and the evidence supporting the role of vestibular rehabilitation in the remediation of imbalance and gaze instability in older adults.

AGE-RELATED CHANGES IN THE POSTURAL CONTROL SYSTEM

The ability to maintain postural stability under different environmental conditions is critical to the ability to safely perform activities of daily living. Postural control is a sensory-motor process that involves the dynamic interplay between multiple body systems, including the central nervous system and both sensory and musculoskeletal systems. Postural stability refers to the ability to maintain the center of mass of the body positioned over the small base of support provided by the feet, either of which may be moving. Age-related changes are evident in all of the systems, both sensory and motor, that contribute to postural control (reviewed in the sections below); thus, an accumulation of nonspecific changes distributed across body systems result in a multifactorial problem that requires assessment of and rehabilitation for multiple systems.

Age Effects on Vestibular System

Postural stability is a multisensory motor task that depends on reliable input from the vestibular, somatosensory and visual systems, and the vestibular system, particularly the otolith organs, provide important information about self-motion and gravity. The two types of vestibular sensory organs (the semicircular canals and otolith organs) contribute to gaze and postural stability. When functioning normally, the vestibulo-ocular reflex (VOR) generates eye movements that are equal and opposite to head rotation, which enables images to remain stable on the fovea during head motion and ensures gaze stability during head motion. The otolith organs, the utricle and saccule, sense linear acceleration, head tilt, and gravity. Vestibular input for postural control is modulated via the vestibulospinal reflexes (VSRs). The lateral vestibulospinal tract receives a majority of input from the otolith organs and cerebellum and aids in tonic contractions of the antigravity muscles in the lower extremities. The VOR is better understood as it is relatively simple and for excitatory input involves a three-neuron arc, whereas the VSR is much more complex involving inputs from both semicircular canal and otolith organs and multiple connections to neck, trunk, and leg muscles.

The effects of aging on the vestibular system are well documented both anatomically and physiologically for all vestibular sensory organs (semicircular canals and otolith organs), although the functional impact of these age-related changes is less well understood. Morphological studies reveal that sensory hair cells degenerate with age in both the semicircular canals as well as both of the otolith organs (Johnsson, 1971; Velazquez-Villasenor et al., 2000). A parallel reduction occurs in fibers of the vestibular nerve and the vestibular nuclei, such that the number of vestibular sensory hair cells and nerve cells decreases by approximately 20% to 40% between the ages of 40 and 75 years (Lopez, Honrubia, & Baloh, 1997; Park, Tang, Lopez, & Ishiyama, 2001; Richter, 1980; Rosenhall, 1973). Some studies report a similar age-related effect on VOR function evidenced by reduced VOR gain at higher velocities in older versus younger subjects (Baloh, Jacobson, & Socotch, 1993), whereas other studies have shown minimal influence of age on the VOR response (Furman & Redfern, 2001; Wall & Black, 1984).

Age-related changes to the otolith organs have been consistently demonstrated across studies using vestibular evoked myogenic potential (VEMP) testing. The cervical VEMP test, a test of saccular/inferior vestibular nerve function, demonstrated reduced amplitude in individuals over the age of 60 (Akin, Murnane, Tampas, & Clinard, 2011; Su, Huang, Young, & Cheng, 2004). Similar age-related reductions in amplitude have been reported for the ocular VEMP test, a test of utricular/superior vestibular nerve function (Tseng, Chou, & Young, 2010).

One of the primary roles of the VOR is to stabilize gaze during head movement. Measurement of visual acuity during head movements provides a functional assessment of gaze stability and can be performed using either clinical or computerized tests. During the dynamic visual acuity (DVA) test the head moves at a predetermined velocity and the target size is systematically decreased. The DVA score is the difference between static visual acuity and visual acuity during head movements. The computerized DVA test is a highly reliable test in adults ($r = 0.79 - 0.83$) (Herdman et al., 1998; Rine et al., 2013). During the computerized gaze stabilization test (GST) the target size remains fixed at a predetermined size and head velocity is systematically increased. The computerized GST has demonstrated fair to good reliability (Ward, Mohammad, Whitney, Marchetti, & Furman, 2010). Both the DVA and GST differentiate vestibular patients from normal controls providing support that these measures give estimates of the VOR contribution to gaze stability (Goebel et al., 2007; Herdman et al., 1998). Furthermore, both DVA and GST tests have demonstrated a significant relationship with age indicating worse performance with increasing age (Herdman et al., 1998; Honaker & Shepard, 2010; Ward, Mohammad, Whitney, et al., 2010). Herdman and colleagues (1998) found that 42% of the variance in yaw plane DVA scores was accounted for by age alone. Conflicting findings regarding an age effect for GST have been shown perhaps as a result of small sample sizes, high variability in performance, or differences in optotype presentation time (Honaker & Shepard, 2010; Pritcher, Whitney, Marchetti, & Furman, 2008).

Age Effects on the Visual System

Multiple changes in vision occur with aging: reduced acuity, depth perception, contrast sensitivity, adaptation, and ability to detect motion in the visual field (Elliott, Yang, & Whitaker, 1995; Gilmore, Wenk, Naylor, & Stuve, 1992; Weale, 1975). Visual acuity decreases by 0.01 LogMAR per year from the seventh decade on and is weakly correlated with impaired functional balance (Baloh et al., 1993). Additionally,

poor visual acuity has been found to predict falls in older adults (Lord, Rogers, Howland, & Fitzpatrick, 1999). Some studies have suggested that visual measures other than static visual acuity (e.g., reduced contrast sensitivity or depth perception) are stronger correlates of impaired postural control (Lord & Dayhew, 2001; Lord & Menz, 2000; Turano, Rubin, Herdman, Chee, & Fried, 1994). For example, in a cohort of community-dwelling older adults (age 63 to 90 years), whereas both visual acuity and contrast sensitivity were individually correlated with postural sway while standing on a compliant surface, in multiple regression, contrast sensitivity, depth perception, and quadriceps strength were independent predictors of postural sway (Lord & Menz, 2000). Of note, this model explained only 21% of the variance and the authors concluded that other variables such as vestibular function, tactile sensitivity, and strength of other muscle groups were needed to fully explain postural sway. Given the contribution of both motor and sensory systems to balance control, it is to be expected that more complex models of postural control are needed. Era and colleagues (1996) demonstrated that good visual acuity, vibration sense, strength, and reaction times explained reduced postural sway (i.e., better postural stability) in a large sample of community-dwelling older adults.

An increased reliance on vision for postural control is evident by an increased postural sway in older versus younger subjects when proprioceptive information is reduced and the visual environment is modified (Peterka & Black, 1990; Poulain & Giraudet, 2008). Furthermore, when peripheral vision is occluded along with reduced proprioceptive inputs, older adults exhibit more postural sway than young adults (Manchester, Woollacott, Zederbauer-Hylton, & Marin, 1989).

Cataracts are common in older adults, and other eye conditions, such as glaucoma and macular degeneration, are associated with increasing age. These diseases can negatively affect postural control. Elderly subjects with visual impairment demonstrate more postural sway during challenging balance tasks than those with no visual impairment (Chen, Fu, Chan, & Tsang, 2012). Studies in healthy older adults show that when vision is blurred experimentally with lenses designed to simulate a cataract, mediolateral instability is induced during stepping up or down indicating the importance of vision for the control of precision in stepping (Buckley, Heasley, Scally, & Elliott, 2005).

Older adults are less able to deal with inaccurate sensory information suggestive of an inability to integrate and re-weight sensory input centrally and produce an appropriate response (Gauchard, Lion, Perrin, & Parietti-Winkler, 2012; Wade, Lindquist, Taylor, & Treat-Jacobson, 1995). There is evidence that central processing is slowed leading to longer latencies in postural responses to perturbations, particularly when sensory input is novel (Peterka & Black, 1990; Stelmach, Teasdale, Di Fabio, & Phillips, 1989; Sundermier, Woollacott, Jensen, & Moore, 1996; Woollacott, Shumway-Cook, & Nashner, 1986). Not only do older adults sway more in response to visual flow (Haibach, Slobounov, & Newell, 2009; Wade et al., 1995), but the effect of visual flow is amplified in older adults with impaired balance placing them at even greater risk for falls when vision is inaccurate (Sundermeier et al., 1996).

It may be that the increased reliance on vision for postural sway is due to a decline in proprioceptive ability. Toledo and Barela (2014) compared postural sway in healthy young and older persons under the moving room paradigm, in which the walls move and the floor remains still resulting in inaccurate visual input. Older participants swayed more than younger participants. Moreover, a multivariate analysis of the contributions of visual and motor systems to the increased sway revealed that proprioceptive ability (measured by sensitivity to passive motion) was the main contributor to postural sway.

Age Effects on the Somatosensory System

Several changes have been identified in proprioceptive function with aging. Increased muscle spindle capsule thickness, loss of total intrafusal muscle fibers, and impaired muscle spindle sensitivity have been reported; however, these changes can be highly individualized (see Goble, Coxon, Wenderoth, Van Impe, & Swinnen, 2009, for review). An age-related decrease in cutaneous sensation due to a loss of Pacinian and Meissner's receptors results in reduced deep tendon reflex responses and decreased vibration sense at the ankles (Baloh, Ying, & Jacobson, 2003). Cutaneous afferents are known to be

important in postural control. If the plantar surface of the foot is anaesthetized, the amplitude of muscle responses is reduced in the soleus muscles (Do, Bussel, & Breniere, 1990). Kristinsdottir and colleagues (2001) demonstrated the effect of decreased vibration sense on postural control by comparing healthy younger adults (mean age = 37.5 years) with healthy older adults stratified by vibration sense (mean age = 74.6 years). In general, older age was correlated with greater sway; however, reduced vibration sensation resulted in significantly greater sway compared to older and younger adults with intact vibration perception. Vision attenuated sway in all individuals, but to a lesser extent in older subjects with diminished vibratory sensation. Interestingly, one-third of the older subjects exhibited head shaking-induced nystagmus suggesting that vestibular impairment may have been a contributing factor to impaired postural stability.

Age Effects on the Neuromuscular System

Aging results in decreased muscle mass and strength (sarcopenia). Numerous mechanisms are thought to be responsible for sarcopenia including changes in protein synthesis, proteolysis, neuromuscular integrity, muscle fat content, as well as lifestyle factors (physical activity and nutrition) (Doherty, 2003). There is a nearly 40% reduction in muscle fiber numbers, especially Type II fast twitch fibers, between the ages of 20 and 89 years resulting in loss of muscle strength and power (Narici & Kayser, 1995; Porter, Vandervoort, & Lexell, 1995). Muscle strength peaks in the third decade and begins to decline in the fourth (Metter, Conwit, Tobin, & Fozard, 1997). Studies have measured a 1% to 3% per year decline in skeletal muscle maximum voluntary contraction in healthy adults with a steeper decline after the fifth and sixth decades, although there is considerable heterogeneity among older adults (Goodpaster et al., 2006; Hurley, 1995; Rantanen et al., 1998).

Strength of the lower extremities is important in postural control. Reduced ankle muscle strength is associated with decreased ability to recover from induced postural perturbations (Carty, Barrett, Cronin, Lichtwark, & Mills, 2012; Fujimoto, Hsu, Woollacott, & Chou, 2013), and reduced plantar flexor strength has been found to be associated with a reduction in the limits of stability (Melzer, Benjuya, Kaplanski, & Alexander, 2009) and increased postural sway (Bok, Lee, & Lee, 2013). Fukagawa, Wolfson, Judge, Whipple, and King (1995) found that lower limb strength was a predictor of loss of balance during the sensory organization test and an independent predictor of falls. Quadriceps strength was found to be one of the three best predictors of increased mediolateral sway in a modified tandem Romberg test with eyes closed (Lord et al., 1999). Both reduced quadriceps and hip abduction strength have been associated with an increased likelihood of taking multiple protective steps during balance testing as well as future fall risk (Hilliard et al., 2008; Lord et al., 1999).

Older adults demonstrate a loss of postural control and lateral stability appears to be most affected (Lord et al., 1999). Longer onset latencies in distal muscles, disorganized muscle recruitment, and longer periods of coactivation have also been found during perturbations in older subjects when compared to younger subjects (Manchester et al., 1989; Tang & Woollacott, 1998; Woollacott et al., 1986). Elderly subjects at risk of falling have been found to use stepping, reaching, and hip strategies more than those not at risk of falling who tend to use the ankle strategy (Mille et al., 2013; Maki & McIlroy, 2006). Older adults initiate stepping at lower amplitudes of instability than younger adults. For example, Mille and colleagues (2013) found that when a mediolateral perturbation was provided by a motorized waist pull system, older subjects took multiple steps, often directed laterally, to regain balance, whereas younger subjects regained balance with a single step. The loss of mediolateral control may be due in part to inability to produce hip muscle torque and increased trunk stiffness when an unexpected perturbation is induced (Rogers & Mille, 2003). As well as taking multiple steps, older adults more frequently initiate arm movements and use a reach and grasp strategy to recover balance after a perturbation (Maki & McIlroy, 2006).

Age and Attentional Demands of Postural Control

A common complaint voiced by individuals with vestibular dysfunction is difficulty concentrating (Jacobson & Newman, 1990). This effect may be the result of increased utilization of attentional resources due to impaired balance and has been explored using the dual-task paradigm. The dual-task methodology assumes that limited attentional capacity can be allocated to activities at any given time and that performance of any task requires a given proportion of that capacity (Abernethy, 1988). Therefore, multiple tasks performed simultaneously compete for available resources and when the available attentional resources are exceeded, performance degrades in one or both of the activities (Abernethy, 1988). Using the dual-task paradigm, researchers have demonstrated that the processes used to maintain balance require attentional resources (Kerr, Condon, & McDonald, 1985). Not only does postural control require attentional resources, but also the demands on attentional resources increase in the presence of increased age and impaired balance (Shumway-Cook & Woollacott, 2000). In older individuals with impaired balance control, performing even simple cognitive tasks leads to further impairments of balance (Shumway-Cook, Woollacott, Kerns, & Baldwin, 1997). Older adults with balance impairment demonstrated significantly more postural sway (i.e., greater instability) than either young or old healthy subjects under dual-task conditions (Kerr et al., 1985; Shumway-Cook & Woollacott, 2000). More importantly, some older adults with impaired balance who had been able to maintain balance under single-task condition fell under dual-task conditions (Shumway-Cook & Woollacott, 2000).

Studies involving individuals with vestibular deficits also demonstrate interference between postural control and cognitive task performance. Redfern, Talkowski, Jennings, and Furman (2004) tested healthy controls and well-compensated patients with surgically induced unilateral vestibular loss. For both groups, postural sway increased during the dual-task conditions. However, reaction times for patients were slower than controls under all postural conditions, including sitting as well as standing. This is a surprising finding given the minimal balance requirements involved in sitting and may indicate a general increase in attentional resource utilization required to integrate multiple sensory inputs for spatial orientation. Yardley et al. (2001) also found poorer cognitive performance for patients with uncompensated vestibular dysfunction of various etiologies versus healthy control subjects under all postural conditions including sitting and standing. Reaction time for both groups increased with increasing postural demands (from sitting to standing on stable surface to standing on sway-referenced surface) (Yardley et al., 2001); although in this study, in contrast to Redfern's findings, there were no additional dual-task costs for patients with vestibular dysfunction compared to healthy controls.

FUNCTIONAL IMPACT OF VOR ON POSTURAL CONTROL

As demonstrated in the previous section, age-related changes in the vestibular system are well documented. However, the specific contributions of reduced VOR and VSR to balance deficits in older adults are less clear. The increase in postural sway with aging is well known and was first demonstrated by Peterka and Black (1990). In their study of healthy subjects across a wide range of ages (7 to 81 years) the correlation between VOR gain and postural sway was weak; however, otolith organ function was not assessed. Recently, Serrador, Lipsitz, Gopalakrishnan, Black, and Wood (2009) found a significant correlation between age-related reduction in otolith organ response and increased postural sway.

Hall, Schubert, and Herdman (2004) first identified dynamic visual acuity as an important predictor of the degree of fall risk reduction in individuals with unilateral vestibular deficits. More recently Honaker and Shepard (2011, 2013) have examined the use of computerized DVA and GST testing to identify fall risk in older adults. In a small sample of older adults with a history of recurrent falls ($n = 16$; 4 of 16 had unilateral vestibular hypofunction), a cut-point of >0.25 logMAR during DVA testing demonstrated good sensitivity (87% for rightward head movement and 80% for leftward head movement) and specificity (61%) for identifying fallers (Honaker & Shepard, 2011). In addition, the DVA test and Dynamic Gait Index (total scores <20/24 indicate fall risk) demonstrated perfect correlation in identifying the same individuals as fallers. Based on history of falls, the study demonstrated that a unit increase of 0.1 logMAR from the DVA cut-point score increased the odds of being a faller by 3.90. This study is limited by small study sample and the confounding factor of vestibular hypofunction in a quarter of the subjects.

It has been demonstrated that older adults with reduced GST performance also have reduced mobility and balance (Ward, Mohammed, Brach, et al., 2010). In these older adults, GST performance in the yaw plane was significantly associated with the short performance physical battery (SPPB), gait speed, 15-s sit to stand, and standing balance; however, after adjusting for age and sex, only standing balance remained significant (Ward, Mohammed, Whitney, et al., 2010). In the pitch plane GST was associated only with 15-s sit to stand, and this relationship remained significant after adjusting for age and sex. Additionally, those unable to generate a minimum head velocity of 90°/s in either pitch or yaw plane were significantly older, had slower gait speed, and worse SPPB than those able to achieve this threshold. A significant relationship was found between GST scores and gait performance during the Dynamic Gait Index in older patients with vestibular disease; however, a similar relationship was not noted between GST scores and DGI in the older control subjects (Whitney, Marchetti, Pritcher, & Furman, 2009). Honaker and Shepard (2013) demonstrated a significant association between history of falls and GST performance in older adults as well as an association between scores DGI and GST performance. A criterion value of 100.5°/s or less for GST velocity demonstrated good sensitivity and specificity for identifying recurrent fallers based on history of falls and fall risk based on DGI (Honaker & Shepard, 2013). Whitney and colleagues (2009) also identified a criterion value for GST (78°/s) based on DGI, although it is different to that identified by Honaker and Shepard. Differences in the studies, thus differences in cutoff values, may be related to the grouping criteria (i.e., recurrent fallers versus healthy controls, Honaker; vestibular deficits versus healthy controls, Whitney). Further research is warranted with larger sample sizes to better determine whether GST is a useful screening tool to identify fall risk in community-dwelling older adults and appropriate cutoffs.

It is not clear what contribution that a loss of VOR function makes to balance impairments. A recent study provides evidence that gaze stability is important in corrective postural responses following balance perturbations (Diehl & Pidcoe, 2010). Subjects looking at a visual target (compared to no visual target) had faster stepping reactions in response to a perturbation. Individuals with the greatest percentage of foveal fixation had the quickest responses allowing for better recovery of stability. Older subjects were less successful maintaining visual fixation and had slower stepping response times than younger subjects suggesting that decreased gaze stability during balance recovery contributes to postural instability. Although these data suggest a relationship between gaze stabilization and postural stability in older adults, cross-sectional designs cannot determine causality.

Utilization of visual acuity during head movement (either DVA or GST) demonstrates usefulness as screening for fall risk in older adults; this may lead to recommendations for vestibular rehabilitation with an emphasis on gaze stabilization exercises for reduction in falling risk. Hall, Heusel-Gillig, Tusa, and Herdman (2010) recently demonstrated that the inclusion of gaze stability exercises led to the reduction in falling risk in a group of older adults with a history of falls and normal vestibular function as measured by caloric and bedside vestibular testing. Thus, inclusion of objective vestibular measures, such as DVA or GST, in a fall risk screening protocol may be warranted.

IMPACT OF VESTIBULAR AND BALANCE REHABILITATION

Uncompensated vestibular hypofunction results in subjective complaints of dizziness, imbalance and visual blurring, and postural and gaze instability resulting in decreased activity and avoidance or modification of driving (Cohen & Kimball, 2003; Yardley, Verschuur, Masson, Luxon, & Haacke, 1992). The goals of vestibular rehabilitation are to reduce symptoms, improve gaze and postural stability particularly during head movements, and to return the individual to normal activities, including regular physical activity, driving, and work. A number of randomized controlled trials (RCTs) provide compelling evidence in support of vestibular rehabilitation as an effective treatment for patients with unilateral and bilateral vestibular loss. A recent Cochrane Review (Hillier & McDonnell, 2011) included 27 RCTs and concluded that there is moderate to strong evidence that vestibular rehabilitation is both well

tolerated and effective for patients with unilateral vestibular hypofunction (UVH); however, there was insufficient evidence to compare the effectiveness of different treatment approaches. A recent systematic review (Porciuncula, Johnson, & Glickman, 2012) based on seven cohort and case-control studies concluded that there is moderate evidence to support exercise-based vestibular rehabilitation to improve gaze and postural stability for patients with bilateral vestibular hypofunction (BVH); however, there was insufficient evidence to support effectiveness of sensory prosthetics (e.g., vibrotactile feedback) in vestibular rehabilitation.

Elements of Vestibular Rehabilitation

Vestibular rehabilitation typically consists of different exercise approaches to address the impairments and functional limitations identified during initial evaluation: (1) exercises to habituate symptoms, (2) exercises to promote gaze stability, and (3) exercises to improve balance and gait, including walking for endurance. Habituation as a treatment approach involves repeated exposure to the specific stimulus that provokes dizziness. Habituation exercises are chosen based on particular movements or situations (e.g., busy visual environments) that provoke symptoms. The individual performs several repetitions of two to three of the motions that caused moderate symptoms on evaluation. This systematic repetition of provocative movements leads to a reduction in symptoms and has been found to reduce disability in patients with peripheral or central vestibular deficits; however, habituation has not been found to be effective in individuals with BVH (Telian, Shepard, Smith-Wheelock, & Hoberg, 1991; Telian, Shepard, Smith-Wheelock, & Kemink, 1990).

Gaze stability exercises were developed based on the concepts of adaptation and substitution. Adaptation refers to long-term change in the neuronal response with the goal of reducing symptoms and normalizing gaze and postural stability. A critical signal to induce adaptation is retinal slip during head movements (Shelhamer, Tiliket, Roberts, Kramer, & Zee, 1994); thus, adaptation exercises involve head movement while maintaining focus on a target, which may be stationary or moving. Adaptation exercises alone have been found to reduce symptoms of disequilibrium and to improve balance while walking in individuals who are postsurgery for resection of acoustic neuroma (Herdman, Clendaniel, Mattox, Holliday, & Niparko, 1995). The goal of substitution exercises is to substitute alternative strategies (e.g., use of cervical ocular reflex, smooth pursuit eye movements, or central preprogramming of eye movements for VOR and use of visual and/or somatosensory cues for VSR) for missing vestibular function (Herdman, Schubert, & Tusa, 2001; Horak, Jones-Rycewicz, Black, & Shumway-Cook, 1992; Schubert, Das, Tusa, & Herdman, 2004). For example, during active eye-head exercise between targets, a large eye movement to a target is made prior to the head moving to face the target, potentially facilitating use of preprogrammed eye movements.

Balance and gait exercises under challenging sensory and dynamic conditions are typically included as part of vestibular rehabilitation. Static exercises include balancing under conditions of altered visual and somatosensory input. Dynamic conditions include walking with head turns, walking with quick turns, or performing a secondary task while walking. Many individuals with vestibular hypofunction limit regular physical activities; thus, while general conditioning alone does not reduce symptoms or improve postural stability (Horak et al., 1992), including physical activity is an important element of rehabilitation.

Age and Vestibular Rehabilitation Outcomes

Several studies have investigated whether age is a factor predicting outcomes following vestibular rehabilitation. In a case-control study (matched by gender, vestibular function, and diagnoses), Whitney, Wrisley, Marchetti, and Furman (2002) reviewed rehabilitation outcomes and found that age did not influence the proportions of patients demonstrating improvement after vestibular rehabilitation. Herdman, Hall, and Delaune (2012) investigated predictors of outcome of vestibular rehabilitation in a large sample of patients with unilateral vestibular loss and found that age did not predict improvement in function or reduction in dizziness; however, age was associated with fall risk and gait speed at discharge. Additionally, age does not predict improvements in

dynamic visual acuity after vestibular rehabilitation (Herdman, Schubert, Das, & Tusa, 2003) or recovery after vestibular schwannoma resection (Cohen, Kimball, & Jenkin, 2002).

Gauchard and colleagues (2012) divided patients with acoustic neuromas into three age categories (30 to 44, 45 to 59, and 60 to 75 years) and followed them postsurgery. All of the patients received post-op rehabilitation. The elderly group had significantly worse balance (based on computerized dynamic posturography) than the younger group prior to surgery and immediately following surgery. By 3-months post-op, the differences were reduced and all groups improved their balance performance relative to presurgery. The authors suggested this was indicative both of a benefit of removal of the neuroma and of neuroplasticity which were still evident with advancing age. Vereeck, Wuyts, Truijen, De Valck, and Van de Heyning (2008) dichotomized patients post acoustic neuroma resection into two groups (above and below 50 years of age). They compared customised vestibular rehabilitation to general instructions to get physically active. The results indicated a superior benefit of customized vestibular rehabilitation over general instructions, but only for the older group. The authors concluded that differential approaches to treatment may be needed; for those under 50 years of age general instructions for physical activity may suffice, but in patients over 50 years a customized program should be implemented.

Effect of Age on Fall Risk Reduction

General findings from several studies reveal that age does not affect rehabilitation outcomes: older adults improve to a similar extent as younger adults with vestibular deficits, although older adults may need more treatment sessions perhaps because of multiple comorbidities (Cohen & Kimball, 2003; Shepard, Telian, Smith-Wheelock, & Raj, 1993; Whitney, Wrisley, Marchetti, & Furman, 2002). Whereas older and younger adults demonstrate similar improvements in DGI scores following vestibular rehabilitation, one retrospective study showed that a greater proportion of older adults remained at risk for falls at discharge (45% of older adults versus 11% of younger adults) (Hall, Schubert, & Herdman, 2004). Older adults may remain at risk for falls at discharge due to comorbidities or polypharmacy and their effects on balance and may need an assistive device to prevent falls.

Impact of Newer Technologies on Rehabilitation

In the past decade, the availability of low-cost technology to provide biofeedback, virtual reality, and gaming systems (such as the Nintendo Wii) has resulted in a proliferation of studies investigating their effectiveness in rehabilitation. Care needs to be taken when incorporating technology in the rehabilitation of older adults, because older adults are generally less confident in using technology and are also less likely to use technology (Czaja et al., 2006). However, initial case studies and uncontrolled studies suggest that older adults are open to technology in rehabilitation (Meldrum, Glennon, Herdman, Murray, & McConn-Walsh, 2012; Taylor et al., 2012; Williams, Doherty, Bender, Mattox, & Tibbs, 2011) and a recent systematic review has further clarified the role that technology may play in rehabilitation (Booth et al., 2014).

Randomized controlled trials (RCTs) have found conflicting results in the use of gaming for balance rehabilitation (Szturm, Betker, Moussavi, Desai, & Goodman, 2011; Toulotte, Toursel, & Olivier, 2012). Toulotte and colleagues (2012) found that community-dwelling older adults who played the Nintendo Wii Fit over a period of 20 weeks improved static balance, but a combination of the Wii Fit plus additional exercise conferred the most benefit to dynamic balance. On the other hand, Stzurm et al. (2011) demonstrated a superior effect in the gaming group on Berg Balance Scores and Activities Balance Confidence Scores compared to conventional therapy in frail elderly. This finding was supported by Griffin, McCormick, Taylor, Shawis, and Impson (2012) who found that the Wii Fit Plus when combined with conventional physical therapy conferred an additional improvement in timed up and go (TUG) and functional reach scores. A recent systematic review of the effectiveness of virtual reality interventions in improving balance concluded that evidence to support the use of gaming to improve impairments, activity limitations, and participation in older adults is weak at present (Booth, Masud, Connell, & Bath-Hextall,

2014). Adherence and acceptability were generally positive, but initial training and monitoring for safety in the home were factors that needed attention in the trials. Importantly, no evidence for superiority of virtual reality over conventional therapy was found using meta-analysis (Booth et al., 2014). The role of technology in rehabilitation for older adults is far from clear at present but appears to achieve similar outcomes to conventional rehabilitation.

Studies specific to vestibular-impaired elderly are lacking at present. but a recent trial (Meldrum et al., 2014) in patients with unilateral peripheral vestibular loss that included elderly subjects found no evidence of superiority of a Nintendo Wii Fit vestibular rehabilitation program compared to conventional rehabilitation (both home based). In this study, adherence was similar between the two groups, and there was evidence that the Nintendo Wii Fit group enjoyed the treatment more and found the balance exercises less difficult and less tiring. The systems described above pertained mainly to retraining balance and mobility, but more recently, systems incorporating the Wii remote controller (Chen, Hsieh, Wei, & Kao, 2012) and the iPod (Huang, Sparto, Kiesler, Siewiorek, & Smailagic, 2014) have been designed to track head velocity in order to retrain gaze stability. These systems are likely to become commercially available for future rehabilitation.

Impact of Fear of Falling on Outcomes

Psychological factors such as fear of falling, anxiety, and depression have an added negative effect on physical impairments and evidence suggests that these factors are more prevalent in older individuals with vestibular impairment. Fear of falling (FOF) is defined as "low perceived self-efficacy at avoiding falls during essential, nonhazardous activities of daily living" (Tinetti, Richman, & Powell, 1990) and is commonly measured using a dichotomous yes/no question of "are you afraid of falling?" or indirectly with balance efficacy scales (e.g., Activities-specific Balance Confidence Scale or Falls Efficacy Scale). Fear of falling has been found in approximately 30% of community-dwelling older adults in longitudinal studies of aging and has a negative impact of mobility (Donoghue, Cronin, Savva, O'Regan, & Kenny, 2013; Reelick, van Iersel, Kessels, & Rikkert,

2009; Rochat et al., 2010). For example, when anxiety, number of previous falls, number of medications, and level of activity were controlled for, FOF was independently associated with reduced gait speed in a sample of older adults (Reelick et al., 2009). This finding has been confirmed by two large longitudinal studies which also controlled for physical, mental, and cognitive health (Donoghue et al., 2013; Rochat et al., 2010). These findings are important given that slow gait speed has been implicated in falls (Ambrose, Paul, & Hausdorff, 2013; Dunlap, Perera, VanSwearingen, Wert, & Brach, 2012) and a 7% increase in fall risk occurs for every 0.1 m/s reduction in gait speed (Verghese, Holtzer, Lipton, & Wang, 2009).

Dizziness is associated with an increase in FOF in older adults. Two case-control studies (Burker et al., 1995; Perez-Jara et al., 2012) found a significantly greater prevalence of FOF (47% and 71%, respectively) in older patients attending dizzy clinics compared to age-matched healthy controls (3% and 31.2%, respectively). In a cross-sectional study of elderly patients with vestibular impairment Marchetti, Whitney, Redfern, and Furman (2011) found that 42% of elderly vestibular-impaired patients had fear of falling and impaired balance and gait that were significantly associated with lower Activities-specific Balance Confidence scores. Significant associations were also found with anxiety, depression, and general health. A recent qualitative study on older patients with dizziness and fear of falling uncovered themes such as embarrassment, depression, and anxiety and the perception of being a burden on family members. Almost all patients reported feeling anxious about falling and dizziness, with many reporting they were more sedentary and limited the places they went as a result of the fear of falling (Honaker & Kretschmer, 2014).

That fear of falling is independently associated with reduced gait and balance raises the question of causative factors. Slower gait speed with shorter stride lengths is associated with a more cautious gait pattern and is found in healthy controls in conditions where postural threat is perceived, for example, walking on an elevated walkway (Brown, Gage, Polych, Sleik, & Winder, 2002). Gait during this task is modified to a greater extent in older individuals and even more so when healthy older are compared

with older adults who have fear of falling (Delbaere, Sturnieks, Crombez, & Lord, 2009). Postural threat is also associated with a generalized stiffening of the body indicated by increased co-contraction and decreased sway (Carpenter, Adkin, Brawley, & Frank, 2006; Nagai et al., 2012; Osler, Tersteeg, Reynolds, & Loram, 2013). It is postulated that the modification of the postural response reflects an adaptive response to control the body's momentum and exert more control over the center of mass in order to prevent falls. Studies specifically investigating gait in vestibular impaired populations have shown that while gait speed is slower in these populations, it appears to be *chosen*, as evidenced by an ability to walk at greater cadences when asked to do so (Krebs, Gill-Body, Parker, Ramirez, & Wernick-Robinson, 2003) lending support to an adaptive theory.

In conclusion, the changes in gait seen in the elderly with fear of falling or vestibular impairment (or both) may reflect a conscious modification of gait to avoid falls (Delbaere et al., 2009). Anxiety and depression are closely linked to both fear of falling and vestibular impairment and should be taken into account when planning vestibular rehabilitation in this population.

Does Therapy Have to Be Individualized or Can Group Therapy Work?

The question of whether individualized or group therapy is superior when rehabilitating older patients with vestibular dysfunction is not clear. A recent systematic review found five studies that exclusively investigated vestibular rehabilitation in older subjects (Ricci et al., 2010). Group rather than individualized therapy was the most common mode of administration in the clinical setting. Only one study compared two types of vestibular rehabilitation (Cawthorne-Cooksey–based exercises versus adaptation exercises) and no differences were found between the two treatments. The other four studies in the review compared vestibular rehabilitation to no treatment and found significant improvement in most measures of balance, gait, and dizziness. In four of the five studies, exercises were performed at home with weekly visits to a therapist for progression; in the other, exercises were performed exclusively at home. The review concluded that in middle-aged and older patients receiving vestibular rehabilitation, there is insufficient evidence at present to recommend one form of rehabilitation over another or individual exercise versus group exercise.

Strength training is rarely included as a component of vestibular rehabilitation. Two retrospective reviews of vestibular rehabilitation in older populations incorporated lower limb strengthening (Cronin & Steenerson, 2011; Macias, Massingale, & Gerkin, 2005). However, no study seems to have measured the specific impact of the strength training on outcomes. This would be of interest given the role of strength in postural stability discussed above and the positive effect of strengthening on gait stability in elderly who have functional limitations (Hausdorff et al., 2001; Krebs, Jette, & Assmann, 1998).

CONCLUSION

There are many factors involved in postural stability and many of the systems involved undergo age-related changes. Assessment and treatment of dizziness and imbalance in older adults require a multidimensional approach, but there is sufficient evidence to support successful outcomes in older adults. The use of technology in vestibular rehabilitation is rapidly evolving, and there is evidence that older adults will adopt such technology.

REFERENCES

Abernethy, B. (1988). Dual-task methodology and motor skills research: Some applications and methodological constraints. *Journal of Human Movement Studies, 14,* 101–132.

Adams, P. F., Martinez, M. E., Vickerie, J. L., & Kirzinger, W. K. (2011). Summary health statistics for the U.S. population: National Health Interview Survey, 2010. National Center for Health Statistics. *Vital Health Statistics, 10*(251).

Akin, F. A., Murnane, O. D., Tampas, J. W., & Clinard, C. (2011). The effect of age on the vestibular evoked myogenic potential and sternocleidomastoid muscle tonic EMG level. *Ear and Hearing, 32,* 617–622.

Ambrose, A. F., Paul, G., & Hausdorff, J. M. (2013). Risk factors for falls among older adults: A review of the literature. *Maturitas, 75,* 51–61.

Baloh, R. W., Jacobson, K. M., & Socotch, T. M. (1993). The effect of aging on visual-vestibuloocular responses. *Experimental Brain Research, 95,* 509–516.

Baloh, R. W., Ying, S. H., & Jacobson, K. M. (2003). A longitudinal study of gait and balance dysfunction in normal older people. *Archives of Neurology, 60,* 835–839.

Bok, S. K., Lee, T. H., & Lee, S. S. (2013). The effects of changes of ankle strength and range of motion according to aging on balance. *Annals Rehabilitation Medicine, 37,* 10–16.

Booth, V., Masud, T., Connell, L., & Bath-Hextall, F. (2014). The effectiveness of virtual reality interventions in improving balance in adults with impaired balance compared with standard or no treatment: A systematic review and meta-analysis. *Clinical Rehabilitation, 28,* 419–431.

Brown, L. A., Gage, W. H., Polych, M. A., Sleik, R. J., & Winder, T. R. (2002). Central set influences on gait. Age-dependent effects of postural threat. *Experimental Brain Research, 145,* 286–296.

Buckley, J. G., Heasley, K., Scally, A., & Elliott, D. B. (2005). The effects of blurring vision on medio-lateral balance during stepping up or down to a new level in the elderly. *Gait & Posture, 22*(2), 146–153.

Burker, E. J., Wong, H., Sloane, P. D., Mattingly, D., Preisser, J., & Mitchell, C. M. (1995). Predictors of fear of falling in dizzy and nondizzy elderly. *Psychology Aging, 10,* 104–110.

Carpenter, M. G., Adkin, A. L., Brawley, L. R., & Frank, J. S. (2006). Postural, physiological and psychological reactions to challenging balance: does age make a difference? *Age and Ageing, 35,* 298–303.

Carty, C. P., Barrett, R. S., Cronin, N. J., Lichtwark, G. A., & Mills, P. M. (2012). Lower limb muscle weakness predicts use of a multiple- versus single-step strategy to recover from forward loss of balance in older adults. *Journals of Gerontology Series A: Biological Sciences and Medical Sciences, 67,* 1246–1252.

Chen, E. W., Fu, A. S., Chan, K. M., & Tsang, W. W. (2012). Balance control in very old adults with and without visual impairment. *European Journal of Applied Physiology, 112,* 1631–1636.

Chen, P. Y., Hsieh, W. L., Wei, S. H., & Kao, C. L. (2012). Interactive wiimote gaze stabilization exercise training system for patients with vestibular hypofunction. *Journal of Neuroengineering and Rehabilitation, 9,* 77.

Cohen, H. S., & Kimball, K. T. (2003). Increased independence and decreased vertigo after vestibular rehabilitation. *Otolaryngology-Head and Neck Surgery, 128,* 60–70.

Cohen, H. S., Kimball, K. T., & Jenkin, H. A. (2002). Factors affecting recovery after acoustic neuroma resection. *Acta Oto-Laryngologica, 122*, 841–850.

Colledge, N. R., Wilson, J. A., Macintyre, C. C., & MacLennan, W. J. (1994). The prevalence and characteristics of dizziness in an elderly community. *Age and Ageing, 23*, 117–120.

Cronin, G. W., & Steenerson, R. L. (2011). Disequilibrium of aging: Response to a 3-month program of vestibular therapy. *Physical and Occupational Therapy in Geriatrics, 29*, 148–155.

Czaja, S. J., Charness, N., Fisk, A. D., Hertzog, C., Nair, S. N., Rogers, W. A., & Sharit, J. (2006). Factors predicting the use of technology: Findings from the Center for Research and Education on Aging and Technology Enhancement (CREATE). *Psychology and Aging, 21*, 333–352.

Deandrea, S., Lucenteforte, E., Bravi, F., Foschi, R., La Vecchia, C., & Negri, E. (2010). Risk factors for falls in community-dwelling older people: A systematic review and meta-analysis. *Epidemiology, 21*, 658–668.

Delbaere, K., Sturnieks, D. L., Crombez, G., & Lord, S. R. (2009). Concern about falls elicits changes in gait parameters in conditions of postural threat in older people. *Journal of Gerontology Series A: Biological Sciences and Medical Sciences, 64*, 237–242.

Diehl, M. D., & Pidcoe, P. E. (2010). The influence of gaze stabilization and fixation on stepping reactions in younger and older adults. *Journal of Geriatric Physical Therapy, 33*, 19–25.

Do, M. C., Bussel, B., & Breniere, Y. (1990). Influence of plantar cutaneous afferents on early compensatory reactions to forward fall. *Experimental Brain Research, 79*, 319–324.

Doherty, T. J. (2003). Invited review: Aging and sarcopenia. *Journal of Applied Physiology, 95*, 1717–1727.

Donoghue, O. A., Cronin, H., Savva, G. M., O'Regan, C., & Kenny, R. A. (2013). Effects of fear of falling and activity restriction on normal and dual task walking in community dwelling older adults. *Gait & Posture, 38*, 120–124.

Downton, J. H., & Andrews, K. (1991). Prevalence, characteristics and factors associated with falls among the elderly living at home. *Aging (Milano), 3*, 219–228.

Dunlap, P., Perera, S., VanSwearingen, J. M., Wert, D., & Brach, J. S. (2012). Transitioning to a narrow path: The impact of fear of falling in older adults. *Gait & Posture, 35*, 92–95.

Elliott, D. B., Yang, K. C., & Whitaker, D. (1995). Visual acuity changes throughout adulthood in normal, healthy eyes: Seeing beyond 6/6. *Optometry and Visual Science, 72*, 186–191.

Era, P., Schroll, M., Ytting, H., Gause-Nilsson, I., Heikkinen, E., & Steen, B. (1996). Postural balance and its sensory-motor correlates in 75-year-old men and women: A cross-national comparative study. *Journal of Gerontology Series A: Biological Sciences and Medical Sciences, 51*, M53–M63.

Fujimoto, M., Hsu, W. -L., Woollacott, M. H., & Chou, L. -S. (2013). Ankle dorsiflexor strength relates to the ability to restore balance during a backward support surface translation. *Gait & Posture, 38*, 812–817.

Fukagawa, N. K., Wolfson, L., Judge, J., Whipple, R., & King, M. (1995). Strength is a major factor in balance, gait, and the occurrence of falls. *Journals of Gerontology Series A: Biological Sciences and Medical Sciences, 50*, 64–67.

Furman, J. M., & Redfern, M. S. (2001). Effect of aging on the otolith-ocular reflex. *Journal of Vestibular Research, 11*, 91–103.

Gauchard, G. C., Lion, A., Perrin, P. P., & Parietti-Winkler, C. (2012). Influence of age on postural compensation after unilateral deafferentation due to vestibular schwannoma surgery. *Laryngoscope, 122*, 2285–2290.

Gilmore, G. C., Wenk, H. E., Naylor, L. A., & Stuve, T. A. (1992). Motion perception and aging. *Psychology and Aging, 7*, 654–660.

Goble, D. J., Coxon, J. P., Wenderoth, N., Van Impe, A., & Swinnen, S. P. (2009). Proprioceptive sensibility in the elderly: Degeneration, functional consequences and plastic-adaptive processes. *Neuroscience and Biobehavioural Reviews, 33*, 271–278.

Goebel, J. A., Tungsiripat, N., Sinks, B., & Carmody, J. (2007). Gaze stabilization test: A new clinical test of unilateral vestibular dysfunction. *Otology and Neurotology, 28*, 68–73.

Goodpaster, B. H., Park, S. W., Harris, T. B., Kritchevsky, S. B., Nevitt, M., Schwartz, A. V., & Newman, A. B. (2006). The loss of skeletal muscle strength, mass, and quality in older adults: The health, aging and body composition study. *Journals of Gerontology Series A: Biological Sciences and Medical Sciences, 61*, 1059–1064.

Griffin, M., McCormick, D., Taylor, M. J., Shawis, T., & Impson, R. (2012). Using the Nintendo Wii as an intervention in a falls prevention group. *Journal of the American Geriatric Society, 60*(2), 385–387.

Haibach, P., Slobounov, S., & Newell, K. (2009). Egomotion and vection in young and elderly adults. *Gerontology, 55*, 637–643.

Hall, C. D., Heusel-Gillig, L., Tusa, R. J., & Herdman, S. J. (2010). Efficacy of gaze stability exercises in older adults with dizziness. *Journal of Neurologic Physical Therapy, 34*, 64–69.

Hall, C. D., Schubert, M. C., & Herdman, S. J. (2004). Prediction of fall risk reduction as measured by dynamic gait index in individuals with unilateral vestibular hypofunction. *Otology and Neurotology, 25*, 746–751.

Hausdorff, J. M., Nelson, M. E., Kaliton, D., Layne, J. E., Bernstein, M. J., Nuernberger, A., & Singh, M. A. F. (2001). Etiology and modification of gait instability in older adults: A randomized controlled trial of exercise. *Journal of Applied Physiology, 90,* 2117–2129.

Herdman, S. J., Blatt, P., Schubert, M., & Tusa, R. (2000). Falls in patients with vestibular deficits. *American Journal of Otology, 21,* 847–851.

Herdman, S. J., Clendaniel, R. A., Mattox, D. E., Holliday, M. J., & Niparko, J. K. (1995). Vestibular adaptation exercises and recovery: Acute stage after acoustic neuroma resection. *Otolaryngology-Head and Neck Surgery, 113,* 77–87.

Herdman, S. J., Hall, C. D., & Delaune, W. (2012). Variables associated with outcome in patients with unilateral vestibular hypofunction. *Neurorehabilitation and Neural Repair, 26,* 151–162.

Herdman, S. J., Schubert, M. C., Das, V. E., & Tusa, R. J. (2003). Recovery of dynamic visual acuity in unilateral vestibular hypofunction. *Archives Otolaryngology-Head and Neck Surgery, 129,* 819–824.

Herdman, S. J., Schubert, M. C., & Tusa, R. J. (2001). Role of central preprogramming in dynamic visual acuity with vestibular loss. *Archives Otolaryngology-Head and Neck Surgery, 127,* 1205–1210.

Herdman, S. J., Tusa, R. J., Blatt, P., Suzuki, A., Venuto, P. J., & Roberts, D. (1998). Computerized dynamic visual acuity test in the assessment of vestibular deficits. *American Journal of Otology, 19,* 790–796.

Hilliard, M. J., Martinez, K. M., Janssen, I., Edwards, B., Mille, M. L., Zhang, Y., & Rogers, M. W. (2008). Lateral balance factors predict future falls in community-living older adults. *Archives of Physical Medicine and Rehabilitation, 89,* 1708–1713.

Hillier, S. L., & McDonnell, M. (2011). Vestibular rehabilitation for unilateral peripheral vestibular dysfunction. *Cochrane Database Systematic Review.* Issue 2, Art. No.: CD005397.

Honaker, J. A., & Kretschmer, L. W. (2014). Impact of fear of falling for patients and caregivers: Perceptions before and after participation in vestibular and balance rehabilitation therapy. *American Journal Audiology, 23,* 20–33.

Honaker, J. A., & Shepard, N. T. (2010). Age effect on the Gaze Stabilization test. *Journal of Vestibular Research, 20,* 357–362.

Honaker, J. A., & Shepard, N. T. (2011). Use of the Dynamic Visual Acuity Test as a screener for community-dwelling older adults who fall. *Journal of Vestibular Research, 21,* 267–276.

Honaker, J. A., & Shepard, N. T. (2013). Clinical use of the gaze stabilization test for screening falling risk in community-dwelling older adults. *Otology and Neurotology, 34,* 729–735.

Horak, F. B., Jones-Rycewicz, C., Black, F. O., & Shumway-Cook, A. (1992). Effects of vestibular rehabilitation on dizziness and imbalance. *Otolaryngology-Head and Neck Surgery, 106,* 175–180.

Huang, K., Sparto, P. J., Kiesler, S., Siewiorek, D. P., & Smailagi, A. (2014). iPod-based in-home system for monitoring gaze-stabilization exercise compliance of individuals with vestibular hypofunction. *Journal of Neuroengineering and Rehabilitation, 11,* 69.

Hurley, B. F. (1995). Age, gender, and muscular strength. *Journals of Gerontology. Series A, Biological Sciences and Medical Sciences, 50,* 41–44.

Jacobson, G. P., & Newman, C. W. (1990). The development of the Dizziness Handicap Inventory. *Archives of Otolaryngology-Head and Neck Surgery, 116,* 424–427.

Johnsson, L. G. (1971). Degenerative changes and anomalies of the vestibular system in man. *Laryngoscope, 81,* 1682–1694.

Kerr, B., Condon, S. M., & McDonald, L. A. (1985). Cognitive spatial processing and the regulation of posture. *Journal of Experimental Psychology. Human Perception and Performance, 11,* 617–622.

Krebs, D. E., Gill-Body, K. M., Parker, S. W., Ramirez, J. V., & Wernick-Robinson, M. (2003). Vestibular rehabilitation: Useful but not universally so. *Otolaryngology-Head and Neck Surgery, 128,* 240–250.

Krebs, D. E., Jette, A. M., & Assmann, S. F. (1998). Moderate exercise improves gait stability in disabled elders. *Archives of Physical Medicine and Rehabilitation, 79,* 1489–1495.

Kristinsdottir, E. K., Fransson, P. A., & Magnusson, M. (2001). Changes in postural control in healthy elderly subjects are related to vibration sensation, vision and vestibular asymmetry. *Acta Oto-Laryngologica, 121*(6), 700–706.

Lopez, I., Honrubia, V., & Baloh, R. W. (1997). Aging and the human vestibular nucleus. *Journal of Vestibular Research, 7,* 77–85.

Lord, S. R., & Dayhew, J. (2001). Visual risk factors for falls in older people. *Journal of the American Geriatrics Society, 49,* 508–515.

Lord, S. R., & Menz, H. B. (2000). Visual contributions to postural stability in older adults. *Gerontology, 46,* 306–310.

Lord, S. R., Rogers, M. W., Howland, A., & Fitzpatrick, R. (1999). Lateral stability, sensorimotor function and falls in older people. *Journal of the American Geriatrics Society, 47,* 1077–1081.

Macias, J. D., Massingale, S., & Gerkin, R. D. (2005). Efficacy of vestibular rehabilitation therapy in reducing falls. *Otolaryngology-Head and Neck Surgery, 133,* 323–325.

Maki, B. E., & McIlroy, W. E. (2006). Control of rapid limb movements for balance recovery: Age-related changes and implications for fall prevention. *Age and Ageing, 35*(Suppl 2), 12–18.

Manchester, D., Woollacott, M., Zederbauer-Hylton, N., & Marin, O. (1989). Visual, vestibular and somatosensory contributions to balance control in the older adult. *Journal of Gerontology, 44*, M118–M127.

Marchetti, G. F., Whitney, S. L., Redfern, M. S., & Furman, J. M. (2011). Factors associated with balance confidence in older adults with health conditions affecting the balance and vestibular system. *Archives of Physical Medicine and Rehabilitation, 92*, 1884–1891.

Meldrum, D., Glennon, A., Herdman, S., Murray, D., & McConn-Walsh, R. (2012). Virtual reality rehabilitation of balance: Assessment of the usability of the Nintendo Wii® Fit Plus. *Disability and Rehabilitation, Assistive Technology, 7*, 205–210.

Melzer, I., Benjuya, N., Kaplanski, J., & Alexander, N. (2009). Association between ankle muscle strength and limit of stability in older adults. *Age and Ageing, 38*, 119–123.

Metter, E. J., Conwit, R., Tobin, J., & Fozard, J. L. (1997). Age-associated loss of power and strength in the upper extremities in women and men. *Journals of Gerontology. Series A, Biological Sciences and Medical Sciences, 52*, B267–B276.

Mille, M. L., Johnson-Hilliard, M., Martinez, K. M., Zhang, Y., Edwards, B. J., & Rogers, M. W. (2013). One step, two steps, three steps more . . . Directional vulnerability to falls in community-dwelling older people. *Journals of Gerontology. Series A, Biological Sciences and Medical Sciences, 68*, 1540–1548.

Nagai, K., Yamada, M., Uemura, K., Tanaka, B., Mori, S., Yamada, Y., . . . Tsuboyama, T. (2012). Effects of fear of falling on muscular coactivation during walking. *Aging Clinical Experimental Research, 24*, 157–161.

Narici, M. V., & Kayser, B. (1995). Hypertrophic response of human skeletal muscle to strength training in hypoxia and normoxia. *European Journal of Applied Physiology and Occupational Physiology, 70*, 213–219.

Osler, C. J., Tersteeg, M. C., Reynolds, R. F., & Loram, I. D. (2013). Postural threat differentially affects the feedforward and feedback components of the vestibular-evoked balance response. *European Journal of Neuroscience, 38*, 3239–3247.

Park, J, J., Tang, Y., Lopez, I., & Ishiyama, A. (2001). Unbiased estimation of human vestibular ganglion neurons. *Annals of the New York Academy of Sciences, 942*, 475–478.

Peel, N. M., Kassulke, D. J., & McClure, R. J. (2002). Population based study of hospitalised fall related injuries in older people. *Injury Prevention, 8*, 280–283.

Perez-Jara, J., Olmos, P., Abad, M. A., Heslop, P., Walker, D., & Reyes-Ortiz, C. A. (2012). Differences in fear of falling in the elderly with or without dizzines. *Maturitas, 73*(3), 261–264.

Peterka, R. J., & Black, F. O. (1990–1991). Age-related changes in human posture control: Sensory organization tests. *Journal of Vestibular Research, 1*, 73–85.

Porciuncula, F., Johnson, C. C., & Glickman, L. B. (2012). The effect of vestibular rehabilitation on adults with bilateral vestibular hypofunction: A systematic review. *Journal of Vestibular Research, 22*, 283–298.

Porter, M. M., Vandervoort, A. A., & Lexell, J. (1995). Aging of human muscle: Structure, function and adaptability. *Scandinavian Journal of Medicine & Science in Sports, 5*, 129–142.

Poulain, I., & Giraudet, G. (2008). Age-related changes of visual contribution in posture control. *Gait and Posture,27*, 1–7.

Pritcher, M. R., Whitney, S. L., Marchetti, G. F., & Furman, J. M. (2008). The influence of age and vestibular disorders on gaze stabilization: A pilot study. *Otology and Neurotology, 29*, 982–988.

Rantanen, T., Masaki, K., Foley, D., Izmirlian, G., White, L., & Guralnik, J. M. (1998). Grip strength changes over 27 yr in Japanese-American men. *Journal of Applied Physiology, 85*, 2047–2053.

Redfern, M. S., Talkowski, M. E., Jennings, J. R., & Furman, J. M. (2004). Cognitive influences in postural control of patients with unilateral vestibular loss. *Gait and Posture, 19*, 105–114.

Reelick, M. F., van Iersel, M. B., Kessels, R. P., & Rikkert, M. G. (2009). The influence of fear of falling on gait and balance in older people. *Age and Ageing, 38*(4), 435–440.

Ricci, N. A., Aratani, M. C., Doná, F., Macedo, C., Caovilla, H. H., & Ganança, F. F. (2010). A systematic review about the effects of the vestibular rehabilitation in middle-age and older adults. *Revista Brasileira de Fisioterapia, 14*, 361–371.

Richter, E. (1980). Quantitative study of human Scarpa's ganglion and vestibular sensory epithelia. *Acta Oto-Laryngologica, 90*, 199–208.

Rine, R. M., Schubert, M. C., Whitney, S. L., Roberts, D., Redfern, M. S., Musolino, M. C., . . . Slotkin J. (2013). Vestibular function assessment using the NIH Toolbox. *Neurology, 80*, S25–S31.

Rochat, S., Bula, C. J., Martin, E., Seematter-Bagnoud, L., Karmaniola, A., Aminian, K., . . . Santos-Eggimann, B. (2010). What is the relationship between fear of falling and gait in well-functioning older persons aged 65 to 70 years? *Archives of Physical Medicine and Rehabilitation, 91*, 879–884.

Rogers, M. W., & Mille, M. L. (2003). Lateral stability and falls in older people. *Exercise and Sport Sciences Reviews, 31*, 182–187.

Rosenhall, U. (1973). Degenerative patterns in the aging human vestibular neuro-epithelia. *Acta Oto-Laryngologica, 76*, 208–220.

Schubert, M. C., Das, V., Tusa, R. J., & Herdman, S. J. (2004). Cervico-ocular reflex in normal subjects and patients with unilateral vestibular hypofunction. *Otology and Neurotology, 25*, 65–71.

Serrador, J. M., Lipsitz, L. A., Gopalakrishnan, G. S., Black, F.O., & Wood, S.J. (2009). Loss of otolith function with age is associated with increased postural sway measures. *Neuroscience Letters, 465*, 10–15.

Shelhamer, M., Tiliket, C., Roberts, D., Kramer, P. D., & Zee, D. S. (1994). Short-term vestibulo-ocular reflex adaptation in humans. II. Error signals. *Experimental Brain Research, 100*, 328–336.

Shepard, N. T., Telian, S. A., Smith-Wheelock, M., & Raj, A. (1993).Vestibular and balance rehabilitation therapy. *Annals of Otology, Rhinology, and Laryngology, 102*, 198–205.

Shumway-Cook, A., & Woollacott, M. H. (2000). Attentional demands and postural control: The effect of sensory context. *Journals of Gerontology. Series A, Biological Sciences and Medical Sciences, 55A*, M10–M16.

Shumway-Cook, A., Woollacott, M., Kerns, K. A., & Baldwin, M. (1997). The effects of two types of cognitive tasks on postural stability in older adults with and without a history of falls. *Journals of Gerontology. Series A, Biological Sciences and Medical Sciences, 52A*, M232–M241.

Stelmach, G. E., Teasdale, N., Di Fabio, R. P., & Phillips, J. (1989). Age related decline in postural control mechanisms. *International Journal of Aging and Human Development, 29*, 205–223.

Stevens, J. A., Ballesteros, M. F., Mack, K. A., Rudd, R. A., DeCaro, E., & Adler, G. (2012). Gender differences in seeking care for falls in the aged Medicare population. *American Journal of Preventive Medicine, 43*, 59–62.

Su, H. -C., Huang, T. -W., Young, Y. -H., & Cheng, P. -W. (2004). Aging effect on vestibular evoked myogenic potential. *Otology and Neurotology, 25*, 977–980.

Sundermier, L., Woollacott, M. H., Jensen, J. L., & Moore, S. (1996). Postural sensitivity to visual flow in aging adults with and without balance problems. *Journals of Gerontology. Series A, Biological Sciences and Medical Sciences, 51*, M45–M52.

Szturm, T., Betker, A. L., Moussavi, Z., Desai, A., & Goodman, V. (2011). Effects of an interactive computer game exercise regimen on balance impairment in frail community-dwelling older adults: A randomized controlled trial. *Physical Therapy, 91*, 1449–1462.

Tang, P. F., & Woollacott, M. H. (1998). Inefficient postural responses to unexpected slips during walking in older adults. *Journals of Gerontology. Series A, Biological Sciences and Medical Sciences, 53*, M471–M480.

Taylor, M. J., Shawis, T., Impson, R., Ewins, K., McCormick, D., & Griffin, M. (2012). Nintendo Wii as a training tool in falls prevention rehabilitation: Case studies. *Journal of the American Geriatrics Society, 60*(9), 1781–1783.

Telian, S. A., Shepard, N. T., Smith-Wheelock, M., & Hoberg, M. (1991). Bilateral vestibular paresis: Diagnosis and treatment. *Otolaryngology-Head and Neck Surgery, 104*, 67–71.

Telian, S. A., Shepard, N. T., Smith-Wheelock, M., & Kemink, J. L. (1990). Habituation therapy for chronic vestibular dysfunction: Preliminary results. *Otolaryngology-Head and Neck Surgery, 103*, 89–95.

Tinetti, M. E., Richman, D., & Powell, L. (1990). Falls efficacy as a measure of fear of falling. *Journal of Gerontology, 45*, P239–P243.

Toledo, D. R., & Barela, J. A. (2014). Age-related differences in postural control: Effects of the complexity of visual manipulation and sensorimotor contribution to postural performance. *Experimental Brain Research, 232*, 493–502.

Toulotte, C., Toursel, C., & Olivier, N. (2012). Wii Fit® training vs. Adapted Physical Activities: which one is the most appropriate to improve the balance of independent senior subjects? A randomized controlled study. *Clinical Rehabilitation, 26*, 827–835.

Tromp, A. M., Pluijm, S. M., Smit, J. H., Deeg, D. J., Bouter, L. M., & Lips, P. (2001). Fall-risk screening test: A prospective study on predictors for falls in community-dwelling elderly. *Journal of Clinical Epidemiology, 54*, 837–844.

Tseng, C. L., Chou, C. H., & Young, Y. H. (2010). Aging effect on the ocular vestibular-evoked myogenic potentials. *Otology and Neurotology, 31*, 959–963.

Turano, K., Rubin, G. S., Herdman, S. J., Chee, E., & Fried, L. P. (1994). Visual stabilization of posture in the elderly: Fallers vs. nonfallers. *Optometry and Vision Science, 71*, 761–769.

Velázquez-Villaseñor, L., Merchant, S. N., Tsuji, K., Glynn, R. J., Wall, C., 3rd, & Rauch, S. D. (2000). Temporal bone studies of the human peripheral vestibular system. Normative Scarpa's ganglion cell data. *Annals of Otology, Rhinology and Laryngology Supplement, 181*, 14–19.

Vereeck, L., Wuyts, F. L., Truijen, S., De Valck, C., & Van de Heyning, P. H. (2008). The effect of early customized vestibular rehabilitation on balance after acoustic neuroma resection. *Clinical Rehabilitation, 22*, 698–713.

Verghese, J., Holtzer, R., Lipton, R. B., & Wang, C. (2009). Quantitative gait markers and incident fall risk in older adults. *Journals of Gerontology. Series A, Biological Sciences and Medical Sciences, 64*, 896–901.

Wade, M. G., Lindquist, R., Taylor, J. R., & Treat-Jacobson D. (1995). Optical flow, spatial orientation, and the control of posture in the elderly. *Journals of Gerontology. Series B, Psychological Science and Social Science, 50*, P51–P58.

Wall, C., 3rd, & Black, F. O. (1984). Intersubject variability in VOR responses to 0.005–1.0 Hz sinusoidal rotations. *Acta Oto-Laryngologica Supplementum, 406*, 194–198.

Ward, B. K., Mohammed, M. T., Brach, J. S., Studenski, S. A., Whitney, S. L., & Furman, J. M. (2010). Physical performance and a test of gaze stabilization in older adults. *Otology and Neurotology, 31*, 168–172.

Ward, B. K., Mohammad, M. T., Whitney, S. L., Marchetti, G. F., & Furman, J. M. (2010). The reliability, stability, and concurrent validity of a test of gaze stabilization. *Journal of Vestibular Research, 20*, 363–372.

Weale, R. A. (1975). Senile changes in visual acuity. *Transactions of the Ophthalmological Societies of the United Kingdom, 95*, 36–38.

Whitney, S. L., Marchetti, G. F., Pritcher, M., & Furman, J. M. (2009). Gaze stabilization and gait performance in vestibular dysfunction. *Gait and Posture, 29*, 194–198.

Whitney, S. L., Wrisley, D. M., Marchetti, G. F., & Furman, J. M. (2002). The effect of age on vestibular rehabilitation outcomes. *Laryngoscope, 112*, 785–790.

Williams, B., Doherty, N. L., Bender, A., Mattox, H., & Tibbs, J. R. (2011). The effect of nintendo wii on balance: A pilot study supporting the use of the wii in occupational therapy for the well elderly. *Occupational Therapy and Health Care, 25*, 131–139.

Woollacott, M. H., Shumway-Cook, A., & Nashner, L. M. (1986). Aging and posture control: Changes in sensory organization and muscular coordination. *International Journal of Aging and Human Development, 23*, 97–114.

Yardley, L., Gardner, M., Bronstein, A., Davies, R., Buckwell, D., & Luxon, L. (2001). Interference between postural control and mental task performance in patients with vestibular disorder and healthy controls. *Journal of Neurology, Neurosurgery, and Psychiatry, 71*, 48–52.

Yardley, L., Verschuur, C., Masson, E., Luxon, L., & Haacke, N. (1992). Somatic and psychological factors contributing to handicap in people with vertigo. *British Journal of Audiology, 26*, 283–290.

Multifactorial Assessment of Falls Risk in the Elderly[1]

Gary P. Jacobson and Devin L. McCaslin

INTRODUCTION

The area of assessment of falls risk is a relatively young area of practice for clinical audiologists. This area is within the audiologist's scope of practice as defined by both the American Speech-Language-Hearing Association (ASHA, 1992, 1999) and the American Academy of Audiology (AAA; http://www.audiology.org/publications/documents/practice/default.htm?PF=1). The audiologist scope of practice as defined by ASHA states, "Audiologists are professionals . . . engaged in autonomous practice to promote . . . quality of life . . . through the . . . identification, assessment, and rehabilitation of balance systems." The audiologist scope of practice as stated by the AAA states that the areas of practice can include, "identification, assessment, diagnosis and treatment of individuals with impairment of . . . vestibular function, and . . . the prevention of (vestibular) impairments."

The topic of falls in the elderly is appearing regularly in the popular press and in textbooks that either address falls in the elderly directly (Downton, 1993; Lord, Sherrington, Menz, & Close 2007) or in general audiology and physical therapy textbooks that address balance function assessment (e.g., Herdman, 2000; Luxon, Furman, Martini, & Stephens, 2003).

The reduction in falls in the elderly and the attendant morbidity and mortality has become a national goal as stated in the National Action Plan of the Falls Free Coalition. Additionally, there was legislation introduced that addressed the issue of falls in the elderly. This legislation, the Keeping Seniors Safe from Falls Act of 2007 Senate Bill 845 (House Bill 845) (2007) passed and passed both houses of Congress and was signed into law. Among other objectives this bill states that the Secretary of Health and Human Services shall . . .

(A) conduct and support research to—
  (i) improve the identification of older adults who have a high risk of falling;
  (ii) improve data collection and analysis to identify fall risk and protective factors;
  (iii) design, implement, and evaluate the most effective fall prevention interventions;
  (iv) improve strategies that are proven to be effective in reducing falls by tailoring these strategies to specific populations of older adults;
  (v) conduct research in order to maximize the dissemination of proven, effective fall prevention interventions;
  (vi) intensify proven interventions to prevent falls among older adults;

[1]Portions of this chapter have been published previously in Jacobson, G. P. (2002). Development of a clinic for the assessment of risk of falls in elderly patients. *Seminars in Hearing, 23*(2).

(vii) improve the diagnosis, treatment, and rehabilitation of elderly fall victims and those at high risk for falls; and

(viii) assess the risk of falls occurring in various settings; . . .

Finally, since January of 2005, Medicare has subsidized the cost of every new enrollee's first medical examination. This "Welcome to Medicare Visit" includes an initial preventive physical examination (IPPE) that includes assessments of depression, hearing, activities of daily living, home safety, and an assessment of falls risk.

Falls, particularly for the elderly person (i.e., persons ≥65 years of age), are a significant health risk. Data collected in the United States suggest that 20% of patients over 65 years of age will fall in the next year amounting to approximately 7 million falls annually. Approximately 33% of these falls will occur at home (Rubenstein et al., 1988). Between 45% and 70% of the falls will occur in nursing homes (Thapa & Wray, 1996). Of those elderly people who have fallen, 10% of this group will experience two or more falls, and only half of those individuals will survive the next year of life (Cumming, 1998).

Unintentional injury, which almost always results from a fall, ranks as the sixth leading cause of death in the elderly population. Besides mortality there is significant morbidity associated with falls. The greatest fall risk is that of hip fracture. It has been estimated 350,000 hip fractures will occur annually as a result of falls (Watters & Moran, 2006). At a cost of $35,000 to repair these fractures, the total cost excluding rehabilitation is estimated to be $1.2 billon. In this country 20% of elderly people who sustain a hip fracture from a fall will die within a year. Another 20% will be moved to an inpatient long-term care center for the first time. In contrast, in the United Kingdom it has been reported that of those elderly people who sustain an injury from falling that is sufficient to require medical attention 17% to 25% will die within 12 months (Wild, Nayak, & Isaacs, 1981). Of those who sustain hip fractures, 49% will die within 6 months (Grimley-Evens, Prudham, & Wandess, 1979). Elderly people who fall are 10 times more likely to be hospitalized and are eight times more likely to die than are children who fall. Seventy-five percent of the deaths due to falls that occur each year involve elderly individuals, who constitute 12% of the population (Rubenstein et al.,

1988). The cost of caring for elderly patients who fall has been estimated to be between $10 and $20 billion per year (Tibbits, 1996; Tinetti, Williams, & Gill, 2000). Accordingly, falls in the elderly population are associated with significant morbidity (and reductions in quality of life), mortality, and, expense to our health care system. It is possible that the human and monetary costs associated with falls could be reduced if those at greatest risk for falling were identified ahead of time and measures were implemented to reduce or eliminate the risk(s).

PURPOSE OF THE RISK OF FALLS CLINIC

The goal of a risk of falls (ROF) assessment clinic is to identify those elderly people at greatest risk for falling by administering a set of evaluations aimed at the assessment of specific risk factors known to be associated with falling. The long-term objective is to keep independent elderly independent for as long as possible. It was our assumption that a finding of normal function on these examinations would not necessarily guarantee that a patient would not fall. That is, accidental falls are, by nature of the term, accidental. However, a number of exogenous and endogenous factors are known to place elders at a heightened risk for falling. By evaluating patients across these factors and comparing their performance to established normative data it might be possible to identify future fallers and intervene to reduce the risk.

Unfortunately, in the elderly population there is a high likelihood that a patient will show not a single risk factor, but instead, multiple risk factors. The assessment of total risk in these cases is not simply additive as there may be overlap between risk factors. For example, depression may be a risk factor for falls in the elderly population. Depression may be treated with antidepressant medications that carry an inherent risk for falling. For example, we assume the risk of falling for a depressed patient is 1.4 times greater than that for a nondepressed patient. Furthermore, let us assume that the risk of falling for a patient who is taking anxiolytic medications is 2.0 times greater than that of a patient who is not taking anxiolytic medications. The cumulative increased risk for that patient would not be 3.4 times greater, that is, because depressed patients might be treated with anxiolytic medications, the two risk factors probably are not truly independent. Another example would be patients who report dizziness. These patients are at greater risk of falling than patients who do not report dizziness. Patients who take antidepressant medications often report dizziness as a side effect. Therefore, in this case, dizziness and antidepressant medications would not be independent predictors of falls.

The multidimensional ROF assessment does not yield a single number reflecting a patient's relative risk. Such an expectation would imply that we understand not only the effect each individual risk factor has on the determination of odds ratios, but also the interactions that multiple risk factors have on the determination of risk. Accordingly, a more empirical approach is to determine the numbers of risk factors for each patient with the expectation that risk would be greater as numbers of risk factors increased. Thus, a patient with seven risk factors would be more at risk for falling than a patient with two risk factors. Therefore, the objective of a ROF assessment is not to determine precise risk values but, instead, to quantify the number of risk factors demonstrated by a given patient.

The final report generated for the referring physician should include a general impression of how much at risk it is felt the patient is for falling (e.g., low, moderate, high) and a description of those subtests where the patient's performance deviated from normal. It is an objective not only to identify those at increased risk for falls but also to recommend to the referring physician appropriate interventions, where possible, to decrease the fall risk. Medical interventions might include a reassessment of medications by the primary care physician, adjustment of dosages of antihypertensive medications, and referral to ophthalmology for assessment of vision impairment. Nonmedical interventions could range from referral to physical therapy for assistance in overall strengthening, to assistance with ambulation (e.g., through the dispensing of assistive devices), to balance rehabilitation therapy.

ASSESSMENT OF RISK OF FALLS IN THE ELDERLY

There are many known risk factors for falls in the elderly population. These include specific diseases and conditions such as Parkinson's disease (i.e., the associated movement disorder), osteoporosis (i.e., in severe cases, the changes in posture that result in changes in center of gravity of the body during ambulation that places that patient at increased risk), heart disease (including cardiac arrhythmias and atherosclerotic heart disease), diabetes (and associated polyneuropathy that reduces proprioception in the lower extremities), cerebrovascular diseases including stroke and drop attacks, and postural hypotension that is either disease or medication induced (i.e., medications may cause postural hypotension either by impairing homeostatic mechanisms of blood pressure regulation, e.g., antipsychotics and antidepressants, or by reducing blood volume, e.g., diuretics).

Gender also influences the ROF. For example, in a study where subjects' postural stability was challenged artificially, Pavol, Owings, Foley, and Grabiner (1999) reported that women were four times more likely to fall than men. Alternately, van Dijk, Meulenberg, van de Sande, and Habbema (1993) have reported that men older than 75 years of age were approximately twice as likely to fall as women the same age. Age also shows a positive relationship with falls risk (Pavol et al., 1999). More general risk factors that increase ROF include age-related reductions in physiologic functions for maintenance of postural control that directly or indirectly result in loss of balance. These factors include reduction of visual functions (e.g., visual acuity, contrast sensitivity, darkness adaptation), somatosenses (e.g., vibration, proprioception), vestibular function, and muscle tone. Use of anxiolytic or sedative drugs is associated with a high risk of falling. In fact, the use of four or more prescription drugs, of any type, is associated with a correct prediction of a fall in that year (Tibbits, 1996). This probably occurs as the number of prescription medications a patient is taking serves as an index of the patient's overall health. Also, specific environmental factors (e.g., poor lighting, loose rugs, unstable furniture, stairs with poor railings, low beds, and toilets) are associated with increased falls risk (Tibbits, 1996).

The following are descriptions of specific risk factors associated with ROF, and, examinations that may be used to assess each risk factor.

The reader will note that an assessment of auditory sensitivity is not included as part of the ROF assessment. The relationship between falls, fractures, and auditory sensitivity was considered by

Purchase-Helzner and colleagues (2004). The sample included 6,480 women (mean age 77 years) and 40% of these individuals had significant hearing impairments. The annual rate of falling was .59 in the normal-hearing group (i.e., <1 fall/per person/per year), and ranged between .54 and .59 in the hearing impaired group (i.e., the investigators included individuals with mild and "significant" hearing impairments). These differences were not significant.

The test battery described herein is based on constraints of current knowledge, scope of practice, and the practicalities of performing these assessments on an elderly patient. Lord, Sherrington, and Menz (2001) stated that from their perspective a ROF assessment should (1) be simple to administer, (2) have a short administration time, (3) be feasible for elderly people to undertake, (4) provide valid and reliable measurements, (5) be low-tech and robust, (6) be portable, and (7) provide quantitative results. The battery described herein fails to satisfy four of these criteria. It is not simple to administer, it is not entirely low tech, and, it is not entirely portable. However, it is believed that this group of assessments yields reliable and quantifiable data that are missing in the low-tech assessments. Ultimately, it is likely that what is chosen to be included in a preferred group of assessments will be an evolutionary process.

Finally, patients are encouraged to bring with them family members/caregivers who remain in the examination room during testing. This creates an environment where patients are more comfortable and where caregivers have first-hand experience observing situations where the patient's performance differs from normal.

Risk Factor: General (e.g., History of Falls, Number of Concurrent Medications)

Directed Case History

It is best to have, at the very least, a family member or significant other attend the case history taking. This is important because recall of falls history has been shown to be affected by age. Cummings, Nevitt, and Kidd (1988) evaluated prospectively over a 12-month period 304 ambulatory men and women over the age of 60 years. Of this cohort, 179 fell dur-

ing the evaluation period. At the end of the study, all participants were interviewed by telephone and asked whether they had fallen during the previous 3, 6, or 12 months. Depending on the interval, they were asked to remember (i.e., the previous 3, 6, or 12 months). Between 13% and 32% of those with confirmed falls failed to remember they had fallen. Patients with poor scores on a standardized screening measure of cognitive impairment (i.e., the Mini-Mental Status Examination—MMSE, see below) were more likely to have forgotten they had fallen.

A representative case history form developed by Tibbits (1994) is shown in Figure 33–1. This case history focuses on those areas that are associated with increased risk of falling in the elderly population. The questionnaire targets six major areas and is administered prior to formal testing. The six major areas include history of previous falls (i.e., the risk of sustaining a fall increases if the patient has sustained previous falls), medication use, gait impairment or muscle weakness, dizziness/vertigo/loss of consciousness, environmental problems (i.e., safety of home environment), and major illnesses. With respect to environmental variables, the results of a meta-analysis of falls literature has suggested that, on average, 37% of falls are accidental and/or environment-related (e.g., poor lighting, objects on the floor such as throw rugs, etc.) (Rubenstein et al., 1988). The rest of the falls were attributable to either medical conditions (55%) as noted above, or, unknown causes.

Risk Factor: Impaired Cognitive Function

Mental Status (Mini-Mental Status Examination)

The reported increased risk for falling that a patient with impaired cognitive function may demonstrate has ranged from 1.42 times (Liu, Topper, Reeves, Gryfe, & Maki, 1995) to 3.4 or 3.5 times (Nygaard, 1998; Poor, Atkinson, O'Fallon, & Melton, 1995). Impaired mentation can result in a lack of awareness of one's immediate environment and the dangers contained therein (Horikawa et al., 2005; van Dijk et al., 1993). The result may be a patient who engages in risky behavior (e.g., walking down stairs without wearing glasses or grasping the banister if one exists) that he or she might not have considered

Office Staff Evaluation of Patient Falls
(From Tibbits, 1996)

Patient name _____ Date _____

Risk factors (circle answers)

1. Previous falls:

yes (last fall date: _____)
no

2. Medications:

1. four or more prescriptions
2. new prescription (last 2 weeks)
3. any of the following types: tranquilizers, sleeping pills, antidepressants, antihypertensives, antidiabetic agents.

3. Gait problem or weakness:

Yes
No

4. Dizziness, vertigo, loss of consciousness:

Yes
No

5. Environmental problems:

Lighting
Flooring
Other

6. Major illnesses:

CNS
Musculoskeletal
Neurologic
Heart
New acute illness
Other

Questions to ask patient or family:

What was happening before the fall occurred?

Any injuries?   Cut   pain   sprain/strain   fracture   other:

Check temperature _____ pulse _____ BP _____

Who is available to help the patient?   Spouse   family member   friend   none

Figure 33-1. Representative falls case history form. From Tibbits, G. M. (1996). Patients who fall: How to predict and prevent injuries. *Geriatrics, 51,* 24–28. Reprinted with the permission of the author.

when mental functions were intact. Thus, a patient who might have held onto a handrail when walking down a stairway might forget or decide not to do so. Or, a patient who awakens in the night may forget to turn on a bedroom light and, as a result, trip and fall in the process of navigating to the bathroom.

Mental status can be screened with a standardized instrument called the Mini-Mental Status Examination (MMSE) (Folstein, Anthony, Parhad, Duffy, & Gruenberg, 1985; Folstein, Folstein, & McHugh, 1975). This instrument consists of 11 sections (e.g., date orientation, place orientation, serial sevens, short-term memory). The maximum score on this assessment is 30 points representing normal function. A score of 23 points or less is considered abnormal. An abnormal score on the MMSE is not diagnostic for dementia but instead suggests that additional testing is indicated. Although the MMSE is ubiquitous in the medical environment, it has some significant flaws. For example, there is only a cursory assessment of memory and there is a notable ceiling effect (Huppert, Cabelli, & Matthews, 2005). Despite these problems, the MMSE has been well studied and has been included in the ROF assessment. The MMSE has been reported to demonstrate 87% sensitivity and 82% specificity for impaired mentation (Anthony, LeResche, Niaz, Von Korff, & Folstein, 1982).

Risk Factor: Impaired Reaction Time

A number of investigators have established a link between simple and complex reaction time and an increased risk for falling. It is empirically obvious that the longer it takes for a significant event (e.g., an impending fall) to be perceived and interpreted as significant, and the longer it takes a person to react to this event the greater the falls risk they will be. There are a number of methods to assess reaction time. These include both simple reaction time which describes the interval between the presentation of a single stimulus and the response from the observer. A second type of reaction time referred to as choice reaction time involves a task similar to that for simple reaction time; however, instead of one stimulus, two are presented in a randomized manner. The listener is directed to respond quickly to only one of the two. Thus, for choice reaction time the listener must not only respond but must quickly classify

the stimulus as either a "target" or "nontarget." For purposes of this chapter only simple reaction time is addressed.

Simple Reaction Time

Simple reaction time can be evaluated by calculating the interval between when a stimulus, such as a light, is presented and when a patient responds to the stimulus by pressing a button. Such a device was developed by Stephen R. Lord, Ph.D., and is shown in Video 33–1. The device is a footswitch containing a light and a controller/counter. At randomized intervals the light is illuminated and the patient is instructed to depress the footswitch as quickly as possible after the light illuminates. The number that is registered on the device represents the interval in milliseconds between the presentation of the light and the patient's response. Reaction times can be calculated for upper extremities (i.e., the patient presses a button or mouse key when a light is presented) and lower extremities. Normative data for both collected by Lord, Menz, and Tiedemann (2003) are shown in Table 33–1.

Another method of measuring reaction time is from data collected during the Motor Control Test (MCT) of computerized dynamic poturography. In this case what is measured is the latency between the onset of platform perturbation and onset of postural correction for the perturbation. There are age-normed data for that measurement. (See Chapters 17 and 18 by Nashner for further information about the MCT.)

Risk Factor: Depression

Depression may serve as a risk factor in different ways. Significant clinical depression may make a

Table 33–1. Normative Data for Lower Extremity Simple Reaction Time

Reaction Time (ms)	Interpretation
Excellent	<250 ms
Good	250 ≤300 ms
Fair	300 ≤350 ms
Poor	>350 ms

Source: Lord et al., personal communication.

patient less aware of his or her environment. That is, they may be more internally and less externally aware. Also, some patients who are placed on psychoactive medications including antidepressants and anxiolytics may be more sensitive than others to these medications and experience significant side effects. For example, Neutel, Hirdes, Maxwell, and Patten (1996) evaluated the risk of falls for men and women who were prescribed benzodiazepine medications. They reported a fourfold increased ROF for men and a 2.5-fold increased ROF for women. Koski, Luukinen, Laippala, and Kivela (1996) and Herings, Stricker, DeBoer, Bakker, and Sturmans (1995) evaluated falls risk for patients taking benzodiazepines that were either short or long acting. The expectation was that patients taking long-acting benzodiazepine medications would experience a greater ROF. In fact, patients taking long-acting benzodiazepine medications experienced a 3.4-fold risk of falling compared to 1.6-fold increased risk for patients taking short-acting benzodiazepines. Herings et al. (1995) reported that both oxazepam and lorazepam in high doses were associated with fivefold increased ROF. Finally, Herings et al. (1995) have underscored the observation that it is important not only to be aware of the medication that is being prescribed but whether there have been recent changes (i.e., increases) in the dosage of that medication. The investigators have reported that sudden increases in the dosage of a benzodiazepine medication are associated with a 3.4-fold increased risk of falling in the elderly within 2 weeks of the increase.

The relationship between depression and gait impairment was evaluated by Hausdorff, Peng, Goldberger, and Stoll (2004). The investigators measured gait in a sample of patients with unipolar major depressive disorder and in a group of patients with bipolar disorder. The performance of the experimental groups was compared to that of a control group. The investigators reported that the experimental groups walked more slowly, with increased stride time, and showed greater swing time variability.

The Geriatric Depression Scale (GDS)
(Yesavage, Brink, Rose, Lum, Huang, Adey, & Leirer, 1983)

The Geriatric Depression Scale is a standardized screening measure for the presence of clinical depres-

sion in the elderly person (Figure 33–2). It consists of 30 statements to which the patient must respond by saying "yes" or "no." A cutoff score of 11 points on the GDS has been reported to yield an 84% sensitivity and 95% specificity for the presence of clinical depression (Koenig, Meador, Cohen, & Blazer, 1988; Mondolo, Jahanshahi, Grana, Biasutti, Cacciatori, & De Bennedetto, 2006; Yesavage et al., 1983). We feel it is important to evaluate patients for the presence of clinical depression as depressed patients may act like patients with impaired cognitive functioning. Accordingly, it is important to be aware of the patient's performance on both the MMSE and the GDS.

Risk Factor: Postural Hypotension

The presence of postural hypotension has been reported by Poor et al. (1995) to place elderly people at a 1.3-fold increased risk for falling. Like hyperventilation syndrome, postural hypotension (i.e., also referred to as orthostatic hypotension) is underdiagnosed in balance function laboratories and may be easiest to remediate. Postural hypotension occurs when patients who have been sitting or lying down for extended periods of time stand quickly and begin to ambulate. Patients will experience dizziness and light-headedness and, in extreme situations, may lose consciousness for a short period of time. During periods of dizziness or loss of consciousness the patient could fall. Postural hypotension is defined as a 20 mm Hg decrease in systolic blood pressure on standing (i.e., the systolic measure represents the pressure exerted by the blood on walls of arteries during contraction of the heart), or a decrease in the systolic blood pressure value to <90 mm Hg on standing. The mechanism of postural hypotension is that during extended periods of sitting and lying down there occurs a pooling of blood in the trunk. On standing, there is an immediate demand for blood to be routed to the brain. If a patient is taking medications designed to reduce blood pressure (i.e., antihypertensive medications), the demand for blood to perfuse the brain will not be met and the patient will become light-headed. Postural hypotension also can occur in patients who are volume depleted (i.e., patients who do not drink enough fluids to replenish the blood volume) and in patients with central nervous system diseases.

Geriatric Depression Scale (GDS)
(Yesavage et al., 1983)

1.	Are you basically satisfied with your life?	Yes	No
2.	Have you dropped many of your activities and interests?	Yes	No
3.	Do you feel that your life is empty?	Yes	No
4.	Do you often get bored?	Yes	No
5.	Are you hopeful about the future?	Yes	No
6.	Are you bothered by thoughts you can't get out of your head?	Yes	No
7.	Are you in good spirits most of the time?	Yes	No
8.	Are you afraid that something bad is going to happen to you?	Yes	No
9.	Do you feel happy most of the time?	Yes	No
10.	Do you often feel helpless?	Yes	No
11.	Do you often get restless and fidgety?	Yes	No
12.	Do you prefer to stay at home, rather than going out and doing new things?	Yes	No
13.	Do you frequently worry about the future?	Yes	No
14.	Do you feel you have more problems with memory than most?	Yes	No
15.	Do you think it is wonderful to be alive now?	Yes	No
16.	Do you often feel downhearted and blue?	Yes	No
17.	Do you feel pretty worthless the way you are now?	Yes	No
18.	Do you worry a lot about the past?	Yes	No
19.	Do you find life very exciting?	Yes	No
20.	Is it hard for you to get started on new projects?	Yes	No
21.	Do you feel full of energy?	Yes	No
22.	Do you feel that your situation is hopeless?	Yes	No
23.	Do you think that most people are better off than you are?	Yes	No
24.	Do you frequently get upset over little things?	Yes	No
25.	Do you frequently feel like crying?	Yes	No
26.	Do you have trouble concentrating?	Yes	No
27.	Do you enjoy getting up in the morning?	Yes	No
28.	Do you prefer to avoid social gatherings?	Yes	No
29.	Is it easy for you to make decisions?	Yes	No
30.	Is your mind as clear as it used to be?	Yes	No

Figure 33-2. The Geriatric Depression Scale (GDS) (see text for explanation). From Yesavage, J. A., Brink, T. L., Rose, T. L., Lum, O., Huang, V., Adey, M., and Leirer, V. O. (1983). Development and validation of a geriatric depression screening scale: A preliminary report. *Journal of Psychiatric Research, 17,* 37–49. Reprinted with permission from the publisher.

The management of postural hypotension can be as simple as (1) attempting to regulate the antihypertensive medications and/or diuretic medications to obtain a minimum effective dosage where the patient is asymptomatic, (2) encouraging patients to consume fluids steadily throughout the day, or (3) teaching patients to stand a few seconds prior to ambulation. The effects of postural hypotension can be exaggerated following meals. The processes associated with the digestion of food require an increased demand for blood. Accordingly, elderly people who sit to eat and then stand to ambulate upon completion of a meal may experience what has been called postprandial, postural hypotension (Maurer, 2001). Interestingly, it has been reported that the effects of postprandial hypotension can be offset if caffeine is consumed before or during the meal (Ahmad & Watson, 1990; Maurer, 2001).

Assessment of Postural Hypotension

Evidence of postural hypotension is tested by having the patient lie supine for a minimum of 5 min. For our purposes, an assessment of postural hypotension is made following the ENG/VNG examination. That examination requires the patient to lie supine for 30 to 45 min. Baseline blood pressure and pulse rate measures are taken. The patient is then asked to stand abruptly (Video 33–2) and blood pressure and pulse measures are repeated. Blood pressure and pulse measures are then repeated over a period of 5 min. Postural hypotension is defined operationally as a drop in systolic blood pressure of ≥20 mm Hg, or, to <90 mm Hg on standing. If there is a reduction in the systolic pressure, pulse rate should increase if autoregulatory systems are intact.

Risk Factor: Impaired Somatosenses (i.e., Proprioception and Vibration Senses)

Proprioception and vibratory senses are two of the somatosenses (e.g., pain, pressure, temperature, touch, vibration, and position sense). People use the proprioceptive information that arrives from muscle spindles and joints in the ankles, knees, and hips and pressure sensors in the feet to tell them about their rate and direction of movement. It is accepted that the somatosenses, and especially vibration and proprioceptive senses, are most important for mainte-

nance of standing balance. It is also well accepted that these somatosenses augment visual and vestibular system information that is processed on a moment-to-moment basis by the brain during ambulation. In this regard, Krittinsdottir, Fransson, and Magnusson (2001) reported their findings from 10 normal adults (mean age 37.5 years) and 40 elderly subjects (mean age 74.6 years) with varying degrees of vibratory sense loss in the lower extremities. The results of their study showed that postural control of elderly patients with intact vibration sense was similar to that of younger adult subjects. The magnitude of postural sway was correlated with the magnitude of impairment of the vibratory sense. Interestingly, allowing subjects with impaired vibration sensation access to vision did not reduce their sway to that of their elderly peers with intact somatosenses. These findings suggest that when the lower extremity somatosenses are impaired, the less efficient sense of vision is not an effective substitute.

Proprioception represents a person's position sense and can be assessed grossly by asking a supine patient to close his or her eyes and report what direction the examiner is moving the big toe (e.g., up, down, left, right). Using tibial nerve somatosensory evoked potentials as the gold standard, we have found this to be an insensitive test for the intactness of the peripheral sensory nerves and central somesthetic pathway. A more quantitative but complicated method of assessing the functional integrity of the proprioceptive pathway is through the use of somatosensory-evoked potentials (SEPs). SEPs represent electrical events emanating from peripheral nerve, spinal cord, brainstem, and cortex that occur following the electrical depolarization of a peripheral nerve in either the upper or lower extremity. In the ROF assessment the posterior tibial nerve posterior to the medial malleolus (i.e., ankle bone) is electrically stimulated and evoked potentials are recorded. The latencies of the evoked potential components provide information about the functional integrity of the peripheral nerve, dorsal column pathways, and brain pathways that mediate (primarily) proprioception.

Tibial Nerve Somatosensory Evoked Potentials (SEPs)

Surface electrodes are placed at the popliteal fossas bilaterally and on the scalp at Cz' (2-cm posterior to true Cz), C3', C4' (2-cm posterior to C3 and C4, respectively), and at Fpz, using conventional, clean, surface electrode preparation techniques. Brief electrical pulses (0.1 ms) are delivered superficially to the tibial nerve posterior to the medial malleolus at a stimulus intensity capable of generating an antidromic response (i.e., a toe twitch) and at a rate of 4.6/s. A signal averaging computer is used to resolve both peripherally (i.e., recorded from the popliteal fossa), and cortically generated (i.e., recorded from two pairs of electrodes placed at Cz and Fpz, and C3' and C4') somatosensory-evoked responses. The distance from the stimulating location to the popliteal fossa is measured in millimeters and the latency of this peripherally generated action potential is then divided into the distance between stimulating and recording sites. The resulting value is an estimate of posterior tibial nerve conduction velocity (i.e., specified in meters/second). Furthermore, a side-to-side comparison of the absolute peak latencies of the cortically generated P40 potential is made. Finally, absolute P40 latency values are evaluated against height-corrected nomograms (Chiappa, 1990). The taller the patient, the longer is the normal latency of the P40 potential.

Measurement of Vibratory Thresholds

Our experience with SEPs was such that invariably when tibial nerve SEPs were absent, so was the perception of a 250-Hz vibratory source applied to the lower extremity. Accordingly, since 2003 we have assessed vibration thresholds using an audiometric bone vibrator held in place at the great toe, medial malleolus, and tuberosity of the tibia (i.e., bony prominence just caudal to the knee cap (Figure 33–3).

These thresholds are compared to those obtained from the thumb, wrist, and ulna (i.e., elbow) (Figure 33–4). In neurologically intact young subjects, there is clear perception of vibration at the lower extremity sites (not just touch) at levels below 40 to 45 dBHL. Perception in the upper extremities occurs in the range of 25 dB HL. Our procedure is to increase stimulus intensity from subthreshold and increase the stimulus intensity until the patient reports perception of the vibration. Thresholds are measured three times at each location. Since we implemented these procedures we have become aware of reports describing methods similar to

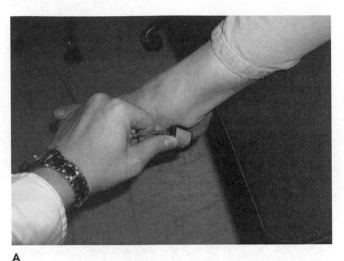

A

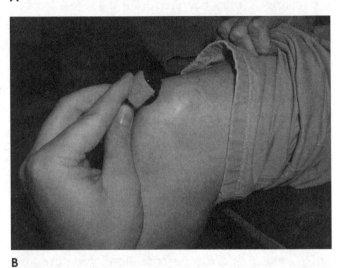

B

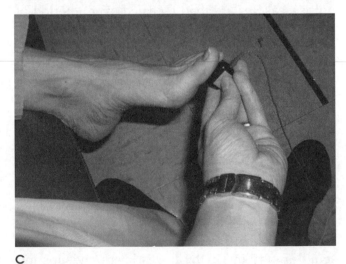

C

Figure 33–3. Locations for placement of bone oscillator for assessment of vibration thresholds in the lower extremities: Bone oscillator placed at the medial malleolus (**A**), tuberosity of the tibia (**B**), great toe (**C**).

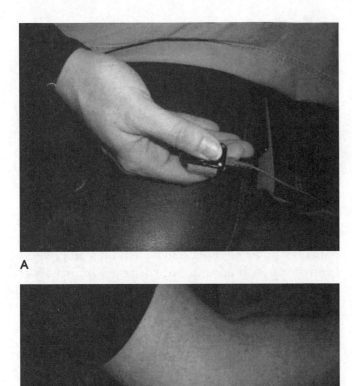

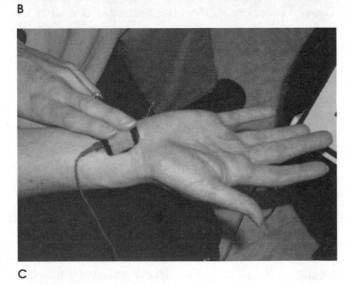

Figure 33-4. Locations for placement of bone oscillator for assessment of vibration thresholds in the upper extremities. Bone oscillator placed at the thumb (**A**), ulna (elbow) (**B**), wrist (**C**).

ours (Bergin, Bronstein, Murray, Sancovic, & Zeppenfeld, 1995; Bronstein, 1996, 2003). These investigators compared the results of vibration threshold measurement conducted with a neuroasthesiometer (i.e., a calibrated vibration meter) and an audiometric bone vibrator generating a 250-Hz stimulus. The investigators found agreement between the two techniques. Additionally, the authors reported thresholds of vibration using the audiometric bone vibrator occurred at or about 35 dB HL for their normal controls and for their patients occurred at about 55 dB HL. The poorer vibration thresholds correlated with increased body sway whether the patient was standing on a fixed surface with eyes open or closed (e.g., Romberg) or whether standing on foam with eyes open or closed. The investigators reported that vibration thresholds increased with age and showed a closer correlation with functional state (i.e., postural stability in everyday life) than electroneurodiagnostic tests (e.g., EMG).

Risk Factor: Impaired Postural Stability

Impaired postural stability and postural control are known risk factors for falling. Slow standing from sitting in a chair and disturbed gait and incomplete step continuity are all associated with a 1.4- to 1.9-fold increased ROF (Davis, Ross, Nevitt, & Wasnich, 1999; Koski et al., 1996). Impairments that have an effect on postural control and gait such as hemiparesis and paraplegia are associated with a 2.6- to 3.0-fold greater risk of fall (Poor et al., 1995). Patients with diseases such as Parkinson's disease have a reported eightfold increased ROF (Northridge, Nevitt, & Kelsey, 1996).

Activity-based testing may be useful at predicting falls, and static and dynamic posturography may be most useful (Topper, Maki, & Holliday, 1993). Maki, Holliday, and Topper (1994) performed computerized posturographic studies of patients and then followed the patients prospectively for a 1-year period. The authors demonstrated that spontaneous lateral sway was among the best predictors of a future fall. For any fall that is not directly related to an endogenous event (e.g., transient ischemic attack), there is usually a perturbation of the support surface (the ground) and a failure of the postural control system to respond appropriately to the challenge (Maki et al., 1994). Computerized dynamic posturography (CDP—Equitest Neuro-Com, Clackamas, OR) has provided us with the technology to analyze, in detail, and in a controlled, safe environment, the response of patients to a postural challenge. Despite what would seem to be high face validity for conducting computerized dynamic posturography for all patients who are perceived to be at risk for falls, Baloh, Spain, Socotch, Jacobson, and Bell (1995) and Baloh, Jacobson, Enrietto, Corona, and Honrubia (1998) have argued that posturography fails to provide sufficient detail to contribute useful information pertinent to prevention of future falls in the elderly. The investigators have been evaluating over time 100 elderly patients (i.e., >75 years of age) who have reported dizziness or disequilibrium and 100 age-matched controls without these complaints. The authors found that, as others had reported, postural sway was greater in older subjects and those reporting disequilibrium. Neither sway velocity nor sway amplitude was a good indicator of those who reported falls either in the year before, or after, testing. Also, the posturography data did not correlate with frequency of falls and did not provide data about the cause of the falls that would have been useful for intervention. In fact, some of the most severe falls were reported by control subjects who fell probably because they were more active than the patients and more likely to take chances. Despite these controversies, CDP has the ability to (1) document postural instability, (2) serve as a cross-check for patients with vestibular impairments on quantitative vestibular testing, (3) provide supportive evidence for patients with vestibular system disease affecting the otolith system, and (4) present evidence of impaired compensation of the vestibulospinal reflex following unilateral peripheral vestibular system impairment.

Computerized Dynamic Posturography (CDP)

Computerized dynamic posturography (CDP) is described in detail in Chapters 17, 18, and 19. CDP at its most basic consists of a battery of two subtests known as the sensory organization test (SOT) and the motor control test (MCT). The SOT is most useful in the ROF assessment. The patient is prepared for testing by being placed in a parachute harness that is suspended loosely from a frame. This harness is designed to prevent the patient from injuring himself or herself should the patient fall during testing. The patient is placed on a platform constructed with load sensors beneath. The information from the load sensors makes it possible to record over time changes in the patient's center of mass. The patient is confronted with a series of six conditions where vestibular, visual, and proprioceptive inputs are either present and undistorted, absent, or present but distorted. The patient must remain as stable as possible for 1 min for each condition. The product of this subtest is an age-adjusted profile that suggests that patients are, or are not, able to remain stable when confronted with accurate or distorted information from vestibular, visual, and proprioceptive senses.

For the MCT the patient is placed on the same force platform. This time, the platform either translates unpredictably in the anterior-posterior direction, or in the posterior-anterior direction. The Equitest program is capable of calculating the latency from onset of the translation to the beginning of the postural correction for the destabilization and what type of strategy the patient is using to restabilize (i.e., are patients adjusting to the destabilization by adjusting their posture at the ankle or hip).

Timed "Up and Go" Test (TUGT)

Though there are many other more detailed devices that have been developed to assess functional balance (e.g., Berg, Wood-Dauphinee, Williams, & Maki, 1992; Tinetti, 1986), the Timed "Up and Go" test (TUGT) has been recommended by both the American Geriatric Society (AGS) and the British Geriatric Society (BGS) as a simple method for the identification of older patients at risk for falling (Kenny, Rubenstein, Martin, & Tinetti, 2001).

The TUGT (Podsiadlo & Richardson, 1991) is a timed version of the "Get-up and Go" test (Mathias, Nayak, & Issacs, 1986). This simple assessment consists of determining the time required for a patient to rise to standing from an armchair, walk 3 m, turn, walk back to the chair, and sit (Video 33–3). Patients are instructed that, "on the word 'go' they are to get up and walk at a comfortable pace to a line on the floor 3 meters away, turn, return to the chair, and sit down again. The patient walks through the test once before being timed in order to be familiar with the test." Although deceptively simple, the TUGT is designed to assess the patient's ability to lift himself or herself out of a chair (i.e., relying on both quadriceps and hamstring muscles), walk a short distance, turn without falling, return to the chair, and sit. These actions are basic to many activities of daily living (e.g., transferring). Several upper limits of normal have been recommended for this assessment. For example, Shumway-Cook, Brauer, and Woollacott (2000) reported that they were able to achieve sensitivity and specificity of 87% using a 13.5-s upper limit of normal. Dite and Temple (2002) reported that a cutoff value of 13 s produced a sensitivity of 89% and specificity of 93%. Rose, Jones, and Lucchese (2002) reported 71% sensitivity and 86% specificity using a 10-s upper limit. Whitney, Lord, and Close (2005) reported that patients requiring longer than 13.5 s to complete the TUGT were 3.7 times more likely to have reported a fall in the previous 6 months, and those with scores greater than 11.1 s were five times more likely to have reported a fall in the past 6 months. Whitney, Marchetti, Schade, and Wrisley (2004) reported 81% sensitivity and 39% specificity using a 15-s upper limit. In light of these findings, and in the current iteration of the falls assessment clinic, a 13.5-s upper limit has been adopted.

Risk Factor: Impaired Vestibular System Function

The reported increased ROF associated with patients who report vertigo has ranged from 1.09-fold (Liu et al., 1995) to 6.0-fold (Poor et al., 1995). It has been estimated in retrospective investigations that the percent of total falls associated with vertigo ranges from 7% to 19% (Downton & Andrews, 1989; Rubenstein et al., 1988). Herdman, Blatt, Schubert, and Tusa (2000) examined the fall frequency of patients with unilateral and bilateral vestibular deficits. They compared the numbers of falls observed to that of community-dwelling adults. The investigators observed that the incidence of falls for patients with unilateral deficits was not significantly different from that of community-dwelling adults. However, for patients with bilateral vestibular deficits, the frequency of falling was significantly greater

than that observed for patients with unilateral deficits. Because age often is associated with incremental loss of peripheral vestibular system sensitivity, the assessment of vestibular system function is an important component of the ROF test battery. It is noteworthy that quantitative vestibular testing is missing from low-tech ROF test batteries (Lord et al., 2001) largely because of the increased cost associated with quantitative testing and the erroneous assumption that patients often become ill during testing.

Dizziness Handicap Inventory (DHI)

The Dizziness Handicap Inventory (DHI) (Jacobson & Newman, 1990) is a 25-item standardized assessment scale of self-perceived impact of dizziness and unsteadiness on a patient's quality of life (see Chapter 8). The DHI consists of 25 questions that are designed to assess the impact that dizziness and unsteadiness have on the patient's ability to carry out everyday activities and their psychosocial function. The patient responds to each item by answering either "yes," "no," or "sometimes." A "yes" is scored 4 points, a "sometimes" response is scored as 2 points, and a "no" response is scored as zero points. A total score of zero points indicates minimal impact of dizziness/unsteadiness on well-being. A score of 100 points indicates a maximum self-report dizziness disability/handicap. Jacobson and McCaslin (2005, unpublished observations) have calculated interquartile ranges from a set of more than 300 patients with different types of vestibular system impairments and from this analysis have created grades of dizziness disability/handicap as presented in Table 33–2.

Table 33–2. Interquartile Ranges That Define Levels of Dizziness Disability/Handicap as Calculated From the Dizziness Handicap Inventory (DHI)

Total DHI Score	Interpretation
0–14 points	No self-report dizziness disability handicap
16–26 points	Mild disability/handicap
28–44 points	Moderate disability/handicap
≥46 points	Severe disability/handicap

Video/Electronystagmography—ENG

The ENG has become the "gold-standard" assessment of the integrity of semicircular canal function. The ENG consists of a set of subtests that evaluate ocular motor subsystem integrity (e.g., saccadic, smooth pursuit, optokinetic subsystems), search for evidence of positional or positioning-induced vertigo, and evaluate the symmetry of function of the left and right lateral semicircular canals. The product of this examination may be evidence of ocular motor system impairment, the presence of positional nystagmus (e.g., benign paroxysmal positioning vertigo), and evidence of unilateral or bilateral end organ damage (i.e., unilateral or bilateral loss of semicircular canal function). Loss of peripheral vestibular function either unilaterally or bilaterally as indicated by the caloric test (see Chapters 12 and 13) in addition to other coexisting impairments may place an elderly patient at greater risk of falling than elderly people with intact peripheral vestibular system function.

Rotary Chair Testing

Rotational testing is performed using electro- or video-nystagmographic recording techniques (see Chapters 14 and 15). Instead of a caloric stimulus the patient is oscillated at calibrated frequencies, velocities, and accelerations, in a chair, in darkness. The product of this examination is an input/output function showing performance characteristics of the horizontal (or "yaw") vestibulocular reflex (i.e., compensatory eye movement phase, gain, and symmetry following left versus right oscillations) at input frequencies exceeding two orders of magnitude of that assessed with caloric testing on ENG. This makes it possible to predict better how a patient will perform under physiological conditions (i.e., ambulating) if all other supporting systems are intact (i.e., visual and proprioceptive systems).

Risk Factor: Impaired Vision

Visual functions that change in the elderly person include visual acuity, darkness adaptation, contrast sensitivity, and smooth pursuit function. Ophthalmic diseases of the elderly population that result

in visual impairments include cataracts, glaucoma, and macular degeneration. The specific impairments caused by these diseases include cloudy vision, impaired peripheral vision, and impaired central vision. Impaired visual function could make it difficult for patients to identify edges (e.g., edges of stairs or changes in surface of a sidewalk) that may result in trips or falls. In this regard, Poor et al. (1995) has reported that patients with severe visual impairments are, on average, 5.5-fold at increased risk for falling than are patients who have normal vision. Koski et al. (1996) reported that patients with poor distance visual acuity (e.g., patients who are nearsighted) have a 1.4-fold increased ROF than do patients with normal distance vision.

Accordingly, it is important to determine whether visual function is normal. Brandt, Paulus, and Straube (1985) have reported that visual acuity poorer than 20/50 can result in measurable decrements in postural control. Finally, Anand, Buckley, Scally, and Elliott (2003) have evaluated the extent that refractive error (i.e., refractive blur induced by magnifying lenses) and refractive error combined with reduced proprioceptive and vestibular information result in postural instability. Subjects were 15 elderly individuals (mean age 71 years). Both anterior-posterior and medial-lateral sway were quantified during six conditions of increasing difficulty. The six conditions consisted of varying combinations of standing still on the platform with eyes open and standing either on the platform or on a foam block placed on the platform, and either standing quietly or holding a tray containing cups, and either conducting or not conducting a mental task. Also, the subject's head was either oriented straight ahead or was inclined upward by 45 degrees. In all conditions where vision was permitted subjects were asked to view a target. The subject's vision was degraded over a range of 0 to 8 diopters (i.e., 0 diopters would represent the subject's undegraded vision). Not surprisingly, the authors reported that postural instability was poorest when vestibular and proprioceptive senses were distorted. Additionally, an increase in the blurring of vision caused increased postural instability. Performing a mental task also increased postural instability. The authors suggested that these findings supported the contention that instability in the elderly is multifactorial in origin. That is, postural instability resulting from impairments in senses we use for orientation increases as the number of distorted senses increase. Furthermore, the authors suggested that correcting visual impairments in the elderly (i.e., refractive error) would represent a simple means of decreasing falls risk.

Visual Acuity

A conventional Snellen chart is used to test visual acuity. The chart is placed at a distance of 20 feet from the patient. The patient is tested separately under monocular and binocular, and in uncorrected (i.e., to estimate acuity when corrective lenses are not being worn) and best-corrected conditions. Visual impairments may disrupt contrast perception (i.e., the ability of a patient to appreciate junctions of light and dark) and make it difficult or impossible for patients to appreciate where edges begin when walking downstairs. For many, impaired vision represents a correctable sensory impairment that may contribute to improved postural stability.

Corneoretinal Potential

The corneoretinal potential (CRP) is a bioelectrical signal that is measured during electroculography (EOG) and electronystagmography (ENG). When electrode wires are placed at the outer canthus of the left and right eyes (i.e., for bitemporal horizontal eye recordings), and/or above and below an eye (i.e., for vertical eye movement recordings), the electrical potential that is measured is the CRP. The origin of the CRP is metabolic activity in the retina and primarily in the retinal pigment epithelium. The potential difference between the cornea and the retina occurs as a function of the tight connections between pigment epithelial cells (Carl, 1997).

When measured at the cornea, the strength of this potential is approximately 1 mV (Carl, 1997), and the magnitude of this potential decreases by the inverse square as distance is doubled from the source of the potential. Contemporary, computerized ENG systems (such as the ICS MASTR system) use automated eye movement calibration routines to ensure that 1 degree of eye deviation results in the equivalent of a 1-mm pen deflection. These automated calibration routines result in a gain value that can be used to determine the number of microvolts of CRP associated with 1 degree of eye deviation. It was our empirical observation (Jacobson & McCaslin, 2004) that occasionally patients were evaluated who demonstrated very "noisy" calibration traces. When the calibration values were obtained it was clear that the "noisiness" occurred as a result of the recording system increasing its gain to a maximum to compensate for a very small CRP. The resulting traces represented the eye movement superimposed on the noise floor of the recording system. Accordingly, it is not surprising that we have observed a high correspondence between the magnitude of the CRP and the presence of retinal impairment. Table 33–3 shows our gender-specific lower limits for the CRP.

SUMMARY OF DATA OBTAINED FROM COHORT OF 180 CONSECUTIVE PATIENTS

Over a 7-year period, we compiled data from 180 patients who were evaluated at both Henry Ford Hospital and Vanderbilt University Medical Center. The data are summarized herein and in a publication (Jacobson, McCaslin, Grantham, & Piker, 2008). What follows is a summary of findings we have observed in the falls assessment clinic.

Table 33–3. Gender-Specific Percentile Values for the Corneo-Retinal Potential (CRP)

Gender	1st	5th	10th	15th	20th	50th	80th	85th	90th	95th	99th
Male	7.1	8.2	9.2	9.5	10.4	13.8	17.3	19.1	19.9	21.8	25.8
Female	9.0	10.8	11.4	13.0	13.2	17.2	21.7	22.2	24.5	27.3	28.2

Note. These data were generated from the "review calibration" routine from the ICS MASTR electro/video-nystagmography system. The units of measure of microvolts was CRP correspond to a 1-degree eye deviation. The measurements were made in a dark-adapted condition. Data adopted from Jacobson and McCaslin (2004).

Thus far we have observed two distinct patterns of referral to this clinic. There is a subgroup of patients who are referred because they have fallen and there is a desire on the part of the referring physician to know why the patient has fallen. A second group of patients have reported that they are concerned they will fall in the future, or they have had close calls in the recent past, or their physicians are concerned, for various reasons, that the patient will fall in the future.

The mean age of this cohort was 76 years (*SD* = 11 years) with a range of 40 to 93 years. It is noteworthy that the mean age of our dizzy clinic patients is 57 years, a full 20 years younger. There were 122 women (68%) in this sample; 61% of the patients in this sample had a previous history of falls either occurring inside or outside the home. This means that 39% of the sample had no previous history of falls but were considered by their referral sources to either be at risk, or were worried themselves about falling. The majority of our referrals were from otolaryngologists in our medical center and in the community. The rest of the patients were referred by a combination of primary care physicians and neurologists both within and outside our medical center.

A summary of the data derived from the directed case history is presented in Figure 33–5. From the case history it was discovered that 41% of patients complained of disequilibrium, 21% were insulin-dependent diabetics, 29% were hypertensive, 17% had histories of cerebrovascular accidents (CVA), 17% had osteoporosis, 29% had heart disease, and 41% had osteoarthritis. The fact that these percentages total over 100% implies that it was not uncommon for patients to have multiple conditions revealed in the case history.

In this regard, the risk of falls assessment showed that most patients demonstrated multiple falls risk factors (Figure 33–6). In fact, only 2% had a single risk factor, 10% had two risk factors, 8% had three risk factors, 33% had four risk factors, 18% had five risk factors, 18% had six risk factors, and 11% had seven risk factors. The fact that 80% of our sample had four or more risk factors attests to the contention that falls are complicated events often occurring as a function of the interaction of multiple causes.

The group mean value obtained on the MMSE was 27 points (range: 13 to 30 points). In fact, abnormal performance (i.e., <23 points) was observed only for 11% of the cohort. This was somewhat surprising to us given that this was a predominately elderly sample. However, the cohort consisted of independent, community-dwelling elderly and this implies that the health of our cohort was generally good.

The group mean score on the geriatric depression scale was 10 points (range: 0 to 24 points). Abnormal performance was observed for 37% of the sample. Although finding evidence of clinical depression in slightly less than one out of every four patients seems high, this is approximately proportional to that observed in groups of elderly seeking medical care (e.g., 22%, McCrea, Arnold, Marchevsky, & Kaufman, 1994; 22%, Cankurtaran et al., 2005; 42%, Yohannes, Baldwin, & Connolly, 2000; 39%, Ellis, Robinson, & Crawford, 2006).

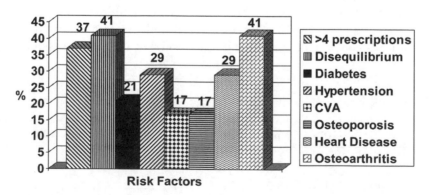

Figure 33–5. Percent of total patients (*ordinate*) demonstrating disorders and diseases (*abscissa*) derived from the structured case history.

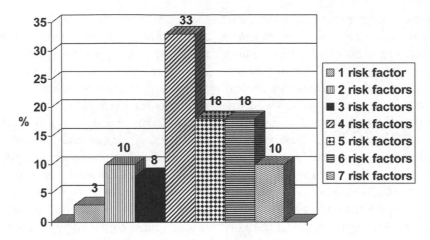

Figure 33-6. Percent of total patients (*ordinate*) demonstrating abnormal performance on each of the components of the multidimensional falls risk assessment.

Orthostatic hypotension (OH) was observed in 24% of the sample. Again, the observation of OH in roughly one out of four patients seems high; however, this is in proportion to that observed in community-dwelling elderly (e.g., 4% to 33%; Applegate et al., 1991; Atkins, Hanusa, Sefcik, & Kapoor, 1991; Caird, Andrews, & Kennedy, 1973; Mader, 1989). This may be one of the most "fixable" of the risks for falling as postural hypotension in many instances occurs as a direct effect of antihypertensive medications. Often, changes in dosage, or patient counseling (i.e., advising patients not to rise from lying down or sitting and immediately begin ambulating, or advising patients to drink caffeine during meals where postprandial postural hypotension is suspect) are sufficient to decrease or eliminate this risk factor.

The group mean for the Timed Up and Go test was 14.25 s (range: 6 to 50 s). Abnormal performance was observed for 50% of our sample.

Best corrected, binocular visual acuity was better than 20/50 in 73% of the sample, poorer than 20/50 in 20% of the sample, and poorer than 20/100 in 7% of the sample. The sources of the visual impairments ranged from cataracts, to glaucoma, to diabetic retinopathies. As reported previously (Brandt et al., 1985), postural stability begins to become affected when visual acuity becomes poorer than 20/50. This is a significant finding as poor visual acuity reduces a patient's ability to perceive contrast (i.e., edges) such as changes in light and shadow when walking

down stairs and may contribute to falls. Also, refractive errors represent another correctable risk factor.

On average, lower extremity simple reaction time was 342 ms (SD: 147 ms, range: 191 to 1435 ms). From the data set developed by Lord et al. (2001), this represents "fair" average reaction time for the cohort.

The most surprising findings were obtained from the results of vestibular function studies and assessments of somesthetic system function. The mean DHI total score was 44 points (SD: 22 points, range: 0 to 98 points) representing moderate to severe self-report dizziness handicap. Of the sample 11% reported no dizziness disability/handicap, 12% reported mild handicap, 31% reported moderate handicap, and 46% reported severe disability handicap. On ENG testing, the mean group caloric asymmetry was 21% (*SD* = 24%) with a range of 0 to 100%. A clinically significant unilateral weakness was observed for 36% of the cohort. Rotary chair abnormalities were observed for 60% of the sample. When combined, abnormal vestibular system function was observed in 76% of the patients referred to our Risk of Falls Assessment Clinic. In this sample 27% demonstrated normal caloric and rotational test results (i.e. no quantitative evidence of peripheral or central vestibular system impairment) and 30% showed both abnormal caloric and abnormal rotational test results (i.e. many of these patients had unilateral, peripheral impairments that were in an uncompensated state). Thus, for only 57% of the group was there agreement for the findings of the two tests. Of the total, 30% of the patients demonstrated normal performance on caloric testing and abnormal performance on rotational testing. Many of these patients demonstrated evidence of central vestibular system impairments. Lastly, 13% of the sample showed unilaterally abnormal caloric test results and normal rotational testing. These patients had unilateral peripheral impairments in a compensated state. These data should be compared to those collected by Agrawal et al. (2009) who used a balancing test (i.e., standing on a firm surface eyes open, eyes closed and then the same protocol standing on moderate to thick foam with eyes open and then eyes closed) to make inferences about the status of the vestibular system (i.e., if the patient fell off of the foam it suggested the presence of a vestibular system impairment). None of the subjects in the Agrawal et al. (2009) had caloric testing, the gold standard test of peripheral vestibular system function. While we agreed with the percent of unsteady patients with vestibular system impairments (~75%), we disagreed with how that value was derived. For us, the ~75% represented the proportion of patients seen in a risk of falls clinic with vestibular system impairment identified with a caloric test and sinusoidal harmonic acceleration testing, For Agrawal et al. that number represented the proportion of individuals >80 years who could not balance themselves. As we know, balance requires the integration of information routed to the brain by the three interdependent senses (i.e., vision, proprioception, and vestibular senses) so it represents a broader concept than vestibular function. It is possible to have unsteady gait, normal vestibular function, and insensate lower extremities that can lead to unsteadiness when standing at rest with eyes open, or when standing at rest with eyes closed. The same investigators (Agrawal et al., 2010) have made similar comments about vestibular function in diabetic patients (i.e., a greater proportion of patients with "vestibular dysfunction" who have had diabetes for a longer period). Accordingly, we question the accuracy of the assertions about vestibular function the authors have made based on their use of a balancing test.

Initially we assessed somesthetic system function in the lower extremities using tibial nerve somatosensory-evoked potential test techniques. We found that fully 93% of the sample failed to generate tibial nerve SEPs. By far, the most common abnormality was the absence of an action potential recorded at the popliteal fossa. These findings supported the contention that more than 90% of elderly patients demonstrate impaired neural conduction in the lower extremities (i.e., they had evidence of a peripheral neuropathy). Moreover, the pattern of abnormality suggested a conduction impairment that affected at least the large diameter heavily myelinated peripheral nerve fibers that carry proprioceptive information up to the lumbar plexus. More recently, this conventional electrodiagnostic test has been replaced with a simpler and less noxious test of vibration threshold. We have found that when there is no perception of a 250-Hz vibratory stimulus presented to great toe or medial malleolus at 40 dBHL, these patients do not generate a tibial nerve SEP.

Of the total, 46 patients (25%) could not complete computerized dynamic posturography because they were too unsteady to test. Of those who could be tested, 22% demonstrated a normal result and 78% demonstrated an abnormal result. When those who were too unsteady to test are combined with those with abnormal posturographic examinations, fully 84% of the cohort demonstrated abnormal performance. Whereas only about 10% of the patients showed abnormal performance on Conditions 1 through 3 of the sensory organization test, 34% showed abnormal performance on Condition 4 (sway-referenced platform, eyes open), and 50% of the patients were unsteady on Conditions 5 and 6 (i.e., sway-referenced platform, eyes closed, and both sway-referenced surround and sway-referenced platform with eyes open, respectively). It is likely that the combination of impaired vestibular and proprioceptive senses and the inability for the slower visual sense to compensate for these impairments explain why these patients were unsteady on Conditions 4 through 6. The most commonly observed SOT "patterns" were the "vestibular" and the combination of "visual" and "vestibular" patterns (Figure 33–7). We interpret the "visual" pattern as suggesting that patients are "proprioceptive-deficient" and therefore "vision-dependent."

When we evaluated the data set, in total, to determine how often patients demonstrated multisensory modality impairments, we found a single sensory modality impairment in 13% of the sample.

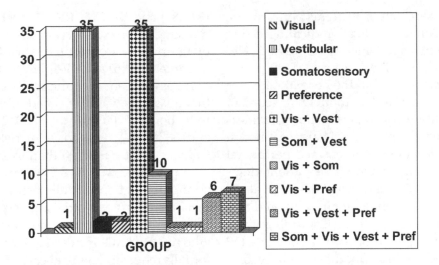

Figure 33–7. Summary of patterns of abnormality observed during sensory organization testing for the falls cohort.

Impairments of the visual and proprioceptive senses were observed 15% of the time. Abnormalities in visual and vestibular senses occurred in 3% of the sample. Abnormalities affecting proprioceptive and vestibular senses occurred 50% of the time (i.e., the most common observation). Finally, impairments affecting visual, proprioceptive, and vestibular senses occurred in 19% of the sample. It is significant that Drachman and Hart (1972) first coined the term "multisensory system impairment" to describe the common phenomenon of disequilibrium (not vertigo) that affects elderly patients. This occurs when impaired sensory information normally used by the brain for orientation is processed by an impaired central processor (the brain), which then generates an inappropriate output (if the input senses are impaired) to stabilize the head and body during movement. Tinetti et al. (2000) consider dizziness in the elderly to be a geriatric syndrome (i.e., its origin is multifactorial), much like delirium and falling.

We were surprised by the number of patients with unsuspected vestibular and somesthetic system impairments. It is known that of the somatosenses, impairments of proprioception and vibration are most predictive of those who fall (e.g., Bergin et al., 1995; Lord, Caplan, Colagiuri, & Ward, 1993; Lord, Clark, & Webster, 1994; Lord & Ward, 1991). In this regard, Richardson, Ching, and Hurvitz (1992), and Horak, Earhart, and Dietz (2001) have commented on the relationship between peripheral neuropathy,

loss of somesthesia, and postural instability and falls. In the absence of intact somesthetic information, the elderly have been shown to rely on the slower visual sense to remain upright (Pyyko, Jantti, & Aalto, 1990). Camicioli, Panzer, and Kaye (1997) reported their elderly were more unstable on Condition 4 of SOT where vision is nondistorted and somesthetic information is distorted. This is, in fact, what we observed.

CLINICAL VIGNETTE

The following clinical case report is characteristic of what might be observed in a falls risk assessment clinic.

The patient is an 84-year-old female who was seen for a ROF assessment. She demonstrates a history of six previous falls, one resulting in rib fractures. Two of the falls occurred in the bathtub. The patient's medical history is significant for osteoarthritis and osteoporosis.

The patient demonstrated uncorrected visual acuity of 20/15 for the right eye, and 20/20 for the left eye. She demonstrated 20/20 uncorrected binocular visual acuity. Postural hypotension was assessed, and she showed a lying down blood pressure of 150/70 and a standing blood pressure of 140/80 at 1 min and 5 min following standing. The patient demonstrated 7 out of 30 points performance on the Geriatric Depression Scale indicating it was unlikely the patient was clinically depressed. Her Mini-Mental State Examination was 30/30 points indicating performance within the normal range.

The patient generated a total DHI score of 56 points representing severe, self-report dizziness disability/handicap. Assessment of balance function revealed evidence of an uncompensated peripheral vestibular system impairment. The patient demonstrated a 35% left unilateral weakness on caloric testing, phase leads at multiple frequencies on rotary chair testing, and fell repeatedly on Conditions 5 and 6 of the Sensory Organization subtest of the CDP examination. Based on these findings, it was recommended to the referring physician that the patient be referred for vestibular rehabilitation in an attempt to improve central vestibular system compensation for this unilateral peripheral vestibular system deficit. If the neural circuitry is not intact enough to make it possible to improve compensation for this deficit, it was our recommendation that the patient be evaluated for an assistive device during ambulation and that she install grab bars in her shower as this is where two of her falls occurred.

INTERVENTION FOR FALLS RISK

There is no need to identify patients at risk for injurious falls if there is no means to intervene and mitigate the risk. There have been a few high quality investigations beginning with Tinetti et al. (1994). Studies that have considered risk reduction usually report their data in terms of risk ratios (e.g., RR = number of events occurring for the group of interest/number of events occurring for the control group * 1) where a RR of 1.0 means there is no difference in risk between the two groups (e.g., a treatment versus control group). A number less than 1.0 means the experimental group is showing a lower risk and number greater than 1.0 means the experimental group is demonstrating a greater risk than the control group. There have been a few very good systematic reviews of this area in recent years. Gillespie, Gillespie, Robertson, et al. (2001) and more recently, Gillespie et al. (2012) have examined interventions for reducing fall risk for community-dwelling elders. It probably was not surprising that exercise

(RR .85) and Tai Chi (RR .71) were both effective at reducing fall risk. Also effective was reassessment of the patient's current medications and dosages of same (RR .61) (Gillespie et al., 2012). Interestingly, assessment of home safety by an occupational therapist (OT) was associated with a significant risk reduction in 2000 but not in 2012 (RR in 2000 = .64 and .88 in 2012). Likewise, the risk reduction for Tai Chi was greater in 2000 than in 2012 (RR in 2000 = .51 and in 2012 was .71). The importance of exercise as an intervention for falls risk was supported by a meta-analysis (i.e., 17 trials, 4,305 participants) by El-Khoury, Cassou, Charles, and Dargent-Molina (2013) who reported rate ratios of .63 for injurious falls, .51 for falls requiring medical care, .57 for severe injurious falls, and .39 for falls resulting in fractures. That is, in general, exercise reduced by half the falls rate. Similarly, Chang, Morton, Rubenstein, et al. (2004) conducted a systematic review and meta-analysis that showed exercise alone had a significant effect on the risk of falling (RR = .86) although a multifactorial falls risk assessment and management (RR = .82) was most effective at reducing the risk of falling. Despite this evidence, the results of the meta-analysis conducted by Gates, Fisher, Cooke, et al. (2008) suggested that when multifactor falls risk testing is combined with targeted interventions, there is no significant reduction in falls and/or fall related injuries. These findings are similar (i.e., nonsignificant reduction in falls for those who underwent a multifactorial assessment with targeted interventions) to those reported by Healthy Quality Ontario (2008), although there are others who disagree (e.g., Fields, 2008) calling into question the heterogeneity of the studies included in the meta-analysis. Part of the problem may be the poor adherence to recommendations which, after a year, has been estimated to be up to half of community-dwelling elders and as many as a third of those in nursing care facilities (Nyman & Victor, 2011, 2012).

SUMMARY

Unintentional injury, which almost always results from a fall, ranks as the sixth leading cause of death in the elderly population. As patients who are "dizzy" are often referred to audiologists for vestibular assessments, we have a unique opportunity to communicate back to the referral source that the patient's disequilibrium may require a more in-depth and multifactorial assessment. In much the same way that we "identify" and then "intervene" for hearing impairments, audiologists have the opportunity to assume a leadership role in the iden-tification of unsteady elderly who are at greatest risk for falling and to suggest to referral sources other professionals who might intervene to reduce the risk and help independent elderly remain independent. There are two general approaches to the assessment and intervention for falls in elders: (1) the multifacto-rial assessment of patients for known risks and then referral to other medical specialties to address those impairments identified (e.g., cataracts, peripheral neuropathy) that may influence the risk of future injurious falls, and (2) enroll all elders who are capa-ble into exercise programs that may be general or targeted. In all cases, systematic review of the exis-tent literature has shown the effects to be a reduction in falls (e.g., Gillespie et al., 2009; El-Khoury et al., 2013; Health Quality Ontario, 2008; Michael et al., 2010,). The current chapter should serve as a guide for clinicians who are interested in developing a multifactorial falls risk assessment clinic.

 ## VIDEOS ASSOCIATED WITH THIS CHAPTER

Video 33–1. Testing simple reaction time.

Video 33–2. Assessment of postural hypertention.

Video 33–3. The Timed Up and Go Test.

REFERENCES

Agrawal, Carey, J. P., Santina, C. D., Schubert, M. C., & Minor, L. B. (2009). Disorders of balance and vestibular function in US adults. *Archives of Internal Medicine, 169,* 938–944.

Agrawal , Carey, J. P., Santina, C. D., Schubert, M. C., & Minor, L. B. (2010). Diabetes, vestibular dysfunction, and falls: Analyses from the National Health and Nutrition Examination Survew (2010). *Otology and Neu-rotology, 31,* 1445–1450.

Ahmad, R. A., & Watson, R. D. (1990). Treatment of pos-tural hypotension. A review. *Drugs, 3,* 74–85.

American Speech-Language-Hearing Association. (1992, March). Balance system assessment. *Asha, 34*(Suppl. 7), 9–12.

American Speech-Language-Hearing Association. (1999, March). Role of audiologists in vestibular and balance rehabilitation: Position statement, guidelines, and tech-nical report. *Asha, 41*(Suppl. 19), 13–22.

Anand, V., Buckley, J. G., Scally, A., & Elliott, D. B. (2003). Postural stability in the elderly during sensory pertur-bations and dual tasking: The influence of refractive blur. *Investigative Ophthalmology and Visual Science, 44,* 2885–2891.

Anthony, J. C., LeResche, L., Niaz, U., von Korff, M. R., & Folstein, M. F. (1982). Limits of the "Mini-Mental State" as a screening test for dementia and delirium among hospital patients. *Psychological Medicine, 12,* 397–408.

Applegate, W. B., Davis, B. R., Black, H. R., Smith, W. M., Miller, S. T., & Burlando, A. J. (1991). Prevalence of pos-tural hypotension at baseline in the Systolic Hyperten-sion in the Elderly Program (SHEP) Cohort. *Journal of the American Geriatric Society, 39,* 1057–1064.

Atkins, D., Hanusa, B., Sefcik, T., & Kapoor, W. (1991). Syncope and orthostatic hypotension. *American Journal of Medicine, 91,* 179–185.

Baloh, R. W., Jacobson, K. M., Enrietto, J. A., Corona, S., & Honrubia, V. (1998). Balance disorders in older persons: Quantification with posturography. *Otolarygology-Head and Neck Surgery, 119,* 89–92.

Baloh, R. W., Spain, S., Socotch, T. M., Jacobson, K. M., & Bell, T. (1995). Posturography and balance problems in older people. *Journal of the American Geriatric Society, 43,* 266–278.

Berg, K., Wood-Dauphinee, S., Williams, J. I., & Maki, B. (1992, July/August). Measuring balance in the elderly: Validation of an instrument. *Canadian Journal of Public Health* (Suppl. 2), S7–S11.

Bergin, P. S., Bronstein, A. M., Murray, N. M. F., Sancovic, S., & Zeppenfeld, K. (1995). Body sway and vibration perception thresholds in normal aging and in patients with polyneuropathy. *Journal of Neurology and Neurosur-gical Psychiatry, 58,* 335–340.

Brandt, T., Paulus, W., & Straube, A. (1985). Visual acu-ity, visual field and visual scene characteristics affect postural balance. In M. Igarashi & F. O. Black (Eds.), *Vestibular and visual control on posture and locomotor equi-librium* (p. 93). Basel, Switzerland: Karger.

Bronstein, A. M. (1996). "Audiometry of the ankles": A quick check on the single most important sensory input for balance control. *British Journal of Audiology, 30,* 63.

Bronstein, A. M. (2003). Posturography. In L. Luxon, J. M. Furman, A. Martini, & D. Stephens (Eds.), *Textbook of audiological medicine* (p. 753). London, UK: Martin Dunitz.

Caird, F. I., Andrews, G. R., & Kennedy, R. D. (1973). Effect of posture on blood pressure in the elderly. *British Heart Journal, 35,* 527–530.

Camicioli, R., Panzer, V. P., & Kaye, J. (1997). Balance in the healthy elderly: Posturography and clinical assessment. *Archives of Neurology, 54*(8), 976–981.

Cankurtaran, M., Halil, M., Yavuz, B. B., Dagli, N., Cankurtaran, E. S., & Ariogul, S. (2005). Depression and concomitant diseases in a Turkish geriatric outpatient setting. *Archives of Gerontology and Geriatrics, 40,* 307–315.

Carl, J. R. (1997). Practical anatomy and physiology of the ocular motor system. In G. P. Jacobson, C. W. Newman, & J. Kartush (Eds.), *Handbook of balance function testing* (pp. 53–68). San Diego, CA: Singular.

Chang, J. T., Morton, S. C., Rubenstein, L. Z., Mojica, W. A., Maglione, M., Suttorp, M. J., . . . Shekelle, P. G. (2004). Interventions for the prevention of falls in older adults: Systematic review and meta-analysis of randomised clinical trials. *British Medical Journal, 328*(7441), 680.

Chiappa, K. (1990). *Evoked potentials in clinical medicine.* New York, NY: Raven Press

Cumming, R. G. (1998). Epidemiology of medication-related falls and fractures in the elderly. *Drugs and Aging, 12,* 43–53.

Cummings, S. R., Nevitt, M. C., & Kidd, S. (1988). Forgetting falls: The limited accuracy of recall of falls in the elderly. *Journal of the American Geriatric Society, 36,* 613–616.

Davis, J. W., Ross, P. D., Nevitt, M. C., & Wasnich, R. D. (1999). Risk factors for falls and serious injuries among older Japanese women in Hawaii. *Japanese American Geriatric Society, 47,* 792–798.

Dite, W., & Temple, V. A. (2002). A clinical test of stepping and change of direction to identify multiple falling older adults. *Archives of Physical Medicine and Rehabilitation, 83,* 1566–1571.

Downton, J. H. (1993). *Falls in the elderly.* London, UK: Edward Arnold.

Downton, J. H., & Andrews, K. (1989). Prevalence, characteristics and factors associated with falls among the elderly living at home. *Aging, 3,* 219–228.

Drachman, D. A., & Hart, C. W. (1972). An approach to the dizzy patient. *Neurology, 22,* 323–334.

El-Khoury, F., Cassou, B., Charles, M. A., & Dargent-Molina, P. (2013). The effect of fall prevention exercise programmes on fall induced injuries in community dwelling older adults: Systematic review and meta-analysis of randomized controlled trials. *British Medical Journal, 347,* f6234. doi:10.1136/bmj.f6234

Ellis, G. P., Robinson, J. A., & Crawford, G. B. (2006). When symptoms of disease overlap with symptoms of depression. *Australian Family Physician, 35,* 647–649.

Fields, S.D. (2008). Commentary. *Evidence Based Medicine, 13,* 116.

Folstein, M., Anthony, J. C., Parhad, I., Duffy, B., & Gruenberg, E. M. (1985). The meaning of cognitive impairment in the elderly. *Journal of the American Geriatric Society, 33,* 228–235.

Folstein, M. F., Folstein, S. E., & McHugh, P. R. (1975). "Mini-Mental State": A practical method for grading the cognitive state of patients for the clinician. *Journal of Psychiatric Research, 12,* 189–198.

Gates, S. (2008). Review; lack of evidence that multifactorial risk assessment and targeted interventions prevent falls in elderly people. *Evidence Based Medicine, 13,* 116.

Gates, S., Fisher, J. D., Cooke, M. W., Carter, Y. H., & Lamb, S. E. (2008). Multifactorial assessment and targeted intervention for preventing falls and injuries among older people in community and emergency care settings: Systematic review and meta-analysis. *British Medical Journal, 336*(7636), 130–133.

Gillespie, L. D., Gillespie, W. J., Robertson, M. C., Lamb, S. E., Cumming, R. G., & Rowe, B. H. (2001). Interventions for preventing falls in the elderly. *Cochrane Database of Sytematic Review,* (3), CD000340.

Gillespie, L. D., Robertson, M. C., Gillespie, W. J., Lamb, S. E., Gates, S., Cumming, R. G., & Rowe, B. H. (2009). Interventions for preventing falls in older people living in the community. *Cochrane Database of Systematic Reviews, 15*(2), CD007146. doi:10.1002/14651858

Gillespie, L. D., Robertson, M. C., Gillespie, W. J., Sherrington, C., Gates, S., Clemson, L. M., & Lamb, S. E. (2012). Interventions for preventing falls in older people living in the community. *Cochrane Database of Systematic Reviews, 12;* 9: CD007146. Pub 3.

Grimley-Evans, J., Prudham, D., & Wandess, I. (1979). A prospective study of falls in an elderly population: I. Incidence and morbidity. *Age and Ageing, 6,* 201–210.

Hausdorff, J. M., Peng, C. K., Goldberger, A. L., & Stoll, A.L. (2004). Gait unsteadiness and fall risk in two affective disorders: A preliminary study. *BMC Psychiatry, 24,* 39.

Health Quality Ontario. (2008). Prevention of falls and fall-related injuries in community-dwelling seniors: An evidence-based analysis. *Ontario Health Technology Assessment Series, 8,* 1–78.

Herdman, S. J. (2000). *Vestibular rehabilitation* (2nd ed.). Philadelphia, PA: F. A. Davis.

Herdman, S. J., Blatt, P., Schubert, M. C., & Tusa, R. J. (2000). Falls in patients with vestibular deficits. *American Journal of Otology, 21,* 847–851.

Herings, R. M. C., Stricker, B. H. C, deBoer, A., Bakker, A., & Sturmans, F. (1995). Benzodiazepines and the risk of falling leading to femur fractures. *Archives of Internal Medicine, 155,* 1801–1807.

Horak, F. B., Earhart, G. M., & Dietz, V. (2001). Postural responses to combinations of head and body displacements: Vestibular-somatosensory interactions. *Experimental Brain Research, 141,* 410–414.

Horikawa, E., Matsui, T., Arai, H., Seki, T., Iswasaki, K., & Sasaki, H. (2005). Risk of falls in Alzheimer's disease: A prospective study. *Internal Medicine, 44,* 717–721.

Huppert, F. A., Cabelli, S. T., & Matthews, F. E. (2005). Brief cognitive assessment in a UK population sample—Distributional properties and the relationship between the MMSE and an extended mental state examination. *BMC Geriatrics, 5,* 7.

Jacobson, G. P., & McCaslin, D. L. (2004). The detection of retinal deficits through indirect measurement of the corneoretinal potential. *Journal of the American Academy of Audiology, 15,* 258–263.

Jacobson, G. P., McCaslin, D. L., Grantham, S. L., & Piker, E. G. (2008). Significant vestibular system impairment is common in a cohort of elderly patients referred for assessment of falls risk. *Journal of the American Academy of Audiology, 19,* 799–807.

Jacobson, G. P., & Newman, C. W. (1990). The development of the Dizziness Handicap Inventory. *Archives of Otolaryngology-Head and Neck Surgery, 116,* 424–427.

Kenny, R. A., Rubenstein, L. Z., Martin, F. R., & Tinetti, M.E. (2001). Guideline for the prevention of falls in older people. *Journal of the American Geriatric Society, 49,* 664–672.

Koenig, H. G., Meador, K. G., Cohen, H. J., & Blazer, D. G. (1988). Self-rated depression scales and screening for major depression in the older hospitalized patient with medical illness. *Journal of the American Geriatric Society, 36,* 699–706.

Koski, K., Luukinen, H., Laippala, P., & Kivela, S. -L. (1996). Physiological factors and medications as predictors of injurious falls by elderly people: A prospective population-based study. *Age and Ageing, 25,* 29–38.

Krittinsdottir, E. K., Fransson, P. -A., & Magnusson, M. (2001). Changes in postural control in health elderly subjects are related to vibration sensation, vision and vestibular asymmetry. *Acta Oto-Laryngologica, 121,* 700–706.

Liu, B. A., Topper, A. K., Reeves, R. A., Gryfe, C., & Maki, B. E. (1995). Falls among older people: Relationship to medication use and orthostatic hypotension. *Journal of the American Geriatric Society, 43,* 1141–1145.

Lord, S. R., Caplan, G. A., Colagiuri, R., & Ward, J. A. (1993). Sensori-motor function in older persons with diabetes. *Diabetic Medicine, 10,* 614–618.

Lord, S. R., Clark, R. D., & Webster, I. W. (1994). Age-associated difference in sensori-motor function and balance in community dwelling women. *Age and Ageing, 23,* 452–460.

Lord, S. R., Menz, H. B., & Tiedemann, A. (2003). A physiological profile approach to falls risk assessment and prevention. *Physical Therapy, 83,* 237–252.

Lord, S. R., Sherrington, C., & Menz, H. B. (2001). *Falls in older people* (pp. 200–201). Cambridge, UK: Cambridge University Press.

Lord, S. R., Sherrington, C., Menz, H. B., & Close, J. C. (2007). *Falls in older people: Risk factors and strategies for prevention.* New York, NY: Cambridge University Press.

Lord, S. R., & Ward, J. A. (1991). Postural stability and associated physiological factors in a population of aged persons. *Journal of Gerontology, 46,* M69–M76.

Luxon, L., Furman, J. M., Martini, A., & Stephens, D. (Eds.). (2003). *Textbook of audiological medicine* (p. 753). London, UK: Martin Dunitz.

Mader, S. L. (1989). Orthostatic hypotension. *Medical Clinics of North America, 73,* 1337–1349.

Maki, B. E., Holliday, P. J., & Topper, A. K. (1994). A prospective study of postural balance and risk of falling in an ambulatory and independent elderly population. *Journal of Gerontology, 49,* M72–M84.

Mathias, S., Nayak, U. S., & Isaacs, B. (1986). Balance in elderly patients: The "get-up and go" test. *Archives of Physical Medicine and Rehabilitation, 67,* 387–389.

Maurer, M. (2001). Hypotension (low blood pressure) in the elderly. *The Health Report.* Radio National. Broadcast, March 12, 2001. Retrieved from http://www.abc.net.au/rn/talks/8.30/helthrpt/stories/s259120.htm

McCrea, D., Arnold, E., Marchevsky, D., & Kaufman, B.M. (1994). The prevalence of depression in geriatric medical outpatients. *Age and Ageing, 23,* 465–467.

Michael, Y. L.,Whitlock, E. P., Lin, J. S.,. Fu, R., O'Connor, E. A., Gold, R., & US Preventive Services Task Force. (2010). Primary care-relevant interventions to prevent falling in older adults: A systematic evidence review for the U.S. Preventive Services Task Force. *Annals of Internal Medicine, 153,* 815–825.

Mondolo, F., Jahanshahi, M., Grana, A., Biasutti, E., Cacciatori, E., & Di Benedetto, P. (2006). The validity of the hospital anxiety and depression scale and the geriatric depression scale in Parkinson's disease. *Behavioral Neurology, 17,* 109–115.

Neutel, C. I., Hirdes, J. P., Maxwell, C. J., & Patten, S. B. (1996). New evidence on benzodiazepine use and falls: The time factor. *Age and Ageing, 25,* 273–278.

Northridge, M. E., Nevitt, M. C., & Kelsey, J. L. (1996). Non-syncopal falls in the elderly in relation to home environments. *Osteoporosis International, 6,* 249–255.

Nygaard, H. A. (1998). Falls and psychotropic drug consumption in long-term care residents: Is there an obvious association? *Gerontology, 44,* 46–50.

Nyman, S. R., & Victor, C. R. (2011). Older people's recruitment, sustained participation, and adherence to falls prevention, and adherence to falls prevention interventions in institutional settings: A supplement to the Cochrane systematic review. *Age and Aging, 40*, 430–436.

Nyman, S. R., & Victor, C. R. (2012). Older people's participation in and engagement with falls prevention interventions in community settings: An augment to the Cochrane Systematic Review. *Age and Aging, 41*, 16–23.

Pavol, M. J., Owings, T. M., Foley, K. T., & Grabiner, M. D. (1999). The sex and age of older adults influence the outcome of induced trips. *Journal of Gerontology, 54A*, M103–M108.

Podsiadlo, D., & Richardson, S. (1991). The timed "up and go": A test of basic functional mobility for frail elderly persons. *Journal of the American Geriatric Society, 39*, 142–148.

Poor, G., Atkinson, E. J., O'Fallon, W. M., & Melton, L. J. (1995). Predictors of hip fractures in elderly men. *Journal of Bone and Mineral Research, 10*, 1900–1907.

Purchase-Helzner, E. L., Cauley, J. A., Faulkner, K. A., Pratt, S., Zmuda, J. M., Talbott, E. O., . . . Newman, A. (2004). Hearing sensitivity and the risk of incident falls and fracture in older women: The study of osteoporotic fractures. *Annals of Epidemiology, 14*, 311–318.

Pyyko, I., Jantti, P., & Aalto, H. (1990). Postural control in elderly subjects. *Age and Ageing, 19*, 215–221.

Richardson, J., Ching, C., & Hurvitz, E. (1992). The relationship between electromyographically documented peripheral neuropathy and falls. *Journal of the American Geriatric Society, 40*, 1008–1012.

Rose, D. J., Jones, C. J., & Lucchese, N. (2002). Predicting the probability of falls in community-residing older adults using the 8-foot up-and-go: A new measure of functional mobility. *Journal of Physical Activity and Aging, 10*, 466–475.

Rubenstein, L. Z., Robbins, A. S., Schulman, B. L., Rosado, J., Osterweil, D., & Josephson, K. R. (1988). Falls and instability in the elderly. *Journal of the American Geriatric Society, 36*, 266–278.

Shumway-Cook, A., Brauer, S., & Woollacott, M. (2000). Predicting the probability of falls in community-dwelling older adults using the Timed Up and Go Test. *Physical Therapy, 80*, 896–903.

Thapa, P. B., & Wray, W. A. (1996). Gait disorders and falls in the elderly. In A. M. Bronstein, T. Brandt, & M. Woollacott (Eds.), *Clinical disorders of balance, posture and gait* (pp. 301–325). New York, NY: Oxford University Press.

Tibbits, G. M. (1996). Patients who fall: How to predict and prevent injuries. *Geriatrics, 51*, 24–28.

Tinetti, M. E. (1986). Performance-oriented assessment of mobility problems in elderly patients. *Journal of the American Geriatric Society, 34*, 119–126.

Tinetti, M. E., Baker, D. I., McAvay, G., Claus, E. B., Garrett, P., Gottschalk, M., . . . Horwitz, R. I. (1994). A multifactorial intervention to reduce the risk of falling among elderly people living in the community. *New England Journal of Medicine, 331*, 821–827.

Tinetti, M. E., Williams, C. S., & Gill, T. M. (2000). Dizziness among older adults: A possible geriatric syndrome. *Annals of Internal Medicine, 132*, 337–344.

Topper, A. K., Maki, B. E., & Holliday, P. J. (1993). Are activity-based assessments of balance and gait in the elderly predictive of risk of falling and/or type of fall? *Journal of the American Geriatric Society, 41*, 479–487.

van Dijk, P. T. M., Meulenberg, O. G. R. M., van de Sande, H. J., & Habbema, J. D. F. (1993). Falls in dementia patients. *Gerontologist, 33*, 200–204.

Watters, C. L., & Moran, W. P. (2006). Hip fractures— A joint effort. *Orthopedic Nursing, 25*, 157–165.

Whitney, J. C., Lord, S. R., & Close, J. C. T. (2005). Streamlining assessment and intervention in a falls clinic using the Timed Up and Go Test and Physiological Profile Assessments. *Age and Ageing, 34*, 567–571.

Whitney, S. L., Marchetti, G. F., Schade, A., & Wrisley, D. M. (2004). The sensitivity and specificity of the Timed "Up and Go" and the Dynamic Gait Index for self-reported falls in persons with vestibular disorders. *Journal of Vestibular Research, 14*, 397–409.

Wild, D., Nayak, U. S. L., & Isaacs, B. (1981). How dangerous are falls in old people at home? *British Medical Journal, 282*, 2132–2133.

Yesavage, J. A., Brink, T. L., Rose, T. L., Lum, O., Huang, V., Adey, M., & Leirer, V. O. (1983). Development and validation of a geriatric depression screening scale: A preliminary report. *Journal of Psychiatric Research, 17*, 37–49.

Yohannes, A. M., Baldwin, R. C., & Connolly, M. J. (2000). Depression and anxiety in elderly outpatients with chronic obstructive pulmonary disease: Prevalence, and validation of the BASDEC screening questionnaire. *International Journal of Geriatric Psychiatry, 15*, 1090–1096.

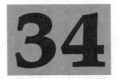

34

Within and Between Measure Relationships Between Balance Function Tests—Illustrative Cases

Gary P. Jacobson, Devin L. McCaslin, Sarah L. Grantham, and Neil T. Shepard

INTRODUCTION

During a balance function assessment a beginning clinician usually is hard pressed to do more than collect high-quality data using a standardized clinical protocol. At the end of an examination, clinicians are often confronted with a series of test results they must make fit into a coherent diagnostic picture. The end objective of training is the mastery of concepts and skills underlying balance function testing. This includes not only the ability to acquire high quality data but also the ability to interpret these data.

In balance function assessment it should be the clinician's end goal to be "one step ahead" during the assessment. Thus, for example, the clinician should be capable of formulating hypotheses of what the end result of quantitative testing will be based on the clinical case history (see Chapter 6) and informal assessment of the patient (i.e., "bedside tests"; see Chapter 7). Moreover, the hypothesis generating process should continue as each bit of new information is acquired through quantitative testing. Thus,

the patient who shows a right-beating head-shake nystagmus (i.e., resulting in a hypothesis of a left, peripheral vestibular system impairment) and a left-deviating Fukuda stepping test may be expected to demonstrate a left, unilateral weakness on caloric testing. This is, in fact, an example of how a master clinician processes information continuously so that a coherent report can be generated promptly at the end of testing. Additionally, the master clinician should be aware of how test results on one assessment, the VNG examination for example, predict the results of both rotational testing and computerized dynamic posturography. In that way the clinician is able to identify quickly disparate pieces of information and make a determination whether additional tests will add to the information needed for an individual patient. The identification of disparate data makes it possible to determine whether tests need to be repeated, or whether it is necessary to formulate new diagnostic hypotheses. For example, a patient who appears with a right-beating spontaneous nystagmus might be hypothesized to have a left-sided impairment. However, the finding of a 25% right unilateral weakness on caloric testing should cause the clinician to suspect that the spontaneous nystagmus is in fact recovery nystagmus. A left deviation on the Fukuda stepping test would help support the hypothesis. As a second example, take the patient with a classic vestibular crisis-style history, a positive head thrust to the right, spontaneous left-beating nystagmus throughout the VNG with a 45% right caloric, reduced vestibular response and normal ocular motor testing, and mild pattern of increased sway on condition 5 and 6 from sensory organization testing on posturography. The presentation to this point indicates an uncompensated right peripheral lesion; therefore, in this patient the use of rotational chair would not be indicated. Chair results would not add any new information to the patient's overall clinical picture. Whereas in this example the VNG results are not dramatic enough to fully predict rotational chair findings, the chair findings, normal or abnormal, will not provide any information about the patient's condition that is not already known.

In this chapter we provide the reader with data showing how the results of the foundation assessments of the balance function tests correlate with one another. That is, in the same way that a Type B tympanogram and absent stapedial reflexes on the probe side predict a conductive hearing loss, we see that a 100% unilateral caloric weakness predicts a phase lead and reduced VOR gain at 0.01 Hz. We then provide the reader with case study examples of how the results of one test, do, in fact, predict the results of another test.

CORRELATIONAL STUDY OF BALANCE FUNCTION TESTS

The authors of this chapter conducted a correlational examination of data derived from VNG, rotational, and computerized dynamic posturography (CDP) tests. The sample consisted of 147 patients (58 male) who were seen for balance function evaluations conducted at the Vanderbilt Bill Wilkerson Center, Balance Disorders Laboratory. The mean age of the subject sample was 62 years (SD = 17 yrs) with an age range from 21 to 96 years.

All of the patients completed the Dizziness Handicap Inventory (DHI; Jacobson & Newman, 1990). Most of the patients received either VNG or ENG examinations and rotational tests. The conventional ENG or videonystagmography (VNG) examination consisted of the following subtests: (1) saccade system testing, (2) horizontal and vertical gaze-evoked nystagmus, (3) optokinetic nystagmus, (4) pursuit system testing, (5) spontaneous nystagmus testing, (6) positioning testing (Dix-Hallpike maneuver) inclusive to all subjects without pathology involving the cervical vertebrae, (7) position testing for the detection of "position-induced" nystagmus in the supine, right and left lateral, and/or the head-hanging positions, (8) alternate binaural bithermal caloric testing, in accordance with the Fitzgerald and Hallpike (1942) procedure (N = 133) as described by Barber and Stockwell (1980) or if indicated monothermal warm caloric testing (N = 14) as described by Jacobson and Means (1985) and Jacobson et al. (1995).

Computerized rotational testing was conducted using either bitemporal ENG or VNG recording techniques. Patients were oscillated at the frequencies of 0.01 Hz, 0.02 Hz, 0.04 Hz, 0.08 Hz, 0.16 Hz, and/or 0.32 Hz (maximum velocity, 50 deg/sec; maximum acceleration, 3 deg/sec, 6 deg/sec, 13 deg/sec, 26 deg/sec, 50 deg/sec, 101 deg/sec for frequencies 0.01 Hz, 0.02 Hz, 0.04 Hz, 0.08 Hz, 0.16 Hz, and 0.32 Hz, respectively). Phase, gain, and asymmetry values of the vestibulo-ocular reflex (VOR) were quantified.

A smaller sample received computerized dynamic posturography (CDP) examinations. Only sensory organization test (SOT) stability scores were included in the present correlational analyses.

The total DHI score was tabulated. Additionally, the following values from alternate binaural bithermal or monothermal warm caloric testing conducted during ENG/VNG examinations were tabulated: total caloric response (i.e., the summation of maximum peak slow phase velocity [SPV] for left and right warm caloric irrigations and left and right cool caloric irrigations), total warm maximum SPV, total cool maximum SPV, monothermal warm percent difference, percent unilateral weakness, and directional preponderance. Additionally, for rotational testing VOR phase (in degrees), gain (in percent), and asymmetry (in percent) for octave frequencies 0.01 Hz, 0.02 Hz, 0.04 Hz, 0.08 Hz, 0.16 Hz, and/or 0.32 Hz were tabulated.

Pearson product-moment correlations were calculated to determine the degree of relationship within and between semiobjective measures of vestibular system impairment and dizziness disability/handicap. Bonferroni adjusted probabilities are reported herein, as multiple comparisons were made during the analysis. Adjusted probability levels of ≤0.05 were accepted as significant.

Within Measure Correlations

Electro/Videonystagmography (ENG/VNG)

The maximum cool slow phase velocity (SPV) was significantly correlated with both the maximum warm SPV ($r = 0.79$, $p \leq 0.01$) and total caloric maximum SPV response ($r = 0.93$, $p \leq 0.01$). Total warm maximum SPV also demonstrated a strong correlation with total caloric response ($r = 0.97$, $p \leq 0.01$). This means that low cool caloric maximum slow phase velocities predict low warm maximum slow phase velocities. Lastly, monothermal warm caloric percent difference demonstrated a strong correlation with percent UW ($r = 0.89$, $p \leq 0.01$) and a significant correlation with percent DP ($r = 0.36$, $p \leq 0.05$). This finding underscores the value of the monothermal warm caloric test when the underlying assumptions for its implementation are fulfilled.

Rotational Testing

VOR phase at 0.01 Hz demonstrated a significant negative correlation with gain at 0.01 Hz ($r = -0.37$, $p \leq 0.05$). That is, as VOR gain (i.e., nystagmus velocity) decreased, phase leads (i.e., phase abnormalities) increased. Phase at 0.02 showed significant negative correlations with gain at 0.01, 0.02 and 0.04 Hz ($r = -0.40$, $p \leq 0.01$; $r = -0.45$, $p \leq 0.01$; $r = -0.38$, $p \leq 0.05$; for gain at 0.01, 0.02, and 0.04 Hz, respectively). Phase at 0.04 Hz demonstrated significant negative correlations with gain at 0.01, 0.02, and 0.04 Hz ($r = -0.47$, $p \leq 0.01$; $r = -0.44$, $p \leq 0.01$; $r = -0.42$, $p \leq 0.05$; for gain at 0.01, 0.02, and 0.04 Hz, respectively). Phase at 0.08 Hz demonstrated significant nega-

tive correlations with gain at 0.01, 0.02, and 0.04 Hz ($r = -0.42$, $p \leq 0.01$; $r = -0.44$, $p \leq 0.01$, $r = -0.51$, $p \leq 0.01$; for gain at 0.01, 0.02, and 0.04 Hz, respectively). Phase at 0.16 Hz showed a significant negative correlation with gain at 0.02 Hz ($r = -0.46$, $p \leq 0.05$). In general, phase leads were negatively correlated with gain values at 0.01–0.04 Hz.

These findings support the contention that end organ impairments have an impact on the velocity storage system, which is reflected in a reduction in time constant. Furthermore, this effect on velocity storage is reflected in greater impairments for frequencies ≤0.10 Hz (Barin & Durrant, 2000). This means that it is not unusual for rotational test results at 0.01 Hz to be uncorrelated with test results at 0.16 Hz and 0.32 Hz.

Additionally, adjacent data points tend to be correlated with one another (e.g., low gain at 0.01 Hz is associated with low gain at 0.02 Hz) and gain and phase tend to be negatively correlated in the presence of disease. Thus, as the magnitude of the electrical drive initiated at the end organ and terminating at the eye muscles decreases (i.e., because of unilateral or bilateral end organ impairment), the timing of the compensatory eye movement in response to the movement of the head deviates further and further from normal. These data also attest to the fact that phase leads accompany gain reductions and that agreement between these measures may be used as a cross-check.

The presence of rotational asymmetries correlates only with other asymmetry values at adjacent octave frequencies. VOR gain asymmetries are an expected finding where there is an existing spontaneous nystagmus which results in a directional preponderance on caloric testing.

Computerized Dynamic Posturography (CDP)

Conditions 4, 5, and 6, demonstrated significant positive correlations with the composite stability score ($r = 0.68$, $p = 0.001$ for condition 4, $r = 0.84$, $p = 0.001$ for condition 5; $r = 0.86$, $p = 0.001$ for condition 6). The condition 1 stability score was correlated only with the condition 2 stability score ($r = 0.41$, $p = 0.009$). The condition 2 stability score was correlated with the stability scores for condition 1 and condition 3 ($r = 0.45$, $p = 0.001$). The condition 3 stability score was correlated only with condition 2. The condition 4 stability score was correlated with the stability scores for conditions 5 and 6 ($r = 0.47$, $p = 0.001$ for condition 5; $r = 0.52$, $p = 0.001$ for condition 6). The condition 5 stability score was correlated with condition 6.

Thus, values representing performance on "easier" trials (e.g., conditions 1, 2, and 3) were correlated with one another, as was performance on "difficult" trials (e.g., conditions 4, 5, and 6). Thus, if a patient is unsteady on condition 4 of the SOT, one might predict they probably will be unstable on conditions 5 and 6 as well.

Summary

The within measure correlations make it possible to identify inconsistencies that may denote technical errors. For example, as cool and warm maximum slow phase eye velocities are correlated, 4 deg/sec maximum slow phase eye velocities for right and left cool calorics should not be followed by 90 deg/sec warm caloric maximum slow phase eye velocities (i.e., the cool caloric stimulus might be out of calibration, or the first irrigations might have been poorly performed). Similarly, it would be unusual for a zero gain at 0.01 Hz on rotational testing to be followed by 1.0 gain at 0.02 Hz. Furthermore, an abnormal increase in phase lead at 0.04 Hz should be followed by an abnormal increase in phase lead at 0.01 Hz of an equal or greater magnitude. A lowering of the phase angle as the frequency is decreased would not follow from these results or from modeling of the physiology of the peripheral vestibulo-ocular reflex (Wall, 1990).

Between Measures Correlations

Between Measures of Impairment

Total cool SPV demonstrated significant negative correlations with phase at 0.01, 0.02, 0.04, and 0.08 Hz ($r = -0.36$, $p \leq 0.05$; $r = -0.38$, $p = 0.05$; $r = -0.43$, $p = 0.05$; $r = -0.40$, $p = 0.01$; for phase at 0.01, 0.02, 0.04, and 0.08 Hz, respectively). That is, as total cool SPV decreased VOR phase increased. The same relationship was observed between total warm SPV and VOR phase at 0.02, 0.04, 0.08, and 0.16 Hz (Total warm SPV: $r = -0.41$, $p \leq 0.01$; $r = -0.45$, $p \leq 0.01$; $r = -0.43$, $p = 0.01$; $r = -0.55$, $p = 0.01$; for phase at 0.02, 0.04 and 0.08 Hz, respectively). Total caloric response also demonstrated significant negative correlations with phase at 0.02, 0.04, 0.08, and 0.16 Hz (Total caloric response: $r = -0.39$, $p = 0.05$; $r = -0.45$; $p = 0.01$; $r = -0.43$, $p = 0.01$; $r = -0.44$, $p = 0.05$; for phase at 0.02, 0.04, 0.08, and 0.16 Hz, respectively). Additionally, significant correlations with gain at 0.01 Hz and 0.02 Hz were observed for total cool SPV ($r = 0.58$, $p = 0.01$ at 0.01 Hz; $r = 0.51$, $p = 0.01$ at 0.02 Hz) total warm SPV ($r = 0.54$, $p = 0.01$ at 0.01 Hz; $r = 0.61$, $p = 0.01$ at 0.02 Hz) and total caloric response ($r = 0.57$, $p = 0.01$ at 0.01 Hz; $r = 0.55$, $p = 0.01$ at 0.02 Hz). Thus, as vestibular responsiveness as reflected in the caloric test results decreased, aberrations in the timing and magnitude of the compensatory eye movement increased.

These data suggest that measures of responsiveness of the peripheral vestibular system are correlated. This means that the adept clinician should predict that reductions in maximum slow phase eye velocities on caloric testing should be accompanied by reductions in at least low and possibly mid-frequency VOR gains. Additionally, as VOR gains and the timing of the compensatory eye movements are correlated, low caloric maximum velocities (e.g., a bilateral caloric weakness, or total absent caloric response) should be accompanied by increases in phase leads on rotational testing. Thus, if, for example, the vestibular end organ is weak on both sides, the electrical drive to the eye muscles during rotation will be less than normal. This will result in lesser contraction of the extraocular muscles that will result in a lower VOR gain and a resulting temporal delay (i.e., a phase abnormality because the decrease in electrical drive to the muscles coupled with the viscoelastic restoring forces keep the eyes from moving until a sufficient electrical drive is generated).

CDP measures correlated only with rotational test results. For example, SOT conditions 4 and 6 demonstrated significant negative correlations with phase measures at 0.01 Hz ($r = -0.39$, $p = 0.03$ for condition 4; $r = -0.39$, $p = 0.03$ for condition 6). This suggests that the loss of the velocity storage function (resulting in the phase lead at 0.01 Hz) affected changes in postural stability in situations where patients were relying on vision (predominately) for orientation.

Between Measures of Impairment and Disability/Handicap

No significant relationships were observed between measures of vestibular system impairment (e.g., ENG, rotational testing, computerized dynamic posturography [i.e., sensory organization test]) and dizziness disability/handicap (e.g., DHI total score).

This finding underscores the contention that dizziness-related activity limitation and participation restriction represents unique information that is not captured by other quantitative measures of balance function testing.

Final Comments Regarding Intermeasure Relationships

Relationship Between VEMP Data and Both Self-Report Handicap and Other Quantitative Measures

We are just beginning to understand the relationships between VEMP test results and other balance function measures. For, example, from unpublished observations (J. L. Augusto, personal communication, 2005) we know that patients who demonstrate evidence of, at least, impairment affecting one horizontal semicircular canal (and/or superior vestibular nerves), do not experience greater self-report handicap compared to patients who demonstrate an additional impairment of the saccule or saccules (and/or inferior vestibular nerves). Patients with isolated evidence of unilateral or bilateral saccular (or inferior vestibular nerve) impairment do not volunteer greater self-report handicap than those with unilateral horizontal semicircular canal impairment (or superior vestibular nerve impairment).

Additionally, one investigation has reported that patients with unilateral or bilateral absence of VEMP demonstrate abnormal postural sway on at least condition 5 of the SOT of the Equitest protocol (de Waele et al., 1999).

Relationships Between Results of the Dix-Hallpike/Head Roll Tests and the Bithermal Caloric Test

Benign paroxysmal positional vertigo (BPPV) may occur either due to otologic disease (i.e., second-ary or symptomatic BPPV) or it can occur without concommitant disease (i.e., idiopathic BPPV). It is easy to explain how, when disease is present, BPPV could occur. For example, otologic disease might be expected to result in deterioration of the otolith membrane. This might increase the likelihood that otoliths would float free into the semicircular canal system.

The proportion of patients who have both BPPV and otologic disease is controversial. Karlberg et al. (2000) have reported that 3% of their 2,847 patients with posterior semicircular canal BPPV (pBPPV) had ipsilateral inner ear disease. Alternately, it has been reported by Roberts et al. (2005) that pBPPV occurred in 53% (i.e., 26/49) of patients with a positive history of otologic disease and 31% (i.e., 33/108) of those without an otologic disease history. In our experience, approximately 30% of patients demonstrating either horizontal or posterior semicircular canal BPPV will demonstrate a significant unilateral weakness, and/or an absent VEMP on the ipsilesional side.

Relationships Between Measures of Central Vestibular System Impairment

The dependence on the midline cerebellum for both gaze maintenance and for orchestrating central compensation for unilateral vestibular system impairment means that the presence of gaze-evoked nystagmus should predict also a failure in VOR suppression. This, in fact, is true.

Summary

Between measures correlations provide the clinician with the ability to predict, with accuracy, given the result of one examination what will be the results of others. In that way it is possible to generate hypotheses about what will be the final result of a vestibular test battery. For example, the observation of a 90-degree leftward deviation on the Fukuda stepping test might predict a left peripheral vestibular system impairment in an acute patient. If present, for the same patient, a right-beating spontaneous nystagmus would predict a right directional preponderance and a unilateral weakness. The finding of a 100% left unilateral weakness would predict a low-frequency phase lead and reduced VOR gain at, at least, 0.01 Hz. This patient might also be predicted to demonstrate a VEMP abnormality on the left side. If the predicted findings on bedside testing, ENG/VNG, rotational, and VEMP tests are observed, it might be predicted that the patient would show a vestibular pattern (e.g., abnormal condition 5 or conditions 5 and 6) on the sensory organization subtest of computerized dynamic posturography.

In a less quantitative manner, a correlation study using over 2,200 patients all of whom had completed ENG, rotational chair, and both SOT and MCT of dynamic posturography resulted in impressions similar to the prospective quantitative findings just described (Shepard & Telian, 1996). The case examples in the chapter on the interpretation of posturography utilize these findings in establishing a staged approach to what tests should be used on a given patient. The findings given above also support the contention that, based on a core set of studies, rational decisions can be made as to potential contribution of rotational chair or formal postural control evaluations for a given patient. Given the demand on a clinician's time and the need to be as fiscally responsible as possible with each medical dollar spent, using information such as that presented herein in the clinical decision process as to how to evaluate the complex dizzy patient is critical. Practical examples of how this information on linkage can be used clinically are provided in the next section.

CASES THAT ILLUSTRATE HOW THE VARIOUS MEASURES LINK TOGETHER

Lesson: Spontaneous Nystagmus, and the Associated Unilateral Peripheral Vestibular System Impairment, Produces Predictable Findings on Quantitative Tests

This patient was evaluated after a 3-day spell of vertigo that was incapacitating on the first day and gradually improved over the next 2 days. The patient fell to the right on Romberg testing, and, although very unsteady, deviated to the right on the Fukuda stepping test.

Figure 34–1 shows that when the patient was examined with eyes open and staring at a midline target he generated a fine left-beating nystagmus. This nystagmus increased in intensity, over that observed at midline, when he gazed in the direction of the fast phase of the nystagmus (i.e., gaze toward the left; Figure 34–2) and diminished when his gaze was directed toward the slow phase (i.e., toward the right; Figure 34–3). In the vision-denied condition (Figure 34–4), the left-beating nystagmus is augmented. The attenuation of the nystagmus in the vision-present condition, the augmentation of the nystagmus in the vision-denied condition, coupled with the finding that the nystagmus follows Alex-

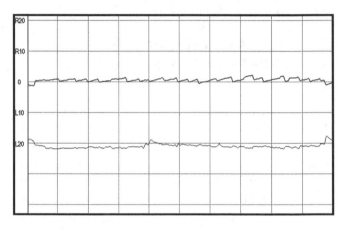

Figure 34–1. Spontaneous nystagmus for patient at center gaze position. Notice the fine left-beating nystagmus.

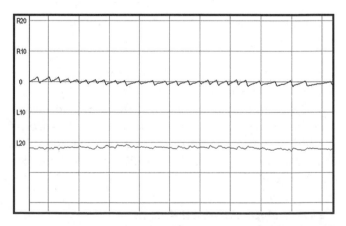

Figure 34–2. Patient 1 is gazing toward the left. Notice that the nystagmus has increased in intensity when gaze is directed toward the fast phase of the nystagmus (Alexander's law).

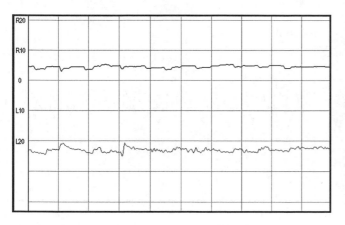

Figure 34-3. Patient is gazing toward the right (i.e., gaze is directed away from the fast phase). The nystagmus is now absent.

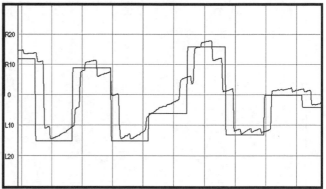

Figure 34-5. Saccade test results for the patient showing the normal saccade velocities but with the overlaid left-beating spontaneous nystagmus.

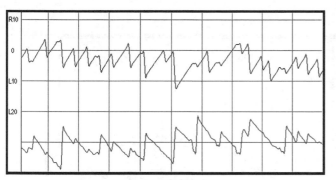

Figure 34-4. Spontaneous nystagmus test results (vision denied, patient alerted) showing augmentation of nystagmus velocity over that observed in the center gaze position.

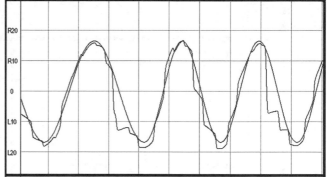

Figure 34-6. Effect of left-beating spontaneous nystagmus on pursuit test results. Note that pursuit gain is normal when the target is moving in a synergistic way with the slow phase of the spontaneous nystagmus. Alternately, pursuit is saccadic when the target is moving in the direction of the fast phase of the spontaneous nystagmus (i.e., toward the left).

ander's law argues for the nystagmus occurring as a result of an abnormal asymmetry in the tonic discharge of the right peripheral vestibular system.

As the patient is generating continuous left-directed saccades (i.e., the fast phase of the left-beating spontaneous nystagmus), the eye movement system will be unable to generate a pursuit eye movement in that direction (i.e., the ocular motility system cannot integrate a saccade and a pursuit signal simultaneously). Thus, when a clinician observes spontaneous nystagmus he or she may hypothesize (correctly) that saccade testing probably will be normal (Figure 34–5), and that both pursuit (Figure 34–6) and optokinetic nystagmus testing (Figure 34–7) will be unilaterally impaired (i.e., impaired when the

patient is pursuing targets in the direction of the fast phase of the spontaneous nystagmus, to the left in this case).

Additionally, as the eye movement system is "biased" to generate a left-beating nystagmus, the presence of a spontaneous nystagmus should serve as predictor of both a left directional preponderance on caloric testing (i.e., Figure 34–8, the spontaneous nystagmus results in stronger caloric nystagmus when it beats in the same direction as the spontaneous nystagmus) and a unilateral weakness in the direction opposite the fast phase of the spontaneous

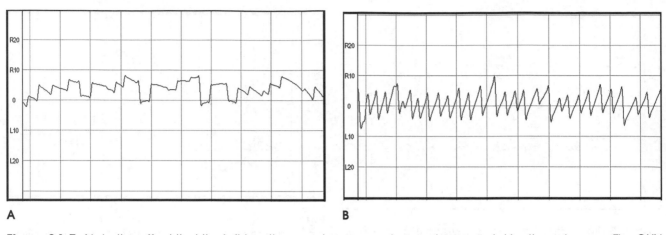

A   **B**

Figure 34-7. Note the effect that the left-beating spontaneous nystagmus has on optokinetic nystagmus. The OKN is impaired when the (pursuit) targets are moving in the direction of the fast phase of the left-beating spontaneous nystagmus (A) and OKN is normal when pursuit of the targets is in the direction of the spontaneous nystagmus slow phase (B).

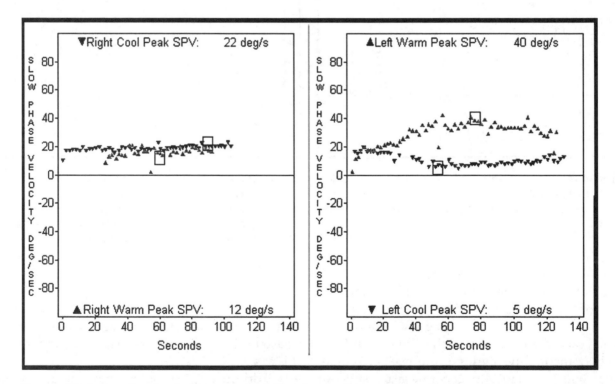

Figure 34-8. Results of caloric testing for the patient with the left-beating spontaneous nystagmus. Note the "bias" in the direction of the left-beating responses (i.e., the directional preponderance).

nystagmus (i.e., a right UW in this case). After correction for the DP (i.e., correction for the bias) the caloric examination showed that the patient had a total loss of function on the right side. The loss of the

right end organ, and its contribution to velocity storage, resulted in a reduction of low-frequency VOR gain and an associated abnormality in the timing of the VOR (i.e., low-frequency phase impairment,

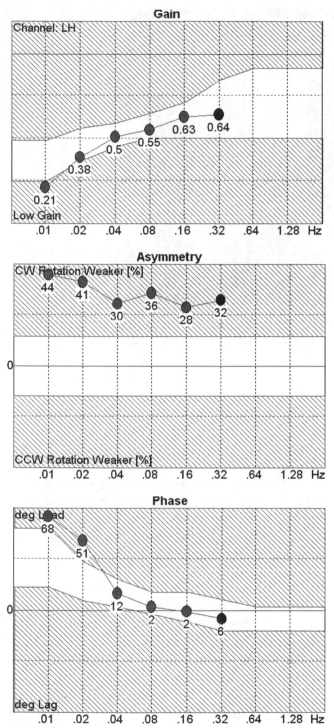

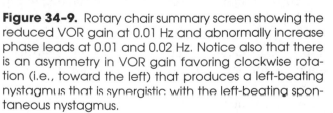

Figure 34-9. Rotary chair summary screen showing the reduced VOR gain at 0.01 Hz and abnormally increase phase leads at 0.01 and 0.02 Hz. Notice also that there is an asymmetry in VOR gain favoring clockwise rotation (i.e., toward the left) that produces a left-beating nystagmus that is synergistic with the left-beating spontaneous nystagmus.

Figure 34–9). The left DP on caloric testing resulted in a right gain asymmetry on rotational testing. That is, when the patient was oscillated to the left (i.e., toward the healthy side) the nystagmus slow phase to the right was greater than the nystagmus slow phase to the left when the patient was oscillated toward the impaired ear. As compensation of the VOR is dependent on the intactness of the midline cerebellum and its neural connections with the vestibular nuclei it was a very positive prognosticating sign that this patient's VOR suppression was normal (Figure 34–10).

Finally, it was not surprising that the patient's posturography scores were consistent with vestibular system impairment (i.e., a 5, 6 pattern on the sensory organization test; Figure 34–11).

Thus, from the moment that the patient entered the laboratory, and the left-beating (i.e., peripheral, vestibular) spontaneous nystagmus was identified, hypotheses could have been generated as to what would be the expected results for the rest of the examinations in the test battery.

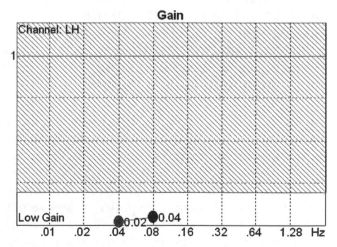

Figure 34-10. VOR suppression as measured using rotary chair techniques. Notice that any nystagmus slow phase velocity that exists during oscillation with a visual target is within the normal range. This suggests that central pathways underlying central compensation are intact.

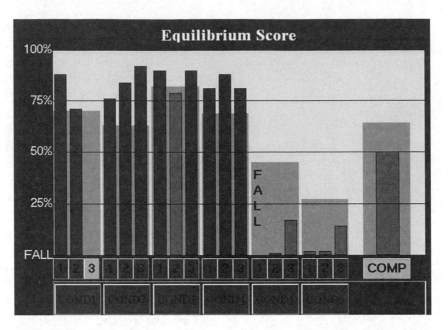

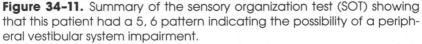

Figure 34–11. Summary of the sensory organization test (SOT) showing that this patient had a 5, 6 pattern indicating the possibility of a peripheral vestibular system impairment.

Lesson: The Presence of a Bilateral Caloric Weakness Should Predict Reduced Low and Mid-Frequency VOR Gain, and Phase. The Loss of the Low-Frequency VOR Should Produce a Patient Who Is Unsteady on Posturography Tasks Requiring Intact Vestibular System Inputs

The patient presented with a history of exposure to gentamicin for treatment of a kidney infection. The patient has few complaints when sitting still. However, he states that when he ambulates, the environment appears to move around him (i.e., the patient complains of oscillopsia). The patient scores 48 out of 100 points on the DHI (i.e., reflecting severe, self-report, dizziness handicap). He shows a catch-up saccade for head-thrust testing both to the right and left. There is no head-shake nystagmus and no spontaneous or gaze-evoked nystagmus. He is too unsteady to perform both the Romberg with eyes closed and the Fukuda stepping test. He is steady with eyes open on the Romberg test.

Spontaneous, gaze, saccade, pursuit, and posi-

tional/positioning tests all were normal (Figures 34–12 and 34–13).

Optokinetic nystagmus testing showed that the patient was capable of generating nystagmus (Figure 34–14). The patient experienced circular vection during full-field OKN stimulation and this suggested some function still existed in the vestibular system.

The total caloric maximum slow phase eye velocity was 12 deg/sec for the bithermal test (Figure 34–15). This result supported the contention that this patient was demonstrating a bilateral caloric weakness and an associated bilateral peripheral vestibular system impairment.

As the caloric examination is akin to a rotational frequency of approximately 0.003 Hz, and based on the correlational analyses reported at the beginning of this chapter, it was predicted that this patient would demonstrate reduced VOR gain at, at least, the lowest rotational frequencies and these reduced gains would also produce phase abnormalities at these frequencies as well. Indeed, this patient demonstrated abnormally low gains at 0.01 Hz through 0.16 Hz with associated phase leads (Figure 34–16).

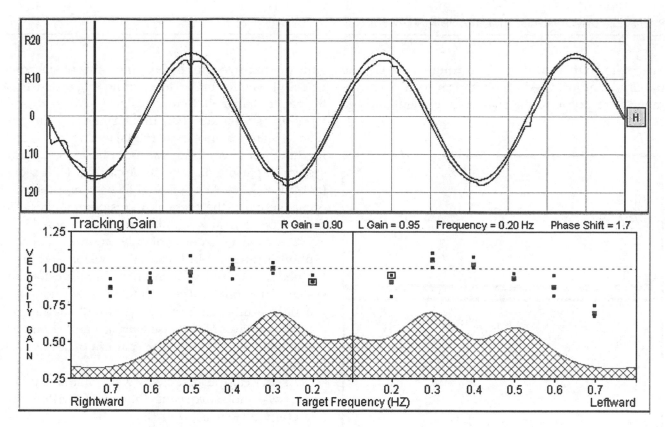

Figure 34-12. Summary data showing pursuit function is normal.

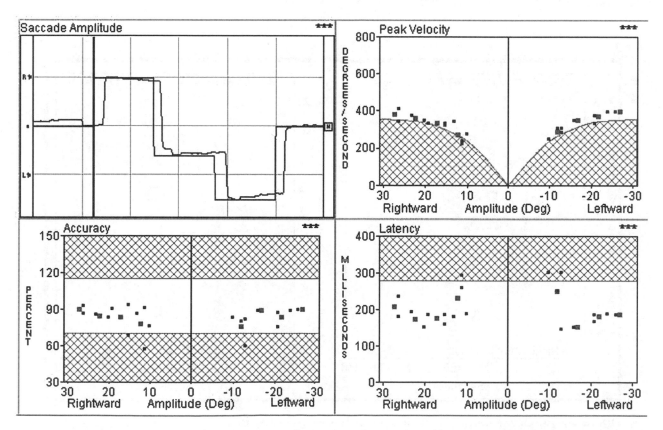

Figure 34-13. Summary data showing that saccade subsystem function was normal.

Note that from 0.16 Hz through 0.64 Hz the patient demonstrated a compensatory eye movement in response to the chair's movement and the

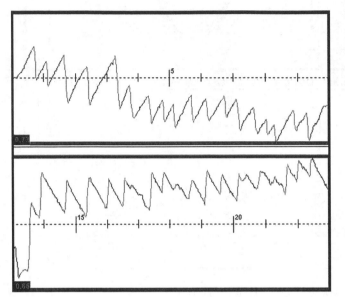

Figure 34–14. Data illustrating that the patient was capable of generating nystagmus from full-field stimulation.

gain of that eye movement, (i.e., the nystagmus velocity) was normal. This finding suggested that the patient had a bilateral, *subtotal* loss of peripheral vestibular system function and, furthermore, underscores the importance of rotational testing for assessing how dense are bilateral, peripheral vestibular system impairments. The 48-point total DHI score (as opposed to a 96-point total DHI score) probably occurred due to the presence of residual, higher frequency, peripheral vestibular system function.

Static balance relies not only on intact proprioception (primarily) but also intact vision and low-frequency sensitivity of the peripheral vestibular system. Thus, bilateral impairment of low-frequency function resulted in impaired postural stability on conditions 5 and 6 of the sensory organization test (i.e., producing a "vestibular" pattern of abnormality; Figure 34–17).

As the caloric responses were bilaterally absent it was not surprising that the VEMPs were bilaterally absent as well (Figure 34–18). That is, we can say that the gentamicin therapy damaged, at least, the horizontal semicircular canals and the saccule.

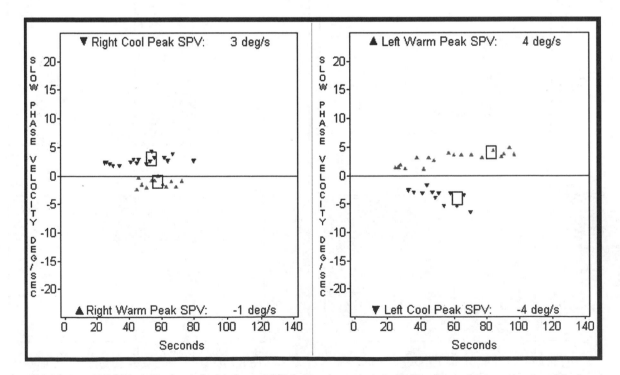

Figure 34–15. Caloric test results for the patient showing a total caloric slow phase velocity of 8 deg/sec (i.e., a bilateral caloric weakness).

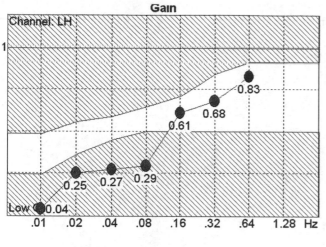

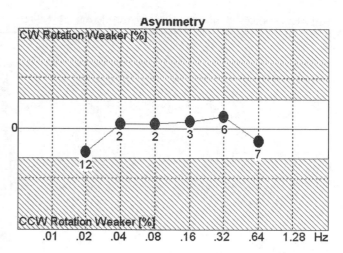

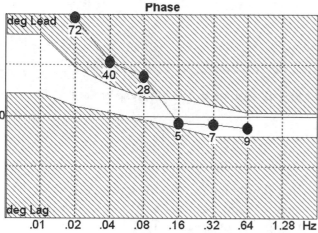

Figure 34-16. Results of rotational testing for the patient with bilateral peripheral vestibular system impairment. Note that gain is abnormally reduced from .01 Hz through .16 Hz and that these gain reductions were associated with phase (timing) impairments.

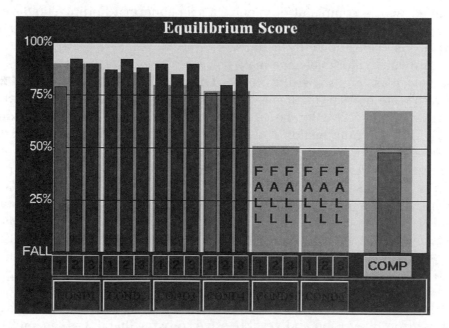

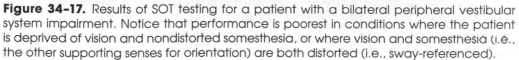

Figure 34-17. Results of SOT testing for a patient with a bilateral peripheral vestibular system impairment. Notice that performance is poorest in conditions where the patient is deprived of vision and nondistorted somesthesia, or where vision and somesthesia (i.e., the other supporting senses for orientation) are both distorted (i.e., sway-referenced).

845

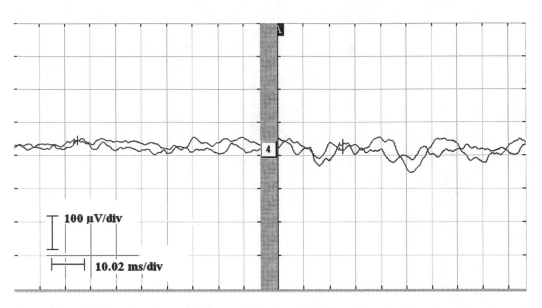

Figure 34–18. VEMP results for patient with bilateral peripheral vestibular system impairment resulting from exposure to vestibulotoxic medications.

Lesson: Unilateral Absence of a VEMP Is Reflected in Abnormal Postural Stability on Conditions Requiring Intact Vestibular System Function?

The patient presented with a complaint of vague unsteadiness. The patient showed normal ocular motility, no spontaneous or positional nystagmus, and symmetric warm water caloric average maximum slow phase velocities (Figure 34–19). Rotational test results also were normal (Figure 34–20). However, the patient showed a VEMP for the left ear only (Figure 34–21). The CDP examination showed abnormal performance conditions 5 and 6 of the sensory organization test (SOT) resulting in a pattern of abnormality typical of that seen in patients with vestibular system impairments (Figure 34–22).

Static postural stability requires the receipt by the brain of intact sensory signals emanating from the pressure sensors in the feet, ankles, and knees that are routed through the dorsal columns (i.e., the proprioceptive system) to subcortical, multisensory integration centers. Additional sensory inputs to these centers include those from the vision and vestibular sensory systems. It is the saccule the responds to linear up-and-down movement and this probably is the vestibular end organ that contributes most

to standing balance. It follows that if the saccule is damaged, then patients will be less steady when standing on CDP testing. This, in fact, was the finding of de Waele et al. (1999). Accordingly, a unilaterally, and more often bilaterally absent VEMP as a sole abnormal finding should be expected to be accompanied by poor postural stability on CDP.

Lesson: Evidence of Central Eye Movement Impairment Affecting the Cerebellum Should also Be Associated with Impairments of the VOR That Rely on the Same Centers

The patient was seen in clinic for "intractable positional vertigo." The patient complained of oscillopsia during movement. The patient's vision was blurry during horizontal versional eye movements.

On informal examination, the patient demonstrated a characteristic bidirectional gaze-evoked nystagmus-GEN (i.e., left-beating on leftward gaze and right-beating on rightward gaze). True to the nature of GEN, it abated with loss of a fixation point (i.e., proving that it was "gazing" that "evoked" the nystagmus). Neither Romberg, nor Fukuda stepping tests could be conducted as the patient's postural stability was so poor.

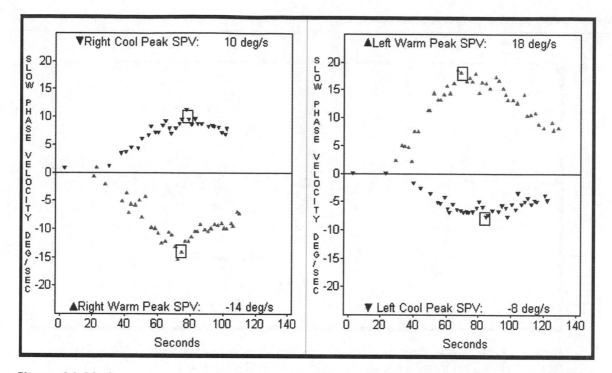

Figure 34-19. Summary screen showing normal, bithermal caloric test for a patient with vague unsteadiness.

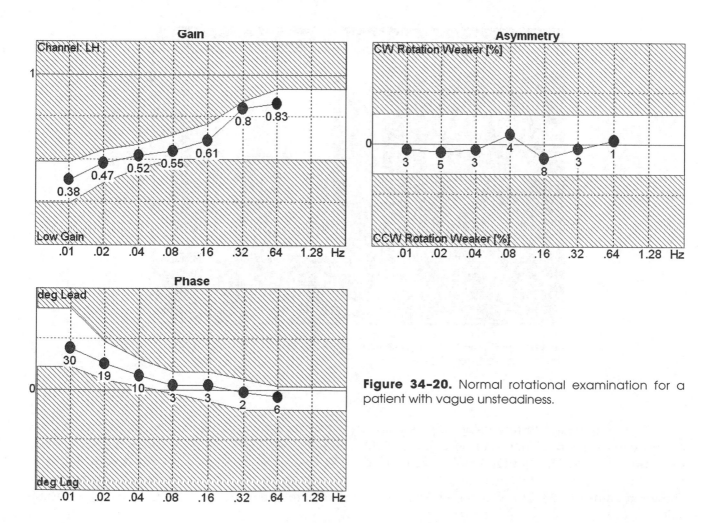

Figure 34-20. Normal rotational examination for a patient with vague unsteadiness.

847

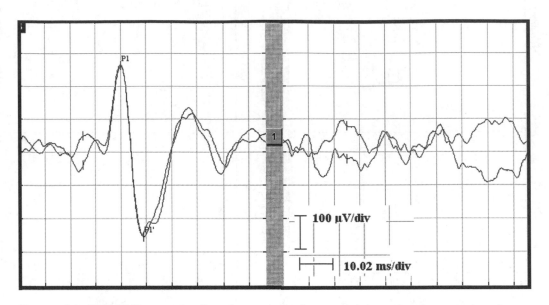

Figure 34-21. VEMP examination for a patient complaining of vague unsteadiness. Notice that the left VEMP is present and the right VEMP is absent.

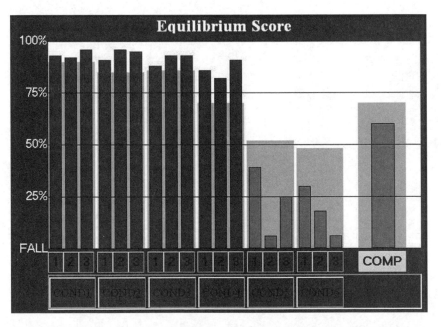

Figure 34-22. Sensory organization test (SOT) results for a patient with an isolated absent right VEMP.

Quantitative gaze testing using targets placed at 30 degrees left deviation and 30 degrees right deviation evoked the bidirectional gaze-evoked nystagmus. These eye movement abnormalities are shown in Figure 34–23. This nystagmus was absent when vision was denied. The patient generated normal saccades (Figure 34–24). As the patient was predisposed to generate saccades at both right and leftward gaze (i.e., the GEN) both the pursuit test and optokinetic nystagmus tests were abnormal

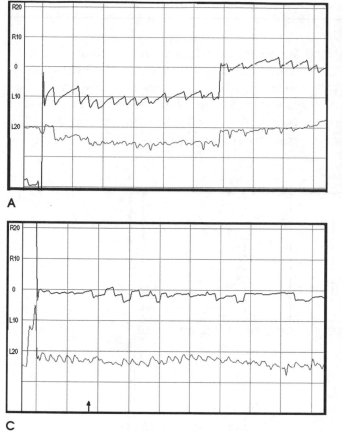

A

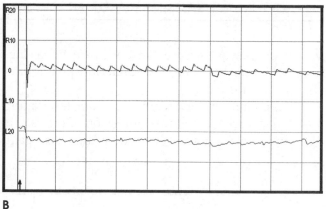

B

C

Figure 34-23. Results of gaze testing to the left (**A**), right (**B**) and up (**C**) for the patient with bidirectional gaze-evoked nystagmus.

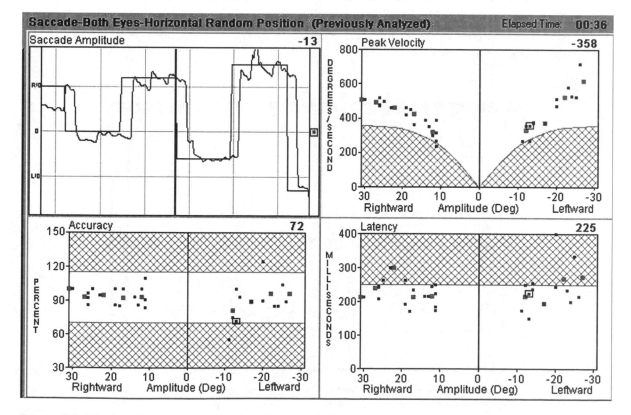

Figure 34-24. Results of saccade testing for a patient with gaze-evoked nystagmus. Notice that the saccade function is essentially normal.

(i.e., pursuit was saccadic in both directions; Figures 34–25 and 34–26). Positional and positioning testing was normal.

The patient showed a normal caloric test (Figure 34–27). However, fixation suppression of the caloric nystagmus was abnormal (Figure 34–28). Phase, gain, and symmetry measures on rotary chair testing all were normal for this patient (Figure 34–29). Noteworthy though was the patient's inability to suppress rotational nystagmus when she attempted to maintain her gaze on a stable target (i.e., she showed impaired VOR suppression/fixation suppression, Figure 34–30).

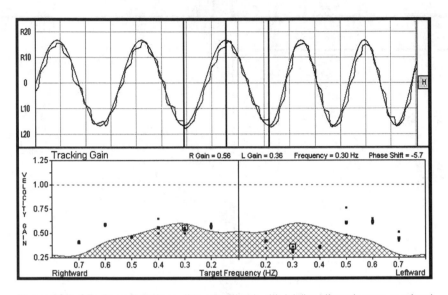

Figure 34–25. Pursuit test result in a patient with bidirectional gaze-evoked nystagmus. Notice that the superimposed GEN produces bidirectionally impaired pursuit.

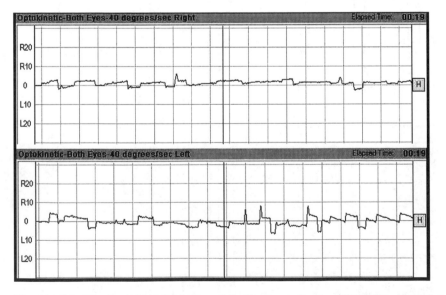

Figure 34–26. Optokinetic test results for a patient with bidirectional gaze-evoked nystagmus. Notice that, as was seen in Figure 34–25, the superimposed GEN produces bidirectionally impaired pursuit (i.e., absent OKN in this case).

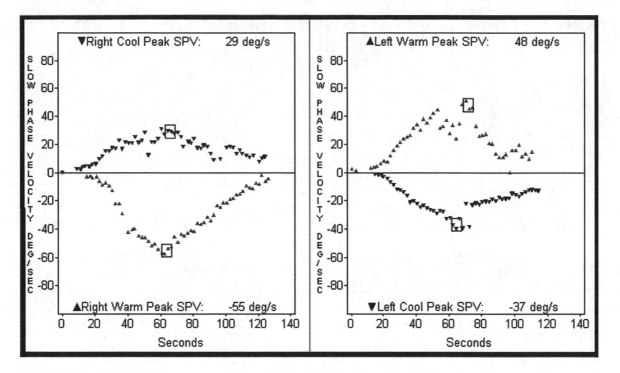

Figure 34–27. Caloric test summary for a patient with bidirectional GEN. There is no asymmetry present.

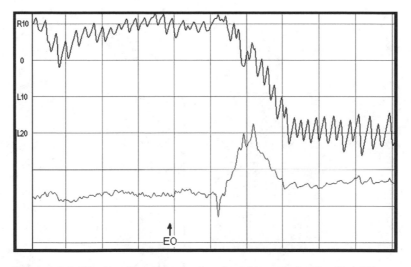

Figure 34–28. Fixation suppression test for a patient with bidirectional GEN. Notice that the patient is unable to suppress the caloric-induced nystagmus.

The presence of bidirectional GEN implies damage has occurred (either permanent or transient) to the connections between the vestibular nuclei and cerebellum. These are the same pathways that must be intact for vestibular compensation to take place after a unilateral peripheral vestibular system impairment and, consequently, are the same pathways that must be intact for visual suppression of the VOR to occur. Thus, the presence of bidirectional GEN is a predictor for both impaired pursuit testing and impaired VOR suppression during caloric testing and rotational testing.

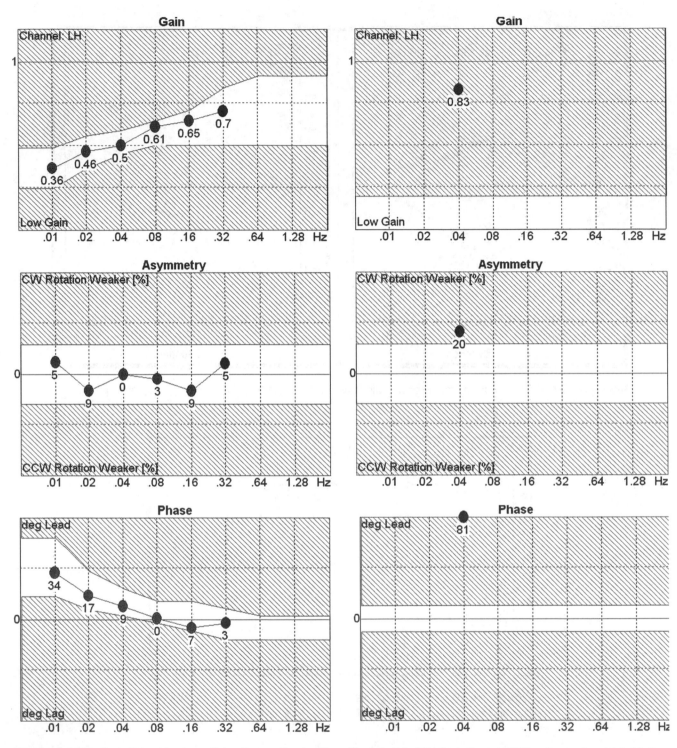

Figure 34–29. Rotational test result for the patient with bidirectional GEN. Notice that phase, gain, and symmetry of the VOR are normal.

Figure 34–30. Rotational VOR suppression test. Notice that, consistent with the caloric findings, the patient is unable to suppress the rotary chair-induced nystagmus (i.e., the patient is generating a gain of 83% (i.e., 42 deg/ sec nystagmus velocity if the chair is moving at a velocity of 50 deg/sec)).

Lesson: The Presence of a Unilateral Peripheral Vestibular Impairment May Predict 13 to 53% of the Time a Benign Paroxysmal Positional Vertigo (BPPV)

The patient has had recurring short duration spells of vertigo lasting 30 to 60 seconds, precipitated by sudden changes in position and accompanied by nausea. The patient has a past medical history of closed head injury that occurred when the patient was an unrestrained passenger in a motor vehicle accident.

Quantitative testing showed the patient to have normal gaze, saccade, pursuit, and optokinetic subsystem function. There was no spontaneous nystag-

mus. However, whereas the Dix-Hallpike maneuver failed to elicit nystagmus and vertigo in the head-dependent left position (Figure 34–31B), evidence of a posterior semicircular canal, canalithiasis was observed when the patient was placed in the head-dependent right position (Figure 34–31A). The bithermal caloric test (Figure 34–32) revealed a significant 58% right unilateral weakness. The VEMP was absent on the ipsilesional (right) side (Figure 34–33). The SOT test revealed a pattern of postural instability consistent with that observed in patients with peripheral vestibular system impairment (Figure 34–34).

Evidence of peripheral vestibular system impairment as revealed by the bithermal caloric test may accompany BPPV between 13 and approximately

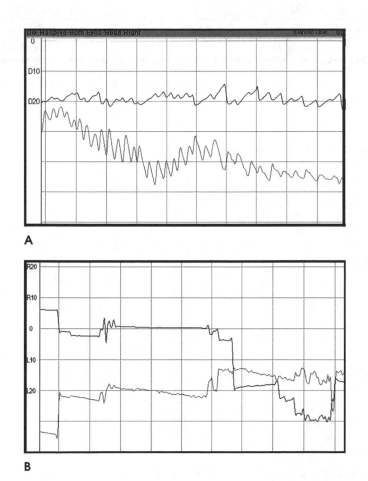

Figure 34–31. Dix-Hallpike positioning result for a patient with a right, posterior semicircular canal, canalithiasis. Notice in the top tracing (*HHR*, **A**) the patient is generating a nystagmus with a primary up-beating component. The patient does not show evidence of BPPV in the Dix-Hallpike HHL positioning (**B**).

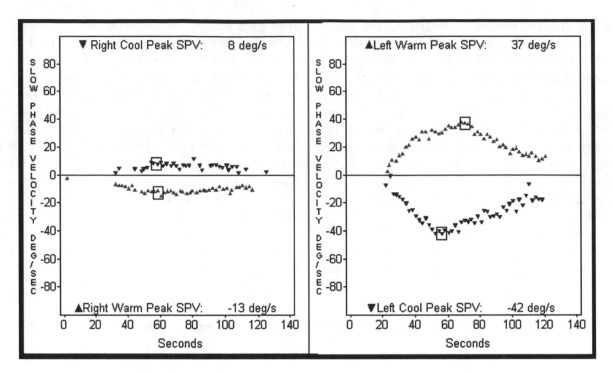

Figure 34–32. Caloric summary showing that this patient with right posterior semicircular canal BPPV also has a right unilateral weakness.

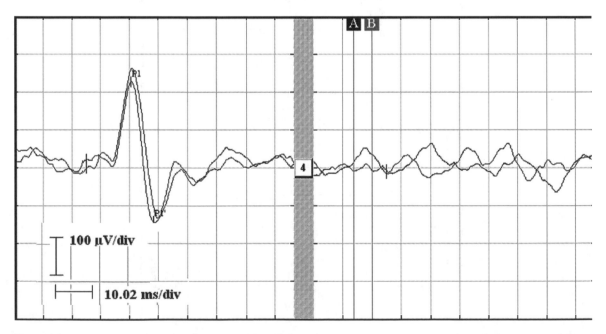

Figure 34–33. VEMP result for patient with a right BPPV. The patient shows a VEMP that is present on the left side (*left side of figure*) and absent on the right side (*right side of figure*).

50% of the time (Karlberg et al., 2000; Roberts et al., 2005). Our experience has suggested that the two coexist approximately 30% of the time. This means that when a BPPV is observed, it may be predicted that as many as 1:2 to 1:3 patients will have a significant UW. The UW on caloric testing also predicts

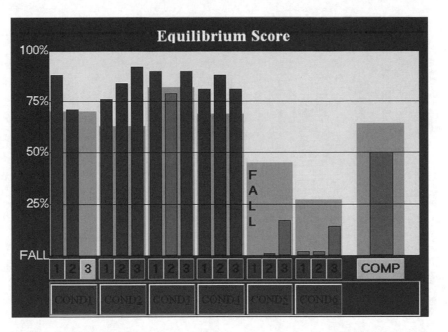

Figure 34–34. Computerized dynamic posturography (*CDP*) results in a patient with right BPPV, right unilateral weakness, and an absent VEMP on the right side. The sensory organization test (*SOT*) shows abnormal function on trials where the patient must depend on vestibular system input for postural stability.

low-frequency phase and gain impairment on rotational testing and a "vestibular" pattern of postural instability on the SOT. The ipsilesional absent VEMP suggests that the function of the saccule may also be impaired.

REFERENCES

Barber, H. O., & Stockwell, C. (1980). *Manual of electronystagmography* (pp. 159–187). St. Louis, MO: C.V. Mosby.

Barin, K., & Durrant, J. D. (2000). Applied physiology of the vestibular system. In R. F. Canalis & P. R. Lambert, *The ear: Comprehensive otology* (pp. 113–140). Philadelphia: Lippincott Willams & Wilkins.

de Waele, C., Huy, P. T., Freyss, G., & Vidal, P. P. (1999). Saccular dysfunction in Mèniére's disease. *American Journal of Otology, 20,* 223–232.

Fitzgerald, G., & Hallpike, C. S. (1942). Studies in human vestibular function. I. Observations on directional preponderance (Nystagmusbereitschaft) of caloric nystagmus resulting from cerebral lesions. *Brain, 65,* 115–137.

Jacobson, G. P., Calder, J. A., Shepard, V. A., Rupp, K. A., & Newman, C. W. (1995). Reappraisal of the monothermal warm caloric screening test. *Annals of Otology, Rhinology and Larygnology, 104,* 942–945.

Jacobson, G. P., & Means, E. D. (1985). Efficacy of a monothermal warm water caloric screening test. *Annals of Otology, Rhinology and Larygnology, 94,* 377–381.

Jacobson, G. P., & Newman, C. W. (1990). The development of the Dizziness Handicap Inventory (DHI). *Archives of Otolaryngology-Head and Neck Surgery, 116,* 424–427.

Karlberg, M., Hall, K., Quickert, N., Hinson, J., & Halmagyi, G. M. (2000). What inner ear diseases cause benign paroxysmal positional vertigo? *Acta Oto-Laryngologica, 120,* 380–385.

Roberts R. A., Gans, R. E., Kastner, A. H., & Lister, J. J. (2005). Prevalence of vestibulopathy in benign paroxysmal positional vertigo patients with and without prior otologic history. *International Journal of Audiology, 44,* 191–196.

Shepard, N. T., & Telian, S. A. (1996). *Practical management of the balance disorder patient.* San Diego, CA: Singular.

Wall, C. (1990). The sinusoidal harmonic acceleration rotary chair test—theoretical and clinical basis. *Neurologic Clinics, 8,* 269–285.

Index

Summating potential (SP)
 cochlear nerve, 596
 elevation of, 609, **610**
 in SSCD, 607–609
Summating potential to action potential (SP/AP) ratio, 602–603
 in Ménière's disease, 604
 reduction of, 609–610
 in SSCD, 607
Superior canal dehiscence (SCD), 679
 cVEMP sensitivity and specificity for, 556, **557**
 cVEMP threshold in, 556, **557**
 Dizziness Handicap Inventory (DHI) for, 199, **201**
 oVEMP sensitivity and specificity for, 556, **557**, 570, **571**
 VEMP recordings in, 556, **557**
Superior colliculus (SC), 33
Superior oblique muscle, 21–22, **22**
Superior rectus muscle, 21–22, **22**
Superior semicircular canal dehiscence (SSCD)
 associated symptoms, 122–123, **125**
 audiographic findings, 702–703, **703**
 case reports, 702–703, **703**, **704**, **705**, **706**
 cVEMPs in, 702–703, **705**
 ECochG findings in, 606–609, **608**, **609**, 702–703, **704**
 exacerbating factors, 124, **125**
 repair of, 609–610, **611**
 surgical repair of, 702–706
 time course, 122, **125**
Superior semicircular canal dehiscence syndrome (SSCDS), 570–571, **571**, 606
Superior vestibular nerve (SVN), 614–615, **615**
 impaired, 617, 621, **621**, **622**, **623**
 normal, 617, **619**
Superior vestibular nerve (SVN) impairment, 627, **629**
Supine head-hanging technique, 262–263, **264**
Supine position, 270, **270**
 ice water caloric testing in, **337**, 337–338, **339**
Supplementary eye fields (SEFs), 33, **34**, 35
Supranuclear saccadic palsies, **31**
Surface electromyography, 453
Surgery
 ablative vestibular, 708–713
 for BPPV, 700–701
 endolymphatic sac procedures, 706–707
 intraoperative ECochG monitoring, 609–610, **611**
 for Ménière's disease, 706–708
 past medical and surgical history, 124–125
 for perilymphatic fistula, 701–702
 rationale for, 699–700
 for SSCD, 609–610, **611**, 702–706
 for vertigo that is otologic in origin, 699–717

SVN. *See* Superior vestibular nerve
SVV. *See* Subjective visual vertical
Sway, 433, **434**
Sway energy scores, **478**
Sway-referencing, 465–466
Syncope
 characteristics of, 120
 in children, 632
 differential diagnosis of, **743**
 neurocardiogenic, 120
 vasovagal, 120

T

Tandem Romberg position, 771–772
TC. *See* Time constant
Technology, 801
Tegretol (carbamazepine), 693–694
Temperature effects, 310, **311**
Temporal bones, 360, **361**
Tenormin (atenolol), 693–694
Terminology, **165**, 165–166, **166**
Test-retest reliability, 167
Tests and testing
 bedside tests, 137, 833
 head impulse test, 11–12
 head-shaking induced nystagmus (HSN), 12–13
 linear acceleration tests, 581–587, **582**
 otolith testing, 581–589
 pediatric vestibular testing, 631–652
 perceptual tests of vestibular function, 589–592
 positional testing, 12, 251–282
 for spontaneous vestibular nystagmus, 137–140
 tools, 168
 velocity perception test, 591, **591**
 of vertical semicircular canals, 412–416
 of vestibular perception, 581–594
 wheel test, 591, **591**
Third window conditions, 609, **610**, 610–611
Third window phenomenon, 702
Threat, perceived, 732, **733**
3-D oculography, 585–586
3-D video-oculography, 583–585, 585–586, **586**
TIAs. *See* Transient ischemic attacks
Tibial nerve somatosensory evoked potentials (SEPs), 817–818
Tilt suppression protocol, 388–389
Time constant (TC), 379
Time course of attacks, 121–122
Timed "Up and Go" Test (TUG or TUGT), 187, **188**, 778–779, 820–821
Tinnitus, 123
Tip-trode electrodes, 598–600, **600**